FUNDAMENTALS OF HIV MEDICINE
2019 EDITION

FOR THE HIV SPECIALIST™

FUNDAMENTALS OF HIV MEDICINE 2019 EDITION

FOR THE HIV SPECIALIST™

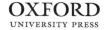

OXFORD
UNIVERSITY PRESS

Oxford University Press is a department of the University of Oxford. It furthers
the University's objective of excellence in research, scholarship, and education
by publishing worldwide. Oxford is a registered trade mark of Oxford University
Press in the UK and certain other countries.

Published in the United States of America by Oxford University Press
198 Madison Avenue, New York, NY 10016, United States of America.

CIP data is on file at the Library of Congress
ISBN 978–0–19094249–6

1 3 5 7 9 8 6 4 2

Printed by Sheridan Books, Inc., United States of America

TARGET AUDIENCE

This resource has been designed to meet the educational needs of physicians, nurse practitioners, physician assistants, registered nurses, and pharmacists involved in the care of patients with HIV disease.

OVERALL LEARNING OBJECTIVES

After reviewing this educational resource, readers should be better able to:

- Describe the evolving epidemiology of HIV disease in the U.S., with an emphasis on age, gender, sexuality, race/ethnicity, socioeconomic status, emerging subtypes and viral resistance;

- Implement appropriate laboratory HIV testing methods for screening and diagnosing HIV infections;

- Adapt pre- and post-testing patient counseling to best meet patient needs in a variety of situations;

- Provide up-to-date HIV care to a broad spectrum of infected patient populations, including pediatrics, adolescents, injection-drug users, incarcerated individuals, and an aging population;

- Review the clinical presentation, diagnosis, treatment and treatment complications of hepatitis B and C in HIV-infected patients;

- Adjust treatment based upon the various co-morbities that are often found in HIV-infected individuals including cardiovascular, renal, and neurologic disease;

- Discuss the ethics and legal issues related to caring for HIV-infected individuals.

EDITORS AND CONTRIBUTORS

LEAD EDITOR

W. David Hardy, MD, AAHIVS
Senior Director, Evidence-based Practices
Whitman-Walker Health
Adjunct Professor of Medicine
Johns Hopkins University School of Medicine
Washington, DC

CO-EDITORS

Jonathan S. Appelbaum, MD, FACP, AAHIVS
Florida State University College of Medicine

Roberto C. Arduino, MD
Professor of Medicine
Department of Internal Medicine
Division of Infectious Diseases
McGovern Medical School, University of Texas Health
Sciences Center at Houston

Laurie L. Dozier Jr., MD
Education Director and Professor of Internal Medicine
Interim Chair, Department of Clinical Sciences
Florida State University College of Medicine

Jeffrey T. Kirchner, DO, FAAFP, AAHIVS
Medical Director, Penn Medicine/LGHP
Comprehensive Care
Lancaster General Hospital
Lancaster, PA

William R. Short, MD, MPH
Associate Professor of Medicine
Division of Infectious Diseases
Perelman School of Medicine
University of Pennsylvania

WRITERS

Saira Ajmal, MD
Advocate Healthcare Illinois

Kevin Alby, MD
University of North Carolina Hospitals

Benjamin Alfred, NP-C
Family Health Center of Worcester

Jonathan Appelbaum, MD, FACP, AAHIVS
Florida State University College of Medicine

Lisa Armitige, MD, PhD
Heartland National TB Center

Renata Arrington-Sanders, MD, MPH, ScM
Johns Hopkins School of Medicine

Jason V. Baker, MD, MS
University of Minnesota

Ben J. Barnett, MD
McGovern Medical School at University of Texas at Houston

Tamara Bininashvili, MD
University of California, San Francisco

Jatandra Birney, PharmD
Ascension Via Christi Hospital

Emily Blumberg, MD
Hospital of the University of Pennsylvania

Philip Bolduc, MD, AAHIVS
Family Health Center of Worcester

Christopher M. Bositis, MD, AAHIVS
Greater Lawrence Family Health Center

Christian Brander, PhD
IrsiCalxa AIDS Research Institute
University of Vic-Central Catalonia
Hospital Universitari Germans Trias i Pujol

Christopher Brendemuhl, DMD
Maricopa Integrated Health System
McDowell Dental Clinic

John P. Casas, MD
Albany Stratton VA Medical Center

Elizabeth Chiao, MD, MPH
Michael E. DeBakey VA Medical Center

Carolyn Chu, MD, MSc, FAAFP, AAHIVS
University of California at San Francisco

Joseph A. Church, MD
Children's Hospital Los Angeles
Keck School of Medicine of University of Southern
    California

Eva Clark, MD, PhD, DTM&H
Baylor College of Medicine

Jennifer Cocohoba, PharmD, BCPS, AAHIVP
University of California, San Francisco, School of Pharmacy
University of California, San Francisco, Women's HIV
    Program

Dagan Coppock, MD
Drexel University College of Medicine

Vishal Dahya, MD
Florida State University College of Medicine

Elizabeth David, MD
Baylor College of Medicine

Trew Deckard, PA-C, MHS, AAHIVS
Medical Practice of Dr. Steven M. Pounders

Alejandro Delgado, MD
Einstein Medical Center Philadelphia

Paul W. DenOuden, MD, AAHIVS
Multnomah County Health Department

Madeline B. Deutsch, MD, MPH
University of California, San Francisco

Quentin Doperalski, MD
University of California, San Francisco

Richard Dunham, PhD
GlaxoSmithKline
HIV Cure Center, University of North Carolina at
    Chapel Hill

James P. Dunn, MD
Wills Eye Hospital
Sidney Kimmel Medical College at Thomas Jefferson
    University

Derek M. Fine, MD
Johns Hopkins Hospital

Anna Forbes, MSS
American Academy of HIV Medicine

Rajesh Gandhi, MD
Massachusetts General Hospital
Harvard Medical School

Taylor K. Gill, PharmD, BCPS, AAHIVP
Ascension Via Christi Hospital

Michelle K. Haas, MD
Denver Public Health
University of Colorado-Anschutz Medical Campus

Dennis J. Hartigan-O'Connor, MD, PhD
University of California, Davis

Rodrigo Hasbun, MD, MPH
McGovern Medical School at University of Texas at Houston

Emily L. Heil, PharmD, BCIDP, BCPS, AAHIVP
University of Maryland School of Pharmacy

Margaret Hoffman-Terry, MD, FACP, AAHIVS
Milton S. Hershey Medical Center
Pennsylvania State University College of Medicine
Lehigh Valley Hospital

Jennifer Husson, MD, MPH
University of Maryland School of Medicine

Nikyati Jakharia, MD
University of Maryland

Boris D. Juelg, MD, PhD
Massachusetts General Hospital

Joseph S. Kass, MD, JD, FAAN
Baylor College of Medicine

Jeffrey T. Kirchner, DO, FAAFP, AAHIVS
Penn Medicine/LGHP Comprehensive Care
Lancaster General Hospital

David E. Koren, PharmD
Temple University School of Pharmacy
Temple University Hospital

Carolyn Kramer, MD, MHS
Sidney Kimmel Medical College at Thomas Jefferson
    University

Doris Kung, DO
Baylor College of Medicine

Sally Spencer Long, ANP C
Bay State Medical Center

Eurides Lopes, MD
Loma Linda University Healthcare

Adrian Majid, MD
Weill Cornell Medicine
New York-Presbyterian Hospital

Poonam Mathur, DO, MPH
University of Maryland Medical Center

Jessica A. Meisner, MD, MS
University of Pennsylvania Health System

Steven Menez, MD
Johns Hopkins School of Medicine

Ana Monczor, MD
McGovern Medical School at University of Texas at Houston

Kudakwashe Mutyambizi, MD
MD Anderson Cancer Center
The University of Texas Medical School at Houston

Puja H. Nambiar, MD
Assistant Professor, Department of Medicine/Infectious
    Diseases
Louisiana State University Health

Naiel Nassar, MD, FACP
University of California, San Francisco

Karin Nielsen-Saines, MD, MPH
David Geffen School of Medicine
University of California, Los Angeles

Karen Nunez-Wallace, MD
Baylor College of Medicine

Babafemi Onabanjo, MD, AAHIVS
Family Health Center of Worcester

Edgar T. Overton, MD
University of Alabama School of Medicine

Bruce J. Packett II
American Academy of HIV Medicine

Neha Sheth Pandit, PharmD, AAHIVP, BCPS
University of Maryland School of Pharmacy

Rachel A. Prosser, PhD, APRN, CNP, FAANP, AAHIVS
Hennepin County Medical Center
University of Minnesota School of Nursing
Metropolitan University School of Nursing
Centurion
RAAN
Positive Healthcare LLC

Christian B. Ramers, MD, MPH, AAHIVS
Family Health Centers of San Diego
University of San Diego School of Medicine
San Diego State University School of Public Health

Brandon H. Samson, PharmD, MPW
Vaniam Group LLC

Aroonsiri Sangarlangkarn, MD, MPH
HIV Netherlands Australia Thailand Research
    Collaboration Clinic
Thai Red Cross

**Jason J. Schafer, PharmD, MPH, BCPS
AQ-ID, BCIDP, AAHIVP**
Jefferson College of Pharmacy
Thomas Jefferson University

Hans P. Schlecht, MD, MMSc
Baystate Health

Jeffrey T. Schouten, MD
Fred Hutchinson Cancer Research Center

**James D. Scott, PharmD, Med, APh,
FCCP, FASHP, AAHIVP**
Western University of Health Sciences College of Pharmacy

Rajagopal V. Sekhar, MD
Baylor College of Medicine

Lydia J. Sharp, MD
Baylor College of Medicine

Kalpana D. Shere-Wolfe, MD
University of Maryland Medical System

Elizabeth M. Sherman, PharmD, AAHIVP
Nova Southeastern University

William R. Short, MD, MPH, AAHIVS
University of Pennsylvania

Daniel J. Skiest, MD
Baystate Medical Center

Anthony C. Speights, MD, FACOG, AAHIVS
Florida State University College of Medicine

Gary F. Spinner, PA, MPH, AAHIVS
Southwest Community Health Center

Rohit Talwani, MD
University of Maryland Medical Center

Zelalem Temesgen, MD, FIDSA
Mayo Clinic

Karen J. Vigil, MD
McGovern Medical School at University of Texas at Houston

Sana Waheed, MD
University of Wisconsin Hospitals and Clinics

Rakel Beall Wilkins, MD
Magellan Health

Amanda L. Willig, PhD, RD
The University of Alabama at Birmingham

Daniel Wlodarczyk, MD
University of California, San Francisco
San Francisco General Hospital
San Francisco Department of Public Health

David A. Wohl, MD
University of North Carolina at Chapel Hill
NC AIDS Training and Education Center

Hojoon You, MD
Einstein Medical Center Philadelphia

Barry Zevin, MD
San Francisco Department of Public Health

CONTENTS

CONTRIBUTOR DISCLOSURES

As part of the development of this educational resource, all contributors were asked to disclose financial relationships or relationships to products or devices they or their spouse/life partner have with commercial interests related to this resource.

Name of Resource Contributor	Reported Financial Relationship
Saira Ajmal	Nothing to disclose
Kevin Alby	Nothing to disclose
Benjamin Alfred	Nothing to disclose
Jonathan Appelbaum	Consulting fees: Merck, ViiV Healthcare
Lisa Armitage	Nothing to disclose
Roberto C. Arduino	Contracted Research Viiv Healthcare, Inc.
Renata Arrington-Sanders	Nothing to disclose
Jason Baker	Nothing to disclose
Ben J. Barnett, MD	Consulting fees: Gilead, BMS Fees for non-CME/CE services: Gilead, Merck
Rakel Beall Wilkins	Nothing to disclose
Tamara Bininashvili	Nothing to disclose
Jatandra Birney	Nothing to disclose
Saira Ajmal	Nothing to disclose
Emily Blumberg	Nothing to disclose
Philip Bolduc	Nothing to disclose
Christopher Bositis	Nothing to disclose
Christian Brander	Salary: Aelix Therapeutics Consulting fees: Gritstone Inc, GLG Contracted research: Aelix Therapeutics Ownership interest: Aelix Therapeutics
Christopher Brendemuhl	Nothing to disclose
John Casas	Nothing to disclose
Elizabeth Chiao	Nothing to disclose
Carolyn Chu	Nothing to disclose
Joseph Church	Nothing to disclose
Eva Clark	Nothing to disclose
Jennifer Cocohoba	Nothing to disclose
Dagan Coppock	Nothing to disclose
Vishal Dahya	Nothing to disclose
Elizabeth David	Nothing to disclose
Trew Deckard	Fees for non-CME/CE services received directly from a commercial interest or their agents (e.g., speakers bureau): Gilead Sciences, Janssen
Alejandro Delgado	Nothing to disclose
Paul DenOuden	Nothing to disclose
Madeline Deutsch	Contracted Research: Gilead
Quentin Doperalski	Nothing to disclose
Richard Dunham	Nothing to disclose
James Dunn	Fees for non-CME/CE services received directly from a commercial interest or their agents (e.g., speakers bureau): AbbVie
Derek Fine	Nothing to disclose
Anna Forbes	Nothing to disclose
Rajesh Gandhi	Consulting fees: Merck, Gilead Research support: Gilead, Theratechnologies, ViiV, Janssen
Taylor Gill	Nothing to disclose
Michelle Haas	Nothing to disclose
Dennis Hartigan-O'Connor	Nothing to disclose
W. David Hardy	Consulting fees: Gilead, Merck, ViiV/GSK Contracted research: Amgen, Gilead, Janssen, Merck, ViiV/GSK
Rodrigo Hasbun	Consulting fees: Gilead Fees for non-CME/CE services received directly from a commercial interest or their agents (e.g., speakers bureau): Biofire Contracted research: Biofire
Emily Heil	Nothing to disclose
Margaret Hoffman-Terry	Consulting fees: Gilead, ViiV Fees for non-CME/CE services received directly from a commercial interest or their agents (e.g., speakers bureau): Gilead Contracted research: ViiV
Jennifer Husson	Contracted research: Merck, Sharpe, Dome Inc., Intercept Pharmaceuticals
Niyati Jakharia	Nothing to disclose
Boris Juelg	Research support: Gilead Sciences
Joseph Kass	Contracted research: Alzheimer's Disease Clinical Trial supported by Biogen, Takeda, Roche/Genentech, Novartis
Jeff Kirchner	Nothing to disclose

David Koren	Consulting fees: Gilead Sciences, ViiV Healthcare Contracted research: Gilead Sciences
Carolyn Kramer**	Nothing to disclose
Doris Kung	Nothing to disclose
Eurides Lopes	Nothing to disclose
Adrian Majid	Nothing to disclose
Poonam Mathur	Nothing to disclose
Jessica Meisner	Nothing to disclose
Steven Menez	Nothing to disclose
Ana Monczor	Nothing to disclose
Kudakwashe Mutyambizi Maloney	Nothing to disclose
Puja Nambiar	Nothing to disclose
Naiel Nassar	Nothing to disclose
Karin Nielsen-Saines	Nothing to disclose
Karen Nunez-Wallace	Nothing to disclose
Babafemi Onabanjo	Nothing to disclose
Edgar Overton	Consulting fees: ViiV Healthcare, Merck, Thera Technologies
Bruce Packett	Nothing to disclose
Rachel Prosser	Consulting fees: Gilead Contracted research: Gilead, ViiV, GSK
Christian Ramers	Consulting fees: Gilead Sciences, AbbVie Commercial interest or their agents (e.g., speakers bureau): Gilead Sciences, AbbVie, ViiV, Merck Contracted research: Gilead Sciences
Brandon Samson	Nothing to disclose
Aroonsiri Sangarlangkarn	Nothing to disclose
Jason Schafer	Consulting fees: Theratechnologies Inc. Contracted research: Merck Sharp and Dohme, Gilead Sciences
Hans Schlecht	Nothing to disclose
Jeffrey Schouten	Nothing to disclose
James Scott	Nothing to disclose
Rajagopal Sekhar	Nothing to disclose
Lydia Sharp	Nothing to disclose
Kalphana Shere-Wolfe	Nothing to disclose
Elizabeth Sherman	Nothing to disclose
Neha Sheth Pandit	Nothing to disclose
William Short	Consulting fees: ViiV, Gilead Sciences Fees for non-CME/CE services received directly from a commercial interest or their agents (e.g., speakers bureau): Janssen
Daniel Skiest	Nothing to disclose
Anthony Speights	Nothing to disclose
Sally Spencer Long	Nothing to disclose
Gary Spinner	Consulting fees: Gilead Sciences Ownership interest: Gilead Sciences
Rohit Talwani	Nothing to disclose
Zelalem Temesgen	Consulting fees: ViiV Healthcare
Karen Vigil	Consulting fees: Viiv, Gilead, Napo Pharmaceuticals Consulting research: Merck
Sana Waheed	Nothing to disclose
Amanda Willig	Nothing to disclose
Daniel Wlodarczyk	Nothing to disclose
David Wohl	Consulting fees: Gilead, ViiV, Janssen, Merck Contracted research: Gilead, Merck, ViiV
Hojoon You	Nothing to disclose
Barry Zevin	Nothing to disclose

DISCLOSURE OF UNLABELED USE

This educational resource may contain discussion of published and/or investigational uses of agents that are not indicated by the FDA. The contributors to this resource do not recommend the use of any agent outside of the labeled indications.

The opinions expressed in the educational resource are those of the faculty and do not necessarily represent the views of the American Academy of HIV Medicine. Please refer to the official prescribing information for each product for discussion of approved indications, contraindications, and warnings.

DISCLAIMER

Readers have an implied responsibility to use the newly acquired information to enhance patient outcomes and their own professional development. The information presented in this resource is not meant to serve as a guideline for patient management. Any procedures, medications, or other courses of diagnosis or treatment discussed or suggested in this resource should not be used by clinicians without evaluation of their patient's conditions and possible contraindications and/or dangers in use, review of any applicable manufacturer's product information, and comparison with recommendations of other authorities.

1.

EPIDEMIOLOGY AND THE SPREAD OF HIV

Philip Bolduc, Benjamin Alfred, and Babafemi Onabanjo

CHAPTER GOALS

Upon completion of this chapter, the reader should be able to

- Provide an overview of the global AIDS pandemic and the US epidemic

- Demonstrate and apply knowledge about the evolving epidemiology of HIV to both individual and population-wide aspects of clinical practice

- Educate clinicians and patients about factors driving HIV transmission so that they will understand who is at greatest risk of infection

---

OVERVIEW OF WORLDWIDE PANDEMIC

LEARNING OBJECTIVE

Discuss the global prevalence and geographic distribution of HIV-1 and HIV-2 infections.

WHAT'S NEW?

The World Health Organization/Joint United Nations Programme on HIV and AIDS (WHO/UNAIDS) estimates that, in 2017, nearly 40 million people worldwide were infected with HIV (UNAIDS, 2018). Although the numbers of new HIV infections and AIDS-related deaths continue to decline in many regions of the world, including sub-Saharan Africa, there are still certain regions where the incidence of HIV is rising, most notably in the eastern European and eastern Mediterranean areas. In his foreword to the UNAIDS Global AIDS Update 2018, executive director Michel Sidibe writes "The global AIDS response is at a precarious point—partial success in saving lives and stopping new HIV infections is giving way to complacency. At the halfway point to the 2020 targets, the pace of progress is not matching the global ambition" (Sidibe, 2018).

KEY POINTS

- UNAIDS identified several demographic subgroups at high risk for HIV infection and in danger of being left behind by the global AIDS response, including adolescent girls and young women, men who have sex with men (MSM), transgender people, people who inject drugs, prisoners, and sex workers.

- HIV occurs as types 1 and 2, with several groups and subtypes comprising HIV-1. Subtype B predominates in the Western Hemisphere and Western Europe, whereas other subtypes and recombinant forms are more prevalent elsewhere. Introduction of other subtypes and recombinant strains is occurring in the Western Hemisphere and Western Europe.

OVERVIEW OF GLOBAL PANDEMIC

Data from the WHO and UNAIDS show global estimates of HIV as a continuing pandemic, with increasing overall prevalence (36.9 million) but fewer new infections each year (1.8 million), more people on antiretroviral therapy (ART; 21.7 million), and fewer annual deaths (0.9 million) (Figures 1.1 and 1.2) (UNAIDS, 2018).

Africa remains the continent most heavily affected by HIV/AIDS, accounting for 70% of persons living with HIV in 2017 (Figure 1.3). However, due to several global initiatives, there has been a dramatic decline in the annual number of new HIV infections (−24%) and deaths (−35%) in 2017 compared to 2000 (UNAIDS, 2018). Annual infections and deaths have also declined over this period in the Americas (−5% and −20%, respectively) and Southeast Asia (−27% and −40%), but trends in Europe (+20% and −5%) and the Western Pacific areas (+7% and −45%) are mixed, and the Eastern Mediterranean area saw increases in both infections and deaths (+27% and +59%) (UNAIDS, 2018).

Across all countries, several key demographic subgroups continue to be most impacted by the HIV/AIDS epidemic. UNAIDS has identified six populations at higher risk of HIV infection that are in danger of being left behind by the global AIDS response: adolescent girls and young women, MSM, transgender people, people who inject drugs, prisoners, and sex workers. The risk of acquiring HIV is 27 times higher among MSM; 23 times higher among people who inject drugs; 13 times higher for female sex workers; and 12 times

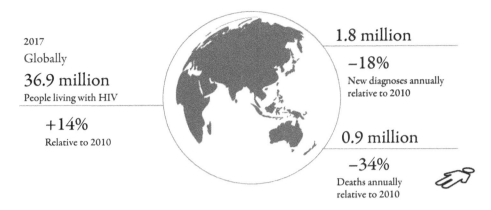

2017
Globally
36.9 million
People living with HIV

+14%
Relative to 2010

1.8 million
−18%
New diagnoses annually
relative to 2010

0.9 million
−34%
Deaths annually
relative to 2010

Figure 1.1 Global HIV epidemic since 2010—prevalence, incidence and mortality trends.   SOURCE: UNAIDS/WHO estimates, 2017.

higher for transgender women compared to other adults in the general population (UNAIDS, 2018).

The importance of each of these populations varies by region and within countries. For example, in southern Africa, age-disparate intergenerational sexual relationships and transactional sex place adolescent girls and young women at extremely high risk for HIV; in Eastern Europe and Central Asia, most new HIV infections are associated with people who inject drugs; and in the Latin American and Caribbean regions, the largest proportion of new HIV infections is among MSM. These six key populations and their sexual partners account for 47% of new HIV infections globally, but with wide geographic differences: just 16% in eastern and southern Africa but an incredible 95% in Eastern Europe, central Asia, the Middle East, and North Africa (UNAIDS, 2018).

As of 2017, 21.7 million people living with HIV were accessing ART, an increase of 2.3 million since 2016 and 13.7 million from 2010. Additionally, in 2017, 80% of pregnant women living with HIV had access to antiretrovirals to prevent mother-to-child transmission (UNAIDS, 2018). With better access to testing, 75% of all people living with HIV knew their HIV status in 2017 compared with ~50% of those living with HIV in 2014. Despite these significant achievements in the global HIV response, there is still much work to be done. The 2017 global HIV testing and care continuum (Figure 1.4) demonstrates that more than half of the world's people living with HIV are still not on antiretroviral treatment and that significant gaps remain to reach the UNAIDS 90-90-90 goal by 2020 (90% of infected persons will be diagnosed, 90% of those will be on treatment, and 90% of those will be virally suppressed).

HIV DIVERSITY

There are two major types of HIV, designated HIV-1 and HIV-2. Each has a similar but distinct genome with a genetic difference of approximately 60%. The vast majority of clinical cases are caused by HIV-1, with HIV-2 comprising only 1–2 million of the 36.9 million HIV cases living in 2016 (Campbell-Yesufu, 2011). HIV-2 is found almost exclusively in persons from or living in West Africa and is transmitted at lower rates than HIV-1. It appears to have a longer incubation

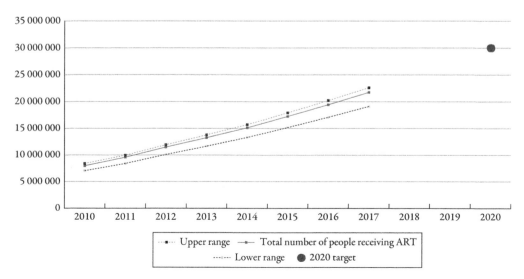

Figure 1.2 Increase in people receiving ART over time.   SOURCE: UNAIDS/WHO estimates, 2017. WHO HIV Update 2018. Available at http://www.who.int/hiv/data/en/. Accessed August 13, 2018.

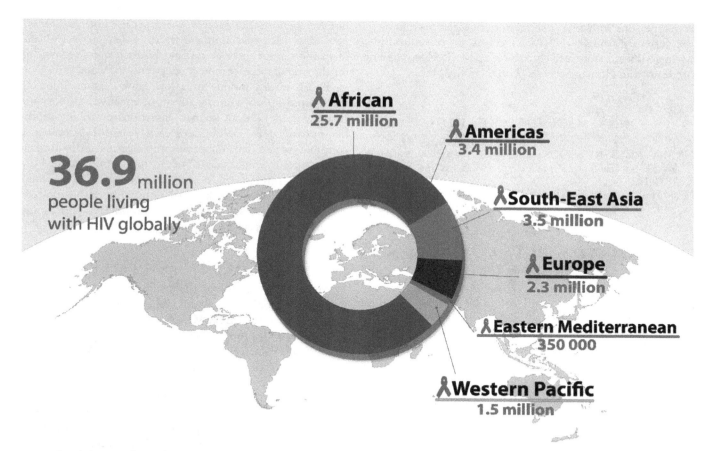

Figure 1.3 People living with HIV by WHO region (2017). SOURCE: UNAIDS/WHO estimates, 2017.

period, produce lower plasma viral load, and lead to AIDS in fewer patients (Apetrei, 2004). HIV-1 is classified into three genetically related subtypes based on the coding sequence of the envelope gene. Group M (Main) is the most common, and groups O (Outlier) and N (Not-M, Not-O or New) remain rare (Apetrei, 2004). Group M has at least 11 subtypes, or clades, designated A–K.

HIV subtype (i.e., group) variability may eventually influence how ART is used, although studies to date suggest that most antiretroviral agents appear to be equally effective regardless of the viral subtype. Certain subtypes may be less sensitive to or have a greater propensity to develop resistance to antiretroviral drugs or classes of these drugs (Spira, 2003; Gomes, 2002; Wainberg, 2004). A study from Thailand found that discordant viral load results were obtained in persons with non-B subtypes (Hackett, 2004).

There is limited clinical trial information on the effect of ART for HIV-2 infection. An in vitro study found that although the HIV-2 isolates tested were susceptible to the antiviral activities of nucleoside reverse transcriptase inhibitors and most protease inhibitors, they were highly resistant to non-nucleoside reverse transcriptase inhibitors (NNRTIs) (Witvrouw, 2004). Older studies of patients infected with HIV-2 receiving ART found mutations in HIV-2 reverse transcriptase and protease genes associated with HIV-1 drug resistance for each major drug class, including enfuvirtide, although HIV-2 also appears to have reverse transcriptase mutations that are not found in HIV-1 (Witvrouw, 2004; Colson, 2005; Damond, 2005; Rodes, 2000).

A 2013 in vitro study found that HIV-2 showed susceptibility to several newer antiretroviral agents, including tenofovir, emtricitabine, and the integrase inhibitor elvitegravir (Andreatta, 2013). A small study of five patients with HIV-2 found effective virologic responses and CD4+ cell increases when raltegravir was part of their ART regimen (Peterson, 2012). The net clinical implication of these findings

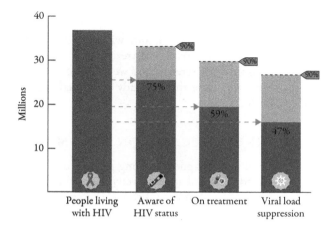

Figure 1.4 HIV testing and care continuum (2017). SOURCE: UNAIDS/WHO estimates, 2017. WHO HIV Update 2018. Available at http://www.who.int/hiv/data/en/. Accessed August 13, 2018.

is that persons with HIV-2 should not be treated with any of the currently available NNRTI medications or enfurvitide, whereas other classes are likely to be effective (US Department of Health and Human Services [USDHHS], 2018).

RECOMMENDED READING

UNAIDS. Global HIV & AIDS statistics—2018 fact sheet. Available at http://www.unaids.org/en/resources/fact-sheet. Accessed September 28, 2018.
World Health Organization. HIV/AIDS data and statistics. Available at http://www.who.int/hiv/data/en/ Accessed September 28, 2018.

OVERVIEW OF US EPIDEMIC

LEARNING OBJECTIVE

Describe current demographic trends in HIV disease in the United States, especially regarding gender, sexuality, race/ethnicity, age, injection-drug use, socioeconomic status, and recent initiatives.

WHAT'S NEW?

HIV, originally concentrated in the urban areas of the Northeast and California, continues its shift into the southeastern United States.

KEY POINTS

- HIV incidence among young black and Latino MSM continues to increase.

- The leading mode of HIV transmission continues to be male same-sex sexual contact.

- Nearly flat overall incidence rates and declining death rates continue to drive up HIV prevalence and workforce demands.

OVERALL US HIV PREVALENCE, INCIDENCE, AND DEATHS

(NB: at the time of this writing, the majority of available US HIV epidemiologic data from the US Centers for Disease Control and Prevention [CDC] was published in 2016, covering through 2015.)

According to the CDC, which reports on the prevalence and incidence of HIV and AIDS in the 50 US states and six territories, in 2015, an estimated 1.1 million persons aged 13 years or older were living with HIV, including 15% who were unaware of their diagnosis (CDC HIV/AIDS Resource Library Slideset, 2016). The year 2016 saw 39,782 new diagnoses, up from 38,500 in 2015. From 2011 through 2015, the annual number of new HIV diagnoses decreased in people who inject drugs (−16%), heterosexuals (−15%), and white gay and

bisexual men (−10%). However, within this same time period, new cases increased among African American (+4%) and Hispanic/Latino (+14%) gay and bisexual men, accounting for the overall increase in new infections (HIV.gov, 2016).

Death rates continue in a low, slow decline following the sharp drop-off with the advent of effective antiretroviral treatments in 1996. With new infections outpacing deaths by approximately 25,000 cases each year, HIV prevalence continues to rise. Two important implications of this are that more clinicians will be needed to care for the burgeoning HIV population, and more must be done to prevent HIV transmission by targeting high-risk populations with interventions of proven efficacy, such as preexposure prophylaxis (PrEP) and treatment-as-prevention.

HIV DEMOGRAPHICS ACROSS THE STATES

To take a regional look at these statistics, Figure 1.5 shows the rates of people living with HIV by state in 2015, showing clear weighting toward the West Coast, Northeast, and South. The South is disproportionally affected, comprising half of the new HIV infections in 2015, 46% of HIV prevalence, and 53% of deaths among HIV patients, despite having only 38% of the US population. Despite this unequal impact, Figure 1.5 also demonstrates that HIV is now also widely distributed throughout the United States. Consequently, HIV clinicians will be needed in new geographic locations to reach underserved areas. In addition, HIV prevention and education must expand beyond historically high-prevalence areas to virtually every state and county in the United States to reduce new infections in a way that we have not been able to do thus far.

AIDS REMAINS COMMON

Despite CDC and US Preventive Task Force recommendations for routine, opt-out, non−risk factor-based HIV screening since 2006, AIDS remains disappointingly common, with 18,160 persons receiving a new AIDS diagnosis in 2016, comprising 46% of the number of new HIV infections in 2016. New AIDS diagnoses follow a geographic trend similar to HIV diagnoses, with the heaviest impact in the South (53%), followed by the West (17%), Northeast (17%), and Midwest (13%). The high rate of AIDS despite widespread availability of effective, tolerable antiretroviral treatment highlights the need for improved HIV screening as well as care linkage, retention, and treatment for those already diagnosed with HIV (HIV.gov, 2016).

THE US HIV CARE CONTINUUM

The US rates of HIV diagnosis among persons estimated to be HIV-infected, care linkage and retention, and viral suppression are represented in the CDC's HIV care continuum (Figure 1.6). Since the National HIV/AIDS Strategy release in 2010, the HIV treatment community has focused on the care continuum as the leading quality indicator in our healthcare system's response to HIV. As ART has become

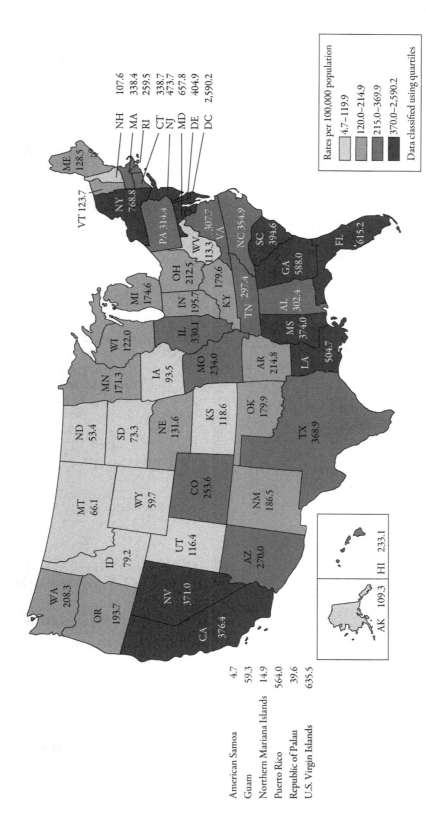

American Samoa   4.7
Guam   59.3
Northern Mariana Islands 14.9
Puerto Rico   564.0
Republic of Palau   39.6
U.S. Virgin Islands   635.5

Rates per 100,000 population

☐ 4.7–119.9
☐ 120.0–214.9
☐ 215.0–369.9
■ 370.0–2,590.2

Data classified using quartiles

NH 107.6
MA 338.4
RI 259.5
CT 338.7
NJ 473.7
MD 657.8
DE 404.9
DC 2,590.2

VT 123.7

ME 128.5

NY 768.8

PA 314.4

WV 113.3

VA 307.7

NC 354.9

SC 394.6

FL 615.2

GA 588.0

AL 302.4

MS 374.0

LA 504.7

TN 297.4

KY 179.6

OH 212.5

IN 195.7

MI 174.6

WI 122.0

IL 330.1

MO 234.0

AR 214.8

IA 93.5

MN 171.3

ND 53.4

SD 73.3

NE 131.6

KS 118.6

OK 179.9

TX 368.9

NM 186.5

CO 253.6

WY 59.7

MT 66.1

ID 79.2

UT 116.4

AZ 270.0

NV 371.0

WA 208.3

OR 193.7

CA 376.4

AK 109.3   HI 233.1

Figure 1.5 Rates of adults and adolescents living with diagnosed HIV infections, year-end 2015 (United States and 6 Dependent Areas).   N = 988,955, Total Rate = 364.3. CDC HIV/AIDS Resource Library Slide Sets. Available at http://www.cdc.gov/hiv/library/slidesets/index.html. Accessed August 14, 2018.

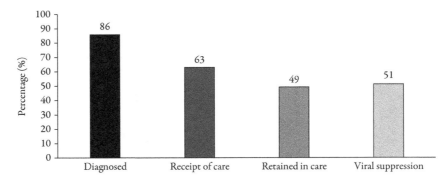

Figure 1.6 Persons living with diagnosed or undiagnosed HIV infection HIV care continuum outcomes, 2015 (United States). CDC HIV/AIDS Resource Library Slide Sets. Available at http://www.cdc.gov/hiv/library/slidesets/index.html Accessed August 14, 2018.

increasingly potent, less toxic, and easier to take, the greatest challenges in suppressing "community viral load" now exist primarily in the first two steps of the continuum, which in 2015 were the percentage of undiagnosed patients (14%) and the additional percentage of diagnosed patients who were not receiving medical care (23%). Only minor progress was made from 2009 to 2012 in these measures, and in 2012 fewer than one-third of persons with HIV in the United States were virally suppressed. However, by 2016, 76% of persons receiving an HIV diagnosis were linked to care within 1 month, improving the overall viral suppression rate to 51%. Providing HIV care across a variety of settings, particularly community health centers and other medical homes that serve affected populations with cultural competence, is critical to further improving the HIV care continuum. This supports the National HIV/AIDS Strategy goals, which include reducing new HIV infections, increasing access to care and improving health outcomes for people living with HIV infection, and reducing HIV-related health disparities (National HIV/AIDS Strategy, 2015 Accessed August 13, 2018).

TRANSMISSION BY MODE AND AGE

Efforts at HIV screening and prevention must target those at greatest risk for HIV infection by understanding how HIV transmissions are occurring and among what age groups. MSM continue to make up the majority of new HIV infections (68%), easily outpacing all other transmission modes combined (Figure 1.7). Another distinct trend is that the decreasing incidence in all age groups older than 34 years is now outweighed by increases in HIV incidence among 13- to 24-year-old and 25- to 34-year-old individuals (Figure 1.8). Of the 39,782 new HIV diagnosis in the United States in 2016, 41% were 13–29 years old; however, 17% of new infections were in the 50+ age group, reminding clinicians to screen for HIV well outside the peak demographic (HIV.gov, 2016).

RECOMMENDED READING

Centers for Disease Control and Prevention. HIV Surveillance Report, 2016. Available at http://www.cdc.gov/hiv/library/reports/surveillance.

SPREAD OF HIV AMONG WOMEN, CHILDREN, AND ADOLESCENTS

WHAT'S NEW?

Nineteen percent of HIV diagnoses in 2015 in the United States were among women, which represents a decrease from 2013 (24%). With widespread utilization of ART, transmission of HIV from mother to child has decreased to less than 1% in the United States.

KEY POINTS

- High-risk heterosexual contact remains the most common risk factor for HIV acquisition among adult women.

- The CDC recommends opt-out testing for all pregnant women in the first trimester and repeat testing in the third trimester for women at risk for infection. Adolescent HIV transmission mirrors adult patterns, with large majorities

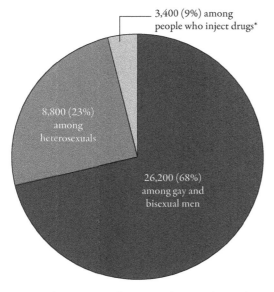

Figure 1.7 Estimated New HIV Infections in the United States by Transmission Category, 2015. SOURCE: CDC, 2017.

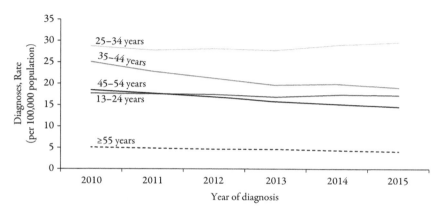

Figure 1.8 Rates of Diagnoses of HIV Infection among Adults and Adolescents by Age at Diagnosis, 2010–2015 (United States). SOURCE: CDC, 2017. CDC HIV In the United States At A Glance. Available at https://www.cdc.gov/hiv/statistics/overview/ataglance.html. Accessed August 15, 2018. CDC HIV/AIDS Resource Library Slide Sets. Available at http://www.cdc.gov/hiv/library/slidesets/index.html Accessed August 14, 2018.

of males infected via same-sex contact and females via heterosexual contact.

WOMEN

Worldwide in 2016, women continue to account for more than half (51%) of all HIV-infected persons and 43% of new infections largely through heterosexual transmission (American Foundation for AIDS Research [amfAR], 2017). In sub-Saharan Africa, three of four new infections are among girls aged 15–19 years, and young women aged 15–24 years are twice as likely as men to be living with HIV (UNAIDS, 2018). However, in the United States, women represented only 19% of HIV diagnoses in 2015, down from 24% in 2013, comprising an estimated 7,529 newly diagnosed infections. This disparity is due to the preponderance of male-to-male HIV transmission in the United States. Of these new diagnoses, approximately 4,271 were stage 3 (AIDS) classifications, a number that has been declining since 1996, but remains stubbornly fixed around one-quarter of all HIV diagnoses among women, highlighting the need to improve testing to find patients before progression to AIDS. HIV incidence among US women continues to be highest in the South, followed by the industrial states of the Northeast. Louisiana, with a rate of 15.3 infections per 100,000 population, is hardest hit, with a rate nearly three times the national average.

From 2007 through 2015, black/African American women accounted for the majority of new HIV diagnoses in US females (59% vs. 17% white). The seropositivity rate of these women (26.2 per 100,000 persons) was 15 times higher than that of white females (1.7/100k) and 5 times higher than that of Hispanic females (5.3/100k). Although black/African American women comprised only 13% of the female population, they accounted for 61% of diagnoses of HIV infection among women. Hispanic/Latino women made up 16% of the female population and accounted for 16% of diagnoses. White women encompassed 63% of the US female population and yet accounted for only 19% of HIV diagnoses in women overall (CDC, 2016).

Factors that increase a woman's risk of acquiring HIV include not knowing her partner's risk factors for HIV infection, having a lack of HIV knowledge, and having a decreased awareness of risk (CDC, 2011). Women's relationships with their partners play a pivotal role as well: in relationships in which women are physically abused, vulnerability to HIV is increased because they may not insist on condom use due to fear of being harmed. Women with a history of sexual abuse are more likely to engage in high-risk sexual activity and use drugs compared to women without such behaviors. This includes exchanging sexual activities for drugs and money as well as having difficulty refusing unwanted sex.

The most common mode of transmission for women is high-risk heterosexual contact (84–88% across various groups), followed by injection drug use. These rates, current through 2016, may change with the deepening national opioid crisis and outbreaks of HIV transmission among needle-sharing networks (CDC, 2016).

Sexual HIV transmission occurs through unprotected vaginal or anal sex, with receptive anal sex posing the highest risk and insertive vaginal sex the lowest. Oral sex is a theoretical risk if there are breaks in the oral and genital mucosa through which blood or genital secretions may pass. Similarly, sexually transmitted infections that disrupt genital mucosa and stimulate a local immune response increase the likelihood of acquiring or transmitting HIV. Because gonorrhea and syphilis in particular have a higher rate in women of color compared to white women, this likely plays a role in their heightened risk of HIV acquisition. Socioeconomic status also plays a role in HIV risk. In states with higher rates of poverty and limited access to healthcare, women are more likely to use drugs and exchange sex for drugs or money. These risk factors have been shown to increase risk of HIV, directly or indirectly (CDC, 2017).

CHILDREN

The reduction of mother-to-child HIV transmission in the United States is a major success of the antiretroviral era. Although the CDC does not publish a similar graph showing perinatal HIV transmission rates over time, Figure 1.9 shows the dramatic

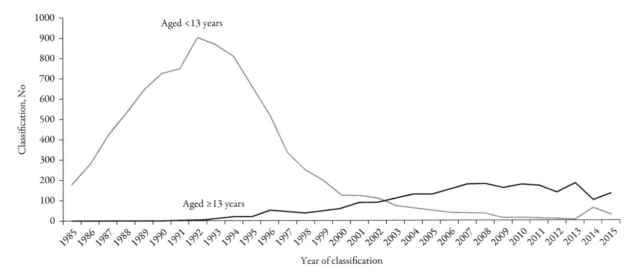

Figure 1.9 Stage 3 (AIDS) classifications among persons with perinatally acquired HIV infection, 1985—2015 (United States and 6 Dependent Areas).   SOURCE: CDC, 2017.

decline in perinatal AIDS diagnoses. In 1992, an estimated 952 pediatric HIV transmissions were reported in the United States. By 2004, the number declined to 177. In 2011, there were only 53 reported perinatal infections, but this has since stabilized to around 100 infections per year through 2016 (CDC, 2017). The overall rate of perinatal HIV infections reported by the CDC for 2015 was 1.5 per 100,000 live births, surpassing the CDC's goal of 5.1 by the end of 2015 (CDC, 2017).

The recent persistence of the number of transmissions in the face of declining rates is due to an increasing number of pregnancies among HIV-positive women as the powerful role of ART in preventing both horizontal and vertical transmission has been promoted among persons living with HIV. However, it bears noting that of all HIV diagnoses in children younger than age 13 years during 2010–2015, only 30% tested positive during their first year of life (Figure 1.10), which is closely linked to data showing that only 20% of these

children's mothers were tested for HIV during their pregnancy (Figure 1.11). Vertical transmission cannot be prevented if the mother's HIV status is not known, thus highlighting the importance of screening all pregnant women for HIV at least once during pregnancy.

HIV disproportionately affects black/African American children. While accounting for 64% of diagnoses, they comprised only 14% of the population of US children in 2016, whereas Hispanic (26% of population, 13% of HIV diagnoses) and white (50% of population, 13% of HIV diagnoses) children are infected far less often than their population percentages (CDC, 2016).

ADOLESCENTS

Adolescents aged 13–24, along with 25- to 34-year-old young adults, account for the only two age groups in which

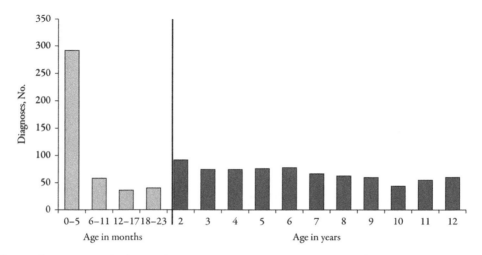

Figure 1.10 Diagnoses of HIV infection among children aged < 13 Years, by age at diagnosis, 2010—2015 (United States and 6 Dependent Areas).   N = 1,179. CDC, 2017.

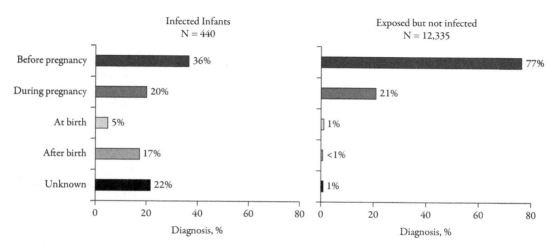

Figure 1.11 Time of maternal HIV testing among children with diagnosed perinatally acquired HIV infection and children exposed to HIV, birth year 2010-2014 (United States and Puerto Rico). SOURCE: CDC, 2016. SOURCE: CDC HIV/AIDS Resource Library Slide Sets. Available at https://www.cdc.gov/hiv/pdf/library/slidesets/cdc-hiv-surveillance-women-2016.pdf. Accessed August 02, 2018.

HIV incidence is rising in the United States, being driven in particular by infections among black and Latino MSM youth. Of all adolescents and young adults aged 13–24 years diagnosed with HIV infection, the CDC reported in 2015 that 54% were black/African Americans, again far outpacing their percentage of the general population. Another striking disparity for black/African American children is that their percentage of all children with AIDS increases dramatically with decreasing age, as seen moving right to left in Figure 1.12.

Transmission rates through male same-sex contact increased from 72% to 92.7% of all transmission from 2009 to 2016 in the adolescent and young adult population, whereas heterosexual infections decreased from 20% to 3%. Infections from injection drug use decreased among adolescents over this period from 4% to 1% (CDC, 2016).

In 2016, females comprised 16% of the HIV diagnoses in adolescents (13–19 years) and 11% in young adults (20–24 years) compared to 21% of adults older than 24 years. The mode of HIV transmission varies between sexes in this age group, as it does in adults: whereas 84% of adolescent and young adult females are infected through heterosexual contact, more than 90% of males contract HIV through male-to-male sexual contact (CDC, 2016).

RECOMMENDED READING

Centers for Disease Control and Prevention. HIV surveillance report: Diagnoses of HIV infection and AIDS in the United States and dependent areas. 2016. Vol. 28. Available at https://www.cdc.gov/hiv/pdf/library/reports/surveillance/cdc-hiv-surveillance-report-2016-vol-28.pdf.

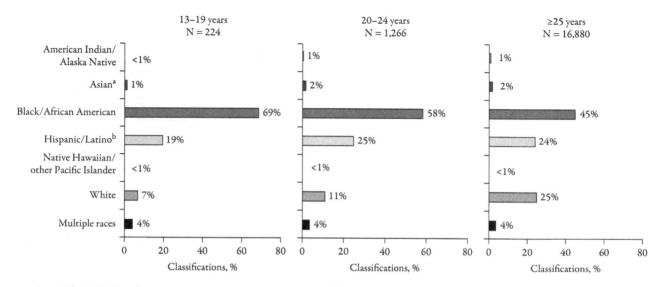

Figure 1.12 Stage 3 (AIDS) Classifications among persons aged 13 years and older with diagnosed HIV infection, by race/ethnicity and age group, 2016 (United States and 6 Dependent Areas). SOURCE: CDC, 2017. SOURCE: CDC HIV/AIDS Resource Library Slide Sets. Available at https://www.cdc.gov/hiv/pdf/library/slidesets/cdc-hiv-surveillance-women-2016.pdf. Accessed August 02, 2018

Centers for Disease Control and Prevention. Adolescents and young adult surveillance. Available at https://www.cdc.gov/hiv/pdf/library/slidesets/cdc-hiv-surveillance-adolescents-young-adults-2016.pdf.

Center of Disease and Prevention. Pediatric surveillance. Available at https://www.cdc.gov/hiv/pdf/library/slidesets/cdc-hiv-surveillance-pediatric.pdf.

SPREAD OF HIV AMONG MEN AND WOMEN IN COMMUNITIES OF COLOR

WHAT'S NEW?

Young black/African American MSM have the highest risk for HIV infection of any demographic group in the United States.

KEY POINTS

- Black/African Americans are HIV-infected at nearly four times higher rates than their percentage of the US population, with rates highest in the southeastern United States.

- AIDS and AIDS-related deaths among black/African Americans and Hispanics are higher than population norms, indicating poorer outcomes with HIV infection.

UNEQUAL BURDENS

Another important perspective of US HIV epidemiologic data is to recognize the ethnic and racial groups hardest hit by HIV infection and deaths, particularly blacks/African Americans. Figure 1.13 shows how this group steadily increased its percentage among AIDS diagnoses early in the epidemic while cases among Caucasians steadily declined, overtaking them in 1995 before leveling off in 2000, continuing to far exceed all other racial groups. Blacks/African Americans continue to be vastly overrepresented among persons living with HIV than in the general population in 2016 (44% vs. 12%). This is also true, but to a lesser extent, for Hispanics (25% vs. 18%). These numbers for whites, by comparison, are 61% and 26%, respectively.

Results from CDC's Young Men's Survey (1994–2000) found that many young black, African American, and Latino MSM outwardly identify as heterosexual, with female spouses or partners, but also engage in same-sex encounters with other men, and that this high-risk group represents a bridge for transmitting HIV to women (Fitzpatrick, 2004; Millett, 2004; Valleroy, 2004). In addition, many poor and/or minority women lack the agency—whether economic, cultural, or otherwise—to use condoms with or separate from abusive or unfaithful men who engage in high-risk sex with other partners or commercial sex workers. HIV prevention efforts must account for such factors to make inroads against HIV transmission in these groups.

The current highest risk demographic in the United States is young black MSM who live in the South, driving the epidemic in this population overall in the United States, such that the

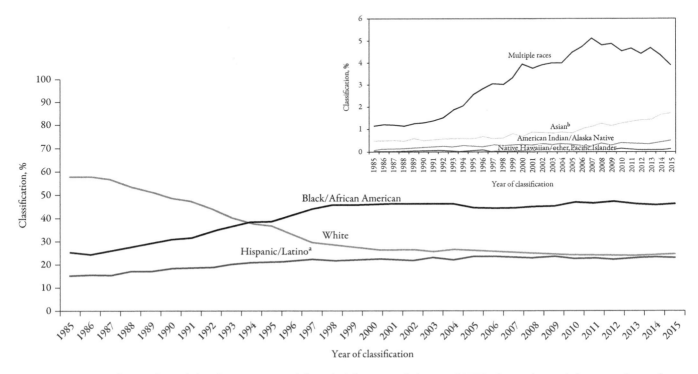

Figure 1.13 Percentages of stage 3 (AIDS) classifications among adults and adolescents with diagnosed HIV infection, by race/ethnicity and year of classification, 1985-2015 (United States and 6 Dependent Areas). SOURCE: CDC, 2017. CDC HIV/AIDS Resource Library Slide Sets. Available https://www.cdc.gov/hiv/pdf/library/slidesets/cdc-hiv-surveillance-race-ethnicity-2016.pdf. Accessed August 3, 2018.

CDC announced in 2016 that if current demographic trends continue, fully one-half of black, male MSM (and one-quarter of Latino MSM) will be HIV-infected in their lifetime. Black/African American women are also heavily disproportionately impacted by HIV, accounting for 61% of all new diagnoses among women, which is 4.7 times the expected population-adjusted rate. Similarly, 64% of all HIV-infected children younger than age 13 years are black/African American. Death rates are also heavily skewed against blacks/African Americans with HIV, with a sevenfold higher death rate than that of HIV-infected whites. The Hispanic death rate is almost twice that of whites, whereas other groups fare the same or better.

Regardless of how these data are examined—whether considering HIV diagnoses, AIDS, or deaths—there is a strikingly excessive burden of HIV shouldered in the United States by blacks/African Americans and, to a lesser extent, by Hispanics as well. The National HIV/AIDS Strategy recognized this in its call to reduce racial disparities in HIV care, which should be incorporated into the mission of all local, regional, and national HIV programs.

Such efforts must address the stigma, fear, discrimination, homophobia, distrust, and socioeconomic issues associated with poor access to care in these at-risk populations. The CDC and its partners are pursuing a high-impact prevention approach, increasing awareness about testing, prevention (including PrEP), and retention in care among populations disproportionately affected by HIV, particularly gay or bisexual men of color (HIV Surveillance Supplemental Report, 2017).

SPREAD OF HIV AMONG IMMIGRANT POPULATIONS

WHAT'S NEW?

- The percentage of new AIDS diagnoses in the United States comprised by minority races/ethnicities continues to climb.

- HIV-2 infection, while still uncommon in the United States, may rise as more persons emigrate from West Africa.

Race/Ethnicity	No.	Rate	%
American Indian/Alaska Native	2,904	122.6	0.3
Asian[a]	12,887	74.8	1.3
Black/African American	405,857	1,017.8	41.7
Hispanic/Latino[b]	213,736	379.4	21.9
Native Hawaiitan/other Pacific Islander	891	160.3	0.1
White	298,670	150.9	30.7
Multiple races	37,934	577.3	3.9
Total[c]	973,846	303.5	100

Figure 1.14 Adults and adolescents living with diagnosed HIV infection by race/ethnicity year-end, 2015 (United States). SOURCE: CDC, 2017.

KEY POINTS

- Different immigrant populations have widely varying rates of HIV infection, and differences within foreign and US-born racial/ethnic minorities are not fully understood.

- Immigrants, legal or not, face many barriers to engagement with the healthcare system.

For several years, the CDC has published data on the incidence and prevalence of HIV, AIDS, and HIV-related deaths among blacks/African Americans, Latinos/Hispanics, Asians, Native Americans, and Pacific Islanders. These data are summarized in Figures 1.14 and 1.15, showing the wide range of impact of HIV in these different groups and the growing overrepresentation of racial and ethnic minorities as a whole among AIDS diagnoses (71%) (Figure 1.16). However, in these data, the CDC does not separate African-born from US-born black/African Americans, or foreign-born versus US-born Latinos/Hispanics, making it difficult to track the HIV epidemic among these different immigrant populations. Despite this, a 2013 review found HIV incidence among African-born versus US-born blacks to be two-thirds higher, presentation with AIDS more frequent (30 vs. 22%), and progression to AIDS within 12 months of an HIV diagnosis more likely (45% vs. 37%), this despite the already high rates of these indicators among blacks/African Americans as a whole. Paradoxically, survival was better among African-born versus US-born blacks (7.1 deaths vs. 19.5 deaths per 1,000/year), possibly due to better engagement in care (Blanas, 2013).

Since January 4, 2010, refugees are no longer tested for HIV infection upon arrival to the United States. However, since 2006, CDC guidelines have recommended universal screening for all persons 13–64 years of age regardless of risk factors or country of origin (Branson, 2006). Given that the chaotic and vulnerable conditions of refugee flight and refugee camps create high risk for HIV transmission, HIV screening of all refugees is encouraged. The CDC-recommended fourth-generation testing algorithm will differentiate between HIV-1 and HIV-2, whereas older-generation HIV antibody screening tests generally do not. Therefore if fourth-generation testing is not available, refugees or immigrants native to or who have transited through countries with high HIV-2 prevalence should have specific testing for HIV-2.

The CDC's 2014 surveillance case definition for HIV and AIDS applies to both variants of HIV and has specified criteria for defining HIV-2. From 1988 to June 2010, only 242 HIV-2 cases were reported to the CDC, but, of these, only 166 met the case definition for HIV-2. These cases were concentrated in the Northeast (66%), including 46% in New York City, occurring primarily among persons born in West Africa (81%) (CDC, 2011). Nevertheless, most HIV infections in the United States are HIV-1, with HIV-2 comprising less than 1% of infections and largely confined to persons from West Africa (CDC, 2014).

Data from King County, Washington, show the percentage of new HIV cases that were foreign-born rising from 23% to 34% from 2006 to 2015. The leading countries of origin were Africa (34%), Latin America (32%), and Asia (22%).

Race/Ethnicity	No.	Rate	%
American Indian/Alaska Native	49	2.1	0.4
Asian[a]	62	0.4	0.5
Black/African American	5,586	14.0	44.7
Hispanic/Latino[b]	2,100	3.7	16.8
Native Hawaiitan/other Pacific Islander	4	0.7	<1
White	3,879	2.0	31.0
Multiple races	817	12.4	6.5
Total[c]	12,497	3.9	100

Figure 1.15 Deaths of persons with diagnosed HIV infection ever classified as stage 3 (AIDS), by race/ethnicity, 2015—United States. SOURCE: CDC, 2017. Accessed August 19, 2018.

Africans with HIV were more likely to be female and heterosexual, while Latin Americans and Asians were similar to US-born individuals by HIV risk factor and gender (male MSM) (Kerani, 2018).

Multiple factors contribute to HIV infection among immigrants. Migration within and across national borders in search of work may contribute to increased HIV risk situations. In addition, change in residence can result in loneliness, isolation, and disruption of social, familial, and sexual relationships that can lead to risk-taking behavior (Organista, 2004). In another study, the authors found lack of knowledge regarding HIV risk, social stigma, secrecy, and symptom-driven health-seeking behavior (as opposed to routine preventive care) as factors in delayed HIV presentation in immigrants. Furthermore, compared to US-born patients, immigrants were significantly younger; more likely to present with indicators of more advanced HIV disease, including opportunistic infections; had lower CD4[+] counts; and were more likely to be hospitalized at the time of HIV diagnosis,

consistent with findings specific to African-born HIV patients, as mentioned earlier (Levy, 2007).

RECOMMENDED READING

Centers for Disease Control and Prevention. HIV slidesets: HIV surveillance by race/ethnicity (through 2016). Available at: https://www.cdc.gov/hiv/library/slidesets/index.html.
Blanas DA, Nichols K, Bekele M, et al. HIV/AIDS among African-Born residents in #the United States. *J Immigr Minor Health* 2013 Aug;15(4):718–724.

THE EVOLVING ROLE OF THE GAY COMMUNITY IN THE SPREAD OF HIV

WHAT'S NEW?

The CDC estimated in February 2016 that, based on current trends, 1 in 2 gay black/African American MSM would become HIV-infected in their lifetime and that one-half of black/African American transgender women already are HIV-infected.

KEY POINTS

- Individuals who identify as gay, bisexual, or as other MSM are the only population group in the United States in which new HIV infections have steadily increased since the 1990s, with young black MSM being disproportionally affected.

- Transgender individuals are at extremely high risk for HIV infection, particularly transgender women of color.

Since the beginning of the HIV/AIDS epidemic in the United States, MSM have constituted the largest percentage

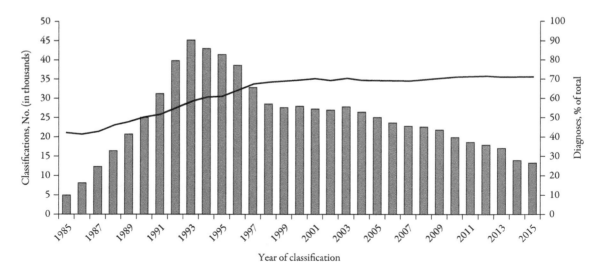

Figure 1.16 Diagnosed HIV infections classified as stage 3 (AIDS) among racial/ethnic minorities, 1985–2015 (United States and 6 Dependent Areas). SOURCE: CDC, 2017. SOURCE: CDC HIV/AIDS Resource Library Slide Sets. Available https://www.cdc.gov/hiv/pdf/library/slidesets/cdc-hiv-surveillance-race-ethnicity-2016.pdf. Accessed August 5, 2018.

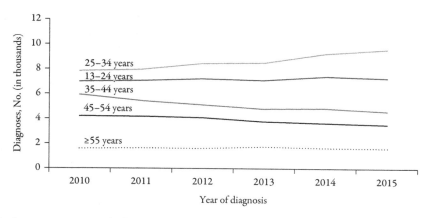

Figure 1.17 Diagnoses of HIV infection among men who have sex with men, by age at diagnosis, 2010–2015 (United States and 6 Dependent Areas).
SOURCE: CDC, 2017. CDC HIV/AIDS Resource Library Slide Sets. Available https://www.cdc.gov/hiv/library/slidesets/index.html. Accessed August 5, 2018

of persons diagnosed with HIV/AIDS, whereas HIV transmission among women who have sex with women has been exceedingly rare. Individuals who identify as gay, bisexual, or other MSM are the only population group in the United States in whom new infections have steadily risen since the early 1990s (CDC, 2016). In 2015, an estimated 82% (31,023) of all diagnosed HIV infections among adult and adolescent males were attributed to male-to-male sexual contact. Conversely, among male adults and adolescents, the number of diagnoses of HIV infection attributed to heterosexual contact from 2010 through 2015 decreased by 22%; diagnoses attributed to injection drug use decreased by 34%; and diagnoses attributed to male-to-male sexual contact and injection drug use decreased by 22% (CDC, 2016).

The percentage of HIV cases diagnosed in the gay community differs based on race/ethnicity and age. In 2015, the estimated percentage of MSM diagnosed with HIV infection who were black/African American, Latino, white and Asian were 38%, 29%, 28%, and 3%, respectively. Native American and Pacific Islander MSM each accounted for less than 1% of new infections, and persons of mixed race 2%. Among those aged 13–24, these disparities were more pronounced, with incidence rates of 54%, 24%, and 16%, respectively, among black/African American, Latino, and white MSM (CDC, 2016).

Differentiating between age groups among MSM, from 2010 to 2015, the largest numbers of diagnoses of HIV infection attributed to male-to-male sexual contact were seen in those aged 25–34 years, an increase of 23% over this period and more than any other MSM age group. From 2010 to 2015, new infections among MSM decreased 22% and 15% among those aged 35–44 and 45–54, respectively; infections in those 55 years and older and aged 13–24 years remained stable (Figure 1.17).

With the high prevalence of HIV in the MSM community, the cumulative risk of contracting or transmitting the virus becomes greater as these individuals age. Being unaware of one's HIV status, especially common among MSM of color and young MSM, increases the risk of transmitting HIV infection as well. According to CDC guidelines, MSM who are high risk for HIV infection should be screened at least annually; this includes those with more than one sex partner since their last HIV test and MSM who are injection drug users. Data are insufficient to recommend more frequent screening, but "each clinician can consider the benefits of offering more frequent screening (e.g., once every 3 or 6 months) to individual MSM at increased risk for acquiring HIV infection, weighing their patients' individual risk factors, local HIV epidemiology, and local testing policies" (CDC, 2017).

Transgender individuals are one of the highest-risk groups in the United States for acquiring HIV infection, and epidemiological data on this group are now available from the CDC. From 2009 to 2014, of the 2,351 transgender people diagnosed with HIV in the United States, 84% were transgender women, 15% were transgender men, less than 1% had another gender identity, and half of these infected persons lived in the South. One-quarter of transgender women are estimated to have HIV; among black/African Americans, this figure rises to one-half.

Despite these worrisome trends, nearly two-thirds of transgender men and women in the Behavioral Risk Factor Surveillance System from 2014 to 2015 were never tested for HIV. This clearly represents an opportunity for improved outreach, education, and testing, as well as for addressing the many factors that put transgender people at risk for HIV infection (multiple sexual partners, condomless sex, commercial sex work, mental illness and substance abuse, homelessness, unemployment, targeted violence, and lack of family support; CDC, 2018).

RECOMMENDED READING

Centers for Disease Control and Prevention. HIV surveillance special report vol. 28, 2016. https://www.cdc.gov/hiv/library/reports/hiv-surveillance.html. Accessed August 19, 2018.

Centers for Disease Control and Prevention. HIV among transgender people in the United States. April 2018. Available at https://www.cdc.gov/hiv/group/gender/transgender/index.html. Accessed August 19, 2018.

REFERENCES

American Foundation for AIDS Research (amfAR). Statistics: Women and HIV/AIDS. Available at http://www.amfar.org/about-hiv-and-aids/facts-and-stats/statistics--women-and-hiv-aids. Accessed August 3, 2018.

Andreatta K, Miller MD, White KL. HIV-2 antiviral potency and selection of drug resistance mutations by the integrase strand transfer inhibitor elvitegravir and NRTIs emtricitabine and tenofovir in vitro. *J AIDS*. 2013;62(4):367–374.

Apetrei C, Marx PA. Simian retroviral infections in human beings. Lancet 2004;364(9429):137–138.

Blanas DA, Nichols K, Bekele M, et al. HIV/AIDS among African-born residents in the United States. *J Immigr Minor Health*. 2013 Aug;15(4):718–724.

Branson BM. To screen or not to screen: is that really the question? *Ann Intern Med*. 2006;145(11):857–859.

Campbell-Yesufu OT, Gandhi RT. Update on human immunodeficiency virus (HIV)-2 infection. *Clin Infect Dis*. 2011;52:780–787.

Centers for Disease Control and Prevention (CDC). HIV/AIDS resource library slide sets (last updated in 2016). Available at https://www.cdc.gov/hiv/library/slideSets/. Accessed August 14, 2018.

Centers for Disease Control and Prevention (CDC). Diagnoses of HIV infection in the United States and dependent areas, 2016. HIV Surveillance Report 2017; vol. 28. Available at https://www.cdc.gov/hiv/library/slidesets/index.html. Accessed January 16, 2018.

Centers for Disease Control and Prevention (CDC). Monitoring selected national HIV prevention and care objectives by using HIV surveillance data—United States and 6 dependent areas, 2015. *HIV Surveillance Supplemental Report* 2017;22(No. 2). Available at http://www.cdc.gov/hiv/library/reports/hiv- surveillance.html. Published July 2017. Accessed August 15, 2018.

Centers for Disease Control and Prevention (CDC). HIV among transgender people in the United States. April 2018. Available at https://www.cdc.gov/hiv/group/gender/transgender/index.html. Accessed August 19, 2018.

Centers for Disease Control (CDC). MMWR recommendations for HIV screening of gay, bisexual, and other men who have sex with men—United States, 2017. Available at https://www.cdc.gov/mmwr/volumes/66/wr/mm6631a3.htm. Accessed August 19, 2018.

Centers for Disease Control and Prevention (CDC). HIV-2 infection surveillance—United States, 1987–2009. *MMWR Morb Mortal Wkly Rep*. 2011;60:985–988.

Centers for Disease Control and Prevention (CDC). Revised surveillance case definition for HIV infection—United States, 2014. Available at https://www.cdc.gov/mmwr/preview/mmwrhtml/rr6303a1.htm. Accessed August 18, 2018.

Colson P, Henry M, Tivoli N, et al. Polymorphism and drug-selected mutations in the reverse transcriptase gene of HIV-2 from patients living in southeastern France. *J Med Virol*. 2005;75:381–390.

Damond F, Brun-Vezinet F, Matheron S, et al. Polymorphism of the human immunodeficiency virus type 2 (HIV-2 protease gene and selection of drug resistance mutations in HIV-2-infected patients treated with protease inhibitors. *J Clin Microbiol*. 2005;43:484–487.

Fitzpatrick LK, Grant L, Eure C, et al. Investigation of HIV transmission among young black men who have sex with men (MSM) in North Carolina: implications for prevention. In: *Program and Abstracts of the XV International AIDS Conference*, July 11–16, 2004; Bangkok, Thailand. Abstract C10746.

Gomes P, Diogo I, Gonca Ives MF, et al. Different pathways to nelfinavir genotypic resistance in HIV-1 subtypes B and C. In: *Program and Abstracts of the 9th Conference on Retroviruses and Opportunistic Infections*, February 24–28, 2002; Seattle, WA. Abstract 46.

Hackett Jr J, Holzmayer V, Swanson P, et al. Analysis of HIV-1 genetic diversity in London and its impact on the performance of viral load assays. In: *Program and Abstracts of the XV International AIDS Conference*, July 11–16, 2004; Bangkok, Thailand. Abstract 3419.

HIV.gov. US HIV statistics. Available at https://www.hiv.gov/hiv-basics/overview/data-and-trends/statistics. Accessed August 14, 2018.

Kerani R, Bennett AB, Golden M, et al. Foreign-born individuals with HIV in King County, WA: a glimpse of the future of HIV? *AIDS Behav*. 2018 Jul;22(7):2181–2188.

Levy V, Prentiss D, Balmas, G, et al. Factors in the delayed HIV presentation of immigrants in Northern California: implications for voluntary counseling and testing programs. *J Immig Minor Health*. 2007;9(1):49–54.

Millett G. Men on the "down low": more questions than answers. In: *Program and Abstracts of the 11th Conference on Retroviruses and Opportunistic Infections*, February 8-11, 2004; San Francisco, California. Abstract 83.

National HIV/AIDS Strategy for the United States. Update to 2020. https://www.aids.gov/federal-resources/national-hiv-aids-strategy/overview. Accessed November 30, 2015.

Organista KC, Carillo H, Avala G. HIV prevention with Mexican migrants: review, critique, and recommendations. *J AIDS*. 2004;37(Suppl 4):S227–S239.

Peterson K, Ruelle J, Vekemans M, et al. The role of raltegravir in the treatment of HIV-2 infections: evidence from a case series. *Antivir Ther*. 2012;17(6):1097–1099.

Rodes B, Holguin A, Soriano V, et al. Emergence of drug resistance mutations in human immunodeficiency virus type 2-infected subjects undergoing antiretroviral therapy. *J Clin Microbiol*. 2000:1370–1374.

Sidibe, M. UNAIDS global AIDS update 2018: miles to go: closing gaps, breaking barriers, righting injustices. Available at http://www.unaids.org/en/resources/documents/2018/global-aids-update   Accessed August 13, 2018.

Spira S, Wainberg MA, Loemba H, et al. Impact of clade diversity on HIV-1 virulence, antiretroviral drug sensitivity and drug resistance. *J Antimicrob Chemother*. 2003;51:229–240.

UNAIDS. Fact Sheet July 2018. Available at: http://www.unaids.org/sites/default/files/media_asset/UNAIDS_FactSheet_en.pd. Accessed August 13, 2018.

US Department of Health and Human Services (USDHHS). Panel on Antiretroviral Guidelines for Adults and Adolescents. Guidelines for the use of antiretroviral agents in adults and adolescents living with HIV. Available at http://www.aidsinfo.nih.gov/ContentFiles/AdultandAdolescentGL.pdf. Accessed August 13, 2018.

Valleroy LA, MacKellar D, Behel S, Secura G. The bridge for HIV transmission to women from 15- to 29-year-old men who have sex with men in 7 US cities. In: *Program and Abstracts of the XV International AIDS Conference*, July 11–16, 2004; Bangkok, Thailand. Abstract 1367.

Wainberg MA. HIV-1 subtype distribution and the problem of drug resistance. *AIDS*. 2004;18(Suppl 3):S63–S68.

Witvrouw M, Pannecouque C, Switzer VM, et al. Susceptibility of HIV-2, SIV and SHIV to various anti-HIV-1 compounds: implications for treatment and postexposure prophylaxis. *Antivir Ther*. 2004;9:57–65.

2.

THE ORIGIN, EVOLUTION, AND EPIDEMIOLOGY OF HIV-1 AND HIV-2

Jeffrey T. Kirchner

CHAPTER GOAL

Upon completion of this chapter, the reader should be able to

- Explain how HIV evolved from cross-species transmission of strains of simian immunodeficiency virus (SIV) to humans (viral zoonosis), spread out of Africa in the early twentieth century, and ultimately resulted in the global AIDS pandemic

---

LEARNING OBJECTIVES

- Discuss the distinct origins of HIV-1 and HIV-2 from SIVs and the multiple cross-transmission events from apes to humans

- Describe the origin of the initial HIV infections in south-central Africa, the key reasons for viral dissemination to other areas of sub-Saharan Africa, and the ultimate global spread of HIV

- Discuss the diversity of HIV, including viral groups, viral clades, and recombinant forms and their implications for future transmission of HIV, as well as treatments and vaccine developments

ORIGIN OF HIV AND ENTRY INTO HUMANS

The origin of HIV-1 can be traced to the early 1920s from southern Cameroon and then to Kinshasa in what is now the Democratic Republic of Congo. The combination of rapid population growth, changes in sexual behaviors, and the use of unsterilized needles likely contributed to the rapid spread of HIV, especially groups M and O.

KEY POINTS

- All strains of HIV-1 and HIV-2 are genetic descendants of simian immunodeficiency viruses (SIVs). Initial cross-species transmission of the virus occurred from butchering and eating of bush meat.

- HIV-1 group M ("Main") and associated viral subtypes (A–K) account for approximately 95% of infections globally, with a much smaller number caused by groups N, O, and P.

- HIV-2 and its groups (A–H) are mainly limited to West Africa, but since the discovery of HIV-2 in 1986, cases have been reported in Europe and the United States. HIV-2 represents approximately 3% of all HIV infections, although its prevalence appears to be declining.

- Genetic diversity of HIV, including recombination between subtypes, may continue to present challenges to the development of a globally effective vaccine.

HIV, a retrovirus and member of the lentivirus family, was identified as the cause of AIDS 2 years after the first cases were reported in 1981 (Gottlieb, 1981). Dr. Luc Montaigner in France and Dr. Robert Gallo in the United States are both credited with identifying HIV-1 (Gallo, 2003). The pandemic form of HIV, also referred to as group M (for "Main"), is responsible for the majority of infections globally, currently estimated to be approximately 75 million. Since the discovery of HIV-1, followed by HIV-2 in 1986, the reasons for its emergence during the twentieth century, its transmission to humans, its genetic diversity, and the pathogenesis of the virus have been the subjects of extensive research.

It was first noted in 1999, via genetic sequencing, that the chimpanzee *Pan troglodytes troglodytes* infected with SIV_{cpz} was likely the primary natural reservoir for HIV-1 (Gao, 1999). Later work by Keele determined that HIV-1 in humans began with cross-species transmission and recombination of two SIVs (from red-capped mangabeys [*Cercocebus torquatus*] and greater spot-nosed monkeys [*Cercopithecus nictitans*]) to chimpanzees that preyed on these animals (Keele, 2006). Keele and his group analyzed mitochondrial DNA and viral-specific antibody from 599 fecal samples from chimpanzees. These samples exhibited a strong and broad cross-reactive western blot profile indistinguishable from that of HIV-1 human controls. To date, serologic evidence for SIV infection has been identified in more than 45 non-human primate species (NHPS) (Sharp, 2011; Peeters, 2014). The genetic diversity of these viral species is complex and includes coevolution of virus–host, cross-species transmission, and viral recombination.

Like HIV, SIV is sexually transmitted in NHPS and can also be transmitted vertically. In deference to previous thinking, SIV is indeed pathogenic in most NHPS, causing

CD4+ T-cell depletion (Keele, 2009). Chimpanzees infected with SIV have a 10- to 16-fold increased risk of death compared to those that are uninfected. Fertility and survival of offspring are also decreased in SIV-positive female chimpanzees.

WHAT'S NEW?

Solid evidence indicated that the first cross-species transmission of HIV to humans that predates emergence of group M occurred in southeast Cameroon (Sharp, 2011). It is not known how humans acquired the zoonotic precursors of HIV-1. However, based on the recognized biology of these viruses, transmission likely arose from cutaneous or mucous membrane exposure to infected chimpanzee blood or body fluid. These exposures often occur in the context of hunting, butchering, and eating of bush meat (Sharp, 2011).

THE SPREAD OF HIV THROUGHOUT AFRICA AND THE WORLD

A 2014 study by Faria and colleagues using phylogenetic analysis and "molecular clocks" (based on the assumption that retroviruses mutate over time at a constant rate) confirmed previous work by Hahn and others regarding the dissemination routes of HIV-1 in West Africa (Sharp, 2011; Cohen, 2014; Faria, 2014). They have also largely determined how group M became the driver of the AIDS pandemic. It is well established that the first known infections with HIV-1 emerged from Kinshasa (formerly called Leopoldville) in the Democratic Republic of the Congo in approximately 1920. Many refer to Leopoldville/Kinshasa as the cradle of the AIDS pandemic. From this area, the virus spread eastward to other communities via railway lines that carried up to 1 million passengers yearly to other areas of Africa, including the three largest population centers—Brazzaville, Mbuji-Mayi, and Lubumbashi (Cohen, 2014; Faria, 2014). Rivers were major travel and commerce routes and are believed to have enabled the spread of HIV geographically (Figure 2.1).

Sexual transmission is thought to be the primary mode and driver of new HIV infections and resultant dissemination of the virus at this time. Unsterilized injections at clinics in the area may have greatly contributed to the spread of HIV. According to Jaques Pepin, well-intended public health interventions by authorities in the Belgian Congo from 1921 to 1959 to treat trypanosomiasis, syphilis, yaws, malaria, and leprosy resulted in the administration of millions of injections to residents of these communities (Pepin, 2011). The majority of injections were intravenous and administered with syringes that clinicians used repeatedly without sterilization of the needles (Pepin, 2011). Consequently, thousands of these individuals may have acquired HIV iatrogenically. Data suggest similar transmission of hepatitis B and C viruses.

The epidemic histories of HIV-1 groups M and O were similar until approximately 1960, when group M infections underwent an epidemiologic transition and exponential increase, outpacing regional population growth (Faria, 2014). It is unknown why the growth rate of infections with HIV group M nearly tripled at approximately this time, but current explanations include

virus-specific factors, population growth factors, and the widespread use of injections (Sharp, 2011; Pepin, 2011).

Tissues samples collected from two patients in Kinshasa in 1959 and 1960 showed that HIV-1 had diversified into different subtypes much earlier than previously believed. Viral sequencing done on plasma from a sailor who died in 1959 is the oldest case of documented HIV-1 infection (Zhu, 1998). Worobey and colleagues amplified and identified HIV-1 from a lymph node specimen obtained in 1960 from a female in Kinshasa (Worobey, 2008). The sizable genetic difference between these two HIV specimens demonstrated that diversification of HIV-1 occurred in Kinshasa at least 20 years before the first AIDS cases were observed in the United States. As HIV-1 group M spread globally, its dissemination led to population bottlenecks ("founder events") that resulted in different lineages, viral subtypes or clades, and circulating recombinant forms (CRFs) (Peeters, 2014).

How and when HIV first arrived in the United States remains debatable. The virus first appeared in Haiti between 1960 and 1966. The probable source was Haitian professionals who returned from working in the newly independent Congo. It is estimated that during the 1960s, approximately 4,500 skilled Haitian workers were employed by the Congolese government. However, Pepin states that "a single technical assistant infected with HIV-1 subtype B went back to Haiti and stayed long enough to start a local chain of sexual transmission" (Pepin, 2011). Some authorities believe that the selling of sex to American tourists in Haiti led to HIV infection in individuals who in turn brought the virus back to the United States. Pepin states, "American gay and bisexual men infected Haitian male sex workers."

Work done by Gilbert and colleagues using HIV-1 *gag* gene sequences from five Haitian AIDS patients determined that HIV-1 subtype B definitely arrived in Haiti before it spread to the United States and other Western countries (Gilbert, 2007). The same group of researchers noted that the most recent common ancestor of HIV-1 subtype B virus appeared in Haiti in 1966, but not in the United States until 1969. Consequently, these data suggest that HIV-1 was circulating cryptically in the United States for approximately 12 years before the 1981 cases of AIDS were recognized and reported (Gottlieb, 1981). The virus was spreading slowly among the heterosexual population before entering the higher risk men who have sex with men (MSM) population, in which it spread much more extensively and began to be recognized clinically. The actual scientific facts will likely never be known; however, Pepin believes that the blood trade in Port-au-Prince exponentially amplified the number of HIV infections in Haiti and possibly other countries in which blood products were sold, including the United States (Pepin, 2011).

HIV-1 AND HIV-2 GROUPS AND SUBTYPES AND THEIR GEOGRAPHIC DISTRIBUTIONS

HIV-1 comprises four distinct lineages termed groups M, N, O, and P. Each has resulted from a distinct and independent cross-species transmission event of SIVs infecting African apes.

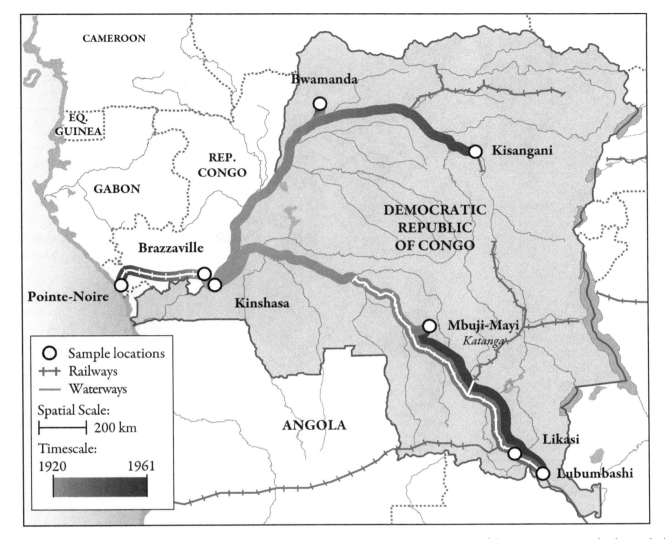

Figure 2.1 Spatial dynamics showing the spread of HIV-1 group 1 from Kinshasa in the Democratic Republic of the Congo via rivers and railways which were operational until about 1960.   Faria NR, Rambaut A, Suchard MA, et al. Science 2014 Oct 3: 346(6205):56-61.

Using molecular clocks, the most recent common ancestor of group M has been dated to approximately 1920 (Sharp, 2011). The four known HIV-1 groups share approximately 50–60% homology in their nucleotide sequences.

HIV-1 group M was the first lineage discovered and represents the pandemic form of HIV-1. It has a widespread global distribution and accounts for 90–95% of HIV-1 infections (Sharp, 2011). The genetic diversity within HIV-1 group M is the result of subsequent evolution and spread in humans. Bases on phylogenic analysis, HIV-1 group M can be further divided into nine pure subtypes or clades (A–D, F–H, J, and K) and additional sub-subtypes (A1–A4 and F1–F2). The subtypes share 80% homology in their genetic sequences, meaning they differ genetically by approximately 20%. Subtypes and sub-subtypes can form additional mosaic forms through recombination of different strains inside dually or multiply infected individuals. Some recombinant forms may further achieve epidemic relevance, giving rise to known CRFs. To date, researchers have identified more than six CRFs and unique recombinant strains. Globally, subtype C, found

mainly in sub-Saharan Africa, represents approximately 50% of HIV-1 infections. This is followed by subtype A (12%), found mainly in central and east Africa. Viral subtype B (11% of infections) is the predominant subtype in the United States and the most geographically dispersed subtype worldwide. Subtypes G and D respectively account for 5% and 2% of infections worldwide (Peeters, 2014) (Figure 2.2 and Box 2.1).

HIV-1

Group N

Group N ("N" for "non-M, non-O," or "new") was isolated in 1995 from a woman in Cameroon who had AIDS (Pepin, 2011). To date, fewer than 20 cases of group N infection have been identified, and all except one were from Cameroon. Similar to group M, it is the result of chimpanzee-to-human transmission. The small number of infections resulting from this group and limited genetic diversity suggest that its introduction into humans did not occur until approximately 1963 (Peeters, 2014).

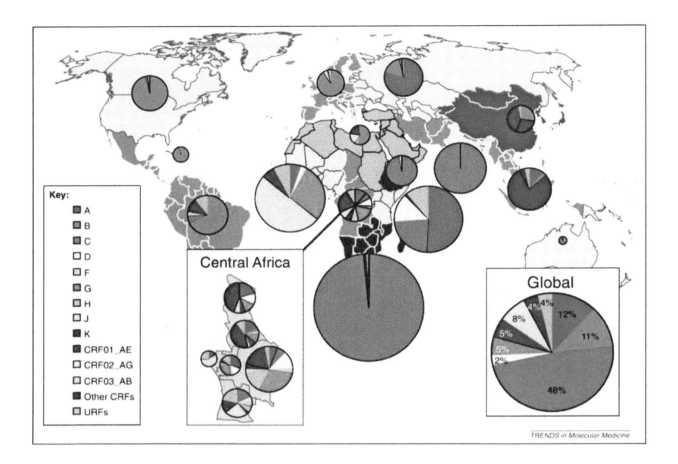

Historically, the distribution of subtypes followed the geographic patterns listed below.

- **Subtype A:** Central and East Africa as well as East European countries that were formerly part of the Soviet Union.

- **Subtype B:** West and Central Europe, the Americas, Australia, South America, and several Southeast Asian countries (Thailand, and Japan), as well as northern Africa and the Middle East.

- **Subtype C**: Sub-Saharan Africa, India, and Brazil.

- **Subtype D**: North Africa and the Middle East.

- **Subtype F**: South and Southeast Asia.

- **Subtype G**: West and Central Africa.

- **Subtypes H, J, and K**: Africa and the Middle East.

Figure 2.2 The global distribution of HIV-1 Group M Sub-types. Hemelaar J. Trends in Molecular Medicine. Mar 1, 2012; 18(3):182-192.

Group O

Group O ("O" for "outlier") was first discovered in 1990 in two Cameroonians living in Belgium (De Leys, 1990) and is thought to represent only approximately 1% all HIV infections. Recent studies have determined that group O originated by cross-species transmission from western lowland gorillas (*Gorilla gorilla*) instead of chimpanzees (D'arc, 2015). Like the other groups, it underwent adaptations to the human hosts. A recent study found the prevalence of HIV-1 group O in Cameroon to be approximately 0.6%, indicating that the frequency of group O has been stable during the past few decades. However, the current distribution of the circulating viral strains still does not allow classification as subtypes (Villabona-Arenas, 2015). There are also some reports of dual infections with HIV-1 group M and group O but no recombinant forms in coinfected patients (Ngoupo, 2016). Natural resistance to HIV medications, including integrase inhibitors, has not been identified. This suggests that infection with HIV-1 group O can be adequately managed in countries in which the virus circulates, but this group remains challenging in regard to diagnostic and monitoring strategies.

Group P

Group P was discovered in 2009, isolated from a Cameroonian woman living in France (Plantier, 2009). Despite subsequent screening for more infections caused by this group, only two cases have been identified. It is uncertain when group P virus entered the human population; it is estimated to be any time from 1845 to 1989 (Peeters, 2014). In addition, it remains unclear if the source was a chimpanzee or gorilla. The inability to antagonize tetherin protein (human restriction factor) may explain the limited spread of HIV-1 group P in the human population (Sauter, 2011).

HIV-2

In 1986, a morphologically similar but antigenically distinct virus was found to cause AIDS in persons living in western Africa and was termed HIV-2 (Clavel, 1986, 1987). This virus has only approximately 30–40% genetic homology with HIV-1; thus, it is considered a different virus and not another HIV-1 group (Pepin, 2011). It was determined that HIV-2 originated in sooty mangabeys (*Cercocebus atys*) with bloodborne transmission to humans, similar to HIV-1 (Chen, 1997; Gao, 1992). Molecular clock research has determined that the most common recent ancestor for HIV-2 dates to 1940 and 1945 for the first two groups—A and B (Pepin, 2011), respectively.

HIV-2 has been found mainly in Guinea-Bissau, Gambia, Senegal, Cote d'Ivoire, Mali, Nigeria, Senegal, and Sierra Leone. With widespread immigration, cases have been reported throughout Europe, the United States, and other areas of the world (Campbell-Yesufu, 2011).

Since its initial discovery, phylogenic analysis has identified eight different lineages of HIV-2 (groups A–H). As for HIV-1, each group represents a different host transfer of SIV from nonprimate species (mangabeys) to humans. However, unlike HIV-1, only types A and B have spread to humans to any significant degree. The other groups only represent individual human cases. Of note clinically, persons infected with HIV-2 often have lower viral loads compared to those with HIV-1 (Campbell-Yesufu, 2011). There is also less genital shedding in semen and cervical secretions. This likely accounts for decreased infectivity. It has also been observed that persons infected with HIV-2 have a longer asymptomatic phase and slower progression to AIDS than those with HIV-1. However, in the absence of treatment, the same progressive decline in immune function and resultant disease complications will occur.

THE FUTURE OF HIV REGIONAL AND GLOBAL GENETIC DIVERSITY

By combining historical, phylogenetic, molecular evolutionary, and epidemiological perspectives, researchers have been able to reconstruct the history of the AIDS pandemic and many unique aspects of HIV-1 and HIV-2. It is hoped that this information will be of value for HIV vaccine research and development that takes into account the genetic diversity discussed previously. It may also determine how strains of HIV may continue to spread and colonize new geographic regions and host populations. It also raises numerous questions: Given the fact that there are many other non-human primates infected with SIV, should there be concern for future zoonotic infections from cross-species transmissions? Will the growing prevalence of sexually transmitted infections continue to facilitate the dissemination and adaptation of HIV-1 and HIV-2? May there be a therapeutic role for host-restriction factors? Will it be possible to develop an HIV vaccine that will be effective against all HIV groups and subtypes?

RECOMMENDED READING

Pepin J. *The Origins of AIDS*. New York: Cambridge University Press; 2011.

Quammen D. *The Chimp and the River: How AIDS Emerged from an African Forest*. New York: Norton; 2015.

REFERENCES

Campbell-Yesufu OT, Gandhi RT. Update on human immunodeficiency virus (HIV)-2 infection. *Clin Infect Dis*. 2011;52(6):780–787. doi:10.1093/cid/ciq248

Chen Z, Lucky A, Sodora DL, et al. Human immunodeficiency virus type 2 (HIV-2) seroprevalence and characterization of a distinct subtype within the range of SIV-infected sooty mangabeys. *J Virol.* 1997;71:3953–3960.

Clavel F, Guétard D, Brun-Vézinet F. Isolation of a new human retrovirus from West African patients with AIDS. *Science.* 1986;233(4761):343–346.

Clavel F, Mansinho K, Chamaret S. Human immunodeficiency virus type 2 infection associated with AIDS in West Africa. *N Engl J Med.* 1987;316:1180–1185.

Cohen, J. Early AIDS virus may have ridden Africa's rails. *Science.* October 2014;346:21–22.

D'arc, M, Ayouba A, Esteban A, et al. Origin of the HIV-1 group O epidemic in western lowland gorillas. *Proc Natl Acad Sci USA.* 2015 March 17;112(11):E1343–E1352.

De Leys R. Isolation and partial characterization of an unusual HIV retrovirus from two persons of west-central Africa origin. *J Virol.* 1990;64:1207–1216.

Faria, NR, Rambaut A, Suchard MA, et al. The early spread and epidemic ignition of HIV-1 in human populations. *Science.* 2014;346(6205):56–61.

Gallo RC, Montagnier L. The discovery of HIV as the cause of AIDS. *N Engl J Med.* 2003;349:2282–2285.

Gao F, Bailes E, Robertson DL, et al. Origin of HIV-1 in the chimpanzee *Pan troglodytes troglodytes. Nature.* February 4, 1999;397:436–441.

Gao F, Yue L, White AT, et al. Human infection by genetically diverse SIVsm-related HIV-2 in West Africa. *Nature.* 1992;358:495–499.

Gilbert MTP, Rambaut A, Wlasiuk G, et al. The emergence of HIV/AIDS in the Americas and beyond. *Proc Natl Assoc Sci USA.* November 20, 2007;104(47):18566–18570.

Gottlieb MS, Schanker HM, Fan PT, et al. *Pneumocystis* pneumonia–Los Angeles. *MMWR.* June 5, 1981;30(21):1–3.

Keele BF, Jones JH, Terio KA, et al. Increased mortality and AIDS-like immunopathology in wild chimpanzees infected with SIV_{cpz}. *Nature.* July 2009;460:515–519.

Keele BF, Van Heuverswyn F, Li Y, et al. Chimpanzee reservoirs for pandemic and nonpandemic HIV-1. *Science.* July 28, 2006;313(5786):523–526.

Ngoupo PA, Sadeu, MB, Alain S, et al. First evidence of transmission of an HIV-1 M/O intergroup recombinant virus. *AIDS.* January 2016;30(1):1–8.

Peeters M, D'Arc M, Delaporta E. The origin and diversity of human retroviruses. *AIDS Rev.* 2014;16(1):23–34.

Pepin J. *The Origins of AIDS.* New York: Cambridge University Press; 2011.

Plantier JC, Leoz, M, Dickerson JE. A new immunodeficiency virus derived from gorillas designated group "P." *Nature Med.* 2009;15:871–872.

Sauter D, Hué S, Petit S, et al. HIV-1 group P is unable to antagonize human tetherin by Vpu, Env or Nef. *Retrovirology.* 2011;8:103.

Sharp PM, Hahn BH. Origins of HIV and the AIDS pandemic. *Cold Spring Harbor Perspect Med.* 2011;1:1–22.

Villabona-Arenas CJ, Domyeum J, Mouacha F, et al. HIV-1 group O infection in Cameroon from 2006–2013: prevalence, genetic diversity, evolution, and public health challenges. *Infect Gener Evo.* 2015;36:210–216. Epub September 11, 2015.

Worobey M, Gemmel M, Teuwen DE, et al. Direct evidence of extensive diversity of HIV-1 in Kinshasa by 1960. *Nature.* October 2, 2008;455(7213):661–664.

Zhu T, Korber BT, Nahmias AJ, et al. An African HIV-1 sequence from 1959 and implications for the origin of the epidemic. *Nature.* 1998;391(6667):594–597.

3.

MECHANISMS OF HIV TRANSMISSION

Puja Nambiar and William R. Short

CHAPTER GOALS

Upon completion of this chapter, the reader should be able to

- Describe the relative risk of acquiring HIV infection based on various types of sexual activity, occupational exposures, drug use, and vertical transmission

- Discuss the significance of viral load quantity and its relationship to transmission risk

- Explain the impact of co-occurring sexually transmitted diseases in HIV transmission

INTRODUCTION

With 20 years of experience demonstrating that ART is highly effective in reducing the transmission of HIV, there is now clear evidence that individuals living with HIV with an undetectable viral load cannot transmit HIV sexually.

WHAT'S NEW?

- U = U campaign: Undetectable viral load equals untransmittable

- Clinical trial data demonstrate that treatment of HIV infection is also prevention.

- It has been shown that occupational transmission is extremely rare in the United States.

KEY POINTS

- The risk of HIV transmission to a receptive partner remains higher than that to an insertive one; however, both carry a risk.

- Anything that compromises the integrity of mucous membranes, such as sexually transmitted infections, may increase the risk of transmission.

- Keeping an infected partner's viral load persistently suppressed to an undetectable level reduces the risk of transmission to an HIV-negative partner.

- Maternal transmission is a larger concern in developing countries due to lack of access to perinatal treatment with antiretroviral drugs.

SEXUAL TRANSMISSION

HIV can be transmitted through infected body fluids—blood, seminal fluid, vaginal fluid, rectal fluid, and breast milk. Sexual contact is the most common mode of HIV transmission worldwide. In the United States, HIV is mainly transmitted by anal or vaginal sex and less commonly by other modes such as oral sex; mother-to-child transmission either during pregnancy, birth, or breastfeeding; needle injury; blood transfusion; or organ transplants (Centers for Disease Control and Prevention [CDC], 2010). In 2016, 70% of HIV diagnosed infection was attributed to male-to-male sexual contact and injection drug use and 24% to high-risk heterosexual activity (CDC, 2017).

Acutely infected individuals, often with very high viral loads, are at the highest risk of transmitting the virus. HIV can be readily found in semen and in vaginal fluid from HIV-positive persons. There is a strong correlation between high plasma viral load and the amount of virus in genital secretions (Zhang, 1998). However, discordance, although rare, can exist between levels of HIV in the plasma and genital secretions. HIV-positive men on antiretroviral therapy (ART) with undetectable virus in plasma can infrequently have detectable HIV in their seminal fluid (Zhang, 1998).

Unprotected anal sex has the highest risk for HIV transmission, with the receptive partner being at higher risk than the insertive partner. The person receiving the infected semen is at highest risk of contracting the infection. This is believed to be the case because of the single cell layer of epithelium lining the rectum, which can be easily disrupted and permit entry of the virus across the rectal mucosa. The insertive partner is also at significant risk because HIV can enter the penis through the urethra; the mucosa of the nonkeratinized portions of foreskin; or through cuts, abrasions, or open sores on the penis. Circumcision has been demonstrated to significantly reduce the risk of HIV acquisition but not of transmission (Dosekun, 2010).

Worldwide, the AIDS epidemic is being driven by new infections occurring in women of childbearing age. During unprotected vaginal intercourse, both partners are at risk of contracting HIV, although there is a higher risk of a woman contracting HIV from an infected man than a man contracting HIV from an infected woman. HIV can enter the body through the vaginal and cervical mucous membrane linings. HIV-1 replicates and persists in the vaginal epithelial dendritic cells (Pena-Cruz, 2018), which provides a readily understandable mechanism for transmission via the vaginal mucosa. Although the risk of men acquiring HIV through heterosexual vaginal or anal intercourse is lower, HIV is abundantly present in vaginal secretions, and the anatomic sites of potential infection in the penis are the same as those described previously for anal intercourse (Dosekun, 2010).

Sexually transmitted infections (STIs) have a significant role in HIV transmission. Genital ulcer disease (i.e., syphilis, chancroid, and herpes simplex infections), and diseases causing mucosal inflammation (i.e., gonorrhea and chlamydia) have been shown to increase HIV transmission threefold. This increase is most likely due to both heightened infectivity and susceptibility. Open ulcers aid HIV entry, and inflammation recruits increased numbers of $CD4^+$ cells that serve as targets for HIV. Early diagnosis of STIs has the potential to significantly reduce HIV incidence in general, especially if applied to high-risk populations. Another potential factor is the use of hormonal contraception in women because it may thin the vaginal mucosa, making it more susceptible to tears and trauma. However, large randomized clinical trials have provided conflicting results, and currently it is not clear whether hormonal contraception has any effect on HIV transmission.

Limiting viral replication in genital secretions is a logical approach to preventing HIV acquisition. Already well-known but of critical historical importance are the data from HPTN 052, in which sexual HIV transmission was shown to be dramatically reduced in HIV serodiscordant couples in which the seropositive partner was receiving suppressive ART along with monthly HIV prevention counseling, provision of and encouragement to use condoms, and regular STI testing and treatment. This unique clinical trial showed that HIV-positive men and women had a 96% reduced risk of transmitting the virus to their original linked, HIV-negative sexual partners through early initiation of ART (Cohen, 2011). Longer term results of the study showed a sustained, overall 93% reduction of HIV transmission among linked couples when the HIV-positive partner was taking ART and had a suppressed viral load (Cohen, 2016). The results of this historic study provided the initial data to support treatment as prevention (TasP).

Taking evaluation of TasP even further, the prospective, observational PARTNER-1 (Partners of people on ART: a New Evaluation of the Risks) study, although of limited follow-up time (median = 1.3 years per couple) showed no linked HIV transmissions with thousands of episodes of condomless anal and vaginal sex among serodiscordant heterosexual and men who have sex with men (MSM) couples in which the HIV-positive partner was virologically suppressed on ART (Rodger, 2016). More recently, the PARTNER-2 study reinforced and extended these data for MSM couples showing no cases of linked HIV transmissions in MSM couples where the HIV-positive partner had fully suppressed virus despite thousands of occurrences of condomless anal sex with or without ejaculation or with or without an STI. Of note, these data were collected without the use of preexposure prophylaxis (PrEP) or post-exposure prophylaxis (PEP) (Rodger, 2018).

Developing novel approaches for the rapid detection and diagnosis of HIV infection and increasing ART coverage are the next important steps in realizing the potential public benefits of these discoveries.

TRANSMISSION IN THE HEALTHCARE SETTING

The risk of occupational transmission of HIV is relatively small, but it has occurred in a variety of settings. Needle stick and other sharp instrument injuries are relatively common in healthcare. However, in developed countries, only a small fraction of these involve HIV-infected blood. In settings in which HIV incidence is high, such as sub-Saharan Africa, this risk is significantly higher, thus increasing the potential for transmission. Other types of healthcare-related procedures that can potentially cause transmission involve the use of vascular cannulas and introducers, suture needles, scalpels, and other sharp or cutting instruments. The risk of HIV transmission after puncture with a large-gauge, hollow-bore needle contaminated with HIV-positive blood has been estimated to be 0.3%. There is virtually no risk of HIV transmission via contact of HIV-infected body fluids with intact skin. However, there is an increased risk of transmission when nonintact skin or mucus membranes is involved. The risk of transmission after exposure of a mucous membrane has been estimated to be 0.09% (CDC, 2008).

In addition to blood, other bodily fluids, such as cerebrospinal, synovial, amniotic, pleural, peritoneal, and pericardial fluids, are considered potentially infectious. Of significance, urine, feces, sputum, vomitus, and saliva are not considered to be infectious. Semen and cervicovaginal secretions have been shown to contain both infectious-free virus and virus-infected cells, and they should be considered infectious.

The major factors influencing the possibility of transmission include type and severity of exposure and magnitude of viremia. Transmission risk is expected to be higher when there are higher levels of virus in blood or body fluids, as in those from persons during or suspected of having acute HIV infection, as well as from those at late stages of disease with unsuppressed viremia (CDC, 2008).

Although not common, there have been several documented transmission events from healthcare workers to patients during routine medical or dental care, the most likely cause being poor adherence to infection control procedures. Furthermore, although increasingly less frequent, there have been documented cases of patient-to-patient transmission, most of which involved the use of contaminated instruments or syringes. Use of universal precautions during all healthcare procedures and encounters cannot be overemphasized.

Since 1991, the US Center for Disease Control and Prevention (CDC) has investigated all cases of HIV infection reported as acquired occupationally by healthcare workers. As of December 31, 2017, there have been a total of 58 confirmed occupationally acquired HIV infections. The majority were in nurses (41%), followed by laboratory clinicians (35%), physicians (10%), and other health-related workers (14%). Since 1999, there has been only one case of occupationally acquired HIV (a laboratory technician who sustained a needle puncture while working with high-titer HIV cultures in 2008) (Joyce, 2015).

In cases in which risk of HIV transmission can be determined, specific guidelines exist for the use of antivirals for PEP.

Occupational exposures require urgent medical evaluation and initiation of PEP, ideally within 2–6 hours after exposure. Prospective, well-controlled clinical data supporting PEP do not exist. By extrapolation from well-controlled animal model studies, it has been estimated that PEP reduces the risk of infection by approximately 80% and that it becomes less effective as time lapses (>72 hours). The preferred initial PEP regimen (three or more antiretroviral drugs) is tenofovir/emtricitabine plus raltegravir (TDF/FTC + RAL) because of its ease of administration, proven potency against established HIV, and good tolerability. It is recommended to start PEP with this regimen following exposure to a source patient who is known to have HIV or for whom there is a reasonably high suspicion of having HIV. If the source person is determined to be HIV-negative, PEP can be discontinued. There is no documented transmission during the window period and hence rapid testing would suffice. PEP is also recommended for nonoccupational exposures. The recommended duration of PEP is 28 days. With the preceding modern, recommended PEP regimen (TDF/FTC + RAL), the medications have fewer serious side effects that can make it difficult to complete the program. CDC recommendations indicate that PEP should be considered only in settings in which HIV exposure is known. Most important, based on strong animal model data indicating time-dependent efficacy, PEP administration should not be delayed for HIV test results but rather should be started empirically and discontinued later if tests are negative (Kuhar, 2013).

TRANSMISSION THROUGH THE USE OF INJECTION DRUGS

Injection drug users (IDUs) accounted for 9% of HIV diagnosis and 13% of AIDS diagnosis in the United States in 2016. Blacks/African Americans and Hispanics/Latinos account for more than two-thirds of all diagnoses of HIV infection due to injection drug use in the United States. Among women, injection drug use accounts for more than 20% of all infections.

The high-risk practices of sharing needles/syringes and engaging in risky sexual behavior, the opioid/heroin epidemic, and social/economic factors limiting access to HIV prevention and care and to substance abuse programs are some of the prevention challenges currently identified by the CDC.

The CDC is pursuing a prevention approach by distributing funds to health departments for surveillance and by supporting intervention programs such as community PROMISE (Peers Reaching Out and Modeling Intervention Strategies); syringe exchange programs that provide access to sterile syringes and needles and thereby reduce transmission of HIV, hepatitis C, hepatitis B virus, and other blood-borne infections; and PrEP and PEP programs, to name a few. Providing comprehensive prevention services and medical and/or addiction treatment referrals for IDUs can help increase access to healthcare and substance use treatment (CDC, 2008).

Individuals who use recreational crystal methamphetamine are at increased risk of contracting HIV. However, there is no clear evidence that methamphetamine itself increases HIV transmission or acquisition. Amphetamine users, in general, report several behaviors known to be risk factors for HIV transmission, including greater numbers of sex partners, reduced use of condoms, exchange of sex for money or drugs, sex with IDUs, and/or a history of STDs. Furthermore, they are more likely to have unprotected anal or vaginal sex with partners of unknown HIV status. Individuals abusing other mind-altering drugs, such as alcohol, can also be at increased risk for HIV infection (CDC, 2007).

MOTHER-TO-CHILD-TRANSMISSION

Perinatal HIV transmission, also known as mother-to-child-transmission, can occur at any time during pregnancy, labor, delivery, and/or breastfeeding. Advances in HIV research, prevention, and treatment have led to a remarkable 90% decline in annual cases of perinatal transmission.

Pediatric HIV infection is associated with an accelerated course of disease and high mortality. In the absence of ART, only 65% of HIV-positive children survive until their first birthday, and less than half will reach 2 years of age. In the absence of breastfeeding and with no ART, the risk of perinatal transmission is 25%. Up to 20% more children can become infected through breastfeeding. In the United States, the rate of perinatal transmission of HIV has drastically declined to less than 2% with the implementation of prenatal HIV screening; the use of antiretrovirals before, during, and after pregnancy; scheduled cesarean delivery when necessary; and the avoidance of breastfeeding. These interventions are not available worldwide, and in areas such as sub-Saharan Africa, AIDS remains a major cause of infant death.

Most children acquire HIV from their mother in utero, intrapartum, or during breastfeeding. In developed countries, the incidence of mother-to-child transmission of HIV is extremely low (< 1%). In these countries, HIV-positive women receive ART before and during pregnancy and delivery, and they are advised to abstain from breastfeeding. Furthermore, their children receive antiretroviral prophylaxis at birth and for several weeks thereafter. The majority of HIV-positive children live in sub-Saharan Africa, where HIV-positive women have limited access to antiretroviral drugs and the health benefits of breastfeeding outweigh the risk of HIV transmission.

Despite the presence of innate factors in human breast milk that display strong HIV inhibitory activity in vitro, up to 44% of HIV infections in children can be attributed to breastfeeding. The risk of acquiring HIV after a single day of breastfeeding is extremely low (0.00028 per day of breastfeeding) (Richardson, 2003). However, after ingesting liters of breast milk over a span of several months to years (~250 liters per year), 5–20% of infants born to HIV-positive women will eventually become infected with HIV in the absence of any preventative measures (WHO, 2008). Elevated levels of HIV particles (cell-free virus) and HIV-infected cells (cell-associated virus) in the breast milk of HIV-positive women are associated with an increased risk of HIV transmission during breastfeeding. Although it has been reported that a tenfold increase in cell-free or cell-associated HIV in breast milk is associated with a threefold increase in transmission, it is still unclear whether cell-free virus and/or cell-associated virus are transmitted during breastfeeding. Furthermore, it is not known if the frequency of cell-free and cell-associated HIV transmission varies at different stages of lactation (i.e., colostrum, early breast milk, and mature breast milk).

REFERENCES

Centers for Disease Control and Prevention (CDC). Methamphetamine use and risk for HIV/AIDS. January 2007. http://www.cdc.gov/hiv/resources/factsheets/meth.htm. Accessed December 20, 2015.

Centers for Disease Control and Prevention (CDC). Recommendations for post-exposure interventions to prevent infection with hepatitis B virus, hepatitis C virus, or human immunodeficiency virus, and tetanus in persons wounded during bombings and other mass-casualty events—United States, 2008. *MMWR*. August 1, 2008;57(RR06):1–19.

Centers for Disease Control and Protection (CDC). HIV transmission. March 25, 2010. http://www.cdc.gov/hiv/resources/qa/transmission.htm. Accessed December 20, 2015.

Centers for Disease Control and Prevention (CDC). HIV Surveillance Report, 2016; vol. 28. http://www.cdc.gov/hiv/library/reports/hiv-surveillance.html. Published November 2017. Accessed August 2018

Cohen MS, Chen YQ, McCauley M, et al. Prevention of HIV-1 infection with early antiretroviral therapy. *N Engl J Med*. 2011;365:493–505.

Cohen MS, et al. Final results of the HPTN 052 randomized controlled trial: antiretroviral therapy prevents HIV transmission. *N Engl J Med*. 2016;375:830–839.

Dosekun O, Fox J. An overview of the relative risks of different sexual behaviours on HIV transmission. *Curr Opin HIV AIDS*. 2010;5:291–297.

Joyce MP, Kuhar D, Brooks JT. Occupationally acquired HIV infection by healthcare personnel—United States, 1985–2013. In *22nd Conference on Retroviruses and Opportunistic Infections*, Seattle, Abstract 1027, Feb 23–26, 2015.

Kuhar DT, Henderson DK, Struble KA, et al. Updated US Public Health Service guidelines for the management of occupational exposures to human immunodeficiency virus and recommendations for postexposure prophylaxis. *Infect Control Hosp Epidemiol*. 2013 November;34(11):1238.

Pena-Cruz V, Agosto, Akiyama et al. HIV replicates and persists in vaginal epithelial dendritic cells. *J Clin Invest*. 2018. https://doi.org/10.1172/JCI98943.

Richardson BA, John-Stewart GC, Hughes JP, et al. Breast-milk infectivity in human immunodeficiency virus type 1-infected mothers. *J Infect Dis*. 2003;187:736–740.

Rodger AJ, Cambiano V, Bruun T, et al. Sexual activity without condoms and risk of HIV transmission in serodifferent couples when the HIV-positive partner is using suppressive antiretroviral therapy. *JAMA*.2016;316(2):171–181. doi: 10.1001/jama.2016.5148

Rodger A, Cambiano V, Bruun T, et al. Risk of HIV transmission through condomless sex in MSM couples with suppressive ART: the PARTNER 2 study extended results in gay men. IAC 2018: Abstract WEAX0104LB.

WHO, UNICEF, UNFPA, and UNAIDS. *HIV Transmission Through Breastfeeding: A Review of Available Evidence: 2007 update*. Geneva: World Health Organization; 2008. http://programme.aids2018.org/Abstract/Abstract/13470

Zhang H, Dornadula G, Beumont M, et al. Human immunodeficiency virus type 1 in the semen of men receiving highly active antiretroviral therapy. *N Engl J Med*. December 17, 1998;339(25):1803–1809.

4.

HIV TRANSMISSION PREVENTION

Carolyn Chu and Christopher M. Bositis

INTRODUCTION

HIV prevention encompasses a vast range of approaches and tools across various biomedical and nonbiomedical (i.e., behavioral and social) as well as structural dimensions. Recent notable developments include (1) ongoing identification of best clinical practices with regard to HIV preexposure prophylaxis (PrEP) and HIV "treatment as prevention" (TasP), two interventions with a firmly established scientific evidence base; (2) further tailoring of behavioral risk reduction strategies for specific at-risk groups; and (3) increased access to and integration of substance use–related services and HIV prevention. Similar to combination HIV treatment using multiple medications, combination HIV prevention remains necessary to effectively reduce transmission. Important structural challenges continue to affect HIV prevention efforts and outcomes in resource-limited as well as resource-rich settings; these include stigma and discrimination, criminalization of HIV- and substance use–associated behaviors, and health inequities involving (but not limited to) race, gender, and socioeconomic status.

BEHAVIORAL INTERVENTIONS

LEARNING OBJECTIVES

Provide an overview of behavioral factors and opportunities surrounding HIV prevention, including strategies to reduce HIV exposure risk and special considerations for unique populations.

WHAT'S NEW

Behavioral interventions continue to be refined and evaluated to determine their effectiveness in preventing HIV and associated risk behaviors. Combination interventions targeted to specific at-risk groups are as important as, if not more than, broad measures for the general population due to (1) multiple and varied social and cultural subtleties and (2) HIV-related health disparities unique to particular communities.

KEY POINTS

- Providers should elicit comprehensive and detailed sociobehavioral histories in a patient-centered, sensitive, and respectful manner to identify risk areas so that appropriate HIV testing can occur and targeted, effective prevention strategies can be shared.

- Various combinations of behavioral strategies will be effective for different populations and should be tailored to an individual's and community's needs and wishes.

Behavioral interventions to prevent HIV transmission include both general educational campaigns about sexual health, substance use, and risk reduction and tailored messages for special at-risk populations and individuals living with HIV ("prevention with persons with HIV"). Condom promotion and skills training for condom use negotiation/strategies, as well as condom distribution services have been mainstays for many sex education and HIV prevention programs. Others have encouraged sexual abstinence or monogamy and fidelity. When used consistently and correctly, condoms are estimated to reduce HIV transmission by more than 70% (Giannou, 2015; Smith, 2015; Weller, 2002). Sexual partnering practices such as partner concurrency and age-discrepant partnering are also underrecognized drivers of HIV risk, particularly in specific communities (Adimora, 2014; Anema, 2013; Harrison, 2008). "Serosorting" and "seropositioning"—collectively termed "seroadaptive"—strategies have also been described and may be popular risk reduction approaches for certain groups (i.e., men who have sex with men [MSM]) (Vallabhaneni, 2012). They encompass a wide variety of practices that utilize knowledge of an individual's HIV status, self-reported or confirmed, to inform decision-making when selecting partners or engaging in particular sexual practices. Although in theory such strategies should prevent infection, in practice each carries a different and uncertain level of risk due to a range of biological and contextual factors (Vallabhaneni, 2012; Wei, 2011), including low rates of accurate HIV status representation between individuals.

Adolescents/young adults and women may be especially vulnerable to HIV not only from socioeconomic-cultural factors (e.g., sexual coercion, partner substance use, trafficking and violence, economic inequality, challenges with condom negotiation) but also from biological considerations. Mucosal and immunological features unique to the female genital tract as well as vaginal microbial dysbiosis may increase HIV susceptibility (Kaushic, 2010; Eastment, 2018). Two recent studies also found that HIV transmission risk (per sex act) increased throughout pregnancy and was highest postpartum, even after accounting for condom use, HIV viral load, and PrEP use, suggesting susceptibility unique to the antenatal and postpartum periods (Thompson, 2018). Behavioral interventions targeted to young people have attempted to reduce risk by delaying sexual debut, promoting condom use, ensuring regular sexually transmitted infection (STI) screening, increasing HIV-related knowledge, and reducing partner concurrency and/or changes (Protogerou, 2014). Methods include school-based and/or peer-led approaches as well as novel cash transfer and incentive programs and social media campaigns aimed at reducing stigma and discrimination (Pettifor, 2013). Similarly, interventions targeted to at-risk women have utilized group-based skills training sessions focused on healthy decision-making, relationship building, and overall wellness.

Older adults also warrant unique consideration. Some exhibit risk behaviors similar to younger people but may be less knowledgeable about HIV, less likely to use condoms, more isolated, and less inclined to discuss sex and substance use with healthcare providers. Additionally, providers may not regularly inquire about risk behaviors with older adults—by doing so, clinicians underestimate HIV risk and subsequently might not recommend screening and prevention measures, including PrEP, in the same manner as they would for younger populations (Adekeye, 2012; Franconi, 2018). Age-related physiologic changes such as vaginal epithelial thinning and decreased vaginal lubrication can also put older, postmenopausal women at especially high risk. Older men using erectile dysfunction medications may demonstrate increased capacity for risky activities (Brooks, 2012). In general, older adults are more likely to be diagnosed with HIV late in the course of disease. Recent data indicate HIV diagnosis delays remain significantly longer among persons who were older at time of diagnosis (Dailey, 2017). Lower initial $CD4^+$ T-cell counts have been described among older adults (one study estimated approximately 15% lower) and a greater proportion of older adults develop AIDS-defining diagnoses at/within 3 months of initial presentation (Althoff, 2010). Importantly, older adults living with—or at risk for—HIV are more likely to have multiple comorbid chronic diseases and geriatric syndromes (i.e., frailty) and unique physical functioning challenges that clinicians should recognize and address where possible (Greene, 2017). They are also more likely to receive multiple medications, thus introducing additional challenges such as drug interactions, polypharmacy, and antiretroviral therapy (ART)-related toxicity (Franconi, 2018; Blaylock, 2015).

In 2011, the US Centers for Disease Control and Prevention (CDC) released a report announcing its pursuit of "High-Impact Prevention." This utilizes combinations of "scientifically proven, cost-effective, and scalable interventions targeted to the right populations in the right geographic areas" (US Centers for Disease Control [CDC], 2011). Similar to other agencies and various organizations (e.g., the National LGBT Health Education Center), the CDC maintains educational resources that offer guidance on best practices for HIV prevention. The CDC's *Compendium of Evidence-Based Interventions and Best Practices for HIV Prevention* includes almost 100 interventions and practices spanning behavioral (for individuals, couples, groups, and communities) to system-level interventions. Many are rooted in the "health belief model," one of several social psychological frameworks used to develop behavioral interventions (Bonell, 2001; Kaufman, 2014).

Despite a growing number of evidence-informed HIV prevention strategies overall, transgender communities remain critically understudied and underrepresented, although they experience some of the highest rates of HIV infection globally: prevalence estimates range from 8% to 68%. Transwomen have an almost 50-fold increase in HIV prevalence compared to the general population (Baral, 2013;

BEHAVIORAL STRATEGIES FOR INDIVIDUAL RISK REDUCTION

HIV testing and risk reduction counseling

Behavior change communication to promote partner reduction and consistent condom use

HIV/STI and sexuality education

Interpersonal communication training, including peer education

Social marketing campaigns focusing on prevention commodities

Cash incentives for individual risk avoidance

SOCIAL AND CULTURAL INTERVENTION STRATEGIES

Community dialogue and coalition-building to increase services/capacity, community-level knowledge

Stigma reduction programming

Advocacy for social justice

Media and interpersonal communication to clarify/share values, change harmful social norms

Education curriculum reform, expansion, and standardization

Leadership training and development

Addressing gender inequality and violence, racism

POLITICAL, LEGAL, AND ECONOMIC STRATEGIES

Human rights programming

Engagement with political leadership, advocacy for legal reform

Community microfinance/microcredit programming

Addressing unemployment and poverty

Training/advocacy with various elements of criminal justice system (police, judges, etc.)

Policies/legislation to increase access to condoms and other harm reduction measures

Stakeholder analysis and alliance-building

Decriminalization of sex work, addressing homophobia, decriminalizing substance use (i.e. IDU)

INTERVENTION STRATEGIES ADDRESSING PHYSICAL ENVIRONMENTS

Housing policy and standards

Infrastructure development – transportation, communications, etc.

Enhance farming/business development and other modes of subsistence/food security

Figure 4.1 Key non-biomedical HIV prevention strategies. Adapted from Figure 8, http://www.unaids.org/sites/default/files/media_asset/JC2007_Combination_Prevention_paper_en_0.pdf

Caceres, 2011). Transgender communities often face social and legal exclusion or marginalization, economic and employment vulnerabilities, stigma, and transphobia, and are at much higher risk of experiencing violence (especially gender-based violence). Transwomen who engage in transactional sex, in particular, face unique individual, interpersonal, and structural susceptibilities and challenges that confer extremely high HIV risk—especially in jurisdictions that criminalize same-sex relationships and/or transactional sex. Additionally, unsafe injection practices for hormone therapy administration and elevated rates of substance use increase risk of HIV transmission (Reback, 2014).

Finally, many behavioral interventions emphasize regular HIV and STI screening as an important cornerstone of prevention for all. Widespread efforts to expand and facilitate HIV/STI counseling and testing along with partner outreach services, coupled with advances in testing technologies, can help decrease transmission risk through a number of mechanisms. These include (1) ensuring that people living with HIV (PLWH) know their status, (2) identifying early HIV infection more reliably, (3) supporting safe disclosure to sex and injection partners, (4) encouraging condom use and other risk reduction measures, and (5) assisting with timely linkage to HIV care and treatment, including consideration of "rapid start" ART soon after diagnosis if feasible.

Over the past several years, accumulating evidence has confirmed that PLWH are central to HIV prevention. Interventions inclusive of PLWH are likely to have a greater and more immediate impact on reducing HIV incidence than changing the behaviors of millions of people who are negative but at risk (CDC, 2014). "Prevention with persons with HIV" includes acknowledgment of related health inequalities. Recommended opportunities for intervention are also framed around the HIV Care Continuum and include goals such as improving linkage to (and retention in) care, initiating early ART, screening for and treating concurrent STIs, addressing mental health and substance use, providing family planning and partner notification counseling, and achieving durable virologic suppression (TasP; see Chapter 25).

RECOMMENDED READING

Buchbinder SP, Liu AY. CROI 2018: epidemic trends and advances in HIV prevention. *Top Antivir Med*. 2018;26(1):1–16.

Globerman J, Mitra S, Gogolishvili D, et al. HIV/STI prevention interventions: a systematic review and meta-analysis. *Open Med (Wars)*. 2017;12:450–467.

Kaufman M, Cornish F, Zimmerman RS, et al. Health behavior change models for HIV prevention and AIDS care: practical recommendations for a multi-level approach. *J Acquir Immune Defic Syndr*. 2014;66(Suppl. 3):S250–S258.

STRUCTURAL AND SYSTEMS-LEVEL INTERVENTIONS

LEARNING OBJECTIVES

- Describe the safety and monitoring of the US blood supply.

- Recognize HIV risk associated with injection drug use (IDU) and interventions that prevent IDU-related HIV transmission.

- Share background on the "Undetectable = Untransmittable" campaign and how it has helped inform new public health messaging around HIV TasP.

- Discuss additional structural/systems-level considerations and interventions that aim to decrease HIV transmission.

Complex issues surround injection and noninjection substance use and their collective effect on HIV transmission. Biomedical and health system advances in treatment (e.g., integrated substance use and HIV care, improved access to medications for substance use disorders) and renewed public health efforts are promising strategies to address these overlapping epidemics. Laws and policies against illicit substance use, particularly IDU, also play a pivotal role in influencing health outcomes. Evidence strongly suggests that criminalization of substance use adversely affects HIV prevention efforts. Recently, the highly visible "U = U" campaign was launched to help overcome negative public perception, reduce stigma, and address misbeliefs regarding HIV transmission risk.

KEY POINTS

- The US blood supply remains extremely safe, largely as a result of multiple layers of safeguards involving comprehensive screening, testing, and quality assurance practices.

- Clinicians should be able to recognize HIV transmission risks associated with both injection- and noninjection-related substance use, as well as use involving prescription medications and nonprescription substances. Widespread application of effective preventive measures is needed: these include harm reduction services, substance use disorder treatment, and integrated HIV and viral hepatitis testing and care.

SAFETY OF THE BLOOD SUPPLY

Multiple organizations (e.g., the American Red Cross, hospital and community blood banks) contribute to population-level and local procurement and donation of blood products. Establishments that collect and process blood are ultimately responsible for product safety; however, the US Food and Drug Administration (FDA) regulates how donations are collected and products are transfused. It does so by ensuring that recipients are protected through multiple, overlapping safeguards. These measures encompass five main "layers" of safety: (1) donor screening, (2) approval of all testing platforms that evaluate donated blood for key blood-borne pathogens, (3) quarantine of donated specimens until testing verifies suitability, (4) donor deferral registries, and (5) required reporting and subsequent investigations and corrective actions when product/process deviations occur. The FDA also regularly inspects collection centers to confirm adherence to quality standards and best practices. Additionally, the CDC helps monitor safety by assisting health departments and hospitals investigate reports of potential infectious disease transmission.

Widespread HIV-1 antibody screening began in the United States in 1985, and HIV-2 antibody screening was introduced in 1992. Since 1999, donations have also been pooled and tested for HIV-1 RNA. This allows for more reliable detection of acute HIV because antibodies typically do not develop until approximately 3 weeks after infection. By routinely incorporating HIV-1 RNA testing, often using high-performing assays, centers can improve identification of donors who might have been recently infected (Busch, 2003; Kleinman, 2009). The modeled risk for HIV infection from blood product transfusion in the United States declined from 1 in 450,000–600,000 donations in 1995 to 1 in 2,135,000 donations in 2001. The most recent population-based estimate for acquiring HIV infection through transfusion in the United States is 1 in 1,467,000 (Zou, 2010).

PREVENTION OF HIV RELATED TO SUBSTANCE USE

IDU has long been linked to HIV transmission, with risk estimates ranging from 0.63% to 2.4% per act (Baggaley, 2006). Although estimated annual HIV infections among people who inject drugs declined more than 30% from 2010 to 2014, increasing IDU in nonurban areas has created new prevention challenges. In 2016, people who inject drugs accounted for 9% of new HIV diagnoses in the United States (CDC, 2016), and IDU remains an important risk factor worldwide. Equipment used for injecting, as well as drug/excipient residue left in needles and syringes, can be effective vectors for spreading virus. HIV generally degrades rapidly outside the body under ambient conditions; however, studies indicate it can survive for longer periods of time (up to 6 weeks) within a sealed syringe (Heimer, 2000). Higher levels of HIV present in the blood injected, larger volume of injected blood, and/or higher injection frequency can all increase risk. In addition to direct sharing of needles/syringes and drug preparation equipment (e.g., cookers, filters), various drug preparation practices can "indirectly" lead to HIV transmission. These include sharing water that has been used to flush blood out of a needle/syringe and reusing equipment that hasn't been sufficiently sterilized. HIV risk has been demonstrated most clearly for intravenous administration of illicit (or prescribed) substances; however any parenteral exposure to virus-containing material/equipment can potentially lead to transmission: this includes subcutaneous and intramuscular injections. Finally, although IDU remains the principal substance use–related behavior leading to HIV transmission, elevated risk has also been connected to use of alcohol, stimulants (especially methamphetamine), and sedatives/hypnotics—all of which can affect decision-making and negotiation around condom use and other sex practices (Berry, 2018; Hoenigl, 2016; Ickowicz, 2015; Shoptaw, 2006).

Prevention of IDU-related HIV transmission has reemerged as a national public health priority recently, in part due to HIV and hepatitis C (HCV) outbreaks attributed to IDU in rural areas and communities previously thought to be at low risk. Experts advocate for a multifaceted public health prevention strategy rather than a "one size fits all" approach (Strathdee, 2015). Elements should include (1) increased access to needle exchange and other harm reduction-oriented programs/services including naloxone, (2) improved recognition of substance use along with increased HIV and viral hepatitis screening, (3) expanded access to health services and providers who offer medications (i.e., opioid agonists, HIV pre- and postexposure prophylaxis) and other therapies that can help mitigate negative clinical consequences associated with IDU, and (4) multidisciplinary care that is colocated/integrated and tailored to specific community needs, including behavioral health programs (Rich, 2018; Perlman, 2018). Many leaders and organizations have also called attention to the harmful effects of opioid marketing, lack of housing and economic opportunity, aggressive policing practices, mass incarceration, and prohibitive legislation/policies on the syndemic of opioid misuse, HIV, and viral hepatitis (Perlman, 2018). See the section "Legal Considerations Surrounding HIV Prevention with People Who Inject Drugs."

Harm Reduction Approaches to IDU and HIV Prevention

Harm reduction is a concept whereby the prevention or reduction of adverse effects associated with certain behaviors is prioritized over absolute cessation of the behavior itself. As applied to substance use (particularly IDU), harm reduction values minimizing substance-related impairment as much as, if not more than, eliminating substance use altogether. Since the early 1990s, multiple harm reduction strategies—both biomedical and nonbiomedical—have effectively decreased IDU-related HIV transmission risk. Needle and syringe exchange programs (NSEPs), peer-based education and outreach, substance use disorder treatment, and pre- and postexposure HIV prophylaxis have all been evaluated (Abdul-Quader, 2013; Aspinall, 2014; Garfein, 2007; MacArthur, 2012; Medley, 2009; US Public Health Service, 2017). NSEPs provide new needles/syringes, generally at no cost, in exchange for used equipment. Programs sometimes also distribute alcohol swabs, sterile water/saline, mixing vessels, filters, and condoms. Various distribution models have been employed including pharmacy-based sales and vending machines (MacArthur, 2014). An extensive 2004 World Health Organization (WHO) report stated that "there is compelling evidence that increasing the availability and utilization of sterile injecting equipment . . . reduces HIV infection substantially" and is cost-effective (Wodak, 2004). Since then, multiple agencies, including the Institute of Medicine and US Department of Health and Human Services/CDC, have also supported NSEPs as integral to comprehensive HIV prevention, especially during new HIV and viral hepatitis outbreaks (Institute of Medicine, 2007; CDC, 2018). In 2016, the first-ever US Surgeon General's Report on Alcohol, Drugs, and Health stated: "studies have clearly shown that needle/syringe exchange programs are effective in reducing HIV transmission and do not increase rates of community drug use" (US Department of Health and Human Services, 2016). Another established prevention strategy, outreach and education, offers HIV education and risk reduction counseling; training on safer injecting and sexual practices; overdose prevention education/training (sometimes with naloxone distribution); substance use treatment counseling; and, occasionally, treatment referrals. Peer-driven and community-based models may be highly useful for engaging difficult to reach populations including those with mistrust of healthcare organizations and professionals. Such models have led to decreased substance use, reduced equipment sharing, increased condom use, increased HIV testing, and increased treatment enrollment (Garfein, 2007; Latkin, 2009; Medley, 2009; Needle, 2005). Researchers have recently begun to describe how social capital and social contact network/relationship-level characteristics shape substance use–related attitudes/beliefs, behaviors, and outcomes (Kumar, 2016; Smith, 2017). Finally, evidence consistently verifies that medically supervised, safe injection facilities (SIFs, also referred to as supervised injection or consumption facilities) are feasible and can play a meaningful role in reducing health-related harms among people who inject drugs (Kennedy, 2017). SIFs have been found to (1) reduce overdose/death and unsafe injection behaviors, (2) effectively connect people who inject drugs to treatment and other services, (3) reduce "public disorder" associated with illicit use (i.e., public injecting, publicly discarded injection-related material), and (4) be cost-effective. In 2017–18, Seattle and Philadelphia city officials announced that SIFs would be allowed to operate as part of jurisdictional efforts to reduce fatal opioid overdoses, increase linkage to treatment, and increase HIV and viral hepatitis screening. Other cities that have been heavily impacted by overdose deaths, such as New York, Miami, and San Francisco, are also considering opening supervised injection sites.

Substance Use Screening and Expanded HIV Testing

Screening, brief intervention, and referral to treatment (SBIRT) is a widely adopted approach to facilitate early identification and linkage to substance use services. Although overall treatment effects are modest, SBIRT has been demonstrated to reduce alcohol misuse and smoking. However, findings regarding its application to other substance use—in particular opioid use disorders—have not been conclusive (Saitz, 2014; Bernstein, 2017). As of mid-2018, the US Preventive Services Task Force (USPSTF) remains in the process of updating its guidance on substance use screening among adolescents and adults (in 2008, the Task Force stated that "evidence is insufficient to assess the balance of benefits and harms of screening"). Nevertheless, some proponents cite a growing body of supporting evidence and encourage continued efforts to identify optimal approaches for screening in routine clinical practice, especially primary care and "safety net" clinics and other settings that serve at-risk populations (Agerwala, 2012; Humeniuk, 2008; Substance Abuse and Mental Health Services Administration, 2011). US HIV PrEP guidelines advise that clinicians briefly screen all patients for alcohol abuse and use of illicit substances (e.g., amyl nitrite, stimulants) that may affect sexual risk behavior, in addition to identifying injection practices that increase HIV risk (US Public Health Service, 2017). The HIV Medicine Association's 2013 primary care guidelines recommend "regular assessment of depression and substance use," given their potential impact on adherence to HIV care and treatment (Aberg, 2014). New York State's AIDS Institute recommends that clinicians screen all PLWH for alcohol and other substance use at baseline and at least annually (New York State Department of Health AIDS Institute, 2007); such practices may identify opportunities to decrease HIV transmission risk to others.

Since 2006, the CDC has recommended that people who inject drugs be screened for HIV at least annually: data consistently indicate that more than 20% of HIV-positive injection drug users are not linked to and retained in care (CDC, 2017; Chen, 2012; Branson, 2006). People who inject drugs also tend to have lower virologic suppression rates (CDC, 2017; Gupta, 2017; Lourenco, 2014), highlighting important health disparities and opportunities. Interventions (including public health and social media campaigns) that reinforce the importance of regular screening and facilitate timely disclosure of results are key to identifying and linking HIV-positive injection drug users with care. Testing can also help prevent additional transmissions, as people who know their status are more likely to reduce risky behaviors (Marks, 2005). Furthermore, testing integrated with services that are already attuned to the needs of people who inject drugs—for example, NSEPs and substance use treatment programs—offers a patient-centered alternative to testing in "traditional" settings (Heimer, 2007; Strathdee, 2012). Improved access to PrEP may also be beneficial.

Medical Management of Substance Use and HIV Prevention

Substance use treatment can be challenging and often requires a comprehensive, coordinated approach involving multicomponent interventions across various dimensions (behavioral, psychological, social, and biomedical). Despite these complexities, multiple pharmacologic therapies effectively reduce substance use and HIV transmission (MacArthur, 2012; Metzger, 2010; Vlahov, 2010). It is unlikely that the benefits of these therapies will be fully realized, however, until access to comprehensive services, including pharmacotherapy provision, is universally implemented. Access to—and coverage of—substance use treatment remains uneven across payers and communities, both geographically and socioeconomically. Provider-level barriers such as stigma and lack of prescriber comfort also contribute to high levels of unmet need with regard to substance use treatment (Haffajee, 2018).

Opioids remain the most commonly injected drugs overall, and there are an estimated 2.1 million persons with opioid use disorder (OUD) in the United States. Multiple medications are available to treat OUD: options include opioid agonist therapies (OAT) and antagonists. Methadone, an agonist, is the most widely used agent internationally. It has been the mainstay of OAT for decades in the United States and is available from federally regulated programs that have attained special accreditation. However, the relatively low number of licensed programs is one factor limiting the ability to treat OUD (at a population level) exclusively with methadone (SAMHSA, 2017). Furthermore, many access-related barriers to methadone programs have been described—these include long waiting lists for program entry, limited geographic availability, variable insurance coverage, and requirements for daily administration. In comparison, buprenorphine (a partial agonist) can be offered across diverse clinical settings including primary care clinics, hospitals, and emergency departments by any eligible prescriber who has completed training and obtained a special designation ("DATA 2000 waiver") from the Drug Enforcement Administration. With buprenorphine, patients can receive care in practices not publicly identified as substance use treatment centers or narcotic treatment programs—this may help alleviate concerns regarding stigma. Despite efforts to educate providers and new legislation attempting to address workforce limitations (e.g., the Comprehensive Addiction Treatment and Recovery Act), large gaps between treatment need and capacity, as well as high state-by-state variability, will likely persist for the foreseeable future (Jones, 2015). Naltrexone (an antagonist) is FDA-approved for relapse prevention and also available to treat OUD. It requires complete detoxification prior to initiation and can be administered at monthly intervals via an extended-release formulation or prescribed for daily oral use. Challenges to completing induction (for the extended-release formulation), low adherence rates, and early treatment discontinuation have generally limited its effectiveness (Jarvis, 2018). Naloxone is another antagonist and is commonly used to reverse the effects of opioids; namely, in overdose. It is also coformulated with buprenorphine (trade names: Suboxone, Zubsolv, Bunavail) to discourage product misuse (i.e., medication injection/inhalation). For people living with HIV who inject drugs, substance use treatment can facilitate adherence to care and viral load suppression (Metzger, 2010). A recent multinational, systematic review found that OAT increased ART coverage by more than 50% and reduced ART discontinuation by approximately 20%, suggesting a positive TasP role for integrated substance use and HIV care delivery (Low, 2016).

Non-opioid substances are frequently used and have also been implicated in HIV transmission. Crystal methamphetamine is a highly habit-forming stimulant that increases sexual arousal while also decreasing social inhibitions. Similar to cocaine, exposure to methamphetamine elevates risk for HIV transmission and acquisition not only through sharing equipment but also via specific sexual practices (e.g., frequently engaging in condomless and/or transactional sex, having multiple partners). Although methamphetamine use and HIV risk have been predominantly described among MSM, the population of people who use methamphetamine is varied. Novel approaches to its treatment and HIV prevention are needed to address the unique complexities and challenges surrounding clinical management of patients who use methamphetamine (Degenhardt, 2010; HRSA, 2009).

Legal Considerations Surrounding HIV Prevention with People Who Inject Drugs

As stated in the WHO's 2004 report, "HIV infection [among injection drug users] is more likely to occur in legal environments where sterile injection equipment is more severely restricted." Some US state laws have expressly prohibited possession of injecting equipment whereas others require a prescription for syringe purchase/possession. Over time, some states have decriminalized syringe possession, and a few states now allow for trace amounts of controlled substances, including residue on syringes. Public facilitation of access to sterile equipment has faced significant controversy from US law enforcement agencies and policymakers for decades. Historically, the United States has had among the most severe restrictions of any country, viewing opioid misuse largely through a punitive criminal justice framework rather than as a public health issue. Use of federal funds for NSEPs was banned in 1988, lifted in 2009, and reinstated in 2011; lack of a central funding mechanism has hampered widespread scale-up of NSEPs which are then ultimately supported through a mix of state and local government monies with some private donations. The Consolidated Appropriations Act of 2016 includes language that gives states and local communities the opportunity to use federal funding to support certain components of NSEPs under limited circumstances. In areas where carrying used needles/syringes could be a prosecutable offense, people who inject drugs are often disincentivized from utilizing NSEPs despite their availability. NSEPs also represent a highly diverse mix of structure and access: they can be fixed or mobile, with differing hours of operation. As of June 2018, exchange programs exist in 42 states and the District of Columbia (Community Access National Network, 2018).

Beyond the presence of drug control laws themselves, enforcement of these laws influences individual behaviors, community stigma, and the overall risk environment for people who inject drugs. In areas and situations perceived to be threatening, people who inject drugs may respond in ways that actually increase the risk of acquiring or transmitting HIV—for example, injecting in a hurried manner, visiting unsupervised "shooting galleries," and improperly disposing of used equipment that can then expose other person(s) to potentially infectious material (Burris, 2011; Perlman, 2018). Although injection drug users might often try to balance risks and opportunities associated with obtaining sterile equipment, significant economic, sociocultural, and political/regulatory limitations in the local environment undoubtedly impact decision-making and subsequently influence a person's actions. A 2017 systematic review concluded that the vast majority of scientific data suggest drug criminalization has negative effects on HIV prevention and treatment; based on this previously undescribed evidence base, the review's authors call for international policy initiatives to "reform legal and policy frameworks criminalizing drug use" (Figure 4.2) (DeBeck, 2017).

In 2016, the Prevention Access Campaign launched their "Undetectable = Untransmittable (U = U)" campaign. This health equity initiative was based on many years of multinational clinical research involving several thousands of monogamous couples which, collectively, did not identify any cases of sexual transmission of HIV from a partner who had achieved durable virologic suppression on ART. Prior to 2016, the paradigm of HIV TasP had been accepted by many in the scientific,

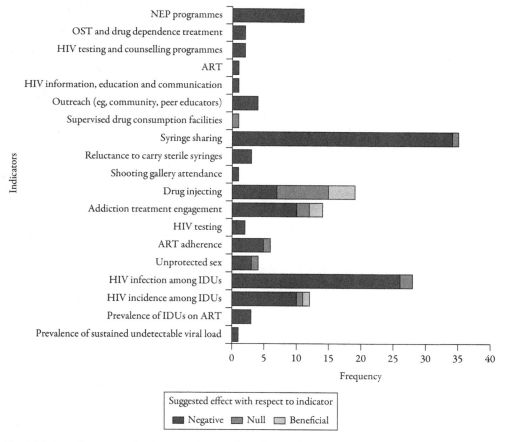

Figure 4.2 Criminalization of drug use among people who inject drugs and its effects on HIV-related treatment and prevention indicators.
Note: "Negative" indicates drug criminalization has a negative, i.e. adverse, effect on HIV prevention and treatment efforts. https://s100.copyright.com/AppDispatchSer vlet?publisherName=ELS&contentID=S2352301817300735&orderBeanReset=true&orderSource=Phoenix

public health, and HIV clinical provider communities. Most clinical guidelines had also already removed specific CD4+ thresholds for ART initiation by then, signaling a universal movement favoring early ART for all PLWH. Among the general population, however, high levels of stigma and skepticism have remained and negatively affected public perception of PLWH since the early epidemic. Through rapid coalition-building efforts, the Prevention Access Campaign engaged a large community of HIV advocates, researchers, and partners across several countries to support and share the "U = U" message and related information. In September 2017, the CDC officially endorsed the campaign. Specific goals of "U = U" include reducing fears of sexual transmission among PLWH; addressing HIV stigma at the community, clinical, and individual levels; encouraging PLWH to start and remain on ART; and achieving universal access to HIV testing, treatment, and care. Early research examining the implementation and impact of "U = U" has attempted to identify factors that correlate with the perceived accuracy of its message to identify additional opportunities for education and intervention (Rendina, 2018).

ADDITIONAL STRUCTURAL AND SYSTEMS-LEVEL CONSIDERATIONS

Several other structural factors should be considered to determine how they influence HIV risk: these represent an extensive landscape of physical, sociocultural, organizational, economic, and policy-related dynamics. Physical factors such as proximity to—and convenience of—HIV services can be primary drivers in determining motivation to seek care. Stigma and HIV-related discrimination often affect decision-making related to testing and engagement, as well as disclosure to family, social contacts, and healthcare providers (Valdiserri, 2002). Care settings that discreetly offer colocated services and open access/expanded hours can help facilitate linkage to and retention in care (Rothman, 2007). Stable housing, as well as community development and mobilization, are other important physical and social determinants of health and HIV risk (Latkin, 2013; Mahajan, 2008). Unsafe and inadequate/unstable housing are significant barriers to care and also increase HIV transmission risk (Aidala, 2015; Garcia, 2015). Beyond specific substance use-associated concerns described previously, the intersections between behavioral/mental health and HIV have also been well-documented (HRSA, 2015; Sikkema, 2010). Integrated behavioral/mental health and HIV prevention and treatment may help ensure coordinated delivery of comprehensive care for vulnerable populations. Providers should elicit a thorough mental health history as well as screen for prior/current trauma and violence when caring for at-risk individuals and PLWH and do so in a sensitive and respectful manner.

Economic factors are closely intertwined with HIV: resource-limited settings are disproportionately affected by high rates of HIV often due to deindustrialization and unemployment. Such disparities directly and indirectly involve inequalities in poverty, gender, and education; economic instability; labor migration patterns; access to health resources and health literacy; unmet substance use and mental health needs; drug policies and enforcement, and more (Zanakis, 2007). Despite efforts to expand testing and prevention broadly across the United States, HIV diagnosis rates continue to be higher for individuals in lower socioeconomic positions, with larger disparities affecting minority groups (An, 2013). Potential contributors to these findings include earlier sexual debut, less frequent condom use, and the exchange of sex for money (Adler, 2006).

Health insurance status is a major economically related determinant affecting access to primary care and preventive services. In 2010, the Affordable Care Act (ACA) was signed into law, with major provisions taking effect in 2014—one principal outcome has been the significant reduction in number of individuals without health insurance coverage. A few notable HIV-related implications resulted from the ACA: (1) coverage could not be denied based on preexisting health conditions including HIV, (2) states were given an option to expand Medicaid eligibility, (3) community health centers received increased support to provide HIV care, and (4) USPSTF-recommended HIV screening became reimbursable. Although there have been efforts to repeal the ACA since its implementation, these efforts have (to date) been unsuccessful.

The epidemiology of incarceration closely reflects that of HIV, and the complex interplay of racial and economic disparities in arrest/incarceration rates, substance use, and HIV is well-described (Csete, 2016; Iroh, 2015; Shubert, 2013; Wirtz, 2018). There is considerable variation in access to and types of HIV prevention, testing, and treatment services offered at correctional facilities; some of this may in part be due to lack of a comprehensive policy on HIV-related care delivery (Valera, 2017). Outcomes along the HIV Care Continuum also reflect important gaps in the application of evidence-based guidelines: incarcerated and recently released individuals generally have low rates of HIV awareness and testing, engagement, and retention (Belenko, 2013). Multiple challenges unique to correctional settings include rapid turnover and transfers, lack of testing and treatment resources (both in correctional facilities as well as in home communities), limited access to condoms and harm reduction services, low utilization of HIV pre- and postexposure prophylaxis, overcrowding and violence, low levels of staff training, and lack of coordination regarding post-release care. Nevertheless, prisons and jails are in unique and important positions to positively impact HIV-related public health outcomes. Novel solutions have included "local change teams," telemedicine/teleconsultation, and transitions programs/navigators to facilitate engagement in post-release care (Young, 2014; Belenko, 2017; Dong, 2017; Hammett, 2015).

Finally, broad dissemination of advocacy efforts and implementation of antidiscrimination policies and laws are critical achievements that can help reduce HIV-related stigma and advance universal human rights. At the Twenty-Second International AIDS Conference in 2018, an expert consensus statement was released advising that "more caution should be exercised when considering criminal prosecution, including careful appraisal of current scientific evidence on HIV-related risks and harms. This is instrumental to reduce stigma and discrimination and to avoid miscarriages of justice" (Barre-Sinoussi, 2018).

RECOMMENDED READING

Jacquot C, Delaney M. Efforts toward elimination of infectious agents in blood products. *J Intensive Care Med.* January 1, 2018;885066618756589. doi: 10.1177/0885066618756589

Perlman D, Jordan AE. The syndemic of opioid misuse, overdose, HCV, and HIV: structural-level causes and interventions. *Current HIV/AIDS Reports.* 2018;15:96–112.

Rich KM, Bia J, Altice FL, Feinberg J. Integrated models of care for individuals with opioid use disorder: how do we prevent HIV and HCV? *Curr HIV/AIDS Rep.* 2018;15(3):266–275.

MEDICAL INTERVENTIONS FOR HIV TRANSMISSION PREVENTION

LEARNING OBJECTIVES

- Define what it means to be at high risk for HIV acquisition and identify patients who meet these criteria.

- Describe the screening and evaluation process necessary prior to starting PrEP, occupational postexposure prophylaxis (oPEP), and nonoccupational postexposure prophylaxis (nPEP).

- Describe the monitoring process for patients on PrEP, nPEP, and oPEP, including visit, laboratory, and counseling recommendations, and describe the common side effects, toxicities, and other potential risks associated with their use.

WHAT'S NEW

- The US Public Health Service (USPHS), New York State Department of Health AIDS Institute, and International AIDS Society-USA (IAS-USA) have recently updated their clinical practice guidelines on PrEP.

- Although uncommon, cases of HIV transmission to patients fully adherent to PrEP have been reported.

- In May, 2018 the FDA approved the use of tenofovir DF/emtricitabine for PrEP in at-risk adolescents.

- In spite of significant increases in the number of patients taking PrEP, significant gaps remain in PrEP uptake, with at-risk African Americans, Latinos, and persons who inject drugs far less likely to be on PrEP than white MSM.

KEY POINTS

- Daily PrEP, consisting of tenofovir DF (300 mg) alone or in combination with emtricitabine (200 mg), has been shown to be safe and effective for preventing HIV acquisition in a variety of at-risk patient groups, including MSM, transgender women, coupled (serodiscordant) and single heterosexual women and men, and people who inject drugs.

- PrEP should not be prescribed as a sole prevention intervention but rather should be used as part of a comprehensive HIV prevention plan, including behavioral and other prevention strategies such as condom use, voluntary medical male circumcision, and STI treatment and prevention.

- Research continues on other potential HIV transmission strategies, including on-demand PrEP, vaccines, broadly neutralizing antibodies, long-acting injectable formulations of PrEP, and microbicides, promising to expand the available armamentarium of such strategies.

INTRODUCTION

Medical interventions used to prevent HIV transmission and acquisition among patients at risk include PrEP, oPEP and nPEP, STI screening and treatment, voluntary medical male circumcision, vertical transmission prevention, and TasP.

PREEXPOSURE PROPHYLAXIS

PrEP is the use of antiretroviral medications before HIV exposure as a means to prevent HIV acquisition in at-risk, HIV-negative individuals. For the purposes of this section, PrEP should be understood to mean daily oral antiretroviral prophylaxis. Other routes and schedules (e.g., vaginal ART-containing gel and intermittent PrEP) have been and/or are being studied but are discussed in the section "Investigational Interventions."

Data: Clinical Trials and Real-World Effectiveness

Studies evaluating this strategy have found that, when taken consistently, PrEP is highly effective at reducing the rate of HIV acquisition in those at highest risk, including MSM, transgender women who have sex with men, people who inject drugs, and coupled and single women and men engaging in heterosexual sex (see Table 4.1). Although the benefit varied slightly across the various studies, with reductions in the rate of HIV infection ranging from 44% to 75%, several common features should be highlighted. First, it was most effective among those who were most adherent. In the iPrEx study, for example, the relative risk of HIV infection was 92% lower among those with detectable levels of study drug compared to those without (Grant, 2010), and in the Bangkok Tenofovir study it was 70% lower (Choopanya, 2013). Furthermore, in the two negative PrEP trials to date, adherence was extremely

Table 4.1 SUMMARY OF EARLY RANDOMIZED, CONTROLLED PREEXPOSURE PROPHYLAXIS (PREP) TRIALS

TRIAL	*N*, STUDY POPULATION; SETTING	INTERVENTION	EFFECT–HAZARD RATIO [ESTIMATED REDUCTION IN HIV ACQUISITION] (95% CI)	REFERENCE
iPrEX	2499 MSM, transgender women, United States, South America, Thailand, South Africa	TDF/FTC	0.56 [44%] (15–63)	Grant (2010)
Partners PrEP	4747 heterosexual women and men; Kenya and Uganda	TDF TDF/FTC	0.33 [67%] (0.19–0.56) 0.25 [75%] (0.13–0.45)	Baeten (2012)
TDF 2	1219 heterosexual women and men; Botswana	TDF/FTC	0.38 [62%] (0.22–0.83)	Thigpen (2012)
Thai IDU	2413 PWIDs; Thailand	TDF	0.51 [49%] (0.1–0.72)	Choopanya (2013)
FemPrEP	2120 heterosexual women; Africa	TDF/FTC	0.94 [6%] (0.59–1.52)	Van Damme (2012)
VOICE	5029 heterosexual women; Africa	TDF TDF/FTC	1.49 [−49%] (0.97–2.29) 1.04 [−4%] (0.73–1.49)	Marrazzo (2015)

FTC, emtricitabine; MSM, men who have sex with men; PWID, people who inject drugs; TDF, tenofovir disoproxil fumarate.

poor (<30%) based on drug-level testing (Marrazzo, 2015; van Damme, 2012), again underscoring the importance of adherence for PrEP to be beneficial. Second, it was generally well tolerated, with fewer than 10% of participants reporting serious adverse events (US Public Health Service, 2017). Third, risk behaviors generally decreased during the study period; in both the iPrEx and the Partners PrEP studies, for example, the percentage of participants who reported unprotected intercourse decreased significantly during the study period (Baeten, 2012; Grant, 2010).

Since the publication of these initial study data, the number of at-risk patients taking PrEP has increased substantially (Figure 4.3), although the number of eligible patients greatly exceeds the number who are actually taking PrEP. Data on the effectiveness of PrEP in the "real world" have been encouraging. The Kaiser group in San Francisco reported no new infections among 657 PrEP initiators in an 18-month period, encompassing 388 person-years of follow-up, despite the fact that data from similar populations would predict an infection rate of 8.9/100 person-years—suggesting that as many as 34 new infections may have been averted through PrEP use (Volk, 2015). In addition, data from the PROUD study in the United Kingdom, which was designed to mimic real-world settings, showed a relative reduction in HIV incidence among MSM receiving PrEP of 86%, corresponding to a number needed to treat of just 13 in order to prevent 1 new HIV infection (McCormack, 2015). Importantly, data from New South Wales, Australia, and San Francisco demonstrate that the rapid scale-up of PrEP in at-risk populations has coincided with population-level reductions in the number of new HIV diagnoses in these communities (Grulich, 2018; Buchbinder, 2018). Despite these substantial gains, it should be underscored that significant gaps remain in PrEP uptake, with PrEP use greatest among white MSM and substantially lower among racial/ethnic minorities, people who inject drugs, and high-risk heterosexuals (Giler, 2017; Buchbinder, 2018; Mayer, 2018; Kuo, 2018).

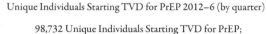

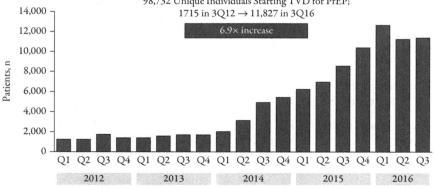

Figure 4.3 Number of New PrEP Starts Over Time. SOURCE: Giler (2017).

It should also be noted that PrEP "failures" can occur, even in those who are taking it consistently and correctly. Although uncommon, three individuals have acquired HIV in spite of high PrEP adherence: two who acquired multiclass/PrEP-resistant HIV infection, and one who acquired wild-type infection and reported condomless anal sex with a median of 2–5 partners per day in the months after he initiated PrEP (Knox, 2017; Grossman, 2016; Hoorneborg, 2017).

Eligibility

Multiple guidelines on PrEP eligibility and use have been released since initial clinical trial results reporting its efficacy were first released. For the purposes of this chapter, specific recommendations are taken from the most recent USPHS guidelines, which were revised in 2017. Other guidelines of interest include those from the World Health Organization (WHO, 2014); the International Antiviral Society–USA (Saag, 2018); and the New York State Department of Health AIDS Institute (New York State Department of Health, 2017).

According to the USPHS's 2017 guidelines, PrEP (once daily tenofovir disoproxil fumarate/emtricitabine [TDF/FTC]) is recommended as a prevention option for adults at substantial risk of acquiring HIV infection, including MSM, heterosexually active women and men, and people who inject drugs (US Public Health Service, 2017). Specific indications based on risk are listed in Table 4.2.

While the USPHS guidelines do not specifically define what it means to be in a "high prevalence area or network," the majority of PrEP studies were conducted in populations in which the background HIV incidence was at least 3 per 100 person-years, and the International Antiviral Society–USA panel therefore recommends PrEP for those in which the background incidence is greater than 2% (Saag, 2018).

Although not yet reflected in the USPHS guidelines, in May 2018 the FDA approved the use of TDF/FTC as PrEP in adolescents weighing at least 35 kg and at substantial risk of HIV acquisition. This approval was based on data from Project PrEPare, which found that TDF/FTC use was both safe and well-tolerated for MSM aged 15–17 in the United States (Hosek, 2017).

It is important to emphasize that PrEP should not be prescribed as a sole prevention intervention in those at risk, but, rather, it should be part of a comprehensive HIV prevention plan, including behavioral and other prevention strategies.

Prescribing PrEP: Baseline Assessment and Follow-Up

Prior to initiating PrEP in eligible patients, providers must document the following:

- Absence of acute or chronic HIV infection

- Normal renal function (creatinine clearance [CrCl] ≥ 60 mL/min)

- Hepatitis B (HBV) immunity or infection and vaccination status

To document absence of acute or chronic HIV infection, the USPHS recommends following the algorithm shown in Figure 4.4. Oral rapid HIV testing should not be used due to its lower sensitivity for detecting HIV compared to blood tests (US Public Health Service, 2017), and a negative test result (preferably a combination antigen/antibody) should be documented within the week before initiating PrEP. For individuals who report signs or symptoms of acute HIV infection within the previous 4 weeks, and for those with high-risk exposures within 4 weeks prior to initiating PrEP, the most recent testing algorithm suggests that the combined

Table 4.2 SPECIFIC INDICATIONS FOR PREEXPOSURE PROPHYLAXIS USE BASED ON RISK FACTOR

MEN WHO HAVE SEX WITH MEN	HETEROSEXUALLY ACTIVE WOMEN AND MEN	PERSONS WHO INJECT DRUGS (PWID)
Adult men	Adult person	Adult person
Without acute or chronic HIV	Without acute or chronic HIV	Without acute or chronic HIV
Any male partner in last 6 months	Any sex with opposite sex partners in past 6 months	Any injection of drugs not prescribed by a clinician in past 6 months
Not in a monogamous partnership with a recently tested, HIV-negative man	Not in a monogamous partnership with a recently tested HIV-negative partner	AND at least one of:
AND at least one of:	AND at least one of:	Any sharing of injection or drug preparation equipment in past 6 months
Any anal sex without condoms (receptive or insertive) in past 6 months	A man who has sex with both women and men (behaviorally bisexual)	Risk of sexual acquisition (see columns to the left)
A bacterial STI (syphilis, gonorrhea, or chlamydia) diagnosed or reported in past 6 months	Infrequently condom use during sex with 1 or more partners of unknown HIV status who at substantial risk of HIV infection (PWID or bisexual male partner)	
	In an ongoing sexual relationship with an HIV-positive partner	
	A bacterial STI (syphilis, gonorrhea in women or men) diagnosed or reported in past 6 months	

SOURCE: Adapted from US Public Health Service (2017).

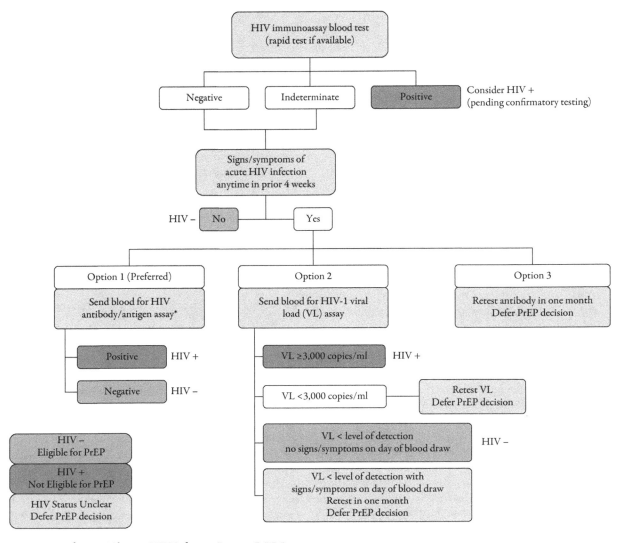

Figure 4.4 Assessment of Acute/Chronic HIV Infection Prior to PrEP Initiation. SOURCE: Centers for Disease Control and Prevention: US Public Health Service: Preexposure prophylaxis for the prevention of HIV infection in the United States—2017 Update: a clinical practice guideline. https://www.cdc.gov/hiv/pdf/risk/prep/cdc-hiv-prep-guidelines-2017.pdf. Published March 2018.

antigen/antibody test alone is acceptable; others would recommend sending an HIV viral load in addition to the combined test to determine the person's baseline HIV status (New York State Department of Health, 2017; US Public Health Service, 2017).

Eligible patients meeting appropriate clinical criteria should receive tenofovir DF/emtricitabine (TDF 300 mg/ FTC 200 mg) once daily. Whereas the USPHS states that daily TDF alone may be given as an alternative to people who inject drugs and heterosexually active women and men, the WHO lists daily TDF as the preferred PrEP regimen (CDC, 2017; WHO, 2015). The USPHS recommends that patients be given no more than a 3-month supply of medications at one time. Recommended follow-up and testing for PrEP toxicity and comorbid conditions are detailed in Table 4.3. While not specifically stated in the table, testing for HCV infection is recommended at baseline in all persons who inject drugs, those born between 1945 and 1965, and MSM. Annual retesting should be performed in those at ongoing risk for exposure (US Public Health Service, 2017).

PrEP Risks

PrEP has generally been very well tolerated in both clinical studies and real-world settings, with fewer than 10% of recipients experiencing serious adverse events (US Public Health Service, 2017). The most commonly reported side effects are gastrointestinal, such as nausea, flatulence, headache, and weight loss. Sometimes referred to as "start-up syndrome," most symptoms resolve within the first month of treatment and can usually be managed with over-the-counter medications.

More serious potential PrEP toxicities include acute and/ or chronic kidney injury and bone demineralization. Analyses from the iPrEX study indicate that PrEP recipients experience a small but statistically significant decline in CrCl that is nonprogressive and reversible upon PrEP discontinuation (Solomon, 2014). Similarly, patients from the same study who received PrEP experienced a small but statistically significant decrease in bone mineral density (BMD) compared to those who received placebo. However, there was no increase in

Table 4.3 SUMMARY GUIDELINES FOR PREEXPOSURE PROPHYLAXIS (PREP) USE

	MEN WHO HAVE SEX WITH MEN	HETEROSEXUALLY ACTIVE WOMEN AND MEN	PERSONS WHO INJECT DRUGS
Those at substantial risk of acquiring HIV	HIV-infected sexual partner Recent bacterial STI (gonorrhea, chlamydia, syphilis) High number of sex partners Inconsistent or no condom use History of engaging in commercial sex work	HIV-infected sexual partner Recent bacterial STI (gonorrhea, syphilis) High number of sex partners Inconsistent or no condom use History of engaging in commercial sex work Being in a high-prevalence area or network	HIV-positive injecting partner History of sharing injection equipment History of recent substance use disorder treatment (but currently injecting)
Clinically eligible if	Documented negative HIV test No signs/symptoms of acute HIV infection Normal renal function (CrCl ≥60 mL/min) No contraindicated medications Documented hepatitis B virus infection and vaccination status		
Prescription	TDF/FTC (FDC) once daily No more than 3-month supply		
Other services	Follow-up visits at least every 3 months to provide HIV test, medication adherence counseling, behavioral risk reduction support, side effect assessment, and STI symptom assessment At 3 months and every 6 months thereafter, assess renal function Every 6 months, test for bacterial STIs		
	Do oral/rectal STI testing	Assess pregnancy intent; pregnancy test every 3 months	Access to clean needles/syringes and substance use disorder treatment services

FDC, fixed-dose combination; FTC, emtricitabine; STI, sexually transmitted infection; TDF, tenofovir disoproxil fumarate.

SOURCE: Adapted from US Public Health Service (2017).

fracture risk, no one with low BMD, and observed decreases in vertebral BMD were reversible with PrEP discontinuation (Mulligan, 2015).

For patients who acquire HIV while on PrEP, there has been concern about the possible development of drug resistance. Such resistance has been rare to date, and, with the exception of the previously noted PrEP "failures," it has been primarily observed in patients who had acute seronegative HIV infection, underscoring the importance of screening patients for possible acute HIV before initiating PrEP (US Public Health Service, 2017). When it does occur, resistance mutations to FTC appear to be more common than those to TDF (Lehman, 2015).

STI diagnoses are common among PrEP users. Whether this is due to increased frequency of screening, an increase in high risk sexual behaviors, or some combination thereof is not entirely clear. In both the iPrEx and Partners PrEP studies, the percentage of participants who reported having sex without a condom decreased during the study period (Baeten, 2012; Grant, 2010). "Real-world" data from the aforementioned Kaiser Cohort and PROUD studies did not demonstrate evidence of risk compensation based on the number of reported sexual partners, condom use, and rates of STIs (McCormack, 2015; Volk, 2015). Similarly, while adherence to PrEP was greatest among those reporting condomless anal intercourse in the PrEPare study, overall rates of sexual risk behavior as measured by the number of male partners,

instances of condomless receptive anal intercourse, and instances of condom breakage during receptive anal intercourse remained stable (Hosek, 2015). On the other hand, data from a clinic in Seattle demonstrated decreased condom use and increased rates of gonorrhea and chlamydia following PrEP initiation when compared with their pre-PrEP baseline (Montano, 2017).

For patients who are chronically infected with HBV as evidenced by a positive HBV surface antigen (sAg) test, the USPHS recommends evaluation by a clinician experienced in the treatment of chronic HBV. Such patients may be given PrEP but should be counseled that there is a potential risk of a flare in their HBV infection should they abruptly discontinue TDF-containing PrEP, although this has not yet been reported in HBV-positive, HIV-negative patients (US Public Health Service, 2017; Solomon, 2016).

Women of childbearing potential who wish to become pregnant or breastfeed while taking PrEP should be counseled that the PrEP studies to date excluded women who were or who became pregnant. However, data from the Antiviral Pregnancy Registry demonstrate no evidence of harm to fetuses exposed to these medications (Antiretroviral Pregnancy Registry, 2018). Furthermore, it should be emphasized that HIV-uninfected women who wish to conceive with an HIV-infected partner may be at increased risk for HIV acquisition, and current US perinatal guidelines permit the use of PrEP for such patients (US Department of

Health and Human Services, 2018). Although data are limited, the use of PrEP during lactation appears to be safe (US Public Health Service, 2017).

Discontinuing PrEP

PrEP should be discontinued in patients who acquire HIV infection; experience unacceptable side effects or toxicities, including renal disease; are unable to adhere to the prescribed regimen or follow-up visit schedule; or change their risk status such that PrEP is no longer indicated (US Public Health Service, 2017). Patients who acquire HIV while taking PrEP should be initiated on combination ART based on genotypic testing results and in accordance with current HIV treatment guidelines.

Unanswered Questions

Although PrEP has clearly been shown to be beneficial in the appropriate settings, unanswered questions remain. It is not clear, for example, how long PrEP can be safely prescribed. The USPHS guidelines state that it should not be given for life but, rather, only during times of highest risk of HIV acquisition; however, many PrEP-eligible patients can be expected to remain so for extended periods of their lives (US Public Health Service, 2017).

The role of "event-driven" PrEP has also not yet been elucidated. Data from the IPERGAY study conducted in France demonstrated high rates of protection when taken before and after sex (Molina, 2015), a strategy that proved effective in those reporting both frequent and infrequent sex (Antoni, 2017). Furthermore, an interim analysis of the Prevenir study, also in France, found that no transmissions occurred in patients taking either daily or on-demand PrEP (Molina, 2018). On the other hand, this strategy was not as effective as daily PrEP among the US-based cohort of the HPTN 067/ADAPT trial (Mannheimer, 2015). Given these differing data, the USPHS does not currently recommend this strategy, whereas the 2018 IAS-USA guidelines state that event-driven PrEP may be considered for MSM (Saag, 2018).

Last, the role of PrEP for patients in serodiscordant relationships in which the HIV-infected partner is on suppressive ART is not clear. It is now generally accepted that PLWH with an undetectable viral load do not transmit HIV to their sexual partners (see the earlier discussion of the "Undetectable = Untransmittable (U = U)" campaign). However, HIV-negative patients in such relationships may have other partners whose HIV status is unknown or who are HIV infected but not yet on treatment. This possibility was highlighted by the fact that nearly 40% of transmissions in the HPTN 052 study were unlinked (i.e., they came from someone other than their identified serodiscordant partner) (Cohen, 2015). PrEP is likely to be beneficial for such patients.

Healthcare providers seeking clinical guidance on PrEP should contact local experts. The National Clinician Consultation Center (nccc.ucsf.edu) also offers free, telephone-based consultation through its PrEPline: (855) 448-7737 | (855) HIV-PrEP.

OCCUPATIONAL AND NONOCCUPATIONAL POSTEXPOSURE PROPHYLAXIS

Ethical considerations prohibit the evaluation of either oPEP or nPEP using randomized controlled trials. The data to support its use largely derive from animal models, inference from postnatal prophylaxis studies, observational studies, and one retrospective case-control study that showed an 81% reduction in the risk of infection among healthcare workers who took zidovudine after exposure (Cardo, 1997; Lunding, 2015; Otten, 2000; Shih, 1991; Young, 2007).

oPEP

The use of ART to prevent transmission of HIV for healthcare personnel who experience a high-risk occupational exposure was first recommended in 1990, and the US Public Health Service released its most recent oPEP guidelines in 2013 (Kuhar, 2013).

The risk of HIV acquisition after exposure in the healthcare setting appears to be directly related to the size of the viral inoculum, which is in turn influenced by the stage of disease of the source patient, as well as by the quantity of blood to which the worker was exposed (Kuhar, 2013).

Current guidelines emphasize the following:

- The HIV status of the source patient should be determined whenever possible to guide the need for initiating and/or maintaining oPEP.

- When indicated, it should be started as soon as possible, preferably within 72 hours from the time of exposure.

- All oPEP regimens should include three antiretroviral medications and should be taken for 4 weeks (Table 4.4). The preferred regimen should be tenofovir (TDF) plus emtricitabine (FTC) plus either raltegravir (RAL) or dolutegravir (DTG). DTG should not be used in women who are pregnant or with child-bearing potential and not on effective contraception.

- Expert consultation, with either local experts or through the national HIV Post-Exposure Prophylaxis Hotline, is recommended in certain situations (Table 4.5).

- Close follow-up services, including counseling, repeat HIV testing, and monitoring for drug toxicity, should be provided. HIV follow-up testing should be done at 4–6 weeks and 3–4 months (if using a combination HIV antigen/antibody test) or at 6 weeks, 3 months, and 6 months if using an HIV antibody only test (Table 4.6).

It is also important to remember that healthcare workers who experience an occupational exposure should be screened for HBV and HCV infections. All hepatitis B-susceptible individuals should initiate the hepatitis B vaccine series, and those exposed to a patient with known acute or active HBV infection should be given hepatitis B immune globulin as well. There is currently no effective prophylaxis for HCV infection.

Table 4.4 RECOMMENDED OCCUPATIONAL POSTEXPOSURE PROPHYLAXIS (OPEP) REGIMENS: ALL TO BE TAKEN FOR 4 WEEKS

	NRTI BACKBONE	BASE
PREFERRED REGIMEN	TRUVADA 1 PO DAILY (TDF 300 MG/FTC 200 MG FDC)	RALTEGRAVIR 400 MG TWICE DAILY OR DOLUTEGRAVIR 50 MG ONCE DAILY*
Alternatives	One of following Tenofovir DF (Viread; TDF) + emtricitabine (Emtriva; FTC) available as Truvada *or* Tenofovir DF (Viread; TDF) + lamivudine (Epivir; 3TC) *or* Zidovudine (Retrovir; ZDV; AZT) + lamivudine (Epivir; 3TC); available as Combivir *or* Zidovudine (Retrovir; ZDV; AZT) + emtricitabine (Emtriva; FTC) *or* Tenofovir + emtricitabine + elvitegravir + cobicistat (TDF/FTC/EVG/cobi, Stribild)	With one of following Raltegravir (Isentress; RAL) *or* Darunavir (Prezista; DRV) + ritonavir (Norvir; RTV) *or* Etravirine (Intelence; ETR) *or* Rilpivirine (Edurant; RPV) *or* Atazanavir (Reyataz; ATV) + ritonavir (Norvir; RTV) *or* Lopinavir/ritonavir (Kaletra; LPV/RTV)

FDC, fixed-dose combination; FTC, emtricitabine; NRTI, nucleotide reverse transcriptase inhibitor; TDF, tenofovir disoproxil fumarate.

* DTG should not be used in women who are pregnant or with child-bearing potential and not on effective contraception.

SOURCE: Adapted from Kuhar (2013) and New York State Department of Health (2018).

nPEP

The CDC's most recent nPEP guidelines were published in 2016 (Dominguez, 2016). The New York State Department of Health AIDS Institute released comprehensive, updated guidelines on the use of antiretroviral medications following nonoccupational exposures, including for victims of sexual assault, in 2018 (New York State Department of Health, 2018). Key points from these guidelines include the following:

- For sexual assault victims, important considerations before initiating PEP include whether or not a significant exposure occurred during the assault; whether the victim is ready and willing to complete a PEP regimen; and knowledge of the alleged assailant's HIV status, although a lack thereof should not delay PEP initiation when warranted based on the nature of the exposure.

- Exposure types warranting PEP include direct contact of the vagina, penis, anus, or mouth with the semen, vaginal fluids, or blood of the alleged assailant, with or without physical injury, tissue damage, or the presence of blood at the site of the assault; when broken skin or mucous membranes of the victim have been in contact with blood, semen, or vaginal fluids from the alleged assailant; and in cases of bites that result in visible blood.

- Baseline HIV testing should be performed for the victim, as should a pregnancy test for female victims.

- When indicated, PEP should be initiated as soon as possible, and within 72 hours after the exposure.

- Prophylactic treatment to prevent gonorrheal and chlamydial infections should also be offered, as should emergency contraception for female victims.

- For patients with other potential nonoccupational exposures to HIV, determination of the level of risk from the exposure is critical; nPEP is generally only indicated for patients with higher risk exposures (Table 4.7). Other key points include the following:
  - HIV testing of the source patient should be performed when possible.
  - All exposed patients should have the following done at baseline: HIV testing, site-specific testing for gonorrhea and chlamydia, testing for syphilis, and pregnancy testing for women.
  - When indicated, PEP should be initiated as soon as possible, and within 72 hours after the exposure.
  - Risk-reduction counseling should also be provided, including referrals for mental health and/or substance use disorder treatment programs when indicated, as well as discussion of future PrEP use for individuals with ongoing risk behavior.

- Recommended nPEP regimens include TDF/FTC plus either raltegravir (RAL) or dolutegravir (DTG).

- Recent data suggest that infants born to women who become pregnant while on DTG may be at higher risk for neural tube defects (Zash, 2018), so DTG should be avoided in women of childbearing potential who are not on effective contraception.

As with patients who experience occupational exposures, those with nonoccupational exposures should be screened for HBV and HCV infections and be given appropriate treatment and follow-up as described previously.

Table 4.5 SITUATIONS IN WHICH EXPERT CONSULTATION FOR OCCUPATIONAL POSTEXPOSURE PROPHYLAXIS (OPEP) IS RECOMMENDED

SCENARIO	COMMENTS
Delayed (i.e., later than 72 hours) exposure report	Interval after which benefits from PEP are undefined.
Unknown source (e.g., needle in sharps disposal container or laundry)	Use of PEP to be decided on a case-by-case basis. Consider severity of exposure and epidemiologic likelihood of HIV exposure. Do not test needles or other sharp instruments for HIV.
Known or suspected pregnancy in the exposed person	Provision of PEP should not be delayed while awaiting expert consultation.
Breast-feeding in the exposed person	Provision of PEP should not be delayed while awaiting expert consultation.
Known or suspected resistance of the source virus to antiretroviral agents	If source person's virus is known or suspected to be resistant to one or more of the drugs considered for PEP, selection of drugs to which the source person's virus is unlikely to be resistant is recommended. Do not delay initiation of PEP while awaiting any results of resistance testing of the source person's virus.
Toxicity of the initial PEP regimen	Symptoms (e.g., gastrointestinal symptoms and others) are often manageable without changing PEP regimen by prescribing antimotility or antiemetic agents. Counseling and support for management of side effects is very important because symptoms are often exacerbated by anxiety.
Serious medical illness in the exposed person	Significant underlying illness (e.g., renal disease) or an exposed provider already taking multiple medications may increase the risk of drug toxicity and drug–drug interactions.

Expert consultation can be made with local experts or by calling the National Clinician Consultation Center's Post Exposure Prophylaxis Hotline (PEPline) at 1-888-448-4911.

SOURCE: Adapted from Kuhar (2013).

SCREENING AND TREATMENT FOR SEXUALLY TRANSMITTED INFECTIONS

The link between STIs and an increased risk for HIV transmission/acquisition has been established for some time. This is supported by both biologic plausibility (e.g., genital tract inflammation leading to increased viral shedding in infected partners and increased access of HIV to subepithelial target cells) and epidemiologic synergy (Mayer, 2011; Ward, 2010). However, multiple confounders have made it difficult to estimate just how much these contribute to increased risk, and STI treatment studies to date have failed to consistently demonstrate any reduction in HIV transmission (Mayer, 2011; Ward, 2010). The Mwanza study from Tanzania stands out as the one notable exception: it demonstrated a 38% reduction in HIV incidence with syndromic STI management (Grosskurth, 1995). Nonetheless, the strong link between the two argues for the importance of regular screening and treatment for STIs in those at risk because those who screen positive are likely to benefit from PrEP and risk reduction counseling in general. This point is highlighted by an analysis from New York City that demonstrated that 1 in 20 MSM with a new syphilis diagnosis were diagnosed with HIV within 1 year (Prathela, 2015). There are also data from Australia that showed that MSM diagnosed with rectal gonorrhea or chlamydia were 2–3 times more likely to be diagnosed with incident HIV in the following 12 months than those who were not (Cheung, 2016).

VOLUNTARY MEDICAL MALE CIRCUMCISION

Three large randomized trials performed in sub-Saharan Africa demonstrated that voluntary circumcision of HIV-uninfected men led to an approximate risk reduction for heterosexual HIV acquisition of 50% (Auvert, 2005; Bailey, 2007; Gray, 2007; Siegfried, 2009). This prevention benefit does not appear to extend to the female partners of circumcised HIV-infected men (Weiss, 2009). Although observational data suggest that circumcision may be beneficial for MSM who practice primary insertive anal intercourse, there is currently insufficient evidence to determine whether or not this is the case in general for MSM (Wiysonge, 2011).

VERTICAL TRANSMISSION PREVENTION

This is reviewed in detail in Chapter 29.

TREATMENT AS PREVENTION

This is reviewed in detail in Chapter 25.

RECOMMENDED READING

New York State Department of Health AIDS Institute. HIV prophylaxis following non-occupational exposure. Available at https://www.hivguidelines.org/pep-for-hiv-prevention/non-occupational/.

Siegfried N, Muller M, Deeks JJ, et al. Male circumcision for prevention of heterosexual acquisition of HIV in men. *Cochrane Database Syst Rev.* 2009;2:CD003362. doi: 10.1002/14651858.CD003362.pub2.

US Public Health Service. Preexposure prophylaxis for the prevention of HIV infection in the United States–2017 Update: a clinical practice guideline. Available at https://www.cdc.gov/hiv/pdf/risk/prep/cdc-hiv-prep-guidelines-2017.pdf.

INVESTIGATIONAL INTERVENTIONS FOR HIV TRANSMISSION PREVENTION

LEARNING OBJECTIVES

Describe three investigational biomedical interventions for HIV prevention and how they complement existing, proven interventions.

TIME FROM EXPOSURE	RECOMMENDED SERVICES	
	COUNSELING	TESTING
Baseline	Transmission prevention (condom use; avoidance of blood/ tissue donation; avoid breast-feeding if possible) Possible drug toxicities Possible drug interactions Importance of adherence	HIV antibody testing (preferably combined antigen/ antibody test) Complete blood count Liver function tests Renal function tests
72 hours	Even if not taking PEP—to review additional information about exposure or the source patient if available *If on PEP* Transmission prevention (condom use; avoidance of blood/ tissue donation; avoid breast-feeding if possible) Possible drug toxicities Possible drug interactions Importance of adherence	
2 weeks	Transmission prevention Possible drug toxicities Possible drug interactions Importance of adherence	Complete blood count Liver function tests Renal function tests
4–6 weeks	Transmission prevention	HIV testing (preferably combined antigen/antibody test)
If fourth-generation (combined antigen/antibody) HIV testing is used		
3–4 months		HIV antigen/antibody testing (if negative, HIV infection is excluded)
If fourth-generation HIV testing is not used, i.e., HIV antibody-only assay		
12 weeks	Transmission prevention	HIV antibody testing
6 months		HIV antibody testing (if negative, HIV infection is excluded)

PEP, postexposure prophylaxis.

SOURCE: Adapted from Kuhar (2013).

WHAT'S NEW

- The use of on-demand and time-driven dosing strategies for oral PrEP, as well as long-acting injectable formulations, is under active investigation.

- DISCOVER, a randomized phase 3 trial evaluating TAF/FTC for PrEP, is ongoing.

- The drug-eluting dapivirine vaginal ring reduced the risk of HIV infection in African women and offers promise as a novel woman-driven HIV prevention method.

- New vaccine strategies, such as the use of broadly neutralizing antibodies and the use of bioinformatically developed antigens, are also being evaluated.

KEY POINT

- The continued development and evaluation of novel preventative approaches are key to an effective, sustainable reduction in the number of new HIV infections globally.

INTERMITTENT AND ON-DEMAND PREEXPOSURE PROPHYLAXIS

As previously mentioned, currently approved PrEP regimens require the daily use of oral antiretrovirals. Alternative dosing schedules, including on-demand and time-driven use of oral formulations as well as the use of long-acting injectable formulations, are under active investigation. Also, as mentioned previously, mixed results have been obtained from studies evaluating nondaily oral PrEP use. The IPERGAY study conducted in France, Quebec, Canada, and other French-speaking countries evaluated event-driven PrEP in high-risk MSM. Participants in the intervention arm of this prospective, randomized, placebo-controlled trial took two tablets of TDF/FTC 2–24 hours before sex, 1 tablet 24 hours after sex, and an additional tablet 48 hours after the first dose. This on-demand approach was highly effective, with an 86% reduction in the risk of HIV seroconversion among those in the intervention arm compared to placebo (Molina, 2015). These data have subsequently been supported by a substudy of IPERGAY which evaluated PrEP efficacy in men reporting less frequent sex, as well as by recent data from Prevenir; in each

Table 4.7 LEVEL OF RISK BASED ON EXPOSURE TYPE FOR CONSIDERATION OF NONOCCUPATIONAL POSTEXPOSURE PROPHYLAXIS (NPEP)

High-risk exposures—nPEP should be recommended	Receptive and insertive vaginal or anal intercourse with a partner who is HIV positive, or when the partner's HIV status is unknown
	Needle sharing with a partner who is HIV positive, or when the partner's HIV status is unknown
	Injuries with exposure to blood or other potentially infected fluids from a source known to be HIV-infected or HIV status is unknown (including needle sticks with a hollow-bore needle, human bites, and accidents)
Lower risk exposures—require case-by-case evaluation for nPEP	Oral–vaginal contact (receptive and insertive)
	Oral–anal contact (receptive and insertive)
	Receptive penile–oral contact with or without ejaculation
	Insertive penile–oral contact with or without ejaculation
	Factors that increase risk (nPEP should be offered)
	Source person is known to be HIV-infected with high viral load
	An oral mucosa that is not intact (e.g., oral lesions, gingivitis, and wounds)
	Blood exposure
	Presence of genital ulcer disease or other sexually transmitted infections
Exposures that do *not* warrant nPEP	Kissing
	Oral-to-oral contact without mucosal damage (mouth-to-mouth resuscitation)
	Human bites not involving blood
	Exposure to solid-bore needles or sharps not in recent contact with blood (e.g., tattoo needles and lancets)
	Mutual masturbation without skin breakdown or blood exposure

SOURCE: Adapted from New York State Department of Health AIDS Institute (2018).

of these, there were no reported HIV infections in MSM who used event-driven PrEP (Antoni, 2017; Molina, 2018). On the other hand, in the HPTN 067/ADAPT Harlem study, which compared daily PrEP with time-driven (one dose twice weekly plus one dose after sex) and event-driven (one dose before and one dose after sex) dosing schedules among MSM and transgender women in the United States, the daily strategy provided better coverage of reported sex acts and higher overall adherence compared to the other two (Mannheimer, 2015). It is also important to note that there are theoretical concerns about the use of nondaily strategies in different populations based on varying levels of drug penetration into different tissue categories. For example, oral tenofovir appears to concentrate more quickly in rectal compared to vaginal mucosa (Hendrix, 2013), which could potentially limit the applicability of event- and time-driven PrEP in women.

NOVEL ANTIRETROVIRALS FOR PREP

TDF/FTC is currently the only FDA-approved regimen for PrEP. TAF/FTC, with its improved renal and bone safety profile, as well as its smaller pill size, is an attractive alternative. However, there are some concerns that it may not be as effective, primarily because TAF concentrates intracellularly and appears to have lower concentrations in genital mucosal tissue when compared with TDF (Cottrell, 2017). The DISCOVER trial is an ongoing, randomized phase 3 clinical trial that is evaluating the efficacy of daily TAF/FTC versus daily TDF/FTC to prevent new HIV infections in MSM and transgender women (ClinicalTrials.gov.NCT02842086).

Another investigational strategy is the use of long-acting injectable antiretrovirals for PrEP. Cabotegravir, a novel integrase strand transfer inhibitor, has been found to be both safe and well-tolerated in phase 2 studies (Markowitz,

2017; Landovitz, 2017) and consistently met pharmacokinetic targets when given every 8 weeks (Landovitz, 2017). Phase 3 clinical trials evaluating this strategy further, in comparison with daily TDF/FTC for MSM, transgender women, and heterosexual women, are now enrolling (HPTN 083, ClinicalTrials.gov.NCT02720094; HPTN 084, ClinicalTrials.gov.NCT03164564).

MICROBICIDES

Microbicides are products that are applied locally to the vaginal or rectal mucosa to reduce the risk of HIV and other STI acquisition. There was great optimism for this strategy when the results of the CAPRISA 004 trial were released. This study examined the effectiveness and safety of coitally dosed (one dose within 12 hours before sex and a second dose as soon as possible within 12 hours after sex) 1% tenofovir vaginal gel in sexually active South African women aged 18–40 years. It was found that use of this gel resulted in a 39% reduction overall in the risk of HIV acquisition and a 54% reduction in those who used the gel at least 80% of the time (Abdool Karim, 2010). However, this optimism was dampened by the failure of two subsequent studies, VOICE and FACTS 001, to show any reduction in HIV acquisition among women using this same tenofovir gel (Marrazzo, 2015; Rees, 2015). Note that HIV acquisition was reduced by approximately 50% among women who used the gel consistently, as measured by plasma TDF levels in both studies (Dai, 2015; Rees, 2015).

Despite the previously mentioned negative results, the use of microbicides or other local drug-delivery devices such as vaginal rings have several theoretical benefits. First, they deliver high concentrations of the drug to the desired tissue with minimal systemic exposure (Hendrix, 2013). As such, they have the potential to provide on-demand protection, especially considering

Table 4.8 SUMMARY OF HIV VACCINE EFFICACY TRIALS

TRIAL	VACCINE PRODUCT	STUDY POPULATION; SITE	RESULTS	REFERENCE
Vax 003	Recombinant gp120 (B/E)	Male and female PWID; Thailand	No efficacy	Pitisuttithum (2006)
Vax 004	Recombinant gp120 (B/B′)	Heterosexual women and MSM; United States and the Netherlands	No efficacy	Flynn (2005)
HVTN 502	Recombinant Ad5 (Clade B gag/pol/nef)	MSM, heterosexual women and men; North and South America, Caribbean, Australia	No efficacy	Buchbinder (2008)
HVTN 503	Recombinant Ad5 (Clade B gag/pol/nef)	Heterosexual women and men; South Africa	No efficacy	Gray (2011)
HVTN 505	6-plasmid DNA vaccine and rAd5 vector boost	MSM; United States	No efficacy	Hammer (2013)
RV 144	ALVAC: Canarypox (gag, pol, env) + AIDSVAX B/E recombinant gp120	Heterosexual women and men; Thailand	31% reduction in acquisition	Rerks-Ngarm (2009)

SOURCE: Adapted from Tieu, 2013 and Rubens, 2015.

the time delay that occurs between oral TDF dosing and drug penetration of the vaginal mucosa. These products also may be given to women, who comprised almost half of new HIV infections globally in 2014 (WHO, 2015), and represent an additional HIV preventive option that they can control. Last, they have the potential to be coformulated with other medications and as such may provide protection against other STIs and pregnancy. Excitement for this approach was reinvigorated by results of the MTN-020/ASPIRE trial, which evaluated the efficacy of a monthly dapivirine-eluting vaginal ring for HIV prevention in at-risk African women. These demonstrated a 27% reduction in the incidence of new HIV infections among women who received the study ring compared to those who received placebo, with adherence again an important factor, as the efficacy of the ring increased to 37% when data from two study sites with reduced rates of adherence and retention were excluded (Baeten, 2016). More recently, an interim analysis of the open label extension (OLE) trial of the dapivirine ring provided more encouraging results: 92% of women enrolled accepted the ring, most (89%) rings were used, and HIV incidence was less than half that expected based on the infection distribution of the enrolled population (Baeten, 2018).

given the complexities of human behavior and the risk that programs supporting treatment-based interventions could be defunded over time (Fauci, 2014). The ability of a vaccine to elicit broadly neutralizing antibodies (BNAbs), or antibodies that can protect against multiple pathogenic HIV strains by binding to highly conserved regions of the virus, is crucial for its success but thus far has been elusive. Recent advances in the identification and understanding of BNAbs have injected new hope into HIV vaccine development. One such antibody product, VRC01, targets the HIV-1 CD4 binding site and is currently under investigation in the AMP study, a collaborative HVTN/HPTN study that recently began enrollment (see http://ampstudy.org). 3BNC117 is another BNAb that has shown promise for further development (Caskey, 2015). Last, the use of bioinformatically developed mosaic antigens to elicit antibody responses that are protective against all clades of HIV is another novel approach that is under investigation in the HIV-V-A004 trial; phase 1/2a results of this trial were recently released and showed that this product does indeed produce robust immune responses in both humans and rhesus monkeys (Barouch, 2018; see http://www.avac.org/trial/hiv-v-a004ipcavd-009-approach).

VACCINES

Multiple challenges, both biomedical and social, have impeded the development of an effective HIV vaccine. These include HIV viral diversity and pathogenesis, identification of appropriate immune correlates of protection, community preparedness and concerns about vaccine-induced positivity, and, more recently, the expanded use of PrEP (Hammer, 2015). With the exception of the modestly positive Thai vaccine trial, which demonstrated a 31% reduction in new infections among vaccine recipients, clinical trials of HIV preventive vaccines have had disappointing results (Table 4.8). However, the pursuit of an effective vaccine remains as important as ever. Even with the promise of ART-mediated control of the epidemic through TasP and PrEP, an effective vaccine is essential for timely, sustainable control to occur,

RECOMMENDED READING

Baeten JM, Palanee-Phillips T, Brown ER, et al. Use of a vaginal ring containing dapivirine for HIV-1 prevention in women. *N Engl J Med.* 2016;375(22):2121–2132.

Fauci AS, Marston HD. Ending AIDS: is an HIV vaccine necessary? *N Engl J Med.* 2014;370(6):495–498.

CONCLUSION

Tremendous strides continue to be made in the field of HIV prevention. Although much attention has focused on ART-based interventions such as TasP and PrEP, "real-world" application of research findings generates important questions for clinical care delivery, some of which remain unanswered at this time. Importantly, a multifaceted approach that includes behavioral, structural, and established biomedical interventions is still needed to make a significant, lasting impact on the global incidence of HIV.

REFERENCES

Abdool Karim Q, Abdool Karim SS, Frohlich JA, et al. Effectiveness and safety of tenofovir gel, an antiretroviral microbicide, for the prevention of HIV infection in women. *Science*. 2010;329(5996):1168–1174.

Abdul-Quader AS, Feelemyer J, Modi S, et al. Effectiveness of structural-level needle/syringe programs to reduce HCV and HIV infection among people who inject drugs: a systematic review. *AIDS Behav*. 2013;17(9):2878–2892.

Aberg JA, Gallant JE, Ghanem KG, et al. Primary care guidelines for the management of persons infected with HIV: 2013 update by the HIV Medicine Association of the Infectious Diseases Society of America. *Clin Infec Dis*. 2014;58(1):e1–e34.

Adekeye OA, Heiman HJ, Onyeabor OS, Hyacinth HI. The new invincibles: HIV screening among older adults in the US. *PLoS One* 2012;7(8):e43618.

Adimora AA, Hughes JP, Wang J, et al. Characteristics of multiple and concurrent partnerships among women at high risk for HIV infection. *J AIDS*. 2014;65(1):99–106.

Adler NE. Overview of health disparities. In: GE Thompson, F Mitchell, M Williams, eds. *Examining the Health Disparities Research Plan of the National Institutes of Health: Unfinished Business*. Washington, DC: National Academic Press; 2006:129–188.

Agerwala SM, McCance-Katz EF. Integrating screening, brief intervention, and referral to treatment (SBIRT) into clinical practice settings: a brief review. *J Psychoactive Drugs*. 2012;44(4):307–317.

Aidala AA, Wilson MG, Shubert V, et al. Housing status, medical care, and health outcomes among people living with HIV/AIDS: a systematic review. *Am J Public Health*. 2015;106:e1–e23.

Althoff KN, Gebo KA, Gange SJ, et al. CD4 count at presentation for HIV care in the United States and Canada: are those over 50 years more likely to have a delayed presentation? *AIDS Res Ther*. 2010;7:45.

An Q, Prejean J, Harrison KM, and Fang X. Association between community socioeconomic position and HIV diagnosis rate among adults and adolescents in the United States, 2005-2009. *Am J Public Health*. 2013;103(1):120–126.

Anema A, Marshall BD, Stevenson B, et al. Intergenerational sex as a risk factor for HIV among young men who have sex with men: a scoping review. *Curr HIV/AIDS Rep*. 2013;10(4):398–407.

Antiretroviral Pregnancy Registry International Interim Report for 1 January 1989–31 January 2018. Available at http://www.apregistry.com/forms/exec-summary.pdf. Accessed July 22, 2018.

Antoni G, Tremblay C, Charreau I, et al. On-demand PrEP with TDF/FTC remains highly effective among MSM with infrequent sexual intercourse: a sub-study of the ANRS IPERGAY trial. In: *Program and Abstracts of the 9th International AIDS Society Conference on HIV Science*, July 23–26, 2017; Paris, France. Abstract TUAC102.

Aspinall EJ, Nambiar D, Goldberg DJ, et al. Are needle and syringe programs associated with a reduction in HIV transmission among people who inject drugs: a systematic review and meta-analysis? *Int J Epidemiol*. 2014;43(1):235–248.

Auvert B, Taljaard D, Lagarde E, Sobngwi-Tambekou J, Sitta R, et al. Randomized, controlled intervention trial of male circumcision for reduction of HIV infection risk: the ANRS 1265 trial. *PLoS Med*. 2005;2(11):e298.

Baeten JM. Donnell D, Ndase P, et al. Antiretroviral prophylaxis for HIV prevention in heterosexual men and women. *N Engl J Med*. 2012;367:399–410.

Baeten JM, Palanee-Phillips T, Brown ER, et al. Use of a vaginal ring containing dapivirine for HIV-1 prevention in women. *N Engl J Med*. 2016;375(22):2121–2132.

Baeten J, Palanee-Phillips T, Mgodi N, et al. High uptake and reduced HIV-1 incidence in an open-label trial of the dapivirine ring. In: *Program and Abstracts of the 2018 Conference on Retroviruses and Opportunistic Infections*, March 4–7, 2018; Boston, Massachusetts. Abstract 143LB.

Baggaley R, Boily M-C, White RG, et al. Risk of HIV-1 transmission for parenteral exposure and blood transfusion: a systematic review and meta-analysis. *AIDS*. 2006;20(6):805–812.

Bailey RC, Moses S, Parker CB, et al. Male circumcision for HIV prevention in young men in Kisumu, Kenya: a randomised controlled trial. *Lancet*. 2007;369:643.

Baral SD, Poteat T, Stromdahl S, Wirtz AL, Guadamuz TE, Beyrer C. Worldwide burden of HIV in transgender women: a systematic review and meta-analyses. *Lancet Infect Dis*. 2013;13(3):214–222.

Barouch DH, Thomka FL, Wegmann F et al. Evaluation of a mosaic HIV-1 vaccine in a multicentre, randomised, double-blind, placebo-controlled, phase 1/2a clinical trial (APPROACH) and in rhesus monkeys (NHP 13-19). *Lancet*. 2018 Jul 21;392(10143):232–243. doi: 10.1016/S0140-6736(18)31364-3. Epub 2018 Jul 6.

Barre-Sinoussi F, Abdool Karim S, Albert J, et. al. Expert consensus statement on the science of HIV in the context of criminal law. *J Int AIDS Soc*. 2018;27(7):e25161.

Belenko S, Hiller, M, Visher C, et al. Policies and practices in the delivery of HIV services in correctional agencies and facilities: results from a multisite survey. *J Correct Health Care*. 2013;19(4):293–310.

Belenko S, Visher C, Pearson F, et al. Efficacy of structured organizational change intervention on HIV testing in correctional facilities. *AIDS Educ Prev*. 2017;29(3):241–255.

Bernstein SL, D'Onofrio G. Screening, treatment initiation, and referral for substance use disorders. *Addict Sci Clin Pract*. 2017;12:18.

Berry MS, Johnson MW. Does being drunk or high cause HIV sexual risk behavior? A systematic review of drug administration studies. *Pharmacol Biochem Behav*. 2018;164:125–138.

Blaylock JM, Wortmann GW. Care of the aging HIV patient. *Cleve Clin J Med*. 2015;82(7):445–455.

Bonell C, Imrie J. Behavioral interventions to prevent HIV infection: rapid evolution, increasing rigor, moderate success. *Br Med. Bull*. 2001;58(1):155–170.

Branson BM, Handsfield HH, Lampe MA, et al.; Centers for Disease Control and Prevention. Revised recommendations for HIV testing of adults, adolescents, and pregnant women in health-care settings. *MMWR Recomm Rep*. 2006;55(RR-14):1–17.

Brooks JT, Buchacz K, Gebo K, et al. HIV infection and older Americans: the public health perspective. *Am J Public Health*. 2012;102(8):1516–1526.

Buchbinder SP, Mehrotra DV, Duerr A, et al. Efficacy assessment of a cell-mediated immunity HIV-1 vaccine (the Step Study): a double-blind, randomised, placebo-controlled, test-of-concept trial. *Lancet*. 2008;372(9653):1881–1893.

Buchbinder SP, Cohen SE, Hecht J. Getting to zero new diagnoses in San Francisco: what will it take? In: *Program and Abstracts of the 2018 Conference on Retroviruses and Opportunistic Infections*, March 4–7, 2018; Boston, Massachusetts. Abstract 87.

Burris S, Chiu J. Punitive drug law and the risk environment for injecting drug users: understanding the connections. Working paper prepared for the Third Meeting of the Technical Advisory Group of the Global Commission on HIV and the Law, 7–9 July 2011. Available at http://hivlawcommission.org/index.php/working-papers?view=document&id=98&tmpl=component. Accessed November 17, 2015.

Busch MP, Kleinman SF, Nemo GJ. Current and emerging infectious risks of blood transfusions. *JAMA*. 2003;289(8):959–962.

Bush S, Ng L, Magnuson D, et al. Significant uptake of Truvada for pre-exposure prophylaxis (PrEP) utilization in the US in late 2014–1Q2015. In: *Abstracts of the 10th International Conference on HIV Treatment and Prevention Adherence*, Miami, FL, 2015. Abstract 74.

Available at http//iapac.org/AdherenceConference/presentations/ADH10_OA74.pdf. Accessed November 29, 2015.

Caceres CF, Gerbase A, Lo YR, et al. *Prevention and Treatment of HIV and Other Sexually Transmitted Infections Among Men Who Have Sex with Men and Transgender People: Recommendations for a Public Health Approach.* Geneva: World Health Organization Document Production Services, 2011.

Cardo DM, Culver DH, Ciesielski CA, et al.; Centers for Disease Control and Prevention Needlestick Surveillance Group. A case control study of HIV seroconversion in health care workers after percutaneous exposure. *N Engl J Med.* 1997;337(21):1485–1490.

Caskey M, Klein F, Lorenzi JC, et al. Viraemia suppressed in HIV-1-infected humans by broadly neutralizing antibody 3BNC117. *Nature.* 2015 Jun 25;522(7557):487–491. doi: 10.1038/nature14411. Epub 2015 April 8.

Centers for Disease Control and Prevention (CDC). High-impact HIV prevention: CDC's approach to reducing HIV infections in the United States. Centers for Disease Control and Prevention, August 2011. Available at: https://www.cdc.gov/hiv/pdf/policies_NHPC_Booklet.pdf. Accessed June 23, 2018.

Centers for Disease Control and Prevention, Health Resources and Services Administration, National Institutes of Health, American Academy of HIV Medicine, Association of Nurses in AIDS Care, International Association of Providers of AIDS Care, the National Minority AIDS Council, and Urban Coalition for HIV/AIDS Prevention Services. Recommendations for HIV prevention with adults and adolescents with HIV in the United States, 2014. December 11, 2014. Available at: http://stacks.cdc.gov/view/cdc/26062. Accessed June 24, 2018.

Centers for Disease Control and Prevention (CDC). Monitoring selected national HIV prevention and care objectives by using HIV surveillance data—United States and 6 dependent areas, 2015. HIV Surveillance Supplemental Report 2017;22(No. 2). Published July 2017. Available at: http://www.cdc.gov/hiv/library/reports/hivsurveillance.html. Accessed June 24, 2018.

Centers for Disease Control and Prevention (CDC). HIV Surveillance Report, 2016; vol. 28. Published November 2017. Available at: http://www.cdc.gov/hiv/library/reports/hiv-surveillance.html. Accessed June 17, 2018.

Centers for Disease Control and Prevention (CDC). Managing HIV and hepatitis C outbreaks among people who inject drugs: a guide for state and local health departments. March 2018. Available at: https://www.cdc.gov/hiv/pdf/programresources/guidance/cluster-outbreak/cdchiv-hcv-pwid-guide.pdf. Accessed June 24, 2018.

Centers for Disease Control and Prevention (CDC). HIV and injection drug use in the United States. Available at: http://www.cdc.gov/hiv/risk/idu.html. Accessed November 11, 2015.

Chen M, Rhodes PH, Hall HI, et al. Prevalence of undiagnosed HIV infection among persons aged ≥13 years: National HIV Surveillance System, United States, 2005–2008. *MMWR Suppl.* 2012;61(02):57–64.

Cheung KT, Fairley CK, Read TRH, et al. HIV Incidence and predictors of incident HIV among men who have sex with men attending a sexual health clinic in Melbourne, Australia. *PLoS One.* 2016 May 24;11(5):e0156160. doi: 10.1371/journal.pone.0156160. eCollection 2016.

Choopanya K, Martin M, Suntharasamai P, et al. Antiretroviral prophylaxis for HIV infection in injecting drug users in Bangkok, Thailand (the Bangkok Tenofovir Study): a randomised, double-blind, placebo-controlled phase 3 trial. *Lancet.* 2013;381:2083–2090.

Cohen MS, Chen YQ, McCauley M, et al. Antiretroviral treatment prevents HIV transmission: final results from the HPTN 052 randomized controlled trial. In: *Program and Abstracts of the 8th IAS Conference on HIV Pathogenesis, Treatment & Prevention,* July 19–22, 2015; Vancouver, Canada. Abstract MOAC0101LB.

Community Access National Network. HIV/HCV Co-Infection Watch. June 2018. Available at: http://www.tiicann.org/co-infection-watch.html. Accessed June 24, 2018.

Cottrell ML, Garrett, KL, Prince HMA, et al. Single-dose pharmacokinetics of tenofovir alafenamide and its active metabolite in the mucosal tissues. *J Antimicrob Chemother.* 2017;72:1731–1740.

Csete J, Kamarulzaman A, Kazatchkine M, et al. Public health and international drug policy: report of the John Hopkins-Lancet. Commission on Drug Policy and Health. *Lancet.* 2016;387(10026):1427–1480.

Dai JY, Hedrix CW, Richardson BA, et al. Pharmacological measures of treatment adherence and risk of HIV infection in the VOICE study. *J Infect Dis.* 2015; doi: 10.1093/infdis/jiv333. [Epub ahead of print]

Dailey AF, Hoots BE, Hall I, et al. Vital signs: human immunodeficiency virus testing and diagnosis delays—United States. *MMWR Weekly.* 2017;66(47):1300–1306.

DeBeck K, Cheng T, Montaner JS, et al. HIV and the criminalization of drug use among people who inject drugs: a systematic review. *Lancet. HIV* 2017;4(8):e357–e374.

Degenhardt L, Mathers B, Guarinieri M, et al. Meth/amphetamine use and associated HIV: implications for global policy and public health. *Int J Drug Policy* 2010;21(5):347–358.

Dominguez K, Smith DK, Vasavi T, et al. Updated guidelines for antiretroviral postexposure prophylaxis after sexual, injection drug use, or other non-occupational exposure to HIV—United States, 2016. US Centers for Disease Control and Prevention. Available at: http://stacks.cdc.gov/view/cdc/38856. Accessed April 25, 2016.

Dong BJ, William MR, Bingham JT, et al. Outcomes of challenging HIV case consultations provided via teleconference by the Clinician Consultation Center to the Federal Bureau of Prisons. *J Am Pharm Assoc.* 2017;57(4):516–519.

Eastment MC, McClelland RS. Vaginal microbiota and susceptibility to HIV. *AIDS.* 2018;32(6):687–698.

Fauci AS, Martson HD. Ending AIDS: is an HIV vaccine necessary? *N Engl J Med.* 2014;370(6):495–498.

Flynn NM, Forthal DN, Harro CD, et al. Placebo-controlled phase 3 trial of a recombinant glycoprotein 120 vaccine to prevent HIV-1 infection. *J Infect Dis.* 2005;191(5):654–665.

Franconi I and Guaraldi G. Pre-exposure prophylaxis for HIV infection in the older patient: what can be recommended? *Drugs Aging.* 2018. 35(6):485–491.

Garcia J, Parker C, Parker RG, et al. "You're really gonna kick us all out?" Sustaining safe spaces for community-based HIV prevention and control among black men who have sex with men. *PLoS One.* 2015;10(10):e0141326.

Garfein RS, Golub ET, Greenberg AE, et al. A peer-education intervention to reduce injection risk behaviors for HIV and hepatitis C virus infection in young injection drug users. *AIDS.* 2007;21:1923–1932.

Giannou FK, Tsiara CG, Nikolopoulos GK, et al. Condom effectiveness in reducing heterosexual HIV transmission: a systematic review and meta-analysis of studies on HIV serodiscordant couples. *Expert Rev Pharmacoecon Outcomes Res.* 2015;1–11.

Giler RM, Magnuson D, Trevor H, et al. Changes in Truvada (TVD) for HIV pre-exposure prophylaxis (PrEP) utilization in the United States: (2012–2016). In: *Program and Abstracts of the 9th International AIDS Society Conference on HIV Science,* July 23–26, 2017; Paris, France. Abstract WEPEC0919.

Grant RM., Lama JR, Anderson PL, et al. Preexposure chemoprophylaxis for HIV prevention in men who have sex with men. *N Engl J Med.* 2010;363:2587–2599.

Gray GE, Allen M, Moodie Z, et al. Safety and efficacy assessment of the HVTN 503/Phambili Study: a double-blind randomized placebo-controlled test-of-concept study of a clade B-based HIV-1 vaccine in South Africa. *Lancet Infect Dis.* 2011;11(7):507–515.

Gray RH, Kigozi G, Serwadda D, et al. Male circumcision for HIV prevention in men in Rakai, Uganda: a randomised trial. *Lancet.* 2007;369:657–666.

Greene M, Justice AC, Covinsky KE. Assessment of geriatric syndromes and physical function in people living with HIV. *Virulence.* 2017;8(5):586–598.

Grosskurth H, Mosha F, Todd J, et al. Impact of improved treatment of sexually transmitted diseases on HIV infection in rural Tanzania: randomised controlled trial. *Lancet.* 1995;346:530–536.

Grossman H, Anderson P, Grant R, Gandhi M, Mohri H, Markowitz M. Newly acquired HIV-1 infection with multi-drug resistant (MDR) HIV-1 in a patient on TDF/FTC-based PrEP. In: *HIV Research for Prevention (HIVR4P 2016)*, October 17–19, 2016, Chicago. Abstract OA03.06LB.

Grulich A, Guy RJ, Amin J, et al. Rapid reduction in HIV diagnoses after targeted PrEP introduction in NSW, Australia. In: *Program and Abstracts of the 2018 Conference on Retroviruses and Opportunistic Infections*, March 4–7, 2018; Boston, Massachusetts. Abstract 88.

Gupta S, Granich R. National HIV care continua for key populations. *J Int Assoc Provid AIDS Care.* 2017;16(2):125–132.

Haffajee RL, Bohnert ASB, Lagisetty PA. Policy pathways to address provider workforce barriers to buprenorphine treatment. *Am J Prev Med.* 2018;54(6S3):s230–242.

Hammer SM. Advances in preventive HIV vaccines: efficacy trial evolution. In: *ID Week 2015*, October 7–11, 2015; San Diego, California. Oral session 0021.

Hammer SM, Sobieszczyk ME, Janes H, et al. Efficacy trial of a DNA/rAd5 HIV-1 preventive vaccine. *N Engl J Med.* 2013;369:2083–2092.

Hammett TM, Donahue S, LeRoy L, et al. Transitions to care in the community for prison releases with HIV: a qualitative study of facilitators and challenges in two states. *J Urban Health.* 2015;92(4):650–666.

Harrison A, Cleland J, Frohlick J. Young people's sexual partnerships in KwaZulu/Natal, South Africa: patterns, contextual influences, and HIV risk. *Studies Fam Planning.* 2008;39(4):295–308.

Heimer R, Abdala N. Viability of HIV-1 in syringes: implications for interventions among injection drug users. *AIDS Reader.* 2000;10(7).

Heimer R, Grau LE, Curtin E, et al. Assessment of HIV testing of urban injection drug users: implications for expansion of HIV testing and prevention efforts. *Am J Public Health.* 2007;97(1):119–116.

Hendrix CW, Chen BA, Guddera V, et al. MTN-001: randomized pharmacokinetic cross-over study comparing tenofovir vaginal gel and oral tablets in vaginal tissue and other compartments. *PLoS One.* 2013;8(1): e55013. doi: 10.1371/journal.pone.0055013.

Hoenigl M, Chaillon A, Moore DJ, et al. Clear links between starting methamphetamine and increasing sexual risk behavior: a cohort study among men who have sex with men. *J AIDS.* 2016;71(5):551–557.

Hoornenborg E, de Bree GJ. Acute infection with a wild-type HIV-1 virus in PrEP user with high TDF Levels. In: *Program and Abstracts of the 2017 Conference on Retroviruses and Opportunistic Infections*, February 13–16, 2017; Seattle, Washington. Abstract 953.

Hosek S, Rudy B, Landowitz R, et al. An HIV pre-exposure prophylaxis (PrEP) demonstration project and safety study for young men who have sex with men in the United States (ATN 110). In: *Program and Abstracts of the 8th IAS Conference on HIV Pathogenesis, Treatment & Prevention*; July 19–22, 2015; Vancouver, Canada. Abstract TUAC0204LB.

Hosek SG, Landovitz RJ, Kapogiannis B, et al. Safety and feasibility of antiretroviral preexposure prophylaxis for adolescent men who have sex with men aged 15 to 17 years in the United States. *JAMA Pediatr.* November 1, 2017;171(11):1063–1071. doi: 10.1001/jamapediatrics.2017.2007.

HRSA CARE Action [newsletter]. Methamphetamines and HIV. June 2009. Available at: http://hab.hrsa.gov/newspublications/careactionnewsletter/june2009.pdf. Accessed November 15, 2015.

HRSA CARE Action [newsletter]. Impact of mental illness on people living with HIV. January 2015. Available at: http://hab.hrsa.gov/deliverhivaidscare/mentalhealth.pdf. Accessed November 24, 2015.

Humeniuk, R, Dennington V, Ali R; WHO ASSIST Phase III Study Group. The effectiveness of brief intervention for illicit drugs linked to the alcohol, smoking and substance involvement screening test (ASSIST) in primary health care settings: a technical report of phase III findings of the WHO ASSIST randomized controlled trial. Geneva: World Health Organization Document Production Services, 2008.

Ickowicz S, Hayashi K, Dong H, et al. Benzodiazepine use as an independent risk factor for HIV infection in a Canadian setting. *Drug Alcohol Depend.* 2015;155:190–194.

Institute of Medicine. *Preventing HIV Infection Among Injecting Drug Users in High-Risk Countries: An Assessment of the Evidence.* Washington, DC: National Academies Press, 2007.

Iroh PA, Mayo H, Nijhawan AE. The HIV care cascade before, during, and after incarceration: a systematic review and data synthesis. *Am J Public Health.* 2015;105(7): e5–e16.

Jarvis BP, Holtyn AF, Subramaniam S, et al. Extended-release injectable naltrexone for opioid use disorder: a systematic review. *Addiction.* 2018;113(7):1188–1209.

Jones CM, Campopiano M, Baldwin G, and McCance-Katz E. National and state treatment need and capacity for opioid agonist medication-assisted treatment. *Am J Public Health.* 2015;105(8): e55–e63.

Kaufman M, Cornish F, Zimmerman RS, et al. Health behavior change models for HIV prevention and AIDS care: practical recommendations for a multi-level approach. *J AIDS.* 2014;66 (Suppl 3): s250–S258.

Kaushic C, Ferreira VH, Kafka JK, et al. HIV infection in the female genital tract: discrete influence of the local mucosal microenvironment. *Am J Reprod Immunol.* 2010;63(6):566–575.

Kennedy MC, Karamouzian M, Kerr T. Public health and public order outcomes associated with supervised drug consumption facilities: a systematic review. *Curr HIV/AIDS Rep.* 2017;14(5):161–183.

Kleinman SH, Lelie N, Busch MP. Infectivity of human immunodeficiency virus-1, hepatitis C virus, and hepatitis B virus and risk of transmission by transfusion. *Transfusion.* 2009;49(11):2454–2489.

Knox DC, Anderson PL et al. Multidrug-resistant HIV-1 infection despite preexposure prophylaxis. *N Engl J Med.* 2017;376:501–502 doi: 10.1056/NEJMc1611639.

Kuhar DT, Henderson DK, Struble KA et al. Updated USPHS guidelines for the management of occupational exposures to human immunodeficiency virus and recommendations for post-exposure prophylaxis. *Infect Control Hosp Epidemiol.* September 2013;34(9):875–892.

Kumar PC, McNeely J, Latkin CA. "It's not what you know but who you know": role of social capital in predicting risky injection drug use behavior in a sample of people who inject drugs in Baltimore City. *J Subst Use.* 2016;21(6):620–626.

Kuo I, Agopian A, Opoku J, et al. Assessing PrEP needs among heterosexuals and people who inject drugs, Washington, DC. In: *Program and Abstracts of the 2018 Conference on Retroviruses and Opportunistic Infections*; March 4–7, 2018; Boston, Massachusetts. Abstract 1030.

Landovitz R, Li S, Grinsztejn B, et al. Safety, tolerability and pharmacokinetics of long-acting injectable cabotegravir in low-risk HIV-uninfected women and men: HPTN 077. In: *Program and Abstracts of the 9th International AIDS Society Conference on HIV Science*, July 23–26, 2017; Paris, France. Abstract TUAC0106LB.

Latkin CA, Davey-Rothwell MA, Knowlton AR, et al. Social network approaches to recruitment, HIV prevention, medical care, and medication adherence. *J AIDS.* 2013;63 (Suppl 1):s54–S58.

Latkin C, Donnell D, Metzger D, et al. The efficacy of a network intervention to reduce HIV risk behaviors among drug users and risk partners in Chiang Mai, Thailand and Philadelphia, US. *Soc Sci Med.* 2009;68(4):740–748.

Lehman DA, Baeten JM, McCoy CO, et al. Risk of drug resistance among persons acquiring HIV within a randomized clinical trial of single- or dual-agent prophylaxis. *J Infect Dis.* 2015;211:1211–1218.

Lourenco L, Colley G, Nosyk B, et al.;STOP HIV/AIDS Study Group. High levels of heterogeneity in the HIV cascade of care across different population subgroups in British Columbia, Canada. *PLoS One.* 2014;9(12): e115277.

Low AJ, Mburu G, Welton NJ, et al. Impact of opioid substitution therapy on antiretroviral therapy outcomes: a systematic review and meta-analysis. *Clin Infect Dis.* 2016;63(8):1094–1104.

Lunding S, Katzenstein TL, Kronborg G, et al. The Danish PEP Registry: experience with the use of post-exposure prophylaxis following blood exposure to HIV from 1999–2012. *Infect Dis (Lond).* November 3, 2015:1–6. [Epub ahead of print].

MacArthur GJ, Minozzi S, Martin N, et al. Opiate substitution treatment and HIV transmission in people who inject drugs: systematic review and meta-analysis. *BMJ.* 2012;345: e5945.

MacArthur GJ, van Velzen E, Palmateer N, et al. Interventions to prevent HIV and hepatitis C in people who inject drugs: a review of reviews to assess evidence of effectiveness. *Int J Drug Policy.* 2014;25(1):34–52.

Mahajan AP, Sayles JN, Patel VA, et al. Stigma in the HIV/AIDS epidemic: a review of the literature and recommendations for the way forward. *AIDS.* 2008;22(Suppl 2):s67–S79.

Mannheimer S, Hirsch-Moverman Y, Loquere A, et al. HPTN 067 ADPAT study: a comparison of daily and intermittent Pre-exposure prophylaxis (PrEP) for HIV prevention in men who have sex with men and transgender women in New York City. In: *8th IAS Conference on HIV Pathogenesis, Treatment, and Prevention.* July 19–22, 2015; Vancouver, Canada. Abstract MOAAC0305LB.

Markowtiz M, Frank I, Grant RM et al. Safety and tolerability of long-acting cabotegravir injections in HIV-uninfected men (ECLAIR): a multicentre, double-blind, randomised, placebo-controlled, phase 2a trial. *Lancet HIV.* August 2017;4(8):e331–e340. doi: 10.1016/S2352-3018(17)30068-1. Epub May 22, 2017.

Marks G, Crepaz N, Senterfitt JW, et al. Meta-analysis of high-risk sexual behavior in persons aware and unaware they are infected with HIV in the United States: implications for HIV prevention programs. *J AIDS.* 2005;39(4):446–453.

Marrazzo JM, Gita R, Richardson BA, et al. Tenofovir-based preexposure prophylaxis for HIV infection among African women. *N Engl J Med.* 2015;372:509–518.

Mayer KH, Grasso C, Levine K, et al. Increasing PrEP uptake, persistent disparities in at-risk patients in a Boston Center. In: *Program and Abstracts of the 2018 Conference on Retroviruses and Opportunistic Infections*, March 4–7, 2018; Boston, Massachusetts. Abstract 1014.

Mayer KH, Venkatesh KK. Interactions of HIV and other sexually transmitted diseases, and genital tract inflammation facilitating local pathogen transmission and acquisition. *Am J Reprod Immunol.* 2011;65:308–316.

McCormack S, Dunn DT, Desai M, et al. Pre-exposure prophylaxis to prevent the acquisition of HIV-1 infection (PROUD): effectiveness results from the pilot phase of a pragmatic open-label randomised trial. *Lancet.* September 9, 2015;pii: s0140–6736(15)00056-2. doi: 10.1016/S0140-6736(15)00056-2.

Medley A, Kennedy C, O'Reilly K, et al. Effectiveness of peer education interventions for HIV prevention in developing countries: a systematic review and meta-analysis. *AIDS Educ Prev.* 2009;21(3):181–206.

Metzger DS, Zhang Y. Drug treatment as HIV prevention: expanding treatment options. *Curr HIV/AIDS Rep.* 2010;7(4):220–225.

Molina JM, Capitant C, Charreau I, et al. On demand PrEP with oral TDF/FTC in MSM: results of the ANRS Ipergay trial. *N Engl J Med.* 2015;373:2237–2246.

Molina JM, Ghosn J, Béniguel L, et al. Incidence of HIV-infection in the ANRS Prevenir study in Paris region with daily or on-demand PrEP with TDF/FTC. In: *Program and Abstracts of the 22nd International AIDS Conference*; July 23–27, 2018; Amsterdam, The Netherlands. Abstract WEAE0406LB.

Montano MA, Dombrowski JC, Barbee LA, et al. Changes in sexual behavior and STI diagnoses among MSM using PrEP in Seattle, Washington. In: *Program and Abstracts of the 2017 Conference on Retroviruses and Opportunistic Infections*, February 13–16, 2017; Seattle, Washington. Abstract 979.

Mulligan K, Glidden DV, Anderson PL, et al. Effects of emtricitabine/tenofovir on bone mineral density in HIV-negative persons in a randomized, double-blind, placebo-controlled trial. *Clin Infect Dis.* 2015;61(4):572–580.

Needle RH, Burrows D, Friedman SR, et al. Effectiveness of community-based outreach in preventing HIV/AIDS among injecting drug users. *Int J Drug Pol.* 2005;16(Suppl):s45–S57.

New York State Department of Health AIDS Institute. Substance use guidelines, 2007. Available at: https://www.hivguidelines.org/substance-use/. Accessed June 24, 2018.

New York State Department of Health AIDS Institute. PEP for Victims of Sexual Assault, October 2014. Available at: https://www.hivguidelines.org/pep-for-hiv-prevention/after-sexual-assault/. Accessed July 29, 2018.

New York State Department of Health AIDS Institute. Guidance for the use of pre-exposure prophylaxis (PrEP) to prevent HIV transmission, October 2017 revision. Available at: https://www.hivguidelines.org/prep-for-prevention/prep-to-prevent-hiv/. Accessed July 29, 2018.

New York State Department of Health AIDS Institute. HIV prophylaxis following non-occupational exposure, May 2018 revision. Available at: https://www.hivguidelines.org/pep-for-hiv-prevention/non-occupational/. Accessed July 29, 2018.

New York State Department of Health AIDS Institute. PEP for Occupational Exposure to HIV (oPEP), May 2018 revision. Available at: https://www.hivguidelines.org/pep-for-hiv-prevention/occupational/. Accessed July 29, 2018.

Otten RA, Smith DK, Adams DR, et al. Efficacy of postexposure prophylaxis after intravaginal exposure of pig-tailed macaques to a human-derived retrovirus (human immunodeficiency virus type 2). *J Virol.* 2000;74(20):9771–9775.

Panel on Antiretroviral Guidelines for Adults and Adolescents. Guidelines for the use of antiretroviral agents in HIV-1-infected adults and adolescents. Recommendations for use of antiretroviral drugs in pregnant HIV-1-infected women for maternal health and interventions to reduce perinatal HIV transmission in the United States Services. Available at: http://www.aidsinfo.nih.gov/ContentFiles/AdultandAdolescentGL.pdf. Accessed May 22, 2018.

Panel on Treatment of Pregnant Women with HIV Infection and Prevention of Perinatal Transmission. Recommendations for Use of Antiretroviral Drugs in Transmission in the United States. Available at: http://aidsinfo.nih.gov/contentfiles/lvguidelines/ PerinatalGL.pdf. Accessed May 22, 2018.

Perlman D, Jordan AE. The syndemic of opioid misuse, overdose, HCV, and HIV: structural-level causes and interventions. *Current HIV/AIDS Reports.* 2018;15:96–112.

Pettifor A, Bekker L-G, Hosek S, et al. Preventing HIV among young people: research priorities for the future. *J AIDS.* 2013;63(Suppl 2):s155–S160.

Pitisuttithum P, Gilbert P, Gurwith M, et al. Randomized, double-blind, placebo-controlled efficacy trial of a bivalent recombinant glycoprotein 120 HIV-1 vaccine among injection drug users in Bangkok, Thailand. *J Infect Dis.* 2006;194:1661–1671.

Prathela P, Braunstein SL, Blank S, et al. The high risk of an HIV diagnosis following a diagnosis of syphilis: a population-level analysis of New York City men. *Clin Infect Dis.* 2015;61(2):281–287.

Protogerou C, Johnson BT. Factors underlying the success of behavioral HIV-prevention interventions for adolescents: a meta-review. *AIDS Behav.* 2014;18(10):1847–1863.

Reback CJ, Fletcher JB. HIV prevalence, substance use, and sexual risk behaviors among transgender women recruited through outreach. *AIDS Behav.* 2014;18(7):1359–1367.

Rees H, Delany-Moretlwe SA, Lombard C, et al. FACTS 001 phase III trial of pericoital tenofovir 1% gel for HIV prevention in women. In: *Program and Abstracts of the 2015 Conference on Retroviruses and Opportunistic Infections*, February 2015; Seattle, Washington. Abstract 26LB.

Rendina HJ, Parsons JT. Factors associated with the perceived accuracy of the Undetectable = Untransmittable slogan among men who have sex with men: implications for messaging scale-up and implementation. *J Int AIDS Soc.* 2018;21(1). doi: 10.1002/jia2.25055

Rerks-Ngarm S, Pitisuttithum P, Nitayaphan S, et al. Vaccination with ALVAC and AIDSVAX to prevent HIV-1 infection in Thailand. *N Engl J Med.* 2009;361:2209–2220.

Rich KM, Bia J, Altice FL, et al. Integrated models of care for individuals with opioid use disorder: how do we prevent HIV and HCV? *Curr HIV/AIDS Rep.* 2018;15(3): 266–275.

Rothman F, Rudnick D, Slifer M, et al. Co-located substance use treatment and HIV prevention and primary care services, New York State, 1990–2002: a model for effective service delivery to a high-risk population. *J Urban Health*. 2007;84(2):226–242.

Rubens M, Ramamoorthy V, Saxena A, et al. HIV vaccine: recent advances, current roadblocks, and future directions. *J Immunol Res*. 2015. Epub October 22, 2015.

Saag MS, Benson CA, Gandhi RT, et al. Antiretroviral drugs for treatment and prevention of HIV infection in adults: 2018 recommendations of the International Antiviral Society–USA Panel. *JAMA*. 2018;320(4):379–396. doi: 10.1001/jama.2018.8431.

Saitz R. Screening and brief intervention for unhealthy drug use: little or no efficacy. *Front Psychiatry*. 2014;5:121.

Shih CC, Kaneshima H, Rabin L, et al. Post exposure prophylaxis with zidovudine suppresses human immunodeficiency virus type 1 infection in SCID-hu mice in a time-dependent manner. *J Infect Dis*. 1991;163(3):625–627.

Shoptaw S, Reback CJ. Associations between methamphetamine use and HIV among men who have sex with men: a model for guiding public policy. *J Urban Health*. 2006;83(6):1151–1157.

Shubert G; for the National Minority AIDS Council and Housing Works. Mass incarceration, housing instability, and HIV/AIDS: research findings and policy recommendations. February 2013.

Siegfried N, Muller M, Deeks JJ, et al. Male circumcision for prevention of heterosexual acquisition of HIV in men. *Cochrane Database Syst Rev*. 2009;2:CD003362. doi: 10.1002/14651858.CD003362.pub2

Sikkema KJ, Watt MH, Drabkin AS, et al. Mental health treatment to reduce HIV transmission risk behavior: a positive prevention model. *AIDS Behav*. 2010;14(2):252–262.

Smith DK, Herbst JH, Zhang XJ, et al. Condom effectiveness for HIV prevention by consistency of use among men who have sex with men (MSM) in the US. *J AIDS*. 2015;68(3):337–344.

Smith LR, Strathdee SA, Metzger D, and Latkin C. Evaluating network-level predictors of behavior change among injection networks enrolled in the HPTN 037 randomized controlled trial. *Drug Alcohol Dep*. 2017;175:164–170.

Solomon MM, Lama JR, Glidden DV, et al. Change in renal function associated with oral FTC/TDF use for HIV pre-exposure prophylaxis. *AIDS*. 2014;28:851–859.

Solomon MM, Schechter M, Liu AY, et al. The safety of tenofovir–emtricitabine for HIV pre-exposure prophylaxis (PrEP) in individuals with active hepatitis B. *J AIDS*. 2016;71(3):281–286. doi: 10.1097/QAI.0000000000000857.

Strathdee SA, Beyrer C. Threading the needle: how to stop the HIV outbreak in rural Indiana. *N Engl J Med*. 2015;373:397–399.

Strathdee SA, Shoptaw S, Dyer TP, et al.; Substance Use Scientific Committee of the HIV Prevention Trials Network. Towards combination HIV prevention for injection drug users: addressing addictophobia, apathy and inattention. *Curr Opin HIV AIDS*. 2012;7(4):320–325.

Substance Abuse and Mental Health Services Administration (SAMHSA). *White Paper on Screening, Brief Intervention and Referral to Treatment (SBIRT) in Behavioral Healthcare–2011*. Rockville, MD: SAMHSA; 2011.

Substance Abuse and Mental Health Services Administration (SAMHSA). *National Survey of Substance Abuse Treatment Services (N-SSATS): 2016. Data on Substance Abuse Treatment Facilities*. BHSIS Series S-93, HHS Publication No. (SMA) 17-5039. Rockville, MD: SAMHSA; 2017.

Thigpen MC, Kebaabetswe PM, Paxton LA, et al. Antiretroviral prophylaxis for heterosexual HIV transmission in Botswana. *N Engl J Med*. 2012;367:423–434.

Tieu HV, Rolland M, Hammer SM, et al. Translational research insights from completed HIV vaccine efficacy trials. *J AIDS*. 2013;63:S150–S154.

Thompson KA, Hughes JP, Baeten J, et al. Female HIV acquisition per sex act is elevated in late pregnancy and postpartum. In: *Papers and Abstracts of 2018 Conference on Retroviruses and Opportunistic Infections*, March 4–7, 2018; Boston, Massachusetts. Abstract 45.

US Department of Health and Human Services (USDHHS), Office of the Surgeon General, *Facing Addiction in America: The Surgeon General's Report on Alcohol, Drugs, and Health*. Washington, DC: HHS; November 2016.

US Public Health Service. Preexposure prophylaxis for the prevention of HIV infection in the United States–2017 Update: a clinical practice guideline. Available at: https://www.cdc.gov/hiv/pdf/risk/prep/cdc-hiv-prep-guidelines-2017.pdf. Accessed July 29, 2018.

Valdiserri RO. HIV/AIDS stigma: an impediment to public health. *Am J Public Health*. 2002;92(3):341–342.

Valera P, Chang Y, Lian Z. HIV risk inside US prisons: a systematic review of risk reduction interventions conducted in US prisons. *AIDS Care*. 2017;29(8):943–952.

Vallabhaneni S, Li X, Vittinghoff E, et. al. Seroadaptive practices: association with HIV acquisition among HIV-negative men who have sex with men. *PLoS One*. 2012;7(10):e45718.

Van Damme L, Corneli A, Ahmed K, et al. Preexposure prophylaxis for HIV infection among African women. *N Engl J Med*. 2012;367:411–422.

Vlahov D, Robertson AM, Strathdee SA. Prevention of HIV infection among injection drug users in resource-limited settings. *Clin Infect Dis*. 2010;50(Suppl 3):s114–S121.

Volk JE, Marcus JL, Phengrasamy T, et al. No new HIV infections with increasing use of HIV preexposure prophylaxis in a clinical practice setting. *Clin Infect Dis*. 2015;61(10):1601–1603.

Ward H, Rönn M. The contribution of STIs to the sexual transmission of HIV. *Curr Opin HIV AIDS*. 2010;5(4):305–310.

Wei C, Fisher Raymond H, Guadamuz TE, et al. Racial/ethnic differences in seroadaptive and serodisclosure behaviors among men who have sex with men. *AIDS Behav*. 2011;15(1):22–29.

Weiss HA, Hankins CA, Dickson K. Male circumcision and risk of HIV infection in women: a systematic review and meta-analysis. *Lancet Infect Dis*. 2009;9:669–677.

Weller S, Davis K. Condom effectiveness in reducing heterosexual HIV transmission. *Cochrane Database Syst Rev*. 2002;1:CD003255.

Wirtz AL, Yeh PT, Flath N, et al. HIV and viral hepatitis among imprisoned key populations. *Epidemiologic Rev*. 2018;40(1):12–26.

Wiysonge CS, Kongnyuy EJ, Shey M, et al. Male circumcision for prevention of homosexual acquisition of HIV in men. *Cochrane Database Syst Rev*. 2011;6.CD007496. doi: 10.1002/14651858.CD007496.pub2

Wodak A, Cooney, A. *Effectiveness of Sterile Needle and Syringe Programming in Reducing HIV/AIDS Among Injecting Drug Users*. Geneva: World Health Organization Document Production Services; 2004.

World Health Organization. Global summary of the AIDS epidemic, 2014. Available at: http://www.who.int/hiv/data/en. Accessed November 29, 2015.

World Health Organization. Guideline on when to start antiretroviral therapy and on pre-exposure prophylaxis for HIV, 2015. Available at: http://www.who.int/hiv/pub/guidelines/earlyrelease-arv/en. Accessed November 8, 2015.

Young JD, Patel M, Badowski M, et al. Improved virologic suppression with HIV subspecialty care in a large prison system using telemedicine: an observational study with historical controls. *Clin Infect Dis*. 2014;59(1):123–126.

Young TN, Arens FJ, Kennedy GE, et al. Antiretroviral post-exposure prophylaxis (PEP) for occupational HIV exposure. *Cochrane Database Sys Rev*. 2007;1:CD002835.

Zanakis SH, Alvarez C, Li V. Socio-economic determinants of HIV/AIDS pandemic and nations efficiencies. *Eur J Operational Res*. 2007;176:1811–1838.

Zash R, Holmes L, Makhema J, et al. Surveillance for neural tube defects following antiretroviral exposure from conception, the Tsepamo study (Botswana). In: *Program and Abstracts of the 22nd International AIDS Conference*, July 23–27, 2018; Amsterdam, The Netherlands. Session TUSY15.

Zou S, Dorsey KA, Notari EP, et al. Prevalence, incidence, and residual risk of human immunodeficiency virus and hepatitis C virus infections among United States blood donors since the introduction of nucleic acid testing. *Transfusion*. 2010;50(7):1495–1504.

5.

IMMUNOLOGY

Dennis J. Hartigan-O'Connor and Christian Brander

CHAPTER GOALS

Upon completion of this chapter, the reader should be able to

- Describe the processes contributing to CD4⁺ T cell decline and immune activation in untreated HIV infection

- Demonstrate knowledge of the effects of HIV on immune cells other than CD4⁺ T cells

- Demonstrate knowledge of the mechanisms that contribute to T cell activation and chronic inflammation in HIV disease

- Demonstrate knowledge of the effect of antiretroviral therapy (ART) on immune function

- Demonstrate knowledge of the leading hypotheses explaining pathogenesis of immune reconstitution inflammatory syndrome (IRIS), including antigen persistence and immune dysregulation

- Demonstrate knowledge of how some individuals maintain durable control of HIV in the absence of therapy

---

MECHANISMS OF CD4⁺ T CELL DECLINE

LEARNING OBJECTIVE

Describe the processes contributing to CD4⁺ T cell decline and immune activation in untreated HIV infection.

KEY POINTS

- Cytopathic infection alone is insufficient to explain CD4⁺ T cell loss in HIV infection.

- Chronic inflammation is strongly associated with CD4⁺ T cell loss in pathogenic lentiviral infection such as HIV, but it is not seen in nonpathogenic infections.

- Translocation of microbial constituents and lymph node scarring have been recognized as likely contributors to CD4⁺ T cell decline.

The prototypic outcomes associated with HIV infection are progressive CD4⁺ T cell decline, consequent immunodeficiency, and chronic inflammation. In untreated disease, circulating memory CD4⁺ T cells, some of which are infected, are both dividing and dying at an accelerated rate (Hellerstein, 1999). In addition, CD4⁺ T cells that reside in the gastrointestinal mucosa are important early targets of infection that are decimated early in disease (Guadalupe, 2003; Heise, 1994; Veazey, 1998). Although direct cytopathic infection contributes to CD4⁺ T cell loss, many *uninfected* CD4⁺ T cells are dividing and dying in HIV disease; thus, other mechanisms must be invoked to fully explain CD4⁺ T cell decline. The death of infected cells is likely due to exposure to Tat, Gp120, or other viral proteins (some of which can induce apoptosis) and/or adaptive immune clearance of HIV-infected cells (Lenardo, 2002). HIV can also impair CD4⁺ T cell regeneration by destroying the immunologic niches that are required for T cell homeostasis, by depleting essential hematopoietic progenitor cells, and by inhibiting the regenerative process through production of immune mediators (Douek, 2003; Grossman, 2002).

Chronic inflammation and immune activation have also been shown to be associated with CD4⁺ T cell decline. It has been shown, for example, that pathogenic lentiviral infections (such as HIV infection) and nonpathogenic infections (such as lentiviral infections of many non-human primates) are each associated with robust virus replication. Immune activation, however, is observed only in the pathogenic models, suggesting that this mechanism is directly responsible for disease progression (Silvestri, 2003).

Chronic inflammation and CD4⁺ T cell decline have recently been linked in a self-perpetuating cycle that may underlie progressive T cell loss in HIV infection. It has been shown that CD4⁺ Th17 cells are among those cells lost from the gastrointestinal tract in early simian immunodeficiency virus (SIV) and HIV infection (Brenchley, 2008; Favre, 2009). Th17 cells are important for maintenance of the "mucosal barrier" between gut luminal contents and circulation. When these cells are depleted, microbial constituents and even whole microbes can migrate from the gut into circulation (Brenchley, 2006; Raffatellu, 2008). These pro-inflammatory microbial products vigorously activate the immune system, resulting in activation-induced cell death and/or altered homeostasis. This cycle is initiated early in SIV infection (Hirao,

2014) and appears to be an important driver of disease progression as the presence of sufficient Th17 cells before infection can limit viral replication (Hartigan-O'Connor, 2012).

Another increasingly recognized self-perpetuating cycle pertains to the impact of HIV-associated inflammation on lymphoid structures. The inflammatory response generated by HIV results in upregulation of certain countervailing "regulatory" responses, including production of transforming growth factor-β (TGF-β), which stimulates collagen deposition (Estes, 2008). The scarring of the lymph nodes, which appears to be irreversible, prevents normal T cell homeostasis and antigen presentation. The immunodeficiency that results can lead to an excess burden of a variety of microbes, including cytomegalovirus (CMV), gut microbes, and perhaps HIV itself. This microbial burden continues to add to the cycle by causing even more inflammation and scarring (Arthos, 2008).

EFFECTS OF HIV ON THE ENTIRE IMMUNE SYSTEM

LEARNING OBJECTIVE

Demonstrate knowledge of the effects of HIV on immune cells other than CD4+ T cells.

KEY POINTS

- HIV has broad effects on many immune cell types, including many cells that are not infected by the virus.

- HIV disrupts the entire lymphoid system through its effects on secondary lymphoid organs such as lymph nodes.

Although HIV is tropic for CD4+ T cells, it is clear that many manifestations of HIV infection result from direct or indirect effects on other immune cell types. One example is the high death rate and turnover of CD8+ T cells, as well as the numerical depletion of naïve CD8+ T cells even in the asymptomatic phase of infection (Roederer, 1995). HIV also has direct or indirect effects on antigen-presenting cells, B cells, and natural killer (NK) cells (Hamada, 2009; Kader, 2009; Klatt, 2010; Nigam, 2011; Zhou, 2015).

One factor that likely mediates some of the effects of HIV on the broader immune system, particularly in late disease, is the destruction of lymphoid tissue architecture. In early disease, as antigen-presenting cells are activated and initiate immune responses within lymph nodes, CD4+ T cells are retained within the nodes while activated CD8+ T cells migrate into circulation, a process that contributes to CD8+ lymphocytosis and inversion of the CD4:CD8 ratio (Bishop, 1990; Bujdoso, 1989). In later disease, there is structural damage to primary and secondary lymphoid organs resulting from fibrotic scarring (Estes, 2008). Naïve T cells, including CD8+ T cells, require access to lymph node paracortical T cell zones for access to critical homeostatic signals and growth factors, including

interleukin-7 (IL-7) (Link, 2007). Presumably, therefore, lymphoid tissue scarring is one factor that contributes to failure to fully reconstitute CD4+ and CD8+ T cells despite complete virologic suppression.

HIV-1 can also infect myeloid cells including macrophages and dendritic cells, both of which can express C-C chemokine receptor type 5 (CCR5). However, myeloid cells are relatively resistant to *productive* infection with HIV, as compared to CD4+ T cells (Coleman, 2009). The relative inability of SIV and HIV-2 to cause productive infection of these cells is mediated by the cellular restriction factor SAMHD1 (Hrecka, 2011; Laguette, 2011). The viral accessory protein Vpx blocks this cellular response, thus allowing infection. As HIV-1 lacks this accessory protein, it remains unclear how this virus might productively infect macrophages (Hrecka, 2011; Laguette, 2011; Manel, 2010). Surprisingly, it is now appreciated that macrophages and memory CD4+ T cells accumulate in adipose tissue during HIV infection (Damouche, 2017; Hsu, 2017; Koethe, 2018). Replicating virus can be recovered from these adipose tissue-resident cells, indicating that adipose tissue is a reservoir, though probably a minor one compared to lymphoid tissue. Antiviral effector cells, such as CD8+ T cells and NK cells, are also present in large numbers (Couturier, 2015, 2016; Damouche, 2015; Dupin, 2002).

Natural Killer T (NKT) cells are also rapidly and selectively depleted in HIV infection (Sandberg, 2002; van der Vliet, 2002). NKT cells may be broadly divided into those that are CD4+ and those that are CD4−, with the former population secreting both Th1 and Th2 cytokines and likely providing B cell help or carrying out immunoregulatory functions. The latter produces mainly Th1 cytokines and has stronger cytolytic activity. The CD4+ NKT population is depleted more rapidly in HIV infection than is the CD4− population but is restored more slowly after initiating highly active antiretroviral therapy (HAART) (Li, 2008). HIV also interferes with the activation of NKT cells by downregulating expression of CD1d (an MHC-related protein that presents glycolipid antigens to NKT cells) on antigen-presenting cells (Hage, 2005). This downregulation appears to be mediated mainly by the viral Nef protein (Cho, 2005).

There is continued interest in the effect of HIV and other agents of chronic infection on NK cells, particularly subsets with expanded functional capacity including "memory" NK cells (Hwang, 2012; Lee, 2015; Lopez-Verges, 2011; Sun, 2009; Zhang, 2013). Such cells are considered to be innate cells with adaptive features, including more robust and rapid responses to pathogen encounter (Sun, 2009). Limited evidence has been presented so far demonstrating that HIV infection drives expansion of memory NK cells (Zhou, 2015). However, NK cells from SIV-infected macaques or from monkeys vaccinated with an Ad26-vectored candidate SIV/HIV vaccine can lyse targets pulsed with SIV peptides in an antigen- and NKG2-dependent fashion (Reeves, 2015). CMV infection, which is common in HIV-positive people, is thought to be the most important driver of memory NK cell expansion (Brodin, 2015; Lopez-Verges, 2011; Zhang, 2013). People coinfected with HIV and CMV may therefore present unique immunologic features.

MECHANISMS OF CHRONIC INFLAMMATION IN HIV DISEASE

LEARNING OBJECTIVE

Demonstrate knowledge of the mechanisms that contribute to T cell activation and chronic inflammation in HIV disease.

KEY POINTS

- Innate immune responses that result in production of type I interferons are important drivers of inflammation in early disease.

- Early depletion of CD4$^+$ T cells from the gastrointestinal mucosa likely contributes to chronic, persistent immune activation.

- CMV and other chronic infections are important contributors to T cell activation in coinfected individuals.

It was first demonstrated more than 10 years ago that T cell activation was associated with shorter survival in advanced HIV disease (Giorgi, 1999). One might imagine that chronic T cell activation is simply the inevitable consequence of ongoing viral replication and that more T cell activation is indicative of more active disease. However, it is clear from studies of nonpathogenic lentiviral infections that chronic, high-level virus replication can occur without eliciting massive immune activation (Silvestri, 2003); indeed, in the natural hosts of SIV, the rapid reduction in immune activation appears to protect against subsequent CD4$^+$ T cell decline and disease progression. The mechanisms by which HIV-1 causes a sustained and partially irreversible increase in immune activation remains a strong focus of ongoing research.

The virion itself elicits innate immune responses via activation of toll-like receptors 7, 8, and 9 within antigen-presenting cells. Toll-like receptor (TLR) engagement results in production of type I interferons, including IFN-α. Indeed, a spike of IFN-α production is observed in acute HIV and SIV infection (Favre, 2009; Stacey, 2009), which doubtless shapes the ensuing adaptive immune responses. Binding of virion components to signaling molecules such as CD4 and CCR5 may also stimulate cells directly, and viral proteins such as Tat and Nef have been shown to have pro-inflammatory effects (Decrion, 2005). After the first 2 weeks of infection, the adaptive immune response to HIV proteins contributes to T cell activation, although many of these activated T cells are specific for CMV and other chronic pathogens, rather than HIV (Doisne, 2004; Papagno, 2004). Less appreciated is the fact that host genetics, in addition to controlling the adaptive immune response, may modulate the intensity of inflammation induced by these pro-inflammatory influences. Subjects in a Zimbabwean cohort having an IL-10 promoter mutation associated with lower inflammation experienced reductions in both mortality and CD4$^+$ T cell loss (Erikstrup, 2007). Finally, lymphopenia itself can lead to T cell activation. For example, resting T cells spontaneously become activated and proliferate when introduced into T cell deficient hosts (Srinivasula, 2011; Surh, 2008). Thus, the progressive loss of CD4$^+$ T cells can be both a consequence and cause of immune activation (Jones, 2009; King, 2004).

In addition to these general effects of lymphocyte depletion, the field has appreciated the implications of early and profound lymphocyte depletion from the gastrointestinal mucosa (Heise, 1994; Veazey, 1998). Among the lymphocytes lost in early infection are CD4$^+$ Th17 cells, which have an important structural role in maintenance of the tight junctions between intestinal epithelial cells (Brenchley, 2008; Favre, 2009). Loss of these cells contributes to a breakdown in the physical barrier separating the gut lumen from general circulation, which allows bioactive microbial products such as lipopolysaccharides (LPS) to reach the blood (Brenchley, 2006), while maintenance of sufficient Th17 cells is associated with reduced viral replication (Hartigan-O'Connor, 2012). Mucosal barrier breakdown and pro-inflammatory processes such as tryptophan catabolism, in turn, are associated with disturbance ("dysbiosis") of the gut-resident microbial community (Vujkovic-Cvijin, 2013). Persistent microbial dysbiosis may help to drive further immune dysregulation and inflammation.

Occult and symptomatic opportunistic infections also contribute to chronic inflammation in HIV disease. In particular, the prevalence of CMV infection among some populations of HIV-infected persons is at least 90% (Berry, 1988; Lang, 1989). Furthermore, CMV infection has been associated with T cell activation in HIV-uninfected people (Lenkei, 1995). Indeed, CMV-specific T cells account for nearly 10% of the circulating memory T cell pool in CMV-seropositive individuals, suggesting that CMV replication can have a major influence on the immune system even in healthy individuals who are not immunocompromised (Sylwester, 2005). CMV appears to have an even stronger effect on T cell remodeling in untreated and treated HIV infection (Naeger, 2010). A pilot study tested the possibility that chronic immune activation in HIV disease could be reduced by treatment of CMV infection, randomizing 30 individuals on antiretroviral therapy (ART) to treatment with valganciclovir or placebo (Hunt, 2011). A significant 20% reduction in the percentage of activated CD8+ T cells was demonstrated in the valganciclovir group, suggesting that CMV infection (or infection with other valganciclovir-sensitive herpesviruses) is a significant contributor to T cell activation in treated HIV- and CMV-coinfected individuals.

IMMUNOLOGIC EFFECTS OF ANTIRETROVIRAL THERAPY AND ROLE OF PERSISTENT IMMUNE DYSFUNCTION ON CLINICAL OUTCOMES IN PATIENTS ON ART

LEARNING OBJECTIVE

Demonstrate knowledge of the effect of ART on immune function.

ART does not fully restore immune function in many patients despite long-term viral suppression. Suboptimal CD4+ T cell gains and chronic inflammation during treatment have both been implicated in the continued risk for HIV-related complications and subsequent disease progression.

KEY POINTS

- A small but clinically important subset of treated patients exhibit suboptimal CD4+ T cell gains.

- Chronic inflammation, lymphoid fibrosis, hematopoietic progenitor cell loss, and thymic dysfunction all likely contribute to failure of normal T cell homeostasis.

- Chronic inflammation during treated disease has been associated with subsequent disease progression.

Combination ART results in complete or near-complete suppression of HIV replication. As a consequence, many of the factors that cause progressive immunodeficiency are reversed. Prevention of continued CD4+ T cell destruction (via both direct and indirect effects) and homeostatic regeneration results in eventual restoration of CD4+ T cell numbers in blood and tissues. The increase in peripheral CD4+ T cell counts during therapy appears to be biphasic (Pakker, 1998). A robust increase of approximately 50–100 cells/mm³ is often observed in the first several weeks. Because memory cells account for most of the increase, it has long been assumed that the redistribution of cells from tissues to the periphery accounts for this rapid increase. After this early phase, CD4+ T cell counts increase slowly (at a rate of approximately 50 cells/mm³/year) until they achieve a normal range (i.e., >500 cells/mm³; Mocroft, 2007). The augmented CD4+ T cell population includes naïve cells and hence is thought to reflect true immune reconstitution. Although less well-studied, CD4+ T cell gains also occur in tissues during effective therapy.

Although the majority of HIV-infected persons exhibits some degree of immune reconstitution during therapy, the outcome is quite variable. A small but clinically important subset of patients fails to achieve normal peripheral CD4+ T cell counts even after many years of therapy. (Mutoh, 2018) These so-called immunologic failures or "nonresponders" remain at relatively high risk for cancer, heart disease, liver failure, and other non-AIDS-defining complications, but they usually achieve sufficient restoration of immune function to prevent most AIDS-related complications. Patients who are older and who start therapy during late disease are at higher risk of exhibiting suboptimal gains during therapy. In one study, approximately 40% of patients who delayed therapy until their CD4+ T cell count was less than 200 cells/mm³ failed to achieve a normal CD4+ T cell count after several years of viral suppression (Kelley, 2009). In a recent study from Japan, 26% of patients did not attain normalization of CD4 counts or CD4% after more than 4 years of viral suppression (Mutoh, 2018). In this study, 48% of patients who started ART with a CD4 count of less than 100 did not achieve normalization of CD4 counts. Other factors that have been associated with blunted CD4+ T cell

gains include hepatitis C virus coinfection, high levels of T cell activation, the use of certain nucleoside analogues (particularly the combination of stavudine and didanosine), and the use of efavirenz-based regimens (as compared to integrase and protease inhibitor-based ART regimens).

Given its clinical importance, there is intense interest in determining the pathogenesis of immunologic failure (defined variably). In untreated disease, HIV-mediated destruction of hematopoietic stem cells, thymic tissue, lymphoid tissue, and central memory cells all contribute to progressive CD4+ T cell loss. Treatment-mediated suppression of HIV replication partially restores these factors. Persistent lymph node fibrosis, thymic dysfunction, and loss of cells with stem-like properties have all been associated with CD4+ T cell regeneration failure and suboptimal gains during therapy (McCune, 2001; Sauce, 2011; Schacker, 2002; Teixeira, 2001). More recently it has been shown that immunologic nonresponders accumulate CD56bright NK cells with cytotoxicity against autologous activated CD4+ T cells (Giuliani, 2017). Those data suggest that autoreactive NK cells, possibly linked to decreased homeostatic control by a depleted T-reg compartment, contribute to poor immune reconstitution.

Untreated HIV infection is associated with heightened levels of immune activation. Long-term suppression of HIV replication dramatically reduces most measures of immune activation, but this effect is often incomplete as inflammatory markers typically remain higher in treated HIV-infected adults than in age-matched uninfected adults (Neuhaus, 2010). Persistent inflammation during therapy is associated with excess risk of non-AIDS complications, including heart disease, cancer, liver disease, kidney disease, bone disease, and neurologic complications (Deeks, 2011; Kuller, 2008; Phillips, 2008). Persistent CMV replication may be an important cause of continued inflammation while on therapy as higher anti-CMV IgG antibody levels are associated with increased prevalence of carotid artery lesions among HIV-infected women who achieve HIV suppression on ART but not among viremic or untreated women (Parrinello, 2012).

Persistent and possibly irreversible damage to the infrastructure that supports T cell homeostasis may account for much of the persistent immunodeficiency and inflammation often observed during therapy. Theoretically, collagen deposition and scarring of the lymphoid system during untreated disease results in a loss of the regulatory pathways (particularly those involving IL-7) that control T cell regeneration (Zeng, 2012). This disruption results in persistently low CD4+ T cell counts and an inability to generate effective memory T cells in response to acute or chronic infections. Loss of lymphoid structures may also result in loss of immune surveillance and development of cancer, as a well as a loss of key anti-inflammatory regulatory responses and, as a result, autoimmune-related clinical syndromes. In a self-perpetuating vicious cycle that persists in absence of any HIV replication, persistent immunodeficiency results in a reduced capacity of host responses to clear pathogens. The resulting burden of these pathogens contributes to more inflammation, which in turn continues to damage the lymphoid tissues. The collective outcome is a combination of low CD4+ T cell counts and chronic inflammation. It is hoped that knowledge about these pathways will lead to novel interventions aimed at preventing or reversing this immunodeficient and pro-inflammatory environment.

PATHOGENESIS OF IMMUNE RECONSTITUTION INFLAMMATORY SYNDROMES

LEARNING OBJECTIVE

Demonstrate knowledge of the leading hypotheses explaining pathogenesis of immune reconstitution inflammatory syndrome (IRIS), including antigen persistence and immune dysregulation.

KEY POINTS

- IRIS are seen most commonly in patients initiating HAART with low CD4+ T cell counts and preexisting opportunistic infections.

- Many IRIS symptoms are localized to sites of previous infection, suggestive of the presence of persistent microbial antigen.

- Development of IRIS is associated with greater T cell activation before initiation of treatment.

A subset of AIDS patients who are immune-restored with ART develop inflammatory conditions known collectively as IRIS (Price, 2009). A meta-analysis showed that 16% of patients starting ART developed an IRIS event (Muller, 2010). Patients most likely to be affected are those initiating ART with low CD4 counts and preexisting opportunistic infections (Muller, 2010; Price, 2009). The symptoms of IRIS are often localized to sites of previous infection (Lawn, 2007), which led to the thought that IRIS is caused by adaptive immune responses to persistent pathogen-derived antigens (Muller, 2010). For example, IRIS in patients with a history of CMV retinitis can manifest as inflammation of the posterior uveal tract of the eye (Nussenblatt, 1998). The most frequent clinical manifestation of cryptococcal IRIS, by contrast, is aseptic meningitis (Boulware, 2010).

The hypothesis that an IRIS is caused by the host immune response to persistent antigen (in the form of intact organisms, dead organisms, or debris) has the appeal of simplicity, but there are surprisingly few data available to support the idea. One study demonstrated that, among patients with recent cryptococcal meningitis who were placed on ART, those developing cryptococcal IRIS had fourfold higher titers of cryptococcal antigen in serum (Boulware, 2010). In cases of *Mycobacterium tuberculosis* or *Mycobacterium avium* complex–associated IRIS, patients normally convert to skin test positivity, suggesting that, at a minimum, the disease is mediated by pathogen-specific CD4+ T cells (French, 2004).

In the case of CMV immune recovery uveitis, however, the presence of CMV antigens has not been demonstrated in affected patients.

A number of studies have suggested that the pre-therapy inflammatory environment predicts IRIS. For example, Antonelli and colleagues showed that individuals who presented with an IRIS episode had a higher proportion of activated CD4+ T cells before starting ART compared with those who did not develop IRIS (Antonelli, 2010). These activated T cells had a skewed Th1/Th17 cytokine profile before therapy began. Furthermore, IRIS patients displayed higher serum IFN-γ levels near the time of their IRIS events. More recently, understanding of the importance of regulatory CD4+ T cells (T-regs) in controlling immune responses to self-antigens has prompted the suggestion that failure to reconstitute these anti-inflammatory cells predisposes to IRIS (Seddiki, 2009), but data on this hypothesis have been inconsistent (Bourgarit, 2006; Hartigan-O'Connor, 2012). Other groups have argued that poorly regulated innate immune responses may be central to IRIS. Pre-therapy and early treatment-mediated changes in various nonspecific inflammatory biomarkers (including c-reactive protein [CRP], IL-6, tumor necrosis factor-α [TNF-α] and D-dimers) have been associated with increased risk of IRIS and mortality during the first several months of effective ART (Barber, 2012; Boulware, 2011).

In summary, pathogenesis of IRIS seems dependent on the presence of both lymphopenia and antigen-specific CD4+ T cells. These T cells may be responding to persistent pathogen-derived antigens, to self-antigens, or to unrelated foreign antigens. In these latter cases, the opportunistic pathogen may be seen as the trigger rather than the target of the pathogenic T cell response. Lymphopenia establishes a dysregulated environment in which either the response of the antigen-specific T cells or the effect of that response on the host is exaggerated.

MECHANISMS AND CONSEQUENCES OF VIRUS CONTROL IN "ELITE" CONTROLLERS

LEARNING OBJECTIVE

Demonstrate knowledge of how some individuals maintain durable control of HIV in the absence of therapy.

WHAT'S NEW?

Multiple mechanisms contribute to durable "elite" HIV control in untreated individuals.

KEY POINTS

- HIV-specific CD8+ T cells contribute to durable control of HIV in "elite" controllers.

- Despite the lack of readily detectable HIV RNA in plasma, "elite" controllers have higher than normal levels of immune activation, which may contribute to slow disease progression.

Approximately 1% of antiretroviral-untreated, chronically infected adults have no readily detectable HIV RNA in plasma. These individuals are generally referred to as "elite" controllers, although other terms—including "long-term nonprogressors"—have been used to define this or similar groups of individuals keeping viral replication low in the absence of ART. Given that the host mechanisms which might account for virus control in these individuals could inform both vaccine and cure research, there has been long-term interest in enumerating their mechanisms of control as well as in describing the degree to which controllers exhibit any evidence of disease progression.

Most investigators interested in determining the mechanisms of virus control in these individuals have assessed specific candidate host factors in controllers and noncontrollers. These studies have generally been cross-sectional, making it difficult to determine if a given host response is a cause or a consequence of virus control (Deeks, 2007). Some recent efforts have been made to follow individuals closely during the pre-HIV infection period, both to capture information about the earliest events after infection as well as to study dynamic changes that may be important for eventual control (Ndhlovu, 2015). Although no one study design is optimal, the collective data support a central role for potent HIV-specific CD8[+] T cells and, to a lesser degree, CD4[+] T cells in maintaining virus control. This is also supported by the fact that most genetic predictors of virus control are found on chromosome 6 in the HLA region that governs the antigenic specificity of T cells (Pereyra, 2010). Several studies in SIV-infected monkeys further support the importance of virus-specific cytotoxic T lymphocyte (CTL) responses in virus control. In the RhCMV-vectored vaccine setting, their major histocompatibility complex (MHC) class I restriction may not be universal and there may be a significant contribution of MHC class II restricted CD8[+] T cells to virus control (Hansen, 2013a, 2013b). Similarly, the role of the Th17 cell compartment in sustaining viral replication has been highlighted in monkey studies and will need to be investigated in the human HIV setting (Hartigan-O'Connor, 2012).

Other factors that have been associated with virus control include (1) strong NK cell responses (Martin, 2007; Sips, 2012), (2) prevention of apoptosis/cell death in central memory cells (van Grevenynghe, 2008), (3) intrinsic intracellular restriction to HIV replication mediated by p21 (Chen, 2011) and other as yet poorly characterized factors (O'Connell, 2011; Saez-Cirion, 2011), and (4) acquisition of a replication-deficient virus. However, care must be taken not to confuse causative, functional markers of virus control with simple correlates of controlled infection. For instance, biomarkers such as the proliferative capacity of HIV-specific T cells may be the consequence of otherwise controlled/uncontrolled HIV infection rather than its physiological cause. Longitudinal studies, capturing infected people within days of infection and following them in the absence of treatment, may

be ethically challenging but could prove highly informative in defining true mechanisms of in vivo virus control.

Given that controllers are being studied as a potential model for "functional cure," the consequences of long-term, host-mediated virus control on overall health remains of great interest (Migueles, 2010). HIV persists at very low levels in nearly all controllers and appears to be replicating (Hatano, 2009; Mens, 2010). Persistent virus production generates a sustained inflammatory environment (Hunt, 2008), which in turn might cause end-organ damage, including neurological disorders and cardiovascular disease (Hsue, 2009). In addition, potential alterations in the gut microbiota of chronically infected individuals may contribute to or be the result of ongoing viral replication, even in elite controllers, and may impact upon therapeutic vaccine outcomes (Williams, 2015). These considerations suggest that even "elite" controllers might benefit from ART. Studies addressing this hypothesis are ongoing.

REFERENCES

Antonelli LR, Mahnke Y, Hodge JN, et al. Elevated frequencies of highly activated CD4[+] T cells in HIV+ patients developing immune reconstitution inflammatory syndrome. *Blood.* 2010;116:3818–3827.

Arthos J, Cicala C, Martinelli E, et al. HIV-1 envelope protein binds to and signals through integrin alpha4beta7, the gut mucosal homing receptor for peripheral T cells. *Nat Immunol.* 2008;9:301–309.

Barber DL, Andrade BB, Sereti I, Sher A. Immune reconstitution inflammatory syndrome: the trouble with immunity when you had none. *Nat Rev Microbiol.* 2012;10(2):150–156.

Berry NJ, Burns DM, Wannamethee G, et al. Seroepidemiologic studies on the acquisition of antibodies to cytomegalovirus, herpes simplex virus, and human immunodeficiency virus among general hospital patients and those attending a clinic for sexually transmitted diseases. *J Med Virol.* 1988;24:385–393.

Bishop DK, Ferguson RM, Orosz CG. Differential distribution of antigen-specific helper T cells and cytotoxic T cells after antigenic stimulation in vivo. A functional study using limiting dilution analysis. *J Immunol.* 1990;144:1153–1160.

Boulware DR, Hullsiek KH, Puronen CE, et al. Higher levels of CRP, D-dimer, IL-6, and hyaluronic acid before initiation of antiretroviral therapy (ART) are associated with increased risk of AIDS or death. *J Infect Dis.* 2011;203(11):1637–1646.

Boulware DR, Meya DB, Bergemann TL, et al. Clinical features and serum biomarkers in HIV immune reconstitution inflammatory syndrome after cryptococcal meningitis: a prospective cohort study. *PLoS Med.* 2010;7:e1000384.

Bourgarit A, Carcelain G, Martinez V et al. Explosion of tuberculin-specific Th1-responses induces immune restoration syndrome in tuberculosis and HIV co-infected patients. *AIDS.* 2006;20:F1–F7.

Brenchley JM, Paiardini M, Knox KS, et al. Differential Th17 CD4 T cell depletion in pathogenic and nonpayhogenic lentiviral infections. *Blood.* 2008;112:2826–2835.

Brenchley JM, Price DA, Schacker TW, et al. Microbial translocation is a cause of systemic immune activation in chronic HIV infection. *Nat Med.* 2006;12:1365–1371.

Brodin P, Jojic V, Gao T. Variation in the human immune system is largely driven by non-heritable 1. influences. *Cell.* 2015;160:37–47.

Bujdoso R, Young P, Hopkins J. Non-random migration of CD4 and CD8 T cells: changes in the CD4: CD8 ratio and interleukin 2 responsiveness of efferent lymph cells following in vivo antigen challenge. *Eur J Immunol.* 1989;19:1779–1784.

Chen H, Li C, Huang, J, et al. CD4[+] T cells from elite controllers resist HIV-1 infection by selective upregulation of p21. *J Clin Invest.* 2011;121:1549–1560.

Cho S, Knox KS, Kohli LM, et al. Impaired cell surface expression of human CD1d by the formation of an HIV-1 Nef/CD1d complex. *Virology.* 2005;337:242–252.

Coleman CM, Wu L. HIV interactions with monocytes and dendritic cells: viral latency and reservoirs. *Retrovirology.* 2009;6:51.

Couturier J, Agarwal N, Nehete PN, et al. Infectious SIV resides in adipose tissue and induces metabolic defects in chronically infected rhesus macaques. *Retrovirology.* 2016;13:30.

Couturier J, Suliburk JW, Brown JM, et al. Human adipose tissue as a reservoir for memory CD4+ T cells and HIV. *AIDS.* 2015;29:667–674.

Damouche A, Lazure T, Avettand-Fenoel V. Adipose tissue is a neglected viral reservoir and an inflammatory site during chronic HIV and SIV infection. *PLoS Pathog.* 2015;11: e1005153.

Damouche A, Pourcher G, Pourcher V. High proportion of PD-1-expressing CD4(+) T cells in adipose tissue constitutes an immunomodulatory microenvironment that may support HIV persistence. *Eur J Immunol.* 2017;47:2113–2123.

Decrion AZ, Dichamp I, Varin A, Herbein G. HIV and inflammation. *Curr HIV Res.* 2005;3:243–259.

Deeks SG. HIV infection, inflammation, immunosenescence, and aging. *Annu Rev Med.* 2011;62:141–155.

Deeks SG, Walker BD. Human immunodeficiency virus controllers: mechanisms of durable virus control in the absence of antiretroviral therapy. *Immunity.* 2007;27:406–416.

Doisne JM, Urrutia A, Lacabaratz-Porret C, et al. CD8+ T cells specific for EBV, cytomegalovirus, and influenza virus are activated during primary HIV infection. *J Immunol.* 2004;173:2410–2418.

Douek DC, Picker LJ, Koup RA. T cell dynamics in HIV-1 infection. *Annu Rev Immunol.* 2003;21:265–304.

Dupin N, Buffet M, Marcelin AG, et al. HIV and antiretroviral drug distribution in plasma and fat tissue of HIV-infected patients with lipodystrophy. *AIDS.* 2002;16:2419–2424.

Erikstrup C, Kallestrup P, Zinyama-Gutsire RB, et al. Reduced mortality and CD4 cell loss among carriers of the interleukin-10-1082G allele in a Zimbabwean cohort of HIV-1-infected adults. *AIDS.* 2007;21:2283–2291.

Estes JD, Haase AT, Schacker TW. The role of collagen deposition in depleting CD4+ T cells and limiting reconstitution in HIV-1 and SIV infections through damage to the secondary lymphoid organ niche. *Semin Immunol.* 2008;20:181–186.

Favre D, Lederer S, Kanwar B, et al. Critical loss of the balance between Th17 and T regulatory cell populations in pathogenic SIV infection. *PLoS Pathol.* 2009;5: e1000295.

French MA, Price P, Stone SF. Immune restoration disease after antiretroviral therapy. *AIDS.* 2004;18:1615–1627.

Giorgi JV, Hultin LE, McKeating JA, et al. Shorter survival in advanced human immunodeficiency virus type 1 infection is more closely associated with T lymphocyte activation than with plasma virus burden or virus chemokine coreceptor usage. *J Infect Dis.* 1999;179:859–870.

Giuliani E, Vassena L, Di Cesare S, et al. NK cells of HIV-1-infected patients with poor CD4(+) T cell reconstitution despite suppressive HAART show reduced IFN-gamma production and high frequency of autoreactive CD56(bright) cells. *Immunol Lett.* 2017;190:185–193.

Grossman Z, Meier-Schellersheim M, Sousa AE, et al. CD4+ T cell depletion in HIV infection: are we closer to understanding the cause? *Nat Med.* 2002;8:319–323.

Guadalupe M, Reay E, Sankaran S, et al. Severe CD4+ T cell depletion in gut lymphoid tissue during primary human immunodeficiency virus type 1 infection and substantial delay in restoration following highly active antiretroviral therapy. *J Virol.* 2003;77:11708–11717.

Hage CA, Kohli LL, Cho S, et al. Human immunodeficiency virus gp120 downregulates CD1d cell surface expression. *Immunol Lett.* 2005;98:131–135.

Hamada H, Garcia-Hernandez Md, L, Reome JB, et al. Tc17, a unique subset of CD8 T cells that can protect against lethal influenza challenge. *J Immunol.* 2009;182:3469–3481.

Hansen SG, Piatak M, Jr, Ventura AB, et al. Immune clearance of highly pathogenic SIV infection. *Nature.* 2013a;502:100–104.

Hansen SG, Sacha JB, Hughes CM, et al. Cytomegalovirus vectors violate CD8+ T cell epitope recognition paradigms. *Science.* 2013b;340:1237874.

Hartigan-O'Connor DJ, Abel K, Van Rompay KK, et al. SIV replication in the infected rhesus macaque is limited by the size of the preexisting TH17 cell compartment. *Sci Transl Med.* 2012;4:136–169.

Hartigan-O'Connor DJ, Jacobson MA, Tan QX, et al. Development of cytomegalovirus (CMV) immune recovery uveitis is associated with Th17 cell depletion and poor systemic CMV-specific T cell responses. *Clin Infect Dis.* 2011;52:409–441.

Hatano H, Delwart EL, Norris PJ, et al. Evidence for persistent low-level viremia in individuals who control human immunodeficiency virus in the absence of antiretroviral therapy. *J Virol.* 2009;83:329–335.

Heise C, Miller CJ, Lackner A. Primary acute simian immunodeficiency virus infection of intestinal lymphoid tissue is associated with gastrointestinal dysfunction. *J Infect Dis.* 1994;169:1116–1120.

Hellerstein M, Hanley MB, Cesar D, et al. Directly measured kinetics of circulating T lymphocytes in normal and HIV-1-infected humans. *Nat Med.* 1999;5:83–89.

Hirao LA, Grishina I, Bourry O, et al. Early mucosal sensing of SIV infection by paneth cells induces IL-1beta production and initiates gut epithelial disruption. *PLoS Pathol.* 2014;10:e1004311.

Hrecka K, Hao C, Gierszewska M, et al. Vpx relieves inhibition of HIV-1 infection of macrophages mediated by the SAMHD1 protein. *Nature.* 2011;474:658–661.

Hsu DC, Wegner MD, Sunyakumthorn P, et al. CD4+ cell infiltration into subcutaneous adipose tissue is not indicative of productively infected cells during acute SHIV infection. *J Med Primatol.* 2017;46:154–157.

Hunt PW, Brenchley J, Sinclair E, et al. Relationship between T cell activation and CD4+ T cell count in HIV-seropositive individuals with undetectable plasma HIV RNA levels in the absence of therapy. *J Infect Dis.* 2008;197:126–133.

Hunt PW, Martin JN, Sinclair E, et al. Valganciclovir reduces T cell activation in HIV-infected individuals with incomplete CD4+ T cell recovery on antiretroviral therapy. *J Infect Dis.* 2011;203:1474–1483.

Hwang I, Zhang T, Scott JM, et al. Identification of human NK cells that are deficient for signaling adaptor FcRgamma and specialized for antibody-dependent immune functions. *Int Immunol.* 2012;24:793–802.

Jones JL, Phuah CL, Cox AL, et al. IL-21 drives secondary autoimmunity in patients with multiple sclerosis, following therapeutic lymphocyte depletion with alemtuzumab (Campath-1H). *J Clin Invest.* 2009;119:2052–2061.

Kader M, Bixler S, Piatak M, et al. Anti-retroviral therapy fails to restore the severe Th-17: Tc-17 imbalance observed in peripheral blood during simian immunodeficiency virus infection. *J Med Primatol.* 2009;38(Suppl 1):32–38.

Kelley CF, Kitchen CM, Hunt PW, et al. Incomplete peripheral CD4(+) cell count restoration in HIV-infected patients receiving long-term antiretroviral treatment. *Clin Infect Dis.* 2009;48:787–794.

Kuller LH, Tracy R, Belloso W, et al. Inflammatory and coagulation biomarkers and mortality in patients with HIV infection. *PLoS Med.* 2008;5:e203.

King C, Ilic A, Koelsch K, Sarvetnick N. Homeostatic expansion of T cells during immune insufficiency generates autoimmunity. *Cell.* 2004;117:265–277.

Klatt NR, Harris LD, Vinton CL, et al. Compromised gastrointestinal integrity in pigtail macaques is associated with increased microbial translocation, immune activation, and IL-17 production in the absence of SIV infection. *Mucosal Immunol.* 2010;3:387–398.

Koethe JR, McDonnell W, Kennedy A, et al. Adipose tissue is enriched for activated and late-differentiated CD8+ T cells and shows distinct CD8+ receptor usage, compared with blood in HIV-infected persons. *J AIDS.* 2018;77:e14–e21.

Laguette N, Sobhian B, Casartelli N. et al. SAMHD1 is the dendritic- and myeloid-cell-specific HIV-1 restriction factor counteracted by Vpx. *Nature.* 2011;474:654–657.

Lang DJ, Kovacs AA, Zaia JA, et al. Seroepidemiologic studies of cytomegalovirus and Epstein-Barr virus infections in relation to human immunodeficiency virus type 1 infection in selected recipient populations. Transfusion Safety Study Group. *J AIDS.* 1989;2:540–549.

Lawn SD, Myer L, Bekker LG, Wood R. Tuberculosis-associated immune reconstitution disease: incidence, risk factors and impact in an antiretroviral treatment service in South Africa. *AIDS.* 2007;21(3):335–341.

Lenkei R, Andersson B. High correlations of anti-CMV titers with lymphocyte activation status and CD57 antibody-binding capacity as estimated with three-color, quantitative flow cytometry in blood donors. *Clin Immunol Immunopathol.* 1995;77:131–138.

Lee J, Zhang T, Hwang I, Kim A, et al. Epigenetic modification and antibody-dependent expansion of memory-like NK cells in human cytomegalovirus-infected individuals. *Immunity.* 2015;42:431–442.

Lenardo MJ, Angleman SB, Bounkeua V, et al. Cytopathic killing of peripheral blood CD4(+) T lymphocytes by human immunodeficiency virus type 1 appears necrotic rather than apoptotic and does not require env. *J Virol.* 2002;76:5082–5093.

Li D, Xu XN. NKT cells in HIV-1 infection. *Cell Res.* 2008;18:817–822.

Link A, Vogt TK, Favre S, Fibroblastic reticular cells in lymph nodes regulate the homeostasis of naive T cells. *Nat Immunol.* 2007;8:1255–1265.

Lopez-Verges S, Milush JM, Schwartz BS, et al. Expansion of a unique CD57(+)NKG2Chi natural killer cell subset during acute human cytomegalovirus infection. *Proc Natl Acad Sci U S A.* 2011;108:14725–14732.

Manel N, Hogstad B, Wang Y, et al. A cryptic sensor for HIV-1 activates antiviral innate immunity in dendritic cells. *Nature.* 2010;467:214–217.

Martin MP, Qi Y, Gao X. et al. Innate partnership of HLA-B and KIR3DL1 subtypes against HIV-1. *Nat Genet.* 2007;39:733–740.

McCune JM. The dynamics of CD4⁺ T cell depletion in HIV disease. *Nature.* 2001;410:974–979.

Mens H, Kearney M, Wiegand A, et al. HIV-1 continues to replicate and evolve in patients with natural control of HIV infection. *J Virol.* 2010;84(24):12971–12981.

Migueles SA, Connors M. Long-term nonprogressive disease among untreated HIV-infected individuals: clinical implications of understanding immune control of HIV. *JAMA.* 2010;304:194–201.

Mocroft A, Phillips AN, Gatell J, et al. Normalisation of CD4 counts in patients with HIV-1 infection and maximum virological suppression who are taking combination antiretroviral therapy: an observational cohort study. *Lancet.* 2007;370:407–413.

Muller M, Wandel S, Colebunders R. et al. Immune reconstitution inflammatory syndrome in patients starting antiretroviral therapy for HIV infection: a systematic review and meta-analysis. *Lancet Infect Dis.* 2010;10:251–261.

Mutoh Y, Nishijima T, Inaba Y, et al. Incomplete recovery of CD4 cell count, CD4 percentage, and CD4/CD8 ratio in patients with HIV infection and suppressed viremia during long-term antiretroviral therapy. *Clin Infect Dis.* 2018;67(6):927–933.

Naeger DM, Martin JN, Sinclair E, et al. Cytomegalovirus-specific T cells persist at very high levels during long-term antiretroviral treatment of HIV disease. *PLoS One.* 2010;5:e8886.

Ndhlovu ZM, Kamya P, Mewalal N, et al. Magnitude and kinetics of CD8⁺ T cell activation during hyperacute HIV infection impact viral set point. *Immunity.* 2015;43:591–604.

Neuhaus J, Jacobs DR, Baker JV. Markers of inflammation, coagulation, and renal function are elevated in adults with HIV infection. *J Infect Dis.* 2010;201:1788–1795.

Nigam P, Kwa S, Velu V, Amara RR. Loss of IL-17-producing CD8 T cells during late chronic stage of pathogenic simian immunodeficiency virus infection. *J Immunol.* 2011;186:745–753.

Nussenblatt RB, Lane HC. Human immunodeficiency virus disease: changing patterns of intraocular inflammation. *Am J Ophthalmol.* 1998;125:374–382.

O'Connell KA, Rabi SA, Siliciano RF. CD4⁺ T cells from elite suppressors are more susceptible to HIV-1 but produce fewer virions than cells from chronic progressors. *Proc Natl Acad Sci U S A.* 2011;108:E689–E698.

Pakker NG, Notermans DW, de Boer RJ, et al. Biphasic kinetics of peripheral blood T cells after triple combination therapy in HIV-1 infection: a composite of redistribution and proliferation. *Nat Med.* 1998;4:208–214.

Papagno L, Spina CA, Marchant A. Immune activation and CD8(+) T cell differentiation towards senescence in HIV-1 infection. *PLoS Biol.* 2004;2:E20.

Parrinello CM, Sinclair E, Landay AL, et al. Cytomegalovirus immunoglobulin G antibody is associated with subclinical carotid artery disease among HIV-infected women. *J Infect Dis.* 2012;205:1788–1796.

Pereyra F, Jia X, McLaren PJ, et al. The major genetic determinants of HIV-1 control affect HLA class I peptide presentation. *Science.* 2010;330:1551–1557.

Phillips AN, Neaton J, Lundgren JD. The role of HIV in serious diseases other than AIDS. *AIDS.* 2008;22:2409–2418.

Price P, Murdoch DM, Agarwal U, et al. Immune restoration diseases reflect diverse immunopathological mechanisms. *Clin Microbiol Rev.* 2009;22:651–663.

Raffatellu M, Santos RL, Verhoeven DE, et al. Simian immunodeficiency virus-induced mucosal interleukin-17 deficiency promotes Salmonella dissemination from the gut. *Nat Med.* 2008;14:421–428.

Reeves RK, Li H, Jost S, et al. Antigen-specific NK cell memory in rhesus macaques. *Nat Immunol.* 2015;16:927–932.

Rodriguez B. (2014). AIDS 347: IL-6 blockade in treated HIV infection. https://clinicaltrials.gov/ct2/show/NCT02049437.

Roederer M, Dubs JG, Anderson MT, et al. CD8 naive T cell counts decrease progressively in HIV-infected adults. *J Clin Invest.* 1995;95:2061–2066.

Saez-Cirion A, Hamimi C, Bergamaschi A. et al. Restriction of HIV-1 replication in macrophages and CD4⁺ T cells from HIV controllers. *Blood.* 2011;118:955–964.

Sandberg JK, Fast NM, Palacios EH, et al. Selective loss of innate CD4(+) V alpha 24 natural killer T cells in human immunodeficiency virus infection. *J Virol.* 2002;76:7528–7534.

Sauce D, Larsen M, Fastenackels S, et al. HIV disease progression despite suppression of viral replication is associated with exhaustion of lymphopoiesis. *Blood.* 2011;117(19):5142–5151.

Schacker TW, Nguyen PL, Beilman GJ. Collagen deposition in HIV-1 infected lymphatic tissues and T cell homeostasis. *J Clin Invest.* 2002;110:1133–1139.

Seddiki N, Sasson SC, Santner-Nanan B. Proliferation of weakly suppressive regulatory CD4⁺ T cells is associated with over-active CD4⁺ T cell responses in HIV-positive patients with mycobacterial immune restoration disease. *Eur J Immunol.* 2009;39:391–403.

Silvestri G, Sodora DL, Koup RA, et al. Nonpathogenic SIV infection of sooty mangabeys is characterized by limited bystander immunopathology despite chronic high-level viremia. *Immunity.* 2003;18:441–452.

Sips M, Sciaranghella G, Diefenbach T, et al. Altered distribution of mucosal NK cells during HIV infection. *Mucosal Immunol.* 2012;5:30–40.

Srinivasula S, Lempicki RA, Adelsberger JW, et al. Differential effects of HIV viral load and CD4 count on proliferation of naive and memory CD4 and CD8 T lymphocytes. *Blood.* 2011;118:262–270.

Stacey AR, Norris PJ, Qin L, et al. Induction of a striking systemic cytokine cascade prior to peak viremia in acute human immunodeficiency virus type 1 infection, in contrast to more modest and delayed responses in acute hepatitis B and C virus infections. *J Virol.* 2009;83:3719–3733.

Sun JC, Beilke JN, Lanier LL. Adaptive immune features of natural killer cells. *Nature.* 2009;457:557–561.

Surh CD, Sprent, J. (2008). Homeostasis of naive and memory T cells. *Immunity.* 2008;29:848–862.

Sylwester, AW, Mitchell BL, Edgar, JB, et al. Broadly targeted human cytomegalovirus-specific CD4$^+$ and CD8$^+$ T cells dominate the memory compartments of exposed subjects. *J Exp Med.* 2005;202:673–685.

Teixeira L, Valdez H, McCune JM, et al. Poor CD4 T cell restoration after suppression of HIV-1 replication may reflect lower thymic function. *AIDS.* 2001;15:1749–1756.

Williams WB, Liao HX, Moody MA, et al. HIV-1 VACCINES. Diversion of HIV-1 vaccine-induced immunity by gp41-microbiota cross-reactive antibodies. *Science.* 2015;349:aab1253.

van der Vliet HJ, von Blomberg BM, Hazenberg MD, et al. Selective decrease in circulating V alpha 24+V beta 11+ NKT cells during HIV type 1 infection. *J Immunol.* 2002;168:1490–1495.

van Grevenynghe J, Procopio FA, He Z, et al. Transcription factor FOXO3a controls the persistence of memory CD4(+) T cells during HIV infection. *Nat Med.* 2008;14:266–274.

Veazey RS, DeMaria M, Chalifoux LV, et al. Gastrointestinal tract as a major site of CD4$^+$ T cell depletion and viral replication in SIV infection. *Science.* 1998;280:427–431.

Vujkovic-Cvijin I, Dunham RM, Iwai S, et al. Dysbiosis of the gut microbiota is associated with HIV disease progression and tryptophan catabolism. *Sci Transl Med.* 2013;5:193ra191.

Zeng M, Southern PJ, Reilly CS, et al. Lymphoid tissue damage in HIV-1 infection depletes naive T cells and limits T cell reconstitution after antiretroviral therapy. *PLoS Pathogens.* 2012;8:e1002437.

Zhang T, Scott JM, Hwang I. Cutting edge: antibody-dependent memory-like NK cells distinguished by FcRgamma deficiency. *J Immunol.* 2013;190:1402–1406.

Zhou J, Amran FS, Kramski M, et al. An NK cell population lacking fcrgamma is expanded in chronically infected HIV patients. *J Immunol.* 2015;194:4688–4697.

6.

HIV CURE STRATEGIES

Boris Juelg and Rajesh Gandhi

CHAPTER GOAL

Upon completion of this chapter, the reader should be able to

- Identify key hurdles for HIV eradication strategies and explain how the "Kick and Kill" approaches might overcome these challenges.

INTRODUCTION

LEARNING OBJECTIVE

Identify key hurdles for HIV eradication strategies and explain how the "Kick and Kill" approaches might overcome these challenges.

WHAT'S NEW?

Novel strategies to promote HIV latency reversal and approaches to boost HIV-specific immunity are moving into clinical trials aimed at eradicating HIV.

KEY POINTS

- HIV-1 persists quiescently in cellular reservoirs not detected by the immune system due to the lack of active viral replication; these reservoirs represent the biggest obstacle to cure approaches.

- Reversal of HIV-1 latency and induction of virus expression by a variety of interventions may render infected cells susceptible to immune recognition and active clearance.

- Strategies to boost immune responses via vaccination, immunomodulation, or gene therapy are being evaluated with the aim of achieving HIV-1 control without antiretroviral therapy (ART), if not viral eradication.

WHY SHOULD WE TRY TO CURE HIV?

Although current ART is highly effective at controlling HIV-1 replication, it does not eradicate or cure the infection. There are several compelling reasons for trying to cure HIV-1. First,

despite efforts to expand access to treatment, many HIV-1-positive individuals worldwide are not receiving ART, which leads to ongoing transmission of the virus. Second, because current ART does not eradicate HIV-1, infected patients must take ART for many decades, which may eventuate in difficulties with adherence, substantial cost, and the potential for long-term side effects. Third, HIV-1–infected patients have increased rates of cardiovascular disease, liver disease, neurocognitive disorders, and other noninfectious complications that may be driven by elevated levels of inflammation that persist despite suppressive ART. Finally, HIV-1 infection continues to be associated with stigma and social isolation, which adversely affects quality of life. Given the limitations of current ART, there is a renewed and concerted effort to find a cure for HIV-1.

While complete viral eradication, or a "sterilizing cure," is the ultimate goal, the concept of a "functional cure" has been introduced, which includes strategies aimed at achieving host control of the virus without the need for ART. Several clinical observations within the past few years have fueled the belief that one or the other of these types of "cure" might be possible. Certainly, the most compelling example is that of the "Berlin patient," the only person to have been cured of HIV-1. This HIV-1–positive patient with virologic suppression on ART received, as treatment for acute myelogenous leukemia, allogeneic hematopoietic stem cell transplants from a donor who carried a homozygous deletion in CCR5 (Hutter, 2009), the co-receptor for HIV-1, thereby making his new CD4$^+$ T cells resistant to infection. Following discontinuation of ART, no HIV-1 RNA has been detected in the Berlin patient's peripheral blood; moreover, multiple attempts to detect HIV-1 RNA or proviral DNA in cellular reservoirs and other tissue compartments have been negative (Yukl, 2013). Because of the risk of stem cell transplantation, however, this intensive approach is not appropriate in HIV-1–infected patients who do not have a hematologic malignancy. Another notable "proof-of-concept" came from studies of early initiation of ART during acute HIV-1 infection. The Visconti study identified 14 HIV-1–infected patients whose viremia has remained controlled for years after the interruption of ART that had been initiated during primary infection (Saez-Cirion, 2013). Along these lines, the "Mississippi baby," a child born to an HIV-1–infected mother, was started on ART 30 hours after delivery (Persaud, 2013) and quickly achieved virologic suppression. The child was lost to follow-up, however, and ART was discontinued by the caregiver. Despite stopping ART, the virus remained undetectable for 27 months, but the child ultimately suffered virologic rebound (Luzuriaga, 2015). These examples demonstrate that it is possible, under extraordinary circumstances, to eradicate HIV-1 (in the case of the "Berlin patient") or control HIV-1 without ART (in the case of the VISCONTI cohort and, temporarily, the "Mississippi child"). Now, the challenge is to extend the insights from these remarkable cases to the development of practical interventions that will lead to ART-free remission in the large population of people living with HIV-1.

EARLY ESTABLISHMENT AND PERSISTENCE OF THE LATENT HIV-1 RESERVOIR

In 1995, Chun et al. identified integrated provirus as a persistent reservoir of infection in the resting CD4$^+$ T cells of HIV-1–infected patients (Chun, 1995). While most activated memory CD4$^+$ T cells are destroyed during viral replication, a small fraction of infected cells survives to return to a resting and memory state. Once converted to a resting memory state, HIV-1 gene expression is shut down, resulting in latently infected CD4$^+$ T cells (Nabel, 1987). Because these infected cells do not express viral proteins, they remain hidden from the host immune response; moreover, without active replication, antiretroviral drugs cannot act against the virus. While infected resting cells leave the quiescent memory pool at a steady rate, the pool of infected cells persists, perhaps in part because of homeostatic proliferation. It has also been suggested that specific CD4$^+$ T cell memory subsets, including central memory (TCM), transitional memory (TTM), and memory stem cells (TSCM), harbor the majority of integrated HIV-1 DNA and that eradication therapies may require targeting of specific CD4$^+$ T cell populations (Buzon, 2014).

When latently infected cells are reactivated, viral gene expression is renewed and productive infection is reignited. In patients on long-term ART, the frequency of latently infected cells is extremely low: less than 1 per million resting memory CD4$^+$ T cells harbor replication-competent HIV-1 (Finzi, 1997; Wong, 1997). Nevertheless, this latent pool decays very slowly: the mean half-life of this reservoir is approximately 44 months, and, as a result, suppressive antiretroviral therapy would need to be maintained for more than 60 years to achieve viral eradication even if an infected person has only 100,000 latently infected cells (Finzi, 1999). In addition, it is conceivable that latent infection may persist in cells that are not CD4$^+$ T cells; however, this has yet to be proved.

It was initially believed that early suppression of viral replication during primary infection might prevent the reservoir from becoming established. However, Chun et al. demonstrated that ART initiated within 10 days of primary infection did not prevent the generation of latently infected CD4$^+$ T cells (Chun, 1998), pointing toward an early seeding of the reservoir. Newer data from the rhesus macaque model demonstrate that the latent reservoir is established within days of virus exposure, even before virus can be detected in peripheral blood (Whitney, 2014); the implication of this finding is that it will be practically impossible to treat or even diagnose HIV-1 infection early enough to avoid reservoir seeding. Several studies, however, have demonstrated that initiating ART during the acute/early phase of the infection results in a smaller HIV-1 reservoir (Saez-Cirion, 2013; Ananworanich, 2012; Hocqueloux, 2013), suggesting that early treatment could be beneficial by reducing the barrier to cure (Strain, 2005; Henrich, 2013).

The presence and persistence of the HIV-1 latent reservoir represents the biggest obstacle for cure approaches. For this reason, a deeper understanding of how latency is maintained and how this state can be reversed is critical to inform HIV-1 eradication strategies (Richman, 2009).

"KICK AND KILL"

In order to achieve viral eradication, or at least a state of HIV-1 suppression without requiring continuous ART, different strategies have been proposed, including modification of the host immune response to achieve enhanced control of viral replication, interventions to prevent reactivation of virus latency (Mousseau, 2015), and gene therapy to increase the resistance of target cells to HIV-1 infection (Tebas, 2014). Currently, the strategy that is receiving the most attention is the "shock and kill" or "kick and kill" approach. In this strategy, the first step is to flush out HIV-1 from the latent reservoir by activating proviral DNA expression in resting cells, leading to de novo viral protein production (the "shock" or "kick"). If this "kick" is successful, the next step is to enhance immune recognition and elimination of infected cells (the "kill"). This two-step approach, however, requires a latency-reversing strategy and an antiviral immune response in order to clear infected cells; both tasks are encumbered by substantial challenges.

LATENCY REVERSAL APPROACHES

The absence of HIV-1 gene expression in patients on suppressive ART enables evasion of latently infected CD4$^+$ T cells from immune surveillance (Hermankova, 2003). Reversal of HIV-1 latency and induction of virus expression may render infected cells susceptible to attack by cytolytic T lymphocytes or to destruction by viral cytopathic effects (Deeks, 2012; Chun, 1997). Several latency-reversing agents (LRAs) have been identified, perhaps the most promising of which are histone deacetylase inhibitors (HDACi) and toll-like receptor (TLR) agonists. HDACi agents are currently approved as anti-cancer drugs, and several agents have been evaluated in ART-suppressed HIV-1–infected individuals (Archin, 2014; Elliott, 2014; Rasmussen, 2014) for their latency-reversing potential. Vorinostat, the first HDACi to be studied in HIV-1–infected patients on ART, was found to induce HIV-1 RNA expression by an average of 4.8-fold in resting CD4$^+$ T cells after a single dose (Archin, 2014). Two other HDACi agents—panobinostat and romidepsin—have also been found to induce virus expression in HIV-1–infected patients on suppressive ART (Rasmussen, 2014; Sogaard, 2015). Following administration of romidepsin, plasma HIV-1 RNA levels became detectable in some patients, suggesting the LRA was inducing virus production (Sogaard, 2015). However, the size of the HIV-1 reservoir, based on measurements of HIV-1 DNA and virus outgrowth assay, remained unchanged following three weekly infusions of romidepsin, suggesting that additional interventions will be needed. A larger trial of romidepsin is currently enrolling to confirm these results (ClinicalTrials.gov identifier: NCT01933594), and combination studies are being planned.

Another strategy that is being studied is the use of TLR agonists. The TLR7 agonist vesatolimod has been shown to induce transient increases in plasma viral load and decreases in cellular viral DNA levels in simian immunodeficiency virus (SIV)-infected rhesus macaques (Whitney, 2015). In a separate study done in monkeys treated with ART during acute simian-human immunodeficiency virus (SHIV) infection, a combination of a TLR-7 agonist with a broadly neutralizing antibody (PGT121) led to virologic control after the interventions and ART were stopped in 5 of 11 animals (Borducchi, 2018). Trials using vesatolimod in ART-treated HIV-1–infected humans are currently under way (NCT02858401 and NCT03060447). Furthermore, the TLR9 agonist lefitolimod increased HIV-1 transcription and enhanced cytotoxic natural killer (NK) cell activation in a small group of ART-suppressed individuals (Vibholm, 2017). Overall, it remains uncertain whether a single agent will be sufficient to effectively and completely purge the pool of replication-competent, integrated, latent HIV-1; rather a combination of LRAs targeting distinct pathways, and potentially different cell types, might be required (Laird, 2015).

LATENCY SILENCING

In contrast to activating latency, it has been proposed that reinforcing a deep state of latency by permanently silencing HIV transcription could be an alternative approach for a functional cure. This concept, also known as "block and lock" strategy, would apply latency-promoting agents (LPAs) to block the reactivation of latently infected HIV-1 proviruses. Potential agents that have been suggested include the Tat inhibitor didehydro-cortistatin A, which, when added to ART, systemically reduced viral mRNA in tissues of HIV-1–infected humanized mice and significantly delayed viral rebound following ART interruption (Kessing, 2017). More in vivo studies are needed to further determine the role of these concepts in HIV cure.

IMMUNE ENHANCING AND/OR MODULATING STRATEGIES

While latency reversal will be crucial for eradication strategies, inducing viral replication alone will most likely not be sufficient to eliminate the infection. Indeed, in an in vitro model, reversal of latency alone did not result in clearance of infected cells (Shan, 2012). For this reason, it is anticipated that, following reactivation, cells harboring the reservoir will need to be actively cleared, most likely through a second line of attack by the host's immune system. Strategies to enhance immune responses via immunization or immunomodulation have been proposed based on the hypothesis that boosting T cell responses will lead to enhanced viral control—similarly to what is seen in so-called HIV-1 elite controllers, individuals who maintain undetectable viral loads in the absence of ART (Deeks, 2007), where antiviral T cells have been associated with viral suppression (Deeks, 2007; McMichael, 2010).

T Cell Vaccines

The ability to enhance the host's immune responses by therapeutic vaccination faces several key challenges. The majority of HIV-1–infected individuals have dysfunctional HIV-1–specific effector cells (Sauce, 2013) as a result of continuous antigenic stimulation prior to treatment, and ART only incompletely restores T cell functionality. Furthermore, in patients who initiate ART during chronic infection, almost all of the proviral sequences in the latent reservoir contain escape mutations (Papuchon, 2013; Deng, 2015) that prevent killing of infected cells by cytotoxic T lymphocytes. The implication is that an effective vaccination strategy, instead of just expanding preexisting responses that already had failed to control the infection, would need to improve the quality and functionality of HIV-1–specific immune response and elicit CD8+ T cell responses against previously untargeted epitopes or unmutated regions of the virus to avoid escape. To achieve this goal, multiple approaches are currently being tested in preclinical and clinical studies, including:

- Viral-vector–based vaccines, such as adenovirus, poxvirus modified vaccinia Ankara (MVA), and modified cytomegalovirus (CMV). Some of these approaches to deliver HIV-1 antigens have demonstrated robust immunogenicity, inducing broad and durable cellular immune responses which were able to protect monkeys against SIV infection in preclinical challenge studies (Barouch, 2012, 2013a; Hansen, 2011, 2013) but, more importantly, significantly reduced the viral load set points in SIV-infected macaques following ART cessation when combined with a TLR7 agonist (Borducchi, 2016). Studies of the safety and efficacy of therapeutic vaccination with an adenovirus type 26 vector prime and an MVA boost, each with mosaic HIV inserts, are ongoing in people with HIV (ClinicalTrials.gov identifiers: NCT02919306 and NCT03307915).

- Plasmid DNA expressing HIV-1 genes (Hallengard, 2011; Ramirez, 2013; Rodriguez, 2013).

- Dendritic cell–based vaccines to deliver HIV-1 antigens. In one study, this approach was associated with reduced plasma viral load post treatment interruption (Levy, 2014).

Some of these vaccines have been tested already in humans and are safe and immunogenic, but proof of efficacy in reducing the

HIV-1 reservoir has yet to be demonstrated (ClinicalTrials.gov identifiers: NCT02919306, NCT03307915).

Immune Modulation: Checkpoint Inhibitors

Given the challenge that preexisting T cell exhaustion in HIV-1–infected patients poses for therapeutic vaccination strategies, novel immune-modulating concepts have been developed to reverse this state of exhaustion by inhibiting immune checkpoints. During progressive HIV-1 infection with persistent antigen exposure, increased expression of inhibitory receptors like PD-1 on HIV-1–specific T cells is associated with greater immune dysfunction (Day, 2006; Khaitan, 2011). Inhibiting the PD-1 pathway has shown efficacy in reversing T cell exhaustion in the cancer field (Topalian, 2012), and recent data suggest that PD-1 blockade restores the ability of antiviral T cells to inhibit HIV-1 replication in animal models (Palmer, 2013; Velu, 2009). A dose-escalation trial of an anti–PD-L1 antibody in HIV-1–positive patients demonstrated an increase in HIV-specific T cell responses in two out of six participants; however, the trial was stopped prior to full enrollment as there was concern about antibody-associated retinal toxicity in animal studies (Gay, 2017). Intriguingly, repeated doses of the anti–PD-1 antibody pembrolizumab in a single HIV-positive individual with lung cancer were associated with an increase in functional HIV-specific CD8$^+$ T cells and a decline in cell-associated HIV DNA (Guihot, 2018).

Multiple studies of immune checkpoint inhibitors and their effect on the virus reservoir in HIV-positive individuals on ART with concomitant malignant diseases are in progress (ClinicalTrials.gov identifiers: NCT02408861, NCT02595866, NCT03304093, NCT03354936, NCT03367754).

T Cell Trafficking

The intestinal mucosa is a key site for HIV-1 replication, and inhibition of CD4$^+$ T cell trafficking to theses tissues has been suggested as a potential cure strategy. The gut-homing integrin $\alpha_4\beta_7$ is expressed on the surface of CD4$^+$ T cells, and treatment of SIV-infected ART-suppressed macaques with an anti-$\alpha_4\beta_7$ integrin monoclonal antibody resulted in persistent viral control following ART cessation (Byrareddy, 2016). However, the antibody vedolizumab (approved by the US Food and Drug Administration [FDA] for treatment of inflammatory bowel disease), which targets human $\alpha_4\beta_7$ integrin, did not show evidence of delayed viral rebound following cessation of ART in virally suppressed HIV-positive persons (Fauci, 2018) (ClinicalTrials.gov identifiers: NCT03147859 and NCT02788175). In contrast to preventing trafficking of HIV target cells into anatomic sites of high viral replication, an alternative approach is promoting cytotoxic CD8$^+$ T cell migration into lymph node follicles to clear infected cells. In the non-human primate model, administration of an interleukin-15 super-agonist resulted in an increase of CXCR5 expression on CD8$^+$ T cells and increased frequency of such cells in the lymphoid tissues (Webb, 2018). This concept is now being examined in humans (ClinicalTrials.gov identifier: NCT02191098).

Chimeric Antigen Receptor T Cells

An alternative approach, which circumvents the problem of eliciting immune responses in HIV-1–infected patients with immune dysregulation, is the adoptive transfer of T cells with molecularly cloned high-affinity T cell receptors (TCR) and superior antiviral activity (Varela-Rohena, 2008) targeting conserved and vulnerable regions of the virus. A phase 1 study testing the in vivo efficacy of these high-affinity gag-specific T cells in ART-treated patients has been performed; the results of this study are pending (ClinicalTrials.gov identifier: NCT00991224). Furthermore, chimeric antigen receptor transduced T cells, which combine the specificity of an antibody with the signaling of a T cell receptor, have shown promise in the cancer field (Hombach, 2013) and are now being studied in HIV (Lam, 2013; Leibman, 2017).

Broadly Neutralizing Antibodies

The recent identification of novel broadly neutralizing anti–HIV-1 antibodies (bNAbs), which are able to neutralize the majority of viral strains at very low concentrations, may provide another approach to target the HIV-1 reservoir. In preclinical studies, administration of bNAbs was shown to reduce plasma viremia in chimeric SHIV-infected macaques (Barouch, 2013b; Shingai, 2013; Julg, 2017); in fact, one particular bNAb, PGT121, also resulted in substantial reductions of proviral DNA in peripheral blood, lymph nodes, and gastrointestinal mucosa (Barouch, 2013b). As a potential mechanism, it has been suggested that clearance of infected cells expressing viral antigen on their surfaces (Lu, 2016) is mediated through interactions between the Fc component of the antibody and its receptor on innate immune effectors cells like NK cells and macrophages (Bruel, 2016). Three different bNAbs have been tested so far in HIV-1–positive humans and have shown promising reductions in plasma viremia (Caskey, 2015, 2017; Lynch, 2015). Administration of the antibodies 3BNC117 and VRC01 to HIV-positive individuals on ART resulted in delayed viral rebound after ART cessation compared with historical controls, but the effects were modest and generally transient (Bar, 2016; Scheid, 2016). Not surprisingly, rapid selection of archived resistant viral strains reduced the therapeutic efficacy of single bNAbs; for this reason, bNAb combinations are currently being evaluated to overcome this limitation (ClinicalTrials.gov identifiers: NCT03205917, NCT03565315, NCT03526848). In addition, next-generation antibodies that incorporate the antigen specificity of different bNAbs by binding to multiple nonoverlapping sites on the virus or attaching to both virus and CD4$^+$ receptors have been engineered (Huang, 2016; Xu, 2017). It remains to be determined what effect bNAbs will have on the viral reservoir in humans, however, and limitations like the lack of accessibility of antibodies to certain anatomic reservoir sites, such as the central nervous system, will need to be overcome. Nevertheless, the exciting results of a study combining a TLR-7 agonist with the broadly neutralizing antibody PGT121 in a non-human primate study (Borducchi, 2018; see earlier discussion) warrant follow-up in additional animal and human trials.

DUAL-AFFINITY RETARGETING

Finally, a novel method to combine antibody and T cell activity against HIV-1–infected cells is through bispecific protein constructs (dual-affinity re-targeting [DARTs]), which are designed to latch onto HIV-1 envelope proteins on the surface of infected cells while also binding to CD3 on T cells. This approach directs cytotoxic T cells to eliminate infected cells while obviating the need for the T cells to specifically bind to HIV-1 surface antigens (Sung, 2015; Pegu, 2015). Early in vitro studies of this approach are promising, but additional preclinical work is needed to confirm that these immunomodulatory proteins are safe enough to test in human trials.

GENE MODIFICATION

RENDERING THE HOST'S CD4 T CELLS RESISTANT TO INFECTION

The finding that the Berlin patient appears to be cured from HIV-1 after receiving a stem cell transplant from a CCR5-δ-32 homozygous donor has inspired attempts to generate HIV-1–resistant cells through gene therapy. Using bioengineered restriction enzymes like zinc-finger nucleases (ZFN), DNA can be cleaved at specific sites; this approach has been used to disrupt the CCR5 gene (which encodes the HIV-1 co-receptor) in CD4$^+$ T cells (Perez, 2008). Using the ZFN strategy, Tebas et al. modified the CCR5 gene ex vivo in autologous CD4$^+$ T cells in 12 HIV-1–positive study participants and infused the cells back into the autologous donors (Tebas, 2014). The study found that genetically modified cells persisted in vivo with a half-life of nearly a year. While no dramatic difference was seen in viral load set points following interruption of ART in six study participants, the modified cells appeared to be protected from HIV-1 infection as unmodified cells showed a faster depletion. Recent data in SHIV-infected and ART-suppressed pigtail macaques demonstrated that CCR5 gene-edited hematopoietic stem/progenitor cells (HSPCs) persisted following transplantation and expanded through virus-dependent positive selection, resulting in a significant reduction of tissue-associated SHIV DNA and RNA levels in the transplanted animals compared to controls (Peterson, 2018). The safety and feasibility of administration of CRISPR/Cas9 CCR5 gene-modified CD34$^+$ HSPC and ZFN CCR5 modified autologous CD4$^+$ T cells in ART-suppressed HIV-positive individuals is currently being evaluated (ClinicalTrials.gov identifiers: NCT02500849, NCT03164135, respectively).

EXCISING THE HIV-1 PROVIRUS FROM THE HOST CELL GENOME

The clustered regularly interspaced short palindromic repeat (CRISPR)/Cas9 system permits targeted and precise genome editing in diverse cell types and organisms, including human cells (Cong, 2013). Recently, several research groups have successfully applied gene editing technology to excise HIV-1 provirus from the host cell genome (Ebina, 2013; Hu, 2014; Liao, 2015). Importantly, the disruption of provirus expression not only restricted transcriptionally active provirus, but it also blocked the expression of latently integrated provirus (Ebina, 2013). Moreover, inserting the stably expressed CRISPR/Cas9 system into a T cell line conferred long-term protection against HIV-1 infection (Liao, 2015). These results from in vitro cell culture models are promising, and this technology may open new avenues to developing antiviral therapies in the future.

CONCLUSION

Although antiretroviral medications effectively treat HIV-1 infection, there are many compelling reasons to attempt to cure HIV-1, not the least of which is the stigma and isolation experienced by many persons living with HIV. The major barrier to HIV-1 cure is the persistence of a long-lived population of latently infected cells in patients on suppressive treatment; because the latent reservoir is established soon after HIV-1 acquisition, even early initiation of ART cannot cure the infection. Current efforts to cure HIV-1 infection are centered on flushing HIV-1 out of the latent reservoir along with enhancing immune mechanisms to clear infected cells. We are still in the early days of this massively difficult undertaking, and it is too soon to tell whether the approaches being pursued now will be effective. That being said, just as the development of combination ART was based on a series of advances that culminated in our ability to successfully treat HIV-1, the stepwise progress being made today will hopefully lead us to an even greater breakthrough: the capability to eradicate or control HIV-1 without the need for life-long therapy.

ACKNOWLEDGMENTS

This chapter is based on a previous version written by David Margolis MD, University of North Carolina at Chapel Hill.

REFERENCES

Ananworanich J, Schuetz A, Vandergeeten C, et al. Impact of multi-targeted antiretroviral treatment on gut T cell depletion and HIV reservoir seeding during acute HIV infection. *PloS One*. 2012;7(3):e33948.

Archin NM, Bateson R, Tripathy MK, et al. HIV-1 expression within resting CD4++ T cells after multiple doses of vorinostat. *J Infect Dis*. 2014;210(5):728–735.

Bar KJ, Sneller MC, Harrison LJ, et al. Effect of HIV antibody VRC01 on viral rebound after treatment interruption. *N Engl J Med*. 2016;375:2037–2050.

Barouch DH, Liu J, Li H, et al. Vaccine protection against acquisition of neutralization-resistant SIV challenges in rhesus monkeys. *Nature*. 2012;482(7383):89–93.

Barouch DH, Stephenson KE, Borducchi EN, et al. Protective efficacy of a global HIV-1 mosaic vaccine against heterologous SHIV challenges in rhesus monkeys. *Cell*. 2013a;155(3):531–539.

Barouch DH, Whitney JB, Moldt B, et al. Therapeutic efficacy of potent neutralizing HIV-1-specific monoclonal antibodies in SHIV-infected rhesus monkeys. *Nature*. 2013b;503(7475):224–228.

Borducchi E, Abbink P, Nkolola J, et al. PGT121 combined with GS-9620 delays viral rebound in SHIV-infected rhesus monkeys. The Conference on Retroviruses and Opportunistic Infections. Boston, MA, March 4–7, 2018. Abstract 73LB.

Borducchi EN, Cabral C, Stephenson KE, et al. Ad26/MVA therapeutic vaccination with TLR7 stimulation in SIV-infected rhesus monkeys. *Nature*. December 8, 2016;540(7632):284–287.

Bruel T, Guivel-Benhassine F, Amraoui S, et al. Elimination of HIV-1 infected cells by broadly neutralizing antibodies. *Nat Commun*. 2016;7:10844.

Buzon MJ, Sun H, Li C, et al. HIV-1 persistence in CD4++ T cells with stem cell–like properties. *Nat Med*. 2014;20(2):139–142.

Byrareddy SN, Arthros J, Cicala C, et al. Sustained virologic control in SIV+ macaques after antiretroviral and α4β7 antibody therapy. *Science*. 2016;354:197–202.

Caskey M, Klein F, Lorenzi JC, et al. Viraemia suppressed in HIV-1–infected humans by broadly neutralizing antibody 3BNC117. *Nature*. 2015;522(7557):487–491.

Caskey M, Schoofs T, Gruell H, et al. Antibody 10-1074 suppresses viremia in HIV-1-infected individuals. *Nat Med*. 2017;23(2):185–191.

Chun TW, Engel D, Berrey MM, et al. Early establishment of a pool of latently infected, resting CD4+(+) T cells during primary HIV-1 infection. *Proc Natl Acad Sci U S A*. 1998;95(15):8869–8873.

Chun TW, Finzi D, Margolick J, et al. In vivo fate of HIV-1–infected T cells: quantitative analysis of the transition to stable latency. *Nat Med*. 1995;1(12):1284–1290.

Chun TW, Stuyver L, Mizell SB, et al. Presence of an inducible HIV-1 latent reservoir during highly active antiretroviral therapy. *Proc Natl Acad Sci U S A*. 1997;94(24):13193–13197.

Cong L, Ran FA, Cox D, et al. Multiplex genome engineering using CRISPR/Cas systems. *Science*. 2013;339(6121):819–823.

Day CL, Kaufmann DE, Kiepiela P, et al. PD-1 expression on HIV-specific T cells is associated with T cell exhaustion and disease progression. *Nature*. 2006;443(7109):350–354.

Deeks SG. HIV: shock and kill. *Nature*. 2012;487(7408):439–440.

Deeks SG, Walker BD. Human immunodeficiency virus controllers: mechanisms of durable virus control in the absence of antiretroviral therapy. *Immunity*. 2007;27(3):406–416.

Deng K, Pertea M, Rongvaux A, et al. Broad CTL response is required to clear latent HIV-1 due to dominance of escape mutations. *Nature*. 2015;517(7534):381–385.

Ebina H, Misawa N, Kanemura Y, Koyanagi Y. Harnessing the CRISPR/Cas9 system to disrupt latent HIV-1 provirus. *Sci Rep*. 2013;3:2510.

Elliott JH, Wightman F, Solomon A, et al. Activation of HIV transcription with short-course vorinostat in HIV-positive patients on suppressive antiretroviral therapy. *PLoS Pathog*. 2014;10(10):e1004473.

Fauci AS, et al. AIDS 2018. Abstract WESS0102. Durable control of HIV infections in the absence of antiretroviral therapy: Opportunities and obstacles and Jonathan Mann Memorial Lecture: Data to drive equity. Abstract WESS01, 22nd International AIDS Conference 2018, Amsterdam, Netherlands.

Finzi D, Blankson J, Siliciano JD, et al. Latent infection of CD4++ T cells provides a mechanism for lifelong persistence of HIV-1, even in patients on effective combination therapy. *Nat Med*. 1999;5(5):512–517.

Finzi D, Hermankova M, Pierson T, et al. Identification of a reservoir for HIV-1 in patients on highly active antiretroviral therapy. *Science*. 1997;278(5341):1295–1300.

Gay CL, Bosch RJ, Ritz J, et al. Clinical trial of the anti-PDL-L1 antibody BMS-936559 in HIV-1 infected participants on suppressive antiretroviral therapy. *J Infect Dis*. June 1, 2017;215(11):1725–1733.

Guihot A, Marcelin AG, Massiani MA, et al. Drastic decrease of the HIV reservoir in a patient treated with nivolumab for lung cancer. *Ann Oncol*. 2018;29:517–518.

Hallengard D, Haller BK, Maltais AK, et al. Comparison of plasmid vaccine immunization schedules using intradermal in vivo electroporation. *Clin Vaccine Immunol*. 2011;18(9):1577–1581.

Hansen SG, Ford JC, Lewis MS, et al. Profound early control of highly pathogenic SIV by an effector memory T cell vaccine. *Nature*. 2011;473(7348):523–527.

Hansen SG, Piatak M, Jr., Ventura AB, et al. Immune clearance of highly pathogenic SIV infection. *Nature*. 2013;502(7469):100–104.

Henrich TJ, Gandhi RT. Early treatment and HIV-1 reservoirs: a stitch in time? *J Infect Dis*. 2013;208(8):1189–1193.

Hermankova M, Siliciano JD, Zhou Y, et al. Analysis of human immunodeficiency virus type 1 gene expression in latently infected resting CD4+ T lymphocytes in vivo. *J Virol*. 2003;77(13):7383–7392.

Hocqueloux L, Avettand-Fenoel V, Jacquot S, et al. Long-term antiretroviral therapy initiated during primary HIV-1 infection is key to achieving both low HIV reservoirs and normal T cell counts. *J Antimicrobial Chemother*. 2013;68(5):1169–1178.

Hombach AA, Holzinger A, Abken H. The weal and woe of costimulation in the adoptive therapy of cancer with chimeric antigen receptor (CAR)-redirected T cells. *Curr Mol Med*. 2013;13(7):1079–1088.

Hu W, Kaminski R, Yang F, et al. RNA-directed gene editing specifically eradicates latent and prevents new HIV-1 infection. *Proc Natl Acad Sci*. 2014;111(31):11461–11466.

Huang Y, Yu J, Lanzi A, et al. Engineered bispecific antibodies with exquisite HIV-1-neutralizing activity. *Cell*. 2016;165:1621–1631.

Hutter G, Nowak D, Mossner M, et al. Long-term control of HIV by CCR5 Delta32/Delta32 stem-cell transplantation. *N Engl J Med*. 2009;360(7):692–698.

Julg J, Pequ A, Abbink P, et al. Virologic control by the CD4-binding site antibody N6 in simian-human immunodeficiency virus-infected rhesus monkeys. *J Virol*. July 27, 2017;91(16):e00498–17.

Kessing CF, Nixon CC, Li C, et al. In vivo suppression of HIV rebound by didehydro-cortistatin A, a "block-and-lock" strategy for HIV-1 treatment. *Cell Rep*. October 17, 2017;21(3):600–611.

Khaitan A, Unutmaz D. Revisiting immune exhaustion during HIV infection. *Current HIV/AIDS reports*. 2011;8(1):4–11.

Laird GM, Bullen CK, Rosenbloom DI, et al. Ex vivo analysis identifies effective HIV-1 latency-reversing drug combinations. *J Clin Invest*. 2015;125(5):1901–1912.

Lam S, Bollard C. T cell therapies for HIV. *Immunotherapy*. 2013;5(4):407–414.

Leibman RS, Richardson MW, Ellebrecht CT, et al. Supraphysiologic control over HIV-1 replication mediated by CD8 T cells expressing a re-engineered CD4-based chimeric antigen receptor. *PLoS Pathog*. October 12, 2017;13(10):e1006613.

Levy Y, Thiebaut R, Montes M, et al. Dendritic cell-based therapeutic vaccine elicits polyfunctional HIV-specific T cell immunity associated with control of viral load. *Eur J Immunol*. 2014;44(9):2802–2810.

Liao HK, Gu Y, Diaz A, et al. Use of the CRISPR/Cas9 system as an intracellular defense against HIV-1 infection in human cells. *Nat Commun*. 2015;6:6413.

Lu CL, Murakowski DK, Bournazos S, et al. Enhanced clearance of HIV-1–infected cells by broadly neutralizing antibodies against HIV-1 in vivo. *Science*. 2016;352:1001–1004.

Luzuriaga K, Gay H, Ziemniak C, et al. Viremic relapse after HIV-1 remission in a perinatally infected child. *N Engl J Med*. 2015;372(8):786–788.

Lynch RM, Boritz E, Coates EE, et al. Virologic effects of broadly neutralizing antibody VRC01 administration during chronic HIV-1 infection. *Sci Ttransl Med*. 2015;7(319):319ra206.

McMichael AJ, Borrow P, Tomaras GD, The immune response during acute HIV-1 infection: clues for vaccine development. *Nat Rev Immunol*. 2010;10(1):11–23.

Mousseau G, Kessing CF, Fromentin R, et al. The tat inhibitor didehydrocortistatin A prevents HIV-1 reactivation from latency. *MBio*. 2015;6(4).

Nabel G, Baltimore D. An inducible transcription factor activates expression of human immunodeficiency virus in T cells. *Nature*. 1987;326(6114):711–713.

Palmer BE, Neff CP, Lecureux J, et al. In vivo blockade of the PD-1 receptor suppresses HIV-1 viral loads and improves CD4+ T cell levels in humanized mice. *J Immunol*. 2013;190(1):211–219.

Papuchon J, Pinson P, Lazaro E, et al. Resistance mutations and CTL epitopes in archived HIV-1 DNA of patients on antiviral treatment: toward a new concept of vaccine. *PloS One*. 2013;8(7):e69029.

Pegu A, Asokan M, Wu L, et al. Activation and lysis of human CD4 cells latently infected with HIV-1. *Nature Commun*. 2015;6:8447.

Perez EE, Wang J, Miller JC, et al. Establishment of HIV-1 resistance in CD4⁺ T cells by genome editing using zinc-finger nucleases. *Nat Biotechnol*. 2008;26(7):808–816.

Persaud D, Gay H, Ziemniak C, et al. Absence of detectable HIV-1 viremia after treatment cessation in an infant. *N Engl J Med*. 2013;369(19):1828–1835.

Peterson CW, Wang J, Deleage C, et al. Differential impact of transplantation on peripheral and tissue-associated viral reservoirs: implications for HIV gene therapy. *PLoS Pathog*. April 19, 2018;14(4):e1006956.

Ramirez LA, Arango T, Boyer J. Therapeutic and prophylactic DNA vaccines for HIV-1. *Expert Opin Biological Ther*. 2013;13(4):563–573.

Rasmussen TA TM, Brinkmann CR, Olesen R, Erikstrup C. Panobinostat, a histone deacetylase inhibitor, for latent-virus reactivation in HIV-infected patients on suppressive antiretroviral therapy: a phase 1/2, single group, clinical trial. *Lancet HIV*. 2014;1(1):e14–e21.

Richman DD, Margolis DM, Delaney M, et al. The challenge of finding a cure for HIV infection. *Science*. 2009;323(5919):1304–1307.

Rodriguez B, Asmuth DM, Matining RM, et al. Safety, tolerability, and immunogenicity of repeated doses of dermavir, a candidate therapeutic HIV vaccine, in HIV-infected patients receiving combination antiretroviral therapy: results of the ACTG 5176 trial. *J Acquir Immune Defic Syndr*. 2013;64(4):351–359.

Saez-Cirion A, Bacchus C, Hocqueloux L, et al. Post-treatment HIV-1 controllers with a long-term virological remission after the interruption of early initiated antiretroviral therapy ANRS VISCONTI Study. *PLoS Pathog*. 2013;9(3):e1003211.

Sauce D, Elbim C, Appay V. Monitoring cellular immune markers in HIV infection: from activation to exhaustion. *Curr Opin HIV AIDS*. 2013;8(2):125–131.

Scheid JF, Horwitz JA, Bar-On Y, et al. HIV-1 antibody 3BNC117 suppresses viral rebound in humans during treatment interruption. *Nature*. 2016;535:556–560.

Shan L, Deng K, Shroff NS, et al. Stimulation of HIV-1-specific cytolytic T lymphocytes facilitates elimination of latent viral reservoir after virus reactivation. *Immunity*. 2012;36(3):491–501.

Shingai M, Nishimura Y, Klein F, et al. Antibody-mediated immunotherapy of macaques chronically infected with SHIV suppresses viraemia. *Nature*. 2013;503(7475):277–280.

Sogaard OS, Graversen ME, Leth S, et al. The depsipeptide romidepsin reverses HIV-1 latency in vivo. *PLoS Pathog*. 2015;11(9):e1005142.

Strain MC, Little SJ, Daar ES, et al. Effect of treatment, during primary infection, on establishment and clearance of cellular reservoirs of HIV-1. *J Infect Dis*. 2005;191(9):1410–1418.

Sung JA, Pickeral J, Liu L, et al. Dual-affinity re-targeting proteins direct T cell-mediated cytolysis of latently HIV-infected cells. *J Clin Invest*. 2015;125(11):4077–4090.

Tebas P, Stein D, Tang WW, et al. Gene editing of CCR5 in autologous CD4 T cells of persons infected with HIV. *N Engl J Med*. 2014;370(10):901–910.

Topalian SL, Hodi FS, Brahmer JR, Gettinger SN, Smith DC, McDermott DF, et al. Safety, activity, and immune correlates of anti-PD-1 antibody in cancer. *N Engl J Med*. 2012;366(26):2443–2454.

Varela-Rohena A, Molloy PE, Dunn SM, et al. Control of HIV-1 immune escape by CD8 T cells expressing enhanced T cell receptor. *Nat Med*. 2008;14(12):1390–1395.

Velu V, Titanji K, Zhu B, et al. Enhancing SIV-specific immunity in vivo by PD-1 blockade. *Nature*. 2009;458(7235):206–210.

Vibholm L, Schleimann MH, Hojen JF, et al. Short-course toll-like receptor 9 agonist treatment impacts innate immunity and plasma viremia in individuals with human immunodeficiency virus infection. *Clin Infect Dis*. June 15, 2017;64(12):1686–1695.

Webb GM, Li S, Mwakalundwa G, et al. The human IL-15 superagonist ALT-803 directs SIV-specific CD8⁺ T cells into B-cell follicles. *Blood Adv* 2018;2:76–84.

Whitney JB, Hill AL, Sanisetty S, et al. Rapid seeding of the viral reservoir prior to SIV viraemia in rhesus monkeys. *Nature*. 2014;512(7512):74–77.

Whitney JB, Osuna CE, Sanisetty S, et al. Treatment with a TLR7 agonist induces transient viremia in SIV-infected ART-suppressed monkeys. Conference on Retroviruses and Opportunistic Infections. Seattle, Washington, 2015.

Wong JK, Hezareh M, Gunthard HF, et al. Recovery of replication-competent HIV despite prolonged suppression of plasma viremia. *Science*. 1997;278(5341):1291–1295.

Xu L, Pequ A, Rao E, et al. Trispecific broadly neutralizing HIV antibodies mediate potent SHIV protection in macaques. *Science*. 2017;358:85–90.

Yukl SA, Boritz E, Busch MB, et al. Challenges in detecting HIV persistence during potentially curative interventions: a study of the Berlin patient. *PLoS Pathog*. 2013;9(5):e1003347.

7.

HIV TESTING AND COUNSELING

Alejandro Delgado and Hojoon You

CHAPTER GOALS

Upon completion of this chapter, the reader should be able to

- List and describe the types of HIV testing.

- Present an overview of HIV counseling, as well as how to adapt counseling to the variety of situations or environments in which these conversations can take place.

- Initiate early HIV therapy.

HIV TESTING: HISTORY AND EVOLUTION

In 1985, when HIV testing first became available, the main goal of testing was for blood banks to screen the US blood supply. When it was discovered that those who simply wished to learn their HIV status were using blood donation testing sites, alternative testing sites were implemented. Because at that time no treatment was available and routes of transmission were still being investigated, opinion was divided about the value of testing. By 1987, the implications of a positive HIV serology were clear, and the US Public Health Service and the Centers for Disease Control and Prevention (CDC) issued the first set of guidelines for HIV testing and counseling (CDC, 1987). Earlier guidelines targeted those in "high-risk groups," but experience taught that a more productive approach focused on behaviors rather than membership in a particular population. Hence, the thrust of the current guidelines is that HIV screening is recommended for all persons aged 13–65 years, regardless of risk factors. Periodic revisions informed by the epidemiology of the pandemic extended the outreach and flexibility of testing, culminating in the "Revised Recommendations for HIV Testing of Adults, Adolescents, and Pregnant Women in Health-Care Settings" (Branson, 2006).

LEARNING OBJECTIVES

- List and describe the types of HIV testing.

- Present an overview of HIV counseling as well as how to adapt counseling to the variety of situations or environments in which these conversations can take place.

WHAT'S NEW?

- During the past decade, the evidence favoring the early institution of therapy for HIV has been steadily growing, showing benefits in virologic control and decreased transmission of HIV. The World Health Organization (WHO) has published data from 2017 showing that the proportion of low- to middle-income countries that have adopted the "Treat All ART initiation" has increased from 33% to 70%.

- The most recent data published in 2015 by the CDC estimate that approximately 14% of people living with HIV are unaware of their diagnosis. In certain states and among men who have sex with men (MSM), who constitute 82% of new yearly diagnoses, the percentage of people who are unaware of their HIV infection may be as high as 25%, prompting the CDC to update its HIV screening recommendations for the MSM population.

- In June 2014, the CDC revised its testing algorithm favoring the use of fourth-generation assays that are capable of early detection of HIV-1 and HIV-2 antibodies as well as the p24 antigen. This has substantially narrowed the window between initial infection and positive test results. For the first time since 1989, the CDC has eliminated the use of confirmation testing with a first-generation western blot or immunofluorescence assay, now recommending that a nucleic acid amplification test (NAAT) be used (Figure 7.1).

KEY POINTS

- HIV testing should be offered as part of routine medical care to all patients. The US Preventive Services Task Force put forth recommendations in 2013 that clinicians screen all patients between the ages of 15 and 65 years. Testing in younger and older patients should be offered when special circumstances deem this appropriate.

- The CDC recommends that clinicians screen asymptomatic sexually active MSM at least annually and more frequently (i.e., every 3 or 6 months) for MSM patients at increased risk for HIV infection

- All persons screened for HIV should be counseled regarding risk-reduction strategies including preexposure

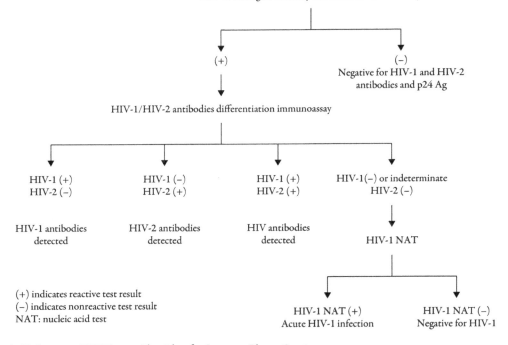

Figure 7.1 Recommended Laboratory HIV Testing Algorithm for Serum or Plasma Specimens. SOURCE: CDC Laboratory Testing Guidance. Available at: HIV-1/-2 testing algorithm. Accessed September 27, 2018.

prophylaxis (PrEP) and other prevention methods depending on test results.

- All pregnant women should be screened for HIV at the earliest instance possible.

HIV TESTING TERMINOLOGY, TYPES, AND ALGORITHM

Initially, the CDC guidelines focused on the diagnosis of HIV-1 using a sensitive antibody immunoassay with validation of those results by a more specific test such as the western blot or indirect immunofluorescence assay. By 1992, the guidelines also included testing recommendations for the diagnosis of HIV-2. In 2004, protocols for rapid antibody test results were issued with recommendations that all rapid testing be confirmed with either western blot or immunofluorescence assay. With the advent of improved immunoassays and tests, recommendations regarding HIV diagnostic testing have undergone changes.

The CDC's guidelines for laboratory testing for HIV are outlined in an algorithm (Figure 7.1). Initial testing should be done with an antigen/antibody combination immunoassay that detects both HIV-1 and HIV-2 antibodies and HIV-1 p24 antigen. If a positive result is obtained, the specimen should be tested with an antibody immunoassay that differentiates HIV-1 and HIV-2 antibodies. In the situation of a reactive antigen/antibody combination immunoassay with a nonreactive or indeterminate HIV-1/HIV-2 antibody differentiation immunoassay, the specimen should be further tested with an HIV-1 nucleic acid test. If the nucleic acid test is reactive, then it indicates acute HIV infection if the antibody differentiation immunoassay was negative. If the antibody differentiation immunoassay was indeterminate and the nucleic acid test is reactive, this indicates confirmed infection. A negative nucleic acid test indicates a false-positive result of the initial immunoassay.

Table 7.1 enumerates the various types of HIV testing.

LABORATORY MARKERS FOR HIV

There is a brief period immediately after HIV infection where there are no laboratory markers that can be detected in plasma; this is termed the *eclipse period*. After about 5–10 days of infection, HIV RNA can be detected by nucleic acid tests, followed by HIV-1 p24 antigen within 4–10 days after RNA is detected. HIV-1 p24 antigen is detected by fourth-generation immunoassays, but, as antibodies begin developing, the p24 antigens begin forming immune complexes with the antibodies and become no longer detectable. Immunoglobulin M antibodies start to be expressed about 3–5 day after the p24 antigen is detected, which are detected by third- and fourth-generation immunoassays. This is followed by immunoglobulin G antibodies, which will remain throughout the course of the infection (Branson, 2014).

WHO SHOULD BE TESTED?

HIV testing should be undertaken in anyone who has symptoms and signs of acute or chronic HIV infection.

In the healthcare setting, every individual between the ages 13 and 65 should be offered testing once in their lifetime. For

Table 7.1 TESTING TERMINOLOGY

TEST TYPE	DESCRIPTION
Anonymous testing	No identifying information links the patient to the test sample. At the time of testing, the patient is handed a code number, and a matching code number is affixed to the sample. No institutional record of the code is kept. Results are given only verbally because no medical record is created. Treatment cannot be instituted based on this form of testing. Useful for personal informational purposes.
Confidential testing	Test is linked to patient identifiers, and access to results is available for review only by those identified within "need to know" medical standards, including local, state, and national (e.g., CDC) public health agencies.
Screening	Performing an HIV test for all persons in a defined population. For individual patients, screening is most cost-effective through an antibody-based test, the most common of which is the enzyme-linked immunosorbent assay (ELISA).
Opt-in screening	Patient approaches the provider and requests HIV testing.
Opt-out screening	Healthcare provider offers routine HIV testing to all patients unless refused by patient.
Point-of-care or rapid testing	Simplified antibody- or antibody- and antigen-based testing procedure that can give a screening-level result in approximately 20 minutes or less and that can be implemented by a trained non-healthcare individual.
Diagnostic testing	Testing prompted by the presence of clinical signs or symptoms. The term may also refer to the antigen-based confirmation of a positive ELISA. In the United States, the validation test formerly used most often was the western blot analysis. New CDC guidelines now recommend using a fourth-generation HIV Ag/Ab enzyme immunoassay test or HIV RNA test for diagnostic confirmation. The validation testing may also be referred to as *confirmatory testing*.
Targeted testing	Performing an HIV test on persons perceived to be at higher risk, as defined by behavioral, clinical, or demographic characteristics. Formerly the main strategy for HIV testing, it has been supplanted by the recommendation to treat HIV screening as a routine part of medical care.

higher risk groups, repeat testing may be indicated. Healthcare providers should offer yearly testing to at-risk groups such as persons who inject drugs, people who engage in sex with an HIV-positive partner, people who exchange money for sex, MSM, or heterosexual persons who have had one more sex partner since their last HIV test. These individuals should be offered annual testing or more frequently if indicated by their risk factors.

Unless recent HIV test results are immediately available, any person whose blood or body fluid is the source of an occupational exposure for a healthcare provider should be informed of the incident and tested for HIV infection at the time the exposure occurs.

Any person seeking testing or having been diagnosed with any sexually transmitted infection (STI) should be offered HIV testing.

PRE- AND POSTTEST COUNSELING ELEMENTS

PRETEST COUNSELING

According to the CDC's 2006 recommendations for HIV testing in the healthcare setting, written consent and prevention counseling is not required. A meta-analysis of 27 published studies saw that HIV counseling and testing was effective in secondary prevention but not an effective strategy for primary prevention (Weinhardt, 1999). However, randomized controlled studies suggest that the quality and delivery of the counseling affects its efficacy on primary prevention. (Kamb, 1998; Koblin, 2004). As such, HIV testing in itself can offer the opportunity to refer patients for prevention counseling especially in those with high-risk behaviors.

Effective pretest counseling is an interactive process of assessing risk, recognizing specific risk-inducing behaviors, and reviewing risk-reduction strategies. This may be done in a variety of ways—through written material, films, or orally by a variety of trained staff. Of greatest importance is setting a nonjudgmental atmosphere, imparting accurate information in a useful format, offering an opportunity for questions, and maintaining strict confidentiality of personal information.

If deemed to be appropriate, elements of pretest counseling should include the following:

- A functional assessment of the patient's decision-making capacity

- The meaning, sensitivity, and specificity of the test

- The potential ramifications of a positive test result

- A discussion about confidentiality and disclosure of test results by the healthcare providers to public health authorities and by the patient to sexual and/or drug partners

- A frank discussion of risk-reduction behaviors

- Specific instructions about accessing treatment in the event of a positive result

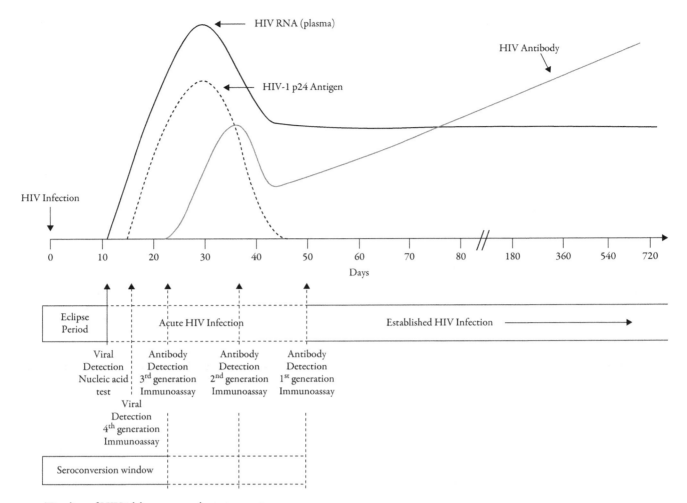

Figure 7.2 Timeline of HIV-1 laboratory markers.   Adapted from Branson 2014.

POSTTEST COUNSELING

Elements of posttest counseling should include the following:

- For a negative result:
  - The validity of the negative result
  - Possible retesting if indicated
  - Reinforcement of transmission reduction behaviors (US Department of Veterans Affairs, 2002)
  - Prevention strategies including PrEP, condom use, safer sex practices, and clean needle and syringe services
- For a positive result:
  - Optimally given during a face-to-face meeting
  - Review of the availability and effectiveness of treatment
  - Reinforcement of disclosure to spouse and/or sexual and/or drug-using partners
  - Reinforcement of transmission reduction behaviors
  - An assessment of any intent to harm self or others

SPECIAL POPULATIONS AND ENVIRONMENTS

BLOOD SUPPLY SCREENING

Since 1990, all persons desiring to donate blood or plasma are required to undergo testing, as are those donating sperm for artificial insemination or tissue or organs for transplantation. The donor is notified only if the specimen tests positive. The laboratory assays used for testing blood, blood products, tissues, and organs have evolved along with those used to screen individuals (and often are the same). However, because the volume of testing is larger, pooled testing using nucleic acid tests is commonly done to improve testing and to possibly detect blood or blood products from acutely infected persons.

PERINATAL SCREENING

HIV screening should be a routine component of prenatal testing and should be performed during the first trimester or at entry into care. Retesting in the third trimester (preferably <36 weeks of gestation) is recommended for women at high risk for HIV exposure, for those who receive healthcare in high-incidence areas, and for those with signs or symptoms consistent with acute HIV infection. Women with undocumented HIV status at the time of labor or delivery should be screened with a point-of-care (POC) HIV test unless they opt out. If a mother's HIV status is unknown postpartum, POC testing of the newborn is recommended (and is legally mandated in many states) as soon as possible so that antiretroviral prophylaxis can be offered to HIV-exposed infants. The mother should be informed that the identification of

HIV antibodies in the newborn indicates that the mother is infected (Branson, 2006).

MSM

MSM have been identified as a population that is at high risk for HIV infection as well as STIs. Disproportionately higher rates of HIV infection are seen within the black and Hispanic population compared to white and Asian MSM, with up to 44% being unaware of their serostatus (CDC, 2009). Due to the high-risk nature of the MSM population, the CDC recommends screening for HIV and syphilis at least annually. In addition, it is recommended to screen for urethral and rectal gonorrhea and chlamydia along with pharyngeal gonorrhea in sexually active patients.

In the 2015 (most current version), CDC Sexually Transmitted Disease (STD) Screening and Treatment Guidelines, it is now recommended to do more frequent STD screening (i.e., for syphilis, gonorrhea, and chlamydia) at 3- to 6-month intervals with MSM, including those with HIV infection, if risk behaviors persist or if they or their sexual partners have multiple partners. Evaluation for HSV-2 infection with type-specific serologic tests also can be considered if infection status is unknown in persons with previously undiagnosed genital tract infection.

TESTING SETTINGS

There are two primary models of HIV testing as per the CDC: routine testing in a standard medical setting and targeted testing in nonclinical settings. Nonclinical settings are sites where medical services are not routinely provided but select diagnostic services are offered, such as HIV testing. Examples of nonclinical settings include mobile testing units, churches, shelters, syringe services programs, and homes. The essential elements for HIV testing are the same for both a standard medical setting and a nonclinical setting. An important principle with HIV testing in a nonclinical setting to link any HIV-positive patients into medical care.

HOME TESTING

Currently, there are only two home HIV tests: the Home Access HIV-1 Test System and the OraQuick In-home HIV test. While these tests seek to empower patients and allow them to seek testing outside of the healthcare settings, the limitations of oral swab testing especially should be emphasized.

The Home Access HIV-1 Test System is a home collection kit that involves pricking the finger to collect a blood sample, sending the sample to a licensed laboratory, and then calling in for results as early as the next business day. This test is anonymous. If the test is positive, a follow-up test is performed by the lab right away, and the results include the follow-up test. The manufacturer provides confidential counseling and referral for treatment. The tests conducted on the blood sample collected at home find infection later after exposure than most lab-based tests using blood from a vein but earlier than tests conducted with oral fluid.

The OraQuick In-Home HIV Test provides rapid results in the home. The testing procedure involves swabbing the gums or mucosal surface for an oral fluid sample and using a kit to test it. Results are available in 20 minutes. Those who test positive need a follow-up test. The manufacturer provides confidential counseling and referral to follow-up testing sites. Because the level of antibody in oral fluid is lower than it is in blood, oral fluid tests detect infection later after exposure than do blood tests. Up to 1 in 12 infected people may test falsely negative with this test.

STRATEGIES TO IMPROVE UPTAKE OF HIV TESTING

HIV screening should be voluntary and undertaken only with the person's knowledge and understanding. Testing is optimally undertaken with the goal of preventing newly acquired infection in those found to be negative and of providing linkage to care in those found to be positive. The knowledge imparted and self-reflection on the part of the person during testing is an essential part of the screening process. Without knowledge of risk reduction for those who are negative and linkage to care for those who are positive, screening is of little benefit to the persons being tested (CDC, 2011). The commonality of concurrent STDs in HIV practices argues against the notion that safer sex practices are promoted through knowledge of one's positive status alone. In the highly structured, technical, reimbursement-driven healthcare environment, a truly successful screening program is not one that is measured by the number of tests performed but, rather, one that takes into account that HIV screening deals with the most elemental and intimate aspects of human existence.

AREAS FOR IMPROVEMENT

Recently published data have demonstrated that, despite current recommendations by various medical organizations including the CDC, an important percentage of at-risk individuals goes untested annually.

In a recent survey, high-risk individuals were anonymously interviewed and tested for HIV infection. Of the MSM population interviewed, 22% had a positive test result, and 8% of people who injected drugs had a positive test result. Of those who were HIV-positive, 8% of MSM and 12% of people who injected drugs were unaware of their infection. Most notably, the majority of people surveyed reported visiting a clinician but fewer than 50% were offered HIV testing.

Clearly, an opportunity for education and increased testing is still present.

RECOMMENDED READING

Centers for Disease Control and Prevention (CDC). 2015 Sexually Transmitted Diseases Treatment Guidelines: Special populations.

January 25, 2017. Available at https:// www.cdc.gov/ std/ tg2015/ specialpops.htm. Accessed July 10, 2018.

Hall HI, Tang T, Espinoza L. Late diagnosis of HIV infection in metropolitan areas of the United States and Puerto Rico. *AIDS Behav.* 2016;20(5):967–972. Available at http:// www.ncbi.nlm.nih.gov/ pubmed/ 26542730.

Kelen GD, Hsieh YH, Rothman RE, et al. Improvements in the continuum of HIV care in an inner-city emergency department. *AIDS.* 2016;30(1):113–120. Available at http:// www.ncbi.nlm.nih.gov/ pubmed/ 26731757.

Truong H. Sentinel surveillance of HIV- 1 transmitted drug resistance, acute infection, and recent infection. *PLoS One.* October 6, 2011;6:e25281.

Weeks BS, Alcamo EL. AIDS: *The Biological Basis.* Sudbury, MA: Jones & Bartlett;2010.

Wejnert, Prejean. Prevalence of missed opportunities for HIV testing among persons unaware of their infection. *JAMA.* 2018;319(24):2555.

REFERENCES

Branson BM, Hansfield HH, Lampe MA, et al. Revised recommendations for HIV testing of adults, adolescents, and pregnant women in health-care settings. CDC MMWR Recommendations and Reports, September 22, 2006. Available at https://www.cdc.gov/mmwr/preview/mmwrhtml/rr5514a1.htm. Accessed July 9, 2018.

Branson BM, Owen SM, Wesolowski LG, et al. Laboratory testing for the diagnosis of HIV infection: updated recommendations. June 27, 2014. Available at https://stacks.cdc.gov/view/cdc/23447. Accessed July 15, 2018.

Centers for Disease Control and Prevention (CDC). Perspectives in disease prevention and health promotion public health service guidelines for counseling and antibody testing to prevent HIV infection and AIDS. August 14, 1987. Available at https://www.cdc.gov/mmwr/preview/mmwrhtml/00015088.htm. Accessed July 10, 2018.

Centers for Disease Control and Prevention (CDC). HIV infection among young black men who have sex with men: Jackson, Mississippi, 2006–2008. February 6, 2009. Available at https://www.cdc.gov/mmwr/preview/mmwrhtml/mm5804a2.htm. Accessed July 18, 2018.

Centers for Disease Control and Prevention (CDC). Vital signs: HIV prevention through care and treatment, November 29, 2011. Available at https://www.cdc.gov/mmwr/preview/mmwrhtml/mm6047a4.htm. Accessed February 25, 2012.

Centers for Disease Control and Prevention (CDC). Implementing HIV testing in nonclinical settings: a guide for HIV testing providers. Published March 2, 2016. Available at https://www.cdc.gov/hiv/pdf/testing/cdc_hiv_implementing_hiv_testing_in_nonclinical_settings.pdf. Accessed July 18, 2018.

Kamb ML, Fishbein M, Douglas JM, et al. Efficacy of risk-reduction counseling to prevent human immunodeficiency virus and sexually transmitted diseases. *JAMA.* 1998;280:1161–1167.

Koblin B, Chesney M, Coates T, et al. Effects of a behavioural intervention to reduce acquisition of HIV infection among men who have sex with men: the EXPLORE randomised controlled study. *Lancet.* 2004;364 (9428):41–50. Available at https://www.ncbi.nlm.nih.gov/pubmed/15234855.

US Department of Veterans Affairs. *The VA Prevention Handbook: A Guide for Clinicians.* Washington, DC: Veterans Health Administration; 2002.

Weinhardt LS, Carey MP, Johnson BT, et al. Effects of HIV counseling and testing on sexual risk behavior: a meta-analytic review of published research, 1985–1997. *Am J Public Health.* 1999;89 (9):1397–1405. Available at https://www.ncbi.nlm.nih.gov/pmc/articles/PMC1508752.

8.

LABORATORY TESTING STRATEGIES DETECTION AND DIAGNOSIS

Jessica A. Meisner and Kevin Alby

CHAPTER GOALS

Upon completion of this chapter, the reader should be able to

- Understand the various laboratory testing methods used for screening and diagnosis of HIV infections.

- Explain how available immunoassays can be used for screening and diagnosing most early and primary HIV infections.

- Discuss when virologic assays should be considered as complementary diagnostics to immunoassays for screening and confirmation of HIV-1 and HIV-2 infections.

- Explain the rationale behind the HIV testing algorithm.

- Describe how HIV infection can be diagnosed in newborns and children younger than age 18 months.

SEROLOGIC TESTING METHODS

LEARNING OBJECTIVE

Explain how available immunoassays can be used for screening and diagnosing most early and primary HIV infections.

WHAT'S NEW?

- Fifth-generation immunoassays are approved for screening and diagnosing HIV infections in the United States.

- These assays detect both antibodies to HIV-1 and HIV-2 and HIV p24 antigen and differentiate between them, thereby allowing earlier detection of acute and primary HIV infections.

KEY POINTS

- Laboratory confirmation of HIV infection is primarily through the detection of HIV antibodies and/or the p24 antigen in an individual.

- The western blot is no longer used as a confirmation test.

- The prevalence of HIV-2 is increasing in the United States, so it is important to use immunoassays approved for

detecting HIV-2 (as well as other non–group M HIV-1 viruses).

- Using the current immunoassays and confirmatory testing, false-positive results are exceedingly rare. However, providers should use clinical judgment when interpreting test results and consider additional follow-up testing when appropriate.

- False-negative immunoassays are also exceedingly rare except for individuals who are early in their infection and have yet to produce HIV antibodies that are detectable by current assays.

- Rapid HIV tests can be useful testing options for settings such as health fairs, nonclinical locations, and other situations in which quickly receiving preliminary test results would be beneficial (e.g., pre- and/or postexposure prophylaxis).

IMMUNOLOGY BEHIND TESTING

The timelines for viremia and antibody seroconversion following initial HIV infection have been well characterized (Fiebig, 2003). Figure 8.1 shows the curves for viral RNA, p24 antigen, and HIV antibody development. Following HIV infection, there is a seroconversion "window" that includes an "eclipse period" and an acute infection period in which an HIV infection may not be detectable by immunological or virologic assays. Although there is no accepted laboratory definition for an acute HIV infection, a current operational definition is the detection of HIV RNA or p24 antigen in the blood before antibodies have formed (Cohen, 2010). In these individuals, nonserologic assays should be used or follow-up serological testing should be performed after several weeks. In addition, it is important to understand that viral kinetics and serologic markers may not always be as accurate with non-clade B subtype infections. Additional testing may be necessary to fully understand what is occurring with regard to these markers (Hackett, 2012; Swenson, 2014).

HISTORY OF TESTING

The first enzyme immunoassay (EIA) was licensed in 1985 (CDC, 1990). HIV EIAs are typically described as being from

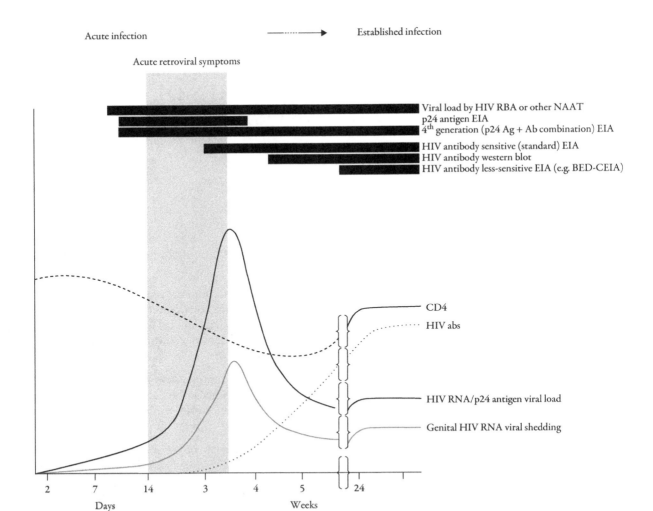

Figure 8.1 Sequence of appearance of laboratory markers for HIV infection.   SOURCE: Branson (2010).

particular "generations," which helps to classify them based on technological advancements throughout the years. These advancements have shortened the detection window significantly, as seen in Figure 8.2. The first-generation EIAs used HIV lysate as an antigen to capture antibodies present in a blood sample but could only detect HIV-1. However, these had a significant number of false positives due to cellular protein contamination (Houn, 1987; Louie, 2006). The second-generation EIAs used recombinant viral proteins or peptides, which limited cellular protein contamination (Chappel,

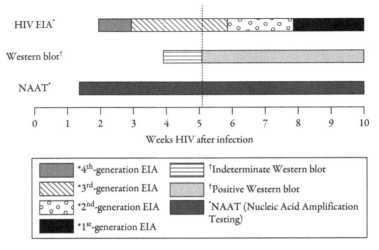

Figure 8.2 Time to detection differences for various generations of EIAs.   SOURCE: Modified from Branson (2007) and Patel (2010); data from Fiebig (2003) and Hecht (2011).

2009). This generation was used to screen blood donations in the 1980s. Third-generation EIAs in the 1990s used a technique that was able to bind both immunoglobulin G (IgG) and IgM antibodies so even further reduced the window period.

The first western blot assay was approved in 1987; thereafter, it was recommended as a confirmatory assay for positive immunoassays (CDC, 1988). A western blot separates the individual proteins of the HIV-1 lysate into bands that allow for capturing antibodies specific to selected HIV antigens in an individual's blood or urine (Healey, 1992). Assays are reported positive if the bands present meet an established criterion; assays are reported as indeterminate if bands are detected, but those detected do not meet the criteria for a positive test (CDC, 1989). Western blots are no longer used for confirmation of positive immunoassays.

ENZYME IMMUNOASSAYS

Enzyme immunoassays are currently the most reliable and cost-effective testing method for most individuals in the United States. Screening and testing for HIV-2 infections has become more common in the United States and require the use of assays that are specifically approved to detect this virus type. HIV-2 assays are essential in locations outside the United States (Hackett, 2012; Swenson, 2014). EIAs are still not completely reliable for screening and diagnostic testing for individuals with acute HIV infections (see the section "Virologic Assays") or for screening and diagnostic testing for infants and newborns (see the section "Alternative Algorithms for Screening and Diagnosing HIV Infections").

Antigen/antibody combination assays are also known as *fourth-generation EIAs*. These assays act as both a third-generation assay and a capture immunoassay, directly detecting the p24 antigen (Weber, 1998). Thus, fourth-generation EIAs reduce the detection window period even further while maintaining the third generation's accuracy (Pandori, 2009; Rosenberg, 2015; Sickinger, 2004). It is important to note that fourth-generation EIAs may have a second window period in some patients (Speers, 2005).

The fifth-generation test detects both the p24 antigen and antibodies but can separate results for HIV-1 p24 antigen, HIV-1 antibody, and HIV-2 antibody. The only fifth-generation test approved by the US Food and Drug Administration (FDA) is the Bio-Rad Bio Plex.

Current FDA-approved HIV antigen/antibody screening tests include:

- Abbott Architect HIV Ag/Ab Combo Assay
- ADVIA Centaur HIV Ag/Ab combo
- Alere Determine HIV-1/2 Ag/Ab combo
- Bio-Rad BioPlex 2200 HIV Ag-Ab
- Bio-Rad GS HIV Combo Ag/Ab EIA
- Ortho VITROS HIV Combo Test on the VITROS 3600 Immunodiagnostic System
- Roche Elecsys HIV combi PT

RAPID HIV TESTS

Rapid HIV tests detect HIV antibodies present in an oral fluid, finger-stick blood, or venipuncture whole blood/plasma sample. Fourth- and fifth-generation EIAs have shorter detection windows compared to the currently available rapid tests, but rapid tests are as accurate and test results are available in less than 30 minutes (Branson, 2007). Individuals with a potential exposure and those with on-going high risk for HIV infection who have negative rapid test results should be counseled to be retested or considered for testing that is more sensitive for detecting acute HIV infections in these situations. There are currently more than 15 rapid HIV tests approved by the FDA. Several of these rapid tests have received Clinical Laboratory Improvement Amendment (CLIA) waivers, making them available for point-of-care testing and screening in settings in which transporting specimens to a laboratory is either not possible or not practical.

Examples of CLIA waived rapid tests include:

- Chembio DPP HIV-1/2
- Chembio SURE CHECK HIV ½ Assay
- Clearview HIV ½ STAT-Pak
- Determine HIV-1/2 Ag/Ab combo test
- INSTI HIV-1/HIV-2 Antibody Test
- OraQuick ADVANCE Rapid HIV-1/2 Antibody Test
- Uni-Gold Recombigen HIV-1/2

When determining whether to use an approved rapid HIV test or EIA testing for screening and/or diagnosing HIV infections, one should consider the setting in which testing will occur, the cost, and the population being tested. Rapid tests generally cost more compared to EIA assays, especially if large numbers of tests are being performed. Rapid testing can be particularly useful for public health testing programs outside of clinical settings, such as during health fairs or at social venues where high-risk individuals may be located. Testing women who are in labor is another situation in which rapid HIV testing may be a more suitable choice for compared to EIAs (Merhi, 2005).

RECOMMENDED READING

Branson BM. The future of HIV testing. *J AIDS*. 2010;55:S102–S105.
Busch MP, Satten GA. Time course of viremia and antibody seroconversion following human immunodeficiency virus exposure. *Am J Med*. 1997;102:117–124.
Centers for Disease Control. Laboratory testing for the diagnosis of HIV infection. 2014. Available at http://www.cdc.gov/hiv/pdf/hivtestingalgorithmrecommendation-final.pdf.
Masciotra S, Luo W, Westheimer E, et al. Performance evaluation of the FDA-approved Determine HIV-1/2 Ag/Ab Combo assay using plasma and whole blood specimens. *J Clin Virol*. 2017;91: 95–100.

VIROLOGIC ASSAYS

LEARNING OBJECTIVE

Discuss when virologic assays should be considered as complementary diagnostics to immunoassays for screening and confirmation of HIV-1 and HIV-2 infections.

KEY POINTS

- Virologic assays should be used in diagnosing acute HIV infections and infections in newborns and infants younger than age 18 months.

- Compared to immunoassays, virologic assays are more expensive and have an increased rate of false-positive results; virologic assays may also be falsely negative in individuals with chronic infections, undetectable viral loads, and non–clade B infections.

- To improve cost-effectiveness, several public health laboratories in the United States are pooling negative immunoassay samples and testing the pooled samples using a nucleic acid amplification test (NAAT). This method increases a screening program's overall accuracy by detecting individuals with acute infections who would have otherwise received a negative test result.

Virologic assays include qualitative and quantitative DNA and RNA assays as well as p24 antigen assays. Fourth- and fifth-generation antigen/antibody combination immunoassays use the HIV p24 core protein as the antigen component and thus can be considered both a serologic and a virologic assay (Weber, 1998). Stand-alone p24 antigen assays are available, however the p24 antigen rapidly becomes undetectable after antibodies develop, thereby limiting the period during which a p24 antigen assay uniquely provides diagnostic information (see Figure 8.1).

Virologic assays should be considered for the following:

- Diagnosing HIV infection in newborns and infants younger than age 18 months
- Diagnosing acute HIV infections in cases in which patients would likely not yet have detectable antibodies (see Figure 8.2)

Because infection transmission risk correlates well with an individual's plasma viral load (Chan, 2012; Quinn, 2000), considerable attention has been given to detecting acute HIV infections (Cohen, 2010; Hecht, 2002; Patel, 2006, 2010; Pilcher, 2005). Individuals acutely infected will typically have relatively high viral loads before seroconverting (Daar, 1991) and are likely unaware of their infection (Hecht, 2002). Studies have shown that recently infected individuals are likely the source of transmission for up to 50% of all new infections (Yerly, 2012).

QUANTITATIVE ASSAYS FOR DETECTING HIV-1 RNA (VIRAL LOAD ASSAYS)

Several commercially available assays reliably quantify HIV-1 RNA in plasma.:

- NGI UltraQual Multiplex PCR Assay for HCV, HIV-1, HIV-2 and HBV
- NucliSens HIV-1 QT bioMérieux, Inc
- Procleix HIV-1/HCV Assay
- UltraQual HIV-1 RT-PCR Assay
- VERSANT HIV-1 RNA 3.0 Assay (bDNA)
- Procleix Ultrio Assay
- Human Immunodeficiency Virus, Type 1 (HIV-1) Reverse Transcription (RT) Polymerase Chain Reaction (PCR) Assay Manufacturer: BioLife Plasma Services, L.P.
- Abbott RealTime HIV-1 Amplification Reagent Kit,
- COBAS AmpliPrep/COBAS TaqMan HIV-1 Test
- Aptima HIV-1 Test

All of these tests quantify plasma HIV-1 RNA within variable dynamic range. These assays detect most HIV-1 subtypes, and, although they have become increasingly effective at detecting non–subtype B infections, there is some variability based on clade variations and each assay's performance characteristics. Both kPCR and RT-PCR assays are proficient at quantitation of many non–clade B strains of HIV-1 (Alvarez, 2015; Elbeik, 2002; Karasi, 2011; Peter, 2004).

Because of the rate of false positives, these quantitative assays must be used with caution as a diagnostic test. In an acute HIV infection, plasma HIV-1 RNA levels are typically very high, whereas levels of false positives tend to be very low (Hecht, 2002).

QUALITATIVE ASSAYS FOR DETECTING HIV-1 RNA

Currently, there is one qualitative virologic assay, frequently referred to as NAAT, approved for use as an aid in the diagnosis of HIV-1 (APTIMA; Gen-Probe, San Diego, CA). This assay can be used to assist with diagnosing an acute HIV infection and as an additional test to confirm an HIV-1 infection when an EIA or a rapid test is repeatedly reactive for HIV-1 antibodies. Qualitative assays are not commonly used because quantitative assays are the preferred detection for HIV RNA.

HIV-2 VIROLOGIC ASSAYS

An approved HIV-2 virologic assay is not currently available in the United States. Although some assays may detect a viral load, caution should be exercised when utilizing these results to monitor response to treatment because underquantification is common when viremia is detected (Campbell-Yesufu, 2011). A number of international laboratories use in-house (or laboratory-developed) HIV-2 viral load assays. Some reference laboratories in the United States maintain in-house qualitative HIV-2 polymerase chain reaction (PCR) assays, but variances between results have been observed, thus limiting their interpretation (Damond, 2011; Gottlieb, 2013). Reference

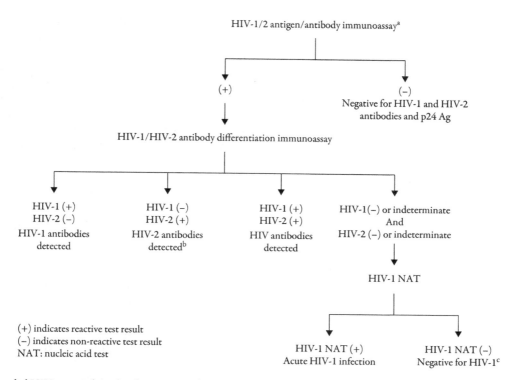

Figure 8.3 Recommended HIV testing algorithm for serum or plasma specimens. Updated testing algorithm for US HIV diagnosis. CDC. 2018. The 2018 Quick reference guide: Recommended laboratory HIV testing algorithm for serum or plasma specimens. January 2018. Available at: https://stacks.cdc.gov/view/cdc/50872. Accessed September 1, 2018.

laboratory resources are available through the US Centers for Disease Control and Prevention (CDC) for public health laboratories evaluating HIV-2–reactive specimens.

ALGORITHMS FOR SCREENING AND DIAGNOSING HIV INFECTIONS

LEARNING OBJECTIVE

Explain the rationale behind the HIV testing algorithm.

WHAT'S NEW?

Because newer serologic and virologic assays are available, new algorithms have replaced the western blot as a confirmatory assay.

KEY POINTS

- The algorithm removes the use of the western blot assay because of its limitations, particularly in confirming acute or recent HIV infections.

- The algorithm recommends using the most sensitive immunoassay (fourth-generation EIA) as a screening test, as well as following any repeatedly positive results with a different immunoassay that can discriminate between HIV-1 and HIV-2.

- Samples with a positive screening assay but negative confirming assay should be tested using a NAAT.

Key factors driving the evolution of the current algorithms are the availability of NAAT and the increasing prevalence of HIV-2 infection in the United States (Owen, 2008). In 2014, an updated testing algorithm was recommended by the CDC and the Association of Public Health Laboratories (APHL) that recommends the use of the most sensitive immunoassays for primary screening along with a confirmatory test that discriminates HIV-1 from HIV-2 after a repeatedly positive screening test (Wesolowski, 2014). In this algorithm, if the confirmatory test is negative, HIV NAAT should be performed. A positive NAAT would be confirmatory for HIV infection. Figure 8.3 shows the recommended HIV testing algorithm (CDC, 2018).

RECOMMENDED READING

Centers for Disease Control and Prevention and Association of Public Health Laboratories. Laboratory Testing for the diagnosis of HIV infection: updated recommendations. Published June 27, 2014. Available at http://dx.doi.org/10.15620/cdc. 23447.

Delaney KP, Wesolowski LG, Owen SM. The evolution of HIV testing continues. *Sex Transm Dis.* 2017;44(12):747–749. doi: 10.1097/OLQ.0000000000000736.

Murphy G, Parry JV. Assays for the detection of recent infections with human immunodeficiency virus type 1. *Eurosurveillance.* 2008;13:4–10.

Rosenberg NE, Pilcher CD, Busch MP, et al. How can we better identify early HIV infections? *Curr Opin HIV AIDS.* 2015;10(1):61–68. doi: 10.1097/COH.0000000000000121.

Wesolowski LG, Parker MM, Delaney KP, Owen SM. Highlights from the 2016 HIV diagnostics conference: the new landscape of HIV testing in laboratories, public health programs and clinical practice. *J Clin Virol.* 2017;91:63–68. doi: 10.1016/j.jcv.2017.01.009.

SCREENING AND DETECTING HIV IN NEWBORNS AND CHILDREN

LEARNING OBJECTIVE

Describe how HIV infection can be diagnosed in newborns and children younger than age 18 months.

WHAT'S NEW?

Virologic assays must be used for detecting HIV infection in newborns and infants younger than 18 months with perinatal and postnatal HIV exposure.

KEY POINTS

- Maternal antibodies passed in utero are detectable in a newborn's blood using current immunoassays, so ruling out HIV infections in newborns requires virologic assay testing.

- DNA- and RNA-based assays show similar performance so either can be used.

- HIV testing should be performed within 48 hours of birth, at 14–21 days, at 1 or 2 months of age, and at 3–6 months of age in infants who are born of HIV-positive women.

- Laboratory confirmation of HIV infection requires that more than one test be positive; infections typically can be diagnosed by the age of 1 month and definitively in almost all children at age 6 months.

Maternal-to-child transmission of HIV infection can occur in utero, at the time of labor and delivery, and through breastfeeding (Kourtis, 2001). Because maternal antibodies passed in utero can be detected in uninfected newborns, immunoassays may be positive in uninfected newborns until 18 months of age. Children aged 18–24 months with perinatal exposure occasionally can have residual maternal antibodies to HIV. Figure 8.4 depicts the HIV RNA levels and antibody response for exposed infants with or without infection.

Thus, when interpreting immunoassay results for an infant, it is important to consider serological window periods after each of these potential exposure events, as well as the presence of maternal antibodies. Non–breastfed children can be considered presumptively uninfected if there is at least one negative HIV-1 antibody test result at 6 months of age or older, and they can be considered definitively uninfected if there are at least two negative HIV antibody tests from separate specimens obtained at age 6 months or older (CDC, 2008). Virologic assays, however, represent the gold standard for diagnostic testing of infants and children younger than 18 months (Read, 2007).

Virologic assays should be performed at birth on infants born to HIV-infected mothers who meet the following criteria: did not receive prenatal care, did not receive antepartum or intrapartum antiretroviral (ARV) drugs, received intrapartum ARV drugs only, initiated antiretroviral therapy (ART) late in pregnancy, diagnosed with acute HIV during pregnancy, had detectable HIV viral load close to delivery, received ARV combination drugs and did not have viral suppression (Momplaisir, 2015).

Additionally, testing should occur at 14–21 days, at 1 or 2 months of age, and at 4–6 months of age. Testing should also be performed 2–4 weeks after cessation of ARV prophylaxis. Some experts also recommend serologic testing to confirm the absence of infection between 12 and 18 months. If any tests are positive, repeat testing is recommended, and the diagnosis of HIV infection can be made based on two separate positive results.

The schematic in Figure 8.4 depicts the timing of positive HIV-1 antibody testing and RNA levels among HIV-exposed infants. The horizontal axis shows infant age in months. The left vertical axis shows mean HIV-1 RNA level on a logarithmic scale and corresponds to the green lines on each graph. The right vertical axis shows the proportion of infants for whom an HIV antibody test would likely return positive and corresponds to the red lines on each graph. The proportion of infants with a positive antibody test mean RNA levels in all panels are approximate. (a) Results for an HIV-exposed infant who is born without HIV infection and remains uninfected throughout breastfeeding. In this case, HIV RNA level remains zero, and maternal HIV antibody fades with time. (b) Results for infants infected before birth, either during the intrauterine period (IU; resulting in a high RNA level immediately after birth) or during the intrapartum period (IP; resulting in a 1- or 2- week delay before viremia is detectable). Maternal HIV antibody is present at birth; although maternal antibody fades with time, endogenous infant antibody production begins in response to infant infection. (c) Results for an HIV- exposed infant who is uninfected at birth but becomes infected at approximately 6 months of age through breastfeeding. HIV RNA is undetectable while the infant is uninfected but rises rapidly within the first few weeks after infection. Maternal antibody is present at birth and begins to fade with time, but infant antibody production begins after infant infection occurs (Ciaranello, 2011).

For surveillance purposes, in non–breastfeeding children age 18 months or younger, definitive exclusion of HIV infection can be based on at least two negative virologic test results from separate specimens, both obtained at age 1 month or younger, and one obtained at age 4 months or older. A presumptive exclusion of HIV infection can be based on two negative virologic tests from separate specimens, both obtained at age 2 weeks or older, and one obtained at age 4 weeks or older. One negative virologic test result obtained at age 8 weeks or older also presumptively excludes HIV infection.

For children with a single positive HIV virologic test result, the presumptive exclusion of HIV infection can be based on two subsequent negative virologic test results with at least one performed at age 8 weeks or older. Definitive exclusion of HIV infection is based on two negative virologic tests with one obtained at age 1 month or older and one obtained at age 4 months or older (CDC, 2008).

Infants born to HIV-2–infected mothers should be tested with HIV-2–specific virologic assays at time points similar to those used for HIV-1 testing. HIV-2 virologic

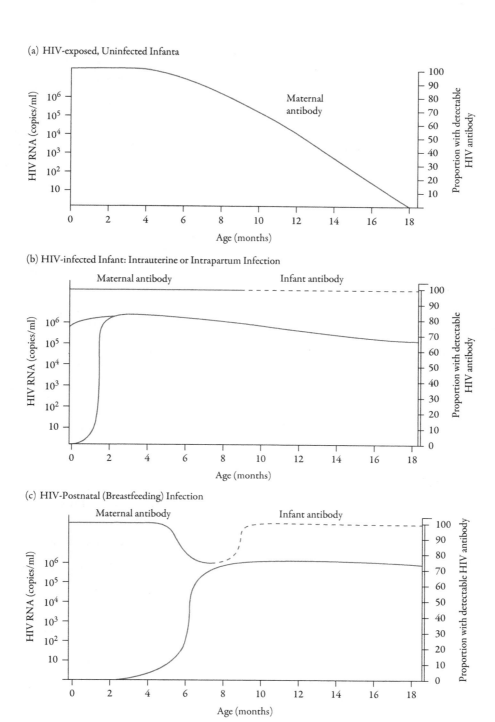

(a) HIV-exposed, Uninfected Infanta

(b) HIV-infected Infant: Intrauterine or Intrapartum Infection

(c) HIV-Postnatal (Breastfeeding) Infection

Figure 8.4 HIV-RNA levels and anti-HIV antibody responses among HIV-exposed infants with and without HIV infection.   Ciaranello, 2011.

assays are not commercially available, but the National Perinatal HIV Hotline (1-888-448-8765) can provide a list of sites that perform this testing (Panel on Treatment of HIV-Infected Pregnant Women and Prevention of Perinatal Transmission, 2011).

TESTING NEWBORNS IN RESOURCE-LIMITED SETTINGS

Access to early infant diagnosis of HIV infection is improving in resource-limited settings (Ciaranello, 2011), but key barriers continue to exist. Virologic assays are generally more expensive than immunoassays, and additional barriers such as accurate specimen collection, transport, and laboratory processing can limit their use in these settings. However, multiple RNA and DNA PCR assays are currently being used, and the use of dried blood spots has decreased the phlebotomy requirements. Dried blood spots may be obtained through a finger or heel stick, are heat stable, are noninfectious, and can be shipped via mail or courier (Ciaranello, 2011).

Because breastfeeding may be recommended for children born in resource-limited settings through the age of

12 months, provided the mother and/or child is receiving ARV prophylaxis, clinical and laboratory monitoring for HIV transmission should take into consideration this ongoing exposure risk (World Health Organization, 2010).

RECOMMENDED READING

Centers for Disease Control and Prevention and Association of Public Health Laboratories. Laboratory testing for the diagnosis of HIV infection: updated recommendations. Published June 27, 2014. Available at http://stacks.cdc.gov/view/cdc/23447. Accessed May 22, 2016.

Jourdain G, Mary JY, Coeur SL, et al. Risk factors for in utero or intrapartum mother-to-child transmission of human immunodeficiency virus type 1 in Thailand. *J Infect Dis.* 2007;196(11):1629–1636. Available at http://www.ncbi.nlm.nih.gov/pubmed/18008246.

Read JS, Committee on Pediatric Aids AAoP. Diagnosis of HIV-1 infection in children younger than 18 months in the United States. *Pediatrics.* 2007;120(6):e1547–1562. Available at http://www.ncbi.nlm.nih.gov/pubmed/18055670.

Wessman MJ, Theilgaard Z, Katzenstein TL. Determination of HIV status of infants born to HIV-infected mothers: a review of the diagnostic methods with special focus on the applicability of p24 antigen testing in developing countries. *Scand J Infect Dis.* 2012;44(3):209–215. Available at http://www.ncbi.nlm.nih.gov/pubmed/22074445.

REFERENCES

Alvarez P, Martin L, Prieto L, et al. HIV-1 variability and viral load technique could lead to false positive HIV-1 detection and to erroneous viral quantification in infected specimens. *J Infect.* 2015;71(3): 368–376. doi: 10.1016/j.jinf.2015.05.011.

Branson BM. State of the art for diagnosis of HIV infection. *Clin Infect Dis.* 2007;45:S221–S225.

Campbell-Yesufu OT, Gandhi RT. Update on human immunodeficiency virus (HIV)-2 infection. *Clin Infect Dis.* 2011;52(6):780–787.

Centers for Disease Control and Prevention (CDC). Serologic testing for antibody to human immunodeficiency virus. *MMWR Morb Mortal Wkly Rep.* 1988;36:509–515.

Centers for Disease Control and Prevention (CDC). Interpretation and use of the Western blot assay for serodiagnosis of human immunodeficiency virus type 1 infections. *MMWR Morb Mortal Wkly Rep.* 1989;38:1–7.

Centers for Disease Control and Prevention (CDC). Update: serologic testing for HIV-1 antibody—The United States, 1988 and 1989. *MMWR Morb Mortal Wkly Rep.* 1990;39:380–383.

Centers for Disease Control and Prevention (CDC). Revised surveillance case definitions for HIV infection among adults, adolescents, and children aged <18 months and for HIV infection and AIDS among children aged 18 months to <13 years—United States, 2008. *MMWR Rec Reports.* 2008;57(RR10):1–8.

Centers for Disease Control and Prevention (CDC). The 2018 Quick reference guide: recommended laboratory HIV testing algorithm for serum or plasma specimens. January 2018. Available at https://stacks.cdc.gov/view/cdc/50872. Accessed September 1, 2018.

Chan DJ. Can HIV-1 Incidence be estimated from plasma viral load and sexual behavior. *Int J STD AIDS.* 2012;23(10):724–728.

Chappel RJ, Dax EM, Wilson KM. Immunoassays for the diagnosis of HIV: meeting future needs by enhancing quality of testing. *Fut Microbiol.* 2009;48:963–982.

Ciaranello AL, Park JE, Ramirez-Avila L, et al. Early infant HIV-1 diagnosis programs in resource-limited settings: opportunities for improved outcomes and more cost-effective interventions. *BMC Medicine.* 2011;9:1–15.

Cohen MS, Gay CL, Busch MP, et al. The detection of acute HIV infection. *J Infect Dis.* 2010;202:S270–S277.

Daar E, Moudgil M, Meyer R, et al. Transient high levels of viremia in patients with primary human immunodeficiency virus type 1 infection. *N Engl J Med.* 1991;324:961–964.

Damond F, Benard C, Jurg Boni M, et al. An international collaboration to standardize HIV-2 viral load assays: results from the 2009 ACHIEV2E quality control study. *J Clin Microbiol.* 2011;49:3491–3497.

Elbeik T, Alvord G, Trichavaroj R, et al. Comparative analysis of HIV-1 viral load assays on subtype quantification: Bayer Versant HIV-1 RNA 3.0 versus Roche Amplicor HIV-1 Monitor Version 1.5. *J AIDS.* 2002;29:330–339.

Fiebig EW, Wright DJ, Rawal BD, et al. Dynamics of HIV viremia and antibody seroconversion in plasma donors: implications for diagnosis and staging of primary HIV infection. *AIDS.* 2003;17:1871–1879.

Gottlieb, GS. Changing HIV epidemics: what HIV-2 can teach us about ending HIV-1. *AIDS.* 2013;27(1):135–137.

Hackett J Jr. Meeting the challenge of HIV diversity: strategies to mitigate the impact of HIV-1 genetic heterogeneity on performance of nucleic acid testing assays. *Clin Lab.* 2012;58(3–4):199–202.

Healey D, Maskill W, Howard T, et al. HIV-1 Western blot: development and assessment of testing to resolve indeterminate reactivity. *AIDS.* 1992;6:629–633.

Hecht F, Busch M, Rawal B, et al. Use of laboratory tests and clinical symptoms for identification of primary HIV infection. *AIDS.* 2002;16:1119–1129.

Hecht F, Wellman R, Busch M, et al. Identifying the early post-HIV antibody seroconversion period. *J Infect Dis.* 2011;204:526–533.

Houn HY, Pappas AA, Walter EM. Status of current clinical tests for human immunodeficiency virus (HIV): applications and limitations. *Ann Clin Lab Sci.* 1987;17:279–285.

Karasi JC, Dziezuk F, Quennery L, et al. High correlation between the Roche COBAS AmpliPrep/COBAS TaqMan HIV-1, v2.0 and the Abbott m2000 RealTime HIV-1 assays for quantification of viral load in HIV-1 B and non-B subtypes. *J Clin Virol.* November 2011;52(3):181–186. doi: 10.1016/j.jcv.2011.07.002.

Kourtis AP, Bulterys M, Nesheim SR, et al. Understanding the timing of HIV transmission from mother to infant. *JAMA.* 2001;285:709–712.

Louie B, Pandori M, Wong E, et al. Use of an acute seroconversion panel to evaluate a third-generation enzyme-linked immunoassay for detection of human immunodeficiency virus-specific antibodies relative to multiple other assays. *J Clin Microbiol.* 2006;44:1856–1858.

Merhi Z, Minkoff H. Rapid HIV screening for women in labor. *Exp Rev Mol Diagnostics.* 2005;5:673–679.

Momplaisir FM, Brady KA, Fekete T, Thompson DR, Diez Roux A, Yehia BR. Time of HIV diagnosis and engagement in prenatal care impact virologic outcomes of pregnant women with HIV. *PLoS One.* 2015;10(7):e0132262. Available at http://www.ncbi.nlm.nih.gov/pubmed/26132142.

Murphy G, Parry JV. Assays for the detection of recent infections with human immunodeficiency virus type 1. *Eurosurveillance.* 2008;13:4–10.

Owen SM, Yang C, Spira T, et al. Alternative algorithms for human immunodeficiency virus infection diagnosis using tests that are licensed in the United States. *J Clin Microbiol.* 2008;46:1588–1595.

Pandori MW, Hackett J Jr, Louie B, et al. Assessment of the ability of a fourth-generation immunoassay for human immunodeficiency virus (HIV) antibody and p24 antigen to detect both acute and recent HIV infections in a high-risk setting. *J Clin Microbiol.* August 2009;47(8):2639–2642. doi: 10.1128/JCM.00119-09. Epub 2009 June 17.

Panel on Treatment of HIV-infected Pregnant Women and Prevention of Perinatal Transmission 2011. Recommendations for use of antiretroviral drugs in pregnancy HIV-1 infected women for maternal health and interventions to reduce perinatal HIV transmission in the United States. 2001.

Patel P, Klausner J, Bacon O, et al. Detection of acute HIV infections in high-risk patients in California. *J AIDS.* 2006;42:75–79.

Patel P, Mackellar D, Simmons P, et al. Detecting acute human immunodeficiency virus infection using 3 different screening immunoassays and nucleic acid amplification testing for human immunodeficiency virus RNA, 2006–2008. *Arch Int Med.* 2010;170:66–74.

Peter JB, Sevall JS. Molecular-based methods for quantifying HIV viral load. *AIDS Patient Care.* 2004;18:75–79.

Pilcher C, Fiscus S, Nguyen T, et al. Detection of acute infections during HIV testing in North Carolina. *NEJM.* 2005;352:1873–1883.

Quinn, TC. Viral load, circumcision and heterosexual transmission. *Hopkins HIV Rep.* 2000;12(3):1,5,11.

Read JS; Committee on Pediatric AIDS. Diagnosis of HIV-1 infection in children younger than 18 months in the United States. *Pediatrics.* 2007;120:e1547–e1562.

Rosenberg NE, Pilcher CD, Busch MP, et al. How can we better identify early HIV infections. *Curr Opin HIV AIDS.* January 2015;10(1): 61–68. doi: 10.1097/COH.0000000000000121.

Sickinger E, Steiler M, Kaufman B, et al. Multicenter evaluation of a new, automated enzyme-linked immunoassay for detection of human immunodeficiency virus-specific antibodies and antigen. *J Clin Microbiol.* 2004;42:21–29.

Speers D, Phillips P, Dyer J. Combination assay detecting both human immunodeficiency virus (HIV) p24 antigen and anti-HIV antibodies opens a second diagnostic window. *J Clin Microbiol.* 2005;43(10):5397–5399. doi:10.1128/JCM.43.10.5397-5399.2005.

Swenson LC, Cobb B, Geretti AM, et al. Comparative performances of HIV-1 RNA load assays at low viral load levels: results of an international collaboration. *J Clin Microbiol.* February 2014;52(2):517–523. doi: 10.1128/JCM.02461-13.

Weber B, Fall EH, Berger A, et al. Reduction of diagnostic window by new fourth-generation immunodeficiency virus screening assays. *J Clin Microbiol.* 1998;36:2235–2239.

Wesolowski LG, Parker MM, Delaney KP, Owen SM. Highlights from the 2016 HIV diagnostics conference: the new landscape of HIV testing in laboratories, public health programs and clinical practice. *J Clin Virol.* 2017;91, 63–68. doi:10.1016/j.jcv.2017.01.009

Yerly S, Hirschel B. Diagnosing acute HIV infection. *Expert Rev Ant Infect Ther.* 2012;10:31–41.

9

THE MEDICAL HISTORY AND PHYSICAL EXAMINATION OF THE PATIENT WITH HIV

Hans P. Schlecht and Daniel J. Skiest

CHAPTER GOAL

Upon completion of this chapter, the reader should be able to
- Describe key elements of the HIV-oriented history and physical.

LEARNING OBJECTIVE

Describe key elements of the HIV-oriented history and physical.

WHAT'S NEW?

This chapter discusses additional questions to pose in the history-taking of patients infected with HIV.

KEY POINTS

- Fostering a strong and empathetic patient–physician relationship is essential for the success of the therapeutic plan.

- A comprehensive understanding of all medical and psychiatric comorbidities, medication history, risk behaviors, and current state of physical and emotional health is fundamental in caring for the HIV-infected individual.

- The physical exam needs to be comprehensive both for the assessment of current complaints and for baseline comparison with future findings.

THE HIV-ORIENTED MEDICAL HISTORY

The initial office or clinic visit with a new HIV-infected patient, either newly diagnosed or chronically infected, represents a unique opportunity to establish an ongoing beneficial relationship. Establishing a trusting provider–patient relationship is an important factor in retention in care and medication adherence and is predictive of future therapeutic success (Doshi, 2015; Flickinger, 2013). It is important for the provider to be supportive and nonjudgmental. If the patient is accompanied by another person (friend, spouse,

partner, relative), do not assume the other person is aware of the HIV diagnosis and other medical history. It is best to ask the patient if he or she wants the person to leave the room and if you can speak freely about "everything" in front of the person.

The following items should be addressed in the initial history of the patient with HIV:

- What is the emotional status of the patient? How is he or she coping with the diagnosis of HIV (especially if newly diagnosed)?

- Has the patient disclosed his or her HIV status to anyone (partner, family member(s), or friends)? Nondisclosure may lead to lower adherence to therapy.

- Which sexual partners (or needle-sharing partners) may have been exposed and are potentially at risk for HIV? Have they been notified and tested? If not, would the patient benefit from assistance in contacting past sexual or needle-sharing partners?

A full history, physical examination, and complete review of systems should be performed during the initial visit (Box 9.1 and Table 9.1). Certain elements of the history, review of systems, and exam that are unique to the HIV-infected patient should be emphasized.

THE MORE THE PATIENT KNOWS, THE BETTER HE OR SHE CAN CARE FOR HIM- OR HERSELF

Knowledge matters, especially for the patient with HIV infection, as studies have demonstrated that patients with more knowledge of their disease status do better over time. Assessing the patient's level of understanding of his or her disease, medications, and risks is essential in the comprehensive care of the individual with HIV. The level of sophistication will obviously be different depending on a person's background, level of education, health literacy, years of infection, and other factors, but any opportunity to emphasize education, understanding, and knowledge of the disease state should be fully embraced. However, lower educational level does not correlate with lower adherence.

- *Chief complaint*

- *HIV history*: date of probable/possible seroconversion, risk factor(s) for transmission, date of initial HIV diagnosis, CD4$^+$ cell count nadir (if known), pretreatment CD4$^+$ cell count and viral load, detailed antiretroviral therapy history as well as medication-related side effects, HLA-B5701 testing, all prior HIV resistance tests (if any)

- *Hospitalization history*

- *Comorbidities*: thorough understanding of all concurrent diseases (dermatological conditions, cancer, diabetes mellitus, hypertension, hyperlipidemia, heart disease, cerebrovascular disease, kidney disease, endocrine disease, liver disease, etc.)

- *Childhood illnesses* (e.g., varicella)

- *Surgical history*: operations, dates, type, reason, outcome, complications

- *Psychiatric history* (concomitant mental health diagnoses are common)

- *Full medication list*, including over-the-counter and herbal supplements and alternative medications

- *Drug allergies* with specific reactions

- *Sexual history*, including specific practices and history of sexually transmitted diseases (STDs), reproductive history, HIV status of partner(s), plans for future pregnancy or adoption, gender of sexual partner(s)

- *Detailed social history*, including domestic status; history of abuse; occupational history; travel history; use of tobacco, ethyl alcohol, and/or recreational drugs; employment status; relationship status; sleep habits; hobbies

- *Animal exposures and pets*

- *Complete family history*, including children (and their HIV status)

- *Complete immunization history*

- *Health maintenance*: last cervical Pap, mammogram, purified protein derivative (PPD) or interferon-γ releasing assay, colonoscopy, anal Pap smear, dual-energy X-ray absorptiometry (DXA) scans

- *Prior healthcare providers*, HIV providers, specialists, and contact information

- *Healthcare proxy*, advance directives, primary contact person in case of emergency, disclosure information

Review of Systems

- *Constitutional*: intentional/unintentional weight change, fever, chills, night sweats, fatigue, malaise

- *Head, eyes, ears, nose, and throat (HEENT)*: hearing changes, ear pain, nasal congestion, sinus pain, hoarseness, sore throat, rhinorrhea, swallowing difficulty, oral lesion, eye pain, swelling, redness, foreign body, discharge, vision changes

- *Cardiovascular*: chest pain, dyspnea, orthopnea, claudication, edema, palpitations

- *Respiratory*: cough, sputum, blood in phlegm, wheezing, smoke exposure

- *Gastrointestinal*: nausea, vomiting, diarrhea, constipation, pain, heartburn, anorexia, dysphagia, hematochezia, melena, flatulence, jaundice

- *Genitourinary*: dysmenorrhea, bleeding, dyspareunia, dysuria, urinary frequency, hematuria, urinary incontinence, urgency, flank pain, urinary flow changes, hesitancy, genital lesion

- *Musculoskeletal*: arthralgias, myalgias, joint swelling, joint stiffness, back pain, neck pain, injury history

- *Skin*: skin lesion, pruritus, hair changes, breast/skin changes, nipple discharge

- *Neurologic*: weakness, numbness, paresthesias, loss of consciousness, syncope, dizziness, headache, coordination changes, recent falls

- *Psychiatric*: anxiety/panic, depression, insomnia, personality changes, delusions, rumination, suicidal ideation, homicidal ideation, hallucinations, social issues, memory changes, violence/abuse history, eating concerns

- *Hematologic*: bruising, bleeding, transfusion history, lymphadenopathy

- *Endocrine*: polyuria, polydipsia, heat or cold intolerance

Do not assume that the patient has a thorough understanding of HIV, even in patients with long-standing infection. Open-ended questions such as the following are recommended: "What do you know about HIV?" "What do you think you can do to maintain your health long term?" The "teach back" method may be useful to demonstrate the patient's level of understanding.

COMMUNICATION IS KEY

Both HIV infection and the treatments for it will impact other medical conditions. For example, many medications used to treat HIV and its comorbid conditions have drug interactions. Thus, it is essential for the HIV provider (if he or she is not the primary care provider) to be in close communication with the patient's primary care provider and other healthcare providers involved in the care of the patient. The medication list should be updated at each visit and after hospitalization. Both the patient and the other healthcare providers should be aware of the potential for drug interactions before prescribing any new medications, including herbal and over-the-counter products.

Table 9.1 PHYSICAL EXAM OF THE HIV-INFECTED PATIENT

BODY ORGAN/ SYSTEM	BE ESPECIALLY ATTENTIVE TO
Vital Signs	Weight loss, body mass index, fat distribution, blood pressure, pulse, respiration rate, temperature Pain/tenderness
General	Body habitus, nutritional status, obvious disabilities
Skin	Rash, seborrheic dermatitis, folliculitis, moles, psoriasis, lichen planus, Kaposi sarcoma lesions Warts, vesicular lesions, dermatophytes, molluscum contagiosum Needle marks
HEENT	Visual acuity Retinal CMV (hemorrhages and exudates) HIV retinopathy (cotton-wool spots) Oral exam: thrush, oral hairy leukoplakia, Kaposi's lesions, gingivitis, aphthous ulcers, chancres, dentition, herpetic lesions, angular cheilitis Thyroid exam
Hemolymphatic	Regional versus generalized lymphadenopathy Splenomegaly
Cardiac	Heart sounds, murmurs, gallop
Pulmonary	Focal or generalized abnormalities
Gastrointestinal	Jaundice, hepatomegaly Abdominal masses Anorectal exam (ulcers, vesicles, chancres, masses, hemorrhoids, warts)
Genitourinary	Ulcers, warts, chancres, herpetic vesicles Gender-specific exam: For women: pelvic exam, cervical exam, cervical Pap smear For men: testicular exam For either: if indicated, anal Pap
Neurologic	Mental status, cognitive function—consider baseline HIV cognitive assessment (e.g., Montreal Cognitive Assessment test) Cranial nerves, motor strength, sensation, gait, vibratory/proprioceptive exam
Psychiatric	Depression screen should be done at baseline (PHQ-2 as a screen or other validated tools) Evidence of self-injury or self-mutilation Evidence of abuse

SENSITIVE, RESPECTFUL, AND NONJUDGMENTAL

HIV providers frequently care for patients with a wide variety of sexual practices, patients who have been victims of abuse, patients who are or have been commercial sex workers, patients who have used intravenous drugs, and individuals in the gay/lesbian/transgender/bisexual communities. Issues of privacy and cultural sensitivity are especially relevant in these encounters. Fostering trust—encouraging truthfulness and openness in the patient–provider relationship—requires special attention to cultivating a nonjudgmental and approachable demeanor. It is important to be sensitive to patients' priorities, be respectful of their individuality, and be aware of their self-perception.

THE HIV-ORIENTED PHYSICAL EXAMINATION

Sir William Osler is credited with the saying, "He who knows syphilis knows medicine." The modern-day equivalent of the old adage is "He who knows HIV knows medicine," because indeed HIV infection and its sequelae can affect every organ system and can present in every clinical way possible. The HIV-oriented exam, therefore, needs to be especially comprehensive, both for the assessment of current complaints and for establishing a baseline to compare with future findings.

CULTURAL COMPETENCY ISSUES

In an increasingly globalized and diverse society, clinicians are caring for patients from very different backgrounds, cultures, and places of origin.

The first step to cultural competency is to avoid generalizations, stereotyping, and assumptions. Not all Latino/ Hispanic individuals necessarily share the same culture. All Muslim patients do not have the same needs. The many different Asian cultures are not interchangeable. Explore each individual's sensitivities, expectations, and perspectives. Build trust by developing understanding, showing curiosity, and respecting limits. Maintaining a patient-centered approach is important. One should ask transgender patients what is their preferred pronoun.

TRADITIONS, BELIEFS, AND FAMILY INVOLVEMENT

Different cultures bring to the table different degrees of family and individual involvement in patient care. Negotiating through a balance of autonomy, informed decision-making, and a culturally acceptable degree of family participation may be fundamental for successful outcomes. Explore beliefs and spirituality, inquire about the use of alternative or non-Western medical approaches, and ask about disease understanding in terms of cultural value systems. Prior experiences and culture of the provider and patient may differ, and thus discussion of expectation is important.

LANGUAGE

Language barriers may account for significant misunderstandings in diagnosis and treatment, as well as errors in medication administration, follow-up, and overall clinical care in minorities and immigrants. Clinicians should explore the language competency and literacy of all patients and proactively check for feedback in terms of understanding and comfort with instructions. Providing HIV care through an independent interpreter (e.g., not a friend or relative) is important in order to ensure understanding by both the provider and the patient.

RECOMMENDED READING

Aberg JA, Gallant JE, Ghanem KG, et al. Primary care guidelines for the management of persons infected with HIV: 2013 update by the HIV Medicine Association of the Infectious Disease Society of America. *Clin Infect Dis*. 2014;58:1–34.

REFERENCES

Doshi RK, Milberg J, Isenberg D, et al. High rates of retention and viral suppression in the US HIV safety net system: HIV care continuum in the Ryan White HIV/AIDS Program, 2011. *Clin Infect Dis*. 2015;60(1):117–125.

Feinberg J, Keeshin S. Management of newly diagnosed HIV infection. *Ann Intern Med*. 2017;167:ITC1–ITC16. doi: 10.7326/AITC201707040.

Flickinger TE, Saha S, Moore RD, Beach MC. Higher quality communication and relationships are associated with improved patient engagement in HIV care. *J Acquir Immune Defic Syndr*. 2013;63(3):362–366z.

10.

INITIAL LABORATORY EVALUATION AND RISK STRATIFICATION OF THE PATIENT WITH HIV

Hans P. Schlecht and Daniel J. Skiest

CHAPTER GOALS

Upon completion of this chapter, the reader should be able to

- describe the core baseline laboratory evaluation of the recently diagnosed HIV-infected patient.

- Describe the core baseline laboratory evaluation of the recently diagnosed HIV-infected patient.

WHAT'S NEW?

Baseline resistance testing is indicated, but integrase resistance is not indicated as it is remains rare.

KEY POINT

- Essential tests include CD4+ count, HIV viral load, HIV resistance assay, and serologic evaluation for certain opportunistic and latent infections.

To adequately understand the stage of disease, risk profile, and management needs of a patient with HIV, a series of laboratory tests must be performed (Table 10.1). The availability and indication for many of these may be influenced by cost considerations, especially in resource-limited settings.

RECOMMENDED READING

Aberg JA, Gallant JE, Ghanem KG, et al. Primary care guidelines for the management of persons infected with HIV: 2013 update by the HIV Medicine Association of the Infectious Disease Society of America. *Clin Infect Dis*. 2014;58:1–34.

US Department of Health and Human Services, Panel on Antiretroviral Guidelines for Adults and Adolescents. Guidelines for the use of antiretroviral agents in HIV-1-infected adults and adolescents. Available at http://www.aidsinfo.nih.gov/ContentFiles/AdultandAdolescentGL.pdf. Accessed July 25, 2018.

ACKNOWLEDGMENTS

The authors thank Jose Martagon Villamil, MD, a contributing author of previous editions for this chapter.

Table 10.1 **BASELINE LABORATORY AND DIAGNOSTIC TESTING FOR THE NEWLY DIAGNOSED HIV-INFECTED PATIENT**

TEST	COMMENTS
HIV antibody testing* (4th generation Ab-Ag testing)	Consider repeating if no prior documentation available.
CD4+ count (absolute and percentage)	Establishes the clinical stage of HIV infection. Identifies the risk of complications and opportunistic infections, as well as the indications for prophylaxis. Initially, monitor every 3–6 months; in clinically stable patients with consistent virologic suppression for 2 years and CD4 300-500 cells/mm^3, monitoring every 12 months is adequate and if CD4 >500 cells/mm^3, monitoring is optional.
HIV RNA level (viral load)	Helps predict the rate of CD4 loss and risk of clinical progression. Consider obtaining two values to establish a firm baseline (viral set point) prior to therapy. Initially obtain 2–8 weeks after starting or changing ART, and then monitor every 3 or 4 months; can increase intervals to 6 months in clinically stable, adherent patients with consistent virologic suppression.

(continued)

Table 10.1 CONTINUED

TEST	COMMENTS
Drug resistance testing	A baseline resistance test should be part of the initial evaluation due to the possibility of transmission of drug-resistant virus (~5–15% in developed countries). Genotypic tests preferred initially, however, screening for integrase strand transfer resistance is generally not recommended as it is rare and not cost effective. May influence the components of ART. May be useful in guiding future antiretroviral choices in the event of treatment failure. Repeat in the event of treatment failure or prior to antiretroviral modification.
Complete blood count with differential	Screen for anemia, thrombocytopenia, or leukopenia. Essential for future comparison during therapy. Eosinophilia may be a clue to parasitic infection, allergy or atopy, eosinophilic folliculitis, drug-related reactions or may reflect the immune dysregulation of untreated HIV. In resource-limited settings, the absolute lymphocyte count may be a surrogate marker for CD4+ count.
Electrolytes and renal function (BUN, creatinine)	Baseline estimated GFR is essential for adequate drug dosing and choice of initial ART. Elevated BUN/Cr may be a clue to HIV-associated nephropathy, in itself an indication for therapy.
Liver function tests (AST, ALT, bilirubin, alkaline phosphatase)	May be a clue to subclinical hepatitis (e.g., viral, drug induced or steatosis). May influence the choice of ART.
Hepatitis serology profile	Screening for hepatitis A, B and C (HAV IgG, HBV sAb, HBVsAg, HBV cAb, HCV Ab) establishes the need for vaccination and the indication for further workup in terms of active coinfection(s). May influence the choice of ART. Repeat HCV screening should be performed for at-risk patients.
Urinalysis	A baseline is needed to assess the effect of ART on kidney function.
Pregnancy test	In women of childbearing potential
Fasting blood glucose Vitamin D level	May influence the choice of ART. Consider especially if other risks for osteopenia (Feinberg, 2017).
Lipid profile	A baseline is needed to assess the effect of ART on these parameters and to assess risk of future cardiovascular event, which is increased in HIV-infected individuals (Nou, 2016; Triant, 2007).
G6PD screen	Establishes the risk of hemolytic anemia with certain medications, including primaquine and dapsone.
HLA-B5701 screen	Establishes the risk of abacavir hypersensitivity syndrome and, if positive, represents a contraindication for its use. Obtain either at baseline or prior to prescribing abacavir.
Toxoplasma serology (IgG)	Identifies need for *Toxoplasma* prophylaxis, when CD4+ count is <100 cells/mm³. If negative, may be an indication for counselling, to avoid infection.
Varicella serology (IgG)	Identifies need for primary vaccination or vaccination against herpes zoster.
Syphilis serology	Screen for latent syphilis. A positive test may indicate further workup and may be an indication for therapy. Screen yearly in patients at risk for STDs with more frequent screening (i.e., every 3–6 months) for those who have multiple or anonymous partners (Panel on Opportunistic Infections in HIV-Infected Adults and Adolescents).
Tuberculosis screening	A baseline tuberculin skin test (PPD) or IGRA is indicated in all HIV-infected individuals without a history of prior positive test or treatment for latent TB. Note that a PPD result ≥5 mm induration is considered reactive in HIV-infected patients. If positive, a chest X-ray should be obtained to rule out active disease along with a careful ROS and exam to rule out extrapulmonary TB.
Sexually transmitted diseases	Screen all women for trichomoniasis initially and annually thereafter. Screen men and women for gonorrhea and chlamydia initially. Screen yearly in patients at risk for STDs. More frequent testing may be indicated depending on exposure history (Workowski, 2015) If positive, this is an indication for treatment and counselling on prevention of STDs.
Cervical Pap smear	Establishes human papillomavirus infection and risk for neoplastic transformation. All HIV-infected women should receive a cervical Pap smear initially and 6-12 months later (see Chapter 12).

Table 10.1 CONTINUED

TEST	COMMENTS
Anal Pap smear	Consider anal Pap testing in HIV-infected men or women with a history of receptive anal intercourse or abnormal cervical Pap and/or genital warts. However, the optimal follow-up of an abnormal anal Pap has not yet been definitively established.
Age-appropriate health care maintenance	Breast cancer and colon cancer screening should follow age-appropriate guidelines. The US Preventive Services Task Force has recommended against routine prostate cancer screening in men using prostate-specific antigen.
DXA	Baseline bone DXA screening for osteoporosis in postmenopausal women and men age 50 years or older. Consider in others at risk (tenofovir disoproxil based regimens)

ART, antiretroviral therapy; BUN, blood urea nitrogen; DXA, densitometry; GFR, glomerular filtration rate; HAV, hepatitis A virus; HBV, hepatitis B virus; HCV, hepatitis C virus; IGRA, interferon-gamma release assay; PPD, purified protein derivative; ROS, review of systems; STD, sexually transmitted diseases; TB, tuberculosis.

REFERENCES

Nou E, Lo J, Grinspoon SK. Inflammation, immune activation, and cardiovascular disease in *HIV. AIDS*. June 19, 2016;30(10): 1495–1509.

Panel on Opportunistic Infections in HIV-Infected Adults and Adolescents. Guidelines for prevention and treatment of opportunistic infections n HIV-infected adults and adolescents. Centers for Disease Control and Prevention, the National Institutes of Health, and the HIV Medicine Association of the Infectious Diseases Society of America. Available at http://aidsinfo.nih.gov. Accessed July 29, 2018.

Triant VA, Lee H, Hadigan C, Grinspoon SK. Increased acute myocardial infarction rates and cardiovascular risk factors among patients with human immunodeficiency virus disease. *J Clin Endocrinol Metab*. 2007;92,2506–2512.

Workowski KA, Bolan GA; Centers for Disease Control and Prevention. Sexually transmitted diseases treatment guidelines, 2015. *MMWR Recomm Rep*. 2015;64(RR-03):1–137.

11.

RECOGNITION OF ACUTE AND ADVANCED HIV INFECTION

Hans P. Schlecht and Daniel J. Skiest

LEARNING OBJECTIVE

Describe the syndrome complexes of acute (primary) and chronic HIV infection, including HIV wasting syndrome.

WHAT'S NEW?

- Updated nutritional guidelines

KEY POINTS

- Acute retroviral syndrome may present with a "mononucleosis-like" illness. It is often missed, especially atypical presentations. A high index of suspicion and a thorough history, including potential sources of exposure, are essential in diagnosing acute retroviral syndrome; however, not all patients will disclose potential risks.

- Most chronically infected individuals are asymptomatic. However, some patients with chronic HIV infection may present with certain clinical and laboratory abnormalities prior to the diagnosis of an opportunistic infection, which should increase suspicion of HIV infection.

- HIV wasting syndrome is infrequently diagnosed in the era antiretroviral therapy (ART). Recognition of HIV wasting is important because it carries adverse prognostic implications. Management includes a multifaceted approach, including ART, lifestyle and nutritional support, appetite stimulation, and possibly hormonal agents.

CLINICAL PRESENTATION OF ACUTE RETROVIRAL INFECTION

The acute retroviral syndrome (or primary HIV infection) has been variously compared to a "mononucleosis-like" syndrome, a "generalized viral illness," a "prolonged flu, "or a "fever–myalgia–rash" syndrome. In one series, in which patients with suspected mononucleosis who had a negative Monospot test underwent HIV testing, the incidence of acute HIV syndrome was 2% (Rosenberg, 1999). The true incidence of acute HIV illness has been difficult to determine accurately. Published series estimate that the incidence of symptomatic, acute retroviral syndrome ranges from 40% to 90% (Kassutto, 2004), depending on the definition and which symptoms are considered attributable to acute HIV infection.

The clinical presentation of acute HIV may include most commonly fever, myalgia, pharyngitis/sore throat, lymphadenopathy, rash, diarrhea, and headache, in various combinations (Table 11.1). The rash tends to be erythematous/maculopapular, nonpruritic, and involves most commonly the trunk and extremities and, occasionally, the face, palms, or soles. A subset of patients may present with aseptic meningitis. In some cases, patients may present with disease severe enough to warrant hospitalization, including hypotension; ulcerative disease of oral, genital, or rectal areas; hemophagocytic syndrome; and, rarely, a full-blown opportunistic infection, including oropharyngeal candidiasis and/or esophagitis, *Pneumocystis* pneumonia, or gastrointestinal cytomegalovirus disease. In one large series, 30% of patients with acute retroviral syndrome presented with atypical signs and symptoms of an acute opportunistic infection (Braun, 2015).

Laboratory abnormalities that may point to acute retroviral illness include thrombocytopenia, leukopenia/lymphopenia, anemia, a positive Monospot in an unexpected setting, and a mild transaminitis, especially if seen in conjunction with the previously discussed symptoms.

The key factor in diagnosing acute HIV infection remains an accurate and thorough history and exam, especially eliciting a suggestive exposure history—for example, risk behaviors including sexual activity or blood-borne exposure (sharing needles in the case of injecting drug use). Patients

Table 11.1 SIGNS AND SYMPTOMS OF ACUTE RETROVIRAL ILLNESS

SIGNS AND SYMPTOMS	APPROXIMATE INCIDENCE (%)
Fever	48–88
Pharyngitis/sore throat	21–51
Lymphadenopathy	36–45
Rash	12–47
Oral ulcers	12–17
Myalgia/arthralgia	28–46
Diarrhea	17–35
Headache	34–44
Hepatosplenomegaly	10–15
Oral/oropharyngeal or vaginal candidiasis	10
Weight loss	21–39
Neurologic syndromes: Aseptic meningitis Peripheral neuropathy Guillain–Barré syndrome	Approximately 10

with concomitant sexually transmitted diseases are more likely to acquire HIV.

When acute HIV illness is suspected, the clinician should keep in mind that the fourth-generation HIV antibody–antigen complex is sensitive in the setting of recently acquired infection because it measures both HIV antibodies and p24 antigen and can detect HIV within 10–14 days of infection. Currently, this is the screening/diagnostic test recommended by the Centers for Disease Control and Prevention (CDC, 2014, 2018). Therefore, if the HIV antibody test is negative or indeterminate, an HIV RNA should be ordered to rule out the presence of replicating virus.

RECOMMENDED READING

Braun DL, Kouyos RD, Balmer B, et al. Frequency and spectrum of unexpected clinical manifestations of primary HIV-1 infection. *Clin Infect Dis.* 2015;61:1013–1021.
Kassutto S, Rosenberg S. Primary HIV type 1 infection. *Clin Infect Dis.* 2004;38:1447–1453.
Quinn TC. Acute primary HIV infection. *JAMA.* 1997;278:58–62.

CLINICAL PRESENTATION OF CHRONIC INFECTION

In 2006, in response to the high number of undiagnosed people living with HIV (~20%) in the United States, the CDC recommended universal voluntary screening for HIV in adults as part of "usual" medical care. Although the number of undiagnosed individuals has declined since then, the CDC estimates that up to 13% of persons infected with HIV in the United States may be unaware of their status (a decrease from 20% in 2003; Branson, 2006).

As a result of increased awareness and testing, the median CD4$^+$ cell count at time of diagnosis has risen in developed countries including the United States; however, a small number of patients still present with manifestations of advanced AIDS at the time of their initial diagnosis (Haines, 2014; Braunstein, 2016). Clinicians should maintain a high index of suspicion in patients with known risk behaviors, and they should screen for HIV at least annually and potentially more frequently for those at high risk (Branson, 2006). Moreover, specific symptoms and signs that suggest chronic HIV infection should prompt testing in the hopes of early diagnosis; these include the following:

- Any sexually transmitted infection
- Oral ulcers/aphthous stomatitis
- Oral hairy leukoplakia
- Oral candidiasis
- Unexplained weight loss
- Unexplained chronic fatigue
- Persistent or difficult-to-control seborrheic dermatitis
- Persistent or difficult-to-control vaginal candidiasis
- Unexplained/persistent fevers
- Herpes zoster/shingles (especially if more than one dermatome or recurrent, and especially in young people)
- Chronic diarrhea
- Persistent night sweats
- Persistent generalized lymphadenopathy
- Severe or difficult-to-control psoriasis
- Chronic or persistent herpes simplex infection of the genital tract or perianal region

Likewise, some laboratory findings may clue the clinician to the possibility of chronic HIV infection:

- Any sexually transmitted infection
- Chronic thrombocytopenia
- Leukopenia
- Anemia of chronic inflammation, especially without an alternative explanation
- Low lipid levels (low cholesterol, high-density lipoprotein [HDL], and low-density lipoprotein [LDL]), with elevated triglycerides; this has been attributed to chronic inflammatory cytokines (Grunfeld, 1992)
- Elevated globulin:albumin ratio, indicating polyclonal gammopathy

- Persistent or intermittent unexplained transaminitis
- Low albumin or prealbumin, especially if wasting is present
- Decreased renal function with proteinuria (HIV nephropathy)

Also, a new diagnosis of certain diseases should prompt an HIV test because their incidence is increased in individuals with HIV:

- Active tuberculosis
- Non-Hodgkin lymphoma or Hodgkin's disease
- Cervical carcinoma in situ
- Listeriosis in an otherwise non–immune-suppressed or pregnant patient
- Extraintestinal salmonellosis
- Recurrent bacterial pneumonia
- Bacteremic pneumococcal pneumonia
- Pelvic inflammatory disease

HIV WASTING SYNDROME

DIAGNOSIS

HIV wasting syndrome is an AIDS-defining condition and is defined as weight loss of greater than 10%, plus either chronic diarrhea or chronic weakness, for more than 30 days in the absence of an alternative explanation.

In 2004, Polsky et al. published an updated definition describing HIV wasting as any one of the following:

- 10% unintentional weight loss over 12 months
- 7.5% unintentional weight loss over 6 months
- 5% body cell mass (BCM) loss within 6 months
- Body mass index (BMI) of less than 20 kg/m^2
- In men: BCM less than 35% body weight and BMI less than 27 kg/m^2
- In women: BCM less than 23% body weight and BMI less than 27 kg/m^2

BCM (defined as fat-free mass without bone mineral mass and extracellular water) can be measured by body composition testing, either through underwater weighing in research settings or, more commonly in clinical practice, total body potassium or bioelectrical impedance analysis. However, this is rarely done in the ART era. In the pre-ART era, wasting was a common AIDS-related presentation, estimated to occur in approximately 20% of patients. Although much less common in the ART era, when present, it can be an important and challenging condition; its presence has been associated with increased morbidity and mortality and more rapid disease progression (Palenicek, 1995).

The cause of HIV wasting is not known, but it is likely multifactorial. Many patients likely have a combination of inadequate caloric intake and an increased rate of metabolism due to increased resting energy expenditure in untreated HIV infection (Macallan, 1995). When wasting is suspected, treatable causes need to be ruled out, especially opportunistic diseases, infectious causes of diarrhea/malabsorption, thyroid dysfunction, malignancy, protein-calorie malnutrition (especially from economic or financial factors), hypogonadism, and psychiatric disease (especially depression). The workup for these should be tailored according to each person's signs and symptoms. In males, measurement of morning serum testosterone (free and total) is recommended, especially if there are signs of hypogonadism. It is important to differentiate wasting from lipodystrophy or lipoatrophy in the setting of ART. Peripheral lipoatrophy due to nucleoside analogs (especially stavudine, didanosine, and zidovudine, which are currently rarely used) can be confused with wasting. However, neither the presence of lipodystrophy nor the use of ART rule out the possibility of wasting.

MANAGEMENT

The management of HIV-associated wasting should include the following (Polsky, 2004):

- Prompt recognition/diagnosis
- Targeted workup for treatable causes
- Commencement of or optimization of ART

Table 11.2 NONPHARMACOLOGIC INTERVENTIONS FOR HIV-ASSOCIATED WASTING

INTERVENTION	COMMENTS
Treatment of underlying causes	Targeted workup according to each patient's clinical presentation. Infectious and opportunistic diseases should be ruled out.
Dietary assessment and counselling	Micronutrient supplementation is recommended (Willig, 2018). Targeted caloric supplementation is encouraged. Swallowing evaluation may be needed in select cases. Alternative routes of feeding may be considered in select cases (nasogastric, gastric or jejunal tubes, and parenteral nutrition). Glutamine replacement (40 g daily in divided doses) and antioxidants may help patients gain weight and body cell mass (Shabert, 1999).
Addressing psychosocial and life stressors	Financial realities may be an important component to malnutrition in indigent, homeless, migrant, or otherwise vulnerable populations. Depression and anxiety may be significant contributors to weight loss.
Exercise	As an adjunct to nutritional support, may improve function, quality of life, and lean body mass.

- Corrective measures for the weight loss, including dietary/nutritional assessment and support, with supplements as needed (Willig, 2018)
- Additional therapeutic interventions as needed in each individual case to target appetite stimulation and weight gain (specifically lean body mass)
- Proactively addressing psychosocial and lifestyle issues, especially depression, substance abuse, financial stressors, and transportation issues

Nonpharmacologic and pharmacologic interventions for HIV-associated wasting are shown in Tables 11.2 and 11.3, respectively.

ACKNOWLEDGMENTS

The authors thank Jose Martagon-Villamil, MD, a contributing author of previous editions for this chapter.

Table 11.3 PHARMACOLOGIC INTERVENTIONS FOR HIV-ASSOCIATED WASTING

INTERVENTION	DOSE	COMMENTS
ANTIRETROVIRAL THERAPY	Specific to each regimen	The most effective regimen with the least side effects (especially GI-related) should be selected for each individual patient, with the goal of maintaining an undetectable viral load. ART should not be thought of as the sole solution to wasting because weight loss and loss of body mass may still occur despite therapy, with or without adequate virologic control.
APPETITE STIMULANTS Megestrol (Megace) Dronabinol (Marinol)	400–800 mg/day 2.5–10 mg twice a day	Both agents are effective for appetite stimulation and modest weight gain in patients with appetite loss. Not effective in patients with normal appetite. Most weight gain is fat (e.g., not lean body mass). Megace (progestin analogue) can be associated with hyperglycemia, diarrhea, rash, adrenal insufficiency, erectile dysfunction, gynecomastia, and, over longer periods of time, hypogonadism. Marinol can cause fatigue and central nervous system side effects, including confusion, dizziness, euphoria, paranoia, somnolence, and anxiety. There is no benefit to the use of both drugs combined. Megesterol and Dronabinol are US Food and Drug Administration (FDA) approved for weight loss in HIV/AIDS.
TESTOSTERONE REPLACEMENT THERAPY Testosterone cypionate injection Testosterone enanthate injection Transdermal patch (Androderm) 1% gel 1.62% gel Subcutaneous pellet implanted at 3- to 6-month intervals Buccal form	100–200 mg IM every two weeks to 50–100 mg weekly 50–400 mg every 2–4 wks 2–6 mg/day Dose varies No specific dosing data in HIV-positive patients	Indicated for males only because there are minimal data for females. Testosterone free and total levels should be checked in the morning due to diurnal variation. If low, testosterone replacement may be indicated, which improves lean body mass, energy, libido, and quality of life. A digital rectal exam and prostate-specific antigen test are recommended at baseline and every 3–6 months. Not a specific FDA-approved indication.
ANABOLIC STEROIDS Oxandrolone Oxymetholone	2.5–20 mg PO in divided doses 2–4 times/day	May have a role in patients with wasting but normal testosterone levels, but they are not more effective than testosterone (Corcoran 1999). Role in women unclear. Weight gain and improved muscle mass. Long-term use may be associated with decrease in HDL, increase in LDL, prostate hypertrophy, hypogonadism, liver dysfunction, mood swings, increased hematocrit, acne, hair loss, sleep apnea, and, over time, increased risk of breast and prostate cancer. Oxandrolone is FDA approved for weight gain in chronic infections.
GROWTH HORMONE THERAPY Recombinant human growth hormone/rHGH (Serostim) Growth Hormone Releasing Factor/Tesamorelin (Egrifta)	35–45 kg: 4 mg SC daily 45–55 kg: 5 mg SC daily >55 kg: 6 mg SC daily	Multiple trials have documented benefits, including weight gain, increase in lean body mass, decrease in fat, and increased quality of life. No significant changes observed beyond 12 weeks of therapy, although weight gain can be maintained. Adverse effects may include edema, myalgia/arthralgia, glucose intolerance, pancreatitis, and carpal tunnel syndrome. Cost issues may be a barrier to use. FDA approved indication.

Table 11.3 CONTINUED

INTERVENTION	DOSE	COMMENTS
Thalidomide	100–200 mg PO daily	Thought to cause weight gain by cytokine modulation, increase in plasma tumor necrosis factor-α levels in HIV-positive patients. Side effects may include neutropenia, rash, peripheral neuropathy, and severe teratogenicity for the fetus, so its use in women of childbearing age mandates reliable contraception. Access is very restricted, requiring extensive documentation from the prescribing physician. Rarely used. Not an FDA-approved indication.
Cannabis	N/A	Not legal in every state. Limited data on efficacy for HIV wasting syndrome. A Cochrane review (2013) failed to show benefit.
Tesamorelin (Egrifta)	2 mg SC qd	Growth hormone-releasing factor analogue. Not an FDA-approved indication. May cause hyperglycemia.

ART, antiretroviral therapy; FDA, US Food and Drug Administration; HDL, high- density lipoprotein; LDL, low-density lipoprotein.

REFERENCES

Branson BM, Handsfield HH, Lampe MA, et al.; Centers for Disease Control and Prevention (CDC). Revised recommendations for HIV testing of adults, adolescents, and pregnant women in health-care settings. *MMWR Recomm Rep.* 2006;55(RR-14):1–17.

Braun DL, Kouyos RD, Balmer B, et al. Frequency and spectrum of unexpected clinical manifestations of primary HIV-1 infection. *Clin Infect Dis.* 2015;61:1013–1021.

Braunstein SL, Robertson MM, Myers J, et al. Increase in CD4+ T-cell count at the time of HIV diagnosis and antiretroviral treatment initiation among persons with HIV in New York City. *J Infect Dis.* 2016;214(11):1682–1686.

Centers for Disease Control and Prevention (CDC) and Association of Public Health Laboratories. Laboratory testing for the diagnosis of HIV infection: updated recommendations. Published June 27, 2014. Available at http://dx.doi.org/10.15620/cdc.23447. Accessed July 29, 2018.

Centers for Disease Control and Prevention (CDC). 2018 Quick reference guide: Recommended laboratory HIV testing algorithm for serum or plasma specimens. Available at https://stacks.cdc.gov/view/cdc/50872. Accessed July 23, 2018.

Corcoran C, Grinspoon S. Treatments for wasting in patients with the acquired immunodeficiency syndrome. *N Engl J Med.* 1999;340:1740–1750.

Grunfeld C, Pang M, Doerrler WT, et al. Lipids, lipoproteins, triglyceride clearance, and cytokines in human immunodeficiency virus infection and the acquired immunodeficiency syndrome. *J Clin Endocrinol Metab.* 1992;74:1045–1052.

Haines CF, Fleishman JA, Yehia BR, et al; HIV Research Network. Increase in CD4 count among new enrollees in HIV care in the modern antiretroviral therapy era. *J AIDS.* 2014;67(1):84–90.

Kassutto S, Rosenberg S. Primary HIV type 1 infection. *Clin Infect Dis.* 2004;38:1447–1453.

Macallan DC, Noble C, Baldwin C et al. Energy expenditure and wasting in human immunodeficiency virus infection. *N Engl J Med.* 1995;333(2):83–88.

Palenicek JP, Graham NM, He YD, et al. Weight loss prior to clinical AIDS as a predictor of survival. Multicenter AIDS Cohort Study Investigators. *J AIDS Hum Retrovirol.* 1995;10(3):366–373.

Polsky B, Kotler D, Steinhart C. Treatment guidelines for HIV-associated wasting. *HIV Clin Trials.* 2004;5:50–61.

Rosenberg E, Caliendo A, Walker B. Acute HIV infection among patients tested for mononucleosis. *N Engl J Med.* 1999;340:969.

Shabert JK, Winslow C, Lacey J, et al. Glutamine-antioxidant supplementation increases body cell mass in AIDS patients with weight loss: a randomized, double-blind controlled trial. *Nutrition.* 1999;15:860–864.

Willig A, Wright L, Galvin TA. Practice Paper of the Academy of Nutrition and Dietetics: nutrition intervention and human immunodeficiency virus infection. *J Acad Nutr Diet.* March 2018;118(3):486–498.

12.

HEALTH MAINTENANCE

*Jonathan Appelbaum, Michelle K. Haas, Christopher Brendemuhl,
Jason V. Baker, and Anthony C. Speights*

CHAPTER GOALS

Upon completion of this chapter, the reader should be able to

- Describe tuberculosis screening indications (including exposure history) and assessment methods (including selection, interpretation, and limitations of screening tests in HIV-infected patients).

- Discuss the importance of routine dental care for HIV-infected patients and essential information to be included in the treating physician's written referral.

- Discuss the prevention of cardiovascular disease before clinical presentation among individuals with HIV infection.

- Discuss family planning and preconception care considerations in serodiscordant and seroconcordant couples living with HIV.

- Discuss the recommended frequency and specimen collection technique for cervical Pap smears in HIV-infected women, the role of human papillomavirus (HPV) testing, and indications for specialist referral for colposcopy.

HIV HEALTHCARE FLOW SHEETS FOR PRIMARY CARE

Most electronic health record (EHR) systems allow for individually designed disease-specific flow sheets. These flow sheets can be designed to address specific centers' care reporting needs. At minimum, flow sheets should include HIV-specific information such as CD4⁺ cell counts, HIV viral loads, HIV drug resistance test results, vaccine records, and healthcare maintenance reports. Ideally, the EHR flow sheet is designed to trigger clinical reminders regarding the need for opportunistic infection prophylaxis and vaccinations or health maintenance screening based on patients' current CD4⁺ cell counts, serologies, age, and sex.

The following sections describe examples of items that should be included in HIV healthcare flow sheets. Flow sheets should be individualized to the healthcare facilities' and providers' needs. Additional guidelines regarding healthcare maintenance recommendations can be found at https://www.idsociety.org/Guidelines/Patient_Care/IDSA_Practice_Guidelines/Infections_By_Organism-28143/HIV/AIDS/Primary_Care_Management_of_HIV-Infected_Patients/.

RECOMMENDED READING

Aberg JA, Gallant JE, Ghanem KG, et al Primary care guidelines for the management of persons infected with HIV: 2013 update by the HIV medicine association of the Infectious Diseases Society of America. *Clin Infect Dis.* January 2014;58(1):e1–34. doi: 10.1093/cid/cit665. Epub November 13, 2013.

TUBERCULOSIS SCREENING AND ASSESSMENT

LEARNING OBJECTIVE

Describe tuberculosis screening indications (including exposure history) and assessment methods (including selection, interpretation, and limitations of screening tests in HIV-infected patients).

WHAT'S NEW?

Interferon-gamma release assays (IGRAs) are an alternative to tuberculin skin tests (TSTs) for detection of *Mycobacterium tuberculosis* infection and are preferred for individuals aged 5 years or older who are Bacillus Calmette–Guérin (BCG) vaccinated.

KEY POINTS

- Due to immunodeficiency, HIV-positive individuals are at increased risk for developing active tuberculosis (TB) disease and thus should be routinely screened for TB.

- HIV-positive individuals also frequently have other indications for TB screening, including contact with persons from areas of the world where there is a high incidence of TB and high-risk exposures in correctional and residential facilities.

- In HIV-positive individuals, TSTs or IGRAs should be performed at the time of initial HIV diagnosis. For persons who are initially TST or IGRA negative, testing should be repeated in those who have experienced improvement in immune function due to antiretroviral therapy (ART). Annual testing may be considered in persons with ongoing or repeated exposure to TB.

- TST responses of 5 mm or larger induration are considered positive in persons with HIV. However, even negative TST or IGRA results may warrant preventive therapy in the setting of high-risk exposures.

- Chest radiography is indicated regardless of TST or IGRA results in HIV-positive individuals with recent exposure to patients with active TB or with a history of symptoms consistent with TB, as well as in any HIV-infected person with a positive test result.

HIV-associated immune compromise is associated with an increased incidence of TB among HIV-infected individuals, with a relative risk of 10 times that of HIV-negative persons (Horsburgh, 2011). As with other opportunistic infections, there has been a substantial decrease in the incidence of TB among persons receiving ART. However, untreated TB is one of the few opportunistic infections transmissible to others and thus has additional public health implications for control and prevention.

HIV-infected individuals are at increased risk for developing active disease by reactivation of untreated latent TB infection (LTBI), at an estimated rate of 3–16% *per year* compared to 5–10% *lifetime* risk in HIV-negative persons with no other risk factors. Once infection with *M. tuberculosis* occurs, there can be rapid progression of newly acquired infection to disease—for example, within the first month following exposure to an infectious person. Similarly, reactivation disease may also progress rapidly, particularly in highly immunocompromised individuals. The majority of HIV-negative individuals infected with TB who develop active disease in the United States were born, previously lived, or traveled for extended periods of time in TB endemic areas. Currently, 8% of individuals with active TB have underlying HIV disease. However, prior to the advent of ART, in the United States, the proportion of individuals with TB who had underlying HIV was nearly 50%. TB outbreaks were identified among individuals living with HIV in US institutional settings, including healthcare facilities, correctional facilities, and homeless shelters. Although transmission in institutional settings in the United States is now rare, there is substantial risk in resource-limited settings in which TB is endemic in the general population. HIV-infected individuals who are employees or volunteers in settings identified as high risk by local health authorities should be advised of their risk of exposure to TB and offered alternate sites of work. HIV-infected healthcare workers who intermittently work or volunteer in TB endemic countries should be similarly advised about their risk. The healthcare provider should help the patient assess the level of risk by evaluating factors such as the prevalence of TB in that community, the precautions against transmission that are in place, and the patient's specific duties in those settings.

HIV-infected individuals, especially those with CD4$^+$ cell counts of less than 200/μL, are more likely to present with extrapulmonary TB, miliary pulmonary disease, and disseminated TB compared to HIV-uninfected persons. Persons with HIV may have active pulmonary TB with normal chest radiographs. Similarly, HIV–TB coinfected patients may present with negative acid-fast bacilli (AFB) sputum in up to 70% of cases (Getahun, 2007). In a high-incidence setting and active case-finding study of patients with culture-positive TB, up to 32% had normal chest radiographs; of those who were AFB smear-negative and had normal chest radiographs, 8% had TB, 5% had CD4$^+$ cell counts of 350/μL or greater, and 10% had CD4$^+$ cell counts of less than 350/μL (Cain, 2010). Nucleic acid amplification tests such as Gene Xpert MTB/RIF are more sensitive than AFB smear, and they may identify up to 70% of smear-negative, culture-positive cases (Boehme, 2010).

INDICATIONS FOR LATENT TUBERCULOSIS INFECTION SCREENING

Many indications for LTBI screening may be present concurrently in HIV-infected patients, which represent conditions with higher risk of development of TB than those without these conditions, or in situations that pose high risks of exposure or recent infection with *M. tuberculosis*. Indications for screening include the following:

- Foreign-born persons, or persons in close contact with recent immigrants or refugees, from regions with high rates of TB (i.e., Africa, Asia, Latin America, Russia, and countries of the former Soviet Union)

- Other medical conditions, such as diabetes mellitus, silicosis, chronic renal failure, being underweight (≤10% below normal), gastrectomy, injection drug use, malignancies (lymphoma, leukemia, and head and neck cancer), cardiac and renal transplantation, or use of immunosuppressive therapies (especially tumor necrosis factor-α inhibitors)

- Persons from situations with a high risk for person-to-person transmission, such as those working or residing in correctional facilities (3% of TB cases in the United States), homeless shelters (6% of TB cases in the United States), and other congregate settings (American Thoracic Society, Centers for Disease Control and Prevention, and Infectious Diseases Society of America, 2005)

- Close contacts of person with active TB, 30–40% of whom will be found to have LBTI, and 1% or 2% of whom will have active disease

- Children born to HIV-infected mothers who have TB or who are at high risk for possible LBTI (e.g., close contacts of persons with active disease)

- Persons previously treated for latent or active TB who are re-exposed to someone with active TB can become reinfected, particularly in hyperendemic settings.

SCREENING TESTS FOR *MYCOBACTERIUM TUBERCULOSIS* INFECTION

Tuberculin Skin Testing

The time-honored method for diagnosis of *M. tuberculosis* infection is the TST, which measures a polycellular delayed-type hypersensitivity response at the site of injection following the administration of purified protein derivative (PPD), an admixture of mycobacterial antigens. The preferred skin test is the intradermal, or Mantoux, method. It is administered by injecting 0.1 mL of 5 tuberculin units (TU) PPD intradermally into the dorsal or volar surface of the forearm. Tests should be read 48–72 hours after test administration, and the diameter of induration transverse to the long axis of the arm should be recorded in millimeters. Multiple puncture tests (i.e., tine test, Heaf test) and PPD strengths of 1 and 250 TU are not sufficiently accurate and should not be used (American Thoracic Society/Centers for Disease Control and Prevention, 2000). Induration of 5 mm or greater in HIV-infected individuals indicates a positive TST. TSTs require two visits to perform and confirm the results of the test and experience in intradermal placement of the test. There is some subjectivity in its interpretation, and false-positive results may occur from exposure to nontuberculous mycobacteria or prior vaccination with *M. bovis* BCG. A positive TST has been shown to be predictive of progression to active TB in HIV-infected individuals, who benefit from preventive therapy with a reduction in TB incidence.

Interferon-γ Release Assays

IGRAs are blood tests that measure interferon-γ (IFN-γ) secreted by sensitized T lymphocytes after exposure to TB-specific antigens ESAT-6 and CFP-10. Two tests are currently approved by the US Food and Drug Administration (FDA) and in use for the detection of *M. tuberculosis* infection: QuantiFERON-TB Gold In-Tube (QFT) and T-SPOT TB test (T-Spot). QFT measures IFN-γ concentration using an enzyme-linked immunosorbent assay (ELISA), whereas the T-Spot enumerates T cells releasing IFN-γ using an ELISPOT assay. QFT requires fresh blood to be incubated for 18–24 hours with plasma separation, ELISA testing, and comparison to negative and positive mitogen control antigens (phytohemagglutinin). T-Spot assays must be done on fresh blood specimens, processed within 12 hours, and incubated overnight. IGRAs require a single visit, are less subjective in interpretation than TSTs, and are more specific for detection of *M. tuberculosis* infection—that is, less cross-reactivity to nontuberculous mycobacteria (except *M. kansasii*, *M. szulgai*, and *M. marinum*) and BCG (Centers for Disease Control and Prevention [CDC], 2010).

Current evidence suggests that IGRAs have higher specificity (92–97%) compared to TSTs (56–95%) (NIH-CDC-HIVMA/IDSA, 2013). TSTs are more likely to identify persons with long-standing cellular immune responses to TB antigens, and IGRAs are more likely to be positive in persons with recent *M. tuberculosis* infection (Horsburgh, 2011). For diagnosis of LTBI, the correlation between TSTs and IGRAs is poor to moderate among persons with HIV infection (Cattamanchi, 2011). For HIV-infected individuals with active TB, in one study, sensitivity was low for both QFT-GIT and TST (63% and 55%, respectively) and was inversely correlated with low CD4$^+$ cell counts (Raby, 2008). In HIV-infected patients at low risk of TB exposure, false-positive tests with QFT have also been reported, suggesting the need to repeat a positive QFT test to confirm the diagnosis of LTBI when patients are at low risk of exposure (Gray, 2012). There have been no definitive comparisons of TSTs and IGRAs for LTBI screening of persons with HIV infection in low-incidence settings.

Either TSTs or IGRAs are appropriate for TB screening among HIV-infected individuals in the United States. Some experts have suggested using both the TST and an IGRA to screen for LTBI, but the predictive value of this approach is not clear, and use of this strategy would be more expensive and more difficult to implement. The routine use of both TSTs and IGRAs to screen for LTBI in the same patient is not recommended in the United States (NIH-CDC-HIVMA/IDSA, 2013).

Testing Frequency

HIV-infected individuals should receive a test for LTBI at the time of initial HIV diagnosis, with repeat testing considered for those who are TST or IGRA negative initially with advanced HIV infection (CD4$^+$ cell counts <200/μL) and who have improvement in immune function due to ART (CD4$^+$ cell counts ≥200/μL). Annual testing may also be considered in those who have ongoing or repeated exposure to TB, such as individuals who travel for extended periods of time to hyperendemic TB settings. Intercurrent testing should be done based on recent exposure to a case of active TB, including repeat testing 8–12 weeks after the initial negative test for TB infection because it may take this long for the TST or IGRA to become positive following infection.

Anergy Testing

HIV-infected patients are at increased risk to have impaired delayed-type hypersensitivity responses to skin test antigens due to decreased CD4$^+$ cell counts and, therefore, to have a compromised ability to react to tuberculin skin testing (i.e., to have cutaneous anergy). Anergy testing has not been helpful in attempting to distinguish false-negative TST results due to anergy from true-negative results. Anergy testing is not recommended for routine use in HIV-infected individuals due to problems with test standardization and reproducibility, the variable risk for TB in the setting of anergy, and the lack of demonstrated benefit of preventive therapy in anergic HIV-infected individuals.

Chest Radiography and Symptom Screening in HIV-Infected Patients

In asymptomatic persons with positive tests for LTBI, chest radiography should be done to exclude active TB. Persons with symptoms of TB, such as cough, fever, and night sweats, should be evaluated for TB regardless of IGRA or skin test results. The absence of these symptoms has a high negative predictive value for excluding active TB (Cain, 2010). Chest radiography should also be considered following recent exposure to a person with active TB regardless of skin test or IGRA results. HIV-infected individuals with pulmonary TB are more likely to exhibit atypical radiological presentations, especially those with low CD4[+] cell counts and, in some cases, normal chest radiographs (Palmieri, 2002).

Preventive Therapy

Preventive therapy is recommended following exposure to persons with active TB, regardless of initial or repeat TST results, or in persons with TST of 5 mm or greater and who have not been treated for active or latent TB and have no clinical evidence of active TB. Preventive therapy should be considered in persons with a history of potential exposure in high-risk settings (as listed previously) regardless of results of testing for LTBI.

For further information on evaluation and treatment of active TB disease, see Chapter 32.

RECOMMENDED READING

Centers for Disease Control and Prevention. Anergy skin testing and preventive therapy for HIV-infected persons: revised recommendations. *MMWR Morb Mortal Wkly Rep.* 1997;46(RR-15):1–12.

ACKNOWLEDGMENTS

This section is an update from the original version authored by David Cohn, MD, in the previous edition.

DENTAL CARE

LEARNING OBJECTIVE

Discuss the importance of routine dental care for HIV-infected patients and essential information to be included in the treating physician's written referral.

WHAT'S NEW?

A large proportion of HIV-infected patients do not receive needed dental and oral care despite the high prevalence of such disorders in this population. Referrals for dental care should include information about the patient's risk for secondary infection and bleeding, infectious status, and current medications.

KEY POINTS

- HIV-infected patients are at increased risk for oral and dental problems due to immunodeficiency, salivary gland dysfunction, substance use, tobacco use, poor oral hygiene, and limited access to dental care.

- Oral cavity problems can undermine the success of ART by exacerbating existing medical, nutritional, and psychosocial problems; compromising adherence to treatment regimens; and diminishing quality of life.

- Providers should include basic oral screening in their routine clinic visits and advocate for routine dental care for patients.

- Referrals for dental care should include information about the patient's risk for secondary infection and bleeding, infectious status, and current medications.

Oral healthcare is an important component of the management of patients with HIV infection. Oral cavity problems can undermine the success of ART by exacerbating existing medical, nutritional, and psychosocial problems; compromising adherence to treatment regimens; and diminishing quality of life (New York State Department of Health AIDS Institute (NYSDOH), 2001).

Oral disease occurs disproportionately in the same individuals most affected by HIV: those of low socioeconomic status, those with limited healthcare access and use of services, and substance users whose attention to personal health and hygiene is often suboptimal (NYSDOH, 2001). They do not receive the dental care they need. In the HIV Cost and Services Utilization Study, which examined a nationally representative sample of persons in HIV care, 35% of patients had no regular source of dental care, 22% had not received dental care in more than 2 years, 25% had not received needed dental care, and 48% had no dental insurance coverage (Freed, 2005).

Significant proportions of HIV-infected patients have HIV-related oral problems such as untreated caries (39%), gum problems (47%), missing teeth (47%), and xerostomia (dry mouth) (37%) (Freed, 2005). HIV-infected patients with advanced immunosuppression also are at risk for serious systemic opportunistic infections and neoplasms, many of which can manifest in the oral cavity. Examples include candidiasis, hairy leukoplakia, Kaposi's sarcoma, and aphthous ulcerations (Bonito, 2001). The presence of oral candidiasis without medical explanation (e.g., recent antibiotics) is most often related to a low CD4 cell number and is considered a marker for cell-mediated immunodeficiency. Deterioration of oral immunologic functions and changes in salivary flow rate and composition also aid in the development of caries and periodontal diseases, including gingivitis, which can progress to serious necrotizing gingivitis and compromise masticatory functions and nutrition (Bonito, 2001). The presence of necrotizing ulcerative periodontitis, a more aggressive form of periodontal disease, should also be considered a sign of severe immune deterioration. It is a rapidly progressing disease, and treatment should be initiated as early as possible.

Thus, oral healthcare should be an integral component of primary healthcare for persons with HIV disease (NYSDOH, 2001). Providers must become familiar with oral conditions that affect HIV-infected persons and include basic oral screening in routine clinic visit exams. Providers also must be aware of and advocate for oral healthcare and dental services in their communities. Finally, providers must educate patients about the importance of good oral hygiene practices and regular dental care (at least twice annually) (NYSDOH, 2001).

When considering referral to a dental specialist, the main issues of concern are the patient's risk for bleeding, risk for infection, and infectiousness. Accordingly, the following information should be provided in dental referrals:

- *Bleeding risk*: Platelet count (platelet count <60,000/mm³ may require platelet transfusion or steroids prior to dental treatment), liver biochemical tests, history of coagulation or other bleeding disorders, history of liver disease, and current hemoglobin (to ascertain risk of anemia should significant bleeding occur)

- *Infection risk*: Total white blood cell count, absolute neutrophil count, CD4⁺ cell count, history of valvular or congenital heart disease, and other medical risks for infection (e.g., active intravenous drug use posing a risk for endocarditis)

- *Antibiotic prophylaxis*: Based on the individual need of each patient, antibiotic prophylaxis may be indicated prior to dental care. The need for antibiotic prophylaxis is not based on CD4 counts, viral load, or AIDS diagnosis. Patients with severe neutropenia (neutrophil count <500/mm³) should be premedicated with antibiotics prior to dental treatment. Otherwise, antibiotic prophylaxis is recommended based on the standard guidelines set forth by the American Heart Association (http://www.aha.org) for the prevention of bacterial endocarditis.

- *Concurrent infections*: Current HIV viral load, chronic active hepatitis B or hepatitis C infections, and contagious respiratory diseases such as active/untreated TB.

All medications also should be detailed to prevent drug interactions or adverse effects if medications will be used or prescribed as part of the dental care.

RECOMMENDED READING

Freed JR, Marcus M, Freed BA, et al. Oral health findings for HIV-infected adult medical patients from the HIV Cost and Services Utilization Study. *J Am Dental Assoc.* 2005;136:1396–1405.

Greenspan JS, Greenspan D, Winkler JR. Diagnosis and management of the oral manifestations of HIV infection and AIDS. *Infect Dis Clin North Am.* 1988;2:373–385.

Integrating HIV Innovating Practices. Implementing oral healthcare into HIV primary care settings curriculum. December 2013. Available at https://careacttarget.org/library/implementing-oral-health-care-hiv-primary-care-settings-curriculum-0. Accessed November 15, 2015.

Lee KC, Tami TA. Otolaryngologic manifestation of HIV disease. In: Cohen PT, Sande MA, Volberding PA, eds. *The AIDS Knowledge Base.* 3rd ed. Philadelphia, PA: Lippincott Williams & Wilkins; 1999:559–575.

CARDIOPROTECTION AND PREVENTION STRATEGIES

LEARNING OBJECTIVE

Discuss the prevention of cardiovascular disease (CVD) before clinical presentation among individuals with HIV infection.

WHAT'S NEW?

Most patients with HIV infection engaged in clinical care are receiving effective treatment with ART. Prevention of HIV-related CVD entails a comprehensive strategy of minimizing toxicity from specific antiretroviral (ARV) medications, traditional risk factor modification through pharmacotherapies (e.g., blood pressure and cholesterol control), lifestyle modification (e.g., smoking cessation and exercise), and, ultimately, integrating anti-inflammatory strategies as they become available.

KEY POINTS

- HIV-related CVD is a consequence of long-term ART exposure, HIV itself, and associated persistent immune activation, as well as a higher prevalence of traditional CVD risk factors.

- The profile of metabolic abnormalities among patients with HIV infection typically includes many of the same criteria of the metabolic syndrome.

- The breadth of current ARV medication choices allows providers and patients to tailor ART regimens and greatly minimize metabolic complications.

- Exercise has anti-inflammatory benefits in addition to its accepted effects on traditional risk factors.

- Future research should focus on defining the optimal use of established CVD prevention treatments, specifically among individuals with HIV infection.

Epidemiologic data suggest that individuals with HIV infection are at increased risk for atherosclerotic CVD events, such as acute myocardial infarction and sudden cardiac death, compared to uninfected persons (Freiberg, 2011; Tseng, 2012). Reasons for this excess risk are complex but appear to involve a greater prevalence of traditional risk factors as well as consequences more directly attributable to ART and HIV itself (Friis-Moller, 2007; SMART Study Group, 2006). Rates of cigarette smoking among HIV-infected persons in the United States are typically approximately twice those in the general population. Pro-atherosclerotic disturbances in blood cholesterol are now well-described consequences of ART use and HIV itself (Riddler, 2003). Data also suggest that HIV infection is associated with greater vascular stiffness and endothelial dysfunction (Baker, 2009; Solages, 2006), which has been linked to future risk for development of hypertension as well as CVD events (e.g., myocardial infarction and heart failure). Finally, HIV-related immune activation and inflammation appear to persist despite effective treatment with ART, and this has consequences for the development of premature CVD (Longenecker, 2016). Despite the unique aspects of CVD risk in the context of HIV infection, traditional CVD risk factor modification should remain the centerpiece of current CVD prevention strategies for patients with HIV infection (Petoumenos, 2014).

CARDIOVASCULAR DISEASE RISK ASSOCIATED WITH SPECIFIC ANTIRETROVIRAL MEDICATIONS

Findings from the randomized, controlled clinical outcomes START (Strategic Timing of Antiretroviral Therapy) trial have demonstrated the clear net clinical benefit of ART treatment for reducing risk for both AIDS and non-AIDS conditions, even at very high CD4+ counts (INSIGHT START Study Group, 2015). Thus, the vast majority of HIV-infected patients will likely spend many decades exposed to ART, when access permits. When considered together with the sentinel finding from the Data collection on Adverse events of anti-HIV Drugs (D:A:D) cohort that risk for myocardial infarction increases with each additional year of ART exposure (with risk largely restricted to protease inhibitors [PIs] and abacavir use), the CVD-related toxicity from specific ARVs has become a key consideration for both primary and secondary CVD prevention (Worm, 2010). Specifically, much (although not all) of the CVD risk associated with ART use has been attributable to changes in blood cholesterol (Friis-Moller, 2007). Thus, choosing ART regimens associated with the most favorable lipid profiles is one common approach to minimizing CVD risk.

Differences in blood lipid profiles are now an important secondary outcome in trials comparing the effectiveness of specific ARVs. First-line ART medications associated with the most favorable lipid profiles include tenofovir and dolutegravir or raltegravir (Quercia, 2015; Tungsiripat, 2010). Conversely, currently used ARVs associated with the most pro-atherogenic lipid changes include atazanavir or darunavir with ritonavir, or elvitegravir with cobicistat (DeJesus, 2012; Quercia, 2015). Finally, controversy remains with respect to whether current abacavir use increases risk for acute myocardial infarction, with numerous epidemiology studies supporting the presence of an abacavir–CVD link (Choi, 2011; Durand, 2011; INSIGHT/SMART and D:A:D Study Investigators, 2008; Martin, 2009; McComsey, 2012; Obel, 2010; Roget, 2013; Worm, 2010; Elion, 2018) and others showing no association (Bedimo, 2011; Cruciani, 2011; Lang, 2010; Ribaudo, 2011).

TRADITIONAL RISK FACTOR MODIFICATION

Hypertension, dyslipidemia, and insulin resistance (or diabetes mellitus) are strong predictors of CVD risk. Targeting these risk factors remains central to any prevention strategy. The consequences of ART toxicity and/or HIV infection itself on increased risk for these conditions are well known. Specifically, persons with ART-treated HIV infection can have a higher prevalence of many of the key features of the metabolic syndrome: elevated blood pressure, elevated triglycerides, low high-density lipoprotein cholesterol (HDL-C), abdominal obesity, insulin resistance, and a pro-inflammatory state. Comprehensive reviews of these data are available elsewhere (e.g., American Heart Association conference proceedings on CVD risk among patients with HIV/AIDS in *Circulation* 2008; 118). The growing use of integrase strand transfer inhibitors (INSTI) as components of first-line ART regimens will likely result in a reduced prevalence of these previously common metabolic abnormalities in the future. However, when present, the treatment strategies and goals of therapy for HIV-infected persons with metabolic abnormalities tend to follow those recommended for the general population.

Historically, the effects of HIV infection on body composition often resulted in low body mass index (BMI) from a loss in lean mass, with additional toxicities from ART in the early era of therapy, resulting in lipodystrophy with losses in subcutaneous fat and accumulation of visceral fat. Toxicities have greatly improved with contemporary ARV medications, and HIV-related wasting is much less common with a high proportion of patients receiving effective ART in the United States. However, data suggest that impaired fasting glucose (>100 mg/dL) and, ultimately, type 2 diabetes mellitus is prevalent among patients with HIV infection and is associated with ART exposure (Betene, 2014). Persons at risk of disorders of glucose metabolism should have their ART regimen tailored to minimize any ARV-related toxicity while still maintaining suppression of HIV replication. Ultimately, although the mechanisms of insulin resistance in the context of HIV infection may have unique features, once present, the application of lifestyle modification and pharmacotherapies (e.g., insulin-sensitizing agents and insulin) in clinical practice is similar to those for uninfected persons.

The dyslipidemia associated with ART-treated HIV infection is characterized both by an increase in pro-atherogenic lipids, including low-density lipoprotein cholesterol (LDL-C) and triglycerides, and by a decline in the anti-atherogenic HDL-C that does not fully reverse with ART (Riddler, 2003). Currently, there are no pharmacologic strategies to raise HDL-C that have been associated with corresponding reductions in clinical risk, and the association between triglycerides and CVD risk (when adjusting for other lipoproteins) is believed to be modest at best. Therefore, although unproven, the lipid-lowering properties of HMG-CoA reductase inhibitors (i.e., "statins") are assumed to be at least as clinically protective in the context of HIV-related dyslipidemia as they are in the general population. When also considering their anti-inflammatory effects, statin therapy may be particularly beneficial in the context of HIV-related CVD—a hypothesis that is currently being testing in the Randomized Trial to Prevent Vascular Events in HIV (REPREIVE) clinical trial. Until data from REPREIVE are available, goal LDL-C targets applied in the management of HIV-positive individuals remain similar to those established for the general population in the third report of the Adult Treatment Panel III (NIH, 2001): (1) less than 100 mg/dL for those with known coronary heart disease or risk equivalent, (2) less than 130 mg/dL for patients with two or more risk factors, and (3) less than 160 mg/dL for those with one or no risk factors.

The Eighth Joint National Committee on the Prevention, Detection, Evaluation and Treatment of High Blood Pressure (James, 2014) defines a normal blood pressure at less than 140/90 mm Hg for persons younger than age 60 years and 150/90 mm Hg for persons aged 60 years or older. Any reading above that is considered hypertension, and the goal of treatment is then to achieve a blood pressure below these parameters, or of less than 140/90 mm Hg among persons with diabetes or chronic kidney disease. Treatment strategies include traditional blood pressure–lowering medications along with lifestyle modifications such as a low-salt diet, weight reduction, physical activity, and/or moderation of alcohol consumption. HIV is not addressed as a special, or high CVD risk, condition in current blood pressure guidelines. However, it is worth noting that the association between lower blood pressure levels and lower CVD risk is present throughout the normotensive range (e.g., systolic blood pressures from 115 to 140 mm Hg). Thus, it follows that if HIV-positive individuals remain at increased CVD risk despite optimizing lipid levels and other traditional risk factors, more aggressive blood pressure goals may be a strategy to study in future clinical trials.

In summary, although some important factors contributing to HIV-related CVD risk are unique to HIV infection and/or ART exposure, strategies that target traditional CVD risk factors remain a highly effective and beneficial prevention approach. For example, smoking cessation or reductions in blood cholesterol levels in middle age (e.g., age ~50 years) may significantly reduce subsequent risk for CVD events during a person's lifetime (Petoumenos, 2014).

CIGARETTE SMOKING

Smoking cessation is a critically important clinical goal for patients with HIV infection, given the broad consequences for CVD, lung disease, cancer, infection risk, and overall higher mortality rates among those who smoke cigarettes. An increasing number of pharmacotherapy aids are now available and are generally believed to be the cornerstone of smoking cessation strategies. Both nicotine replacement therapy and non-nicotine medications (e.g., varenicline) have demonstrated success in clinical trials within the general population, although the durability of smoking cessation may remain a question (Ebber, 2015; Koegelenberg, 2014; Schnoll, 2015). More data are needed to establish effective smoking cessation strategies for persons with HIV infection, for whom unique challenges often exist related to a higher prevalence of socioeconomic barriers, multiple comorbidities, and coadministration of ART. Currently, a simple brief option to effectively start the process of smoking cession in the context of a routine clinic visit entails asking about tobacco use, advising to quit, and referring patients who are receptive to available resources.

LIFESTYLE MODIFICATIONS

Lifestyle factors that are emphasized as potential cardioprevention strategies typically include those related to physical activity, moderation of alcohol intake, smoking cessation, and a healthy diet (e.g., high in fruits and vegetables and low in saturated fats and trans-fatty acids). These factors are also an important component of a broader strategy to counteract obesity and achieve and maintain a desirable weight (e.g., BMI ~19–25 kg/m^2) through caloric restriction and increased energy expenditure. There is also a growing appreciation that psychosocial factors such as depression and anxiety have consequences for CVD risk. Depression is both associated with a physiologic response that may be detrimental for cardiovascular health and may also exacerbate CVD risk through coassociation with unhealthy behaviors. Without question, an emphasis on a healthy lifestyle should be a central component of CVD prevention for patients with HIV infection.

The benefits of exercise may be particularly important for persons with HIV infection. Beyond its role in counteracting obesity, insulin resistance, dyslipidemia, and elevated blood pressure, exercise has anti-inflammatory effects that make it attractive for both preventing and treating HIV-related CVD. This may result from a combination of reducing visceral fat mass (known to be pro-inflammatory) and triggering the release of anti-inflammatory mediators during the exercise event (Gleeson, 2011). Furthermore, beyond CVD, exercise may reduce risk for cancer, dementia, and other end-organ diseases.

CLINICAL QUESTIONS FOR FUTURE RESEARCH

Inflammation is a key factor in the pathogenesis of CVD and a hallmark of HIV infection that persists despite effective treatment with ART. In this context, adjunct anti-inflammatory strategies are needed to improve HIV-related CVD prevention, whether or not they target HIV-specific mechanisms or downregulate inflammatory pathways more broadly. One approach may be to take advantage of the pleiotropic anti-inflammatory properties of traditional CVD medications (e.g., statins). Data from the ongoing randomized, placebo-controlled clinical outcomes trial of pitavastatin (REPREIVE trial) will provide essential information on the absolute and relative CVD benefits of statin therapy at low to moderate LDL-C levels among persons with HIV infection.

In addition to novel pharmacotherapy approaches, an important clinical question is whether individual treatment goals for blood pressure and cholesterol levels should be more aggressive than they are for the general population or whether HIV infection should potentially be approached as a CVD-risk equivalent, analogous to the case that has been made for diabetes. A related question is whether indications for medicines such as aspirin should be expanded for all persons with HIV infection, for whom the antiplatelet and anti-inflammatory properties may be uniquely beneficial, but clinical data from HIV studies are lacking.

Finally, changes in the spectrum of CVD manifestations and the availability of new ARV medications will also be important considerations in managing HIV-related CVD risk in the future. As the armamentarium of ARV agents continues to expand and toxicity improves, ART comparative effectiveness trials will need to include the effects on CVD risk markers, inflammation, and metabolic abnormalities, as well as potential interactions with traditional CVD prevention pharmacotherapies. With reduced ART-related CVD toxicity and improved (and potentially more aggressive) risk factor modification among persons with HIV infection in resource-rich countries, atherosclerotic-related clinical complications may continue to decline. Concurrent with such changes, important questions may arise related to risk for other CVD manifestations such as heart failure, which may increase as a result of preventing clinical myocardial infarctions as well as HIV-associated changes in both systolic and diastolic function (Remick, 2014).

RECOMMENDED READING

Franklin BA, Cushman M. Recent advances in preventive cardiology and lifestyle medicine (a themed series). *Circulation.* 2011;123:2274–2283.

Person TA, Blair SN, Daniels SR, et al. AHA guidelines for primary prevention of cardiovascular disease and stroke: 2002 update. Consensus panel guide to comprehensive risk reduction for adult patients without coronary or other atherosclerotic vascular diseases. *Circulation.* 2002;06:388–391.

Stein JH, Hadigan CM, Brown TT, et al. Prevention strategies for cardiovascular disease in HIV-infected patients: working group 6. *Circulation.* 2008;118(2):e54–e60.

CONTRACEPTION AND PRECONCEPTION CARE

LEARNING OBJECTIVE

Discuss family planning and preconception care considerations in serodiscordant and seroconcordant couples living with HIV.

WHAT'S NEW?

- New recommendations on the use of dolutegravir in women who are currently pregnant and those of childbearing potential have been issued. Updated recommendations for the use of efavirenz (EFV) have also been issued.

- Prior to attempts at conception, maximal viral load suppression should be achieved to decrease the risk of sexual transmission to a partner without HIV and potentially to the infant if conception is achieved.

- In serodiscordant couples who wish to conceive naturally, unprotected (condom-less) intercourse on the day of ovulation, and 2–3 days preceding ovulation may be considered if the person living with HIV (PLWH) is on ART and has maintained sustained viral suppression. This option for conception carries very low risk of transmission to the HIV-negative partner.

- For serodiscordant couples who attempt to conceive naturally through unprotected (condom-less) intercourse

when the PLWH has not maintained sustained viral suppression or their status is unknown, daily use of preexposure prophylaxis (PrEP) is recommended to reduce the risk of HIV transmission to the partner without HIV. Unprotected (condom-less) sex should be limited to days of peak fertility.

- In serodiscordant couples who wish to conceive naturally through unprotected (condom-less) intercourse during peak fertility, it is unclear whether the use of PrEP for the uninfected partner further reduces the risk of sexual transmission when the PLWH has achieved viral suppression.

KEY POINTS

- Healthcare providers need to be proactive in addressing issues related to preconception care and contraception in women living with HIV who are of childbearing age.

- Family planning discussions in women living with HIV should include condoms to prevent transmission of HIV and other sexually transmitted diseases.

- Patients living with HIV should strive to achieve long-term, maximal suppression of viral load prior to attempts at conception. New recommendations have been made to address situations in which maximal suppression has been achieved, has not been achieved, or is unknown in serodiscordant couples.

- HIV infection does not preclude the use of any methods of hormonal contraception; however, providers must make themselves aware of any potential drug–drug interactions between hormonal contraceptive methods and ART.

- Emergency contraception, including emergency contraceptive pills or the copper intrauterine devices (IUDs), may be offered to HIV-infected women when clinically appropriate. Drug–drug interactions must be considered when using hormonal emergency contraception in combination with ART.

Women now account for approximately 30% of the HIV-infected patients in the United States (ACOG, 2015). Because of this, there is continued emphasis placed on family planning and preconception care. The goals of family planning and preconception care are to promote pregnancy planning, reduce unintended pregnancy, and support safer conception and pregnancy for mother, fetus/infant, and partner without HIV. All women of childbearing age who are living with HIV should be offered comprehensive family planning and preconception care as part of routine primary medical care (ACOG, 2015; http://aidsinfo.nih.gov/contentfiles/PerinatalGL.pdf; accessed August 6, 2018).

THE IMPORTANCE OF FAMILY PLANNING AND PRECONCEPTION CARE

It is increasingly important for healthcare providers to be proactive in addressing issues related to preconception care and contraception in persons living with HIV who are of child-bearing age. In areas where ARV drugs are widely available and accessible, HIV has become a chronic disease with life expectancy comparable to that of uninfected persons (van Sighem, 2010), and perinatal transmission rates have been reduced to less than 1% (ACOG, 2015). Fertility desires in women with HIV in many studies show little difference from those in HIV-uninfected women. (Loutfy, 2009; Craft, 2007; Nattabi, 2009; Squires, 2011; Finocchario-Kessler, 2012). In the Women's Interagency HIV Study (WIHS) cohort there was a 150% increase in live birth rates among HIV-infected women in the ART era when compared to the pre-ART era (Sharma, 2007). Studies among women living with HIV suggest that unintended pregnancies are approximately 50% or higher (Massad, 2004; Loutfy, 2009; Craft, 2007) Many pregnancies among women with HIV occur despite use of contraception (Massad, 2004), implying that the pregnancies were unintended and highlighting the importance of adequate and accurate counseling about use of effective birth control. Women living with HIV express the desire to talk about reproductive plans with their healthcare providers; however, data suggest that such counseling does not often occur until after conception (Squires, 2011; Finorcchario-Kessler, 2010; Panozzo, 2003).

COUNSELING AND ASSESSMENT ABOUT CHILDBEARING AND CONTRACEPTION

Because they may change over time, childbearing desires and intentions, including desired timing of pregnancy, should be assessed during the initial evaluation and at intervals throughout the course of care. A comprehensive HIV, medical, and ob/gyn history and understanding of patient goals are important areas on which to focus counseling and assist in decision-making. Women who wish to prevent or delay pregnancy should receive information about contraceptive options, their efficacy, adverse effects, and other advantages or disadvantages, including noncontraceptive benefits. Women who wish to conceive should be given information about risk, rates, and prevention of perinatal transmission and the potential effects of HIV or its treatment on pregnancy course and outcomes. Safer sex practices, including condom use, should be discussed and reinforced both in women who desire to prevent or delay pregnancy and in those wishing to conceive to reduce HIV transmission or superinfection, as well as to prevent transmission and acquisition of other sexually transmitted infections (STIs). A meta-analysis by Weller et al. demonstrated an 80% reduction in the transmission risk of HIV through consistent use of male condoms alone in serodiscordant couples (ACOG, 2015). Also, for couples in serodiscordant relationships, the PLWH should be counseled about the benefits of ART in reducing HIV transmission (Cohen, 2011). Disclosure and/or knowledge of HIV status for both partners is particularly important when conception is planned and should be encouraged and supported. It is also important to reinforce with patients that there may be legal ramifications for nondisclosure in certain jurisdictions.

Knowledge of the disclosure laws in your area is suggested for review with patients during counseling sessions.

CARE FOR WOMEN WISHING TO CONCEIVE

Interventions for women who wish to conceive include the following:

- Overall health should be optimized with attention to standard primary care and management of chronic diseases, as well as treatment of drug and alcohol abuse.

- Benefits of smoking cession and the elimination of other drugs and alcohol for mother and developing fetus should be reviewed and referrals to cessation services should be offered.

- All current medications, including prescription, over-the-counter, and complementary/alternative medications should be reviewed, and potential adverse effects associated with use of these drugs in pregnancy should be assessed.

- The need to initiate or modify an ART regimen should be evaluated for all women living with HIV prior to conception. For women on ART, a stable, maximally suppressed maternal viral load should be achieved prior to conception. The choice of ART regimen should take into account current adult treatment guidelines, what is known about the use of specific drugs in pregnancy, and the risk of teratogenicity or other adverse effects. The current guidelines for ART management during conception and the prenatal period can be found at http://aidsinfo.nih.gov/contentfiles/lvguidelines/PerinatalGL.pdf.

- Both partners should be screened for genital tract infections, and these should be treated if present. Genital tract inflammation is associated with genital tract shedding of HIV, even in the setting of fully suppressed HIV viral load, and may additionally increase plasma viremia (Johnson and Lewis, 2008).

- Immunizations should be reviewed and updated as indicated, and folic acid supplementation should be started.

- Education on the risks of breastfeeding and potential transmission of the HIV virus to the infant should be discussed. It is currently recommended that women living with HIV in the United States not breastfeed their infants due to the availability of sustainable and safe formula alternatives.

Dolutegravir

Data from an ongoing NIH observational study in Botswana has identified neural tube defects in 4 of 426 infants whose mothers initiated dolutegravir (DTG) use prior to becoming pregnant and were still receiving it at conception (World Health Organization [WHO], 2018).

The same study provided data that, of 116 women started on DTG-based regimens in the first trimester, no neural tube defects were identified. Similar findings were noted in 396 women who began a first-trimester EFV-based regimen (Zash, 2017).

In May of 2018, the US Department of Health and Human Services (USDHHS) updated its recommendations on the use of DTG in pregnant women and those of childbearing age. A summary of the recommendations is noted here (http://aidsinfo.nih.gov/contentfiles/PerinatalGL.pdf, 2018).

1. In women of childbearing age who are not pregnant, it is recommended that providers document a negative pregnancy test prior to starting DTG.

2. Women living with HIV who are currently being treated with DTG (or wish to initiate its use) should be counseled on the potential risk of neural tube defects when DTG is taken in approximation to conception. These defects occur within 6 weeks of the last menstrual period (LMP) or within 28 days of conception.

3. Patients should speak to their care provider if they are currently pregnant, within 8 weeks of their LMP, and still taking a DTG-containing regimen about the potential risks and benefits of their regimen. Switching to a regimen without DTG may be considered if other treatment options are available.

4. Pregnant women living with HIV who are 8 weeks or more from their LMP may initiate new therapy with DTG or continue a current DTG-containing regimen. Stopping a DTG-containing regimen after formation of the neural tube is unlikely to show added benefit. As well, changes in the regimen during pregnancy could potentially lead to viremia and transmission of the virus to the infant.

5. Based on data currently available, it is unclear if DTG is the only INSTI that can cause neural tube defects.

6. HIV providers are encouraged to report all DTG exposures in pregnant women to the Antiretroviral Pregnancy Registry.

7. A Perinatal HIV/AIDS Hotline has been setup for additional inquiries at 888-448-8765.

For more details on these recommendations, a table summary of the recommendations, and detailed treatment alternatives, please refer to the original article or most recent DHHS guidelines. (https://aidsinfo.nih.gov/news/2109/recommendations-regarding-the-use-of-dolutegravir-in-adults-and-adolescents-with-hiv-who-are-pregnant-or-of-child-bearing-potential).

Efavirenz

Animal models have suggested an increased risk of neural tube defects with the use of EFV. Prospective follow-up trials have not detected an increased risk when EFV is used in the first trimester of pregnancy (ACOG, 2016). In prior updates to the USDHHS guidelines, the use of EFV prior to 8 weeks of pregnancy was not recommended due to the perceived risk of neural tube defects. Newer data from the Antiretroviral Pregnancy Registry include defects in 29 of 990 first-trimester exposures to the drug (2.4%, 95% CI 1.4, 3.3). The same data revealed defects in 3 of 190 with late exposure (1.6%, 95% CI 0.3, 4.6. (Antiretroviral Pregnancy Registry [APR], 2017). Current data on first-trimester exposures have been enough to rule out a twofold increase neural tube defects with use of the drug (http://aidsinfo.nih.gov/contentfiles/lvguidelines/PerinatalGL.pdf. 2018). This has led to the USDHHS lifting its restriction on the use of EFV prior to 8 weeks gestation. This decision is in line with both the World Health Organization (WHO) and British HIV Association recommendations. It is also recommended that women who are tolerating EFV well and have suppressed viral loads continue its use throughout their pregnancy. It is of note that the caution remains in the package insert of the product.

HIV SEROCONCORDANT COUPLES

In couples where both partners are HIV-positive, a crucial aspect of the reproductive effort is ensuring that both partners have optimized their individual health. This should be accomplished from both the general and HIV perspective. This includes the aforementioned visits to the primary care provider, gynecologist, and HIV specialist for the female partner and evaluation by a primary care provider and HIV specialist for the male partner. In both cases, sustained optimal viral suppression through ART is critical. Each partner should be evaluated and treated for STIs, because their presence can cause inflammation in the genital tract which can lead to shedding of the virus even when the plasma viral load is undetectable (http://aidsinfo.nih.gov/contentfiles/lvguidelines/PerinatalGL.pdf.). Unprotected intercourse should be timed to coincide with ovulation.

A semen analysis should be strongly considered for any HIV-infected male partner prior to attempting conception. Semen abnormalities have been noted in male patients living with HIV. These include motility abnormalities, low sperm count, low volume of ejaculate, and abnormal morphology (Cardona-Maya, 2009). These abnormalities are thought to arise from ART use and/or as a consequence of viral exposure itself. Early detection of semen abnormalities can identify potential infertility issues and thus limit the risk of viral mutation from unprotected intercourse.

Along with discussions aimed at identifying potential fetal risks and benefits during pregnancy, it is also important to counsel patients on psychosocial issues. While there have been advances to allow couples to conceive with significantly lower risk of superinfection or viral mutation, other issues remain. Specifically, although ART has significantly extended life expectancy in HIV-infected patients, it is unclear how well that correlates to life expectancy in the uninfected. Medication adherence, genetics, and other factors may still cause the loss of one or both HIV-infected parents prior to the child becoming an adult (American Society for Reproductive Medicine [ASRM], 2015). This in and of itself is not enough to counsel against conception but should be a part of conversations on the risk and benefits of conception in HIV-positive parents.

HIV SERODISCORDANT COUPLES

In cases where the female partner is living with HIV and is not virologically suppressed, it is advised that artificial insemination is the safest route of conception. This may be achieved through consultation with a physician, or the patient may choose to inseminate herself during her ovulatory window.

In cases where the male partner is living with HIV, consultation with a reproductive health specialist may be beneficial in identifying the options available to the couple. As previously mentioned, a semen analysis is recommended for HIV-affected males prior to attempts at conception to evaluate for abnormalities. The safest option for conception is insemination with a donor sperm. If this method is unacceptable or undesirable, techniques such as intrauterine insemination (IUI) or in-vitro fertilization (IVF) with intracytoplasmic sperm injection (ICSI) utilizing sperm that have gone through preparatory techniques may be a suitable alternative (ASRM, 2015; http://aidsinfo.nih.gov/contentfiles/lvguidelines/PerinatalGL.pdf). Each of these options provides an excellent chance for fertility, with low risk of seroconversion of the mother and fetus. Although ART-related options greatly reduce or eliminate HIV transmission risk between serodiscordant partners, many couples desire more natural options to conceive.

In couples where one partner is HIV-negative and natural conception is desired, the goal is to achieve pregnancy while minimizing the risk of HIV transmission to the unaffected partner and newborn. It is estimated that the risk of transmission to a non-HIV partner is approximately 1 in 500–1,000 episodes of unprotected intercourse. The risk depends on the viral load of the partner with HIV (Mandelbrot, 1997). In light of this, the HIV-affected partner should receive ART to achieve sustained, maximal viral suppression prior to attempting conception (http://aidsinfo.nih.gov/contentfiles/lvguidelines/PerinatalGL.pdf).

The PARTNERS 1 trial was conducted to investigate HIV transmission rates in serodiscordant couples (both heterosexual and MSM) when maximal viral suppression with ART was achieved in the partner living with HIV. A total of 1,166 couples recruited into the trial practiced condomless sex. At the end of 1.3 years, no cases of transmission of HIV to the unaffected partner were demonstrated (Rodger, 2016; http://aidsinfo.nih.gov/contentfiles/lvguidelines/PerinatalGL.pdf). Similar results were found in a study of serodiscordant couples attempting to conceive via natural means. The study included 161 couples. Of the couples attempting to conceive, 144 were successful; 107 babies were born, and no cases of

vertical transmission or transmission of HIV to the uninfected partner were noted (http://aidsinfo.nih.gov/contentfiles/lvguidelines/PerinatalGL.pdf; Del Romero, 2016).

Based on the results of these trials several new recommendations have been made in regard to natural conception between serodiscordant partners. They are summarized here:

1. In serodiscordant couples who wish to conceive naturally, unprotected (condomless) intercourse in the peri-ovulatory period (2–3 days preceding ovulation) and the day of ovulation may be considered if the PLWH is on ART and has maintained sustained viral suppression. This option for conception carries very low risk of transmission to the HIV-negative partner.

2. In serodiscordant couples who wish to conceive naturally through unprotected (condomless) intercourse when the PLWH has not maintained sustained viral suppression or their status is unknown, daily use of PrEP is recommended to reduce the risk of HIV transmission to the partner without HIV. Unprotected (condomless) sex should be limited to days of peak fertility.

3. In serodiscordant couples who wish to conceive naturally through unprotected (condomless) intercourse during peak fertility, it is unclear whether the use of PrEP for the uninfected partner further reduces the risk of sexual transmission when the PLWH has achieved viral suppression.

Providers may present the optional use of ovulation kits to couples in order to better predict peak fertility and assist in timing of unprotected intercourse.

In serodiscordant couples who elect to use PrEP during the conception period, the CDC recommends that the partner without HIV begin treatment with daily combination tenofovir/emtricitabine 1 month prior to attempting conception and continue for 1 month beyond attempted conception (http://aidsinfo.nih.gov/contentfiles/lvguidelines/PerinatalGL.pdf). As in patients who are using PrEP for routine HIV prophylaxis, baseline HIV and pregnancy testing should be drawn and repeated at 3-month intervals and renal function at baseline and 6-month intervals (http://aidsinfo.nih.gov/contentfiles/lvguidelines/PerinatalGL.pdf).

CARE FOR WOMEN WISHING TO PREVENT OR DELAY PREGNANCY

In 2014, an expert panel from the WHO reviewed the evidence on currently available methods of hormonal contraception and reaffirmed their 2009 statement that women living with HIV can potentially use all existing hormonal contraceptive methods without restriction (WHO, 2014). However, special care must still be taken to address any potential drug–drug interactions and alterations in pharmacokinetics that may occur when ART and contraceptives are used together.

The WHO and the CDC state that with use of methods involving spermicides containing nonoxynol-9, risk generally outweighs advantages of the method because of potential disruption of cervical mucosa, which may increase viral shedding and HIV transmission to uninfected partners. Both the copper IUD (Cu-IUD) and levonorgestrel-containing IUD can be initiated or continued in women living with HIV who are clinically doing well on ART therapy. Pharmacokinetic interactions between hormonal contraceptives (primarily studied with combined estrogen-progestin oral contraceptives) and some PIs and non-nucleoside reverse transcriptase inhibitors (NNRTIs) may modify steroid levels and potentially decrease contraceptive effectiveness or increase risk of adverse effects, although the true clinical effect is not clear; an additional or alternative contraceptive method is generally advised if hormonal contraception is considered (El-Ibiary, 2008; Vogler, 2010; Cohn, 2007; http://aidsinfo.nih.gov/contentfiles/PerinatalGL.pdf, 2018). Specifically, women on ritonavir-based PI regimens should be placed on an additional or alternative method of contraception if using ART with combination hormonal contraceptives. These methods include patches, pills, rings, or progestin-only pills. Similarly, in patients taking EFV, an additional barrier contraceptive or alternative regimen can be considered in women using etonogestrel or levonorgestrel contraceptive implants (Patel, 2015; http://aidsinfo.nih.gov/contentfiles/PerinatalGL.pdf, 2018). For a detailed list of contraceptive drugs and their potential interactions with ARVs, please see the table labeled "Drug Interactions Between Antiretroviral Agents and Hormonal Contraceptives" in the most current USDHHS Recommendations for Use of Antiretroviral Drug in Pregnant HIV-1 Infected Women for Maternal Health and Interventions to Reduce Perinatal HIV Transmission in the United States.

Most studies have found no association between the use of hormonal contraception and HIV disease progression (Morrison, 2011; Polis, 2010: Stringer, 2009). There are conflicting data on the role of hormonal contraception in HIV susceptibility or infectiousness. A secondary analysis of data from a large prevention trial found an increased risk of HIV seroconversion (both transmission and acquisition) associated with hormonal contraception (primarily depot medroxyprogesterone acetate) among more than 3,700 serodiscordant African couples (Heffron, 2012). A WHO expert group reviewed all available evidence and concluded that the data were not sufficient to warrant a change in the current guidance on the use of the hormonal contraception for women at risk of HIV infection (WHO, 2012).

Emergency contraception, including emergency oral contraceptives or the copper IUD, may be offered to HIV-infected women if clinically appropriate. When oral contraceptives (either combination or levonorgestrel only) are used with ARVs, the potential for drug interactions seems to be similar to when they are used for routine contraception (http://aidsinfo.nih.gov/contentfiles/lvguidelines/PerinatalGL.pdf).

Currently, there are no data on interactions between ART and ulipristal acetate, but interactions should be anticipated due to the metabolism of ulipristal acetate through the CYP3A4 pathways (http://aidsinfo.nih.gov/contentfiles/lvguidelines/PerinatalGL.pdf).

INFERTILITY

HIV can adversely affect fertility in HIV-infected patients, regardless of symptom status, in terms of reduced pregnancy rates, increased pregnancy loss, and longer intervals between births. A study from Spain found that almost one-third of HIV-infected women undergoing fertility assessment had evidence of tubal occlusion (Coll, 2007), likely reflecting past infection with gonorrhea or chlamydia. Another potential contributing factor to subfertility in HIV-infected women is a possible increase in menstrual dysfunction, particularly with lower $CD4^+$ cell counts (Ezechi, 2010; Harlow, 2000; Massad, 2006). Higher viral loads have also been independently associated with decreased fertility (Ngyuen, 2006). Women living with HIV who are unable to conceive should receive fertility evaluation and management. HIV-infected patients should not be denied access to fertility services solely based on their HIV status (Phelps, 2007).

CONSIDERATIONS FOR RESOURCE-LIMITED SETTINGS

Studies from resource-limited settings show that unmet need for contraception, rates of unintended pregnancy, and HIV serodiscordance rates are high. There is strong cultural and personal value placed on pregnancy. There are also data which demonstrate better maternal and infant outcomes with appropriate birth spacing. With better access to ART, both restoration of fertility and desire for pregnancy may increase, but risk of unintended pregnancy may increase as well. The general principles discussed under preconception counseling and contraception also apply in resource-limited settings.

RECOMMENDED READING

Panel on Treatment of Pregnant Women with HIV Infection and Prevention of Perinatal Transmission. Recommendations for use of antiretroviral drugs in transmission in the United States. Available at https://aidsinfo.nih.gov/news/2109/recommendations-regarding-the-use-of-dolutegravir-in-adults-and-adolescents-with-hiv-who-are-pregnant-or-of-child-bearing-potential.

Panel on Treatment of Pregnant Women with HIV Infection and Prevention of Perinatal Transmission. Recommendations for Use of Antiretroviral Drugs in Pregnant HIV-1–Infected Women for Maternal Health and Interventions to Reduce Perinatal HIV Transmission in the United States. 2018. Available at http://aidsinfo.nih.gov/contentfiles/lvguidelines/PerinatalGL.pdf. Accessed July 30, 2018.

ACKNOWLEDGMENTS

I would like to acknowledge Jean Anderson, MD, FACOG, AAHIVS. She provided the bulk of the material covered in this section in the 2012 edition. I have updated the more recent changes, in line with current treatment goals, strategies, and guidelines published since the last edition. This was an outstanding section, and I hope that my contributions will only make it better.

CERVICAL PAP SMEARS

LEARNING OBJECTIVE

Discuss the recommended frequency and specimen collection technique for cervical Pap smears in HIV-infected women, the role of human papillomavirus (HPV) testing, and indications for specialist referral for colposcopy.

WHAT'S NEW?

The cervical cancer screening guidelines for women living with HIV have been updated by the USDHHS to include new recommendations for follow-up of an atypical squamous cells of undetermined significance (ASCUS) Pap smear with negative reflex HPV and a new recommendation for screening in women living with HIV who are 65 and older.

KEY POINTS

- In HIV-infected patients younger than 21 years, cervical cancer screening (with liquid-based Pap alone) should begin within 1 year of the onset of sexual activity and no later than age 21 years. If normal, the test is repeated in 12 months. If the patient has three consecutive normal screenings, testing interval should be increased to every 3 years.

- In HIV-infected women older than 30 years, cervical cancer screening with either Pap alone or combined with HPV co-testing may be offered. The appropriate interval of follow-up screening is determined by the type of screening performed and the results returned.

- Unlike the general population, women living with HIV who are 65 and older should continue screening with Pap alone or Pap and HPV co-testing.

CERVICAL HPV INFECTION IN HIV-INFECTED WOMEN

In general, infection with HPV, the cause of cervical cancer, is very common in the United States, with an estimated 24.9 million 14- to 59-year-old women infected (Dunne, 2007). Compared with HIV-uninfected women, HIV-infected women have a higher prevalence and incidence of HPV (Ahdieh, 2001; Branca, 2003), longer persistence of HPV (Ahdieh, 2001; Sun, 1997), higher HPV levels (Jamieson, 2002), higher prevalence of multiple HPV subtypes (Firnhaber, 2009; Jamieson, 2002; Sahasrabuddhe, 2007), and higher prevalence of oncogenic subtypes (Firnhaber, 2009; Minkoff, 1998; Volkow, 2001). In addition, there is increased HPV prevalence and persistence of

high-risk HPV with decreasing CD4+ cell counts (Denny, 2008; Palefsky, 1999) and increasing HIV RNA levels (Palefsky, 1999). Also, compared to HIV-uninfected women, HIV-infected women are more likely to have abnormal cervical cytology (Denny, 2008; Ellerbrock, 2000), and both frequency and severity of cervical dysplasia increase with declining CD4+ cell counts (Davis, 2001; Massad, 2001, 2008). Recurrent cervical dysplasia after treatment is more common among HIV-infected women (Boardman, 1999; Fruchter, 1996; Holcomb, 1999; Massad, 2001; Six, 1998). Rates of cervical cancer are also significantly higher among HIV-infected women compared to women in the general population (Chaturvedi, 2009; Clifford, 2005; Dal Maso, 2009; Grulich, 2007). Several HPV subtypes have been associated with the development of squamous intraepithelial lesions and cervical cancer, including most commonly HPV-16 (found in almost half of all cervical cancers) and HPV-18 (found in 10–12% of cervical cancers) and less commonly HPV-31, -33, -35, -39, -45, -51, -52, -56, -58, -59, and -68 (each accounting for <5% of cervical cancers) (Castle, 2009; Schiffman, 2009).

CERVICAL PAP SMEARS

Due to the high level of HPV infection and higher prevalence of oncogenic subtypes, it is critical for HIV-infected women to be regularly screened for cervical dysplasia. Although a single Pap smear has historically been associated with high false-negative rates (10–25%), regular screening can significantly improve accuracy (Anderson, 2012), and Pap smear screening programs have been associated with marked reductions in cervical cancer incidence (Eddy, 1990; Nygard, 2002).

Overall, the frequency and type of testing recommended for HIV-infected women remains consistent with the 2017 edition of *Fundamentals of HIV Medicine*. However, new recommendations for the follow-up of ASCUS with negative high-risk HPV and screening for women older than 65 have been added. The cervical cancer screening recommendations reflect the paradigm shift in testing noted with non–HIV-infected women in the 2012 recommendations. The following sections present a summary of the cervical cancer screening recommendations from the NIH-CDC-HIVMA/IDSA (2018). The recommendations are categorized into two groups: those for HIV-infected women younger than 30 years and those for HIV-infected women older than 30 years.

HIV-INFECTED WOMEN YOUNGER THAN 30 YEARS

Liquid-based Pap screening (with reflex HPV testing if ASCUS) should be the primary method of testing. HPV co-testing is not recommended because of the high prevalence of HPV in this age group.

In patients younger than age 21 years, the initial cervical screening should begin within 1 year of the onset of sexual activity. If a patient has not begun sexual activity by the age of 21 years, routine screening should begin at that time. This recommendation holds true regardless of the method of exposure to the virus. In women aged 21–29 years, a baseline Pap should be done at the time of the patient's initial HIV diagnosis. If the Pap is normal, a repeat screen should be done 12 months later (some experts recommend a test 6 months after the baseline). If the patient has three consecutive normal tests, the screening interval should be increased to every 3 years.

Follow-up of ASCUS Results

If the result of ACSUS with positive HPV co-testing is returned, the patient should be referred for colposcopy. Pap screening should be repeated in 6–12 months for patients in whom HPV results are not available. For any result ASCUS or greater on repeat cytology, the patient should be referred for colposcopy. Regardless of HPV screening results (if done), any result of low-grade squamous intraepithelial lesion (LGSIL) or greater should be referred for colposcopy.

HIV-INFECTED WOMEN OLDER THAN 30 YEARS

Pap screening alone or in combination with HPV testing is acceptable.

If Screening with Pap Alone

Pap should be done as a baseline at the time of diagnosis and then every 12 months. Some experts recommend a repeat screen 6 months after the baseline exam. As with the younger group, if the results are negative on three consecutive exams, then subsequent screens should be carried out every 3 years.

Pap Screen Plus HPV Co-testing

Co-testing (Pap smear plus HPV testing) should begin at the age of 30 years or at the time of diagnosis (if available). When Pap screen and HPV co-testing are performed together, results should be reviewed. If the Pap is normal and HPV is negative, the co-test screening can be repeated in 3 years.

If the Pap screen is normal but HPV is positive, the appropriate follow-up is dictated by the HPV subtype(s) identified. If the subtype is HPV-16 or HPV-16/18, the patient should be referred for colposcopy. If HPV is identified and is of any other subtype, follow-up should be carried out in 1 year with a repeat of Pap and HPV testing. On repeat exam, if HPV testing remains positive or Pap is abnormal, then the patient should be referred for colposcopy.

Follow-up of ASCUS Results

If the result of ASCUS with negative HPV co-testing is returned, the patient has the option for repeat Pap in 6–12 months or repeat co-testing in 1 year. If repeat cytology yields any result of ASCUS or greater, the patient should be referred for colposcopy.

If the result of ASCUS with positive HPV co-testing is returned, the patient should be referred for colposcopy. Pap screening should be repeated in 6–12 months for patients in whom HPV results are not available. For any result ASCUS or greater on repeat cytology, the patient should be referred for colposcopy.

For results LGSIL or greater, the patient should be referred for colposcopy in accordance with American Society for Colposcopy and Cervical Pathology (ASCCP) guidelines, regardless of HPV results.

Unlike the general population who may end cervical cancer screening at the age of 65 years under ideal circumstances,

Table 12.1 ITEMS TO INCLUDE IN HIV HEALTH MAINTENANCE FLOWSHEET

1. HIV diagnostic information
   a. Date of HIV diagnosis
   b. HIV risk group
   c. CD4$^+$ count at diagnosis
2. Current ART and date started
3. Table of CD4$^+$ counts, HIV RNA by dates
4. Annual Screening Flowsheet with dates
   a. Vital signs: weight, BMI, blood pressure
   b. TB (skin test or IGRA)
   c. Pap smear: cervical, anal (for women and men)
   d. Mammogram (for cis- and trans-women)
   e. Eye exam
   f. Dental evaluation
   g. Colon cancer screening (colonoscopy or FIT test)
   h. Risk reduction counseling: smoking, alcohol, substance use, secondary prevention for HIV and STIs
   i. Mental health
   j. Labs:
      i. Urinalysis
      ii. Lipid panel
      iii. Hepatitis C
      iv. STI screen: syphilis, gonorrhea, chlamydia
5. Immunization history with dates
   a. PCV 13 (conjugated pneumococcal)
   b. PPSV23 (polysaccharide pneumococcal)
   c. Influenza
   d. Hepatitis A series (2)
   e. Hepatitis B series (3)
   f. Meningococcal
   g. TD/TDAPp
   h. Zoster, recombinant (2)
6. Antibody/Antigen Titers
   a. Hepatitis A total (IgG and IgM)
   b. HBsAg
   c. HBsAb
   d. Hep B core
   e. HBeAg
   f. HBeAb
7. Problem list
8. HIV Diagnostics Flowsheet
   a. HLA B*5701 allele present or not
   b. HIV genotype(s)
   c. G6PD
   d. Toxoplasma IgG
   e. CMV IgG and/or IgM (not generally recommended)

ART, antiretroviral therapy; CMV, cytomegalovirus; Ig, immunoglobulin; PCV, pneumococcal conjugate vaccine; STI, sexually transmitted infection cervical cancer screening should continue for HIV-infected women throughout their lifetimes. Screening can consist of Pap alone or Pap and HPV co-testing.

RECOMMENDED READING

American College of Obstetricians and Gynecologists. Gynecologic Care for Women and Adolescents with Human Immunodeficiency Virus. *ACOG Practice Bull.* No. 167. October 2016.

Bloomfield GS, Alenezi F, Barasa FA, et al. Human immunodeficiency virus and heart failure in low- and middle-income countries. *JACC Heart Fail.* 2015;3:579–590.

Carten ML, Kiser JJ, Kwara A, et al. Pharmacokinetic interactions between the hormonal emergency contraception, levonorgestrel (Plan B), and Efavirenz. *Infect Dis Obstet Gynecol.* 2012.

Panel on Opportunistic Infections in HIV-Infected Adults and Adolescents. Guidelines for the prevention and treatment of opportunistic infections in HIV-infected adults and adolescents: Recommendations from the Centers for Disease Control and Prevention, the National Institutes of Health, and the HIV Medicine Association of the Infectious Diseases Society of America. Available at http://aidsinfo.nih.gov/contentfiles/lvguidelines/adult_oi.pdf Accessed July 30, 2018.

ACKNOWLEDGMENTS

We acknowledge Jean Anderson, MD, FACOG, AAHIVS. She provided the bulk of the material discussed in this section in the 2012 and 2017 editions.

REFERENCES

American College of Obstetricians and Gynecologists. Gynecologic care for women with human immunodeficiency virus. Practice Bulletin No. 117. *Obstet Gynecol*. 117:1492–1509. Reaffirmed 2015.

American College of Obstetricians and Gynecologists. Gynecologic Care for Women with Human Immunodeficiency Virus. ACOG Practice Bulletin No. 167. October 2016. Reaffirmed 2019.

Ahdieh L, Klein RS, Burk R, et al. Prevalence, incidence, and type-specific persistence of human papillomavirus in human immunodeficiency virus (HIV)-positive and HIV-negative women. *J Infect Dis.* 2001;184:1682–1690.

American Society for Reproductive Medicine (ASRM). Human immunodeficiency virus (HIV) and infertility treatment: a committee opinion. *Fertil Steril.* July 1, 2015;104(1):e1–e8.

American Society for Reproductive Medicine. Recommendations for reducing the risk of viral transmission during fertility treatment with the use of autologous gametes: a committee opinion. *Fertil Steril.* 2013;99:340–346.

American Thoracic Society, Centers for Disease Control and Prevention, and Infectious Diseases Society of America. Controlling tuberculosis in the United States. *Am J Respir Crit Care Med.* 2005;172:1169–1227.

American Thoracic Society/Centers for Disease Control and Prevention. Targeted tuberculin testing and treatment of latent tuberculosis infection: joint statement of the American Thoracic Society and the Centers for Disease Control and Prevention. *Am J Respir Crit Care Med.* 2000;161:S221–S247.

Anderson J. HIV and reproduction. In *A Guide to the Clinical Care of Women with HIV/AIDS*, 2005 ed., Anderson JR, ed. Rockville, MD: Department of Health and Human Services, Health Resources and Services Administration, HIV/AIDS Bureau; 2005. Available at http://hab.hrsa.gov/publications/womencare05. Accessed July 20, 2006.

Anderson, J., Lu, E., Sanghvi, H., Kibwana, S., & Lu, A. (2012). Cervical cancer screening and prevention for HIV-infected women in the developing world. In Cancer Prevention-From Mechanisms to Translational Benefits. IntechOpen.

Anderson J. Gynecologic problems. In Anderson JR, ed., *A Guide for Clinical Care of Women with HIV/AIDS, 2013 Edition*. Rockville, MD: US Department of Health and Human Services, Health Resources and Services Administration, HIV/AIDS Bureau.

Antiretroviral Pregnancy Registry (APR) Steering Committee. Antiretroviral Pregnancy Registry International interim report for 1 January 1989–31 July 2017. Available at www.APRegistry.com. Accessed July 30, 2018.

Baker JV, Duprez D, Rapkin J, et al. Untreated HIV infection and large and small artery elasticity. *J Acquir Immune Defic Syndr.* 2009;52:25–31.

Bedimo RJ, Westfall AO, Drechsler H, et al. Abacavir use and risk of acute myocardial infarction and cerebrovascular events in the highly active antiretroviral therapy era. *Clin Infect Dis.* 2011;53:84–91.

Betene ADC, De Wit S, Neuhaus J, et al. Interleukin-6, high sensitivity C-reactive protein, and the development of type 2 diabetes among HIV-positive patients taking antiretroviral therapy. *J AIDS.* 2014;67:538–546.

Boardman LA, Peipert JF, Hogan JW, et al. Positive cone biopsy specimen margins in women infected with the human immunodeficiency virus. *Am J Obstet Gynecol.* December 1999;181(6):1395–1399.

Boehme CC, Nabeta P, Hillemann D, et al. Rapid molecular detection of tuberculosis and rifampin resistance. *N Engl J Med.* September 9, 2010;363(11):1005–1015.

Bonito AJ. Management of dental patients who are HIV positive. Summary, evidence report/technology assessment: number 37. AHRQ Publication No. 01-E041, March 2001. Rockville, MD: Agency for Healthcare Research and Quality. Available at http://www.ncbi.nlm.nih.gov/books/NBK11965. Accessed November 15, 2015.

Branca M, Garbuglia AR, Benedetto A, et al.; DIANAIDS Collaborative Study Group. Factors predicting the persistence of genital human papillomavirus infections and Pap smear abnormality in HIV-positive and HIV-negative women during prospective follow-up. *Int J STD AIDS.* 2003;14(6):417–425.

Cain KP, McCarthy KD, Heilg CM, et al. An algorithm for tuberculosis screening and diagnosis in people with HIV. *N Engl J Med.* 2010;362:707–716.

Cardona-Maya W, Velilla P, Montoya CJ, Cadavid A, Rugeles MT. Presence of HIV-1 DNA in spermatozoa from HIV–positive patients: changes in the semen parameters. *Curr HIV Res.* 2009;7(4):418–424.

Castle PE, Rodriquez AC, Burk RD, et al. Short term persistence of human papillomavirus and risk of cervical precancer and cancer: population based cohort study. *BMJ.* July 28, 2009;339:b2569. doi: 10.1136/bmj.b2569.

Cattamanchi A, Smith R, Steingart KR, et al. Interferon-gamma release assays for the diagnosis of latent tuberculosis infection in HIV-infected individuals: a systematic review and meta-analysis. *J AIDS.* 2011;56:230–238.

Centers for Disease Control and Prevention (CDC). Trials of pre-exposure prophylaxis for HIV prevention. 2006. Available at http://www.cdc.gov/hiv/resources/factsheets/PDF/prep.pdf. Accessed August 16, 2006.

Centers for Disease Control and Prevention (CDC). US medical eligibility criteria for contraceptive use, 2010. *MMWR Recomm Rep,* 2010;59(RR-4):1–86.

Centers for Disease Control and Prevention (CDC). Updated guidelines for using interferon gamma release assays to detect *Mycobacterium tuberculosis* infection—United States, 2010. *MMWR Morb Mort Wkly Rep.* 2010;59(RR-5):1–26.

Chaturvedi AK, Madeleine MM, Biggar RJ, et al. Risk of human papillomavirus-associated cancers among person with AIDS. *J Natl Cancer Inst.* August 19, 2009;101(16):1120–1230.

Choi AI, Vittinghoff E, Deeks SG, et al. Cardiovascular risks associated with abacavir and tenofovir exposure in HIV-infected persons. *AIDS.* 2011;25:1289–1298.

Clifford GM, Polesel J, Rickenbach M, et al. Cancer risk in the Swiss HIV Cohort Study: associations with immunodeficiency, smoking and highly active antiretroviral therapy. *J Natl Cancer Inst.* March 16, 2005;97(6):425–432.

Cohen MS, Chen YQ, McCauley M, et al. Prevention of HIV-1 infection with early antiretroviral therapy. *N Engl J Med.* 2011;365:493–505.

Cohn, S. E., Park, J. G., Watts, D. H., Stek, A., Hitti, J., Clax, P. A., . . . & Lertora, J. J. L. (2007). Depo-medroxyprogesterone in women on antiretroviral therapy: Effective contraception and lack of clinically significant interactions. *Clinical Pharmacology & Therapeutics,* 81(2), 222–227.

Coll O, Lopez M, Vidal R, et al. Fertility assessment in non-infertile HIV-infected women and their partners. *Reproductive Biomedicine Online.* 2007;14(4):488–494.

Connor EM, Sperling RS, Gelber R, et al. Reduction of maternal-infant transmission of human immunodeficiency virus type 1 with zidovudine treatment. *N Engl J Med.* 1994;331:1173–1180.

Craft, S. M., Delaney, R. O., Bautista, D. T., & Serovich, J. M. (2007). Pregnancy decisions among women with HIV. *AIDS and Behavior,* 11(6), 927–935.

Cruciani M, Zanichelli V, Serpelloni G, et al. Abacavir use and cardiovascular disease events: a meta-analysis of published and unpublished data. *AIDS.* 2011;25:1993–2004.

Dal Maso L, Polesel J, Serraino D, et al. Pattern of cancer risk in persons with AIDS in Italy in the HAART era. *British J Cancer.* 2009;100(5):840.

Davis AT, Chakraborty H, Flowers L, et al. Cervical dysplasia in women infected with the human immunodeficiency virus (HIV): a correlation with HIV viral load and CD4$^+$ count. *Gynecol Oncol.* March 2001;80(3):350–354.

Dejesus E, Rockstroh JK, Henry K, et al. Co-formulated elvitegravir, cobicistat, emtricitabine, and tenofovir disoproxil fumarate versus ritonavir-boosted atazanavir plus co-formulated emtricitabine and tenofovir disoproxil fumarate for initial treatment of HIV-1 infection: a randomised, double-blind, phase 3, non-inferiority trial. *Lancet.* 2012;379:2429–2438.

Del Maso L, Polesel J, Serraino D, et al. Pattern of cancer risk in persons with AIDS in Italy in the HAART era. *Br J Cancer.* March 10, 2009;100(5):840–847. doi: 10.1038/sj.bjc.6604923.Epub February 17, 2009.

Del Romero J, Baza MB, Rio I, et al. Natural conception in HIV-serodiscordant couples with the infected partner in suppressive antiretroviral therapy: a prospective cohort study. *Medicine (Baltimore).* 2016;95(30):e4398.

Denny L, Boa R, Williamson AL, et al. Human papillomavirus infection and cervical disease in human immunodeficiency virus-1-infected women. *Obstet Gynecol.* June 2008;111(6):1380–1387. doi: 10.1097/AOG.0b013e181743327.

Dunne EF, Unger ER, Sternberg M, et al. Prevalence of HPV infection among females in the United States. *JAMA.* 2007;297(8):813–819.

Durand M, Sheehy O, Baril JG, et al. Association between HIV infection, antiretroviral therapy, and risk of acute myocardial infarction: a cohort and nested case–control study using Quebec's public health insurance database. *J AIDS.* 2011;57:245–253.

Ebbert JO, Hughes JR, West RJ, et al. Effect of varenicline on smoking cessation through smoking reduction: a randomized clinical trial. *JAMA.* 2015;313:687–694.

Eddy DM. Screening for cervical cancer. Ann Int. Med. *Ann Intern Med.* August 1, 1990;113(3):214–226.

Elion RA, Althoff KN, Zhang J, North American AIDS Cohort Collaboration on Research and Design of IeDE, et al. Recent abacavir use increases risk of type 1 and type 2 myocardial infarctions among adults with HIV. *J AIDS.* May 1, 2018;78(1):62–72. doi: 10.1097/QAI.0000000000001642.

Ellerbrock TV, Chiasson MA, Bush TJ, et al. Incidence of cervical squamous intraepithelial lesions in HIV-infected women. *JAMA.* February 23, 2000;283(8):1031–1037.

El-Ibiary, S. Y., & Cocohoba, J. M. (2008). Effects of HIV antiretrovirals on the pharmacokinetics of hormonal contraceptives. *The European journal of contraception & reproductive health care,* 13(2), 123–132.

Ezechi, O. C., Jogo, A., Gab-Okafor, C., Onwujekwe, D. I., Ezeobi, P. M., Gbajabiamila, T., . . . & Meschack, E. (2010). Effect of HIV-1 infection and increasing immunosuppression on menstrual function. *Journal of Obstetrics and Gynaecology Research,* 36(5), 1053–1058.

Firnhaber C, Zungu K, Levin S, et al. Diverse and high prevalence of human papillomavirus associated with a significant high rate of cervical dysplasia in human immunodeficiency virus-infected women in Johannesburg, South Africa. *Acta Cytol.* January–February 2009;53(1):10–17.

Finocchario-Kessler, S., Dariotis, J. K., Sweat, M. D., Trent, M. E., Keller, J. M., Hafeez, Q., & Anderson, J. R. (2010). Do HIV-infected women want to discuss reproductive plans with providers, and are those conversations occurring? *AIDS patient care and STDs,* 24(5), 317–323.

Finocchario-Kessler, S., Mabachi, N., Dariotis, J. K., Anderson, J., Goggin, K., & Sweat, M. (2012). "We weren't using condoms because we were trying to conceive": The need for reproductive counseling for HIV-positive women in clinical care. *AIDS patient care and STDs,* 26(11), 700–707.

Freed JR, Marcus M, Freed BA, et al. Oral health findings for HIV-infected adult medical patients from the HIV Cost and Services Utilization Study. *J Am Dental Assoc.* 2005;136:1396–1405.

Freiberg M, McGinnis K, Butt A, et al. HIV is associated with clinically confirmed myocardial infarction after adjustment for smoking and other risk factors. 18th Conference on Retroviruses and Opportunistic Infections, 2011, Boston, MA.

Friis-Moller N, Reiss P, Sabin CA, et al. Class of antiretroviral drugs and the risk of myocardial infarction. *N Engl J Med.* 2007;356:1723–1735.

Fruchter RG, Maiman M, Sedlis A, et al. Multiple recurrences of cervical intraepithelial neoplasia in women with the human immunodeficiency virus. *Obstet Gynecol.* 1996;87:338–344.

Getahun H, Harrington M, O'Brien R, et al. Diagnosis of smear-negative pulmonary tuberculosis in people with HIV infection or AIDS in resource-constrained settings: informing urgent policy changes. *Lancet.* 2007;369(9578):2042–2049.

Gleeson M, Bishop NC, Stensel DJ, et al. The anti-inflammatory effects of exercise: mechanisms and implications for the prevention and treatment of disease. *Nat Rev Immunol.* 2011;11:607–615.

Gray J, Reves R, Johnson S, et al. Identification of false-positive QuantiFERON-TB Gold In-Tube assays by repeat testing in HIV-infected patients at low risk of tuberculosis. *Clin Infect Dis.* 2012;54:e20–e23.

Gray RH, Wawer MJ, Brookmeyer R, et al. Probability of HIV-1 transmission per coital act in monogamous, heterosexual, HIV-1-discordant couples in Rakai, Uganda. *Lancet.* 2001;357:1149–1153.

Grulich AE, van Leeuwen MT, Falster MO, et al. Incidence of cancers in people with HIV/AIDS compared with immunosuppressed transplant recipients: a meta-analysis. *Lancet.* July 7, 2007;370(9581):59–67. Review. PMID:17617273.

Harlow, S. D., Schuman, P., Cohen, M., Ohmit, S. E., Cu-Uvin, S., Lin, X., . . . & Muderspach, L. (2000). Effect of HIV infection on menstrual cycle length. *Journal of acquired immune deficiency syndromes* (1999), 24(1), 68–75.

Heffron, R., Ngure, K., Mugo, N., Celum, C., Kurth, A., Curran, K., & Baeten, J. M. (2012). Willingness of Kenyan HIV-1 serodiscordant couples to use antiretroviral based HIV-1 prevention strategies. *Journal of acquired immune deficiency syndromes* (1999), 61(1), 116.

Holcomb K, Matthews RP, Chapman JE, et al. The efficacy of cervical conization in the treatment of cervical intraepithelial neoplasia in HIV-positive women. *Gynecol Oncol.* September 1999;74(3):428–431.

Horsburgh CR, Rubin EJ. Latent tuberculosis infection in the United States. *N Engl J Med.* 2011;364:1441–1448.

Hoyt MJ, Storm, DS, Aaron E, Anderson J. Preconception and contraceptive care for women living with HIV. *Infect Dis Obstet Gynecol.* 2012.

INSIGHT START Study Group. Initiation of antiretroviral therapy in early asymptomatic HIV infection. *N Engl J Med.* 2015;373:795–798.

INSIGHT/SMART and DAD Study Investigators. Use of nucleoside reverse transcriptase inhibitors and risk of myocardial infarction in HIV-infected patients. *AIDS.* 2008;22:F17–F24.

Jackson JB, Barnett S, Piwowar-Manning E, et al. A phase I/II study of nevirapine for pre-exposure prophylaxis of HIV-1 transmission in uninfected subjects at high risk. *AIDS.* 2003;17:547–553.

James PA, Oparil S, Carter BL, et al. 2014 Evidence-based guideline for the management of high blood pressure in adults: report from the Panel Members Appointed to the Eighth Joint National Committee (JNC 8). *JAMA*. 2014;311(5):507–520.

Jamieson DJ, Duerr A, Burk R, et al. Characterization of genital human papillomavirus infection in women who have or are at risk for having HIV infection. *Am J Obstet Gynecol*. January 2002;186(1): 21–27.

Johnson, L. F., & Lewis, D. A. (2008). The effect of genital tract infections on HIV-1 shedding in the genital tract: a systematic review and meta-analysis. *Sexually transmitted diseases*, 35(11), 946–959.

Koegelenberg CF, Noor F, Bateman ED, et al. Efficacy of varenicline combined with nicotine replacement therapy vs. varenicline alone for smoking cessation: a randomized clinical trial. *JAMA*. 2014;312:155–161.

Lang S, Mary-Krause M, Cotte L, et al. Impact of individual antiretroviral drugs on the risk of myocardial infarction in human immunodeficiency virus-infected patients: a case–control study nested within the French Hospital Database on HIV ANRS cohort CO4. *Arch Intern Med*. 2010;170:1228–1238.

Longenecker CT, Sullivan C, Baker JV. Immune activation and cardiovascular disease in chronic HIV infection. *Curr Opin HIV AIDS*. 2016;11(2):216–225.

Loutfy MR, Blitz S, Zhang Y, et al. Self-reported preconception care of HIV-positive women of reproductive potential: a retrospective study. *J Intl Assoc Prov AIDS Care (JIAPAC)*. 2013(5), 424–433.

Loutfy, M. R., Hart, T. A., Mohammed, S. S., Su, D., Ralph, E. D., Walmsley, S. L., . . . & Angel, J. B. (2009). Fertility desires and intentions of HIV-positive women of reproductive age in Ontario, Canada: a cross-sectional study. *PloS one*, 4(12), e7925.

Mandelbrot L, Heard I, Henrion-Geeant E, Henrion R. Natural conception in HIV-negative women with HIV-infected partners. *Lancet* 1997;349:850–851.

Martin A, Bloch M, Amin J, et al. Simplification of antiretroviral therapy with tenofovir–emtricitabine or abacavir–lamivudine: a randomized, 96-week trial. *Clin Infect Dis*. 2009;49:1591–1601.

Martin HL Jr, Nyange PM, Richardson BA, et al. Hormonal contraception, sexually transmitted diseases, and risk of heterosexual transmission of human immunodeficiency virus type 1. *J Infect Dis*. 1998;178:1053–1059.

Massad LS, Ahdieh L, Benning L, et al. Evolution of cervical abnormalities among women with HIV-1: evidence from surveillance cytology in the Women's Interagency HIV study. *J AIDS*. 2001;27:432–442.

Massad, L. S., Springer, G., Jacobson, L., Watts, H., Anastos, K., Korn, A., . . . & Minkoff, H. (2004). Pregnancy rates and predictors of conception, miscarriage and abortion in US women with HIV. *Aids*, 18(2), 281–286.

Massad, L. S., Evans, C. T., Minkoff, H., Watts, D. H., Greenblatt, R. M., Levine, A. M., . . . & Cohen, M. (2006). Effects of HIV infection and its treatment on self-reported menstrual abnormalities in women. *Journal of Women's Health*, 15(5), 591–598.

Massad LS, Seaberg EC, Wright RL, et al. Squamous cervical lesions in women with human immunodeficiency virus: long-term follow-up. *Obstet Gynecol*. June 2008;111(6):1388–1393.

McComsey GA, Kitch D, Daar ES, et al. Inflammation markers after randomization to abacavir/lamivudine or tenofovir/emtricitabine with efavirenz or atazanavir/ritonavir. *AIDS*. 2012;26:1371–1385.

Minkoff H, Feldman J, DeHovitz J, et al. A longitudinal study of human papillomavirus carriage in human immunodeficiency virus-infected and human immunodeficiency virus-uninfected women. *Am J Obstet Gynecol*. 1998;178:982–986.

Morrison, C. S., Chen, P. L., Nankya, I., Rinaldi, A., Van Der Pol, B., Ma, Y. R., . . . & Salata, R. A. (2011). Hormonal contraceptive use and HIV disease progression among women in Uganda and Zimbabwe. *Journal of acquired immune deficiency syndromes* (1999), 57(2), 157.

Nattabi, B., Li, J., Thompson, S. C., Orach, C. G., & Earnest, J. (2009). A systematic review of factors influencing fertility desires and intentions among people living with HIV/AIDS: implications for policy and service delivery. *AIDS and Behavior*, 13(5), 949–968.

National Institutes of Health (NIH). Adult NCEP Treatment Panel III. Detection, evaluation, and treatment of high blood cholesterol in adults (Adult Treatment Panel III). NIH Publication No. 01-3670, May 2001.

New York State Department of Health AIDS Institute (NYSDOH). HIV and oral health: general principles. 2001. Available at http://www.hivguidelines.org/clinical-guidelines/hiv-and-oral-health/general-principles. Accessed November 15, 2015.

Nguyen, R. H., Gange, S. J., Wabwire-Mangen, F., Sewankambo, N. K., Serwadda, D., Wawer, M. J., . . . & Gray, R. H. (2006). Reduced fertility among HIV-infected women associated with viral load in Rakai district, Uganda. *International journal of STD & AIDS*, 17(12), 842–846.

NIH-CDC-HIVMA/IDSA. Guidelines for prevention and treatment of opportunistic infections in HIV-infected adults and adolescents. 2015. Available at http://aidsinfo.nih.gov/guidelines/html/4/adult-and-adolescent-oi-prevention-and-treatment-guidelines/0.

NIH-CDC-HIVMA/IDSA. Guidelines for prevention and treatment of opportunistic infections in HIV-infected adults and adolescents. 2018. Available at https://aidsinfo.nih.gov/guidelines/html/4/adult-and-adolescent-opportunistic-infection/0. Accessed July 31, 2018.

Nygard JF, Skare GB, Thoresen SO. The cervical cancer screening programme in Norway, 1992–2000: changes in Pap smear coverage and incidence of cervical cancer. *J Med Screen*. 2002;9(2):86–91.

Obel N, Farkas DK, Kronborg G, et al. Abacavir and risk of myocardial infarction in HIV-infected patients on highly active antiretroviral therapy: a population-based nationwide cohort study. *HIV Med*. 2010;11:130–136.

Palefsky, J. M., Minkoff, H., Kalish, L. A., Levine, A., Sacks, H. S., Garcia, P., . . . & Burk, R. (1999). Cervicovaginal human papillomavirus infection in human immunodeficiency virus-1 (HIV)-positive and high-risk HIV-negative women. *Journal of the National Cancer Institute*, 91(3), 226–236.

Palefsky JM, Holly EA, Ralston ML, et al. Effect of highly active antiretroviral therapy on the natural history of anal squamous intraepithelial and anal human papillomavirus infection. *J AIDS*. 2001;28:422–428.

Palefsky JM. Cervical human papillomavirus infection and cervical intraepithelial neoplasia in women positive for human immunodeficiency virus in the era of highly active antiretroviral therapy. *Curr Opin Oncol*. 2003;15:382–388.

Palmieri F, Girardi E, Pellicelli AM, et al. Pulmonary tuberculosis in HIV-infected patients presenting with normal chest radiograph and negative sputum smear. *Infection*. 2002;30(2):68–74.

Panel on Treatment of Pregnant Women with HIV Infection and Prevention of Perinatal Transmission. Recommendations for Use of Antiretroviral Drugs in Transmission in the United States. Available at http://aidsinfo.nih.gov/contentfiles/lvguidelines/PerinatalGL.pdf.

Panozzo, L., Friedl, A., & Vernazza, P. L. (2003). High risk behaviour and fertility desires among heterosexual HIV-positive patients with a serodiscordant partner-two challenging issues. Swiss Medical Weekly, 132(0708).

Patel RC, Onono M, Gandhi M, et al. Pregnancy rates in HIV-positive women using contraceptives and efavirenz-based or nevirapine-based antiretroviral therapy in Kenya: a retrospective cohort study. *Lancet HIV*. 2015;2(11):e474–e482.

Petoumenos K, Reiss P, Ryom L, et al. Increased risk of cardiovascular disease (CVD) with age in HIV-positive men: a comparison of the D:A:D CVD risk equation and general population CVD risk equations. *HIV Med*. 2014;15:595–603.

Phelps, J. Y. (2007). Restricting access of human immunodeficiency virus (HIV)–seropositive patients to infertility services: a legal analysis of the rights of reproductive endocrinologists and of HIV-seropositive patients. *Fertility and Sterility*, 88(6), 1483–1490.

Polis, C. B., Wawer, M. J., Kiwanuka, N., Laeyendecker, O., Kagaayi, J., Lutalo, T., . . . & Gray, R. H. (2010). Effect of hormonal contraceptive use on HIV progression in female HIV seroconverters in Rakai, Uganda. AIDS (London, England), 24(12), 1937.

Quercia R, Roberts J, Martin-Carpenter L, et al. Comparative changes of lipid levels in treatment-naive, HIV-1-infected adults treated with dolutegravir vs. efavirenz, raltegravir, and ritonavir-boosted darunavir-based regimens over 48 weeks. *Clin Drug Invest.* 2015;35:211–219.

Quinn TC, Wawer MJ, Sewankambo N, et al. Viral load and heterosexual transmission of human immunodeficiency virus type 1. *N Engl J Med.* 2000;342:921–929.

Raby E, Moyo M, Devendra A, et al. The effects of HIV on the sensitivity of a whole blood IFN-gamma release assay in Zambian adults with active tuberculosis. *PLOS One.* June 18, 2008;3(6)e2489.

Remick J, Georgiopoulou V, Marti C, et al. Heart failure in patients with human immunodeficiency virus infection: epidemiology, pathophysiology, treatment, and future research. *Circulation.* 2014;129:1781–1789.

Ribaudo HJ, Benson CA, Zheng Y, et al. No risk of myocardial infarction associated with initial antiretroviral treatment containing abacavir: short and long-term results from ACTG A5001/ALLRT. *Clin Infect Dis.* 2011;52:929–940.

Riddler SA, Smit E, Cole SR, et al. Impact of HIV infection and HAART on serum lipids in men. *JAMA.* 2007;289:2978–2982.

Rodger AJ, Cambiano V, Bruun T, et al. Sexual activity without condoms and risk of HIV transmission in serodifferent couples when the HIV-positive partner is using suppressive antiretroviral therapy. *JAMA.* 2016;316(2):171–181.

Rotger M, Glass TR, Junier T, et al. Contribution of genetic background, traditional risk factors, and HIV-related factors to coronary artery disease events in HIV-positive persons. *Clin Infect Dis.* 2013;57:112–121.

Sahasrabuddhe VV, Mwanahamuntu MH, Vermund SH, et al. Prevalence and distribution of HPV genotypes among HIV-infected women in Zambia. *Br J Cancer.* May 7, 2007;96(9):1480–1483.

Schiffman M, Solomon D. Screening and prevention methods for cervical cancer. *JAMA.* October 28, 2009;302(16):1809–1810. doi: 10.1001/jama.2009.1573.

Schnoll RA, Goelz PM, Veluz-Wilkins A, et al. Long-term nicotine replacement therapy: a randomized clinical trial. *JAMA Intern Med.* 2015;175:504–511.

Semprini AE, Levi Setti P, et al. Insemination of HIV-negative women with processed semen of HIV- positive partners. *Lancet.* 1992;340:1317–1319.

Sewankambo N, Gray RH, Wawer MJ, et al. HIV-1 infection associated with abnormal vaginal flora morphology and bacterial vaginosis (erratum in *Lancet.* 1997;350:1036). *Lancet.* 1997;350:546–550.

Sharma, A., Feldman, J. G., Golub, E. T., Schmidt, J., Silver, S., Robison, E., & Minkoff, H. (2007). Live birth patterns among human immunodeficiency virus-infected women before and after the availability of highly active antiretroviral therapy. American journal of obstetrics and gynecology, 196(6), 541–e1.

Six C, Heard I, Bergeron C, et al. Comparative prevalence, incidence and short-term prognosis of cervical squamous intraepithelial lesions amongst HIV-positive and HIV-negative women. *AIDS.* 1998;12:1047–1056.

SMART Study Group. CD4+ count-guided interruption of antiretroviral treatment. *N Engl J Med.* 2006;355:2283–2296.

Smith SM, Mefford M, Sodora D, et al. Topical estrogen protects against SIV vaginal transmission without evidence of systemic effect. *AIDS.* 2004;18:1637–1643.

Solages A, Vita JA, Thornton DJ, et al. Endothelial function in HIV-infected persons. *Clin Infect Dis.* 2006;42:1325–1332.

Squires, K. E., Hodder, S. L., Feinberg, J., Bridge, D. A., Abrams, S., Storfer, S. P., & Aberg, J. A. (2011). Health needs of HIV-infected women in the United States: insights from the women living positive survey. *AIDS patient care and STDs*, 25(5), 279–285.

Stafford MK, Ward H, Flanagan A, et al. Safety study of nonoxynol-9 as a vaginal microbicide: evidence of adverse effects. *J Acquir Immune Defic Syndr Hum Retrovirol.* 1998;17:327–331.

Stringer, E. M., Giganti, M., Carter, R. J., El-Sadr, W., Abrams, E. J., & Stringer, J. S. (2009). Hormonal contraception and HIV disease progression: a multicountry cohort analysis of the MTCT-Plus Initiative. AIDS (London, England), 23(01), S69–77.

Sun XW, Kuhn L, Ellerbrock TV, et al. Human papillomavirus infection in women infected with the human immunodeficiency virus. *N Engl J Med.* November 6, 1997;337(19):1343–1349.

Tovanabutra S, Robison V, Wongtrakul J, et al. Male viral load and heterosexual transmission of HIV-1 subtype E in northern Thailand. *J AIDS.* 2002;29:275–283.

Townsend, C. L., M. Cortina-Borja, et al. (2008). Low rates of mother-to-child transmission of HIV following effective pregnancy interventions in the United Kingdom and Ireland, 2000–2006. *AIDS* 22(8): 973–981.

Tseng ZH, Secemsky EA, Dowdy D. Sudden cardiac death in patients with human immunodeficiency virus infection. *J Am Coll Cardiol.* 2012;59:1891–1896.

Tungsiripat M, Kitch D, Glesby MJ, et al. A pilot study to determine the impact on dyslipidemia of adding tenofovir to stable background antiretroviral therapy: ACTG 5206. *AIDS.* 2010;24:1781–1784.

van Sighem, A., Gras, L., Reiss, P., Brinkman, K., & de Wolf, F. (2010). Life expectancy of recently diagnosed asymptomatic HIV-infected patients approaches that of uninfected individuals. *Aids*, 24(10), 1527–1535.

Vernazza PL, Graf I, Sonnenberg-Schwan U, et al. Preexposure prophylaxis and timed intercourse for HIV-discordant couples willing to conceive a child. *AIDS.* 2011;25:2005–2008.

Volkow P, Rubí S, Lizano M, et al. High prevalence of oncogenic human papillomavirus in the genital tract of women with human immunodeficiency virus. *Gynecol Oncol.* 2001;82:27–31.

Vogler, M. A., Patterson, K., Kamemoto, L., Park, J. G., Watts, H., Aweeka, F., . . . & Cohn, S. E. (2010). Contraceptive Efficacy of Oral and Transdermal Hormones When Co-Administered With Protease Inhibitors in HIV-1–Infected Women: Pharmacokinetic Results of ACTG Trial A5188. *Journal of acquired immune deficiency syndromes* (1999), 55(4), 473.

Wang CC, Reilly M, Kreiss JK. Risk of HIV infection in oral contraceptive pill user: a meta-analysis (erratum in *J AIDS.* 1999;21:428). *J AIDS.* 1999;21:51–58.

World Health Organization (WHO). Hormonal contraceptive methods for women at high risk of HIV and living with HIV: 2014 guidance statement. 2014.

World Health Organization (WHO). *Potential Safety Issue Affecting Women Living with HIV Using Dolutegravir at the Time of Conception.* Geneva, Switzerland: May 18, 2018.

Worm SW, Sabin C, Weber R, et al. Risk of myocardial infarction in patients with HIV infection exposed to specific individual antiretroviral drugs from the 3 major drug classes: the Data Collection on Adverse Events of Anti-HIV Drugs (D:A:D) study. *J Infect Dis.* 2010;201:318–330.

Youle M, Wainberg MA. Pre-exposure chemoprophylaxis (PREP) as an HIV prevention strategy. *J Int Assoc Physicians AIDS Care (Chicago, IL).* 2003;2:102–105.

Zash R, Jacobson D, et al. Dolutegravir/tenofovir/emtricitabine (DTG/TDF/FTC) started in pregnancy is as safe as efavirenz/tenofovir/emtricitabine (EFV/TDF/FTC) in nationwide birth outcomes surveillance in Botswana. Ninth IAS 2017. Paris, France.

13.

ISSUES IN SPECIFIC PATIENT POPULATIONS

Gary F. Spinner, Joseph A. Church, Renata Arrington-Sanders, Aroonsiri Sangarlangkarn, Paul W. DenOuden, Madeline B. Deutsch, Daniel Wlodarczyk, Barry Zevin, Rachel A. Prosser, and Vishal Dahya

CHAPTER GOALS

Upon completion of this chapter, the reader should be able to

- Provide an understanding of the diversity of patients with HIV, the complexity of their unique cultures that are shaped by a multitude of factors, and the importance of becoming competent in developing a clinician–patient relationship across cultural differences.

- Relate how a patient's values, beliefs, and judgments may create barriers to successful treatment if the HIV provider does not competently navigate the cultural differences between patient and provider.

- Recognize the challenges in addressing racial and ethnic disparities in healthcare and in HIV in particular.

- Discuss the impact that culture, ethnicity, immigration status, sexual orientation, religion, gender, and behavioral health problems may have on the care of HIV-infected patients.

- Identify the diagnostic criteria, laboratory markers, epidemiologic patterns, spectrum of disease manifestations, and unique immunization and therapy issues in HIV-infected children.

- Describe the developmental, cognitive, social, and environmental factors that may affect treatment adherence and secondary prevention in adolescents.

- Describe the differences in HIV care and management for patients who are 50 years or older.

- Discuss issues in determining the relative priority of initiating and/or maintaining antiretroviral therapy (ART) in the context of hospitalized HIV patients with significant comorbid conditions, as well as issues of continuity of care after discharge from the inpatient setting.

- Describe important considerations in the perioperative care of an HIV-infected patient.

- Equip providers with the knowledge and skill to develop and provide gender-affirming primary and HIV care and prevention for transgender persons.

- Describe special considerations affecting the medical management of homeless or displaced individuals.

- Discuss the provision of HIV care and release planning in the context of correctional facilities.

- Describe obstacles to optimal HIV care for patients in rural settings.

- Discuss limitations in HIV care and special needs among migrant populations or patients with undocumented citizenship.

DIVERSITY AWARENESS

LEARNING OBJECTIVES

- Relate how a patient's values, beliefs, and judgments may create barriers to successful treatment if the HIV provider does not competently navigate the cultural differences between the patient and the healthcare provider.

- Recognize the challenges in addressing racial and ethnic disparities in healthcare and in HIV in particular.

- Discuss the impact that culture, ethnicity, immigration status, sexual orientation, religion, gender, and behavioral health problems may have on the care of HIV-infected patients.

WHAT'S NEW?

It is estimated that 61% of new HIV infections are transmitted by patients who have either dropped out of care or are not taking their medications. In order to improve patient adherence and retention in care, efforts to enhance trust in healthcare providers require a broader understanding of the diversity and cultures of many different groups of patients with HIV.

KEY POINT

- Patients with HIV come from diverse backgrounds and are often mistrustful of healthcare providers.

LOSS OF RETENTION IN CARE

Retaining patients in care requires culturally competent staff at all levels of an organization. It could be easy for the busy HIV specialist to focus more intensely on the complex medical aspects of HIV medicine and relegate the issues of diversity and cultural competence to "soft areas" that are of lesser importance than learning resistance mutations or developing expertise in the use of the latest antiviral drugs. However, to do so runs the risk of failing to adequately comprehend how a patient's behaviors, beliefs, and the characteristics of his or her unique social, ethnic, racial, religious, gender identity, or country of origin may affect his or her engagement with the healthcare system. Failing to understand the important cultural context within which a patient interacts with the healthcare system often leads to poor patient adherence with treatment, misunderstandings about the treatment plan, or, worse, loss of retention in care. To successfully treat patients and to achieve the goals of treatment, we need to do our best to understand the unique context of our diverse group of patients and to provide care that acknowledges the cultural values that may impact acceptance of treatment.

A recent US Centers for Disease Control and Prevention (CDC) analysis (Skarbinski, 2015) estimated that patients with previously diagnosed HIV infection who were out of care were responsible for 61% of new HIV infections in the United States. Furthermore, a statewide study from North Carolina that analyzed patients with acute HIV infection found that most transmission events (77%) were attributable to partners with previously diagnosed infection, of whom only 23% were reportedly in care and taking antiviral medication within the time that transmission was likely to have occurred (Cope, 2015). This is compelling evidence that the system of HIV care in the United States is failing to treat and retain many patients already diagnosed with HIV. There are likely many reasons for lack of success in patient retention, but it underscores the crucial need to improve the ways healthcare providers interact with patients in order to successfully keep them engaged in care and adherent with their antiviral medications. Developing competence in understanding the attributes of a diverse patient population is challenging, but failure to do so will allow greater numbers of HIV-infected patients to lose contact with care. The greater challenge in becoming culturally competent is for each healthcare provider to develop self-awareness of his or her own values, beliefs, and attitudes and what biases may be inherent in the provider's own culture.

DIVERSITY OF PATIENTS WITH HIV

An HIV provider caring for patients with HIV is likely caring for a diverse population of patients from racial or ethnic groups different from his or her own. In the United States, people with HIV are disproportionately African American and Hispanic, and, regardless of race or ethnicity, they are often affected by poverty, drug or alcohol abuse, mental health problems, lack of employment, lack of permanent housing, histories of incarceration, inadequate education, and sexual preferences different from those of the general population. Some patients may be immigrants or refugees whose language and cultural differences may cause barriers to acceptance of healthcare services from a system of care culturally different from that of their own. Understanding how a patient's spiritual and religious values may impact his or her healthcare decision-making is important when caring for a diverse group of patients. However, in our attempt to develop cultural understanding of their diversity, it is critical to avoid stereotyping patients, which also creates barriers to acceptance of treatment. The values, beliefs, and judgments of patients may differ from those of their healthcare provider, and unless the healthcare provider is able to withhold his or her own judgment of a patient's circumstances, a trusting relationship may never develop.

THE IMPORTANCE OF TRUST

Trust is a critically important component of a successful patient–clinician relationship. Without trust, a patient is less likely to adhere to a treatment plan. Patients who do not trust their healthcare provider or the healthcare system will be less likely to take prescribed medications, keep scheduled appointments, or accept the advice of their clinician.

Mistrust by certain racial and ethnic minorities in the United States is common. A telephone survey by the Kaiser Family Foundation (James, 1999) found that one-third of African Americans and one-third of Hispanics reported experiencing unfair treatment by the healthcare system compared to less than half those numbers of whites (James, 1999). African Americans were used without their informed consent in medical experimentation by the US Public Health Service from 1932 to 1972 in the notorious Tuskegee syphilis study, which created a legacy of mistrust (Skarbinski, 2015). Mistrust has led to conspiracy theories about the origins of HIV. In 2005, a national telephone survey of 500 African Americans (Bogart, 2005) found that 53% agreed that "there is a cure for AIDS, but it is being withheld from the poor," 27% agreed that "AIDS was produced in a government laboratory," and 16% agreed that "AIDS was created by the government to control the black population."

DISPARITIES IN HEALTHCARE

The HIV epidemic in the United States is characterized by significant racial and ethnic disparities. In 2016, the distribution of diagnoses of HIV infection by race/ethnicity was 26% for whites, 25% for Hispanic/Latino, 44% for blacks/African Americans, 3% for Asians, 1% for American Indian/Alaskan Natives, 2% for those of multiple races, and less than 1% for Native Hawaiian/Other Pacific Islanders (CDC, 2017). For many patients, the route of HIV transmission carries significant stigma. Among black/African American men, of whom 79% contracted the disease by male-to-male sexual contact, being gay or bisexual carries a stigma that is prevalent both in the general population and within the African American community. Stigma creates barriers that keep many men from being tested for HIV or connecting to care once identified as being HIV-positive. Understanding the effect of stigma and developing nonjudgmental ways to communicate effectively with patients require that we first acknowledge that patients may enter their relationship with a healthcare provider assuming the healthcare provider harbors the same biases as the general population. Becoming culturally competent requires clinicians to develop strategies with each patient to allay the patient's fear of disapproval by his or her healthcare provider as well as to provide reassurance that the patient's personal health information will be protected and kept confidential.

With significant racial and ethnic disparities concerning who is infected with HIV, the need to provide culturally appropriate care is evident. Failing to adequately understand a patient's culture—best defined as the unique set of beliefs, characteristics, and behaviors formed by the communities in which a patient resides—can create a barrier between patient and healthcare provider. A lack of trust by the patient may prevent successful treatment. Mistrust of healthcare providers occurs particularly if patients believe they will receive unequal treatment. Many studies across all disease states have documented the unequal treatment provided to blacks and Hispanics. According to the Institute of Medicine (Smedley, 2003), racial and ethnic minorities often receive a lower quality of healthcare services even when insurance status and income are the same as those for nonminorities. Blacks are less likely to be referred for coronary artery revascularization compared to whites when the same degree of disease severity exists for both (Sheifer, 2000). Other studies have shown that African Americans are less likely than whites to receive antiviral therapy (ART) (Moore, 1995) or prophylaxis for Pneumocystis pneumonia (Shapiro, 1999).

Sometimes racial and ethnic disparities result from patient choice or socioeconomic situation, as in cases in which minorities are more likely to refuse recommended treatment services or to delay seeking treatment (Mitchell, 1997). Healthcare clinicians need to understand what objections a patient may have to the recommended treatment in an effort to help the patient understand potential consequences that may occur without treatment. Clinicians need to take the time to ask patients open-ended questions. Asking questions such as "What are your concerns about taking this medication?" allows the patient to express his or her concerns and gives the healthcare provider the opportunity to address them.

BIAS IN HEALTHCARE

Cultural competence requires taking time to learn what cultural barriers might exist. The ethnocentric healthcare provider only views a patient's culture from the perspective of his or her own culture and risks losing patient trust. Healthcare providers are not immune from the same biases that exist in the general population. Bias can be subtle and unconscious. Weisse found that white males were twice as likely to be prescribed analgesics for pain as black males, whereas female physicians prescribed higher doses for blacks than for whites (Weisse, 2001). A study examining how patient race affects physician perceptions found that physicians rated black patients as less intelligent, less educated, more likely to abuse drugs and alcohol, and less likely to adhere to treatment even when considering the patient's income and education (van Ryn, 2000). These studies show how racism and personal bias can lead to unequal care.

Bias can be either overt or covert. Derogatory comments made by either providers or office staff about particular "types" of patients are an example of bias. Judgmental comments about "how frequently certain patients develop sexually transmitted infections," "use the emergency room," "look for pain medications," and "had too many uncared-for children" are examples of overt bias and stereotyping. Such comments, in addition to be highly unprofessional and judgmental, may reinforce among medical staff involved in patient care that bias and judgment are an acceptable form of professional conduct. Negative comments about a patient, especially if overheard by other patients, can transmit to patients that they may be the unwanted topic of conversation. Healthcare organizations need to make certain that staff at all levels and functions within the institution become culturally competent. Recognizing the cultural differences that might exist between a patient and a healthcare provider is an essential step to welcoming each patient with acceptance and understanding. Only by attempting to recognize and to understand these differences can a healthcare provider best comprehend what may be needed to best inspire patient trust in the provider, the institution, and the plan of treatment.

WOMEN AND HIV

There are 18 million women worldwide living with HIV, and in the United States, 19% of peoples with HIV are women (UN AIDS, 2015). The vast majority of women diagnosed with HIV (75%) acquire the virus through heterosexual sex (CDC, 2017). African American women are disproportionately infected with HIV, with 58% of US women with HIV being black (CDC, 2017). Women with HIV experience intimate partner violence at twice the national average (Gruskin, 2014). The meta-analysis by Gruskin et al. (2014) showed that 55% of women with HIV in the United States have experienced trauma and violence. HIV-positive women and transgender women who have experienced trauma and violence had a fourfold higher likelihood of nonadherence to ART (Machinger, 2012), The HIV provider should inquire about a history of violence and abuse and should refer the patient to appropriate crisis and domestic violence services as needed. Healthcare providers should understand that many women who are victims of domestic abuse feel powerless and trapped because of economic dependency, primary responsibility for children, and fear of being homeless. Many women may be slow or unwilling to seek help. A careful mental health and depression screening should be done, and referral to appropriate mental health services should be made when indicated.

LESBIAN, GAY, BISEXUAL, AND TRANSGENDER PATIENTS

Many lesbian, gay, bisexual, and transgender (LGBT) patients do not feel welcome by their healthcare providers. Many LGBT people do not seek medical care because they have had bad experiences with healthcare providers (National LGBT Health Education Center, 2015). One recent study of African American men who have sex with men (MSM) found that 29% experienced racial and sexual stigma from their healthcare providers, and 48% reported mistrust of the healthcare system (Eaton, 2015). If patients feel uncomfortable speaking about their sexual orientation, they are far more likely to withhold important information. Ways to help LGBT patients feel more welcome include using gender-neutral pronouns, allowing LGBT patients to be called by their preferred name (even if their legal name may be different), and training staff to have a nonjudgmental attitude. Learning and using the language that patients use may make patients feel more comfortable. For example, patients may use the terms "top" or "bottom" to describe insertive anal sex or receptive anal sex. Asking patients if they "have sex with men, women, or both" is an appropriate way to learn patients' sexual orientation. Avoidance of words that imply a patient has a relationship with someone of the opposite sex is also important. "Do you have a partner?" or "Are you in a relationship?" are more appropriate questions than "Do you have a husband or wife?" A patient who feels accepted by his or her care provider is more likely to return for care. Conversely, a patient who perceives disapproval of his or her lifestyle, sexual orientation, or practices will feel uncomfortable and is much more likely to not return.

BEHAVIORAL HEALTH PROBLEMS

The HIV Costs and Services Utilization Study found that nearly 50% of adults treated for HIV have symptoms of a psychiatric disorder—a four to eight times higher prevalence than the general population (Bing, 2001). In the general population, there is a 10- to 20-year reduction in life expectancy in people with severe mental health disorders (Chang, 2011). According to the World Health Organization (WHO), the vast majority of these deaths are due to chronic illnesses such as cardiovascular, respiratory, and infectious diseases, diabetes, and hypertension (WHO, 2015). Mental illness caries a risk of mortality greater than that of smoking (Chesney, 2014).

Identifying patients with mental illness or addiction is crucial in caring for patients with HIV disease. A careful history followed by referral to mental health services as needed is important because patients with mental illness have been reported to have lower levels of adherence (Paterson, 2000). Stigma about mental health diagnoses may keep many patients from accessing mental health services. On-site behavioral health services increase the likelihood that patients will connect to treatment. Many patients with substance abuse problems may experience a sense of rejection when they reveal that they have chemical dependency or are participating in a substance abuse treatment program. They may assume that mentioning pain will be perceived as drug-seeking by their healthcare provider—a common stereotype of healthcare providers. Cultural competence requires communicating with patients openly and without judgment. It requires efforts to develop trust and to help reduce the stigma that most drug users have about their chemical dependency.

CARING FOR IMMIGRANTS AND REFUGEES

Refugees are people who have experienced or been at risk of being persecuted due to race, religion, nationality, membership in a particular social group, or political opinion and have become emigrants fleeing their home country of origin to seek safety. Of the approximately 42 million displaced people in the world, approximately 16 million have sought asylum. The number of refugees accepted into the United States is projected to increase, and many healthcare providers may see additional refugees in the coming years (Gordon, 2015). Refugees are often victims of physical and emotional trauma. Many immigrants from sub-Saharan Africa have walked hundreds of miles to refugee camps, often while witnessing deaths of family members and becoming victims of violence and sexual trauma. Others have been separated from family. To provide adequate care, it is important for the healthcare provider to understand both the physical and the emotional trauma the patient has experienced and to provide services that respect the culture, gender roles, and family structure of the patient. Finding culturally and linguistically appropriate counseling or specialty care for immigrants and refugees can be difficult. The use of translation services is often necessary when caring for immigrants and refugees. The diagnosis of HIV for many refugees and immigrants carries great stigma. The HIV provider will need to pay particular attention to understanding how the patient's culture may impact the patient's acceptance of his or her illness and the need to take antiviral medications.

LANGUAGE AND COMMUNICATION

Language comprehension and communication are essential to patient understanding and, ultimately, to good adherence. Many HIV patients speak languages other than English. Language barriers can interfere with the success of treatment. Exit interviews of emergency room patients found that Spanish-speaking patients were less likely to understand their discharge instructions or carry out follow-up plans (Crane, 1997). Another survey found that one in five Spanish-speaking patients delayed or refused medical treatment because of language barriers, underscoring the need to provide linguistically appropriate services to HIV patients who will need lifelong care (Bass, 2000).

Hiring bilingual and bicultural staff is important in a culturally competent organization when there are significant numbers of patients in the local population who speak a particular language. The culturally competent clinical practice needs to make use of professional interpreter services for patients who do not speak the language of the healthcare provider. The use of family members or friends may inhibit patient honesty when asked to discuss personal information. Telephone interpreter services, although costly, are a necessary tool when on-site interpretation is unavailable. This is especially important for immigrant populations, for whom linguistic barriers, often combined with significant cultural differences, may greatly impede the delivery of healthcare. Patients who used the interpreter services received significantly more recommended preventive services, made more office visits, and had more prescriptions written and filled (Jacobs, 2004).

RELIGION AND SPIRITUALITY

A 2014 Gallup survey found that 81% of Americans identify with a particular religion (Newport, 2014). Patients turn to religion in times of illness, and this often influences the way a person perceives and copes with his or her situation. Many patients with HIV have strong religious affiliations (Cotton, 2006). A patient's faith may sometimes conflict with medical advice, which can lead to a lack of adherence to treatment. It is important to ask patients about their religious and spiritual beliefs and how those beliefs may affect their perception of illness and acceptance of treatment.

CREATING A CULTURALLY COMPETENT HIV PRACTICE

Racial and ethnic diversity in healthcare leadership and staff is a priority in building culturally competent healthcare organizations. Including community members and consumer representatives on governing boards, as is done at Federally Qualified Health Centers (FQHCs), can help hold an organization accountable for providing culturally competent care to a diverse patient population. Providing materials that are linguistically appropriate to the population being served at a literacy level appropriate to the level of most patients is important.

Changing the model of care from the traditional physician-centered practice to a model that places the patient in the center of the relationship—the patient-centered medical home (PCMH) model—can improve the quality of care. This model relies on reorganizing care to ensure that it is comprehensive, with integrated physical and mental health services. Care that is patient-centered supports patients' efforts to manage their own care to whatever degree they may choose. It is coordinated so that there is a smoother transition across levels of care, such as primary care, hospital care, and specialty care. Services are accessible, with after-hours access to a healthcare provider, along with flexible office hours. Last, there is a focus on quality and safety, using evidence-based standards and data for performance improvement (Agency for Healthcare Research and Quality, 2015). Culturally and linguistically appropriate services are offered. In one study, retention in care for HIV patients was improved with the PCMH model (Sitapati, 2012).

Patients want healthcare providers who communicate with them and who are empathic. Better healthcare outcomes have been associated with providers with whom patients can share their feelings and thoughts. Patients of empathic and communicative healthcare providers are far more likely to comply with their treatment plans (Sitapati, 2012).

The patient-centered approach incorporates cultural competency interventions in order to better address the racial, ethnic, and cultural differences between provider and patient, and it offers training to providers and to all staff who interact with patients in order to make them more culturally competent (Kim, 2004). Healthcare provider training to improve providers' knowledge and attitudes about diverse populations is essential to creating a culturally competent system of care.

Perhaps most important, aspiring culturally competent healthcare providers must raise their individual self-awareness of their own cultural beliefs, values, and attitudes and any biases that may be inherent in them. Consciousness of one's own cultural biases and an honest attempt to transcend them will allow the HIV provider to communicate effectively, with empathy, and without prejudgment, facilitating an improved and mutually satisfying relationship with each patient.

RECOMMENDED READING

Anderson LM, Scrimshaw SC, et al. Culturally competent healthcare systems: a systematic review. *Am J Prev Med*. 2003;24(3S):68–79.

Betancourt JR. Cultural competence in healthcare: emerging frameworks and practical approaches: Field Report 2002. The Commonwealth Fund. Available at http://www.commonwealthfund.org/usr_doc/betancourt_culturalcompetence_576.pdf. Accessed December 1, 2015.

Institute of Medicine. Unequal treatment: what healthcare providers need to know about racial and ethnic disparities in healthcare 2002. National Academy of Sciences. Available at https://www.nationalacademies.org/hmd/~/media/Files/Report%20Files/2003/Unequal-Treatment-Confronting-Racial-and-Ethnic-Disparities-in-Health-Care/Disparitieshcproviders8pgFINAL.pdf. Accessed December 1, 2015.

Institute of Medicine. *Unequal Treatment: Confronting Racial and Ethnic Disparities in Health Care* (full printed version). Washington, DC: National Academies Press; 2003. doi: 10.17226/10260.

CARING FOR HIV-INFECTED CHILDREN

LEARNING OBJECTIVE

Identify the diagnostic criteria, laboratory markers, epidemiologic patterns, spectrum of disease manifestations, and unique immunization and therapy issues in HIV-infected children.

WHAT'S NEW?

In 2014, the CDC revised the definitions for and stage classification of HIV infection in persons of all ages, and, in 2018, the

Panel on Antiretroviral Therapy and Medical Management of Children Living with HIV updated the guidelines for use of antiretroviral (ARV) agents in pediatric HIV infection.

KEY POINTS

- In the United States, the prevalence of perinatally acquired HIV has declined dramatically.

- Pediatric and adult HIV/AIDS differ in the following areas: AIDS-defining conditions, epidemiology and transmission, pathophysiology, diagnostic challenges, clinical manifestations, and management issues.

- In the United States, pediatric HIV/AIDS disproportionately affects ethnic minorities, particularly African Americans.

- Due to pathophysiologic differences, untreated HIV-infected children younger than 2 years of age are uniquely susceptible to encephalopathy and routinely have higher viral loads than adults.

- Normal CD4$^+$ T cell counts are higher in healthy infants and children younger than 6 years of age than in adults.

- Infants born to HIV-positive mothers will test positive on routine anti-HIV antibody tests due to placental immunoglobulin (IgG) transport; sequential nucleic acid test (NAT) analysis can identify infected infants usually by 1 month of age.

- Clinical features more common in children include developmental delay, recurrent otitis media and sinobronchial infections, lymphoid interstitial pneumonia, and severe dental carries.

- In children and adults, the general concepts of ART, opportunistic infection (OI) prophylaxis, and viral load and CD4$^+$ T cell count monitoring are similar, and treatment of all HIV-infected children regardless of age, symptoms, or CD4$^+$ T cell count is now recommended.

- Administration of routine immunizations in HIV-infected children is complicated by the use of live virus vaccines (rotavirus; measles, mumps, and rubella (MMR); varicella) in standard practice.

- Avoidance of breastfeeding by HIV-infected mothers continues to be advised. However, the latest guidelines (USDHHS, 2018) now provide for counseling and managing HIV-infected women in the United States who desire to breastfeed.

- The HIV-infected child's family needs, both material and psychosocial, are often extraordinarily complex, requiring intensive, community, social services utilization.

- Whenever possible, a pediatric HIV specialist should supervise the management of children younger than 16 years.

In the United States, the prevalence of perinatally acquired HIV/AIDS has declined dramatically during the past 30 years due to extraordinary public health investments. Despite this, children continue to be born to HIV-infected women and to be infected with HIV. Pediatric and adult HIV/AIDS differ significantly in the following areas: AIDS-defining conditions, epidemiology, pathophysiology, diagnostic challenges, clinical manifestations, and management issues that are unique to children.

DEFINITION

In 2014, the CDC and the Council of State and Territorial Epidemiologists revised and combined surveillance case definitions and stage classification for HIV infection into a single entity covering persons of all ages (Selik, 2014). Confirmed cases of HIV infection are classified into stages 0, 1, 2, 3, or unknown.

Stage 0 is defined as the presence of early HIV infection with a negative HIV antibody test. The stage includes "acute HIV infection" or "acute retroviral syndrome" that occurs days to weeks postexposure and presents with flu-like or mononucleosis-like signs and symptoms.

Classification of stages 1, 2, and 3 is based on age-specific CD4$^+$ T lymphocyte count or percentage of total lymphocyte count (Table 13.1) or the diagnosis of an opportunistic condition in the case of stage 3 (Table 13.2). Furthermore, clinical features considered as "mild" or "moderate" HIV-related symptoms are listed in the recent guidelines (see https://aidsetc.org/guide/hiv-classification-cdc-and-who-staging-systems).

Table 13.1 HIV INFECTION STAGING BASED ON AGE-SPECIFIC CD4$^+$ T LYMPHOCYTE NUMBERS OR PERCENTAGE

	AGE ON DATE OF CD4$^+$ T LYMPHOCYTE TEST					
	<1 YEAR		1–5 YEARS		≥6 YEARS	
STAGE	CELLS/ML	%	CELLS/ML	%	CELLS/ML	%
1	≥1500	≥34	≥1000	≥30	≥500	≥26
2	750–1499	26–33	500–999	22–29	200499	14–25
3	<750	<26	<500	<22	<200	≤14

SOURCE: Reproduced from Centers for Disease Control and Prevention. Revised surveillance care definition for HIV infection—United States, 2014. *MMWR.* 2014;63(3):1–10.

Table 13.2 STAGE-3/AIDS-DEFINING CONDITIONS

All ages	Opportunistic infections (e.g., PJP and severe or disseminated CMV, toxoplasma HSV, mycobacteria) Selected malignancies (lymphoma, KS) HIV encephalopathy HIV wasting
<1 year old	CD4⁺ T cell count <750 (<26%)
1–5 years old	CD4⁺ T cell count <500 (<22%) Recurrent bacterial infections
≥6 years old	CD4⁺ T cell count <200 (<14%) Cervical cancer, invasive Recurrent pneumonia

SOURCE: Adapted from Centers for Disease Control and Prevention. Revised surveillance care definition for HIV infection—United States, 2014. *MMWR*. 2014;63(3):1–10.

EPIDEMIOLOGY

It is estimated that 70% of HIV-infected women are sexually active and 25–30% of HIV-infected women in North America express a desire to have children (Chen, 2001). In the United States, factors that place children at increased risk for HIV infection include being born to an HIV-infected mother, blood transfusion (outside the United States), being fed premasticated food, sexual abuse, and accidental sharps injury.

Remarkably, in contrast to the modest reduction in the incidence of new HIV infections in adults in the United States from 2010 to 2016 (to an estimated 39,700 new cases per year in 2016; CDC, 2018), the number of HIV-infected children has declined dramatically over the past 20 years (Figure 13.1). This decline has been due to the intense efforts by public health departments and local perinatal HIV centers. Factors contributing to this dramatic change include the following:

- HIV transmission through blood transfusion has been eliminated (except in very rare circumstances) through the screening of all blood products since 1985.

- HIV-infected women are increasingly aware of their HIV-infection status and receive effective ART prior to conception and throughout their pregnancies.

- HIV screening of pregnant women has allowed the implementation of ART during pregnancy and prior to delivery.

- Rapid HIV testing during labor identifies HIV-infected women, allowing initiation of antiviral therapy during labor and delivery and postnatally to the newborn.

- Treatment of newborns exposed to HIV (e.g., in a mother without prenatal care) can still result in a substantial reduction in transmission when the infant alone is treated. This was the first demonstration of effective postexposure prophylaxis.

- HIV-infected infants and children treated prior to the development of clinical symptoms and adherent to their treatment regimens rarely develop AIDS-defining conditions.

Despite this extraordinary progress in reducing maternal-to-child transmission, disturbing racial and ethnic disparities among children persist and generally reflect the prevalence of HIV infection in the respective populations. Black and Hispanic children are disproportionately infected with HIV. African Americans comprise more than 50% of newly infected children (Figure 13.2).

At year's end 2015, 11,847 persons were living with perinatally acquired HIV infection. Figure 13.3 shows that a remarkable 27% of these individuals were older than 24 years.

UNIQUE FEATURES OF PEDIATRIC HIV/AIDS PATHOGENESIS

HIV pathogenesis in children differs from that in adults in several ways. Untreated infection during embryologic or perinatal development has the potential to interfere with normal neurologic and immunologic developmental processes at critical

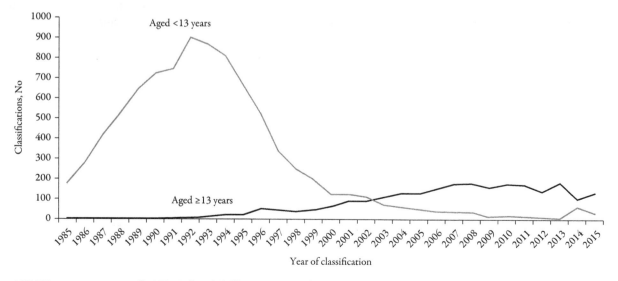

Figure 13.1 AIDS Diagnoses in perinatally HIV-Infected children <13 years of age and >13 years of age by year of diagnosis, 1985–2015.

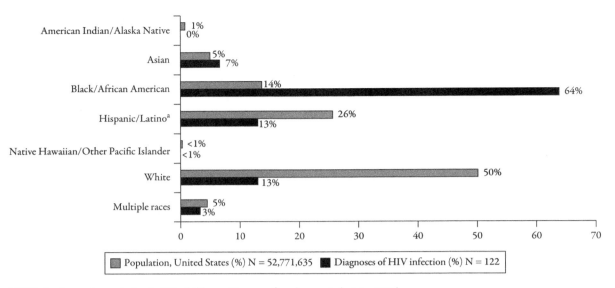

Figure 13.2 HIV Infection and population in U.S. children <13 years of age by race/ethnicity, 2016.

times during ontogeny. In addition, the blood–brain barrier in children is more permissive to viral entry, and the combination of undiagnosed HIV infection and an OI such as *Pneumocystis jirovecii* pneumonia (PCP) may increase trafficking of HIV-infected monocytes to the brain (Nottet, 1996).

HIV infection in infants that occurs prior to the generation of antigen-specific T and B cell repertoires may damage the thymus before these protective immune responses can occur. Furthermore, the "normal" recurrent infection pattern in children may enhance the immunologic activation that is part of the immunopathogenesis of HIV (Sodora, 2008). The combination of these factors can result in unique manifestations of pediatric neuroencephalopathy, immunodeficiency, and pathologic findings.

DIAGNOSIS OF HIV INFECTION IN CHILDREN

Although current fourth-generation HIV antigen/antibody testing algorithms are useful for decreasing the "window" between infection and seropositivity, they are not particularly useful in children. Maternal antibodies are efficiently

transported across the placenta, and infants born to HIV-infected mothers have high levels of HIV antibodies that may persist for more than 15 months. Therefore, interpretation of an HIV test result in a particular infant depends on his or her age. A positive HIV antibody test in an infant younger than age 18 month identifies the infant as being "at risk" for HIV infection but not necessarily infected (Husson, 1990) (Box 13.1).

SELECTED CLINICAL FEATURES OF HIV INFECTION IN CHILDREN

Clinical features of HIV infections that are similar in children and adults include OIs, "opportunistic" malignancies, chronic enteropathy (infectious and noninfectious), hepatosplenomegaly, lymphadenopathy, parotitis, and cardiomyopathy. However, clinical features that are more common in children than in adults include the following (Church, 2000):

- Toxoplasmosis, other agents, rubella, cytomegalovirus, and herpes simplex" (Torch) syndrome

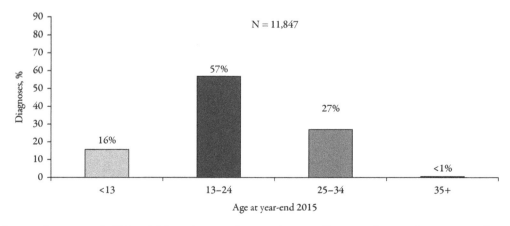

Figure 13.3 Age distribution of persons in the U.S. and 6 dependent areas living with perinatally-acquired HIV infection, year-end 2015.

A. Diagnosis of HIV Infection in Children

<24 months of age	2 positive nucleic acid (NAT) tests; DNA or RNA PCR preferred
>24 months of age	Confirmed positive HIV antibody test

B. Exclusion of HIV Infection in Children

Birth	Negative maternal HIV Ab/Ag test
<18 months of age: Definitive *exclusion* of HIV infection (in absence of breast feeding)	At least 2 negative virologic tests (DNA or RNA PCR): One at > 1 month age, and One at >4 months of age
>24 months of age (in absence of breast feeding)	Negative HIV antibody test

Reproduced from: http://aidsinfo.nih.gov/guidelines/html/2/pediatric-treatment-guidelines—Diagnosis of HIV infection in infants.

Table 13.3 POTENTIAL NEWBORN CONSEQUENCES OF MATERNAL HIV RISK BEHAVIOR AND HIV INFECTION

MATERNAL HIGH-RISK BEHAVIORS WITH NEWBORN CONSEQUENCES
Lack of prenatal care
　↑ risk prematurity
　↑ pregnancy, labor and delivery complications
Compromised intrauterine environment
　Malnutrition
　Illicit drug exposure
Increased risk of non-HIV congenital infections
　Toxoplasmosis – hepatitis B – condylomata (HPV)
　Cytomegalovirus – hepatitis C
　Herpes simplex virus – group B b Streptococci

NEWBORN CONSEQUENCES OF MATERNAL HIV INFECTION
HIV transmission
↑ Early spontaneous abortions
Complications of C-section
Impaired T-cell progenitor function
Exposure to antiretroviral drugs
　Infection with resistant HIV
　↑ Risk prematurity
　Nucleoside analogues
Anemia, neutropenia
Mitochondrial toxicity/encephalopathy
Premature delivery

- Growth failure/short stature

- Developmental delay/mental retardation

- Cerebral palsy

- Aspiration/swallowing dysfunction

- Recurrent otitis media/sinusitis

- Recurrent bacterial pneumonias

- Severe molluscum contagiosum

- Lymphoid interstitial pneumonia

- Bacterial meningitis

- Severe dental caries

- Delayed puberty

Importantly, HIV-infected infants and children without other complicating factors (Table 13.3) treated soon after birth usually will develop few of these features.

MANAGEMENT OF HIV-EXPOSED NEWBORNS

HIV-infected pregnant women are best managed in perinatal centers that are highly experienced with this patient population. For newborns at risk of acquiring HIV, the following are recommended (USDHHS, 2017):

- Avoid breastfeeding and giving premasticated foods

- Obtain pretreatment laboratory studies

  - Complete blood count with differential
  - Liver function tests
  - HIV DNA or RNA polymerase chain reaction (PCR)
  - CD4$^+$ T cell count and percentage (optional).
    - Cytomegalovirus PCR (oral swab or urine) (optional).

- ART

  - All newborn exposed to HIV should receive ART.
  - Newborn ART regimen (at gestational age—appropriate doses) should be initiated 6–12 hours postdelivery.
  - Selection of ART regimen should be based on maternal and infant factors the influence transmission risk.
  - Newborns whose mothers have substantial viral suppression may be given a 4-week zidovudine prophylaxis regimen.
    - Newborns at high risk should receive combination ART. Circumstances that define "higher risk" and ARV management according to risk of HIV infection are detailed in the Guidelines.

- Obtain RNA or DNA PCR within 48 hours of birth; repeat at 2–3 weeks, 1–2 months, and 4–6 months. If HIV exposure continues (breastfeeding), HIV DNA or RNA PCR should be done at similar intervals after exposure is discontinued.

- Consult a specialist in pediatric HIV management.

MANAGEMENT OF HIV-INFECTED CHILDREN

Combination ART has transformed the nature of pediatric HIV/AIDS. When initiated in a timely manner and adherence is maintained, HIV-infected children are now leading near normal lives. Management is best guided at centers experienced in the unique features of pediatric HIV/AIDS.

Revised guidelines for the use of ARV agents in pediatric HIV infection (USDHHS, 2018) now recommend treatment of all HIV-infected children regardless of age, symptoms, or CD4+ T cell count. However, specific social and economic factors may temper the initiation of ARV agents in specific situations.

For treatment of ART-naïve children the Panel on Antiretroviral Therapy and Medical Management of Children Living with HIV has recommended the following:

- The selection of an initial regimen should be individualized based on several factors including characteristics of the proposed regimen, patient characteristics, drug efficacy, potential adverse effects, patient and family preferences, and results of viral resistance testing.

- For treatment-naïve children, ART should be initiated with three drugs, including either an integrase strand transfer inhibitor, a non-nucleoside reverse transcriptase inhibitor, or a boosted protease inhibitor (PI), plus a dual nucleoside/nucleotide reverse transcriptase inhibitor backbone.

- In the Guidelines, table 7 provides a list of Panel-recommended regimens that are designated as *Preferred* or *Alternative;* recommendations vary by age, weight, and sexual maturity.

Although there are similarities between children and adults with regard to regimen selection and the importance of adherence to ART, there are special considerations for the treatment of infants and children:

- There is the additional goal of maintaining normal physical growth and neurocognitive development.

- Medication doses must be monitored in growing children.

- Liquids, particularly PIs, have poor palatability. Gastrostomy tube placement may be necessary in selected patients.

- There is a lack of pharmacokinetic and toxicity data for newer drugs.

MONITORING

Close psychosocial, clinical, and laboratory monitoring of children before and after initiation of ART is critical (Table 13.4).

PREVENTION OF HIV-RELATED INFECTIONS

Primary *Pneumocystis jiroveci* pneumonia (PJP) prophylaxis with trimethoprim–sulfamethoxazole is recommended for all HIV-infected infants from 4 weeks of age to 1 year, regardless of CD4+ T cell counts or percentages. After 1 year, the need for PJP prophylaxis is determined by the level of immune suppression. Secondary prophylaxis is also recommended for selected OIs in HIV-infected infants and children and for others only if episodes are frequent or severe change (Table 13.5).

Finally, the Guidelines provide detailed recommendations for the treatment of OIs in children. However, the effectiveness of ART in children can be remarkable. With consistent adherence, HIV-positive children will rarely experience the types of OIs listed previously.

Primary prophylaxis for PJP and *Mycobacterium avium* complex may be discontinued after CD4+ counts exceed the threshold for initiation of prophylaxis.

IMMUNIZATION IN HIV-INFECTED INFANTS AND CHILDREN

- Rotavirus (live) vaccine may be considered in HIV-infected infants (<6 months of age), but it should be

Table 13.4 SAMPLE OF A MONITORING SCHEDULE FOR PEDIATRIC HIV/AIDS

	PRE-THERAPY	1–2 WEEK ON THERAPY	4–6 WEEKS ON THERAPY	EVERY 3–4 MONTHS
History and physical exam	X	X	X	X
Social and adherence evaluations	X	X	X	X
Complete blood count with differential	X		X	X
Chemistry panel	X		X	X
Urinalysis	X			X
CD4+ T-cell count / %	X		X	X
HIV RNA viral load	X		X	X
Resistance testing	X			

SOURCE: Adapted from http://aidsinfo.nih.gov/guidelines/html/2/pediatrc-treatment-guidelines—Use of antiretroviral agents in Pediatric HIV infection.

Table 13.5 PROPHYLAXIS TO PREVENT OCCURRENCES OR RECURRENCES OF SELECTED OPPORTUNISTIC INFECTIONS AMONG HIV-INFECTED INFANTS AND CHILDREN

	PROPHYLAXIS	
PATHOGEN	INDICATION	FIRST CHOICE AGENT
Pneumocystis jiroveci	Severe immunosuppression	TMP-SMZ
Mycobacterium avium complex	Very severe immunosuppression	Clarithromycin plus ethambutol, plus rifabutin
Toxoplasma gondii	Prior toxoplasma encephalitis	Sulfadiazine plus pyrimethamine plus leucovorin
Cryptococcus neoformans	Prior disease	Fluconazole
Histoplasma capsulatum	Prior disease	Itraconazole
Coccidioides immitis	Prior disease	Fluconazole
Cytomegalovirus	Prior disease	Ganciclovir
Recommended only if subsequent episodes are frequent or severe		
Invasive bacterial infections	>2 infections in a 1-year period	TMP-SMZ or IVIG
Herpes simplex virus	Frequent or severe recurrences	Acyclovir
Candida (oropharyngeal or esophageal)	Frequent or severe recurrences	Fluconazole

withheld if there is a suspicion or confirmation of severely reduced CD4$^+$ T cells.

- Infants should receive the primary immunization series and "boosters" with inactivated vaccines when age appropriate:
  - Diphtheria, tetanus, and pertussis (DTaP)
  - Inactivated polio vaccine (IPV)
  - *Haemophilus influenzae* type b conjugate vaccine (Hib)
  - Pneumococcal conjugate vaccine (PCV)
  - Hepatitis A and B vaccines
  - Meningococcal conjugate vaccine (MCV4) at ages 11 and 16 years
  - Influenza vaccine (annually)
- MMR and varicella (live) vaccines are recommended for HIV-infected children who are asymptomatic and not "severely immunosuppressed."
- Human papillomavirus (HPV) vaccine series should begin at age 9 years (Meites, 2016).
- Children who present with low T cell counts may benefit from ART treatment and immunologic reconstitution before additional vaccine are given.

TYPICAL REFERRAL NEEDS OF HIV-INFECTED INFANTS, CHILDREN, AND THEIR FAMILIES

Most HIV-infected children are born into socially and economically disadvantaged families of color and not infrequently are placed in the foster care setting. These children and families require multiple support services, including the following:

- Medical management for HIV, sexually transmitted diseases, and hepatitis
- AIDS prevention case management
- Drug/alcohol abuse prevention/treatment
- Mental health services for the child and family
- Partner counseling and services for parents
- Legal and immigration services
- Housing, food, and transportation needs
- Child care services
- Domestic violence counseling
- Education programs
- Disclosure counseling
- Adherence counseling

Other issues important to families are illustrated by the following questions:

- When should an HIV-infected child be told of his or her diagnosis?
- Are families obligated, legally or ethically, to disclose their child's diagnosis to other care providers and schools?
- Should HIV-infected children be allowed to participate in contact sports?

- Under what circumstances should postexposure prophylaxis be offered to an HIV-negative child potentially exposed after sexual abuse or needle stick injury?

- When should an HIV-infected child be removed from parental custody if ART adherence is poor?

- Can HIV-infected children safely have children of their own?

UNRESOLVED PEDIATRIC ISSUES

Although ART has dramatically improved the longevity and quality of life for HIV-infected children, there are unresolved, long-term questions that remain to be answered, including the following:

- Is neurocognitive development really normal in children treated early in the course of infection?

- Will inadequate bone mineralization in childhood result in increased bone disease later in life?

- What will be the clinical impact of the mitochondrial dysfunction identified in HIV-infected infants and those exposed to ARV agents in utero?

- Will the cardiovascular complication of dyslipidemia and long-term immune activation (despite effective viral suppression in the peripheral blood) result in early myocardial infarction or stroke?

- What will be the long-term outcome of HIV-infected children with coinfections including tuberculosis, hepatitis B virus, and hepatitis C virus?

RECOMMENDED READING

AIDS Info website. Available at http://www.aidsinfo.nih.gov/guidelines.

American Academy of Pediatrics. Human immunodeficiency virus infection. In Kimberlin DW, Brady MT, Jackson MA, et al., eds., *Red Book: 2015 Report of the Committee on Infectious Diseases*. 30th ed. Elk Grove Village, IL: American Academy of Pediatrics; 2015:453–476.

Centers for Disease Control and Prevention website. Available at http://www.cdc.gov/hiv.

HIV InSite website. Available at http://hivinsite.ucsf.edu.

Lala MM, Merchant RH, eds. *Principles of Perinatal and Pediatric HIV/AIDS*. New York: Jaypee Brothers; 2011.

National Perinatal Hotline. 888-449-8765.

Women, Children, and HIV website. Available at http://www.womenchildrenhiv.org.

CARING FOR HIV-INFECTED ADOLESCENTS

LEARNING OBJECTIVE

Describe the developmental, cognitive, social, and environmental factors that may affect treatment adherence and secondary prevention in adolescents.

WHAT'S NEW?

Worldwide, adolescent women represent the majority of new HIV cases. In the United States, rates of infection have increased among young MSM of color.

KEY POINTS

- Adolescents are at risk for HIV through sexual behaviors; most adolescents acquire HIV through unprotected sex.

- Adolescents in late puberty can be managed according to adult/adolescent guidelines; prepubescent and early pubescent adolescents can be managed according to pediatric guidelines.

- Psychosocial issues that could affect adherence should be addressed before starting treatment.

- Sexual risk behaviors in HIV-infected adolescents should be given special attention.

The period of adolescence (defined as ages 12–24 years) is a critical time of physical, social, emotional, and cognitive growth and development (Sanders, 2013). However, adolescents are the most uninsured and underinsured age group in the United States and the least likely group to use primary care and other outpatient medical services (Kaiser Foundation, 2007). Those with specific health and social problems, as well as those with particular difficulty obtaining appropriate medical care and other services, are at heightened risk for HIV infection. These groups include adolescents who are gay, lesbian, bisexual, or transgender; homeless and runaway individuals; injection drug users; individuals who have a mental illness; and those who have been sexually or physically abused or incarcerated or are in foster care.

Health disparities occur as a result of an individual's interaction with socioenvironmental factors at the interpersonal (e.g., family and social/sexual networks), intermediate structural (e.g., community, social institutions, culture, social norms, and values), and macrostructural (e.g., socioeconomic conditions) levels (McLeroy, 1988) that contribute to high rates of HIV. For example, young black men who have sex with men and bisexual men and other MSM were disproportionately impacted by HIV in the United States between 2010 and 2016 (CDC, 2018) (Figures 13.4 and 13.5) and accounted for the majority of new HIV infections in their age group (CDC, 2018). Worldwide, adolescent girls disproportionately account for new HIV infections (UNICEF). Such high rates do not result from increased individual behavior but rather from the complex interrelationship of multiple social identities—for example, race, ethnicity, gender, socioeconomic status, and sexual orientation—that intersect at the individual's experience and reflect larger social-structural inequities experienced on the macro level (Bowleg, 2013; Crenshaw, 1991; Haltikis, 2013).

Approximately 1 million adult persons living in the United States are transgender (i.e., someone who has a gender identity that differs from the sex they were assigned at birth; Meerwijk, 2017). From 2009 to 2014, 2,351 transgender people were diagnosed with HIV in the United States, and the CDC

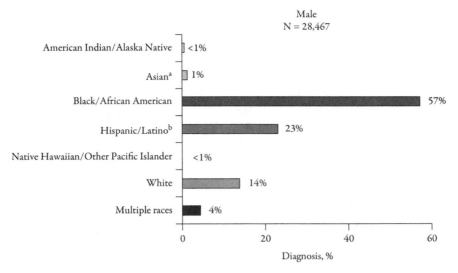

Male
N = 28,467

American Indian/Alaska Native   <1%
Asian[a]   1%
Black/African American   57%
Hispanic/Latino[b]   23%
Native Hawaiian/Other Pacific Islander   <1%
White   14%
Multiple races   4%

0   20   40   60

Diagnosis, %

Figure 13.4 Adolescent and Young Males Aged 13-24 Years Living with Diagnosed HIV Infection by Sex and Race/Ethnicity, Year-end 2015—United States and 6 Dependent Areas. [a] Includes Asian/Pacific Islander legacy cases. [b] Hispanic/Latinos can be of any race.

estimates that 21.6% of transgender women in the United States are living with HIV. More than one-third (36.3%) of these women were adolescents and young adults less than 24 years old (Clark, 2017). This represents a 34-fold increased odds of HIV infection compared to that of all reproductive-age adults (Baral, 2013). Transwomen of color are particularly affected. Data from Washington, DC, suggest that rates of HIV are as high as 32% among black transgender women (Xavier, 2005). Higher rates of HIV are attributed to experiences of stigma, discrimination, negative healthcare encounters, lack of familial support, limited healthcare and housing access, and high mental health diagnoses that contribute to high drug

and alcohol abuse, sex work, incarceration, homelessness, and attempted suicide.

Perinatally infected youth from the 1990s are another group of adolescents and young adults living with HIV. Currently, with near universal maternal screening and treatment, this population is remaining small in most high-income countries. The same cannot be said for low-resource countries, in which perinatal transmission continues to be an ongoing concern. Perinatal youth share many common issues with youth infected behaviorally—namely stigma, sexuality, disclosure, unplanned pregnancy, nonadherence, and substance misuse and abuse. However, this population generally is on more complicated ARV regimens based on the development of resistance mutations during childhood.

The same socioecologic factors (discrimination, isolation, microaggressions, and minority stress) that contribute to HIV risk predispose youth to comorbidities (high rates of mental health and substance use disorders) and medical nonadherence in care. Differences in the treatment cascade of care by age have been hypothesized as an explanation for the increase in HIV infections by at-risk youth nationally (Zanoni, 2014). Less than half (40%) of those aged 13–29 years are aware of their HIV status, and best estimates suggest that only 62% of those are connected to care within their first year of diagnosis (Zanoni, 2014). Other studies have suggested that adolescents have much lower linkage rates, ranging from 29% to 73% successfully linked within the first year of diagnosis (Craw, 2008; Torian, 2008). The CDC and the US Preventive Services Task Force recommend routine HIV screening for all youth (Branson, 2006; Moyer, 2013). Annual screening is recommended based on risk, and gay and bisexual youth should be screened every 3–6 months (CDC, 2015). Venue-based and social networking testing is another effective strategy to reach high-risk youth and increase the identification and linkage of youth into care (Barnes, 2010; Boyer, 2013; Straub, 2011). Once diagnosed with HIV, special

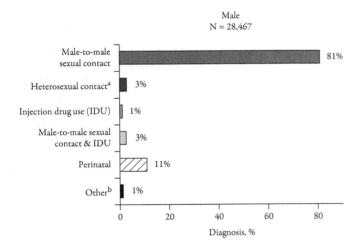

Male
N = 28,467

Male-to-male sexual contact   81%
Heterosexual contact[a]   3%
Injection drug use (IDU)   1%
Male-to-male sexual contact & IDU   3%
Perinatal   11%
Other[b]   1%

0   20   40   60   80

Diagnosis, %

Figure 13.5 Adolescent and Young Adult Males Aged 13-24 Years Living with Diagnosed HIV Infection by Sex and Transmission Category, Year-end 2015—United States and 6 Dependent Area. *Note*: Data have been statistically adjusted to account for missing transmission category. "Other" transmission category not displayed as it comprises less than 1% of cases. [a] Heterosexual contact with a person known to have, or be at high risk for, HIV infection. [b] Includes hemophilia, blood transfusion, and risk factor not reported or not identified.

efforts to improve engagement in care are often necessary to maximize youth accessing care.

DEVELOPMENTAL ISSUES

Adolescents face the same barriers to treatment adherence as adults, but they have additional challenges due to their developmental stage and legal circumstances (Table 13.6). Social stigma, fear of alienation from peer groups, medication side effects, lack of transportation, dependence on parents or other caregivers, growing autonomy, and "feeling fine" are major contributors to nonadherence (Futterman, 2005; Health Resources and Services Administration [HRSA], 2014; Radcliff, 2010).

MEDICAL MANAGEMENT

Currently, most adolescents who acquire HIV are infected through sexual transmission and are unaware of their diagnosis, making them excellent candidates for prevention counseling, linkage to and engagement in care, and initiation of ART (USDHHS, 2018). Adolescents often experience high viral loads at diagnosis (mean HIV viral load in a cohort of adolescents from 15 HIV sites was 94,398 copies/mL [Ellen, 2014] and multiclass resistance at time of diagnosis). Multiclass resistance suggests a transmission dynamic that includes older partners who have been on medications (Agwu, 2012). Data extrapolated from the START and TEMPRANO trials favor initiating ART in all individuals who are able and willing to commit to treatment, understand the benefits and risks of therapy, and understand the importance of adherence (USDHHS, 2018). The course of disease in youth is similar to that in adults, and they generally should be treated according to the same guidelines (USDHHS, 2018).

The newest guidelines recommend ART for all individuals with HIV, regardless of CD4[+] T lymphocyte cell count and age. Therapy should be initiated as soon as possible, and deferred treatment should be determined on a case-by-case basis. Recent guidelines for adolescents and young adults include data on the efficacy and feasibility of immediate ART and recommendations for certain populations. Earlier initiation of ART has been associated with reduced morbidity and mortality associated with HIV.

SEXUAL RISK

Youth living with HIV continue to engage in sexual behavior that may predispose them to sexual risk. Studies suggest that youth living with HIV experience high rates of unintended pregnancy (Nachman, 2009), STIs (Trent, 2007), and condomless sex (Clum, 2009; Weiner, 2007). This, combined with rates of screening for STIs that lag in HIV clinics compared to non-HIV clinics, can promote high rates of STI and transmission of HIV (Barry, 2015). In addition, recent work suggests that in females living with HIV, overall self-efficacy (B = −0.15, p = 0.01), self-efficacy to discuss

Table 13.6 BARRIERS TO ADOLESCENT ADHERENCE

Barriers for the general population

Complexity of medical regimen

Lack of social support

Adverse effects of treatment

Distrust of healthcare providers

Lack of understanding about the medication

Difficulty coming to terms with a life-threatening illness

Sense of invulnerability

Additional barriers: developmental capacities of adolescence

Early adolescence

Concrete, not yet abstract, thinking (undeveloped problem-solving skills)

Preoccupation with self and questions about pubertal changes

Middle adolescence

Need for acceptance from peers (desire not to appear different)

Present orientation (decreased ability to plan for future doses and future implications of disease)

Busy, unstructured lives (difficulty remembering to take pills)

Late adolescence

Establishment of independence (the need to challenge authority figures and restructure regimens)

Feelings of immortality (disbelief that HIV can hurt them)

Simultaneous increase in risk perception with greater emotional satisfaction with risk-taking behavior

Additional barriers for adolescents with HIV

For most, fear of disclosure of their HIV status to family and friends

For many, lack of adult or peer support to reinforce their adherence

For youth establishing independence, the conflict between the need to challenge authority figures and need to depend on adult providers for support in taking antiretroviral therapy (ART)

For asymptomatic adolescents, difficulty accepting the implications of a serious illness when they still feel well

For some who still think concretely, difficulty grasping the concept that there is a connection between strict adherence to ART and prevention of disease progression

For youth who live in the inner city, fear that they will die from violence, not AIDS

For homeless and transient youth, lack of refrigeration or a place to store medicines and lack of a daily routine

Source: Adapted from Schietinger et al., 1999.

safe sex with one's partner (B = −0.14, p = 0.01), and self-efficacy to refuse unsafe sex (B = −0.21, p = 0.01) are related to condomless vaginal and anal intercourse episodes (Boone, 2015). In young men, alcohol may be a key contributor to condomless sex with HIV-negative or unknown status partners (Bruce, 2013). Other studies suggest a complicated relationship with psychological stress, substance use, and mental health that contributes to condomless sex (Nugent, 2009). Disclosure is complicated by HIV stigma and fear of rejection personally with partners and publicly (Toska, 2015).

There is a need to regularly address the risk for pregnancy, acquiring STIs, and the secondary spread of HIV to partners. The CDC recommends screening for STIs in women younger than 25 years because of the high rates of STIs in this age range. In young MSM, screening for STIs is recommended from extragenital body sites because oropharyngeal, rectal, and urethral infections are commonly present in this population (Workowski, 2015). The CDC provides complete screening guidelines for youth living with HIV, and clinic-based motivational interviewing can improve condom use (Chen, 2011; Naar-King, 2006). The CDC also recommends preexposure prophylaxis (PrEP) for persons at high risk for HIV acquisition. PrEP is recommended for adolescents with an HIV-positive partner; HIV-negative gay or bisexual men who report inconsistent condom use or STI diagnosis in the last 6 months; heterosexual adolescents with inconsistent condom use, females with a diagnosis of gonorrhea or syphilis, or high-risk partners; adolescents who inject drugs or have a partner who injects drugs; and adolescents who have engaged in exchange of sex for goods or services. PrEP is approved for use in adolescents and young adults weighing 35 kg or more.

A client-centered approach that includes culturally grounded risk reduction and addresses not only the client's individual risk but also the complicating contextual factors that impact risk is most helpful. For example, to be effective, providers will also need to also address key social factors that may contribute to risk including discrimination, housing, employment, mental health, and substance use. Personalized cognitive counseling (PCC) and Many Men, Many Voices (MMMV) are two evidence-based interventions that have been suggested to address the needs of vulnerable, at-risk communities. PCC uses an individual approach focusing on last sexual risk behavior, while MMMV attempts to address the intersecting factors and identities impacting adolescents.

SUBSTANCE ABUSE

According to the 2017 National Youth Risk Behavior Survey (YRBS), approximately 40% of youth described ever having sex, with 29% of high school students reporting that they were currently sexually active. Among youth who described being currently sexually active, 19% drank alcohol or used drugs prior to last sexual intercourse. Substance use predisposes adolescents to other high-risk sexual behaviors like inadequate condom use, and, for HIV-infected youth, substance use can interfere with clinical care. In a large AIDS Treatment Network (ATN) study of 1,712 youth, 61% of males and 45% of females scored 2 or higher on the CRAFT screener (data presented at

the October 2011 ATN meeting). Daily use of cannabis was 33% for males and 25% for females. Daily use of alcohol was reported for 5% of males and 2.6% of females. Substance use prior to and during sex was commonly described. The regular assessment of substance abuse with appropriate counseling and referral is a key requirement in care.

MENTAL HEALTH

In the ATN study of 1,712 youth, 21% had a positive screen for depression and 15% for anxiety. Fifteen percent of the cohort had reported seriously considering suicide, and 14% were prescribed psychotropics. Seventy percent of the cohort recalled seeing a mental health provider while in care, and 38% of men and 42% of women reported currently wanting to receive mental health services (data presented at the October 2011 ATN meeting). These data suggest that regular screening and referral for mental health disorders is crucial. Stigma is another common concern for youth living with HIV (Dowshen, 2009; Swenderman, 2010) and can relate to HIV status, sexual identity, or racial/ethnic minority. Stigma can lead to risky behaviors, including unsafe sex and nonadherence to medications, and counseling may be required to adequately address this issue.

MEDICATION ADHERENCE

Youth living with HIV are at risk for nonadherence because of the aforementioned psychosocial, developmental, and cognitive factors. Several studies have documented nonadherence in youth living with HIV (Belzer, 1999, 2008; Reisner, 2009). Rates of adherence to HIV medications during the past 30 days range from 28% to 70% (Reisner, 2009). Barriers include medical, psychological, and logistic issues. Medical barriers include an AIDS diagnosis (Martinez, 2012; Murphey, 2003), a difficult ART regimen (Buchanan, 2012), the absence of symptoms, and an unwelcoming medical environment (Philbin, 2014). Psychological barriers include depression, anxiety (Tanney, 2012; Wagner, 2011), stigma associated with the diagnosis or transmission history (Rao, 2007), and lack of social support (Williams, 2006). In addition, behavioral problems impact 50% of youth living with HIV (Bing, 2001). Positive self-efficacy and outcome expectancy were associated with better adherence, and logistical barriers such as lack of housing, insurance, and transportation were associated with poorer adherence (Rudy, 2008). Comprehensive systems of care are required to serve the medical, logistical, and psychosocial needs of youth living with HIV. Individually tailored interventions that address social and psychological factors (e.g., substance use, lack of insurance despite universal access to care, and lack of social support) and structural barriers (e.g., housing and insurance instability) will need to be developed in order to better meet the needs of youth living with HIV. Attention to potential barriers to adherence prior to treatment initiation is likely to improve outcomes.

CARE MODELS

Based on the high rates of psychosocial problems reviewed previously, developmentally based care models that utilize interdisciplinary care teams are preferable. When a one-stop shopping care model is not available, it becomes imperative that the management of complex youth with behavioral problems be facilitated by close communication among physicians, nurses, social workers or case managers, and behavioral health providers. Avoiding potentially catastrophic health outcomes, including rapid HIV progression, multiclass drug resistance, depression and suicide, chronic homelessness, prolonged incarceration, drug addiction, and secondary transmission of HIV, may require intensive attention to psychosocial issues. At times, a temporary approach of delaying early ARV initiation may improve outcomes by allowing time to focus on developmental and social barriers.

TRANSITION TO ADULT CARE

Finally, clinicians must plan for the transition of HIV-infected adolescents into adult care. In a joint statement, the American Academy of Pediatrics, the American Academy of Family Physicians, the American College of Physicians, and the American Society of Internal Medicine affirmed that all adults, including those with special medical needs, benefit from care by doctors who are trained in adult medicine (Cohen, 2002). They recommend that an identified healthcare provider be responsible for the transition, that a portable medical summary be maintained, and that a written transition plan be developed with the patient and family by age 14 years. In addition to these recommendations, Valenzuela et al. (2011) recommends the following:

- Optimizing provider communication between adolescent and adult clinics

- Identifying adult care providers willing to care for adolescents and young adults

- Addressing patient and family resistance to transition of care caused by lack of information, concerns about stigma or risk of disclosure, and differences in practice styles

- Helping youth develop life skills, including counseling them on the importance of appropriate use of a primary care provider, managing appointments, symptom recognition and reporting, and self-efficacy

- Identifying an optimal clinic model based on specific needs

- Implementing ongoing evaluation to measure the success of a selected model

- Engaging adult and adolescent care providers in regular multidisciplinary case conferences

- Implementing interventions that may improve outcomes, such as support groups and mental health consultation

- Incorporating a family planning component into clinical care

- Educating HIV care teams and staff about transitioning

The National Health Alliance also has resources that organize transition into the Six Core Elements. These resources can effectively be used in any clinical setting (see http://www.gottransition.org/providers/index.cfm).

SUMMARY

Adolescents or youth who are living with HIV may have multiple developmental, cognitive, social, contextual, and environmental challenges that impact their identification, linkage, and engagement with care. Attention to the factors noted previously will likely improve the care, treatment, and adherence of youth living with HIV and, potentially, will prevent them from "falling through the cracks."

CARING FOR OLDER HIV-INFECTED PATIENTS

LEARNING OBJECTIVE

Describe the differences in HIV care and management for patients who are 50 years or older.

WHAT'S NEW?

- Recombinant zoster vaccine (RZV) is recommended in adults aged 50 years or older.

- Goal blood pressure in older adults based on the Systolic Blood Pressure Intervention Trial (SPRINT) trial is less than 130/80 mm Hg per the American College of Cardiology (ACC) and the American Heart Association (AHA) guideline.

KEY POINTS

- Each HIV-infected older adult is a unique and complex individual, and disease-centric guidelines should not be applied the same way in every patient.

- Management of diseases in older HIV-infected patients should be individualized based on aging phenotypes, interactions with multimorbidity, and patient preferences.

- The Veterans Aging Cohort Study (VACS) Index may be used to identify aging phenotypes and can provide prognostic information to help prioritize interventions and guide shared decision-making with patients and caregivers.

INTRODUCTION

There are increasing proportions of older individuals living with HIV. It is estimated that at year-end 2015, persons aged 50–54 years made up the largest percentage of those living with HIV (18%). From 2011 to 2015, the largest increase in rates of persons living with HIV was among persons aged 65 years and older (57%, from 94.2 in 2011 to 148.0 in 2015) (CDC, 2016). Part of this group consisted of individuals who have aged with chronic HIV infection, but a large proportion also resulted from new HIV diagnosis, with 17% of all new HIV infection in 2016 diagnosed in patients aged 50 years or older (CDC, 2016).

Although many of the recommendations on the management of HIV infection are not age-specific, HIV-infected patients older than 50 differ from their younger counterparts in many aspects, including diagnostic considerations, immune response to ART, and multimorbidity. In this chapter, we outline these differences, offer a strategy on how to care for this unique population, and provide special considerations for problem-based management of HIV-infected adults older than 50.

DIFFERENCES IN OLDER HIV-INFECTED ADULTS COMPARED TO THE YOUNGER HIV-INFECTED POPULATION

Diagnostic Considerations

The most common mode of HIV transmission among adults 50 years and older is through sexual contact (CDC, 2013a). Among men, male-to-male sexual contact was the most common transmission risk (CDC, 2013b), while heterosexual contact was the most common among women. This may be due to a false sense of security among older patients, who view sexually transmitted disease (STD) as a condition of the young and may forgo safe sex practices based on this perception (Pilowsky, 2015). They may also forgo barrier contraceptives when unwanted pregnancy is no longer a concern. Even though sexual exposure is the most common mode of HIV transmission among HIV-infected patients 50 years and older, prior research has found that healthcare professionals often underestimate the level of sexual activity among older adults and their risk of STD exposure (Pilowsky, 2015; Lindau, 2007).

Moreover, many symptoms of early HIV infection mimic those of old age and may be difficult for clinicians to tease apart. Symptoms of acute HIV infection such as headache, loss of energy, loss of appetite, flu-like symptoms, or weight loss are common in older adults and can be caused by a myriad of conditions associated with old age, such as malignancy or frailty.

With inaccurate perception of HIV exposure risk and symptom mimicry, underdiagnoses and late diagnoses of HIV infection are common among older adults (Pilowsky, 2015; Dai, 2015). Late diagnosis is associated with delayed treatment, impaired response to ART, increased morbidity and mortality, lost opportunity to prevent onward transmission, and increased cost of healthcare (British HIV Association [BHIVA], 2015). As a result, it is essential that clinicians maintain a high suspicion and routinely screen older adults for HIV, regardless of risk perception. Although guidelines from the CDC recommend routine screening up to the age of 64 years (CDC, 2006), the rationale or research evidence for this age cutoff was not included, and we recommend routine screening for all older adults as risk perception may be inaccurate in this population.

IMMUNE RESPONSE TO ANTIRETROVIRAL THERAPY

Despite successful viral suppression with ART, older adults have less robust immunologic recovery compared to their younger counterparts, with associated increased mortality (Semeere, 2014; Vinikoor, 2014). Consequently, early HIV diagnosis and treatment are of great importance.

MULTIMORBIDITY

Older HIV-infected adults are at increased risk of multimorbidity (Guaraldi, 2014), defined as the development of multiple chronic conditions that do not simply coexist, but together interact to worsen health outcomes. Compared to the uninfected, older HIV-infected adults have higher burdens of cardiovascular, metabolic, pulmonary, renal, bone, and malignant diseases (Schouten, 2014). Multimorbidity is likely contributed by both lifestyle risk factors as well as chronic HIV infection, with longer duration of severe immunodeficiency (CD4 counts of <200 cells/μL) correlating with higher comorbidity burden (Schouten, 2014).

Multimorbidity has important ramifications on health outcomes. It is associated with self-reported poor health, declines in self-rated health status, and increased mortality (adjusted odds ratio 11.87, 95% CI 5.72, 24.62) (Koroukian, 2015). With increasing disease burden, HIV-infected patients with multimorbidity are also at risk of fragmentation in care due to involvement of multiple clinicians in multiple settings. Guidelines for one disease may clash with another, as most are disease-centric recommendations based on the ideal patient without multimorbidity (Tinetti, 2012). Treatments for one disease may inadvertently worsen other conditions, and increased treatment burden stemming from efforts to adhere to all relevant disease-centric guidelines without prioritization may not bring improvement in mortality or quality of life.

MANAGEMENT STRATEGY FOR THE CARE OF OLDER HIV-INFECTED ADULTS

Each HIV-infected older adult is a unique and complex individual. They cannot be described fully by one-dimensional classifications, such as chronological age or single disease entities. Aging occurs at different rates in different individuals, and within the same individual in different organs (Emory University, 2015), resulting in different aging phenotypes that cannot be predicted by chronological age alone. Additionally, viewing HIV-infected patients by a single disease entity ignores the importance of multimorbidity and the often-multifactorial nature of their diseases. Most importantly, different patients have different goals and preferences. Consequently, applying disease-centric guidelines uniformly to every patient without taking into account aging phenotypes, multimorbidity, or individual preference ignores the unique care needs of each patient and likely will not lead to desirable patient-centered outcomes.

Understanding that not all 50-year-old HIV-infected patients should be approached the same way, clinicians may utilize the VACS Index (Justice, 2013b) to distinguish between those who are aging well and those who may appear phenotypically older than their chronological age. The VACS index has been shown to correlate with functional status (Malcolm, 2014), provide insight to clinician assessment of severity of illness (Justice, 2013a), and predict cause-specific (Justice, 2012) as well as all-cause mortality (Justice, 2013b). Based on prognosis predicted by the VACS Index, clinicians can elicit patient preferences, identify diseases and risk factors that affect these goals, calculate the likely effects and lag time to benefit (Lee, 2013) of various disease-centric guidelines on these goals, and use this information to prioritize interventions and guide shared decision-making with patients and caregivers (Tinetti, 2012).

SPECIAL CONSIDERATIONS FOR PROBLEM-BASED MANAGEMENT OF HIV-INFECTED ADULTS AGED 50 AND OLDER

Immunizations

Live attenuated varicella vaccination approved prior in uninfected adults over 50 years old can be given to adult HIV-infected patients without evidence of immunity with CD4 counts ≥200 cells/μL (CDC, 2010), as no transmission of vaccine strain varicella-zoster virus (VZV) has been documented in HIV-infected persons with CD4 counts above this threshold (Shafran, 2016).

Although the CDC has no recommendation on zoster vaccine in HIV-infected adults over 60 years old with CD4 count ≥200 cells/μL, it may be reasonable to vaccinate HIV-infected adults aged 60 years or older with CD4 count ≥200 cells/μL (Aberg, 2014).

A recent study showed superior immunogenicity in adults 65 years and older who received high-dose inactivated influenza vaccine (IIV) compared to standard dosing. Similar results were shown in a small clinical trial among HIV-infected patients aged 18 years and older (McKittrick, 2013). Currently, the CDC recommends high-dose IIV as an equivalent option to standard-dose IIV in adults aged 65 years and older regardless of HIV status (CDC, 2010).

HIV-infected adults aged 19 years and older should receive both 13-valent pneumococcal conjugate vaccine (PCV13) and 23-valent pneumococcal polysaccharide vaccine (PPSV23). However, the interval between the two types of vaccine and the number of doses needed differ in HIV-infected adults aged 65 years and older. In pneumococcal vaccine–naïve persons, PCV13 should be given first followed by PPSV23 at least 1 year after. In person who previously received PPSV23 at 65 years or older, only PCV13 should be given, at the interval of least 1 year after the prior dose of PPSV23. In persons who previously received PPSV23 before age 65 years, PCV13 should be given at least 1 year after the prior dose of PPSV23, followed by a second dose of PPSV23 at least 1 year after PCV13 and at least 5 years after the prior dose of PPSV23 (CDC, 2015).

In October 2017, a new shingles vaccine called *recombinant zoster vaccine* was approved by the US Food and Drug Administration (FDA) for the prevention of herpes zoster in adults aged 50 years or older. This is preferred over zoster vaccine live and should be given regardless of whether patients have received zoster vaccine live in the past or not (CDC, 2018).

DIABETES

Although primary care guidelines for the management of persons infected with HIV by the Infectious Disease Society of America (IDSA) did not include age-specific glycemic goals, the American Association of HIV Medicine (AAHIVM) recommends a target hemoglobin A1C of 8% for aging HIV-infected patients with frailty, less than 5-year life expectancy, high risk for hypoglycemia, or high risk for polypharmacy (AAHIVM, 2014). This recommendation mirrors the guideline on standards of medical care in diabetes from the American Diabetes Association (2015).

HYPERTENSION

Goal blood pressure for hypertensive patients in the general population remains controversial and presents a challenge for clinicians, with even less evidence to guide management among the HIV-infected population. SPRINT was halted early in September 2015 due to benefits of lowering systolic blood pressure to below 120 mm Hg (Ambrosius, 2014), and results of SPRINT have affected a change in guidelines in the United States and other countries. The ACC/AHA guideline currently recommends a blood pressure cutoff of 130/80 mm Hg (Whelton, 2017). The 2016 Canadian Hypertension Education Program Guidelines recommend a target systolic blood pressure of 120 mm Hg or lower (Grade B) (Leung, 2016), while the 2016 Australian guideline (National Heart Association, 2016) also recommends a target systolic blood pressure of 120 mm Hg or lower (strong recommendation, Class II) for patients with high cardiovascular risk without diabetes, including patients with chronic kidney disease and those older than 75 years. However, the Eighth Joint National Committee (JNC8) recommendation has not been updated since SPRINT, and the goal remains less than 150/90 mm Hg in hypertensive adults aged 60 years and older, and a blood pressure goal of less than 140/90 mm Hg for all hypertensive adults with diabetes or nondiabetic chronic kidney disease (James, 2014). Current gaps include lack of specific recommendations for the HIV-infected population and lack of consensus among varying guidelines.

POLYPHARMACY

Older HIV-infected adults are at increased risk of polypharmacy (Hughes, 2015), defined as prescribing medications that are inappropriate for the patient's medical condition, using medications that cause adverse drug events, or underutilizing beneficial therapy. Polypharmacy in older HIV-infected adults is contributed by increased multimorbidity, multiple HIV-related factors affecting cytochrome P450 isoenzymes and renal function, and few pharmacokinetic studies conducted in older HIV-infected adults.

To avoid polypharmacy, we recommend a medication review at every visit and a medication reconciliation annually

(AAHIVM, 2014). Routine use of an up-to-date electronic resource such as Epocrates, Lexi-Comp, and Tarascon will help the clinician monitor the array of drug–drug interactions and needed dose modifications based on renal or hepatic function. Of note, although the Chronic Kidney Disease Epidemiology Collaboration (CKD-EPI) glomerular filtration rate (GFR) estimate is the most accurate for use in HIV-infected adults on stable ART (Vrouenraets, 2012), the Cockroft-Gault calculated creatinine clearance remains the standard of care for medication dosing. With growing evidence of improved tolerability and no significant CYP3A4-associated drug interactions, integrase inhibitors are preferred in older adults who are at higher risk of polypharmacy (USDHHS, 2018). Lastly, patients should be encouraged to utilize a single pharmacy, preferably specializing in HIV, with an integrated computer network.

BONE

Certain lifestyle and HIV-related factors put HIV-infected adults at higher risk of osteoporosis, including smoking, alcohol abuse, glucocorticoid therapy, low consumption of calcium and vitamin D, low physical activity, immune dysfunction and persistent inflammation, and side effects of ART (Castronuovo, 2015). Modifiable risk factors should be addressed, and viral suppression should be achieved with ART. The IDSA recommends baseline bone densitometry (DXA) (Aberg, 2014) screening for osteoporosis in HIV-infected postmenopausal women and men aged 50 years and older. If osteoporosis is detected, vitamin D, calcium, and bisphosphonates may be considered, with a follow-up DXA 1 year later to monitor response to therapy.

NEUROCOGNITIVE DISORDERS

Age is a risk factor for cognitive impairment associated with HIV as well as other causes (Chan, 2014). Although the CDC or the IDSA do not offer guidelines on HIV-associated neurocognitive impairment, the European AIDS Clinical Society guideline provides an algorithm for its diagnosis and management (EACS, 2017).

Age is also a risk factor for peripheral neuropathy (Kaku, 2014). As a result, pain should be considered the fifth vital sign and should be assessed at every visit. Currently, trials on symptomatic and disease-modifying treatments for HIV-associated distal symmetric polyneuropathy have had limited success, and there are no FDA-approved treatments at this time.

AGE-RELATED SEXUAL CHANGES

Age-related sexual changes in HIV-infected patients include menopause in women and hypogonadism in men.

The IDSA guideline advises that although hormone replacement therapy may be considered in patients with severe menopausal symptoms, it should be used only for a limited period of time at the lowest effective dose. This is because hormone replacement therapy has been associated with a small increased risk of breast cancer, cardiovascular disease, and thromboembolic morbidity (Aberg, 2014).

Morning serum testosterone level may be assessed in aging HIV-infected men with decreased libido, erectile dysfunction, reduced bone mass or low-trauma fractures, hot flashes, or sweats. Low levels should be confirmed with repeat testing. Full recommendations are included in the IDSA guidelines (Aberg, 2014).

MALIGNANCY

As with the general population, age is a risk factor for multiple types of malignancies among HIV-infected adults. According to the IDSA, mammography should be performed annually in HIV-infected women aged 50 years or older, and colorectal cancer screening should be performed at age 50 years in asymptomatic HIV-infected adult with average risk (Aberg, 2014). The US Preventive Services Task Force recommends annual screening for lung cancer with low-dose computed tomography (CT) in adults aged 55–80 years who have a 30 pack-year smoking history and currently smoke or have quit within the past 15 years. The screening should be discontinued once the patient has not smoked for 15 years or develops a health problem that limits life expectancy or the ability/willingness to have curative lung surgery (Agency for Health Research and Quality, 2018). Although there was concern that HIV-infected patients will have a higher false-positive rate from chronic lung changes related to immunosuppression-related pulmonary infections, a prior study has shown that this may not be true (Sigel, 2014). There was a similar likelihood of pulmonary nodules meeting National Lung Screening Trial (NLST) criteria for a positive CT scan among the HIV-infected and the uninfected population. There were also similar patterns of clinical evaluation triggered by the CT scan, suggesting the follow-up may not be more aggressive among HIV-infected persons (Sigel, 2014).

ADVANCE CARE PLANNING

With increased risk of neurocognitive impairment and debility from multimorbidity, advance care planning is essential among aging HIV-infected adults. Without appropriate documentation of surrogate decision-maker for healthcare and finances, decisions regarding emergent or end-of-life care may be legally deferred to estranged family members who are unaware of the patient's preferences or HIV status (Sangarlangkarn, 2015). Although there are no specific guidelines for HIV-infected patients, the US Department of Health and Human Services recommends advance care planning in all patients with chronic life-limiting illness or anyone over 55 years old regardless of health status (Agency for Health Research and Quality, 2015).

SUMMARY

There are increasing proportions of older individuals living with HIV, and they differ from their younger counterparts in many ways, including the risk for late diagnoses or underdiagnoses, decreased immunologic recovery, and increased multimorbidity. However, each HIV-infected older adult is a unique and complex individual, and disease-centric guidelines should not be applied the same way in every patient. Management of diseases in older HIV-infected patients should be individualized based on aging phenotypes, interactions with multimorbidity, and patient preferences. The VACS Index may be used to identify aging phenotypes and can provide useful prognostic information to help prioritize interventions and guide shared decision-making with patients and caregivers.

RECOMMENDED READING

American Academy of HIV Medicine. Recommended treatment strategies for clinicians managing older patients with HIV. Available at http://hiv-age.org/wp-content/uploads/2013/11/HIVandAgingConsensus Project051815.pdf.

Boyd CM, Lucas GM. Patient-centered care for people living with multimorbidity. *Curr Opin HIV AIDS.* 2014;9(4):419–427.

Calcagno A, Nozza S, Muss C, et al. Aging with HIV: a multidisciplinary review. *Infection.* 2015;43(5):509–522.

ANTIRETROVIRALS DURING AND AFTER HOSPITALIZATION

LEARNING OBJECTIVE

Discuss issues in determining the relative priority of initiating and/or maintaining ART in the context of the hospitalized HIV patients with significant comorbid conditions, as well as issues of continuity of care after discharge from the inpatient setting.

WHAT'S NEW?

- An updated link to a reference table of available ART formulations is provided.

- New ART agents since last publication are incorporated.

- No new large trials have been performed that have changed the current understanding of hospitalized patient management.

KEY POINTS

- Understand the evolving drivers for hospitalization in the ART era.

- Appropriately weigh the decision to start ART in newly diagnosed or nonadherent patients during hospitalization.

- Balance issues of ART continuation in terms of disease severity, tolerability, and drug–drug interactions while hospitalized.

Patients with HIV have higher rates of hospitalization for multiple reasons. In the pre-ART era, progressive OIs and end-stage AIDS were the main causes of recurrent hospitalizations. Hospitalization rates dramatically declined in the ART era, but in the current period there has been evidence that hospitalizations continue to occur at higher than average rates, often for different causes (Crum-Cianflone, 2010). Recent drivers for hospitalization have diversified, with non–AIDS-related comorbidities being the most common causes of admission; examples include methicillin-resistant *Staphylococcus aureus* and other non-AIDS infections; chronic end-organ diseases, particularly liver disease as well as cardiovascular disease; malignancies; and surgical issues. Higher than average rates of substance abuse and psychiatric disorders in the HIV-infected population are also important drivers for hospital admission. There are many considerations in the use of ART during hospitalization, and this issue can be divided into two main categories.

The first category consists of patients not on ART at the time of admission. This may be due to nonadherence or having not been diagnosed with HIV until the hospitalization (usually via presentation with an OI). The main issue in this situation is whether and when to start ART during hospitalization. Concerns regarding additional pill burden, increased potential for side effects and drug interactions, and possible immune reconstitution inflammatory syndrome (IRIS) complications must be weighed against faster OI improvement and ultimate morbidity/mortality benefits. A 2009 randomized controlled trial helped inform the issue, concluding that early ART initiation resulted in less AIDS progression/death with no increase in adverse events or loss of virologic response compared to deferred ART (Zolopa, 2009). A critical additional factor in deciding whether to initiate ART during hospitalization is the importance of ensuring that the patient will be able to access and continue ART upon discharge to prevent lapses in adherence and potential resistance. This issue involves both the immediate availability of ART on discharge (i.e., if the patient has access to outpatient medications via insurance coverage or AIDS Drug Assistance Program [ADAP]) and whether the patient is in a position to continue with successful adherence (i.e., housing stability, substance abuse treatment needs, mental healthcare optimization, and willingness to take ART). In all cases, it is essential to ensure that patients will have streamlined access to ongoing outpatient HIV specialty care and that patients are linked before discharge to prevent adherence lapses.

The second category consists of patients with a known HIV diagnosis who are on ART at the time of admission. Patients who are on stable ART and admitted to the hospital should continue taking their regimen, with few exceptions. Issues that impact ART continuation include the reason for admission and if it impacts the ability to take oral medications—that is, severe gastrointestinal (GI) disturbances such as intractable vomiting, diarrhea, or obstruction, and so on. In such cases, ART use may need to be temporarily suspended until the patient's GI symptoms resolve sufficiently to tolerate oral medications again to avoid intermittent absorption and subtherapeutic drug levels predisposing to resistance. In addition, temporary ART discontinuation may need to be considered in presentations of severe lactic acidosis, pancreatitis, severe hepatic enzyme elevations, obtundation, or emergent surgical issues. ART dosing should be resumed as soon as safely possible when the patient clinically improves from these initial severe presentations.

If possible, patients who are *nihil per os* (NPO) should continue ART with water unless there is an acute GI problem that is rendering them NPO. Patients with nasogastric tubes should be given all ART in liquid form, when available, or crushed and reconstituted if no liquid form is available. An updated reference table based on a literature review for ARVs that can be crushed or sprinkled and also information on liquid formulation availability can be found at http://www.hiv-druginteractions.org/data/ExtraPrintableCharts/ExtraPrintableChartID10.pdf.

Drug interaction issues need to be considered routinely during hospitalization. Any new medications given need to be checked for interactions with the patient's current ART regimen, and dose adjustments or medication changes should be made as needed, ideally in concert with an HIV specialty pharmacist. Particular attention should be paid to proton pump inhibitor (PPI) interactions because PPIs are often started for ulcer prophylaxis or other reasons during hospitalization. Atazanavir and rilpivirine are particularly susceptible to subtherapeutic drug levels due to PPI interaction; therefore, extra care should be taken to mitigate problematic interactions.

Some other ART considerations during hospitalization include formulary availability, especially at smaller hospitals with less HIV/AIDS experience, and adequate stock of all agents because the number and classes of ART medications have dramatically increased. It is important to work with the pharmacy to ensure that correct ART is available without delay in the correct dosing form and that, if there are any supply problems, appropriate class substitutions are given in consultation with an HIV expert. If a patient is on an investigational medication via a research study, it is imperative that the treating physician and the research team administering the investigational drug are notified of the patient's hospital admission because they must make arrangements to bring the drug to the hospital and arrange for its administration by the staff there. Currently, multiple long-acting injectable ART medications are being investigated; if and when these come into clinical use, they may play a significant role in the management of the hospitalized patient in terms of expanding treatment options while decreasing pill burden.

RECOMMENDED READING

Mobula L, Barnhart M, Malati C, et al. Long-acting, injectable antiretroviral therapy for the management of HIV infection: an update on a potential game-changer. *J AIDS Clin Res*. 2015;6:466.

Nyberg C, Patterson BY, Williams MM. When patients cannot take pills: Antiretroviral drug formulations for managing adult HIV infection. *Topics Antiviral Med*. 2011;19(3):126–131.

Zucker J, Mittal J, Jen S, et al. Impact of stewardship interventions on antiretroviral medication errors in an urban medical center: a 3-year, multiphase study. *Pharmacotherapy*. 2016;36(3):245–251.

PERIOPERATIVE CARE AND SURGICAL ISSUES

LEARNING OBJECTIVE

Describe important considerations in the perioperative care of an HIV-infected patient.

WHAT'S NEW?

A 2014 study on perioperative complications after total hip arthroplasty showed a very slight increase in HIV-infected patients (2.9% vs. 2.7%).

KEY POINTS

- The balance of data shows no worsening of operation-associated morbidity and mortality in HIV-infected patients in general.

- Perioperative complications may be more frequent or severe in very immunosuppressed AIDS patients.

- There are some specific anesthesia considerations in HIV-infected patients.

There are evolving data that indicate that overall operation-associated morbidity and mortality in HIV-infected patients are not different from those in uninfected patients. Most of the studies conducted on surgical complications in HIV-infected patients are descriptive, retrospective, and so inconsistent in that many fields of surgery have published reports documenting both favorable and unfavorable postoperative outcomes (Rose, 1998). Given the available data, however, it seems that HIV infection does not increase the postoperative risk for complications or death (Cacala, 2006; Evron, 2004), especially in the ART era. Due to improvements in outcomes and overall OI reduction in the early ART era, the number of operations for AIDS-related surgical illnesses has decreased considerably (Saltzman, 2005). However, given the vastly improved survival and longevity of patients in the current ART era and the ongoing comorbidities that increase with an aging HIV population, the need for surgical operations and anesthesia has become far more commonplace overall.

POSTOPERATIVE COMPLICATIONS AND HIV INFECTION

HIV infection may influence postoperative wound healing and complication rates (Rose, 1998). Advanced HIV infection accompanied by OIs or malignancies may complicate the perioperative course and management. This may be due to debility and wasting as much as immunosuppression. A CD4$^+$ T cell count and viral load measurement are useful when calculating surgical risks and developing a prognosis in the HIV-infected patient (Evron, 2004; Saltzman, 2005). Postoperative CD4$^+$ T cell counts of 200 cells/mm^3 or less are associated with higher mortality rates (Saltzman, 2005). Irrespective of surgical procedure, there is a 13.3% mortality rate with a CD4$^+$ T cell count less than 50 cells/mm^3 and a 0.8% mortality rate with the CD4$^+$ T cell count greater than 200 cells/mm^3 6 months postoperatively (Evron, 2004). Postoperative viral loads greater than 75,000 RNA copies/mL are associated with higher complication and mortality rates (Saltzman, 2005). A 2006 Kaiser retrospective study showed that viral load suppression to less than 30,000 copies/mL reduced surgical complications (Harberg, 2006).

In a comprehensive literature review, wound infection rates varied widely, especially for abdominal, anorectal, and general surgeries and central venous catheter insertions, whereas documented ophthalmologic surgery and splenectomies had consistently low morbidity rates (Rose, 1998). In 33% of the reports, complication rates were significantly higher in patients with late-stage HIV compared to early-stage patients. One study of dental extractions found that complication rates did not significantly differ by CDC stage of disease. A study of cesarean sections found that complication rates were not significantly different between CDC stages of disease but were significantly associated with patients' $CD4^+$ T cell counts (Rose, 1998).

To mitigate operative complications, patients with a history or signs of cardiac or pulmonary dysfunction should undergo a more thorough evaluation prior to surgery (e.g., blood gases, pulmonary function tests, echocardiography, further cardiac testing, or even cardiac catheterization as appropriate). Relevant history of past treatment with potentially cardiotoxic therapies, such as chemotherapy for Kaposi's sarcoma or lymphoma, should be considered in assessing operative risk. HIV-infected patients may be in a relatively hypercoagulable state, with accelerated coronary atherosclerosis and possibly decreased left ventricular contractility (Evron, 2004).

ANESTHETIC CONSIDERATIONS AND DRUG INTERACTIONS

Information about the relative general hazards of anesthesia and surgery for HIV-infected patients is scarce (Evron, 2004). Most ARVs interact directly with anesthetic drugs and can cause side effects that directly influence which anesthetics are used and how they will be administered (Evron, 2004; Hughes, 2004). This issue is continually evolving; currently, there are more than 30 ARVs in six distinct classes.

Specific considerations when administering general anesthesia to HIV-infected patients include the possible effects of anesthesia and opioids on the immune system, the cardiopulmonary and neurologic status of the patient, and possible interactions with ART medications.

- *Opioids*: Although there is laboratory evidence that opioids may detrimentally affect immune function, the clinical significance of short-term opioid administration during general anesthesia is unclear, and not enough clinical data are available to justify its avoidance.

- *Neurologic considerations*: Neurologic manifestations, such as overt dementia, may impair the ability of the patient to provide preoperative consent and may increase brain sensitivity to sedative or psychoactive drugs such as opioids, benzodiazepines, and neuroleptics.

- *General central nervous system (CNS)*: Increased intracranial pressure (ICP) and CNS infections (i.e., meningitis, encephalopathy, or myelopathy) are contraindications to neuraxial anesthesia.

- *Cerebrospinal fluid analysis and nerve or muscle biopsy* may be required, and radiological studies of the spinal cord should be performed as part of the neurological evaluation to exclude compressive lesions in symptomatic patients. OIs may be associated with increased ICP, especially in the case of toxoplasmosis. Because these infections respond rapidly to medical therapy, surgery should be postponed whenever possible if they are present.

- *Pulmonary considerations*: Pulmonary complications can occur as a consequence of many OIs, leading to respiratory distress and hypoxemia.

Regional anesthesia has been shown to be associated with reduced morbidity and mortality in a wide range of patients, including HIV-positive patients having cesarean delivery under spinal anesthesia. However, a high motor block with intercostal muscle paralysis may not be tolerated (Evron, 2004). Regional anesthesia is less likely to interfere with immune function or interact with ARV drugs. Sepsis and platelet abnormalities are contraindications to regional anesthesia, and neuropathy may also interfere. Post-dural puncture headache may occur after regional anesthesia and may necessitate epidural blood patch. No increase in neurologic abnormalities in six HIV patients receiving an epidural blood patch during a follow-up period of 2 years was observed, and there is no evidence to contraindicate the use of blood patch in HIV-infected patients (Evron, 2004; Tom, 1992).

Nevirapine and efavirenz induce cytochrome P450 enzyme (CYP3A3/4) and may decrease serum levels of some anesthetic or sedative drugs, such as midazolam and fentanyl (Evron, 2004), although these antivirals are not used as frequently. Etomidate, atracurium, remifentanil, and desflurane are not dependent on CYP450 hepatic metabolism and may be preferable in patients using ART (Evron, 2004).

PIs are primarily metabolized by the cytochrome P450 isoform 3A4 (CYP3A4). Because PIs often inhibit, but can sometimes also induce, this enzyme, they may increase or decrease the effects of other drugs metabolized by cytochrome P450, so any anesthetics used concomitantly should be carefully titrated. Ritonavir is the most potent inhibitor of CYP3A4 and CYP2D6. Another more recent CYP3A inhibitor, cobicistat, has been approved for use as an ART boosting agent and needs to be taken into consideration when dosing other drugs. Fentanyl is metabolized mainly by CYP3A4 (Evron, 2004). Ritonavir can reduce fentanyl clearance by up to 67%. This strong interaction suggests that fentanyl and other anesthetic dosing should be adjusted in patients on a boosting agent. Also, respiratory monitoring should be maintained because the risk of respiratory depression for a longer period of time will most likely be higher (Hughes, 2004).

HIV AND TRANSGENDER POPULATIONS

LEARNING OBJECTIVE

Equip providers with the knowledge and skill to develop and provide gender-affirming primary and HIV care and prevention for transgender persons.

It is increasingly recognized that the development of transgender-specific programs and interventions and avoiding grouping transgender people with MSM populations results in improved care and prevention outcomes. Biomedical interactions between hormones and ARVs are unlikely, but transgender people may have poorer HIV outcomes or adherence to PrEP due to unique behavioral factors.

KEY POINTS

- Transgender people have a range of identities and sexual orientations as well as transition-related goals; each transgender patient should be approached as an individual.

- Transgender people and programs should not be aggregated with MSM; programs and materials should be developed specifically for transgender populations using a culturally grounded approach.

- Gender-affirming hormone therapy with estrogens and androgen blockers is generally safe and compatible with ART regimens. Hormone therapy and other gender-affirming interventions may improve HIV outcomes and reduce risk.

- Transgender patients require ongoing primary and preventive care, as do non-transgender patients; it is important to tailor such care based on the hormonal status and individual organ inventory of each patient.

- Providers should maintain a high index of suspicion for injected silicone and other fillers and related morbidity.

EPIDEMIOLOGY, DEMOGRAPHICS, AND TERMINOLOGY

"Transgender" is an umbrella term used to describe persons whose gender identity and/or expression of gender is different from the sex they were assigned at birth. Some transgender persons may seek only gender-affirming hormone therapy (HT), whereas others may seek surgical interventions such as genital reassignment surgery or other procedures on the face, breast, or body. Still other transgender persons may present with a more complex gender identity; some may choose to seek HT or surgical treatments but continue to live part- or full-time in their birth gender, whereas others may assume a fluid gender expression that is not categorizable in either polar gender (Deutsch, 2015a). Some transgender people may choose to not pursue any gender-affirming medical or surgical treatments. A 2012 study by the California Department of Mental Health found that 56% of a state-wide transgender sample identified as either "androgynous" or "genderqueer"; that is, neither male nor female (Mikalson, 2012). Table 13.7 presents a description of selected terminology and identities. The sexual orientations of transgender persons also lie on a spectrum, with the same 2012 California study finding 10%

Table 13.7 DESCRIPTION OF SELECTED TERMINOLOGY AND IDENTITIES

TERM	DESCRIPTION
Transgender	Umbrella term for gender-nonconforming persons; more "modern" and inclusive term, preferred by many
Transsexual	Older, more clinical term, some use to identify those seeking medical or surgical treatment
Trans	Colloquial term increasingly used in place of "transgender," especially among younger populations
Cross-dresser	Individual who wears clothing of the opposite gender for personal expression, entertainment, or sexual purposes only. "Transvestite" is now considered a pejorative term
Travestí	Term used by some Latina/Spanish speaking transgender women
Gay	Term used by some Latina/Spanish speaking transgender women with complex gender/sexual identities
Transgender woman	Person with a feminine gender identity who was assigned male birth sex
Transgender man	Person with a masculine gender identity who was assigned female birth sex

identified as heterosexual, 25% as lesbian, 9% as gay, 32% as queer, and 22% as bi/pansexual. In most cases, transgender persons define their sexual orientation based on their affirmed gender. For example, a transgender man who has sex with men would identify as gay. However, this also varies across cultural and linguistic lines, and the most effective method for determining the sexual history and health of a patient is to ask, "What are the gender(s) of people you have sex with? Are any of them transgender people? What kind of genitals do they have? A penis? A vagina?" "What kind of genitals are involved in the sex you have?" (Deutsch, 2018). Allowing transgender persons to define their own identity and experience and viewing them as individuals rather than as a stereotype will enhance the patient–provider relationship and may serve to improve adherence with ART and other care (Melendez, 2009).

The World Professional Association for Transgender Health's *Standards of Care for the Health of Transsexual, Transgender and Gender Non-Conforming People*, seventh version (SOCv7; Coleman, 2012) states,

Gender nonconformity refers to the extent to which a person's gender identity, role, or expression differs from the cultural norms prescribed for people of a particular sex. . . . Gender dysphoria refers to discomfort or distress that is caused by a discrepancy between a person's gender identity and that person's sex assigned at birth (and the associated gender role and/or primary and secondary sex characteristics).

SOCv7 further states (Coleman, 2012),

> Transsexual, transgender, and gender nonconforming individuals are not inherently disordered. Rather, the distress of gender dysphoria, when present, is the concern that might be diagnosable and for which various treatment options are available. The existence of a diagnosis for such dysphoria often facilitates access to healthcare and can guide further research into effective treatments. Research is leading to new diagnostic nomenclatures, and terms are changing in both the [Diagnostic and Statistical Manual of Mental Disorders]DSM . . . and the [International Classification of Disease] ICD.
>
> In order to access covered medical and surgical procedures, transgender people are generally given a billable diagnosis. Historically this has been "Gender Dysphoria" as described in both the DSM-V and the ICD-10 as a state of distress caused by mismatch between gender identity and birth-assigned sex. The need for a diagnosis to access care, including ongoing routine care when dysphoria is absent after gender transition has occurred, has historically forced all transgender people to carry a mental health diagnosis. The World Health Organization has recently announced that the ICD-11 will include a new diagnosis of "gender incongruence" which will be moved from the mental health section to a new section on sexual health. (Gander, 2018)

Epidemiologic surveillance in transgender populations has been limited due to inconsistencies in the collection of gender identity data. Incomplete or inconsistent identification of transgender populations represents a significant structural determinant of the health disparities seen in transgender populations. Best practice for the collection of gender identity data involves the use of the "two-step" method, which records both the current gender identity and the birth assigned sex (Cahill, 2013, 2014; Deutsch, 2013). This method has been found to identify twice as many transgender people as a "one-step" method in which a single "sex/gender" question is asked (Tate, 2012). A population-based statewide telephone survey in Massachusetts found a prevalence of 0.5% (Conron, 2012). The current estimate of the proportion of the transgender population by the UCLA Williams Institute recently doubled from 0.3% to 0.6% (Flores, 2016).

A 2012 meta-analysis found an HIV prevalence of 19.1% among transgender women living in the United States (Baral, 2013). This striking rate is driven by interactions between structural, personal, behavioral, and biological risks unique to transgender women. Structural factors include a lack of legal recognition or protections that often result in survival sex work. Personal factors include the higher rates of mood disorders seen in transgender populations as a result of ongoing discrimination as well as drive for gender affirmation; the model of gender affirmation describes the relationship between denial of gender affirmation (through lack of access to medical interventions or legal rights such as the ability to

change one's name and gender on identity documents) and high-risk sexual behavior (Sevelius, 2013). Other behavioral factors include increased rates of condomless sex with primary male partners and anecdotes of increased earnings from sex work when no condom is used. Biological factors have not been explored in depth, but they could include changes to the anal epithelium in the presence of feminizing hormones, reduced erectile function resulting in impaired condom effectiveness, and unknowns such as HIV transmission through receptive vaginal sex in those who have undergone vaginoplasty (Poteat, 2015).

Transgender women have lower rates of virologic suppression (74% vs. 81% national overall average) in 2014 Ryan White HIV/AIDS Program monitoring data (HRSA, 2016). A study of HIV indicators comparing transgender women to cisgender (non-transgender) male and female controls found significant differences between transgender women and cisgender men in rates of ART adherence (78.4% vs. 87.4%, $p = 0.0143$) for 100% last 3-day adherence and virologic suppression (50.8% vs. 61.4%, $p = 0.0127$), but no difference in these measures when compared to cisgender women (Mizuno, 2015). Another study found that a high rate of adherence to hormone regimens was associated with a positive odds ratio of 34.5 ($p = 0.002$) for reported high ART adherence, though there was no effect on the rate of undetectable viral load. Satisfaction with current gender expression was also associated with higher reported adherence (OR 2.56, $p = 0.03$) but not with undetectable viral load (Sevelius, 2014).

Few data exist on HIV risks and prevalence among transgender men, although some data suggest an increased risk (Green, 2015). A 2010 San Francisco study found that 61% of transgender men engaged in sex with other men (TMSM), with 51% participating in vaginal receptive sex and 39% participating in anal receptive sex. Transgender men have reported feeling that HIV testing was less accessible to them than cisgender (non-transgender) male controls (43.5% vs. 56.9%, $p = 0.04$) (Sevelius, 2014).

INITIATING HORMONE THERAPY

Gender-affirming HT has been found to have a number of benefits on quality of life and on symptoms of depression, anxiety, and poor social functioning (Colton, 2011; Gómez-Gil, 2011). SOCv7 defines hormonal and surgical treatment as medically necessary and states that it is unethical to deny surgical care solely on the basis of HIV or hepatitis B or C serostatus. SOCv7 departs from prior practices that uniformly required a mental health referral "letter" prior to initiating gender-affirming HT. There are no minimums with regard to time spent in psychotherapy prior to HT, and it is also stated that primary care providers with adequate skill and experience may make their own determination of readiness for initiation of HT. This "informed consent" pathway destigmatizes and depathologizes transgender identities, and it overcomes several perceived or actual barriers to accessing HT; a rigorous mental health screening process may neither be available (lack of resources or lack of trained/willing providers) nor culturally applicable (language barriers and cultural differences between

Western-oriented psychotherapy and persons of Latino, African, Aboriginal, or Asian background) (Deutsch, 2012). It is also appropriate to offer physician-supervised HT to those patients who may otherwise turn to unprescribed sources of hormones (Internet and street purchase) or who have already fully adjusted and socially transitioned to the affirmed (new) gender. A 2009 study of transgender women in New York City found that 10% receiving physician-supervised HT were also obtaining hormones from other sources and that patients were frequently taking two or three concomitant hormone regimens. This same study reported as barriers to accessing physician-supervised HT a lack of a knowledgeable provider (32%), lack of a transgender-friendly provider (30%), cost (29%), location (18%), and language (13%) (Sanchez, 2009). It is important that transgender persons have reasonable and realistic expectations about what HT and other treatments can and cannot do. Effectiveness of treatment relates to the age at initiation and the overall health state of the individual, as well as genetic factors. Once gender-affirming hormones have begun, there should be continued monitoring for underlying psychosocial factors or mental health conditions, with interventions as indicated.

Feminizing Hormone Regimens

Feminizing HT involves testosterone blockade in combination with estrogen replacement and also the possible use of a progestogen. The most commonly used testosterone blocker in the United States is spironolactone, a potassium-sparing diuretic taken in divided doses of 50–300 mg twice daily. Caution must be used with patients on angiotensin-converting enzyme (ACE) inhibitors or those with impaired renal function. Concomitant use of ART medications that may affect renal function, such as tenofovir, is a theoretical risk; however, no case reports exist of spironolactone causing or worsening renal function in these patients. Fosamprenavir and amprenavir are the only ARVs known to have interactions with estrogens that result in lower ARV drug levels, but these ARVs are rarely used. Side effects of spironolactone are mainly orthostatic hypotension and polyuria, both of which tend to resolve after several weeks. Routine monitoring of potassium and renal function (baseline, 2–4 weeks, and then every 3–6 months thereafter) is reasonable. Creatinine levels should be compared to the male normal range. In patients with contraindications to spironolactone, 5-α-reductase inhibitors such as finasteride 5 mg daily or dutasteride 0.5 mg daily may be used. Some transgender women, especially those whose only opportunity for income is sustenance sex work, prefer to retain erectile function and may choose to avoid or use lower doses of testosterone blockers (Hembree, 2009).

Estrogen treatment may be via an oral, transdermal, or injectable route. Transdermal routes of estradiol (50- to 200-μg patch changed one or two times per week) has been studied extensively and is very safe with respect to risk of thromboembolic disease: a 2008 meta-analysis of vascular thrombotic events (VTEs) in postmenopausal hormone therapy found a relative risk of VTEs in users of transdermal estradiol of 1.1 versus nonuser controls. This same review found a two- to threefold increased risk of VTEs among users of any type of oral estrogen in the first year of treatment only; however, this increase translates to only an additional 1.5 VTEs per 1,000 woman-years (Canonico, 2008). The transdermal route also delivers fairly constant and physiologic serum estradiol levels, which helps minimize common estrogenic symptoms such as migraine, weight gain, or mood swings; however, transdermal preparations tend to be expensive, may irritate the skin, and are not always included in HIV formularies. Oral 17β-estradiol in divided doses of 2–4 mg twice daily also delivers a constant and physiologic dose and is well-tolerated. Some providers recommend administering oral estradiol sublingually to minimize first-pass metabolism and effects on clotting factors. Prior studies reporting 20- to 40-fold increases in VTE risk in transgender women involved the use of high-dose, highly thrombogenic synthetic ethinyl estradiol, which is no longer used in cross-sex treatment, and did not control for tobacco use (Asscheman, 1989; van Kesteren, 1997). More recent outcome studies of patients using 17β-estradiol have mixed findings, with one cohort of Dutch transgender women using only transdermal estradiol showing no increased risk of VTE and a US cohort of transgender enrollees in a managed health-care plan using estrogen therapy showing a 3.2 fold increased risk (Asscheman, 2011; Nash, 2018).

Many patients may arrive at clinic requesting, or even demanding, injectable estrogens. Although estradiol valerate 20–40 mg intramuscular or estradiol cypionate 2.5–5 mg twice monthly have been used historically, these routes may deliver supraphysiologic estrogen levels that can vary widely over the injection cycle. Almost no data exist on the short- or long-term effects of this route, although anecdotally it is well-tolerated. This route may be useful in a harm-reduction setting in which there is concern that a patient may turn to unprescribed hormone sources if an injected medication is not prescribed. This route may also be useful in patients who have low psychosocial functioning, poor medication adherence, high pill burden, or to provide an opportunity to bundle HIV-related and other care with frequent hormone injection visits (Ickovics, 2008). Fluctuation of levels may be minimized by dividing the dose into weekly injections and, if needed, titrating peak and trough serum estradiol levels to manage any estrogenic side effects. Furthermore, changes in the hormonal milieu can lead to changes in the balance of Th1–Th2 T lymphocyte function and theoretical alterations in cellular immunity, furthering the argument in favor of constant and physiologic dosing of estrogen.

Interactions between estrogen HT and ART medications are complex and inconsistent. Two small, but important studies were presented at the IAS 2018 conference in Amsterdam in July 2018 investigating possible drug–drug interactions between PrEP and feminizing HT. In practice, the results do not show an important concern. Tenofovir/emtricitabine (TDF/FTC; Truvada) does not affect the levels of feminizing HT, and the possible interaction to reduce TDF is not clinically significant (Cotrell, 2018; Hiransuthikul, 2018).

Data from contraceptive studies are mixed with regard to findings that PI and NNRTI medications may cause changes in serum estrogen and progesterone levels (Kearney, 2009;

Marrazzo, 2015). However, should a patient previously on a stable HT regimen begin to experience symptoms of estrogen excess (migraines, weight gain, and mood swings) or deficiency (hot flashes) after a change in ART regimens, it is reasonable to check serum estradiol levels and/or adjust HT dosages empirically. In addition to the previously mentioned tests, monitoring of transgender women using HT should include baseline fasting glucose and lipid profiles, with subsequent monitoring as clinically indicated.

Progestogens have been suggested to enhance breast development and feminization of the body contours, and they may play a role in improving libido and mood. Patients may have a wide range of emotional responses to progestogens, with some patients preferring its effects and others feeling worse. It is reasonable to attempt a trial of oral micronized Prometrium 100–200 mg every night at bedtime or, if unavailable, medroxyprogesterone acetate 5–10 mg orally at bedtime in patients who request this medication, including those with limited breast development or for those experiencing unpleasant mood or libido changes. Although prior studies on medroxyprogesterone combined with conjugated equine estrogens showed increased risk of thrombogenicity, the risk is minimized when, specifically, medroxyprogesterone is used in combination with estradiol via the oral, transdermal, or injected routes.

Masculinizing Hormone Regimens

Female-to-male treatment primarily involves testosterone administration. Routes include intramuscular testosterone cypionate or enanthate at 50–100 mg once a week or transdermal routes such as patches or gel (5–10 mg/d). Recently, many providers have begun using the subcutaneous route, which is less painful and traumatic and has been found to be noninferior (Olson, 2014). Dosing can be adjusted to 100–200 mg every 2 weeks; however, this may result in wide fluctuations in hormone levels. This treatment is well-tolerated, with a minimum of side effects in most cases. Dose is titrated to cessation of menses and progression of virilization. HIV providers familiar with administering testosterone to cisgender (i.e., non-transgender) men with low testosterone should be aware that transgender men in general will require higher and more frequent dosing since they require complete replacement rather than supplementation. Prior concerns about hepatic injury are currently unfounded with the use of non-oral, nonsynthetic androgens. Monitoring should include baseline and periodic (every 6–12 months) fasting serum lipids, glucose, and hematocrit. Due to the lack of menstruation and the hematopoietic influence of testosterone, hematocrit should be compared to male normal ranges. Because testosterone administration alone is not a reliable contraceptive, even in the setting of prolonged amenorrhea, transgender men who are sexually active with someone who has a penis and testes should be counseled on contraceptive use and the teratogenic risks of unplanned pregnancy while using testosterone. The effects of testosterone on the vagino-cervical mucosa with regards to HIV transmission risk are unknown, though transgender men using testosterone do tend to have higher rates of

atrophic vaginitis and inadequate specimens on cervical Pap sampling (Peitzmeier, 2014).

SURGICAL CONSIDERATIONS

SOCv7 requires a readiness and capacity to provide informed consent by a mental health provider prior to most gender-affirming surgical procedures. Common surgical procedures and recommendations from SOCv7 for referral to surgery are listed in Table 13.8. Expanded insurance coverage for gender-affirming surgeries is available under the Affordable Care Act, and in some states Medicaid has made such procedures available to patients with lower levels of psychosocial functioning and health literacy. Providers should consider additional and ongoing assessments of such perioperative essentials as housing, social support, transportation, and ability for self-care, and

Table 13.8 COMMON SURGICAL PROCEDURES AND RECOMMENDATIONS FOR REFERRAL TO SURGERY

SURGERY	REQUIREMENTS
Transgender women	
Vaginoplasty	Referral from two mental health providers, 12 months continuous full-time living in a gender role congruent with their identity
Orchiectomy or oophorectomy/hysterectomy	Referral from two mental health providers
Augmentation mammoplasty	Referral from a single mental health provider (many surgeons waive this requirement)
Facial feminization procedures	No mental health referral required
Rhinoplasty	
Jaw/mandible contouring	
Reduction thryocondroplasty (Adam's apple reduction)	
Forehead reconstruction/hairline advancement	
Female to male	
Mastectomy (male chest reconstruction, "top surgery")	Referral from two mental health providers (many surgeons waive this requirement)
Hysterectomy +/– oophorectomy	Referral from two mental health providers
Metoidioplasty (removal of clitoral hood and ligaments)	Referral from two mental health providers, 12 months continuous full-time living in a gender role congruent with their identity
Phalloplasty	Referral from two mental health providers, 12 months continuous full-time living in affirmed gender role

they should provide resources and support to address identified needs or gaps (Deutsch, 2016). Patients may also present with a history of any number of surgical procedures. In some cases, the surgery may have been performed in another state or even overseas; as such, local primary care providers may be called upon to provide postoperative care. Most surgeons are willing to work with local physicians and when contacted may ask for photographs to be transmitted by email. For those patients with a complex wound care issue and remote surgeon, referral to a local wound care center may be a reasonable alternative approach.

More than 90% of vaginoplasties are performed using a penile-inversion technique; the erectile tissue is removed and a "neovagina" is created by inverting the penile skin into a pocket created in the pelvis. A clitoris is created using the glans penis, and labia are created with scrotal and possibly urethral skin. The neovagina requires lifelong periodic dilation and/or sexual activity to maintain depth and girth, and an artificial lubricant is required for penetration. Diseases of the neovagina are usually a result of remaining or recurrent granulation tissue (which may be cauterized using silver nitrate) or mixed-skin flora or sebum and debris conditions resulting from a deep inverted pocket of keratinized skin. Candidal infections are uncommon, and the pH would not be expected to be acidic as in a natal vagina (Weyers, 2009). Although it is not possible to perform a Pap smear on a neovagina, providers should maintain a reasonable index of suspicion for occult penile conditions such as Bowen's disease. A small minority of transgender patients receive a vaginoplasty in which a self-lubricating vagina is created using a segment of sigmoid colon. These patients must be monitored for possible malignancy or inflammatory bowel disease of the neovagina. Due to the anatomical differences of the surgically constructed neovagina, an anoscope may facilitate improved visualization and better patient tolerance compared to a vaginal speculum. The prostate is not removed during the vaginoplasty procedure; examination of the prostate in a patient who has undergone vaginoplasty may be more effective when performed endovaginally. The risk of transmission of HIV via penile-neovaginal receptive sex in transgender women is unknown. Care of transgender women with a history of silicone or saline implant breast augmentation is identical to that of non-transgender persons.

PRIMARY CARE

Transgender persons require the same general primary and preventive care considerations as do non-transgender persons. However, it is important to take an inventory of organs on a patient-by-patient basis. For example, transgender women will retain their prostate after vaginoplasty, and some transgender men may have a hysterectomy but retain their ovaries or cervix. All organ screening should be based on a combination of age and risk factors, maintaining sensitivity to the patient's anxiety, which may be provoked due to examinations and studies on organs related to the birth sex. Screening for breast cancer in transgender women has not been studied; case series exist showing a possible increased risk above that of non-transgender men but lower risk than

that of non-transgender women (Brown, 2015; Gooren, 2013). Some experts recommend that after 5–10 years of HT, patients should be considered for breast cancer screening, as are their age-matched non-transgender peers. Overall, providers should attribute HT as the etiology of any new health condition only after other more common causes have been excluded. Solid, long-term health outcome data are lacking. The largest population-based study on mortality outcomes to date is a retrospective series in the Netherlands of more than 2,000 transgender men and women. In this study, overall mortality among transgender women was increased by 51% in comparison to that of the general Dutch population; however, besides a 64% increase in risk of death due to cardiovascular disease, most of this increase was due to HIV, suicide, and substance abuse, and the study did not control for tobacco use. Transgender men did not have an increased overall mortality compared to the general population, but they had a 25-fold increased mortality relating to substance abuse (Asscheman, 2011).

HIV CARE AND
PREVENTION CONSIDERATIONS

HIV prevention, care, and research programs have historically grouped transgender women with MSM. This linkage fails to recognize the significant behavioral and social differences between these two groups, not the least of which is that transgender women are not men (Poteat, 2015). Other than the possible negative impact of estrogens on amprenavir and fosamprenavir, and theoretical renal interaction between tenofovir and spironolactone, there are no clear biomedical differences in the prevention or management of HIV in transgender persons (El-Ibiary, 2008). The most important considerations are ensuring that programs and clinic settings are culturally appropriate; electronic medical record systems should have the capacity to record and display preferred name and pronoun, social marketing and recruitment materials should include imaging and messaging appropriate for transgender populations, waiting rooms should have transgender-oriented pamphlets and wall art, and clinic bathroom policies should be inclusive and clearly posted. Providers and clinic staff should have adequate cultural fluency and sensitivity (Sevelius, 2014).

HIV PrEP in transgender women has not been studied in depth. The only published study to date of PrEP in transgender women is a subgroup analysis of the iPrEx trial that found no efficacy on an intention-to-treat basis. However, none of the transgender women who seroconverted had detectible drug levels at the time of HIV detection. Hormone use was associated with lower drug levels overall, as well as lower likelihood of having therapeutic drug levels, but the relationship between specific drug levels and HIV risk was identical between MSM and transgender women. It remains to be determined if reduced drug levels in transgender women using hormones are due to a direct interaction or to other confounders, such as increased pill burden or personal fear of interaction between hormones and ARVs (Deutsch, 2015b).

SILICONE

The use of injected silicone and other soft tissue fillers (pumping) has become an increasingly prevalent practice, particularly among transgender women of color and sex workers. Unscrupulous practitioners, medical assistants, or laypersons will inject up to 1 liter or more of medical- or industrial-grade silicone, lubricant oil, insulating caulk, tire sealant, and other chemicals with the intent of bringing drastic and rapid changes to the physique (Silva-Santisteban, 2013). Most patients are unaware of exactly what is being injected, and the colloquial "silicone" may refer to any one of a number of injected fillers. In addition to the risks associated with the injected material, risks of acute bacterial infections and sepsis as well as transmission of HIV and hepatitis are high under these uncontrolled operating conditions. Some patients may have a sterile systemic inflammatory response mimicking sepsis or suffer embolization syndromes. The free filler substances could serve as an immunoadjuvant that precipitates an IRIS (Alvarez, 2016). Long-term risks include chronic pain and disfigurement as the injected material migrates and calcifies.

This procedure is sought due to a variety of factors; in addition to peer pressure and a lack of understanding of the risks, more complex factors of survival are at play. Patients engaging in survival sex work may believe that they need to obtain a hyperfeminine figure in order to be competitive—and therefore pay for food and rent. Others may place a priority on erectile function and avoid HT, using silicone as their sole method of body feminization. Still others may live in neighborhoods in which they do not feel safe being identified as a transgender person, and they believe that silicone will assist them in blending in as a non-transgender person (Clark, 2008).

Treatment of silicone-related morbidities is limited and mostly supportive. Two case reports describe improved symptoms with subcutaneous etanercept 25 mg twice weekly; however, the applicability of etanercept when chemicals other than silicone are used, as well as its safety in HIV-positive patients, is unclear (Desai, 2006; Pasternack, 2005; Rapaport, 2005). An additional concern is subcutaneous or intramuscular medications used in HIV-positive patients, such as penicillin and enfuvirtide, and how these injections may be affected by or complicate preexisting soft tissue fillers. One case report described the safe and successful use of subcutaneous enfuvirtide in a patient with extensive migratory silicone material under ultrasound guidance (Gabrielli, 2010).

SUMMARY

Most of the special considerations in the care of transgender people living with HIV relate to provider and staff cultural competency, tone and content of messaging, using the correct name and pronoun, and avoiding categorizing transgender women together with MSM. Gender affirmation through hormone and surgical treatment improves quality of life and, when bundled with HIV care or prevention efforts, may have synergistic benefits. More study is needed to evaluate the role of PrEP in transgender communities.

HOMELESS POPULATIONS

LEARNING OBJECTIVE

Describe special considerations affecting the medical management of homeless or displaced individuals.

WHAT'S NEW?

- Four single-pill combination regimens for HIV treatment currently available should enhance adherence and reduce pill burden and complexity.
- Innovative programs for linkage and retention-in-care are operational.
- Text messaging may be an important tool for retention in care.
- Opioid reversal (naloxone) programs are life-saving.
- Needle exchange programs are essential in preventing clusters of HIV and hepatitis infections in injection drug users.

KEY POINTS

- HIV and homelessness are overlapping epidemics.
- Poverty, mental illness, substance use, and discrimination are barriers to care for both.
- Establishing mutual trust is paramount.
- Linkage to care and retention in care require enhanced teamwork.

Homelessness and HIV are two overlapping epidemics that each lead to worse health outcomes. They share many of the same risk factors of poverty, mental illness, substance use, racism, homophobia, stigmatization, and other forms of discrimination. Linkage to care and retention in care are challenging and are best met through the establishment of a trusting relationship, outreach, case management, partnering with supportive housing programs, and client-centered innovative local programs to reduce the barriers to care.

The federal government estimates that there are approximately 578,424 people who are homeless on any given night. Advocates point to 2 to 3 million persons experiencing homelessness annually (National Law Center on Homelessness and Poverty, 2015). HIV prevalence among homeless populations exceeds national averages. It is estimated that 3.4% of homeless people are HIV-infected, compared to less than 1% nationally (Allen, 1994). In certain areas, the HIV prevalence among homeless people is much higher. In San Francisco, 11% of new HIV infections occur in people who are currently homeless. It has also been estimated that one-third to one-half of people with AIDS are either homeless or at imminent risk of homelessness. Rising costs of housing, diminishing stock of single-room occupancies and public housing, and low wages make it nearly impossible to maintain stable housing in many cities.

Obtaining information about housing status and stability should be a routine part of obtaining a psychosocial history for HIV-infected patients. Questions phrased in the vein of "What is your living situation?" are readily understood and are preferable to "Are you homeless?" A follow-up question on the stability of current living arrangements can also give insight into a patient's housing status. If the patient is marginally housed or homeless, knowing how to contact the patient is extremely important. Be aware of any contact phone numbers, as well as places they usually visit, including any agencies that they use, case managers, and food lines and stores that they frequent. This will allow one to contact them in case of abnormal labs, important appointments, and if they are lost to follow-up. Some social service agencies provide free voice mail, which can be a confidential way for the patient to receive messages. Free cell phones, referred to as "Obama phones," are available for low-income individuals. Text messages relaying appointment reminders and motivating messages have been shown to increase attendance at appointments. In Kenya, text messages significantly improved adherence and viral suppression (Lester, 2010). In another African study, text messages were shown to improve attendance to postpartum clinics and early infant diagnosis in HIV-positive pregnant women.

Health status is poorer in homeless populations than in the general population. A recent systematic review that included 152 studies representing 139,757 patients found that worse housing status was independently associated with worse outcomes among people with HIV/AIDS (Aidala, 2016). The issue of tuberculosis (TB) exposure and transmission is a serious problem for HIV-infected homeless people, and transmission in shelters is well-documented (McElroy, 2003). Aggressive screening for TB is recommended. Louseborne and rat-borne infections are probably underrecognized given that the seroprevalence of rickettsial and other related infections is as high as 50% in homeless populations studied both in the United States and in Europe (Brouqui, 2005). Body lice can transmit a variety of bacterial infections, including relapsing fever caused by *Borrelia recurrentis*, trench fever caused by *Bartonella quintana*, epidemic typhus caused by *Rickettsia prowazekii*, and bacillary angiomatosis caused by *Bartonella henselae* and *Bartonella quintana*. Bacillary angiomatosis occurs in severely immunosuppressed HIV-infected individuals; infestation with body lice is an important factor in transmission of *Bartonella*, the causative organism (Foucault, 2006).

PREVENTION, MORTALITY, AND MORBIDITY

Homelessness remains an important risk factor for HIV transmission (San Francisco Department of Public Health, 2015; Sypsa, 2015). Current prevention strategies including postexposure prophylaxis and PrEP have not been well studied in homeless populations, but indications are positive that these would be effective and acceptable (Doblecki-Lewis, 2016). The success of efforts to eliminate transmission by reducing community viral loads will almost certainly pivot on the ability to reach and assure adherence in homeless and multiply diagnosed populations.

Although death rates for HIV have steadily declined since their peak in 1995, homeless people experience excess mortality compared to the general population. Among the homeless in Boston, the mortality rate was 9-fold higher in 25- to 44-year-olds and 4.5-fold higher in 45- to 64-year-olds. One-third of the deaths were due to drug overdoses (Baggett, 2013). Among a cohort of 300 homeless women in San Francisco, half of whom were HIV-infected, the mortality rate was 10 times higher than that of the general population. Cocaine-related intoxication, rather than HIV-related complications, was the leading cause of death in these women. Overall, leading causes of death among HIV-infected persons in high-income countries are AIDS-related (29%), liver-related (13%), cardiovascular disease (11%), non–AIDS-related cancer (15%), invasive bacterial infections (7%), suicide (4%), and overdose (3%) (Smith, 2014). Studies suggest that substance use treatment, opiate reversal programs, treatment of hepatitis C and B, cancer screening, and supportive housing may be life-saving in homeless HIV-infected persons.

Harm reduction measures such as needle exchange programs and naloxone distribution programs can be life-saving. In May 2015, the CDC (2015) reported that in a rural county in Indiana, 135 persons were diagnosed with HIV in a community of 4,200. The cases were linked to syringe-sharing partners injecting oxymorphone. Coinfection with hepatitis C was found in 114 patients. A public health emergency was declared, and a needle exchange program was authorized by the governor. Needle exchange programs are important for reducing the spread of HIV and hepatitis C, as well as for linking persons to substance use programs and methadone treatment. In a report on more than 10,000 opioid reversals, the CDC stated that making training in the use and distribution of naloxone available to opioid drug users is a strategy that reduces overdose deaths (CDC, 2012). Opioid reversal programs using naloxone have been credited with saving numerous lives. Patients who are prescribed opioids or who use them or are on methadone or buprenorphine should have access to naloxone and training on how to use it.

Clearly, team-based care is essential to address the multiple needs of homeless patients. Randomized controlled trials have shown that HIV-infected homeless people randomized to intensive case management linked to housing were more likely to obtain permanent housing and achieve an undetectable viral load than those who received usual hospital discharge planning (Buchanan, 2009). San Francisco has a respite unit with medical and social services. Homeless patients can have their medications administered, wound care provided, and follow-up appointments tracked. They also may be able to transition into permanent housing. Results from the Seattle Eastlake "wet housing" project showed that heavy alcohol users who were admitted and allowed to drink in the housing significantly decreased their heavy drinking days, reduced their daily intake from 21 to 11 drinks per day, had a major decrease in withdrawal tremors, and saved the city $4 million in the first year (Collins, 2012). Street medicine and mobile healthcare programs such as Homeless Outreach Team (SF HOT) and HIV Homeless Outreach Mobile Engagement (HHOME) in San Francisco assertively provide continuity to patients who would otherwise be lost from the healthcare system aside from high-cost acute services. Ironically, cities with budget deficits may find that providing more care and housing can save money. Failure to do so can result in disastrous increases in HIV infection and morbidity and mortality, as has happened as a result of the austerity measures in Athens, Greece (Sypsa, 2015). Some cities have directly observed ART (DOT) as part of methadone maintenance. Researchers in New York City found that the odds of an undetectable viral load were threefold greater in DOT patients compared to those receiving usual care (Berg, 2011). Methadone clinics can also work with HIV providers to track important appointments and represent an easy way to contact otherwise difficult-to-reach patients. Case management programs can coordinate the comprehensive wraparound services that complex patients need; administrators can accompany these patients to important appointments and find them in the field when necessary. Nevertheless, in recognition of the large disparities that continue to exist for homeless HIV-infected individuals, the Health Resources and Services Administration (HRSA) has initiated a multisite demonstration project called Building a Medical Home for Multiply Diagnosed HIV-Positive Homeless Populations that will evaluate and disseminate information on best practices in caring for this population (HRSA, 2015).

Recent research has demonstrated the pervasive occurrence of chronic pain in this population (Miaskowski, 2011) and the complexity of managing pain in these patients (Hansen, 2011). The National Health Care for the Homeless Clinicians Network has developed a useful guideline for care of homeless patients with chronic pain (Wismer, 2011). Efforts to develop innovative and comprehensive programs to manage pain and co-occurring mental health and chemical dependency in this population are under way in San Francisco and other locations.

With the availability of electronic medical records, quality improvement programs can track measures such as missed appointments, lost to follow-up, detectable viral loads, show-up rates for new patients, or various healthcare maintenance measures, including Pap smears, mammograms, and colorectal cancer screening. Causes for poor performance can be studied locally, and solutions can be tested with quality improvement methods.

HIV TREATMENT

Although homeless people may face challenges to adherence and compliance that housed individuals may not face, homelessness should not be a limiting factor in the decision to prescribe ART. A 12-month prospective study of 148 HIV-infected homeless individuals on ART in San Francisco showed that one-third discontinued their medications (Moss, 2004). Predictors of discontinuation were depressive symptoms, injection drug use (IDU), African American ethnicity, and poor early adherence. In the group that continued with ART, the average adherence by unannounced pill count was 74%, and 55% of these patients had an undetectable viral load. Predictors of lower adherence were African American ethnicity and use of crack cocaine, but not IDU; MSM had higher adherence.

These adherence rates, although not optimal, were similar to those of other population-based studies. A study of HIV-infected injection drug users on ART in Miami showed that homeless subjects had higher rates of anxiety and perceived stress, but they had similar rates of depression as housed subjects (Waldrop-Valverde, 2005). In the study, depression was significantly related to lower adherence, although housing status was not. Sixty-three percent of homeless subjects reported 100% adherence. Both studies showed that depression is a potent predictor of nonadherence, suggesting that HIV-infected homeless individuals should be screened and treated for depression (Moss, 2004; Waldrop-Valverde, 2005).

Strategies to improve adherence in homeless people are similar to those recommended for general populations. There are several additional strategies, including building on existing routines, such as those related to shelter, meals, or even drug-using routines. To assist patients, providers must ask about and understand these routines when prescribing and providing adherence counseling.

We recommend single-pill combination (SPC) regimens, if possible, to prevent running out of part of the regimen and to ease pill burden. In choosing an ART regimen, there are some special considerations, such as whether medications should be taken on an empty stomach or have particular food restrictions, requirements for dose timing that may be difficult to maintain, and food times and types that may not be under a person's control. Medications that have CNS side effects, such as efavirenz, may cause sedation and decreased awareness of one's environment and may affect street safety or worsen underlying psychiatric problems. Large numbers of pill bottles or weekly pill boxes are recognizable and difficult to conceal in a shelter setting; as a result, stigmatization, discrimination, or theft of medications may occur. Medication bottles can be kept by a case manager or program director, and small pill boxes that can be refilled frequently may be useful in these cases. Currently, there are four single-pill combination regimens, and more are likely to become available in the future. Coformulated efavirenz, emtricitabine, and tenofovir (Atripla) can cause CNS side effects and can lower methadone levels. The second tri-coformulated pill containing rilpivirine, emtricitabine, and tenofovir (Complera) lacks the CNS side effects of Atripla, but it must be taken with a 500-calorie meal (see Complera website for sample meals) because nutritional supplements are not adequate. Furthermore, PPIs cannot be used, and Complera is less effective than Atripla as an initial treatment regimen in those with a baseline viral load greater than 100,000 copies/mL. A third SPC regimen of quad-coformulated emtricitabine, cobicistat, tenofovir, and elvitegravir (Stribild) is recommended as first-line therapy in the 2015 US guidelines for those with a creatinine clearance of greater than 70 mL/min. Cobicistat is a CYP3A inhibitor, and there are multiple drug interactions; it is also an inhibitor of several of the transporter systems. It is recommended that it be taken with food. The fourth SPC regimen is dolutegravir, lamivudine, and abacavir (Triumeq). The patient must be HLA B5701-negative before starting. It may be taken with or without food.

THE MODEL OF CARE

There are more than 100 healthcare for the homeless (HCH) programs throughout the United States. Linking with a local program or getting advice from a national HCH organization is helpful to HIV providers working with homeless people. Shelter staff are also key resource providers in education and prevention efforts as well as support. Providing housing, particularly supportive housing targeted to formerly homeless people, is a critical health service function.

HIV-infected homeless people have a high prevalence of mental health disorders, especially depression, which is associated with poorer adherence to medications. Histories of both physical and sexual assault are common, especially among homeless women and transgender individuals. In one study, 32% of women and 38% of transgendered persons reported a history of either sexual or physical assault in the previous year. It has also been reported that African American women with a history of childhood abuse have an increased risk of being homeless and using crack cocaine (Wechsberg, 2003).

Building a trusting relationship and providing a nonjudgmental medical home in which patients can feel that they are valued as individuals is of utmost importance. The healthcare team should be able to recognize and treat posttraumatic stress disorder, depression, and other psychiatric disorders. A harm reduction approach is recommended. An effective program will also need to coordinate services with local jails and prisons because incarceration is more common among the homeless and those with HIV. Many homeless people are devoted to their pets and will not take care of their own health needs unless their pets are safe. Some cities have a special arrangement with the local humane society or have special services for pets.

In San Francisco, the Positive Health Access to Services and Treatment (PHAST) team works to encourage testing in the inpatient setting, emergency room, and urgent care and primary care clinics. The PHAST team provides easy linkage to care and actively works with newly HIV-infected people or people who have fallen out of care, meeting them in the emergency room or in their inpatient room. PHAST works to stabilize patients, navigate them through often complex healthcare and benefits systems, and work on their barriers as defined by the patients. Patients are followed closely to link them to and retain them in care. The key is not giving up on the patients; it may take a long time for them to fully engage. The San Francisco Department of Public Health's Linkage, Navigation, Integration, and Comprehensive Services (LINCS) program takes referrals for all San Francisco clients who would benefit from connecting or reconnecting with services. LINCS has outreach workers who search for both newly diagnosed patients and patients lost to follow-up.

RECOMMENDED READING

O'Connell, J. *Stories from the Shadows: Reflections of a Street Doctor.* Boston, MA: BHCHP Press; 2015.

INCARCERATED POPULATIONS

LEARNING OBJECTIVE

Discuss the provision of HIV care and release planning in the context of correctional facilities.

WHAT'S NEW?

In light of the 2015 USDHHS ART guidelines, which recommend treating everyone who is HIV-positive with ART irrespective of pretreatment $CD4^+$ T cell count, correctional facilities may need to reevaluate and prioritize their ARV formulary list. The splitting of coformulated tablets into their respective components and generic drug preferences may become more common practice as part of efforts to treat more HIV-infected inmates while being fiscally prudent. Caution is urged that correctional facilities do not stray from the USDHHS-recommended regimens for treatment-naïve individuals.

KEY POINTS

- The United States has the highest incarceration rate in the world.

- Persons of color are disproportionately incarcerated.

- Rates of HIV infection and AIDS diagnoses are 5 and 2.5 times higher, respectively, in state and federal correctional facilities compared to the general public.

- Correctional facilities pose unique barriers to ART adherence.

- Strategies for successful release planning may include having an appointment with an HIV provider soon after release and working with case managers/social workers to obtain medical coverage and referrals to community HIV organizations.

According to US Department of Justice statistics, approximately 6,937,600 offenders were under the supervision of correctional systems at the end of 2012. Of these individuals, 4,781,300 were supervised via probation or parole systems. The remaining individuals were living in jails or state or federal prisons. The number of individuals who are incarcerated in the United States has been declining slowly since 2009. At the end of 2012, 1 in every 35 adults in the United States was under some form of correctional observation. This is the lowest rate observed since 1997.

The risk factors associated with acquiring HIV infection and having an interaction with the criminal justice system are similar. In 2014, approximately half of federal inmates and 16% of state inmates were serving time for drug-related offenses. Black, non-Hispanic males have a 3.8–10.5 times higher rate of incarceration compared to their white, non-Hispanic counterparts. Similarly, black, non-Hispanic females have a 1.6–4.1 times higher rate of incarceration compared to white, non-Hispanic females. In 2014, women accounted for approximately 7% of the total prison population. White women comprise 50% and black women 21% of all incarcerated women. An estimated 7.3% of black men between the ages of 30 and 34 years were in a state or federal correctional facility (Guerino, 2011).

HIV EPIDEMIOLOGY IN CORRECTIONAL FACILITIES

Within state and federal correctional systems, HIV infection prevalence is 5 times higher than that in the general population. Rates of confirmed AIDS cases in prisons are approximately 2.5 times greater than those of nonincarcerated populations (Marucschak, 2006; Spaulding, 2002). Results from studies conducted with HIV-infected inmates demonstrated that being black or Hispanic, being an MSM, having a history of IDU, having an STI, or having a psychiatric condition were all positive predictors of HIV infection (Beckwith, 2010).

The prevalence of hepatitis C virus (HCV) coinfection among HIV-infected inmates varies greatly depending on region. Rates of HIV/HCV coinfection in correctional settings have been estimated to be as high as 65–70% (Weinbaum, 2005).

PROBLEMS WITH HIV PREVENTION IN PRISONS

Although risk behaviors such as tattooing, drug use, and sex are forbidden in correctional facilities, these activities are common. Condoms are not available and deemed contraband in most facilities. Not surprisingly, clean needles are not provided, and needle exchange programs do not exist. Thus, prevention programs cannot provide the materials necessary to prevent the spread of sexually transmitted diseases and other illnesses. Fortunately, to date, the actual transmission of HIV within correctional facilities is thought to be relatively low, and it is believed to be lower in comparison to the transmission rates in the general public. However, the true rate of HIV acquisition among inmates is difficult to ascertain because routine HIV testing on entry and exit from correctional facilities is poorly documented. Effective treatment of HIV will further decrease the risk of HIV transmission in correctional settings.

BARRIERS TO HIV TREATMENT IN CORRECTIONAL FACILITIES

Policies governing the provision of care and access to medical testing vary across prisons and jails. For example, some state prisons require HIV testing, whereas some merely recommend it. The CDC has recommended routine opt-out testing of inmates (CDC, 2009). In 2005, only 33% of state and federal prisons were performing routine mandatory HIV testing (Hammett, 2007). Not surprisingly, routine opt-out testing strategies yield greater numbers of screening and subsequent HIV diagnoses. Jails, as opposed to prisons, typically have an extremely rapid turnover rate, making routine or opt-out HIV screening and follow-up difficult to implement. According to

Minton and Sabol (2009), the average weekly turnover rate in jails was 66.5% in 2008.

Facilities may or may not meet national standards; they may or may not have access to HIV specialists and to specialty tests, such as coreceptor tropism assays, integrase inhibitor resistance testing, HLA-B*5701 screening and testing, or resistance genotypes (Bernard, 2006).

Similar to the nonincarcerated population, there are many reasons for nonadherence to ART among inmates, but some are unique to correctional facilities. Movement between facilities, being in segregation, and "lockdown" (when officials forbid any departures from the cells of certain wings or halls by inmates for periods of time) can cause disruptions in adherence. Facilities not receiving medications in a timely manner or inmates not being alerted to pick up their medications can serve as barriers to adherence. Inmates cannot always keep their own medication ("keep on person" [KOP]), and some are required to pick up medication daily at the pharmacy or infirmary (DOT). Confidentiality can be a major concern, for example, when picking up medications or going for DOT. Sometimes the exposure of HIV status can have severe consequences in prisons. Getting medications on schedule and meeting food requirements can be difficult. Inmates may be required to attend programs or report for jobs that interfere with the timely ingestion of medication, especially in DOT situations. Meals are served at specific times that may not coincide with the timing for a particular medication. Taking efavirenz at bedtime may not be possible. DOT regimens do not encourage autonomy on the part of the patient. Facilities that require DOT could consider allowing the more real-life KOP system for a specified time before discharge.

Additional barriers unique to correctional facilities stem from limited budgets and the costs of HIV care. Some facilities may have guidelines or restrictions on when providers can initiate ART. Many correctional facilities have formulary restrictions that appear to be cost-effective. Less expensive ART options often result in more pills daily, twice-daily dosing schedules, and greater side effects (all well-documented correlates of nonadherence). Costs incurred as a result of the need for additional medications to counter common ART side effects are difficult to capture and often not included in cost analyses.

ANTIRETROVIRAL THERAPY USE IN CORRECTIONAL FACILITIES

Providers should include the inmate's length of stay and future transfers in the decision-making process of initiating ART. Often, inmates who are released from prison and violate parole will be brought to a jail and then transferred to prison or brought directly back to prison. This movement often results in missed doses of ART. Note that the selection of ART regimens with a higher barrier to resistance will likely provide greater success for persons unable to fill ART prescriptions and for persons who will be in and out of correctional facilities. In the spirit of cost savings, selection of more durable regimens may prevent the development of drug-resistant HIV. Subsequently, avoiding the development of drug-resistant HIV may save on future lab costs and also costs associated with adding agents to effectively treat drug-resistant strains of HIV. Anecdotally, inmates have reported efavirenz-containing regimens as having "street value" in correctional facilities. The drug can be ground up and huffed or snorted for hallucinogenic effects.

RELEASE PLANNING

A key to success of many programs is collaboration among stakeholders—for example, correctional systems, academic institutions, and medical centers in the community (Braithwaite, 1996). A multitude of resources are available for persons living with HIV. It would behoove individuals working with discharge planning and reentry to the community of HIV-positive inmates to become familiar with the resources available. In some communities, housing and food supplies are available to persons based solely on their HIV diagnosis.

Additional considerations for successful release to the community are scheduling appointments with an HIV provider soon after release and assisting inmates with their linkage to HIV care. Some facilities provide inmates 1 week of medication and a 30-day prescription at time of release. Without some type of healthcare coverage in place, many inmates are unable to fill the prescriptions. In fact, only approximately 20% of released inmates fill their ART prescription within 30 days of release (Baillargeon, 2009).

RURAL POPULATIONS

LEARNING OBJECTIVE

Describe obstacles to optimal HIV care for patients in rural settings.

WHAT'S NEW?

Studies have revealed that rural populations may be less likely to receive quality healthcare and HIV treatment compared to urban populations.

KEY POINTS

- Studies have shown that the epidemiology of HIV/AIDS differs in terms of rural versus urban areas, and some studies even show that some rural populations may be less likely to receive quality healthcare and HIV treatment compared to urban populations.

- Rural HIV-infected patients experience barriers to optimal care, including long travel distances to receive expert care, lack of transportation, poor access to substance use treatment programs, and greater stigma associated with an HIV-infected diagnosis. Establishing

optimal care for rural HIV-infected patients will require innovative programs that address all these issues.

Studies suggest that the quality of HIV healthcare services differs by geographic location, and smaller studies have even found that rural populations are less likely to receive quality care compared to their urban counterparts. Although these conclusions are noteworthy, the results from these studies must be examined closely because large research trials typically sample more urban patients than rural patients due to accessibility to patients for large academic center trials. A 2011 study researched the relationship of geographic location—in particular, rural, urban, and peri-urban—to the receipt of quality HIV healthcare services (Wilson, 2011). The study evaluated both clinical outcomes and healthcare utilization in these patients using data from the HIV Research Network, which is a multistate, multisite research cohort. Researchers concluded that patients living in rural and peri-urban areas who received their healthcare in urban areas had high-quality HIV care and favorable HIV outcomes (virologic suppression and incidence of AIDS-defining illnesses) compared to those patients living in urban areas. High-quality HIV care included initiating ART, attaining HIV suppression on ART, and beginning prophylaxis therapy for opportunistic illnesses. The study also found that the proportion of patients receiving ART was higher for rural patients than for urban patients and that outpatient utilization was lower among rural patients. Unfortunately, this study was not able to follow a large number of rural HIV-infected patients accessing their HIV care in rural locations, and further studies are necessary to examine this issue more closely (Wilson, 2011).

To define urban and rural regions, the CDC used the metropolitan statistical areas employed by the US Office of Management and Budget, with nonmetropolitan or rural areas being those with a population less than 50,000. Figure 13.5 shows the reported AIDS cases among adults and adolescents in metropolitan and nonmetropolitan areas in 2013, and although all states have some HIV-infected patients living in rural settings, the southeastern United States continues to have the highest rural AIDS prevalence, followed by Midwestern states. According to the CDC 2013 HIV Surveillance Statistics, 6.9% of diagnosed HIV infections were reported in nonmetropolitan or rural settings (CDC, 2013). This statistic may also underestimate the number of HIV-infected persons living in and accessing care in a rural setting.

Another study found that rural HIV-infected patients were less likely than their urban counterparts to have a provider who had seen more than 10 HIV-infected patients within the past 6 months, less likely to be using effective ARV regimens, and less likely to be using appropriate prophylactic medication for OIs (Cohn, 2001). One strategy that rural HIV-infected patients employ to gain access to expert healthcare is to travel to the closest urban setting. In one study, 75% of rural HIV-infected patients received their care in urban settings. In addition, more than 25% of these clients had put off healthcare visits within the previous 6 months because they did not have a way to travel to the HIV provider (Schur,

2002). Other barriers to accessing HIV/AIDS care in rural settings include long distances to travel for any care, greater stigma associated with HIV-infected diagnosis, and lack of available substance use treatment programs (Reif, 2005). In a study of US veterans, delayed entry into care increased mortality for rural compared to urban HIV-infected veterans (Ohl, 2010).

Clearly, to provide state-of-the-art healthcare to the large rural population of HIV-infected persons, programs are needed that improve social supports and eliminate stigma for HIV-infected patients and that enhance rural providers' access to expert consultation as they provide care for these patients. Several models exist for providing healthcare to rural HIV-infected patients (McKinney, 2002).

- *Community-based physician networks*: Physician-referral networks can be accessed in which family care practitioners may consult with a network of physicians with HIV/AIDS expertise.

- *Urban outreach programs*: Satellite clinics are operated by urban HIV clinics.

- *Shared care models*: HIV specialists are partnered with family care practitioners in rural settings for managing HIV/AIDS patient cases.

- *"Enhanced" clinics*: These clinics use Ryan White Care Act funds (Parts B and C) to allow existing clinics to provide more comprehensive HIV care.

Outside the United States, other successful models exist for providing care to HIV-infected persons, including a program developed in Haiti using *accompagnateurs* (local community health workers) to provide medications with DOT and to support HIV-infected patients (Koenig, 2004).

Unfortunately, the economic downturn after 2008 has resulted in increased poverty and further access problems throughout rural America. Resources for rural HIV care are available through the National Rural Health Association and the Rural Assistance Center. It is hoped that increased interest in community health centers and implementation of the Affordable Care Act will improve access to basic healthcare throughout the United States. A web resource is available to locate nearby federally funded community health centers (US Department of Health and Human Resources; available at http://findahealthcenter.hrsa.gov/Search_HCC.aspx).

RECOMMENDED READING

Centers for Disease Control and Prevention, National Center for HIV/AIDS, Viral Hepatitis, & STD and TB Prevention. HIV/AIDS surveillance in rural and nonurban areas: slide series (through 2013). 2013. Available at https://www.cdc.gov/hiv/pdf/2013-Urban-Nonurban-slides_508-REV-5_6-5.pdf.

Wilson LE, Korthuis T, Fleishman JA, et al. HIV-related medical service use by rural/urban residents: A multistate perspective. *AIDS Care.* 2011;23(8):971–979.

MIGRANT POPULATIONS

LEARNING OBJECTIVE

Discuss limitations in HIV care and special needs among migrant populations or patients with undocumented citizenship.

WHAT'S NEW?

Updated statistics reveal encouraging trends, but more concerted preventative efforts must be made toward at-risk migrant populations.

KEY POINTS

- The CDC only recently began tracking data regarding country of origin, time in the United States, or immigration status, so a more complete picture of the HIV epidemic among immigrants to the United States is just now emerging.

- Research in these populations is challenging due to a myriad of factors, including recruitment issues, ethical challenges, and subgroup differentiation.

- Prevalence and incidence of HIV in Hispanics and African Americans in the United States are higher than those of whites, and these populations have less access to care and treatment than do whites.

- Among HIV-infected immigrant populations, the prevalence and presentation of OIs or coinfections differ from those of US-born HIV-infected individuals.

Migrating populations experience many barriers to accessing appropriate medical care for HIV infection. These barriers include lack of sufficient epidemiologic data on HIV infection among immigrants to the United States, issues of poverty, legal and language barriers to care among undocumented and/or illegal immigrants, and insufficient cultural competence among healthcare providers caring for immigrants. In addition, the medical presentation of HIV infection in the immigrant may differ in striking ways from that of the native-born US citizen.

Developing an accurate picture of the HIV epidemic among immigrants to the United States has been hampered by a lack of national data. The CDC only recently began tracking country of origin in HIV/AIDS, and currently there is no national publication on the topic. Some reports have been published on AIDS and immigrant populations at the county, city, and state levels. An example is a report from the Massachusetts Department of Public Health (MDPH) on the epidemiologic profile of HIV and AIDS in Massachusetts, which addresses emerging populations (MDPH, 2012). Historically, such local epidemiologic studies have been the predominant method for assessing need and planning services for immigrant populations.

A 2005 study detailed the research challenges posed when attempting to study the migrant and the immigrant

Hispanic populations in the United States. These challenges were grouped into four categories: the need to use multilevel theoretical frameworks, the need to differentiate between Hispanic subgroups, challenges to recruitment and data collection, and ethical issues (Deren, 2005). When studying migrant populations, multilevel theoretical frameworks are necessary that incorporate the multiple influences that affect their daily living, including cultural, social, environmental, and individual factors. Differentiation of subgroups is also necessary due to the complexity of each subgroup, including lifestyle behaviors and cultural backgrounds. Recruitment and data collection is a major challenge because follow-up data are difficult to obtain in these populations due to the fact that their residency is commonly transient. Ethical issues are common in conducting these studies because they involve multiethnic populations with communication obstacles, and important consideration should be placed on cultural norms and sensitivities (Deren, 2005).

It is known that Hispanics and African Americans in the United States have higher HIV prevalence and incidence rates than other groups (Kaiser Family Foundation, 2014). In nearly every transmission category, blacks have annual AIDS incidence and prevalence rates up to twice as high as those of whites. Black Americans also account for more new HIV infections and HIV-related deaths than any other racial/ethnic group in the United States (Kaiser Family Foundation, 2014). Despite these disproportionate statistics, there are declining numbers of new HIV infections among black women (Figures 13.6 and 13.7). Although these data correspond to all members of these racial/ethnic groups, the numbers of infections among *immigrants* within these groups are unknown.

According to the Kaiser Family Foundation, Latinos represented approximately 16% of the US population but account for 21% of the new HIV infections and 19% of people living with HIV. In 2012, it was reported by the National Center for Health Statistics (NCHS) that the HIV death rate per 100,000 for Latinos was more than twice the rate for whites (NCHS, 2012). One large study of the Hispanic population in the United States found that up to 28% of Hispanic residents live below the poverty level (Hajat, 2000). Because

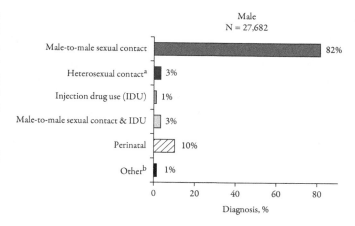

Figure 13.7 Adolescent and Young Adult Males Aged 13-24 Years Living with Diagnosed HIV Infection by Sex and Transmission Category, Year-end 2015—United States and 6 Dependent Area (CDC, 2018). *Note.* Data have been statistically adjusted to account for missing transmission category. "Other" transmission category not displayed as it comprises less than 1% of cases. [a] Heterosexual contact with a person known to have, or be at high risk for, HIV infection. [b] Includes hemophilia, blood transfusion, and risk factor not reported or not identified.

some states require a valid photo identification to receive benefits such as Medicaid, ADAP, or other forms of health insurance, undocumented immigrants are deterred from accessing appropriate HIV care.

Illegal immigrants with HIV infection face additional barriers to accessing healthcare. The Personal Responsibility and Work Opportunity Reconciliation Act of 1996 greatly restricts the provision of many federal, state, and local public services to undocumented immigrants (Kullgren, 2003). Although the intent of such legislation was to reduce illegal immigration, its main effects have been to burden the public healthcare system and to threaten overall public health. The recession of 2008 and improved enforcement of immigration laws have created additional obstacles to the provision of adequate HIV care to many immigrant populations. A positive development was the 2010 lifting of the requirement for HIV testing before immigration to the United States. However, undocumented immigrants are prohibited from accessing the benefits of the Affordable Care Act, including Medicaid and subsidized insurance premiums.

Immigrant HIV-infected populations more often present later in the course of their disease than do US-born patients. The medical presentation of HIV infection is different in immigrants compared with native-born US citizens. For example, the prevalence of infection with *Mycobacterium tuberculosis* is higher among immigrants from Africa, Central America, Southeast Asia, India, and other areas where TB is endemic. Therefore, screening HIV-infected persons for TB infection is essential in many immigrant populations. Active TB often occurs in HIV-infected persons with higher T helper cell counts, has more unusual or atypical presentations, and may be the initial presentation of HIV infection. It is more difficult to successfully treat TB in HIV-infected individuals than in HIV-negative individuals, and HIV-infected patients may require prolonged TB treatment.

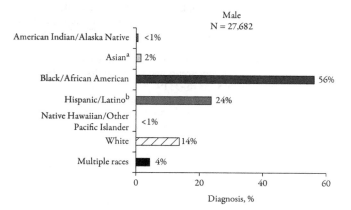

Figure 13.6 Adolescent and Young Males Aged 13-24 Years Living with Diagnosed HIV Infection by Sex and Race/Ethnicity, Year-end 2016—United States and 6 Dependent Areas (CDC, 2018). [a] Includes Asian/Pacific Islander legacy cases. [b] Hispanic/Latinos can be of any race.

Among Asian populations, the prevalence of chronic hepatitis B virus (HBV) infection is higher than that among other populations. ART may be more toxic in persons with chronic hepatitis, so the prevalence of HBV infection in Asian populations may complicate attempts to treat HIV. There is evidence that viral subtypes common in Southeast Asia may respond differently to currently available treatments for HBV. OIs not usually seen in US-born persons may present in HIV-infected immigrants, reflecting the epidemiology of their country of origin. Examples include *Penicillium marnefii* in persons of Southeast Asian origin and a variety of parasitic diseases in persons of African descent.

In summary, immigrants face many barriers to receiving appropriate and affordable HIV care. Efforts to reduce these barriers should include legislation that will support and enhance the public health system, improved access to HIV services, better epidemiologic data on HIV-infected immigrants to the United States, and enhanced training and support for healthcare providers who serve immigrant populations. Often crucial to success in working with immigrant populations is the utilization of a team approach involving interpreters, social workers, and case managers; hiring of cultural-appropriate staff; inclusion of peer navigators; networking with local community-based organizations working with the impacted populations; Ryan White Program and 340B Pharmacy access; and legal services. The CDC has a useful website dedicated to immigrant and refugee health issues (see http://www.cdc.gov/immigrantrefugeehealth).

RECOMMENDED READING

Kaiser Family Foundation. Fact sheet: black Americans and HIV/AIDS. Menlo Park, CA: Henry J. Kaiser Family Foundation; April 2014. Available at http://files.kff.org/attachment/fact-sheet-black-americans-and-hiv-aids.

Kaiser Family Foundation. Fact sheet: Latinos and HIV/AIDS. Menlo Park, CA: Henry J. Kaiser Family Foundation; April 2014. Available at https://kaiserfamilyfoundation.files.wordpress.com/2014/04/6007-11-latinos-and-hiv-aids1.pdf.

Aberg JA, et al. Primary care guidelines for the management of persons infected with HIV: 2013 update by the HIV medicine association of the Infectious Diseases Society of America. *Clin Infect Dis.* 2014;58(1):e1.

Agency for Health Research and Quality: National Guideline Clearinghouse. Advanced care planning guideline. Available at http://www.guideline.gov/content.aspx?id=47803. Accessed October 18, 2015.

Agency for Healthcare Research and Quality. Improving cultural competence to reduce health disparities for priority populations. 2005. Available at http://content.healthaffairs.org/content/24/2/354.full?firstpage=354. Accessed December 1, 2015.

Agency for Healthcare Research and Quality. Defining the PCMH. 2015. Available at https://www.pcmh.ahrq.gov/page/defining-pcmh.

Agency for Health Research and Quality. Recommendations: Screening for Lung Cancer. Available at https://epss.ahrq.gov/ePSS/RecomDetail.do?method=search&sid=256&age=65&sex=Male&sexuallyActive=yes&tobacco=yes. Accessed April 27, 2018.

Agwu AL, Bethel J, Hightow-Weidman LB, et al. Substantial multiclass transmitted drug resistance and drug-relevant polymorphisms among treatment-naive behaviorally HIV-infected youth. *AIDS Patient Care STDS.* April 2012;26(4):193–196.

Aidala AA, Wilson MG, Shubert V, et al. Housing status, medical care, and health outcomes among people living with HIV/AIDS: a systematic review. *Am J Public Health.* 2016;106:e1–e23. Available at http://doi.org/10.2105/AJPH.2015.302905.

Allen DM, Lehman JS, Green TA, et al. HIV infection among homeless adults and runaway youth, United States, 1989–1992. Field Services Branch. *AIDS.* November 1994;8(11):1593–1599.

Alvarez H, Marino A, Garcia-Rodriquez JF, et al. Immune reconstitution inflammatory syndrome in an HIV-infected patient using subcutaneous silicone fillers. *AIDS.* October 23, 2016;30(16):2561–2563.

Ambrosius WT, et al. The design and rationale of a multicenter clinical trial comparing two strategies for control of systolic blood pressure: the Systolic Blood Pressure Intervention Trial (SPRINT). *Clin Trials.* 2014;11(5):532–546.

American Academy of HIV Medicine (AAHIVM). Recommended treatment strategies for clinicians managing older patients with HIV. Available at http://hiv-age.org/wp-content/uploads/2014/02/12.-Diabetes-Mellitus-in-HIV-and-Aging.pdf. Accessed October 18, 2015.

American Academy of HIV Medicine (AAHIVM). Recommended treatment strategies for clinicians managing older patients with HIV. Available at http://hiv-age.org/wp-content/uploads/2014/02/13.-Drug-drug-Interactions-and-Polypharmacy-in-HIV-and-Aging.pdf. Accessed October 18, 2015.

American Diabetes Association. Standards of medical care in diabetes—2015 abridged for primary care providers. *Clin Diabetes.* 2015;33(2):97–111.

Asscheman H, Giltay EJ, Megens JAJ, et al. A long-term follow-up study of mortality in transsexuals receiving treatment with cross-sex hormones. *Eur J Endocrinol.* 2011;164(4):635–642. Available at http://doi.org/10.1530/EJE-10-1038.

Asscheman H, Gooren LJG, Eklund PLE. Mortality and morbidity in transsexual patients with cross-gender hormone treatment. *Metabolism.* 1989;38(9):869–873.

Baggett TP, Hwang SW, O'Connell JJ, et al. Mortality among homeless adults in Boston: shifts in causes of death over a 15-year period. *JAMA Intern Med.* 2013;173:189–195.

Baillargeon J, Giordano T, Rich J, et al. Accessing antiretroviral therapy following release from prison. *JAMA.* 2009;301(8):848–857.

Baral SD, Poteat T, Strömdahl S, et al. (2013). Worldwide burden of HIV in transgender women: a systematic review and meta-analysis. *Lancet Infect Dis.* 2013;13(3):214–222. Available at http://doi.org/10.1016/S1473-3099(12)70315-8.

Barnes W, D'Angelo L, Yamazaki M, et al. Identification of HIV-infected 12–24-year-old men and women in 15 cities through venue-based testing. *Arch Pediatr Adolesc Med.* 2010;164:273–276.

Bass M. Language barriers and illiteracy can affect patient healthcare. 2000; Robert Wood Johnson Foundation. Available at http://www.rwjf.org/en/library/research/2000/12/language-barriers-and-illiteracy-can-affect-patient-heath-care.html. Accessed December 1, 2015.

Beckwith C, Zaller N, Fu J, et al. Opportunities to diagnose, treat, and prevent HIV in the criminal justice system. *J AIDS.* 2010;55(Suppl 1):S49–S55.

Belzer ME, Fuchs DN, Luftman GS, et al. Antiretroviral adherence issues among HIV-positive adolescents and young adults. *J Adolesc Health.* November 1999;25(5):3316–3319.

Belzer ME, Olson J. Adherence in adolescents: a review of the literature. Adolescent medicine: state of the art reviews. Evaluation and management of adolescent issues. *Am Acad Pediatr.* 2008;9:99–117.

Berg KM, Litwin A, Li X, et al. Directly observed antiretroviral therapy improves adherence and viral load in drug users attending methadone maintenance clinics: a randomized controlled trial. *Drug Alcohol Dependence.* 2011;113(2–3):192–199.

Bernard K, Sueker J, et al. Provider perspectives about the standard of HIV care in correctional settings and comparison to the community standard of care: how do we measure up? *Infect Dis Corrections Rep.* March 2006;9(3):1–2, 4–6.

Berry SA, Ghanem KG, Mathews WC, et al. Brief report: gonorrhea and chlamydia testing increasing but still lagging in HIV clinics in the United States. *J AIDS.* 2015;70(3):275–279.

Bing EG, Burnam A, Longshore D, et al. Psychiatric disorders and drug use among HIV-infected adults in the US. *Arch Gen Psychiatry*. 2001;58:721–728.

Bogart LM, Thorburn S. Are HIV/AIDS conspiracy beliefs a barrier to HIV prevention among African-Americans? *J AIDS*. 2005;38(2):213–218.

Boone MR, Cherenack EM, Wilson PA, et al. Self-efficacy for sexual risk reduction and partner HIV status as correlates of sexual risk behavior among HIV-positive adolescent girls and women. *AIDS Patient Care STDS*. June 2015;29(6):346–353.

Bowleg L. "Once you've blended the cake, you can't take the parts back to the main ingredients": black gay and bisexual men's descriptions and experiences of intersectionality. *Sex Roles*. 2013;68(11–12):754–767.

Boyer CB, Hightow-Weidman L, Bether J, et al. An assessment of the feasibility and acceptability of a friendship-based social network recruitment strategy to screen at-risk African American and Hispanic/Latina young women for HIV infection. *JAMA Pediatr*. March 1, 2013;167(3):289–296.

Braithwaite R, Hammett T, Mayberry R. *Prisons and AIDS: A Public Health Challenge*. San Francisco, CA: Jossey-Bass; 1996.

Branson B, Handsfield H, Lampe M, et al. Revised recommendations for HIV testing of adults, adolescents, and pregnant women in health-care settings. *MMWR*. 2006;55(RR14):1–17.

British HIV Association (BHIVA). UK national guidelines for HIV testing. *Public Health*. 2015.

Brooks J, Buchacz K, Gebo KA, et al. HIV infection and older Americans: The public health perspective. *Am J Public Health*. 2012;102(8):1516–1526.

Brouqui P, Stein A, Dupont HT, et al. Ectoparasitism and vector-borne diseases in 930 homeless people from Marseilles. *Medicine (Baltimore)*. January 2005;84(1):61–68.

Brown GR, Jones KT. Incidence of breast cancer in a cohort of 5,135 transgender veterans. *Breast Cancer Res Treat*. 2015;149(1), 191–198. Available at http://doi.org/10.1007/s10549-014-3213-2.

Bruce D, Kahana S, Harper G, et al. Alcohol use predicts sexual risk behavior with HIV-negative or partners of unknown status among young HIV-positive men who have sex with men. *AIDS Care*. 2013;25(5):559–565.

Buchanan AL, Montepiedra G, Sirois PA, et al. Barriers to medication adherence in HIV-infected children and youth based on self- and caregiver report. *Pediatrics*. 2012;129:e1244–e1251.

Buchanan DB, Kee R, Sadowski LS, et al. The health impact of supportive housing for HIV-positive homeless patients: a randomized controlled trial. *Am J Public Health*. 2009;99(6):S675–S680.

Cacala SR, Mafana E, Thomson SR, et al. Prevalence of HIV status and CD4 counts in a surgical cohort: their relationship to clinical outcome. *Ann R Coll Surg Engl*. 2006;88(1):46–51.

Cahill S, Makadon HJ. Sexual orientation and gender identity data collection update: US Government takes steps to promote sexual orientation and gender identity data collection through meaningful use guidelines. *LGBT Health*. 2014. Available at http://doi.org/10.1089/lgbt.2014.0033.

Cahill S, Makadon H. Sexual orientation and gender identity data collection in clinical settings and in electronic health records: a key to ending LGBT health disparities. *LGBT Health*. 2013. Available at http://online.liebertpub.com/doi/abs/10.1089/lgbt.2013.0001.

Canonico M, Plu-Bureau G, Lowe G, et al. Hormone replacement therapy and risk of venous thromboembolism in postmenopausal women: systematic review and meta-analysis. *BMJ*. 2008;336(7655):1227.

Castronuovo D, Pinzone MR, Moreno S, et al. HIV infection and bone disease: a review of the literature. *Infect Dis Trop Med*. 2015;1(2):E116.

Centers for Disease Control and Prevention (CDC). Revised recommendations for HIV testing of adults, adolescents, and pregnant women in health-care settings. *MMWR*. 2006;55(RR14):1–17.

Centers for Disease Control and Prevention (CDC). Recommended adult immunization schedule: United States, 2010. *Ann Intern Med*. 2010;152(1):36–39.

Centers for Disease Control and Prevention (CDC). Community based opioid overdose prevention programs providing naloxone—United States. *MMWR*. 2012;61:101–105.

Centers for Disease Control and Prevention (CDC). Estimated HIV incidence in the United States, 2007–2010. *HIV Surveil Suppl Rep*. 2012;17(4).

Centers for Disease Control and Prevention (CDC). Diagnoses of HIV infection among adults aged 50 years and older in the United States and dependent areas, 2007–2010. *HIV Surveil Suppl Rep*. 2013a;18(3). Available at http://www.cdc.gov/hiv/topics/surveillance/resources/reports/supplemental. Accessed October 18, 2015.

Centers for Disease Control and Prevention (CDC). HIV diagnosis data are estimates from all 50 states, the District of Columbia, and six US-dependent areas. Rates do not include US-dependent areas. *HIV Surveil Rep*. 23;February 2013.

Centers for Disease Control and Prevention (CDC). HIV surveillance report: diagnosis of HIV infection in the United States and dependent areas 2013—HIV by race/ethnicity through 2013; Vol. 25. August 2013.

Centers for Disease Control and Prevention (CDC). HIV Surveillance Report, 2013b; vol. 25. Available at http://www.cdc.gov/hiv/library/reports/surveillance/. Accessed October 18, 2015.

Centers for Disease Control and Prevention (CDC). HIV surveillance report, 2014; vol. 26. Available at http://www.cdc.gov/hiv/pdf/library/reports/surveillance/cdc-hiv-surveillance-report-us.pdf. Accessed January 30, 2016.

Centers for Disease Control and Prevention (CDC). Community outbreak of HIV infection linked to injection drug use of oxymorphone—Indiana. *MMWR*. 2015;64:443–444.

Centers for Disease Control and Prevention (CDC). Intervals between PCV13 and PPSV23 vaccines: recommendations of the Advisory Committee on Immunization Practices (ACIP). *MMWR*. 2015;64(34):944–947.

Center for Disease Control and Prevention (CDC). HIV surveillance data. 2016. Available at https://www.cdc.gov/actagainstaids/pdf/campaigns/hivtw/cdc-new-hiv-diagnoses-infographic-2016.pdf. Accessed August 8, 2018.

Centers for Disease Control and Prevention (CDC). HIV Surveillance Report, 2016; vol. 28. Available at https://www.cdc.gov/hiv/pdf/library/reports/surveillance/cdc-hiv-surveillance-report-2016-vol-28.pdf. Accessed April 27, 2018.

Centers for Disease Control and Prevention (CDC). Diagnoses of HIV infection among adults aged 50 years and older in the United States and dependent areas, 2011–2016. *HIV Surveil Suppl Rep*. 2018;23(5). Published August 2018. https://www.cdc.gov/hiv/pdf/library/reports/surveillance/cdc-hiv-surveillance-supplemental-report-vol-23-1.pdf Accessed August 11, 2018.

Centers for Disease Control and Prevention (CDC). Surveillance report 2016; vol. 28. Published November 2018. Available at http://www.cdc.gov/hiv/library/reports/surveillance/. Accessed July, 21, 2018.

Centers for Disease Control and Prevention (CDC). Recommendations of the Advisory Committee on Immunization Practices for Use of Herpes Zoster Vaccines. *MMWR*. 2018;67(3);103–108.

Centers for Disease Control and Prevention (CDC). US Public Health Service: pre-exposure prophylaxis for the prevention of HIV infection in the United States—2017 Update: a clinical practice guideline. Published March 2018. https://www.cdc.gov/hiv/pdf/risk/prep/cdc-hiv-prep-guidelines-2017.pdf. Accessed August 4, 2018.

Centers for Disease Control and Prevention (CDC). Effective behavioral interventions. https://www.cdc.gov/hiv/research/interventionresearch/ebis/index.html. Assessed August 11, 2018.

Centers for Disease Control and Prevention (CDC). US Public Health Service study of syphilis at Tuskegee. Available at http://www.cdc.gov/tuskegee/index.html. Accessed November 8, 2015.

Chan P, et al. HIV associated neurocognitive disorders in the modern antiviral treatment era: prevalence, characteristics, biomarkers, and effects of treatment. *Curr HIV/AIDS Rep*. 2014;11(3):317–324.

Chang CK, Hayes RD, Perera G, et al. Life expectancy at birth for people with serious mental illness and other major disorders from a secondary mental healthcare case register in London. *PLoS One*. 2011;10:1371.

Chen JL, Philips KA, Kanouse DE, et al. Fertility desires and intentions of HIV-positive men and women. *Family Planning Perspectives*. 2001;33:144–152, 165.

Chen X, Murphy DA, Naar-King S, et al. A clinic-based motivational intervention improves condom use among subgroups of youth living with HIV. *J Adolescent Health*. 2011;49:193–198.

Chesney E, Goodwin GM, Fazel S. Risks all-cause and suicide mortality in mental disorders: a meta-review. *World Psychiatry*. June 2014;13(2):153–160.

Church JA. HIV disease in children: the many ways it differs from the disease in adults. *Postgrad Med*. 2000;107:163–182.

Clark H, Babu AS, Wiewel EW, Opoku J, Crepaz N. Diagnosed HIV infection in transgender adults and adolescents: results from the national HIV surveillance system, 2009–2014. *AIDS Behav*. 2017;21(9):2774–2783.

Clark RF, Cantrell FL, Pacal A, et al. Subcutaneous silicone injection leading to multi-system organ failure. *Clin Toxicol*. 2008;46(9):834–837. Available at http://doi.org/10.1080/15563650701850025.

Clayton, HB, Lowry R, August E, Jones SE. Nonmedical use of prescription drugs and sexual risk behaviors. *Pediatrics*. 2016;137(1):e20152480.

Clum G, Chung S, Ellen J. Mediators of HIV related stigma and risk behavior in HIV infected young women. *AIDS Care*. 2009;21:1455–1462.

Cohen D, Farley T, Taylor S, et al. When and where do youths have sex? The potential role of adult supervision. *Pediatrics*. 2002;110:1–6.

Cohn SE, Berk ML, Berry SH, et al. The care of HIV-infected adults in rural areas of the United States. *J AIDS*. December 1, 2001;28(4):385–392.

Coleman E, Bockting W, Botzer M, et al. Standards of care for the health of transsexual, transgender, and gender-nonconforming people, version 7. *Intl J Transgenderism*. 2012;13(4):165–232. http://doi.org/10.1080/15532739.2011.700873.

Collins SE, Malone DK, Clifasefi SL, et al. Project-based housing first for chronically homeless individuals with alcohol problems: within-subjects analyses of 2-year alcohol trajectories. *Am J Public Health*. 2012;102(3):511–519.

Colton Meier SL, Fitzgerald KM, Pardo ST, et al. The effects of hormonal gender affirmation treatment on mental health in female-to-male transsexuals. *J Gay Lesbian Mental Health*. 2011;15(3):281–299. Available at http://doi.org/10.1080/19359705.2011.581195.

Conron KJ, Scott G, Stowell GS, et al. (2012). Transgender health in Massachusetts: results from a household probability sample of adults. *Am J Public Health*. 2012;102(1):118–122. http://doi.org/10.2105/AJPH.2011.300315.

Conte AH, Esmailian F, LaBounty T, et al. The patient with the human immunodeficiency virus-1 in the cardiovascular operative setting. *J Cardiothorac Vasc Anesth*. February 2013;27(1):135–155.

Cope AB, Power KA, Kuruc JD, et al. Ongoing HIV transmission and the HIV care continuum in North Carolina. *PLoS One*. 2015;10(6):e0127950.

Cotton S. Spirituality and religion in patients with HIV/AIDS. *Gen Intern Med*. 2006;12;21(Suppl. 5):S5–S13.

Cottrell ML, et al. Altered TDF/FTC pharmacology in a transgender female cohort: implications for PrEP. TUPDX0106. Available at http://programme.aids2018.org/Abstract/Abstract/11225.

Crane JA. Patient comprehension of doctor–patient communication on discharge from the emergency department. *Emerg Med*. January–February 1997;15(1):1–7.

Craw JA, Gardner LI, Marks G, et al. Brief strengths-based case management promotes entry into HIV medical care: results of the antiretroviral treatment access study-II. *J AIDS*. 2008;47(5):597–606.

Crenshaw K. Mapping the margins: Intersectionality, identity politics, and violence against women of color. *Stanford Law Rev*. 1991;43:1241–1299.

Crum-Cianflone N, Grandits G, Echols S, et al. Trends and causes of hospitalizations among HIV-infected persons during the late HAART era: what is the impact of CD4+ counts and HAART use? *J AIDS*. 2010;54(3):248–257.

Dai SY, et al. Prevalence and factors associated with late HIV diagnosis. *J Med Virol*. 2015;87(6):970–977.

Deren M, Shedlin M, Decena CU, et al. Research challenges to the study of HIV/AIDS among migrant and immigrant Hispanic populations in the United States. *J Urban Health*. 2005;82(3):iii13–iii25.

Desai AM, Browning J, Rosen T. Etanercept therapy for silicone granuloma. *J Drugs Dermatol*. 2006;5(9):894–896.

Desai DM, Kuo PC. Perioperative management of special populations: immunocompromised host (cancer, HIV, transplantation). *Surg Clin North Am*. 2005;85(6):1267–1282, xi–xii.

Deutsch MB. *J Health Care Poor Underserved*. 2016;27(2):386–391.

Deutsch MB. Use of the informed consent model in the provision of cross-sex hormone therapy: a survey of the practices of selected clinics. *Intl J Transgenderism*. 2012;13(3):140–146. Available at http://doi.org/10.1080/15532739.2011.675233.

Deutsch MB, Bhakri V, Kubicek K. Effects of cross-sex hormone treatment on transgender women and men. *Obstet Gynecol*. 2015a;125(3):605–610. Available at http://doi.org/10.1097/AOG.0000000000000692

Deutsch MB, Glidden DV, Sevelius J, et al. HIV pre-exposure prophylaxis in transgender women: a subgroup analysis of the iPrEx trial. *Lancet HIV*. 2015b. Available at http://doi.org/10.1016/S2352-3018(15)00206-4.

Deutsch MB, Green J, Keatley J, et al. (2013). Electronic medical records and the transgender patient: Recommendations from the World Professional Association for Transgender Health EMR Working Group. *J Am Med Informat Assoc*. 2012, 001472. Available at http://doi.org/10.1136/amiajnl-2012-001472.

Doblecki-Lewis S, Lester L, Schwartz B, et al. HIV risk and awareness and interest in pre-exposure and post-exposure prophylaxis among sheltered women in Miami. *Intl J STD AIDS*. 2016;27(10):873–881. Available at http://doi.org/10.1177/0956462415601304.

Dowshen N, Binns HJ, Garofalo R. Experiences of HIV-related stigma among young men who have sex with men. *AIDS Patient Care STD*. 2009;23:371–376.

Eaton LA, Driffin DD, Kegler C, et al. The role of stigma and medical mistrust in the routine healthcare engagement of black men who have sex with men. *Am J Public Health*. 2015;105(2):75–82.

El-Ibiary SY, Cocohoba JM. Effects of HIV antiretrovirals on the pharmacokinetics of hormonal contraceptives. *Eur J Contraception Reproduc Health Care*. 2008;13(2):123–132. Available at http://doi.org/10.1080/13625180701829952.

Ellen JM, Kapogiannis B, Fortenberry JD, et al. HIV viral load levels and CD4+ cell counts of youth in 14 cities. *AIDS*. May 15, 2014;28(8):1213–1219.

Emory University, Division of Geriatric Medicine and Gerontology. The Emory "big 10" basics in geriatrics. Available at http://medicine.emory.edu/documents/geriatrics-big10.pdfEmory. Accessed July 7, 2015.

European AIDS Clinical Society (EACS). Guidelines Version 9.0 Available at http://www.eacsociety.org/files/guidelines_9.0-english.pdf. Accessed on July 12, 2018.

Evron S, Glezerman M, Harow E, et al. Human immunodeficiency virus: anesthetic and obstetric considerations. *Anesth Analg*. 2004;98(2):503–511.

Flores AR, Herman JL, Gates GJ, et al. How many adults identify as transgender in the United States? The Williams Institute. June 2016. https://williamsinstitute.law.ucla.edu/wp-content/uploads/How-Many-Adults-Identify-as-Transgender-in-the-United-States.pdf. Accessed July 17, 2018.

Futterman D. HIV in adolescents and young adults: half of all new infections in the United States. *Top HIV Med*. August–September 2005;13(3):101–105.

Gabrielli E, Ferraioli G, Ferraris L, et al. Enfuvirtide administration in HIV-positive transgender patient with soft tissue augmentation: US evaluation. *New Microbiologica*. 2010;33:263–265.

Gander K. Being transgender is not a mental illness, World Health Organizations says. Newsweek. June 19, 2018. Available at https://www.newsweek.com/being-transgender-not-mental-illness-world-health-organization-says-983869. Accessed July 18, 2018.

Garofalo R, Deleon J, Osmer E, et al. Overlooked, misunderstood and at-risk: exploring the lives and HIV risk of ethnic minority male-to-female transgender youth. *J Adolesc Health*. 2006;38:230–236.

Gómez-Gil E, Zubiaurre-Elorza L, Esteva I, et al. Hormone-treated transsexuals report less social distress, anxiety and depression. *Psychoneuroendocrinology*. 2012;37(5):662–670.

Gooren LJ, van Trotsenburg MAA, Giltay EJ, et al. Breast cancer development in transsexual subjects receiving cross-sex hormone treatment. *J Sexual Med*. 2013;10(12):3129–3134. Available at http://doi.org/10.1111/jsm.12319.

Gordon MR, Smale A, Lyman R. US will accept more refugees as crisis grows. *New York Times*, September 20, 2015.

Green, N, Hoenigl, M, Morris, S, et al. Risk behavior and sexually transmitted infections among transgender women and men undergoing community-based screening for acute and early HIV infection in San Diego. *Medicine*. 2015;94(41):e1830. Available at http://doi.org/10.1097/MD.0000000000001830.

Gruskin S, Safreed-Harmon K, Moore CL, et al. HIV and gender-based violence: welcome policies and programmes, but is the research keeping up? *Reprod Health Matters*. 2014;22(44):174–184.

Guaraldi G, et al. Multimorbidity and functional status assessment. *Curr Opin HIV AIDS*. 2014;9(4):386–397.

Guerino P, Harrison P, Sabol W. Prisoners in 2010. US Department of Justice, Bureau of Justice Statistics. 2011. Available at http://www.bjs.gov.

Hajat A, Lucas JB, Kington R. Health outcomes among Hispanic subgroups: data from the National Health Interview Survey, 1992–1995. *Adv Data*. February 25, 2000;310:1–14.

Halkitis PN, Wolitski RJ, Millett GA. A holistic approach to addressing HIV infection disparities in gay, bisexual, and other men who have sex with men. *Am Psychologist*. 2013;68(4):261.

Hammet T, Kennedy S, Kuck S. National survey of infectious diseases in correctional facilities: HIV and sexually transmitted diseases. 2007. US Department of Justice. Available at https://www.ncjrs.gov/pdffiles1/nij/grants/217736.pdf.

Hansen L, Penko J, Guzman D, et al. Aberrant behaviors with prescription opioids and problem drug use history in a community-based cohort of HIV-infected individuals. *J Pain Symptom Management*. 2011;42(6):893–902.

Health Resources and Services Administration (HRSA) HIV/AIDS Programs (HRSA SPNS). (n.d.). Building a medical home for multiply diagnosed HIV-positive homeless populations. Available at http://hab.hrsa.gov/abouthab/special/homeless.html. Accessed November 16, 2015.

Hembree WC, Cohen-Kettenis P, Delemarre-van de Waal HA, et al. Endocrine treatment of transsexual persons: an Endocrine Society clinical practice guideline. *J Clin Endocrinol Metabol*. 2009;94(9):3132–3154. Available at http://doi.org/10.1210/jc.2009-0345.

Hiransuthikul A, et al. Drug-drug interactions between the use of feminizing hormone therapy and pre-exposure prophylaxis among transgender women: the iFACT study. TUPDX0107LB. Available at http://programme.aids2018.org/Abstract/Abstract/13177.

Hughes CA, et al. Managing drug interactions in HIV-infected adults with comorbid illness. *Can Med Assoc J*. 2015;187(1):36.

Hughes SC. HIV and anesthesia. *Anesthesiol Clin North Am*. 2004;22(3):379–404.

Husson RN, Comeau AM, Hoff R. Diagnosis of human immunodeficiency virus infection in infants and children. *Pediatrics*. 1990;86:1–10.

Ickovics JR. "Bundling" HIV prevention: Integrating services to promote synergistic gain. *Prevent Med*. 2008;46(3):222–225. Available at http://doi.org/10.1016/j.ypmed.2007.09.006.

Jacobs EA, Shepard D, Suaya JA, et al. Overcoming language barriers in healthcare: costs and benefits of interpreter services. *Am J Public Health*. 2004;94(5):866–869.

James C. Race ethnicity and medical care: a survey of public perceptions and experiences. Kaiser Family Foundation, September 1999.

James PA, et al. 2014 evidence-based guideline for the management of high blood pressure in adults: report from the panel members appointed to the Eighth Joint National Committee (JNC8). *JAMA*. 2014;311(5):507.

Justice AC, et al. Can the Veterans Aging Cohort Study Index improve clinical judgment for both HIV infected and uninfected veterans? *J Gen Intern Med*. 2013a;28:S39–S39.

Justice AC, et al. Predictive accuracy of the Veterans Aging Cohort Study Index for mortality with HIV infection: a North American cross cohort analysis. *J AIDS*. 2013b;62(2)149–163.

Justice AC, et al. Reply to Chow, et al. *Clin Infect Dis*. 2012.

Kaiser Family Foundation. Fact Sheet: black Americans and HIV/AIDS. Menlo Park, CA: Henry J. Kaiser Family Foundation; April 2014. Available at http://files.kff.org/attachment/fact-sheet-black-americans-and-hiv-aids.

Kaiser Family Foundation. Fact sheet: Latinos and HIV/AIDS. Menlo Park, CA: Henry J. Kaiser Family Foundation: April 2014. Available at https://kaiserfamilyfoundation.files.wordpress.com/2014/04/6007-11-latinos-and-hiv-aids1.pdf.

Kaiser Family Foundation. *Key Facts: Race, Ethnicity, and Medical Care*. Menlo Park, CA: Kaiser Family Foundation; 2007.

Kaku M, et al. HIV neuropathy. *Curr Opin HIV AIDS*. 2014;9(6):521–526.

Kann L, McManus T, Harris WA, et al. Youth risk behavior surveillance—United States, 2017. *MMWR Surveillance Summary*. 2018;67(8):1–479.

Kearney BP, Mathias A. Lack of effect of tenofovir disoproxil fumarate on pharmacokinetics of hormonal contraceptives. *Pharmacotherapy*. 2009;29(8):924–929. Available at http://doi.org/10.1592/phco.29.8.924.

Kenagy GP, Bostwick WB. Health and social service needs of transgender people in Chicago. *International J Transgenderism*. 2005;8(2–3):57–66. Available at http://doi.org/10.1300/J485v08n02_06.

Kim SS, Kaplowitz KS. The effects of physician empathy on patient satisfaction and compliance. *Eval Health Prof*. 2004;27(9):237–251.

Koenig SP, Leandre F, Farmer P. Scaling up HIV treatment programmes in resource-limited settings: the rural Haiti experience. *AIDS*. 2004;18(Suppl 3):S21–S25.

Koroukian SM, et al. Multimorbidity redefined: prospective health outcomes and the cumulative effect of co-occurring conditions. *Prev Chronic Dis*. 2015;12:E55.

Kullgren JT. Restrictions on undocumented immigrants' access to health services: the public health implications of welfare reform. *Am J Public Health*. October 2003;93(10):1630–1633.

Lee SJ, Leipzig RM, Walter LC. Incorporating lag time to benefit into prevention decisions for older adults. *JAMA*. 2013;310(24):2609–2610.

Lester RT, Ritvo P, Mills E, et al. Effects of a mobile phone short message service on antiretroviral treatment adherence in Kenya (WelTel Kenya1): a randomized trial. *Lancet*. 2010;376:1838–1845.

Leung AA, Nerenberg K, Daskalopoulou SS, et al. Hypertension Canada's 2016 Canadian Hypertension Education Program guidelines for blood pressure measurement, diagnosis, assessment of risk, prevention, and treatment of hypertension. *Can J Cardiol*. 2016;32:569–588.

Lindau ST, et al. A study of sexuality and health among older adults in the United States. *N Engl J Med*. 2007;357(8):762–774.

Machinger EL, Haberer JE, Wilson TC, et al. Recent trauma is associated with antiretroviral failure and HIV transmission risk behavior among HIV-positive women and female-identified transgenders. *AIDS Behav*. 2012;16(8):2160–2170.

Malcolm J, et al. Veterans Aging Cohort Study (VACS) Index, functional status, and other patient reported outcomes in old HIV-positive (HIV⁺) adults. *Open Forum Infect Dis*. 2014;1(1):S428–S429.

Marrazzo JM, Ramjee G, Richardson BA, et al. Tenofovir-based preexposure prophylaxis for HIV infection among African women. *N Engl J Med*. 2015;372(6):509–518. Available at http://doi.org/10.1056/NEJMoa1402269.

Martinez J, Harper G, Carleton RA, et al. The impact of stigma on medication adherence among HIV-positive adolescent and young adult females and the moderating effects of coping and satisfaction with healthcare. *AIDS Patient Care STDS*. 2012;26:108–115.

Maruschak L. HIV in prisons, 2007–08. US Department of Justice, Bureau of Justice Statics. 2009. Available at http://www.bjs.gov/content/pub/pdf/hivp08.pdf.

Massachusetts Department of Public Health (MDPH). HIV/AIDS Fact sheet: persons born outside the US. 2012. Available at http://www.mass.gov/eohhs/docs/dph/aids/2012-profiles/born-outside-us.pdf.

McKinney MM. Variations in HIV epidemiology and service delivery models in the United States. *J Rural Health*. 2002;18:455–466.

McKittrick N, et al. Improved immunogenicity with high-dose seasonal influenza vaccine in HIV-infected persons: a single-center, parallel, randomized trial. *Ann Intern Med*. 2013;158(1):19–26.

McLeroy KR, Bibeau D, Steckler A, et al. An ecological perspective on health promotion programs. *Health Educ Q*. 1988;15(4):351–377.

Meerwijk EL, Sevelius JM. Transgender population size in United States: a meta-regression of population-based probability samples. *Am J Public Health*. 2017;107(2): e1–e8.

Meites E, Kempe A, Markowitz LE. Use of a 2-Dose Schedule for Human Papillomavirus Vaccination - Updated Recommendations of the Advisory Committtee on Immunization Practices. *MMWR Morb Mortal Wkly Rep* 2016;65:1405–1408. DOIL http//dx.doi.org/10.15585/mmwr.mm6549a5 (http://dx.doi.org/10.15585/mmwr.mm6549a5).

Melendez RM, Pinto RM. HIV prevention and primary care for transgender women in a community-based clinic. *J Assoc Nurses AIDS Care*. 2009;20(5):387–397. Available at http://doi.org/10.1016/j.jana.2009.06.002.

Miaskowski C, Penko JM, Guzman D, et al. Occurrence and characteristics of chronic pain in a community-based cohort of indigent adults living with HIV infection. *J Pain*. 2011;12(9):1004–1016.

Mikalson P, Pardo S, Green J. First, do no harm: reducing disparities for lesbian, gay, bisexual, transgender, queer and questioning populations in California. Published December 2012. Available at http://www.lhc.ca.gov/sites/lhc.ca.gov/files/Reports/225/ReportsSubmitted/CRDPLGBTQReport.pdf. Accessed July 2018.

Minton T, Sabol W. Jail inmates at midyear 2008—Statistical tables. US Department of Justice, Bureau of Justice Statistics. 2009. Available at http://bjs.ojp.usdoj.gov/content/pub/pdf/jim08st.pdf.

Mitchell JB, McCormack LA. Time trends in late-stage diagnosis of cervical cancer: differences by race/ethnicity and income. *Med Care*. 1997;35(12):1220–1224.

Mizuno Y, Frazier EL, Huang P, et al. Characteristics of transgender women living with HIV receiving medical care in the United States. *LGBT Health*. September 2015;2(3):228034. doi: 10.1089/lgbt.2014.0099 Epub April 28, 2015.

Moore RD, Stanton D, Gopalan R, et al. Racial differences in the use of drug therapy for HIV disease in an urban community. *N Engl J Med*. 1995;330(11):763–768.

Moss AR, Hahn JA, Perry S, et al. Adherence to highly active antiretroviral therapy in the homeless population in San Francisco: a prospective study. *Clin Infect Dis*. October 15, 2004;15;39(8):1190–1198.

Moyer VA; US Preventive Services Task Force. Screening for HIV: US Preventive Services Task Force recommendation statement. *Ann Intern Med*. July 2, 2013;159(1):51–60.

Murphy DA, Sarr M, Durako SJ, et al. Barriers to HAART adherence among HIV-infected adolescents. *Arch Pediatr Adolesc Med*. 2003;157:249–255.

Naar-King S, Wright K, Parsons JT, et al. Health choices: Motivational enhancement therapy for health risk behaviors in HIV-positive youth. *AIDS Educ Prevent*. 2006;18:1–11.

Nachman SA, Cheroff M, Gona P, et al. Incidence of noninfectious conditions in perinatally HIV-infected children and adolescents in the HAART era. *Arch Pediatr Adolesc Med*. 2009;163:164–171.

Nash GD, Flanders WD, Baird TC, et al. Cross-sex hormones and acute cardiovascular events in transgender persons: a cohort study. *Ann Intern Med*. August 21, 2018;169(4):205–213. doi: 10.7326/M17-2785. Epub July 10, 2018.

National Alliance to Advance Adolescent Health. Got transition. Available at http://gottransition.org/providers/index.cfm. Accessed January 31, 2016.

National Center for Health Statistics (NCHS). Health, United States, 2012. May 2013.

National Center for Transgender Equality. 2015 US Transgender Survey. Available at http://www.ustranssurvey.org. Accessed August 11, 2018.

National Health Care for the Homeless Council and Clinicians Network. Adapted clinical guidelines. Available at https://www.nhchc.org/resources/clinical/adapted-clinical-guidelines.

National Heart Foundation. Guideline for the diagnosis and management of hypertension in adults—2016. Melbourne: National Heart Foundation of Australia. Available at https://www.heartfoundation.org.au/images/uploads/publications/PRO-167_Hypertension-guideline-2016_WEB.pdf. Accessed April 27, 2018.

National Law Center on Homelessness and Poverty. Homelessness in America: Overview of data and causes. January 2015. Available at http://www.nlchp.org/documents/Homeless_Stats_Fact_Sheet. Accessed November 16, 2015.

National LGBT Health Education Center. Providing welcoming services and care for LGBT people. 2015. Available at http://www.lgbthealtheducation.org/wp-content/uploads/Learning-Guide.pdf. Accessed December 1, 2015.

Naziri Q, Boylan M, Issa K, et al. Does HIV infection increase the risk of perioperative complications after THA? A nationwide database study. *Clin Orthop Relat Res*. 2015;473(2):581–586.

Newport F. Three-quarters of Americans identify as Christian. Gallup.com, December 2014. Available at http://www.gallup.com/poll/180347/three-quarters-americans-identify-christian.aspx. Accessed December 1, 2015.

Nottet, HSLM, Persidsky Y, Sasseville VG, et al. Mechanisms for the transendothelial migration of HIV-1-infected monocytes into brain. *J Immunol*. 1996;156:1284–1295.

Nugent NR, Brown LK, Belzer M, et al. Youth living with HIV and problem substance use: elevated distress is associated with nonadherence and sexual risk. *J Int Assoc Phys AIDS Care*. March–April 2010;9(2):113–115.

Ohl M, Tate J, Duggal M, et al. Rural residence is associated with delayed care entry and increased mortality among veterans with human immunodeficiency virus infection. *Medicare Care*. 2010;48:1064–0170.

Olson J, Schrager SM, Clark LF, et al. Subcutaneous testosterone: An effective delivery mechanism for masculinizing young transgender men. *LGBT Health*. 2014. Available at http://doi.org/10.1089/lgbt.2014.0018.

Panel on Antiretroviral Therapy and Medical Management of HIV-Infected Children. Guidelines for the use of antiretroviral agents in pediatric HIV infection (last updated May 22, 2018). Available at https://aidsinfo.nih.gov/contentfiles/lvguidelines/PediatricGuidelines.pdf. Accessed August 8, 2018.

Panel on Opportunistic Infections in HIV-Exposed and HIV-Infected Children. Guidelines for the prevention and treatment of opportunistic infections in HIV-exposed and HIV-infected children. Available at https://aidsinfo.nih.gov/contentfiles/lvguidelines/oi_guidelines_pediatrics.pdf. Accessed August 8, 2018.

Panel on Treatment of HIV-Infected Pregnant Women and Prevention of Perinatal Transmission. Recommendations for use of antiretroviral drugs in pregnant HIV-1-infected women for maternal health and interventions to reduce perinatal HIV transmission in the United States. Available at https://aidsinfo.nih.gov/contentfiles/lvguidelines/PerinatalGL.pdf. Accessed August 8, 2018.

Pasternack FR, Fox LP, Engler DE. Silicone granulomas treated with etanercept. *Arch Dermatol*. 2005;141(1):13.

Paterson DL Swindells S. Adherence to protease inhibitor therapy and outcomes in patients with HIV infection. *Ann Intern Med*. 2000;133:21–30.

Peitzmeier SM, Reisner SL, Harigopal P, et al. Female-to-male patients have high prevalence of unsatisfactory Paps compared to non-transgender females: Implications for cervical cancer screening. *J Gen Intern Med*. May 2014;29(5):778–784. Published online January 15, 2014.

Philbin MM, Tanner AE, Duval A, et al. Linking HIV-positive adolescents to care in 15 different clinics across the United States: creating solutions to address structural barriers for linkage to care. *AIDS Care.* January 2014;26(1):12–19.

Pilowsky DJ, et al. Sexual risk behaviors and HIV risk among Americans aged 50 years or older: a review. *Subst Abuse Rehabil.* 2015;6:51–60.

Poteat T, Wirtz AL, Radix A, et al. HIV risk and preventive interventions in transgender women sex workers. *Lancet.* 2015;385(9964):274–286. Available at http://doi.org/10.1016/S0140-6736(14)60833-3.

Radcliff J, Doty N, Hawkins LA, et al. Stigma and sexual risk in HIV-positive African American young men who have sex with men. *AIDS Patient Care STD.* 2010;24:493–499.

Rao D, Kekwaletswe TC, Hosek S, et al. Stigma and social barriers to medication adherence with urban youth living with HIV. *AIDS Care.* 2007;19:28–33.

Rapaport MJ. Silicone granulomas treated with etanercept. *Arch Dermatol.* 2005;141(9):1171. Available at http://doi.org/10.1001/archderm.141.9.1171-a.

Reif S, Golin CE, Smith SR. Barriers to accessing HIV/AIDS care in North Carolina: rural and urban differences. *AIDS Care.* July 2005;17(5):558–565.

Reisner S, Mimiaga MJ, Skeer M, et al. A review of HIV antiretroviral adherence and intervention studies among HIV-infected youth. *Int AIDS Soc USA Topics HIV Med.* 2009;17:1425.

Rose D, Collins M, Kelban R. Complications of surgery in HIV-infected patients. *AIDS.* 1998;12:2243–2251.

Rudy BJ, Murphy DA, Harris DR, et al. Patient-related risks for nonadherence to antiretroviral therapy among HIV-infected youth in the United States: a study of prevalence and interactions. *AIDS Patient Care STD.* 2008;23:1–10.

Sabol W, West H, Cooper M. Prisoners in 2008. US Department of Justice, Bureau of Justice Statistics. 2009. Available at http://bjs.ojp.usdoj.gov/content/pub/pdf/p08.pdf.

Saltzman DJ, Williams RA, Gelfand DV, et al. The surgeon and AIDS: twenty years later. *Arch Surg.* 2005;140(10):961–967.

Sanchez NF, Sanchez JP, Danoff A. Health care utilization, barriers to care, and hormone usage among male-to-female transgender persons in New York City. *Am J Public Health.* 2009;99(4):713.

Sanders RA. Adolescent psychosocial, social, and cognitive development. *Pediatr Rev.* August 2013;34(8):354–358; quiz 358–359.

San Francisco Department of Public Health Population Health Division (SFDPH). HIV-Epidemiology Annual Report: 2014. August 2015. Available at https://www.sfdph.org/dph/files/reports/RptsHIVAIDS/AnnualReport2015-20160831.pdf. Accessed November 16, 2015.

Sangarlangkarn A, et al. Advance Care Planning and HIV in the antiretroviral therapy era: a narrative review. *Top Antiviral Med.* 2015.

Schietinger H, Schechter C. Examining medical coverage for Medicare beneficiaries with HIV/AIDS. *AIDS Public Policy J.* Summer 1999;14(2):68–79.

Schouten J, et al. Cross-sectional comparison of the prevalence of age-associated comorbidities and their risk factors between HIV-infected and uninfected individuals: the AGEhIV cohort study. *Clin Infect Dis.* 2014;59(12):1787–1797.

Schur CL, Berk ML, Dunbar JR, et al. Where to seek care: an examination of people in rural areas with HIV/AIDS. *J Rural Health.* Spring 2002;18(2):337–347.

Selik R, Mokotoff E, Branson B, et al. Revised surveillance case definition for HIV infection—United States, 2014. *MMWR.* 2014;63(RR03):1–10.

Semeere AS, et al. Mortality and immunological recovery among older adults on antiretroviral therapy at a large urban HIV clinic in Kampala, Uganda. *J AIDS.* 2014;67(4):382–389.

Sevelius JM. Gender affirmation: a framework for conceptualizing risk behavior among transgender women of color. *Sex Roles.* 2013;68(11–12):675–689. Available at http://doi.org/10.1007/s11199-012-0216-5.

Sevelius JM, Patouhas E, Keatley JG, et al. Barriers and facilitators to engagement and retention-in-care among transgender women living with human immunodeficiency virus. *Ann Behav Med.* 2014;47(1):5–16. Available at http://doi.org/10.1007/s12160-013-9565-8.

Sevelius JM, Saberi P, Johnson MO. Correlates of antiretroviral adherence and viral load among transgender women living with HIV. *AIDS Care.* August 2014;26(8):987–982. Published online March 20, 2014. doi: 10.1080/09540121.2014.896451.

Shafran SD. Live attenuated herpes zoster vaccine for HIV-infected adults. *HIV Med.* 2016;17(4):305–310.

Shapiro MJ, Morton SC, McCaffrey D, et al. Variations in the care of HIV-infected adults in the United States: Results from the HIV Vost and services utilization study. *JAMA.* 1999;281:2305–2375.

Sheifer SE, Escarce JJ. Race and sex differences in the management of coronary artery disease. *Am Heart J.* 2000;139(5):848–857.

Sigel K, Wisnivesky J, Shahrir S, et al. Findings in asymptomatic HIV infected patients undergoing chest computed tomography testing: implications for lung cancer screening. *AIDS.* 2014;28(7):1007–1014.

Silva-Santisteban A, Segura ER, Sandoval C, et al. Determinants of unequal HIV care access among people living with HIV in Peru. *Globalization Health.* 2013;9(1):22. Available at http://doi.org/10.1186/1744-8603-9-22.

Sitapati AM, Limneos J, Bonet-Vázquez M, et al. Retention: building a patient-centered medical home in HIV primary care through PUFF (patients unable to follow-up found). *J Health Care Poor Underserved.* 2012;23(3 Suppl):81–95.

Skarbinski J, Rosenberg E, Paz-Bailey G, et al. Human immunodeficiency virus transmission at each step of the care continuum in the United States. *JAMA Intern Med.* 2015;175(4):596–597.

Smedley D, Stith A, Nelson A (Eds.). *Unequal Treatment—Confronting Racial and Ethnic Disparities in Healthcare.* Washington, DC: Institute of Medicine, The National Academies Press; 2003.

Smith CJ, Ryom L, Weber R, et al. Trends in underlying causes of death in people with HIV from 1999 to 2011 (D:A:D): a multicohort collaboration. *Lancet.* 2014;384:241–248.

Sodora DL, Silvestri G. Immune activation and AIDS pathogenesis. *AIDS.* 2008;22:439–446.

Spaulding A, Stephenson B, Macalino G, et al. Human immunodeficiency virus in correctional facilities. *Clin Infect Dis.* 2002;35:305–312.

Straub DM, Arrington-Sanders R, Harris DR, et al. Correlates of HIV testing history among urban youth recruited through venue-based testing in 15 US cities. *Sex Transm Dis.* August 2011;38(8):691–696.

Subcutaneous administration of testosterone: a pilot study report. *Saudi Med J.* 2006;27(12):1843–1846.

Swenderman D, Rotherman-Borus MJ, Comulada S, et al. Predictors of HIV-related stigma among young people living with HIV. *Health Psychol.* 2006;25:501–509.

Sypsa V, Paraskevis D, Malliori M, et al. Homelessness and other risk factors for HIV infection in the current outbreak among injection drug users in Athens, Greece. *Am J Public Health.* January 2015;105(1):196–204.

Tanney MR, Naar-King S, MacDonnell K. Depression and stigma in high-risk youth living with HIV: a multi-site study. *J Pediatr Health Care.* 2012;26:300–305.

Tate CC, Ledbetter JN, Youssef CP. A two-question method for assessing gender categories in the social and medical sciences. *J Sex Research.* 2012;50, 1–10. Available at http://doi.org/10.1080/00224499.2012.690110.

the Prevention, Detection, Evaluation, and Management of High Blood Pressure in Adults. *J Am Coll Cardiol.* 2017. doi: 10.1016/j.jacc.2017.11.006.

Tinetti ME, et al. Designing health care for the most common chronic condition—multimorbidity. *JAMA.* 2012;307(23):2493–2494.

Torian LV, Wiewel EW, Liu K, et al. Risk factors for delayed initiation of medical care after diagnosis of human immunodeficiency virus. *Arch Intern Med.* 2008;168(11):1181–1187.

Toska E, Cluver LD, Hodes R, et al. Sex and secrecy: how HIV-status disclosure affects safe sex among HIV-positive adolescents. *AIDS Care.* December 2015;27(Suppl 1):47–58.

Trent M, Chung SE, Ellen JM, et al. New sexually transmitted infections among adolescent girls infected with HIV. *Sex Transmitted Infect.* 2007;83:468–469.

UNAIDS. How AIDS changed everything—MDG6: 15 years, 15 lessons of hope from the AIDS response. July 2015. UNAIDS Secretariat, Geneva, Switzerland. Available at https://issuu.com/unaids/docs/mdg6_executivesummary_en. Accessed December 1, 2015.

US Department of Health and Human Services (USDHHS). Panel on Antiretroviral Guidelines for Adults and Adolescents. Guidelines for the use of antiretroviral agents in adults and adolescents living with HIV. Available at https://aidsinfo.nih.gov/contentfiles/lvguidelines/AdultandAdolescentGL.pdf. Accessed April 27, 2018.

US Department of Health of Human Services (USDHHS). Guidelines for the use of antiretroviral agents in HIV-1-infected adults and adolescents. Available at https://aidsinfo.nih.gov/guidelines/html/1/adult-and-adolescent-treatment-guidelines/0. Accessed August 11, 2018.

US Department of Health and Human Services (USDHHS). Guidelines for the use of antiviral agents in Pediatric HIV infection. Updated https://aidsinfo.nih.gov/guidelines. Update 5/22/18. Accessed 3/23/19.

US Department of Health and Human Services (USDHHS). Management of infants born to women with HIV infection. Table 7. https://aidsinfo.nih.gov/guideline/html/3/perinatal/187/antiretroviral-management-of-ne... Accessed 3/23/19.

US Department of Health and Human Services (USDHHS). Guidelines for the use of antiviral agents in Pediatric HIV infection. Updated https://aidsinfo.nih.gov/guidelines. Updated 5/22/18. Accessed 3/23/19.

US Department of Health and Human Services (USDHHA). Guidelines for the Prevention and Treatment of Opportunistic Infections Among HIV-Exposed and HIV-Infected Children (2013). Table 1 and Table 2. https/aidsinfo.nih.gov.guidelines/html/5/pediatric-opportunistic-infection. Accessed 5/2/18.

US Department of Health and Human Services (USDHHA). Guidelines for the Prevention and Treatment of Opportunistic Infections Among HIV-Exposed and HIV-Infected Children (2013). Figure 1 and Figure 2 Immunization Tables. https/aidsinfo.nih.gov.guidelines/html/5/pediatric-opportunistic-infection. Accessed 5/2/18.

US Department of Health and Human Services (USDHHS), Health Resources and Services Administration, HIV/AIDS Bureau. Guide for HIV/AIDS clinical care. 2014. Available at http://hab.hrsa.gov/deliverhivaidscare/2014guide.pdf. Accessed February 12, 2016.

Valenzuela JM, Buchanan CL, Radcliffe J, et al. Transition to adult services among behaviorally infected adolescents with HIV: a qualitative study. *J Pediatr Psychol.* March 2011;36(2):134–140.

van Kesteren PJ, Asscheman H, Megens JA, et al. Mortality and morbidity in transsexual subjects treated with cross-sex hormones. *Clin Endocrinol.* 1997;47(3):337–342.

van Ryn M, Burke J. The effect of patient race and socioeconomic status on physicians' perceptions of patients. *Social Sci Med.* 2000;50:813–828.

Vinikoor MJ, et al. Age at antiretroviral therapy initiation predicts immune recovery, death, and loss to follow-up among HIV-infected adults in urban Zambia. *AIDS Res Hum Retroviruses.* 2014;30(10):949–955.

Vrouenraets SM, et al. A comparison of measured and estimated glomerular filtration rate in successfully treated HIV-patients with preserved renal function. *Clin Nephrol.* 2012;77(4):311–320.

Wagner GJ, Goggin K, Remien RH, et al. A closer look at depression and its relationship to HIV antiretroviral adherence. *Ann Behav Med.* 2011;42:352–360.

Waldrop-Valverde D, Valverde E. Homelessness and psychological distress as contributors to antiretroviral nonadherence in HIV-positive injecting drug users. *AIDS Patient Care STD.* May 2005;19(5):326–334.

Wechsberg WM, Lam WK, Zule W, et al. Violence, homelessness, and HIV risk among crack-using African-American women. *Subst Use Misuse.* February–May 2003;38(3–6):669–700.

Weinbaum C, Sabin K, Santibanez S. Hepatitis B, hepatitis C, and HIV in correctional populations: a review of epidemiology and prevention. *AIDS.* 2005;19(Suppl 3):S41–S46.

Weiner LS, Battles HR, Wood LV. A longitudinal study of adolescents with perinatally or transfusion acquired HIV infection: sexual knowledge, risk reduction self efficacy and sexual behavior. *AIDS Behav.* 2007;11:471–478.

Weisse CS, Sorum PC, Sanders KN, et al. Do gender and race affect decisions about pain management? *J Gen Intern Med.* 2001;16(4):211–217.

Weyers S, Verstraelen H, Gerris J, et al. Microflora of the penile skin-lined neovagina of transsexual women. *BMC Microbiol.* 2009;9(1):102. Available at http://doi.org/10.1186/1471-2180-9-102.

Whelton PK, Carey RM, Aronow WS, et al. ACC/AHA/AAPA/ABC/ACPM/AGS/APhA/ASH/ASPC/NMA/PCNA Guideline for

Williams PL, Storm D, Montepiedra G, et al. Predictors of adherence to antiretroviral medications in children and adolescents with HIV infection. *Pediatrics.* 2006;118:e1745–e1757.

Wilson EC, Garofalo R, Harris DR, et al. Transgender female youth and sex work: HIV risk and a comparison of life factors related to engagement in sex work. *AIDS Behav.* October 2009;13(5):902–913.

Wilson LE, Korthuis T, Fleishman JA, et al. HIV-related medical service use by rural/urban residents: a multistate perspective. *AIDS Care.* 2011;23(8):971–979.

Wismer B, Amann T, Diaz R, et al., eds. *Adapting Your Practice: Recommendations for the Care of Homeless Adults with Chronic Non-malignant Pain.* Nashville, TN: Health Care for the Homeless Clinicians' Network, National Health Care for the Homeless Council; 2011: 119.

Workowski K, Bolan G. Sexually transmitted diseases treatment guidelines, 2015. *MMWR Recomm Rep.* 2015;65(3).

World Health Organization (WHO). HIV/AIDS fact sheet. Available at http://www.who.int/mediacentre/factsheets/fs360/en. Accessed July 15, 2018.

Xavier J, Bobbin M, Singer B, et al. A needs assessment of transgendered people of color living in Washington, DC. *Int J Transgenderism.* 2005;8:31–47.

Zanoni BC, Mayer KH. The adolescent and young adult HIV cascade of care in the United States: exaggerated health disparities. *AIDS Patient Care STD.* 2014;28(3):128–135.

Zolopa AR, Andersen J, Powderly W, et al. Early antiretroviral therapy reduces AIDS progression/death in individuals with acute opportunistic infections: a multicenter randomized strategy trial. *PLoS One.* 2009;4(5):e5575. doi: 10.1371/journal.pone.0005575

14.

COMPLEMENTARY AND ALTERNATIVE MEDICINE/ INTEGRATIVE MEDICINE APPROACHES

Kalpana D. Shere-Wolfe

CHAPTER GOALS

Upon completion of this chapter, the reader should be able to

- Provide HIV providers with general information on complementary and integrative medicine.
- Update HIV providers on the literature pertaining to the use of complementary and integrative modalities for HIV infected patients.

INTRODUCTION

Complementary and integrative medicine, which includes natural products, mind and body practices, and traditional medical systems, is increasing used by patients in the United States and worldwide. As a result of ongoing interest and use, a growing body of research has focused on the potential therapeutic value and safety of these modalities both in the general population and in HIV-infected patients.

LEARNING OBJECTIVES

- Discuss the fundamentals and practice of complementary and integrative medicine as it pertains to HIV medicine.
- Describe the established and evolving science of natural products, mind–body practices, and traditional medical systems.

WHAT'S NEW?

This edition contains updated information on the effects of micronutrient supplementation on CD4+ T cell counts and HIV disease progression; the effects of probiotics, prebiotics, and immunonutrition on inflammatory markers and CD4+ T cell counts; and the effect of mind–body practices on expression of genes, biomarkers of stress, and CD4+ T cell counts. In addition, herb–drug interactions are reviewed, with new data presented on interactions with newer antiretroviral medications.

KEY POINTS

- Complementary and alternative medicine (CAM) use is common in patients with HIV. Physicians caring for HIV-infected individuals should be aware of the high prevalence of CAM use and the failure of most patients to disclose CAM use. Physicians need to routinely ask about CAM use, particularly herbal medicines and supplements.

- Nutritional supplementation with micronutrients— vitamins A, B, C, and E, zinc, and selenium—has been shown to improve markers of HIV progression and, in some studies, to also affect mortality.

- Natural health products (NHPs; herbs, vitamins, and supplements) have the potential for significant drug interactions, which may lower the efficacy or increase the adverse effects of antiretroviral therapy (ART).

- Fish oil supplementation remains controversial. The 2017 American Heart Association advisory recommends fish oil supplementation for secondary prevention of heart disease. However, recent analysis and trials fail to demonstrate benefits of fish oil supplementation for cardiovascular disease (CVD) prevention.

- Studies suggest that probiotics may influence markers of coagulation, inflammation, microbial translocation, and microbiota in HIV-infected individuals.

- Some data suggest that stress, anxiety, and depression can affect HIV progression. Mind–body practices such as meditation, mindfulness, yoga, and tai chi can reduce stress, improve blood pressure, and improve quality of life (QOL). In addition, they may affect adverse health behaviors. The effects of these practices on CD4+ T cell counts and disease progression are currently under investigation.

- Acupuncture may be of benefit in patients with musculoskeletal pain and sleep issues.

WHAT IS CAM AND INTEGRATIVE MEDICINE?

CAM is a group of diverse medical and healthcare systems, practices, and products that are not currently considered part of conventional medicine. Although the terms *complementary* and *alternative* are used simultaneously and interchangeably, they refer to different entities. If a non-mainstream practice is used together with conventional medicine, it is considered "complementary." If a non-mainstream practice is used in place of conventional medicine, it is considered "alternative." True alternative medicine is uncommon in developed countries but may be commonly found in resource-limited settings. Most people who use non-mainstream approaches use them along with conventional treatments (see the National Center for Complementary and Integrative Health (NCCIH) website at https://nccih.nih.gov/health/herbsataglance.htm). Integrative medicine, the increasingly more common term in use, refers to the use of CAM modalities with conventional medicine in an evidence-based integrated manner, with emphasis on the importance of the relationship between practitioner and patient. Cornerstones of integrative medicine—nutrition, stress management, and exercise/movement—overlap those of conventional medicine but vary in their emphasis and approach.

Complementary and integrative health approaches encompass three broad areas: natural products, mind and body practices, and traditional medical systems. *Natural products* are herbs or botanicals, vitamins and minerals, and probiotics. They are widely marketed and available and are typically sold as dietary supplements. *Mind and body practices* include a large and diverse group of techniques typically administered by trained practitioners. They include yoga, chiropractic and osteopathic manipulation, meditation, massage therapy, acupuncture, relaxation techniques (e.g., breathing exercises, guided imagery, and progressive muscle relaxation), tai chi, qi qong, healing touch, movement therapies, and hypnotherapy. *Traditional medical systems* include various types of healers, Ayurvedic medicine, Chinese medicine, homeopathy, and naturopathy. The research on these various modalities varies widely. Although there are many studies on certain herbal products, acupuncture, yoga, spinal manipulation, and meditation, there have been fewer studies on other practices. Moreover, studies using these modalities in HIV-infected patients are limited.

USE OF CAM BY HIV-INFECTED PATIENTS

Historically, CAM was popular in the HIV/AIDS community prior to the development of ART, and it remains popular. This is true in the United States, Canada, Australia, many European countries, Asia, and Africa. Now that effective treatment options exist for people living with HIV/AIDS and the life expectancy of these patients parallels that of people without HIV, CAM therapies are being sought for general wellness, mood disorders, stress reduction, and reduction of medication-associated side effects, as well as for boosting the immune system (Lorenc, 2013; Thompson, 2012). Importantly, one of the key reasons that CAM is being used by patients is because it enables them to have a more active role in their healthcare as well as a sense of control. CAM use is a way to shift the focus away or "demedicalize" HIV management and focus on a sense of wellness and normalcy (Littlewood, 2011). Factors that contribute to the increasingly popular concept of wellness include good nutrition, exercise, physical relaxation, and mental ease.

There is variability in reports of CAM use due to differences in study populations, definitions of CAM, and CAM therapies. CAM is used by approximately 30–60% of HIV-infected patients; however, when restricted to practitioner-based CAM, the prevalence is approximately 15% or 16% (Halpin, 2018; Bahall, 2017; Kelso-Chichetto, 2016; Dhalla, 2006; Greene, 1999; Josephs, 2007; London, 2003; Lorenc, 2013; Standish, 2001; Visser, 2002). CAM use is predicted by higher levels of education, men who have sex with men (MSM), female gender, longer disease duration, symptom severity and time on ART, and financial resources (Halpin, 2018; Agnoletto, 2006; Littlewood, 2008; Lorenc, 2013). In a large recent survey of 1,763 patients enrolled in the Veterans Aging Cohort Study, CAM users were also more likely to be white, have higher CD4$^+$ T cell counts, higher numbers of bothersome symptoms, and more likely to be receiving prescription opioids and benzodiazepines (Halpin, 2018). Similarly, in a study of 803 HIV-infected patients in the Florida Medical Monitoring Project, CAM use was more common in whites ($p = 0.001$) (Kelso-Chichetto, 2016). Vitamins, herbs, and supplements are most common, followed by prayer, meditation, and spiritual approaches. In developing countries and areas with poor access to conventional HIV treatment, traditional culture-based systems are widely used. In general, patients have a high level of satisfaction with CAM modalities, with 50–70% reporting improvement in malaise, various symptoms, and QOL (Agnoletto, 2003; Duggan, 2001).

One study found decreased adherence to ART with CAM use (Owen-Smith, 2007). A more recent study found that CAM users were not only adherent to ART but also likely less likely to have detectable viral load (VL) compared to nonusers (Kelso-Chichetto, 2016). In general, most studies have found that CAM users do not have decreased adherence to conventional medication nor do they reject conventional ART. Rather, they use CAM in an integrated manner with their conventional HIV care (Littlewood, 2008, 2014; Liu, 2009; Milan, 2008).

PHYSICIAN ATTITUDES TOWARD CAM

There are limited data on physician attitudes toward CAM. In a study of 114 physicians, fellows, and residents, the majority of participants expressed a desire to learn more about CAM but were unaware of how to obtain evidence-based information (Patel, 2017). There are also some data showing that physicians are now more willing to use CAM to address patient needs (Wahner-Roedler, 2014). Even less is known about infectious disease (ID) physicians' and HIV providers' attitudes toward CAM. In one study of 89 HIV care providers, 63% believed that CAM and integrative medicine therapies may be helpful for HIV-infected patients, and 36% had personally used one (Wynia, 1999). A national survey of ID physicians demonstrated that they are familiar with various CAM modalities, including vitamin and mineral supplementation, massage, acupuncture, chiropractic, yoga, and herbal medicine. They most recommended vitamin and mineral supplementation (80%) and massage (62%). Data regarding clinical efficacy, drug interactions, and safety appear to be important factors that influence ID physicians' use of these modalities for their patients (Shere-Wolfe, 2013).

PATIENT DISCLOSURE REGARDING CAM USE

Studies have shown that the majority of physicians do not ask their patients about CAM use and that patients may not disclose CAM use for various reasons unless asked directly (Patel, 2017; Wahner, 2014; Wynia, 1999). It is important that clinicians caring for patients with HIV/AIDS ask about CAM use to identify any potential drug interactions and safety issues.

CAM use disclosure rates vary across studies, from 38% to 90% (Littlewood, 2008). In the Women's Interagency HIV Study, CAM use disclosure was associated with women older than age 45 years who had a college degree and health insurance; nondisclosure was associated with minority racial status. Compared to natural products and body-based practices such as acupuncture and massage, mind–body practices have the lowest prevalence of CAM use disclosure. In one study, CAM use disclosure was also significantly associated with higher ART adherence (Liu, 2009).

Discussing CAM use is important, especially with respect to natural products. Concerns regarding drug interactions are paramount; however, also important are issues related to contamination of natural products. One study found that 21% of Ayurvedic medicines purchased via the Internet contained detectable levels of lead, mercury, and arsenic (Saper, 2008). Similarly, Chinese herbal medicines may have microbial and heavy metal contamination (Ting, 2013). Heavy metal toxicity and testing may be considered in patients with new symptoms after initiating Chinese or Ayurvedic medicines. Other safety issues include side effects from taking extremely large doses of vitamins. High doses of vitamin A can cause liver and bone damage as well as increase the risk of birth defects. High-dose vitamin C apparently increases the risk of kidney stones. High doses of zinc (>75 mg/d) have been linked to copper deficiency.

Questions such as "Are you taking any vitamins, supplements, or herbs?" can be asked immediately after inquiring about conventional medications and compliance. For foreign patients, asking "Are you taking any natural medicines from your country?" may elicit information that might not otherwise be offered. A brief statement such as "This is important as many natural products can interfere with your HIV medication" or "I want to make sure what you are using is safe; even simple things like vitamins can hurt you if you take too much" can help elicit information and foster a partnership relationship. With increasing use of electronic medical records, this information can be included and tracked easily. It is important to ask in a nonjudgmental manner that allows the patient to feel comfortable with disclosure. Many patients may not be well-informed about the products they are using. It may be helpful to direct patients to the National Institutes of Health's Medline Plus website for free, easy-to-understand, evidence-based information about many herbal products.

NATURAL HEALTH PRODUCTS TO CONSIDER FOR USE IN HIV-INFECTED PATIENTS

NUTRITIONAL SUPPLEMENTATION

Micronutrients (vitamin and minerals) are important for human development, disease prevention, and well-being. They are not produced in the body and must be derived from the diet. Vitamins A, D, E, C, and B, as well as zinc, iron, and selenium, play an important role in immunity. The HIV-infected population has been found to have various micronutrient deficiencies that are prevalent before symptomatic disease and occur in patients who are ART-naïve and in those taking ART (Baum, 1995; Beach, 1992; Hepburn, 2004; Remacha, 2003a, b). Micronutrient supplementation has been shown to improve markers of HIV progression (CD4$^+$ T cell count and VL) and mortality in both early stages of HIV (Baum, 2013a, b) and late stages of disease (Filteau, 2015; Jiamton, 2003; Kaiser, 2006; Range, 2006), as well as in pregnant women (Fawzi, 2004). There are very limited and conflicting reports regarding whether micronutrient supplementation increases HIV shedding (Jiamto, 2004; McClelland, 2004; Sudfeld, 2014).

In a large randomized clinical trial of Botswanian HIV-infected (subtype C) ARV-naïve individuals with a CD4$^+$ T cell count greater than 350/μL, the effect of multivitamin (MVI; particularly B, C, and E vitamins) with selenium, MVI alone, and selenium alone was compared to placebo in delaying disease progression over 24 months. MVI alone and selenium alone were not statistically different from placebo. MVI plus selenium was found to significantly reduce the risk of reaching a CD4$^+$ T cell count of 250 μL or less and the risk of secondary events of combined outcomes for disease progression (CD4$^+$ T cell count <250/μL, AIDS-defining condition, or AIDS-related death) (Baum, 2013b).

The effects of MVI (vitamins A, B, C, and E) on the health status of HIV-positive pregnant women in Tanzania were studied. A double-blind, randomized controlled trial (RCT) found a significantly lower rate of progression to World Health Organization stage 4 AIDS and a significantly lower death rate in the MVI group compared to the placebo group. Multivitamins also resulted in significantly higher CD4$^+$ T cell counts and significantly lower levels of VL (Fawzi, 2004).

Zinc deficiency is common in HIV-infected adults and is independently associated with disease progression (Baum, 1997, 2003; Beach, 1992; Falutz, 1988; Graham, 1991; Jones, 2006). In a randomized, double-blind, placebo-controlled trial of 231 HIV-infected patients with low plasma zinc levels, zinc supplementation at 12–15 mg of elemental zinc for 18 months resulted in a fourfold decrease in the likelihood of immunological failure, defined as a decrease in CD4$^+$ T cell count to 200 cells/mm^3, compared to placebo. VL was not affected by zinc supplementation. Zinc supplementation also significantly reduced diarrhea compared with placebo. Respiratory diseases and HIV-related mortality were not affected by supplementation. Zinc testing and supplementation should be considered in HIV-infected populations with a high prevalence of zinc deficiency, such as drug users, children, MSM, and populations in developing countries (Baum, 2010).

Another single nutrient that has been studied in the HIV population is selenium. A randomized, double-blind, placebo-controlled trial of 300 HIV-infected individuals in Rwanda with $CD4^+$ T cell counts between 400 and 650 cells/μL demonstrated that selenium supplementation led to a decrease in the rate of $CD4^+$ T cell decline by 43.8% compared to placebo, which was determined to be a difference of approximately 40 cells at the end of 24 months (Kamwesiga, 2015). Another double-blind, randomized, placebo-controlled trial of selenium supplementation in HIV-infected patients showed selenium supplementation to be associated with favorable outcomes on VL and $CD4^+$ T cell count. Selenium responders whose serum level increased significantly had no change in VL compared to placebo and to nonresponders, whose VL increased. Similarly, $CD4^+$ T cell count increased in the selenium responder group by approximately 30 cells compared to a decrease in $CD4^+$ T cell count in the nonresponders and the placebo group (Hurwitz, 2007). HIV-infected pregnant women with selenium deficiency were noted to have eightfold higher risk for preterm delivery ($p = 0.03$) (Okunade, 2018). Selenium supplementation was found to have a significant effect on $CD4^+$ T cell decline and hospital admission rates in a randomized clinical trial of HIV-infected individuals (Burbano, 2002). A randomized trial of nutritional supplementation in ART naïve HIV-infected Botswanan patients demonstrated that Se supplementation, alone and with MVT, decreased the incidence of TB disease in this patient population (Campa, 2017). As already reviewed, Baum et al. found no effect of selenium alone on $CD4^+$ T cell count but did find an effect when it was combined with MVI (Baum, 2010). Selenium supplementation should be used with caution in primiparous women not receiving ART because at least one study has shown increased HIV-1 RNA detection in the breast milk of these women with selenium supplementation (Sudfeld, 2014).

Vitamin D deficiency (VDD) is common among HIV-infected patients but not necessarily more common than in the HIV-negative population. The estimates range widely from 10% to 88% (Sherwood, 2012; Zhang, 2017). The wide range of estimates is likely due to differences in demographics, location, climate/season, and definitions. Etiology of VDD in HIV-infected population is likely multifactorial and includes both traditional risk factors such as dietary deficiency, darker skin, obesity, chronic kidney disease, lack of sun exposure, and malabsorption as well as HIV-related factors and ART, especially regimens with efavirenz, which has been shown to interfere with vitamin D metabolism. Vitamin D plays an important role in osteoporosis, CVD, and the immune system (Eckard, 2014; Shivakoti, 2018). Some but not all data from RCTs in the general population demonstrate that vitamin D supplementation improves bone mineral density (BMD) and decreases fractures (Bischoff-Ferrari, 2005; Dawson-Hughes, 1997; Jackson, 2006). The degree to which VDD contributes to osteopenia and osteoporosis, CVD, and disease progression in the HIV population is unknown. The Endocrine Society recommends that at-risk persons be screened, including all persons receiving ART; the European AIDS Clinical Society recommends screening for VDD in persons with risk factors mentioned earlier or a history of low BMD and/or fracture or high risk for fracture (Holick, 2011; EACS online, 2017).

A recent trial demonstrated that for adolescents and young adults ($n = 214$) aged 16–24 years on a TDF-containing regimen, monthly vitamin D supplementation (50,000 IU) improved vitamin D levels and lumbar spine BMD regardless of baseline vitamin D status (Havens, 2017). Similarly, another study showed that high-dose vitamin D supplementation (120,000 IU/month) decreased bone turnover markers in HIV-infected youth ($n = 165$) on combination ART (c-ART) (Eckard, 2017). In adults 25–47 years of age, supplementation with high-dose vitamin D_3 (4,000 IU) and calcium carbonate (1,000 mg) with ART initiation (efavirenz [EFV], emtricitabine, and tenofovir [TDF]) increased 25-(OH)D levels and attenuated increases in bone turnover markers and bone loss at the hip and lumbar spine by approximately 50% at 48 weeks (Overton, 2015). It is unclear if these results can be extrapolated to non-EFV- and TDF-containing regimens.

VDD may also play a role in risk for tuberculosis (TB) in the HIV-infected population. In a diverse cohort of adults with advanced HIV infection in high-burden TB countries, VDD at ART initiation was found to be independently associated with increased risk of incident TB in next 96 weeks (Tenforde, 2017). Studies show mixed results regarding the role of VDD and CD4 cell count recovery; one trial of vitamin D supplementation in HIV children on c-ART did not show an effect on CD4 cell count (Ezeamama, 2016; Sudfeld, 2012; Kakalia, 2011).

Given the data in the general population that support the use of vitamin D and calcium supplementation to decrease risk of fractures and improve BMD and the increasing number of studies in HIV-infected population, especially those on EFV- and TDF-containing regimens that show improvement in BMD, it seems reasonable to screen high-risk, HIV-infected individuals and provide supplementation to minimize HIV-related complications of osteoporosis and potentially affect immune function and disease progression.

Obviously, macronutrient and micronutrient supplements are no replacement for proper diet. All patients should be counseled with general dietary recommendations that include adequate consumption of fruits, vegetables, whole grains, low-fat dairy products, and seafood and less consumption of foods high in sodium (salt), saturated fats, trans fats, cholesterol, added sugars, and refined grains. However, given the benefits of micronutrients on $CD4^+$ T cell counts and disease progression in a variety of HIV-infected groups, an MVI supplement that has key micronutrients (vitamins A, B, C, and E, selenium, and possibly zinc in certain populations) seems reasonable in all HIV-infected patients. Individuals on integrase strand transfer inhibitor (INSTI)-containing regimens should be counseled on the drug interactions between INSTIs and MVI and minerals and the risk of potential treatment failure. They should be advised to take MVI/minerals either 2 hours before or 6 hours after INSTIs. Vitamin D screening and supplementation should be considered in HIV-infected patients, particularly those who are on ART, which is known to adversely affect BMD.

TEA TREE OIL

Two studies suggest that tea tree oil, *Melaleuca alternifolia*, may be effective in some patients with refractory oral candidiasis. In one study, patients with AIDS and fluconazole-refractory oral candidiasis were treated with melaleuca oral solution. At the 4-week evaluation, 8 of 12 patients showed a response (2 cured and 6 improved), 4 were nonresponders, and 1 had deteriorated (Jandourek, 1998). In a prospective open-label trial of tea tree oil preparations in AIDS patients with fluconazole-refractory oropharyngeal *Candida albicans* infection, 60% of patients showed a clinical response, with 7 patients cured and 8 clinically improved (Vasquez, 2002).

FISH OILS

The HIV-infected population is at increased risk for CVD due to multifactorial reasons. Data show that CVD mortality for the HIV-infected population has increased significantly from 1999 to 2013 (Feinstein, 2016). The use of fish oils for cardioprotection is controversial, and there are to date no studies looking at omega-3 fatty acid use for CVD in HIV-infected population. In the general population, early trials suggested that omega-3 fatty acids offer cardioprotection, with a decrease in mortality to individuals at risk for CVD (Gruppo Italiano per Studio della Sopravivivenza nell'Infarcto miocadrico 1999; Burr, 1989). Later trials as well as several reviews were unable to corroborate these findings (Burr, 2003; Galan, 2010; Kromhout, 2010; ORIGIN Trial Investigators, 2008; Rauch, 2010; Rizos, 2012; Kimmig, 2013). Recent meta-analysis of randomized trials of omega-3 fatty acid supplements involving approximately 78,000 participants in 10 trials with history of coronary heart disease, stroke, or diabetes found no evidence that fish oils have cardioprotective effects (Aung, 2018). One possible explanation for why conflicting data from early and later trials may have to do with the aggressive medical and interventional management of CVD and other factors (Sethi, 2012; Lewis, 2013; Vlachopoulous, 2013; Galli, 2013).

In 2002, the American Heart Association (AHA) recommended that all patients with documented CVD consume 1 g of eicosapentaenoic acid (EPA) + docosahexaenoic acid (DHA) daily either as fish or supplement (Kris-Etherton, 2002). In light of the more recent trials, the AHA reviewed the existing evidence from RCTs and meta-analyses and issued a 2017 scientific advisory which stated that fish oil supplement in patients with recent myocardial infarction or with heart failure with reduced ejection fraction was reasonable for secondary prevention of CHD death, estimating a 9–10% reduction in cardiovascular mortality in these two patient groups (Siscovick, 2017). The difference in AHA advisory and recent meta-analyses conclusions may be due to differences in research method—the AHA looked at outcomes for specific indications rather than pooling of the data and also considered meta-analyses. Four large randomized trials of fish oil supplements are under way, looking at fish oil supplementation in healthy people for primary prevention, in patients with diabetes who do not have arterial disease, and in patients at high risk of CVD on statins with high triglycerides.

There is evidence that inflammation and oxidative stress are important in the pathogenesis of CVD. A randomized, parallel, placebo-controlled trial in Brazilian HIV-infected adults on ART did not show any effect of 3 g of fish oils on high-sensitivity c-reactive protein (hs-CRP), fibrinogen, factor VIII, interleukin-6 (IL6), IL1β, and tumor necrosis factor-α (TNF-α) (Oliveira, 2014). A randomized parallel controlled clinical trial of 70 Mexican HIV-infected adults given 2.4 g of omega-3 fatty acids or placebo did not show a reduction in markers for oxidative stress such as nitric oxide catabolites, lipoperoxides, and glutathione (Amador-Licona, 2016).

Omega-3 fatty acid supplementation has been studied for depression in the general population. The data are unclear as to whether they are helpful for depression due to mixed results. Some analyses have suggested that if omega-3s do have an effect, EPA may be more beneficial than DHA and that omega-3s may best be used in addition to antidepressant medication rather than in place of it (Grosso, 2016). A randomized placebo-controlled trial of 100 HIV patients assigned to either omega-3 fatty acid (720 mg EPA and 480 mg DHA) daily versus placebo showed a reduction of depressive scores within the omega-3 group over time and also in comparison with the placebo group ($P < 0.001$ for both). There were no significant adverse effects (Ravi, 2016).

Fish oils appear to be beneficial for the treatment of hypertriglyceridemia, although the data for modifying CVD risk are inconsistent and further trials are currently ongoing. Fish oils are also relatively safe and do not have significant drug interactions with ART. In 100 HIV-infected patients receiving ART with hypertriglyceridemia, fish oils at doses of approximately 6 g/d significantly reduced triglyceride concentrations. There was no significant effect of fish oils on CD4+ T cell counts or immune function or on lopinavir trough concentrations (Gerber, 2008). This result was confirmed in another RCT study of 48 HIV-infected patients on ART also receiving fenofibrate (Peters, 2012). Fish oils alone have also been shown to decrease triglyceride levels without adverse effects on immune parameters or antiretroviral pharmacokinetics (De Truchis, 2005). In a study of HIV-infected patients on c-ART with elevated fasting triglycerides, the use of 3 g of fish oils combined with diet counseling and exercise resulted in a decrease in triglyceride levels of 25% at 4 weeks versus a 2.8% increase in the control group (Wohl, 2005).

High doses greater than 3 g/d should be used with caution in patients with bleeding disorders or on anticoagulants. Unlike other supplements, fish oils are also available in prescription form as Lovaza (previously Omacor) for use in hypertriglyceridemia. It is reasonable that fish oils—either as supplements or as fatty fish twice a week (salmon, mackerel, herring, lake trout, sardines, and albacore tuna)—be considered in HIV-infected patients with hypertriglyceridemia and possibly those with CVD, especially if they are not medically optimized.

PROBIOTICS

Intestinal microbiota serves to preserve the intestinal barrier, provide resistance to pathogenic colonization, and stimulate the development of gut-associated lymphoid tissue (GALT). Gut microbiota is changed in HIV-infected people compared to the uninfected healthy population (Dillon, 2014; Dinh, 2015; Lozupone, 2013; Mutlu, 2014; Vujkovic-Cvijin, 2013); gut mucosal immunity is not completely restored with ART, leading to microbial translocation which may cause chronic inflammation and incomplete CD4+ T cell recovery. In simian immunodeficiency virus (SIV)-infected macaques treated with ART, probiotic and prebiotic supplementation resulted in enhanced gastrointestinal (GI) immune function, increased reconstitution of colonic CD4+ T cells, and reduced fibrosis of lymphoid follicles in the colon (Klatt, 2013). Recent trials with probiotics in HIV-infected individuals have shown interesting results. They have focused mainly on examining the effect of markers of coagulation (D-dimers), inflammation (IL6), TNF-α, hs-CRP, interferon-γ (IFN-γ), microbial translocation (lipopolysaccharide-binding protein (LBP), soluble CD14, and microbial composition. A few studies have also looked at their effects on CD4+ T cells. Prebiotics, which are nondigestible, selectively fermented carbohydrates that are thought to stimulate the growth and/or activity of gut microbiota, have also been studied in the HIV population.

In a double-blind, randomized, placebo-controlled study, dietary supplementation with a prebiotic mixture in 57 ART-naïve HIV-infected patients with mean CD4+ T cell count of approximately 500 resulted in improvement of gut microbiota composition, reduction of sCD14, CD4+ T cell activation (CD25), and improved natural killer (NK) cell activity (Gori, 2011). Stiksrud et al. demonstrated significantly reduced levels of D-dimer and increases in *Bifidobacteria* spp. and *Lactobacilli* spp. in 15 HIV-infected patients on ART (median CD4+ T cells approximately 350/mm³) treated with multistrain probiotics versus control and placebo groups. There was also a trend toward reduced levels of CRP ($p = 0.05$) and IL6 ($p = 0.06$) (Stiksrud, 2015). In a randomized, double-blind, placebo-controlled trial of 44 HIV-infected patients on stable ART regimen for at least 2 years and undetectable VL (CD4+ T cell were >400/mm³ in half of the participants and <350/mm³ in the other half), *Saccharomyces boulardii* at 6×10^7 yeasts per day for 12 weeks decreased LBP and IL6. The effect persisted for 3 months after treatment (Villar-Garcia, 2015). D'Ettorr et al. demonstrated that HIV-infected patients on ART for at least 3 years ($n = 20$; median CD4+ T cell count was 542) supplemented with probiotics had reduced markers of inflammation and microbial translocation as compared with controls ($n = 11$) (d'Ettorre, 2015). Serrano-Villar et al. also showed that a combination of several prebiotics and glutamine was associated with a beneficial effect on T cell activation in 35 varied HIV-infected individuals (12 viremic untreated with mean CD4+ = 558/mm³ and 23 on ART with varying CD4+ T cell ranging from 230/mm³ to 794/mm³ vs. 9 controls). The effect was more pronounced in the untreated HIV group (Serrano-Villar, 2017).

Several studies have also examined the effect of probiotics and immunonutrition on CD4+ T cell. Cahn et al. showed that a combination of prebiotics, omega-3/-6 fatty acids, bovine colostrum, and cysteine was associated with slower CD4+ T cell decline in ART-naïve, HIV-infected patients. Three hundred and forty patients were randomized but only 143 completed the study treatment. The baseline mean CD4+ T cell count was approximately 400/mm³; the baseline-corrected decline in CD4+ T cells in the treatment group was 28 ± 16 cells/μL compared to 68 ± 15 cells/μL in the control group at 52 weeks $P = 0.03$ (Cahn, 2013). In an open-label study of HIV-infected children in India, the probiotic supplement group showed a significant increase in CD4+ T cell counts compared to the control group ($p = 0.0022$) (Gautam, 2014). In a small trial of 20 patients randomized to probiotic, synbiotic (probiotic + prebiotic), prebiotic, or placebo groups, the synbiotic group was noted to have an increased CD4+ T cell count ($p = 0.05$) and a decreased level of IL6 ($p = 0.016$) (Gonzalez-Hernandez, 2012). In a larger study of 112 HIV-infected patients, the addition of probiotics to a micronutrient-fortified yogurt was well tolerated but was not associated with a further increase in CD4+ T cell count after 4 weeks (Hummelen, 2011). In an African study, probiotic yogurt consumption was reported to improve ability to work, reduce fever incidence, achieve daily nutrient requirements, and have overall lower impact of GI symptoms on routine activities (Irvine, 2011). In contrast to these studies, a recently published double-blind, randomized, placebo-controlled study did not show any improvement in CD4+ T cell and CD4/CD8 ratio recovery, markers of immune activation, inflammation, bacterial translocation, or gut microbiota composition in HIV-infected patients with CD4 counts of less than 350/μL initiating ART with the addition of a mixture consisting of prebiotics, probiotics, omega-3/-6 fatty acids, and amino acids (Serrano-Villar, 2018). Prior studies focused on either ART-naïve population or patients who were on stable ART regimens. It is possible that the effects of ART on immune reconstitution overshadowed any effects by the immunonutrition intervention.

The PROOV IT I and II pilot trials are studying whether probiotics can reduce inflammation and improve gut health in ART-naïve HIV-infected men who are initiating ART as well as in HIV-infected men who are on ART but with CD4+ T cell counts of less than 350/μL by measuring CD8 T cell immune activation, blood inflammatory markers, microbial translocation, blood and gut immunology and HIV levels, microbiota composition, diet, safety, and tolerability (Kim, 2016).

There are a small number of case reports describing bacteremia or fungemia attributed to probiotic administration, including one report of *Lactobacillus acidophilus* bacteremia in a patient with AIDS temporally related to excessive consumption of probiotic-enriched yogurt (Haghighat, 2015). However, this complication has not been reported in any clinical trials with probiotics.

Currently, probiotics cannot be recommended for HIV-infected patients; however, they deserve further investigation, particularly as immunomodulators.

INTERACTION OF NATURAL HEALTH PRODUCTS WITH ANTIRETROVIRAL AGENTS

Concurrent use of NHPs with ART is common among HIV-infected patients. Of all the CAM modalities, herbal supplements have the greatest potential for adverse effects in HIV-infected patients due to potential drug interactions. The following considerations add to the complexity and unpredictability of these interactions (MacDonald, 2009; Stolbach, 2015):

1. Many herbal remedies are complex products made of many different phytochemicals, some of which may not be fully characterized and standardized.

2. Some NHPs induce and inhibit gastrointestinal and hepatic enzymes simultaneously.

3. Many ART medications are substrates, inhibitors, or inducers of the drug-metabolizing enzymes (CYP family) and drug transporters (P-glycoprotein [P-gp]).

4. In vitro experiments may not predict in vivo effects due to various effects of intestinal enzymes, colonic microflora, and other factors.

5. Because of variations in extraction methods, constituents, and plant type and part, results from one study are not generalizable to other brands and formulation of NHPs.

For these reasons, it is difficult to state with absolute certainty that any NHP is free from the possibility of potential drug interactions. However, certain NHPs are known to interact with ART and should be avoided. Most ART drug interactions occur through the cytochrome P450 pathway and through drug transporters, which includes the P-gp efflux drug transporter. These transporters are expressed throughout the body and are increasingly studied for their role in ART drug interactions (Brooks, 2017). The major isoform responsible for protease inhibitor (PI) metabolism is CYP3A4; non-nucleoside reverse transcriptase inhibitors (NNRTIs) are metabolized by CYP3A4 and CYP2B6. PIs tend to inhibit CYP3A4, whereas most NNRTIs induce CYP3A4. Integrase strand transfer inhibitors (dolutegravir and raltegravir) neither induce nor inhibit CYP3A4. Also, PIs are substrates for P-gp, whereas NNRTIs usually are not. Exceptions to this include NRTIs and raltegravir. Raltegravir is primarily metabolized via glucuronidation. It is not an inducer, inhibitor, or substrate of CYPs; therefore, drug interactions with herbal medicines that affect CYPs are unlikely. However, the potential for drug interactions exists with any products that are uridine diphosphate glucuronosyltransferase (UGT) inducers. Any medications, supplements, or herbs that interfere with CYP, P-gp, and other transporters or with UGT have the potential to result in changes in concentration of HIV and non-HIV drugs. In addition, ART–herbal interactions are bidirectional, and ART may affect concentrations, efficacy, and side effects/adverse effects of herbal medicines (Ladenheim, 2008; Lamorde, 2012).

In addition to herbs and supplements, many plant chemicals, especially flavonoids and polyphenols, inhibit CYP3A4. For example, the flavonoids naringenin and furanocoumarin bergamottin, present in grapefruit, interact with CYP3A4. Clinical studies with grapefruit juice and PIs show an increase in saquinavir levels due to an increase in bioavailability but not indinavir or amprenavir (Lee, 2006). Many of the newer ARV agents have 80–100% oral bioavailability so grapefruit juice should not result in serious interactions (Brooks, 2017).

Some commonly used CAM products, such as cod liver oil and flax/flaxseed oil, have no known interactions with ART medications. Kava kava (*Piper methysticum*), black cohosh (*Cimicifuga racemose*), valerian (*Valeriana officinalis*), bitter orange (*Citrus aurantium*), saw palmetto (*Serenoa repens*), and Siberian ginseng (*Eleutheroccus senticosus*) have not been found to interact with CYP3A4. Therefore, it is unlikely that clinically significant pharmacokinetic interactions would

Table 14.1 GUIDE FOR NATURAL HEALTH PRODUCT–DRUG INTERACTION

LIKELY SAFE	USE CAUTION BASED ON IN VITRO AND CASE REPORTS	AVOID	ADJUST TIMING OF SUPPLEMENT
Cod liver oil	Ginseng[a]	Red yeast rice extract	Calcium carbonate in patients on INSTIs[b]
Flaxseed oil/flaxseed	Gingko	St. John's wort	Ferrous fumarate in patients on INSTIs[b]
Fish oils	Cat's claw	Cat's claw in patients on PIs and NNRTIs	MVI in patients on INSTIs[b]
Vitamin C	Goldenseal	Garlic	Other minerals: magnesium, zinc, copper, chromium, selenium[b]
Aloe vera	Evening primrose oil		
	African potato		
	Milk thistle[a]		
	Echinacea[a]		
	Piperine		

[a]Data showing safety with specific ART

[b]separate INSTI from mineral supplement by 2 hours before or 6 hours after.

INSTI, integrase strand transfer inhibitor; NNRTI, non-nucleoside reverse transcriptase inhibitor; PI, protease inhibitor; MVI, multivitamin.

occur with PIs or NNRTIs, but they may affect other ART (Lee, 2006).

Many CAM products have the potential to interact with ART. These are briefly described here and summarized in Table 14.1.

- Red yeast rice extract (RYRE) is sometimes used by patients to lower cholesterol. It is made by fermenting a type of yeast called *Monascus purpureus* over red rice. RYRE contains several compounds known as monacolins, which block the production of cholesterol. One of these, monacolin K, has the same structure as the drugs lovastatin and mevinolin (Ma, 2000). Lovastatin is exclusively metabolized by CYP3A4 and is contraindicated in patients taking PIs. Red yeast rice was marketed in the United States as the dietary supplement Cholestin. The US Food and Drug Administration (FDA) banned it in 1998. However, RYREs are still available, and some of them still contain lovastatin. Patients should be cautioned to avoid RYRE if on PIs or statins.

- St. John's wort or *Hypericum perforatum* is a herbal product used for depression. St. John's wort is known to be an inducer of CYP3A4 and P-gp, and it also contains constituents that can affect other CYPs, including CYP2D6. It has been shown to alter levels of nevirapine, rilpivirine, and indinavir (de Maat, 2001; Hafner, 2010; Piscitelli, 2000). St. John's wort should be avoided by patients on ART.

- Echinacea is commonly used for viral infections and immunologic boosting. The two major forms, *Echinacea angustifolia* and *E. purpurea*, affect CYP3A4 activity. *E. purpurea* has been shown to induce CYP3A4 metabolism of darunavir but without effect on overall darunavir and ritonavir pharmacokinetics (Molto, 2011). Echinacea was also not found to affect etravirine concentrations (Molto, 2012b) or the pharmacokinetics of lopinavir/ritonavir (LPV/RTV) (Penzak, 2010). The potential for drug interactions with other ART still exists.

- Garlic is often taken to prevent heart disease, high cholesterol, and high blood pressure and also to boost the immune system. Garlic may induce intestinal CYP3A4 or P-gp (Berginc, 2010). In one study, garlic markedly reduced the concentration of saquinavir, although the results suggested that it affected the bioavailability of saquinavir rather than its systemic clearance (Piscitelli, 2002a). In single-dose pharmacokinetic (PK) studies garlic extract did not affect the area under the curve (AUC) or C_{max} of ritonavir or saquinavir (Gallicano, 2003; Jacek, 2004). Garlic should be avoided by patients on ART.

- Silybins, the active component of milk thistle, inhibits CYP3A4 and P-gp activity in vitro; however, milk thistle has not been shown to significantly affect darunavir–ritonavir concentrations in one study (Molto, 2012a) or indinavir pharmacokinetics in three separate PK studies (DiCenzo, 2003; Mills, 2005; Piscitelli, 2002b).

- Ginseng may induce CYP3A4 activity in the liver and GI tract. Two multidose PK studies showed no effect of ginseng on ef/RTV or indinavir levels (Calderón, 2014; Andrade, 2008). One case of an HIV-infected patient on RAL + LPV/r therapy who developed liver failure after starting ginseng has been reported (Mateo-Carrasco, 2012).

- *Ginkgo biloba* was not found to significantly alter raltegravir or LPV/RTV pharmacokinetics in healthy volunteers (Blonk, 2012; Robertson, 2008), but it was reported in two patients to potentially affect the efficacy of efavirenz (Naccarato, 2012; Wiegman, 2009).

- Based on a case report, cat's claw (*Uncaria tomentos*), which is used for a wide variety of ailments including inflammatory and infectious diseases, may increase with atazanavir, ritonavir, and saquinavir levels due to CYP3A4 inhibition (Lopez Galera, 2008).

- Goldenseal (*Hydrastis canadensis*) has potent CYP3A4 inhibition properties but was not shown to affect indinavir levels in one study (Sandhu, 2003). Patients taking goldenseal should be monitored for increased toxicity of CYP3A4 substrate drugs.

- Fish oil in combination with LPV/RTV showed no significant decrease in ART level (Gerber, 2008).

- Vitamin C decreased the AUC of indinavir by 15% and its C_{max} by 23% in healthy volunteers. However, another study in healthy individuals found no difference in CYP3A4 activity (Slain, 2005; van Heeswijk, 2005; Jalloh, 2017).

- Two popular African herbs, African potato (*Hypoxis hermerocallidea*) and cancer bush (*Lessertia frutescens*), have been shown to inhibit CY3A4 and P-gp in vitro (Awortwe, 2014). African potato (*H. hemerocallide, Hypoxoside obtuse*) was studied in two PK studies and was found to have no significant effect on AUC or C_{max} with efavirenz and lopinavir/ritonavir (Mogatle, 2008; Gwaza, 2013).

- Evening primrose (*Oenothera biennis*) inhibits CYP3A4 and CYP2D6, and there is one case report of evening primrose increasing LPV levels (Beukel, 2008).

- Calcium carbonate and ferrous fumarate significantly decrease serum levels of dolutegravir; chelation is suspected as the mechanism (Song, 2015). Patients on INSTI-based regimens taking calcium, magnesium, iron, zinc, copper, chromium, or selenium should be educated on this interaction and counseled on separating INSTI from supplement by 2 hours before or 6 hours after calcium or iron supplement (Brooks, 2017).

- MVI decreased dolutegravir levels in healthy volunteers (Patel, 2011).

- Black pepper (*Piper nigrum*) contains the active alkaloid piperine, which is often combined with turmeric to increase absorption. It has been shown to inhibit CYP3A4, P-gp, and UGT isoforms. Nevirapine levels increased significantly in individuals receiving 20 mg/d piperine. Piperine may induce and/or inhibit other ART (Kasibhatta, 2007).

Table 14.2 INTERNET RESOURCES FOR NATURAL HEALTH PRODUCTS INFORMATION AND NATURAL HEALTH PRODUCT–DRUG INTERACTIONS

RESOURCE	WEBSITE
Natural Medicines	http://www.naturalmedicines.therapeuticresearch.com
National Center for Complementary and Integrative Health	https://nccih.nih.gov/health/herbsataglance.htm
HIV–Drug Interaction	http://www.hiv-druginteractions.org
National Institutes of Health, Office of Dietary Supplements Dietary Supplement Label Database	http://www.dsld.nlm.nih.gov/dsld/index.jsp
National Institutes of Health, Office of Dietary Supplements	https://ods.od.nih.gov
National Institutes of Health, MedlinePlus Herbs and Supplements Directory	https://nlm.nih.gov/medlineplus/druginfo/herb_All.html
ConsumerLab	http://www.consumerlab.com

Lack of high-quality studies in humans and lack of standardization of herbal formulations, among other factors, limit our knowledge on ART and herbal interactions. Other than a few herbal products such as St. John's wort, there is no simple guide to which NHP and ARV combinations clearly have significant clinical interactions. In vitro testing may be helpful for identifying products to screen, but it is limited in its clinical extrapolation. Therefore, caution is advised, and consultation with a pharmacist regarding any NHP and ARV interaction is warranted. Resources for information on natural health products for both clinicians and patients are listed in Table 14.2. Particularly useful for clinicians is the Natural Medicines Database website (formerly known as Natural Standard and Natural Medicine Comprehensive Database), which has an extensive database on herbal medicines with in-depth information as well as a drug interaction checker. The database is available through subscription and is usually also available through most academic libraries; it is available as an app for smartphones. ART–herbal interactions can also be checked at http://www.hiv-druginteractions.org. The NCCIH also has concise evidence-based information on common herbs and links for information on herb–drug interactions.

HERBAL MEDICINES FOR HIV TREATMENT

In a meta-analysis of 12 RCTs involving 881 patients with AIDS, traditional Chinese medicine (TCM) interventions were associated with significantly reduced plasma VL compared with placebo ($p = 0.04$). Patients receiving TCM interventions had significantly higher CD4$^+$ T lymphocyte counts compared with those on placebo ($p = 0.002$). In addition, TCM interventions were significantly more likely to result in improved clinical symptoms ($p < 0.00001$). TCM interventions conferred a similar risk of adverse events compared with control interventions ($p = 0.29$). However, the reductions in plasma VL significantly favored conventional Western medical therapy alone over integrated traditional Chinese and Western medical therapy ($p = 0.004$) (Deng, 2014).

MIND–BODY APPROACHES

Mind and body practices include a large and diverse group of procedures or techniques typically administered by trained practitioners or teachers rather than by physicians. They include yoga, chiropractic and osteopathic manipulation, meditation, massage therapy, acupuncture, relaxation techniques (e.g., breathing exercises, guided imagery, and progressive muscle relaxation), tai chi, gi qong, healing touch, and hypnotherapy. Central to these modalities is the elicitation of the relaxation response.

RELAXATION RESPONSE

The relaxation response can be described as a state of deep rest that changes the short- and long-term physical and emotional responses to stress (e.g., decreases in heart rate, blood pressure, rate of breathing, and muscle tension)—it is the opposite of the fight-or-flight response (Benson, 1974). Preliminary studies suggest that this response can affect gene expression and telomere length. One study of 52 healthy people—26 novices and 26 long-term practitioners (yoga/meditation)—showed that one session of relaxation-response practice was enough to enhance the expression of genes involved in energy metabolism and insulin secretion and reduce the expression of genes linked to inflammatory response and stress (Bhasin, 2013). Nobel Laureate Elizabeth Blackburn showed that shortened telomere length and reduced telomerase activity are associated with premature mortality and predict a variety of health risks and diseases (Epel, 2004). She also demonstrated that family dementia caregivers (a typically chronically stressed population) who practiced 12 minutes of daily yogic meditation for 8 weeks had a 43% increase in telomerase activity compared to 3.7% in the passive relaxation group, suggesting an improvement in stress-induced aging (Lavretsky, 2013). A recent analysis of 18 studies of gene expression changes induced by meditation and other mind-body practices found that these practices were associated with a downregulation of the nuclear factor κ-B pathway, which is a key pathway associated with stress. Nuclear factor κ-B pathway translates stress into inflammation by changing the expression of genes which code for inflammatory cytokines. Lower activity of this pathway suggests potential reduction in inflammation (Buric, 2017).

STRESS, DEPRESSION, AND HIV PROGRESSION

HIV infection presents many stresses and challenges—mental, emotional, and physical—that vary from time of diagnosis to coping with adherence and medication-related side effects, aging issues, and dealing with the loss of infected loved ones. Not surprisingly, individuals who are HIV-infected have a higher incidence of depression and anxiety than the uninfected population (Pence, 2006; Whetten, 2008). Psychosocial variables and stress can affect measurable factors such as CD4+ T cell counts and VLs in a variety of ways, including drug adherence, immune function, and health behaviors.

Stress has been shown in prospective human observational studies, animal studies, and laboratory experiments to be associated with depression, CVD, and progression of HIV/AIDS. This effect is generally thought to be mediated by negative affective states such as anxiety and depression, behavioral patterns (adherence, substance abuse, etc.), and stress-elicited endocrine responses mediated by the hypothalamic–pituitary–adrenocortical axis and the sympathetic–adrenal–medullary system (Cohen, 2007). In HIV-infected populations, some studies have shown that stress may be associated with reductions in NK cell and cytotoxic T lymphocyte phenotypes (Leserman, 1997; Evans, 1995).

Results from studies prior to 2000 were inconsistent with respect to the effect of stress and depression on HIV progression. However, several studies after 2000 have suggested a link between stress and HIV progression (Leserman, 2008). Among 96 asymptomatic, HIV-infected gay men not on antiretroviral medication at baseline who were followed every 6 months for up to 9 years, each additional moderately severe stress event increased risk of progression to AIDS by 50% and of developing an AIDS-related clinical condition by 2.5-fold after controlling for demographics, baseline CD4+ T cells and VL, and antiretroviral medications (Leserman, 2002). In a study of 177 HIV-infected men and women, baseline depression and hopelessness predicted slope of CD4+ T cells and VL. High cumulative depression and avoidant coping were associated with approximately twice the rate of CD4+ T cell decline and greater increases in VL (Ironson, 2005).

MEDITATIVE PRACTICES

Meditation is a practice of concentrated focus on a sound, object, visualization, the breath, movement, or attention itself in order to increase awareness of the present moment, reduce stress, promote relaxation, and enhance personal and spiritual growth. Recently the American Heart Association issued a scientific statement on meditation and CVD risk reduction stating that, overall, studies on meditation suggest a possible benefit on cardiovascular risk and that meditation may be considered as adjunctive therapy for cardiovascular risk reduction (Levine, 2017). Examples include mantra meditation and mindfulness meditation. Yoga, tai chi, and chi gong are forms of breath-coordinated movement meditations.

YOGA

Yoga is often practiced for wellness and stress reduction. It has been shown to affect health behaviors. In one large analysis of approximately 35,000 US adults, yoga users reported high rates of health behavior outcomes such as motivation to exercise (~60%), eat healthier (~40%), cut back or stop drinking alcohol (12%), and cut back or stop smoking cigarettes (25%). More than 80% perceived reduced stress as a result of practicing yoga (Stussman, 2015).

Well-designed studies of yoga in the HIV-infected population are lacking. One prospective controlled study of yoga in HIV-infected adults with CVD risk factors showed that 20 weeks of supervised yoga was effective in significantly reducing resting systolic and diastolic blood pressure by an average of 5/3 mm Hg—reductions similar to those achieved with the Dietary Approaches to Stop Hypertension (DASH) diet. Studies suggest that a 10-mm reduction in systolic blood pressure and a 5-mm Hg reduction in diastolic blood pressure predict a 40–50% lower risk of death from coronary artery disease (CAD). Extrapolating from these data in HIV-uninfected adults, yoga intervention would theoretically translate into a decreased risk of death from CAD by 20–25% in HIV-infected patients. Yoga did not affect body weight, fat mass, proatherogenic lipids, glucose tolerance, or immune or virologic status (Cade, 2010).

A 1-month yoga program was found to improve depression, anxiety, and CD4+ T cell counts in 22 HIV-infected individuals on ART compared to 22 HIV-infected controls (Naoroibam, 2016). Mantra meditation (repetition of a word or phrase) was found to be effective in reducing anger, improving QOL, and improving spiritual well-being in a randomized controlled study of HIV-infected adults (Bormann, 2006).

MINDFULNESS-BASED STRESS REDUCTION

Mindfulness-based stress reduction (MBSR) is a technique that uses cultivation of nonjudgmental awareness in the present moment. It is usually taught as an 8-week structured program. MBSR has been shown to decrease the side effects of ART and alleviate symptoms. In one randomized wait-list controlled study of 76 HIV-infected patients with ART-related side effects, MBSR was found to significantly reduce frequency of symptoms and distress related to symptoms (Duncan, 2012). In another RCT of 117 HIV-infected patients, MBSR was found to result in a reduction in avoidance, higher positive affect, and improvement in depression at 6 months (Gayner, 2012). A recent trial in 72 HIV-infected youth aged 14–22 years showed significantly higher levels of mindfulness, problem-solving coping, and life satisfaction as well as lower aggression, and participants were more likely to have or to maintain reductions in HIV VL at 3 months (Webb, 2018).

Few studies have examined the effect of MBSR on $CD4^+$ T cell count. One small randomized controlled short-term study of a diverse group of HIV-infected patients suggested that MBSR could buffer $CD4^+$ T cell decline (Creswell, 2009). In a later RCT of 40 long-term diagnosed and treated HIV-infected patients, mindfulness-based cognitive therapy (which combined elements of MBSR and CBT) patients were found to have decreased stress, anxiety, and depression and also a significantly increased $CD4^+$ T cell count at week 20 compared to placebo ($p < 0.001$), with no change in VL (Gonzalez-Garcia, 2014). In contrast, a recent RCT of MBSR in HIV-infected individuals with $CD4^+$ of greater than 350/ μL not on c-ART, did not show benefit of MBSR with respect to $CD4^+$ T cell counts, CRP, IL-6, VL, or d-dimer (Hecht, 2018).

TAI CHI

In a small study of 38 HIV-infected patients randomized to tai chi, exercise, and control groups, both tai chi and exercise were found to improve physiologic parameters, functional outcomes, and QOL. These patients were also noted to have improved social interactions (Galantino, 2005).

In a large group of 252 HIV-infected patients, those randomized to three 10-week stress management approaches—cognitive–behavioral relaxation training, focused tai chi training, and spiritual growth—were compared to a wait-listed control group. Both the cognitive–behavioral relaxation and tai chi groups used less emotion-focused coping and had augmented lymphocyte proliferative function. Moreover, the tai chi group had an increase in QOL related mainly to an increase in emotional well-being (McCain, 2008).

Meditative practices can increase QOL; reduce stress, anxiety, and depression; and affect health-related behaviors. These practices have not been shown to have harmful side effects, and they should be considered for interested patients with stress, depression, anxiety, and adverse health behaviors. These practices may also be considered for patients who are unwilling to utilize psychological counseling, support, or cognitive–behavioral therapy. Many meditative practices are available. Which one is best depends on patient preference, which may be influenced by cultural factors, convenience, and finances. The practice most likely to be effective is the one that the patient is most likely to do.

ACUPUNCTURE

Pain is a frequently reported symptom in persons living with HIV/AIDS (Vogl, 1999). Pain may be secondary to peripheral neuropathy or to musculoskeletal issues. Results from a number of studies suggest that acupuncture may help with chronic pain syndromes related to low back pain, neck pain, and osteoarthritis/knee pain (Hinman, 2014; Linde, 2009; Manheimer, 2010; Vickers, 2012; Witt, 2006). Acupuncture may also help reduce the frequency of tension headaches and prevent migraine headaches. Clinical practice guidelines issued by the American Pain Society and the American College of Physicians in 2007 recommend acupuncture as one of several nonpharmacologic approaches that physicians should consider when patients with chronic low back pain do not respond to practices such as remaining active, applying heat, and taking pain-relieving medications (Chou, 2007).

Few studies have examined the effect of acupuncture in HIV-infected patients. A large multicenter, modified double-blind, randomized, placebo-controlled study comparing acupuncture and sham acupuncture for symptomatic treatment of HIV-related neuropathy revealed a modest decrease in average pain scores in both groups but no significant improvement with acupuncture (Shlay, 1998). In another small study of 23 HIV-infected participants with sleep disturbances at least three times per week, patients received acupuncture two evening a week for 5 weeks. Both sleep time and sleep quality were reported as improved (Phillips, 2001).

Although studies of acupuncture in HIV-infected patients are limited, it seems reasonable to consider acupuncture in patients with musculoskeletal pain and perhaps those with sleep disturbances, especially in those who are either reluctant to take or intolerant of conventional medications.

EXERCISE

Substantial evidence indicates that regular physical activity contributes to the primary and secondary prevention of several chronic diseases, such as CVD, osteoporosis, and diabetes, and is associated with a reduced risk of premature death (Warburton, 2006). Moreover, studies have shown that in HIV-infected patients, exercise can improve strength, endurance, time to fatigue, and body composition; increase QOL and sense of well-being; mitigate excessive bone loss; and decrease depression and anxiety (Dudgeon, 2004; MacArthur, 1993; Rigsby, 1992; Stringer, 1998; Perazzo, 2018). Given the increased risk of CVD, muscle wasting, and bone disease, it makes sense that some form of physical activity be encouraged for capable HIV-infected patients. Physicians have an important role in educating and encouraging exercise as a measure for well-being and disease prevention.

MANUAL THERAPIES

Manual CAM therapies include massage, shiatsu, reiki, therapeutic touch, acupressure, and chiropractic manipulation. Manual modalities are often used by patients for their purported effects of increasing circulation, pain alleviation, relaxation, and stimulation of immune function (Power, 2002). One small RCT showed that massage therapy combined with stress management resulted in a decrease in medical care usage and an increase in health perceptions in HIV-infected individuals (Birk, 2000). A Cochrane review of massage in HIV-infected patients showed that there appears to be a positive effect on the QOL of affected individuals, particularly when massage is combined with other interventions such as meditation and stress management (Hillier, 2010).

TRADITIONAL MEDICINE

It is beyond the scope of this chapter to review the major traditional medical systems of India, China, and Africa. These systems are broad and complex, and they often combine different therapeutic modalities discussed previously in this chapter, such as a combination of herbal remedies and mind–body practices. Reasons for the use of these traditional systems in the HIV-infected population stem from cultural beliefs, economic considerations, and limited accessibility to ART. Data from well-designed clinical trials regarding efficacy and safety of these systems are sparse.

Traditional Indian medicine consisting of Ayurveda, Unani medicine, Siddha medicine, homeopathy, and naturopathy is used by two-thirds of the Indian population—especially in rural areas—for both primary care needs and HIV. One review found only four RCTs evaluating traditional Indian medicine; the trials had significant methodological flaws (Fritts, 2008).

Similarly, in Africa, a large portion of the population uses herbs for primary health care, HIV/AIDS, and HIV-related health problems (Calitz, 2014). Although there is increasing study of herbal medicines and their potential for drug interactions in vitro, clinical trials are lacking.

TCM has probably been the most studied of the traditional systems, with data showing potential efficacy of TCM herbs for HIV and HIV-associated conditions. Mind–body approaches such as tai chi and acupuncture have also shown benefit for a varieties of health issues; however, many of these studies were performed on the non–HIV-infected population. Many of these were reviewed previously in this chapter.

Given that these systems play such a central role in healthcare delivery in their respective countries and that there are usually many more traditional health practitioners than allopathic practitioners, collaboration and cooperation among traditional and allopathic practitioners seems indicated. However, conflicts often arise between the two. Allopathic physicians frequently regard traditional medicines and practices as untested, possibly unsafe, and likely ineffective. Traditional practitioners, on the other hand, do not necessarily see the need or benefit of rigorously testing their time-honored practices; some also believe that Western-trained physicians misunderstand traditional medical practice because they continue to view it through the scientific lens of biomedicine. Nevertheless, strides toward some form of partnership are being made in these countries. In Africa, many traditional practitioners have been educated and trained on HIV/AIDS transmission and prevention and have served effectively as community educators (Bodeker, 2006).

To date, no data exist to support the use of these systems as primary treatment for HIV. Some data exist on efficacy, especially of TCM on end points such as CD4+ T cells and VL; however, they have been inferior to ART. There may be a role for these systems in the management of symptoms, HIV-associated conditions, and delaying of HIV progression in those not on ART, but more data are needed with respect to their efficacy and herb–drug interactions.

Other aspects of traditional medical systems excluding herbal medicines, such as spiritual and healing practices and attitudes toward sickness and death (provided they do not harm), should be acknowledged and respected by physicians.

SUMMARY

Complementary, integrative, and alternative modalities are widely used by HIV-infected patients. True alternative medicine for HIV is rare in developed countries but widespread in resource-limited areas. Physicians caring for HIV-infected individuals need to be aware of the prevalence of complementary therapies among their patients, the potential for herb–drug interactions, and the potential toxicities of herbal medicines.

Physicians can also play an important role in fostering partnerships with their patients who use CAM modalities by the use of nonjudgmental and open communication about their benefits and risks. Some natural health products, such as fish oils and MVI, should be considered for use in HIV-infected individuals. Strategies to delay HIV progression using micronutrients, probiotics, and traditional natural products in HIV-infected populations with high CD4+ T cell counts deserve further research, particularly in resource-limited settings in which access to ART is limited. Many mind–body techniques are useful for reducing stress, anxiety, and depression—all of which may affect HIV disease progression. These techniques may be especially useful in patients with adverse health behaviors who are unwilling to undergo formal therapy. They should also be considered in resource-limited settings as a self-empowering, low-cost means of coping with the emotional and physical challenges associated with HIV.

Treatment of HIV remains complex and multifactorial. Complementary and integrative modalities with low potential for adverse effects, such as mind–body techniques and certain natural products, should be considered in the balanced approach to dealing with the multidimensional aspects of HIV disease. The use of such practices will likely increase in the future. Therefore, it behooves physicians caring for these patients to understand the range of available options, their potential interactions with standard therapeutic regimens, and the ongoing data regarding their potential efficacy and safety.

RECOMMENDED READING

Abbasi J. Another nail in the coffin for fish oil supplements. *JAMA*. 2018;319(18):1851–1852.

Jiménez-Nácher I, Alvarez E, Morello J, et al. Approaches for understanding and predicting drug interactions in human immunodeficiency virus-infected patients. *Exp Opin Drug Metabol Toxicol*. 2011;7(4):457–477.

REFERENCES

Agnoletto V, Chiaffarino F, Nasta P, et al. Reasons for complementary therapies and characteristics of users among HIV-infected people. *Int J STD AIDS.* 2003;14(7):482–486. doi: 10.1258/095646203322025803.

Agnoletto V, Chiaffarino F, Nasta P, et al. Use of complementary and alternative medicine in HIV-infected subjects. *Complement Therapies Med.* 2006;14(3):193–199.

Amador-Licona N, Díaz-Murillo TA, Gabriel-Ortiz G, et al. Omega 3 fatty acids supplementation and oxidative stress in HIV-seropositive patients. A clinical trial. *PLoS One.* 2016;11(3):e0151637.

Andrade AS, Hendrix C, Parsons TL, et al. Pharmacokinetic and metabolic effects of American ginseng (*Panax quinquefolius*) in healthy volunteers receiving the HIV protease inhibitor indinavir. *BMC Complement Altern Med.* 2008;8:50-6882-8-50. doi: 10.1186/1472-6882-8-50.

Aung T, Halsey J, Kromhout D, et al. Associations of omega-3 fatty acid supplement use with cardiovascular disease risks: meta-analysis of 10 trials involving 77 917 individuals. *JAMA Cardiol.* 2018;3(3):225–234.

Awortwe C, Bouic PJ, Masimirembwa CM, et al. Inhibition of major drug metabolizing CYPs by common herbal medicines used by HIV/AIDS patients in Africa—Implications for herb-drug interactions. *Drug Metabol Lett.* 2014;7(2):83–95. doi: DML-EPUB-58874.

Bahall M. Prevalence, patterns, and perceived value of complementary and alternative medicine among HIV patients: a descriptive study. *BMC Complement Altern Med.* 2017;17(1):422.

Baum MK, Campa A, Lai S, et al. Zinc status in human immunodeficiency virus type 1 infection and illicit drug use. *Clin Infect Dis.* 2013a;37(Suppl. 2):s117–S123. doi: CID30489

Baum MK, Campa A, Lai S, et al. Effect of micronutrient supplementation on disease progression in asymptomatic, antiretroviral-naive, HIV-infected adults in Botswana: a randomized clinical trial. *JAMA.* 2013b;310(20):2154–2163.

Baum MK, Lai S, Sales S, et al. Randomized, controlled clinical trial of zinc supplementation to prevent immunological failure in HIV-infected adults. *Clin Infect Dis.* 2010;50(12):1653–1660. doi: 10.1086/652864

Baum MK, Shor-Posner G, Lu Y, et al. Micronutrients and HIV-1 disease progression. *AIDS.* 1995;9(9):1051–1056.

Baum MK, Shor-Posner G, Lai S, et al. High risk of HIV-related mortality is associated with selenium deficiency. *JAIDS.* 1997;15(5):370–374.

Beach RS, Mantero-Atienza E, Shor-Posner G, et al. Specific nutrient abnormalities in asymptomatic HIV-1 infection. *AIDS.* 1992;6(7):701–708.

Benson H, Beary JF, Carol MP. The relaxation response. *Psychiatry.* 1974;37(1):37–46.

Berginc K, Trdan T, Trontelj J, et al. HIV protease inhibitors: garlic supplements and first-pass intestinal metabolism impact on the therapeutic efficacy. *Biopharmaceut Drug Disposition.* 2010;31(8–9):495–505.

Beukel van den Bout-van den CJ, Bosch ME, Burger DM, et al. Toxic lopinavir concentrations in an HIV-1 infected patient taking herbal medications. *AIDS (London).* 2008;22(10):1243–1244. doi: 10.1097/QAD.0b013e32830261f4.

Bhasin MK, Dusek JA, Chang B, et al. Relaxation response induces temporal transcriptome changes in energy metabolism, insulin secretion and inflammatory pathways. *PLoS ONE.* 2013;8(5):e62817. doi: 10.1371/journal.pone.0062817.

Birk TJ, McGrady A, MacArthur RD, et al. The effects of massage therapy alone and in combination with other complementary therapies on immune system measures and quality of life in human immunodeficiency virus. *J Altern Complement Med.* 2000;6(5):405–414.

Bischoff-Ferrari HA, Willett WC, Wong, JB, et al. Fracture prevention with vitamin D supplementation: a meta-analysis of randomized controlled trials. *JAMA.* 2005;293(18):2257–2264.

Blonk M, Colbers A, Poirters A, et al. Effect of ginkgo biloba on the pharmacokinetics of raltegravir in healthy volunteers. *Antimicrob Agents Chemotherapy.* 2012;56(10):5070–5075. doi: 10.1128/AAC.00672–12.

Bodeker G, Carter G, Burford G, et al. HIV/AIDS: traditional systems of health care in the management of a global epidemic. *J Altern Complement Med.* 2006;12(6):563–576.

Bormann JE, Gifford AL, Shively M, et al. Effects of spiritual mantram repetition on HIV outcomes: a randomized controlled trial. *J Behavior Med.* 2006;29(4):359–376.

Brooks KM, George JM, Kumar P. Drug interactions in HIV treatment: complementary & alternative medicines and over-the-counter products. *Exp Rev Clin Pharmacol.* 2017;10(1):59–79.

Burbano X, Miguez-Bubano MJ, McCollister K, et al. Impact of a selenium chemoprevention trial on hospital admissions of HIV-infected participants. *HIV Clin Trials.* 2002;3(6):483–491.

Buric I, Farias M, Jong J, Mee C, Brazil IA. What is the molecular signature of mind–body interventions? A systematic review of gene expression changes induced by meditation and related practices. *Front Immunol.* 2017;8:670.

Burr ML, Ashfield-Watt PAL, Dunstan FDJ, et al. Lack of benefit of dietary advice to men with angina: results of a controlled trial. *Eur J Clin Nutrit.* 2003;57(2):193–200.

Burr ML, Fehily AM, Gilbert JF, et al. Effects of changes in fat, fish, and fibre intakes on death and myocardial reinfarction: diet and reinfarction trial (DART). *Lancet (London, England).* 1989;2(8666):757–761. doi: s0140-6736(89)90828-3.

Cade W, Reeds DN, Mondy KE, et al. Yoga lifestyle intervention reduces blood pressure in HIV-infected adults with cardiovascular disease risk factors. *HIV Med.* 2010;11(6):379–388.

Cahn P, Ruxrungtham K, Gazzard B, et al. The immunomodulatory nutritional intervention NR100157 reduced CD4 T cell decline and immune activation: a 1-year multicenter randomized controlled double-blind trial in HIV-infected persons not receiving antiretroviral therapy (the BITE study). *Clin Infect Dis.* 2013;57(1):139–146.

Calderón MM, Chairez CL, Gordon LA, et al. Influence of panax ginseng on the steady state pharmacokinetic profile of Lopinavir–Ritonavir in healthy volunteers. *Pharmacotherapy.* 2014;34(11):1151–1158.

Calitz C, Steenekamp JH, Steyn JD, et al. Impact of traditional African medicine on drug metabolism and transport. *Exp Opin Drug Metabol Toxicol.* 2014;10(7):991–1003.

Campa A, Baum MK, Bussmann H, et al. The effect of micronutrient supplementation on active TB incidence early in HIV infection in Botswana. *Nutrition Dietary Suppl.* 2017;2017(9):37.

Chou R, Qaseem A, Snow V, et al. Diagnosis and treatment of low back pain: a joint clinical practice guideline from the American College of Physicians and the American Pain Society. *Ann Inter Med.* 2007;147(7):478–491.

Cohen S, Janicki-Deverts D, Miller GE. Psychological stress and disease. *JAMA.* 2007;298(14):1685–1687.

Creswell JD, Myers HF, Cole SW, et al. Mindfulness meditation training effects on CD4+ T cell T lymphocytes in HIV-1 infected adults: a small randomized controlled trial. *Brain, Behavior, Immunity.* 2009;23(2):184–188.

Dawson-Hughes B, Harris SS, Krall EA, Dallal GE. Effect of calcium and vitamin D supplementation on bone density in men and women 65 years of age or older. *N Engl J Med.* 1997;337(10):670–676.

de Maat MM, Hoetelmans RM, Mathôt RA, et al. Drug interaction between St. John's wort and nevirapine. *AIDS.* 2001;15(3):420–421.

d'Ettorre G, Ceccarelli G, Giustini N, et al. Probiotics reduce inflammation in antiretroviral treated, HIV-infected individuals: results of the "Probio-HIV" clinical trial. *PLoS One.* 2015;10(9):e0137200.

De Truchis P, Kirstetter M, Perier A, et al. Treatment of hypertriglyceridemia in HIV-infected patients under HAART, by (n-3) polyunsaturated fatty acids: a double-blind randomized prospective trial in 122 patients [Abstract 39]. Paper presented at the 12th Conference on Retroviruses and Opportunistic Infections, Boston, February 22–25, 2005.

Deng X, Jiang M, Zhao X, et al. Efficacy and safety of traditional Chinese medicine for the treatment of acquired immunodeficiency syndrome: a systematic review. *J Tradit Chin Med.* 2014;34(1):1–9.

Dhalla S, Chan KJ, Montaner JS, et al. Complementary and alternative medicine use in British Columbia: a survey of HIV positive people on antiretroviral therapy. *Complement Therapies Clin Pract.* 2006;12(4):242–248.

DiCenzo R, Shelton M, Jordan K, et al. Coadministration of milk thistle and indinavir in healthy subjects. *Pharmacotherapy.* 2003;23(7):866–870.

Dillon S, Lee E, Kotter C, et al. An altered intestinal mucosal microbiome in HIV-1 infection is associated with mucosal and systemic immune activation and endotoxemia. *Mucosal Immunol.* 2014;7(4):983–994.

Dinh DM, Volpe GE, Duffalo C, et al. Intestinal microbiota, microbial translocation, and systemic inflammation in chronic HIV infection. *J Infect Dis.* 2015;211(1):19–27. doi: 10.1093/infdis/jiu409.

Dudgeon WD, Phillips KD, Bopp CM, et al. Physiological and psychological effects of exercise interventions in HIV disease. *AIDS Patient Care STD.* 2004;18(2):81–98.

Duggan J, Peterson WS, Schutz M, et al. Use of complementary and alternative therapies in HIV-infected patients. *AIDS Patient Care STD.* 2001;15(3):159–167.

Duncan LG, Moskowitz JT, Neilands TB, et al. Mindfulness-based stress reduction for HIV treatment side effects: a randomized, wait-list controlled trial. *J Pain Sympt Mgmt.* 2012;43(2):161–171.

Eckard AR, McComsey GA. Vitamin D deficiency and altered bone mineral metabolism in HIV-infected individuals. *Curr HIV/AIDS Rep,* 2014;11(3):263–270.

Eckard AR, O'Riordan MA, Rosebush JC, et al. Effects of vitamin D supplementation on bone mineral density and bone markers in HIV-infected youth. *JAIDS.* 2017;76(5):539–546.

Epel ES, Blackburn EH, Lin J, et al. Accelerated telomere shortening in response to life stress. *Proc Natl Acad Sci U S A.* 2004;101(49):17312–17315. doi: 0407162101.

European AIDS Clinical Society (EACS) Guidelines 2017. http://www.eacsociety.org/files/2017_guidelines-9.1-english.pdf.

Evans DL, Leserman J, Perkins DO, et al. Stress-associated reductions in cytotoxic T lymphocytes and natural killer cells in asymptomatic HIV infection. *Am J Psychiatry.* 1995;152(4):543–550.

Ezeamama AE, Guwatudde D, Wang M, et al. Vitamin-D deficiency impairs CD4 T cell count recovery rate in HIV-positive adults on highly active antiretroviral therapy: a longitudinal study. *Clin Nutr.* 2016;35(5):1110–1117.

Falutz J, Tsoukas C, Gold P. Zinc as a cofactor in human immunodeficiency virus-induced immunosuppression. *JAMA.* 1988;259(19):2850–2851.

Fawzi WW, Msamanga GI, Spiegelman D, et al. A randomized trial of multivitamin supplements and HIV disease progression and mortality. *N Engl J Med.* 2004;351(1):23–32.

Feinstein MJ, Bahiru E, Achenbach C, et al. Patterns of cardiovascular mortality for HIV-infected adults in the united states: 1999–2013. *Am J Cardiol.* 2016;117(2):214–220.

Filteau S, PrayGod G, Kasonka L, et al.; NUSTART (Nutritional Support for Africans Starting Antiretroviral Therapy) Study Team (2015). Effects on mortality of a nutritional intervention for malnourished HIV-infected adults referred for antiretroviral therapy: a randomised controlled trial. *BMC Med.* 2015;13, 17-014-0253-8. doi: 10.1186/s12916-014-0253-8.

Fritts M, Crawford CC, Quibell D, et al. Traditional Indian medicine and homeopathy for HIV/AIDS: a review of the literature. *AIDS Res Therapy.* 2008;5, 25-6405-5-25. doi: 10.1186/1742-6405-5-25.

Galan P, Kesse-Guyot E, Czernichow S, et al. Effects of B vitamins and omega 3 fatty acids on cardiovascular diseases: a randomised placebo controlled trial. *BMJ (Clin Res Ed.).* 2010;341:c6273. doi: 10.1136/bmj.c6273

Galantino ML, Shepard K, Krafft L, et al. The effect of group aerobic exercise and t'ai chi on functional outcomes and quality of life for persons living with acquired immunodeficiency syndrome. *J Altern Complement Med.* 2005;11(6):1085–1092.

Galli C, Brenna JH. Omega-3 fatty acid supplementation and cardiovascular disease events [Letter to the Editor]. *JAMA.* 2013;309(1):27.

Gallicano K, Foster B, Choudhri S. Effect of short-term administration of garlic supplements on single-dose ritonavir pharmacokinetics in healthy volunteers. *Br J Clin Pharmacol.* 2003;55(2):199–202. doi:epdf/10.1592/phco.23.7.866.32723

Gautam N, Dayal R, Agarwal D, et al. Role of multivitamins, micronutrients and probiotics supplementation in management of HIV infected children. *Indian J Pediatr.* 2014;81(12):1315–1320.

Gayner B, Esplen MJ, DeRoche P, et al. A randomized controlled trial of mindfulness-based stress reduction to manage affective symptoms and improve quality of life in gay men living with HIV. *J Behav Med.* 2012;35(3):272–285.

Gerber JG, Kitch DW, Fichtenbaum CJ, et al. Fish oil and fenofibrate for the treatment of hypertriglyceridemia in HIV-infected subjects on antiretroviral therapy: results of ACTG A5186. *J AIDS* 2008;47(4):459–466. doi: 10.1097/QAI.0b013e31815bace2

Gonzalez-Garcia M, Ferrer MJ, Borras X, et al. Effectiveness of mindfulness-based cognitive therapy on the quality of life, emotional status, and CD4+ T cell count of patients aging with HIV infection. *AIDS Behav.* 2014;18(4):676–685.

González-Hernández LA, Jave-Suarez LF, Fafutis-Morris, M, et al. Synbiotic therapy decreases microbial translocation and inflammation and improves immunological status in HIV-infected patients: a double-blind randomized controlled pilot trial. *Nutr J.* 2012;11, 90.

Gori A, Rizzardini G, Van't Land B, et al. Specific prebiotics modulate gut microbiota and immune activation in HAART-naïve HIV-infected adults: results of the "COPA" pilot randomized trial. *Nature.* 2011;4(5):554–563.

Graham NM, Sorensen D, Odaka N, et al. Relationship of serum copper and zinc levels to HIV-1 seropositivity and progression to AIDS. *J AIDS.* 1991;4(10):976–980.

Greene KB, Berger J, Reeves C, et al. Most frequently used alternative and complementary therapies and activities by participants in the AMCOA study. *J Assoc Nurses AIDS Care.* 1999;10(3):60–73.

Grosso G, Micek A, Marventano S, et al. Dietary n-3 PUFA, fish consumption and depression: a systematic review and meta-analysis of observational studies. *J Affective Dis.* 2016;205:269–281.

Gruppo italiano per lo studio della sopravvivenza nell'infarto miocardico. (1999) Dietary supplementation with n-3 polyunsaturated fatty acids and vitamin E after myocardial infarction: results of the GISSI-prevenzione trial. *Lancet (London, England).* 1999;354(9177):447–455. doi: s0140673699070725.

Gwaza L, Aweeka F, Greenblatt R, et al. Co-administration of a commonly used Zimbabwean herbal treatment (African potato) does not alter the pharmacokinetics of lopinavir/ritonavir. *Intl J Infect Dis.* 2013;17(10):e857–e861.

Hafner V, Jager M, Matthee AK, et al. Effect of simultaneous induction and inhibition of CYP3A by St John's Wort and ritonavir on CYP3A activity. *Clin Pharmacol Therap.* 2010;8(2):191–196.

Haghighat L, Crum-Cianflone NF. (2015, June 30). The potential risks of probiotics among HIV-infected persons: bacteraemia due to lactobacillus acidophilus and review of the literature. *Intl J STD AIDS.* June 30, 2015. doi: 0956462415590725

Halpin SN, Carruth EC, Rai RP, et al. Complementary and alternative medicine among persons living with HIV in the era of combined antiretroviral treatment. *AIDS Behav.* 2018;22(3):848–852.

Havens PL, Stephensen CB, Van Loan MD, et al. Vitamin D3 supplementation increases spine bone mineral density in adolescents and young adults with human immunodeficiency virus infection being treated with tenofovir disoproxil fumarate: a randomized, placebo-controlled trial. *Clin Infect Dis.* 2017;66(2):220–228.

Hecht FM, Moskowitz JT, Moran P, et al. A randomized, controlled trial of mindfulness-based stress reduction in HIV infection. *Brain Behav Immunity.* 2018. doi: s0889-1591(18)30190-9.

Hepburn MJ, Dyal, K Runser LA, et al. Low serum vitamin B$_{12}$ levels in an outpatient HIV-infected population. *Int J STD AIDS.* 2004;15(2):127–133. doi: 10.1258/095646204322764334.

Hillier SL, Louw Q, Morris L, et al. Massage therapy for people with HIV/AIDS. *Cochrane Library.* 2010;1:CD007502

Hinman RS, McCrory P, Pirotta M, et al. Acupuncture for chronic knee pain: a randomized clinical trial. *JAMA.* 2014;312(13):1313–1322.

Holick MF, Binkley NC, Bischoff-Ferrari HA, et al. Evaluation, treatment, and prevention of vitamin D deficiency: an endocrine society clinical practice guideline. *J Clin Endocrinol Metabol.* 2011;96(7):1911–1930.

Hummelen R, Hemsworth J, Changalucha J, et al. Effect of micronutrient and probiotic fortified yogurt on immune-function of anti-retroviral therapy naive HIV patients. *Nutrients.* 2011;3(10):897–909.

Hurwitz BE, Klaus JR, Llabre MM, et al. Suppression of human immunodeficiency virus type 1 viral load with selenium supplementation: a randomized controlled trial. *Arch Intern Med.* 2007;167(2):148–154.

Ironson G, O'Cleirigh C, Fletcher MA, et al. Psychosocial factors predict CD4+ T cell and viral load change in men and women with human immunodeficiency virus in the era of highly active antiretroviral treatment. *Psychosomatic Med.* 2005;67(6):1013–1021. doi: 67/6/1013

Irvine SL, Hummelen R, Hekmat S. Probiotic yogurt consumption may improve gastrointestinal symptoms, productivity, and nutritional intake of people living with human immunodeficiency virus in Mwanza, Tanzania. *Nutrition Res.* 2011;31(12):875–881.

Jacek H, Rentsch KM, Steinert HC, et al. No effect of garlic extract on saquinavir kinetics and hepatic CYP3A4 function measured by the erythromycin breath test. *Clin Pharmacol Therap.* 2004;75(2):P80–P80. doi: 10.1016/j.clpt.2003.11.304.

Jackson RD, LaCroix AZ, Gass M, et al. Calcium plus vitamin D supplementation and the risk of fractures. *N Engl J Med.* 2006;354(7):669–683.

Jalloh MA, Gregory PJ, Hein D, et al. Dietary supplement interactions with antiretrovirals: a systematic review. *Int J STD AIDS.* 2017;28(1):4–15. doi: 10.1177/0956462416671087.

Jandourek A, Vaishampayan JK, Vazquez JA. Efficacy of melaleuca oral solution for the treatment of fluconazole refractory oral candidiasis in AIDS patients. *AIDS.* 1998;12(9):1033–1037.

Jiamto S, Chaisilwattana P, Pepin J. A randomized placebo-controlled trial of the impact of multiple micronutrient supplementation on HIV-1 genital shedding among Thai subjects (vol 37, pg 1216. 2004). *J AIDS.* 2004;38(2):240–240.

Jiamton S, Pepin J, Suttent R, et al. A randomized trial of the impact of multiple micronutrient supplementation on mortality among HIV-infected individuals living in Bangkok. *AIDS.* 2003;17(17):2461–2469.

Jones CY, Tang AM, Forrester JE, et al. Micronutrient levels and HIV disease status in HIV-infected patients on highly active antiretroviral therapy in the nutrition for healthy living cohort. *J AIDS.* 2006;43(4):475–482. doi: 10.1097/01.qai.0000243096.27029.fe.

Josephs J, Fleishman J, Gaist P, et al. Use of complementary and alternative medicines among a multistate, multisite cohort of people living with HIV/AIDS. *HIV Med.* 2007;8(5):300–305.

Kakalia S, Sochett EB, Stephens D, et al. Vitamin D supplementation and CD4 count in children infected with human immunodeficiency virus. *J Pediatrics.* 2011;159(6):951–957.

Kaiser JD, Campa AM, Ondercin JP, et al. Micronutrient supplementation increases CD4+ T cell count in HIV-infected individuals on highly active antiretroviral therapy: a prospective, double-blinded, placebo-controlled trial. *J AIDS.* 2006;42(5):523–528. doi: 10.1097/01.qai.0000230529.25083.42.

Kamwesiga J, Mutabazi V, Kayumba J, et al. Effect of selenium supplementation on CD4+ T cell recovery, viral suppression and morbidity of HIV-infected patients in Rwanda: a randomized controlled trial. *AIDS (London).* 2015;29(9):1045–1052. doi: 10.1097/QAD.0000000000000673.

Kasibhatta R, Naidu M. Influence of piperine on the pharmacokinetics of nevirapine under fasting conditions. *Drugs Res Dev.* 2007;8(6):383–391.

Kelso-Chichetto NE, Okafor CN, Harman JS, et al. Complementary and alternative medicine use for HIV management in the state of Florida: medical monitoring project. *J Altern Complement Med.* 2016;22(11):880–886.

Kim CJ, Walmsley SL, Raboud JM, et al. Can probiotics reduce inflammation and enhance gut immune health in people living with HIV: study designs for the probiotic visbiome for inflammation and translocation (PROOV IT) pilot trials. *HIV Clin Trials.* 2016;17(4):147–157.

Kimmig LM, Karalis DG. Do omega-3 polyunsaturated fatty acids prevent cardiovascular disease? A review of the randomized clinical trials. *Lipid Insights.* 2013;6:13.

Klatt NR, Canary LA, Sun X, et al. Probiotic/prebiotic supplementation of antiretrovirals improves gastrointestinal immunity in SIV-infected macaques. *J Clin Invest.* 2013;123(2):903–907. doi: 10.1172/JCI66227

Kris-Etherton PM, Harris WS, Appel LJ, American Heart Association Nutrition Committee (2002). Fish consumption, fish oil, omega-3 fatty acids, and cardiovascular disease. *Circulation.* 2002;106(21):2747–2757.

Kromhout D, Giltay EJ, Geleijnse JM. n-3 fatty acids and cardiovascular events after myocardial infarction. *N Engl J Med.* 2010;363(21):2015–2026.

Ladenheim D, Horn O, Werneke U, et al. Potential health risks of complementary alternative medicines in HIV patients. *HIV Med.* 2008;9(8):653–659.

Lamorde M, Byakika-Kibwika P, Merry C. Pharmacokinetic interactions between antiretroviral drugs and herbal medicines. *Br J Hosp Med.* 2012;73(3):132–136.

Lavretsky H, Epel E, Siddarth P, et al. A pilot study of yogic meditation for family dementia caregivers with depressive symptoms: effects on mental health, cognition, and telomerase activity. *Intl J Geriat Psychiatry.* 2013;28(1):57–65.

Lee LS, Andrade AS, Flexner C. Interactions between natural health products and antiretroviral drugs: pharmacokinetic and pharmacodynamic effects. *Clin Infect Dis.* 2006;43(8):1052–1059. doi: CID39658.

Leserman J. Role of depression, stress, and trauma in HIV disease progression. *Psychosomatic Med.* 2008;70(5):539–545. doi: 10.1097/PSY.0b013e3181777a5f.

Leserman J, Petitto J, Gu H, et al. Progression to AIDS, a clinical AIDS condition and mortality: psychosocial and physiological predictors. *Psychological Med.* 2002;32(06):1059–1073.

Leserman J, Petitto JM, Perkins DO, et al. Severe stress, depressive symptoms, and changes in lymphocyte subsets in human immunodeficiency virus-infected men: a 2-year follow-up study. *Arch Gen Psychiatry.* 1997;54(3):279–285.

Levine GN, Lange RA, Bairey-Merz CN, et al. Meditation and cardiovascular risk reduction: a scientific statement from the American Heart Association. *J Am Heart Assoc.* 2017;6(10):e002218.

Lewis E. Omega-3 fatty acid supplementation and cardiovascular disease events [Letter to the Editor]. *JAMA.* 2013;309(1):27.

Linde K, Allais G, Brinkhaus B, et al. Acupuncture for tension-type headache. *Cochrane Database Syst Rev.* 2009;1:CD007587.

Littlewood RA, Vanable PA. Complementary and alternative medicine use among HIV-positive people: research synthesis and implications for HIV care. *AIDS Care.* 2008;20(8):1002–1018.

Littlewood RA, Vanable PA. A global perspective on complementary and alternative medicine use among people living with HIV/AIDS in the era of antiretroviral treatment. *Curr HIV/AIDS Rep.* 2011;8(4):257–268.

Littlewood RA, Vanable PA. The relationship between CAM use and adherence to antiretroviral therapies among persons living with HIV. *Health Psychology.* 2014;33(7):660.

Liu C, Yang Y, Gange SJ, et al. Disclosure of complementary and alternative medicine use to health care providers among HIV-infected women. *AIDS Patient Care STDs.* 2009;23(11):965–971.

London AS, Foote-Ardah CE, Fleishman JA, et al. Use of alternative therapists among people in care for HIV in the united states. *Am J Public Health.* 2003;93(6):980–987.

Lopez Galera RL, Pascuet ER, Mur JE, et al. Interaction between cat's claw and protease inhibitors atazanavir, ritonavir and saquinavir. *Eur J Clin Pharmacol.* 2008;64(12):1235–1236.

Lorenc A, Robinson N. A review of the use of complementary and alternative medicine and HIV: issues for patient care. *AIDS Patient Care STDs.* 2013;27(9):503–510.

Lozupone CA, Li M, Campbell TB, et al. Alterations in the gut microbiota associated with HIV-1 infection. *Cell Host Microbe.* 2013;14(3):329–339.

Ma J, Li Y, Ye Q, et al. Constituents of red yeast rice, a traditional Chinese food and medicine. *J Agricultural Food Chemistry.* 2000;48(11):5220–5225.

MacArthur RD, Levine SD, Birk TJ. Supervised exercise training improves cardiopulmonary fitness in HIV-infected persons. *Med Science Sports Exercise*. 1993;25(6):684–688.

MacDonald L, Murty M, Foster BC. Antiviral drug disposition and natural health products: risk of therapeutic alteration and resistance. *Expert Opin Drug Metab Toxicol*. 2009;5(6):563–578. doi: 10.1517/17425250902942302.

Manheimer E, Cheng K, Linde K, et al. Acupuncture for peripheral joint osteoarthritis. *Cochrane Database Syst Rev*. 2010;1:CD001977.

Mateo-Carrasco H, Gálvez-Contreras MC, Fernández-Ginés FD, Nguyen TV. Elevated liver enzymes resulting from an interaction between raltegravir and panax ginseng: a case report and brief review. *Drug Metabol Drug Interact*. 2012;27(3):171–175

McCain NL, Gray DP, Elswick Jr R, et al. A randomized clinical trial of alternative stress management interventions in persons with HIV infection. *J Consult Clin Psychology*. 2008;76(3):431.

McClelland RS, Baeten JM, Overbaugh J, et al. Micronutrient supplementation increases genital tract shedding of HIV-1 in women: results of a randomized trial. *J AIDS*. 2004;37(5):1657–1663.

Milan FB, Arnsten JH, Klein RS, et al. Use of complementary and alternative medicine in inner-city persons with or at risk for HIV infection. *AIDS Patient Care STDs*. 2008;22(10):811–816.

Mills E, Wilson K, Clarke M, et al. Milk thistle and indinavir: a randomized controlled pharmacokinetics study and meta-analysis. *Eur J Clin Pharmacol*. 2005;61(1):1–7.

Mogatle S, Skinner M, Mills E, Kanfer I. Effect of African potato (Hypoxis hemerocallidea) on the pharmacokinetics of efavirenz. *S Afr Med J*. 2008;98(12):945–949.

Molto J, Valle M, Miranda C, et al. Herb–drug interaction between echinacea purpurea and darunavir–ritonavir in HIV-infected patients. *Antimicrob Agents Chemother*. 2011;55(1):326–330. doi: 10.1128/AAC.01082-10.

Molto J, Valle M, Miranda C, et al. Effect of milk thistle on the pharmacokinetics of darunavir–ritonavir in HIV-infected patients. *Antimicrob Agents Chemother*. 2012a;56(6):2837–2841. doi: 10.1128/AAC.00025-12.

Molto J, Valle M, Miranda C, et al. Herb–drug interaction between echinacea purpurea and etravirine in HIV-infected patients. *Antimicrob Agents Chemother*. 2012b;56(10):5328–5331. doi: 10.1128/AAC.01205-12.

Mutlu EA, Keshavarzian A, Losurdo J, et al. A compositional look at the human gastrointestinal microbiome and immune activation parameters in HIV infected subjects. *PLoS Pathog*. 2014;10(2):e1003829.

Naccarato M, Yoong D, Gough K. A potential drug–herbal interaction between ginkgo biloba and efavirenz. *J Intl Assoc Physic AIDS Care (Chicago)*. 2012;11(2):98–100. doi: 10.1177/1545109711435364.

Naoroibam R, Metri KG, Bhargav H, et al. Effect of integrated yoga (IY) on psychological states and CD4 counts of HIV-1 infected patients: a randomized controlled pilot study. *Intl J Yoga*. 2016;9(1):57–61. doi: 10.4103/0973-6131.171723.

National Center for Complementary and Integrative Health. *What Is Complementary and Alternative Medicine?* https://nccih.nih.gov/health/integrative-health 2018.

Okunade KS, Olowoselu OF, Osanyin GE, et al. Selenium deficiency and pregnancy outcome in pregnant women with HIV in Lagos, Nigeria. *Int J Gynecol Obstet*. 2018;142(2):207–213.

Oliveira JM, Rondó PH, Yudkin JS, et al. Effects of fish oil on lipid profile and other metabolic outcomes in HIV-infected patients on antiretroviral therapy: a randomized placebo-controlled trial. *Int J STD AIDS*. 2014;25(2):96–104.

ORIGIN Trial Investigators. Rationale, design, and baseline characteristics for a large international trial of cardiovascular disease prevention in people with dysglycemia: the ORIGIN trial (Outcome Reduction with an Initial Glargine Intervention). *Am Heart J*. 2008;155(1):26.e1–e26.e13.

Overton ET, Chan ES, Brown TT, et al. Vitamin D and calcium attenuate bone loss with antiretroviral therapy initiation: a randomized trial. *Ann Internal Med*. 2015;162(12):815–824.

Owen-Smith A, Diclemente R, Wingood G. Complementary and alternative medicine use decreases adherence to HAART in HIV-positive women. *AIDS Care*. 2007;19(5):589–593.

Patel P, Song I, Borland J, et al. Pharmacokinetics of the HIV integrase inhibitor S/GSK1349572 co-administered with acid-reducing agents and multivitamins in healthy volunteers. *J Antimicrob Chemother*. 2011;66(7):1567–1572. doi: 10.1093/jac/dkr139.

Patel SJ, Kemper KJ, Kitzmiller JP. Physician perspectives on education, training, and implementation of complementary and alternative medicine. Adv *Med Educ Pract*. 2017;8:499.

Perazzo JD, Webel AR, Alam SK, et al. Relationships between physical activity and bone density in people living with HIV: results from the SATURN-HIV study. *J Assoc Nurses AIDS Care*. 2018;29(4):528–537.

Pence BW, Miller WC, Whetten K, et al. Prevalence of DSM-IV-defined mood, anxiety, and substance use disorders in an HIV clinic in the southeastern United States. *J AIDS*. 2006;42(3):298–306. doi: 10.1097/01.qai.0000219773.82055.aa.

Penzak SR, Robertson SM, Hunt JD, et al. Echinacea purpurea significantly induces cytochrome P450 3A activity but does not alter lopinavir–ritonavir exposure in healthy subjects. *Pharmacotherapy*. 2010;30(8):797–805. doi: 10.1592/phco.30.8.797.

Peters BS, Wierzbicki AS, Moyle G, et al. The effect of a 12-week course of omega-3 polyunsaturated fatty acids on lipid parameters in hypertriglyceridemic adult HIV-infected patients undergoing HAART: a randomized, placebo-controlled pilot trial. *Clin Therapeut*. 2012;34(1):67–76.

Phillips KD, Skelton WD. Effects of individualized acupuncture on sleep quality in HIV disease. *J Assoc Nurses AIDS Care*. 2001;12(1):27–39.

Piscitelli SC, Burstein AH, Chaitt D, et al. Indinavir concentrations and St. John's wort. *Lancet*. 2000;355(9203):547–548.

Piscitelli SC, Burstein AH, Welden N, et al. The effect of garlic supplements on the pharmacokinetics of saquinavir. *Clin Infect Dis*. 2002a;34(2):234–238. doi: CID010586.

Piscitelli SC, Formentini E, Burstein AH, et al. Effect of milk thistle on the pharmacokinetics of indinavir in healthy volunteers. *Pharmacotherapy*. 2002b;22(5):551–556.

Power R, Gore-Felton C, Vosvick M, et al. HIV: effectiveness of complementary and alternative medicine. *Primary Care*. 2002;29(2):361–378.

Range N, Changalucha J, Krarup H, et al. The effect of multi-vitamin/mineral supplementation on mortality during treatment of pulmonary tuberculosis: a randomised two-by-two factorial trial in Mwanza, Tanzania. *Br J Nutrition*. 2006;95(4):762–770.

Rauch B, Schiele R, Schneider S, et al. OMEGA, a randomized, placebo-controlled trial to test the effect of highly purified omega-3 fatty acids on top of modern guideline-adjusted therapy after myocardial infarction. *Circulation*. 2010;122(21):2152–2159. doi: 10.1161/CIRCULATIONAHA.110.948562.

Ravi S, Khalili H, Abbasian L, et al. Effect of omega-3 fatty acids on depressive symptoms in HIV-positive individuals: a randomized, placebo-controlled clinical trial. *Ann Pharmacotherapy*. 2016;50(10):797–807.

Remacha AF, Cadafalch J, Sarda P, et al. Vitamin B-12 metabolism in HIV-infected patients in the age of highly antiretroviral therapy: role of homocysteine in assessing vitamin B-12 status. *Am J Clin Nutr*. 2003;77(2):420–424.

Rigsby LW, Dishman R, Jackson AW, et al. Effects of exercise training on men seropositive for the human immunodeficiency virus-1. *Med Sci Sports Exercise*. 1992;24(1):6–12.

Rizos EC, Ntzani EE, Bika E, et al. Association between omega-3 fatty acids supplementation and risk of major cardiovascular disease events. *JAMA*. 2012;308(10):1024–1033.

Robertson SM, Davey RT, Voell J, et al. Effect of ginkgo biloba extract on lopinavir, midazolam and fexofenadine pharmacokinetics in healthy subjects. *Curr Med Res Opin*. 2008;24(2):591–599. doi: 10.1185/030079908X260871.

Sandhu RS, Prescilla RP, Simonelli TM, et al. Influence of goldenseal root on the pharmacokinetics of indinavir. *J Clin Pharmacol*. 2003;43(11):1283–1288.

Saper RB, Phillips RS, Sehgal A, et al. Lead, mercury, and arsenic in US- and Indian-manufactured Ayurvedic medicines sold via the Internet. *JAMA*. 2008;300(8):915–923.

Serrano-Villar S, Vázquez-Castellanos J, Vallejo A, et al. The effects of prebiotics on microbial dysbiosis, butyrate production and immunity in HIV-infected subjects. *Mucosal Immunol*. 2017;10(5):1279.

Serrano-Villar S, de Lagarde M, Vázquez-Castellanos J, et al. Effects of immunonutrition in advanced HIV disease: a randomized placebo controlled clinical trial (promaltia study). *Clin Infect Dis*.2018;XX(XX):1–11.

Sethi A, Singh M, Arora R. Omega-3 fatty acid supplementation and cardiovascular disease events [Letter to the Editor]. *JAMA*. 2013;309(1):27.

Shere-Wolfe KD, Tilburt JC, D'Adamo C, et al. Infectious diseases physicians' attitudes and practices related to complementary and integrative medicine: results of a national survey. *Evidence-Based Complement Altern Med*. 2013:article ID 294381.

Sherwood JE, Mesner OC, Weintrob AC, et al. Vitamin D deficiency and its association with low bone mineral density, HIV-related factors, hospitalization, and death in a predominantly black HIV-infected cohort. *Clin Infect Dis*. 2012;55(12):1727–1736.

Shivakoti R, Ewald ER, Gupte N, et al. Effect of baseline micronutrient and inflammation status on CD4 recovery post-cART initiation in the multinational PEARLS trial. *Clin Nutr*. 2018.

Shlay JC, Chaloner K, Max MB, et al. Acupuncture and amitriptyline for pain due to HIV-related peripheral neuropathy: a randomized controlled trial. *JAMA*. 1998;280(18):1590–1595.

Siscovick DS, Barringer TA, Fretts AM, et al. Omega-3 polyunsaturated fatty acid (fish oil) supplementation and the prevention of clinical cardiovascular disease. *Circulation*. 2017;135(15):e867–e884.

Slain D, Amsden JR, Khakoo RA, et al. Effect of high-dose vitamin C on the steady-state pharmacokinetics of the protease inhibitor indinavir in healthy volunteers. *Pharmacotherapy*. 2005;25(2):165–170.

Song I, Borland J, Arya N, et al. Pharmacokinetics of dolutegravir when administered with mineral supplements in healthy adult subjects. *J Clin Pharmacol*. 2015;55(5):490–496. doi: 10.1002/jcph.439.

Standish L, Greene K, Bain S, et al. Alternative medicine use in HIV-positive men and women: demographics, utilization patterns and health status. *AIDS Care*. 2001;13(2):197–208.

Stiksrud B, Nowak P, Nwosu FC, et al. Reduced levels of D-dimer and changes in gut microbiota composition after probiotic intervention in HIV-infected individuals on stable ART. *J AIDS*. 2015;70(4):329–337. doi: 10.1097/QAI.0000000000000784.

Stolbach A, Paziana K, Heverling H, et al. A review of the toxicity of HIV medications II: interactions with drugs and complementary and alternative medicine products. *J Med Toxicol*. 2015;11(3):326–341.

Stringer WW, Berezovskaya M, O'Brien WA, et al. The effect of exercise training on aerobic fitness, immune indices, and quality of life in HIV patients. *Med Sci Sports Exercise*. 1998;30(1):11–16.

Stussman BJ, Black LI, Barnes PM, et al. Wellness-related use of common complementary health approaches among adults: United States. 2015. *Natl Health Stat Rep*. 2015;85:1–12.

Sudfeld CR, Wang M, Aboud S, et al. Vitamin D and HIV progression among Tanzanian adults initiating antiretroviral therapy. *PloS One*. 2012;7(6):e40036.

Sudfeld CR, Aboud S, Kupka R, et al. Effect of selenium supplementation on HIV-1 RNA detection in breast milk of Tanzanian women. *Nutrition*. 2014;30(9):1081–1084.

Tenforde MW, Yadav A, Dowdy DW, et al. Vitamin A and D deficiencies associated with incident tuberculosis in HIV-infected patients initiating antiretroviral therapy in multinational case-cohort study. *JAIDS*. 2017;75(3):e71–e79.

Thompson MA, Aberg JA, Hoy JF, et al. Antiretroviral treatment of adult HIV infection: 2012 recommendations of the International Antiviral Society–USA panel. *JAMA*. 2012;308(4):387–402.

Ting A, Chow Y, Tan W. Microbial and heavy metal contamination in commonly consumed traditional Chinese herbal medicines. *J Trad Chinese Med*. 2013;33(1):119–124.

van Heeswijk RP, Cooper CL, Foster BC, et al. Effect of high-dose vitamin C on hepatic cytochrome P450 3A4 activity. *Pharmacotherapy*. 2005;25(12):1725–1728.

Vasquez JA, Zawawi, AA. Efficacy of alcohol-based and alcohol-free melaleuca oral solution for the treatment of fluconazole-refractory oropharyngeal candidiasis in patients with AIDS. *HIV Clin Trials*. 2002;3(5):379–385.

Vickers AJ, Cronin AM, Maschino AC, et al. Acupuncture for chronic pain: individual patient data meta-analysis. *Arch Internal Med*. 2012;172(19):1444–1453.

Villar-Garcia, J, Hernandez JJ, Guerri-Fernandez R, et al. Effect of probiotics (*Saccharomyces boulardii*) on microbial translocation and inflammation in HIV-treated patients: a double-blind, randomized, placebo-controlled trial. *J AIDS*. 2015;68(3):256–263. doi: 10.1097/QAI.0000000000000468.

Visser RD, Grierson J. Use of alternative therapies by people living with HIV/AIDS in Australia. *AIDS Care*. 2002;14(5):599–606.

Vlachopoulos C, Richter D, Stefanadis C. Omega-3 fatty acid supplementation and cardiovascular disease events [Letter to the Editor]. *JAMA*. 2013;309(1):27.

Vogl D, Rosenfeld B, Breitbart W, et al. Symptom prevalence, characteristics, and distress in AIDS outpatients. *J Pain Sympt Mgmt*. 1999;18(4):253–262.

Vujkovic-Cvijin I, Dunham RM, Iwai S, et al. Dysbiosis of the gut microbiota is associated with HIV disease progression and tryptophan catabolism. *Sci Translational Med*. 2013;5(193):193ra91. doi: 10.1126/scitranslmed.3006438.

Wahner-Roedler DL, Lee MC, Chon TY, et al. Physicians' attitudes toward complementary and alternative medicine and their knowledge of specific therapies:8-year follow-up at an academic medical center. *Complement Ther Clin Pract*. 2014;20(1):54–60.

Warburton DE, Nicol CW, Bredin SS. Health benefits of physical activity: the evidence. *Can Med Assoc J*. 2006;174(6):801–809. doi: 174/6/801.

Webb L, Perry-Parrish C, Ellen J, Sibinga E. Mindfulness instruction for HIV-infected youth: a randomized controlled trial. *AIDS Care*. 2018;30(6):688–695.

Whetten K, Reif S, Whetten R, et al. Trauma, mental health, distrust, and stigma among HIV-positive persons: implications for effective care. *Psychosomat Med*. 2008;70(5):531–538. doi: 10.1097/PSY.0b013e31817749dc.

Wiegman DJ, Brinkman K, Franssen, EJ. Interaction of Ginkgo biloba with efavirenz. *AIDS*. 2009;23(9):1184–1185.

Witt CM, Jena S, Brinkhaus B, et al. Acupuncture for patients with chronic neck pain. *Pain*. 2006;125(1):98–106.

Wohl DA, Tien HC, Busby M, et al. Randomized study of the safety and efficacy of fish oil (omega-3 fatty acid) supplementation with dietary and exercise counseling for the treatment of antiretroviral therapy-associated hypertriglyceridemia. *Clin Infect Dis*. 2005;41(10):1498–1504. doi: CID37106.

Wynia MK, Eisenberg DM, Wilson IB. Physician–patient communication about complementary and alternative medical therapies: a survey of physicians caring for patients with human immunodeficiency virus infection. *J Altern Complement Med*. 1999;5(5):447–456.

Zhang L, Tin A, Brown TT, et al. Vitamin D deficiency and metabolism in HIV-infected and HIV-uninfected men in the multicenter AIDS cohort study. *AIDS Res Human Retroviruses*. 2017;33(3):261–270. doi: 10.1089/AID.2016.0144.

15.

HIV CARE COORDINATION

Sally Spencer Long and Daniel J. Skiest

CHAPTER GOAL

Upon completion of this chapter, the reader should be able to
- Demonstrate knowledge and practice of interdisciplinary care coordination in HIV patient care.

IMPORTANCE OF AN INTERDISCIPLINARY APPROACH TO HIV PATIENT CARE

LEARNING OBJECTIVE

Describe the importance of an interdisciplinary team approach to the optimal management of the patient with HIV.

WHAT'S NEW?

- An interdisciplinary team is an essential comprehensive care strategy to approaching the HIV continuum of care—to help diagnose, link, engage, and successfully treat patients with HIV who increasingly have other chronic illnesses. The interdisciplinary HIV team can effectively address the full range of medical, psychosocial, and behavioral comorbidities.

KEY POINTS

- As patients living with HIV are surviving longer, there is an increased prevalence of non–HIV-related comorbidities, which has resulted in an increasing need for chronic disease management.

- The barriers to each of the steps in the HIV continuum of care need to be identified, anticipated, and addressed. Often, addressing these barriers entails medical, psychosocial, and other specialized services.

Currently available antiretroviral therapies (ART) have higher efficacy, are associated with better adherence and have lower side effect profiles compared to ART available in previous decades. This has led to prolonged survival, approaching that of the general population (Samji, 2014; Wada, 2014).

This prolonged survival, coupled with the fact that the US incidence of HIV has decreased only moderately over the past decade (CDC, 2018), has resulted in an increased number of HIV-infected individuals needing medical care.

With the advances in therapy, HIV infection in the United States has become a treatable chronic disease. As patients are being diagnosed earlier and surviving longer, they are more likely to develop chronic illnesses. In addition to developing the same age-related medical issues as the general population, including diabetes, obesity, hypertension and cardiovascular disease, chronic obstructive pulmonary disease, renal disease, cancer, liver disease (both infectious and noninfectious), bone disease, musculoskeletal pain, and other common primary care conditions, patients with HIV have a higher prevalence of certain comorbidities not traditionally considered to be to HIV-related (heart disease, cerebrovascular disease, non–HIV-related cancers). As a result, patients with HIV often require chronic disease management in addition to the treatment of HIV infection (Chu, 2011).

The HIV epidemic disproportionately affects those with less education, lower income, lack of adequate insurance, lack of permanent housing, those with a history of incarceration and those who are members of racial-ethnic minorities. African American men who have sex with men (MSM) have the highest rates of new infection (CDC, 2017). The continued stigma associated with MSM, especially in the African American community, may lead to less HIV testing in these individuals, which results in late presentation to care and more advanced disease. There may be real or perceived personal, cultural, or system-based barriers to care (Bauman, 2013; CDC, 2011; Irvine, 2014; Scanlon, 2013), which in some individuals can result in lower levels of continued engagement and result in suboptimal viral suppression (Gardner, 2011; White House, 2014).

The social determinants of health play an important role in caring for patients infected with HIV. Many patients with HIV suffer from health disparities and often have to deal with nonmedical issues (lack of affordable housing, incarceration, lack of health insurance, etc.) that can impact their engagement in HIV care. These individuals are also likely to have more difficulty navigating the increasingly complicated US healthcare system, which unfortunately can lead to uncoordinated and fragmented medical care. If not addressed, these issues may result in lower levels of continued engagement.

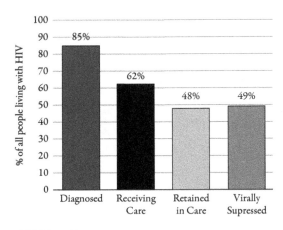

Figure 15.1 HIV Care Continuum. Centers for Disease Control and Prevention. HIV Continuum of Care, U.S., 2014, Overall and by Age, Race/Ethnicity, Transmission-Route and Sex. https://www.cune dc.gov/nchhstp/27, 2018.newsroom/2017/HIV-Continuum-of-Care.html. Accessed June 27, 2018

THE HIV CONTINUUM OF CARE

The goals of HIV clinical care have been defined as suppress viral replication, decrease HIV-related morbidities, improve immune status, prolong survival, improve quality of life, and decrease HIV transmission (USDHHS, 2018). The HIV continuum of care describes the key steps needed to achieve these goals (Figure 15.1).

The first step in the HIV continuum of care is the timely diagnosis of HIV infection. This requires a combination of targeted community outreach to increase testing in high-risk populations as well as routine HIV screening in the general population (CDC, 2006a; US Preventive Services Task Force, 2013). The next step is (prompt) linkage to care, followed by engagement in care, and retention of the patient in care while ART is initiated. Once ART is initiated—and potentially for decades to follow—the patient needs to be effectively followed and supported in care to ensure durable virologic suppression. Each step in the continuum has potential barriers to success that need to be identified, anticipated, and addressed by the clinicians and others providing the care. Achieving the goals in the HIV continuum can be challenging and often requires input and expertise from multiple providers and allied health workers, often as an interdisciplinary HIV care team working together to address potential barriers including depression, substance abuse, lack of housing, lack of medical insurance, and the like (Dombrowski, 2015; Dykeman, 1996).

Optimal management of HIV-infected patients today requires expertise not only in HIV medicine and infectious diseases but also in general medicine, behavioral health, and substance abuse treatment. Many patients also need appropriate ancillary services in order to access medical care and remain engaged throughout the continuum of care. Coordination of often complex care to address these multiple issues is best provided by an interdisciplinary HIV care team.

COMPLEXITY OF HIV PATIENT CARE NEEDS

The following are illustrative case examples of the types of complex comorbidities and chronic conditions that currently characterize the care of patients with HIV infection:

1. A 35-year-old man recently released from jail, where he was diagnosed with HIV/AIDS and a CD4 count of 50 cells/mm^3, is currently homeless and opioid-dependent.

This patient has several immediate needs: ART, stable housing, substance abuse treatment, and opportunistic infection (OI) prophylaxis. The priorities of the patient and the HIV provider may not be in the same order. However, it is likely that by helping the patient with his priorities (housing, substance abuse treatment) the HIV provider will be more successful in meeting the objectives of the provider (engagement in care, antiretroviral therapy, and viral suppression). In order to effectively meet his needs and provide appropriate medical care, the treating clinician will likely require the assistance of multiple HIV team members including a case manager, financial counselor, substance abuse counselor, and social worker. These team members could help the patient navigate complex medical and legal systems to apply for stable housing, obtain medications, receive treatment for substance use disorder, and apply for medical insurance.

2. An obese 55-year-old woman has a history of major depression and prior inconsistent medication adherence, which led to virological failure; she is currently taking ART and has an undetectable HIV viral load.

This patient stopped seeing her therapist and psychiatrist 1 year ago because she felt she no longer required mental health treatment. However, she recently divorced, lost her job (and thus her health insurance), and is not accepting of her new diagnosis of type 2 diabetes mellitus. Although this patient's HIV is currently controlled, the HIV provider is concerned about her recent major life events leading to a depressive episode, which may impact medication adherence, thought to have caused the decreased efficacy of her first HIV regimen. This patient will need several issues addressed simultaneously including treatment of her depression, applying for Medicaid and AIDS Drug Assistance Program (ADAP), and treatment of her obesity and diabetes. She would benefit from prompt referrals to behavioral health for treatment of her depression (both therapist and psychiatrist), to a case manager and financial counselor for assistance with ADAP and Medicaid, and to a nutritionist and endocrinologist for treatment of coexisting medical problems.

3. A perinatally infected 24-year-old pregnant woman with a history of intermittent viral suppression, is in an abusive relationship with her boyfriend. She presents with vaginal bleeding after an episode of domestic violence.

This patient presents unique challenges to the provision of optimal care including obstetrical needs, mental health concerns, and safe housing, and she may require additional efforts to retain in care. A social worker would be helpful to work with the patient to identify housing that would be both safe and supportive (e.g., family shelter) and to provide guidance with implementation of a restraining order to prevent future harmful events. The case manager could assist with linkage to a primary care provider and with transportation needs required to keep appointments for continued engagement in care. A high priority would be arranging prenatal visits as well as primary care and specialist evaluations (e.g., high-risk obstetrician and infectious diseases). Clinicians would need to request assistance from behavioral health specialists to provide ongoing support for the current pregnancy, situational stress/depression, posttraumatic stress, and acceptance of her HIV disease, which will involve life-long engagement in care to maintain optimal health.

RECOMMENDED READING

National Center for HIV/AIDS. Viral hepatitis, STD, and TB prevention 2017. https://www.cdc.gov/hiv/statistics/overview/ataglance.html. Accessed August 29, 2018.

Parry MF, Stewart J, Wright P, et al. Collaborative management of HIV infection in the community: an effort to improve the quality of HIV care. *AIDS Care*. 2004;26:690–699.

Saag M, Benson C, Gandhi R. Antiretroviral drugs for treatment and prevention of HIV infection in adults. *JAMA*. 2018;320(4):379–396.

KEY POINT

- Coordination of care using a patient-centered interdisciplinary team model of care, which usually involves multiple clinicians and healthcare team members working together to meet the needs of the patient, can be an effective strategy for initial and continued engagement in care, especially for complicated patients and/or those with few resources.

HIV PATIENT CARE MODEL

Interdisciplinary Team Care

Due to the complexities of caring for the patient with HIV, including the often concomitant diagnosis of substance use disorder and mental illness, coordinated, patient-centered care is optimally delivered in an ambulatory, chronic disease model by an interdisciplinary (multidisciplinary) team (Chen, 2006; Gallant, 2011; Mayer, 2006; Mugavero, 2011, Ojikutu, 2014, Soto, 2004). In this integrated HIV care model, HIV primary care is combined with mental health and substance abuse services into a single coordinated program. The integrated HIV care model, which has been used effectively to meet the medical and social needs of HIV-positive patients for decades (largely via Ryan White funding; see later discussion), is essentially a patient-centered medical home. In fact, it has been suggested that the HIV integrated care model can be used as a template for primary care clinic medical homes (Beane, 2014). The medical home has been described "as a model or philosophy of primary care that is patient-centered, comprehensive, team-based, coordinated, accessible, and focused on quality and safety." In the integrated or coordinated care model, the goal is to treat the *patient* rather than the *disease* or the *virus*. The team members work together with the patient to clarify goals of care. This leads to improved outcomes by engaging various healthcare workers to work together to help the patient navigate through the complex healthcare system (Bauman, 2013; Boyd, 2014; Chu, 2011).

Studies have demonstrated that shared and coordinated patient care among different disciplines can increase the efficiency of care without duplication of services among multiple healthcare service providers (Gallant, 2011; Horberg, 2012). The interdisciplinary team-based approach has been associated with improved engagement and retention in care (Conviser, 2002; Magnus, 2001; Soto, 2004). It is the model used by Ryan White-funded clinics, which has achieved outcomes superior to non–Ryan White-funded clinics. A recent study of HIV-positive Medicaid patients with HIV and chronic health problems (asthma, chronic obstructive pulmonary disease, diabetes, congestive heart failure) and psychiatric illness and/or substance use disorders found that patients in a medical home model of care had more efficient care which resulted in substantial cost savings compared to patients not cared for in a medical home model (Crits-Christoph, 2018)

RECOMMENDED READING

Knowlton A, Arnstern J, Eldred L, et al. Individual, interpersonal and structural correlates of effective HAART use among urban active injection drug users. *J AIDS*. 2006;41(4):486–492.

Newhouse RP, Spring B. Interdisciplinary evidence-based practice: moving from silos to synergy. *Nurs Outlook*. 2010;58(6):309–317.

Riley TA. HIV-infected client care: case management and the HIV team. *Clin Nurse Spec*. 1992;6(3):136–141.

KEY PRINCIPLES OF THE INTERDISCIPLINARY HIV PATIENT CARE TEAM

LEARNING OBJECTIVES

Describe the roles and responsibilities of the interdisciplinary HIV patient care team.

KEY POINTS

- Effective linkage to and engagement in care can be achieved by interdisciplinary HIV care.

- Each team member has a different area of expertise. The team works together to coordinate comprehensive care, which addresses the medical, mental health, and social issues relevant to each patient. The team is composed of both clinicians and nonclinicians (Box 15.1) (Bauman, 2013; Gallant, 2011; Horberg; 2012). Ideally, decisions are shared among team members.

- The success of an interdisciplinary team depends on effective and open communication and coordination among members.

TEAM MEMBER RESPONSIBILITIES

Roles of HIV Patient Care Team

A comprehensive HIV care team will typically have a physician, nurse, case manager (often a nurse), advanced

Box 15.1 DIFFERENT ROLES OF HIV PATIENT CARE TEAM

KEY ELEMENT(S)	ROLES	RESPONSIBILITIES	POTENTIALLY INVOLVED PERSONNEL
Diagnosis (prevention)	Community outreach	Offer HIV screening Link patients to primary care (Offer Preexposure prophylaxis [PrEP] if HIV negative)	Public health worker Researcher Nurse Health educator
Linkage to Care	Patient navigation	Arrange appointments Function as a liaison between patient and the healthcare provider	Administrative staff Nurse Case manager
Linkage to care Prescribing ART	Insurance/Social support	Link patients to available community resources Apply for medical insurance including ADAP Advocate for patient's needs	Social worker Financial advisor Case manager Advocacy group liaison
Engagement/retention	Retention/Engagement	Outreach to out of care patients Outreach to public health and community-based organizations Gather patient data on retention	Administrative staff Nurse Case manager Public health worker
Engagement/retention	Mental health	Provide counseling Provide mental health treatment Provide psychosocial support	Social worker Psychologist Psychiatrist Substance abuse counselor
Prescribing ART Viral suppression	Medical care	Provide medical management Refer to appropriate specialist(s) Educate on medication adherence	HIV specialist or Primary care clinician Pharmacist/Local pharmacy worker Nurse
Viral suppression	Patient education	Provide education on nutrition, adherence, drug interaction, healthy lifestyle, etc.	Nurse Adherence counselor Nutritionist Health educator Pharmacist HIV specialist or Primary care clinician
Linkage Engagement/ Retention Prescribing ART Viral suppression	Population health management	Gather data on each steps of HIV continuum of care Conduct quality improvement Measure patient outcomes Evaluate projects/programs	Electronic medical record provider Administrative staff Data support staff Researcher HIV specialist or Primary care clinician Public health worker
All stages of care	Team lead	Provide system- based coordination Develop infrastructure	Any team member Commonly done by a clinician

practitioner, mental health provider, social worker, nutritionist, health educator, clinical pharmacist, substance abuse treatment counselor, and financial counselor (Horberg, 2012; Gallant, 2011). The makeup of a particular HIV care team will be specific to the needs of the local patients served and the resources available. Some teams may not have all of the listed positions, and some members of a care team may undertake tasks not traditionally part of their job description. In many cases the roles may overlap (Figure 15.2).

- Physicians and advance practitioners diagnose, treat, refer to other specialists, and often lead interdisciplinary care team.

- Public health workers, nurses, and health educators offer initial HIV screening, provide HIV prevention education including information on preexposure prophylaxis (PrEP)

if HIV negative and link HIV-positive patients to an HIV provider.

- Administrative staff and case managers arrange appointments and serve as liaisons between the patient and healthcare providers.

- Social workers and financial advisors link patients to available community resources (housing, disability, food assistance, etc.) and assist with applications for healthcare insurance, including ADAP.

- Clinical pharmacists and health educators provide assistance with medication information and adherence.

- Nursing staff and nutritionists provide education on nutrition, adherence, and healthy lifestyles.

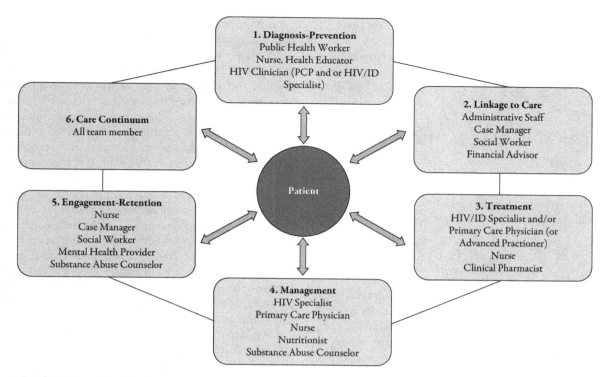

Figure 15.2 Roles of HIV Care Team Members.

- Psychiatrists, therapist/counselors, and substance abuse counselors respectfully provide mental health assessment and treatment, psychosocial support, and treatment of addiction (including substance use disorder).

A team leader is usually designated (physician or advanced practitioner). The team leader should facilitate communication among various team members to support the goal of quality care for patients. Ongoing communication (via electronic health records [EHR], meetings, phone consultation) between the interdisciplinary team and the patient is essential to ensure collaborative and patient-centered care (Gallant, 2011; Nancarrow, 2013). Regular meetings to discuss the needs of patients and to reassess team member roles are important. The complexity of the patient's medical and psychosocial needs can often be overwhelming, and learning the patient's priorities and making partnered decisions with the patient can help interdisciplinary coordination of care among healthcare professionals and the patient (Gallant, 2011; Mugavero, 2011). There are limited data on standardized ways of measuring interdisciplinary team care (Boyd, 2014). However, periodic internal review of the interdisciplinary member responsibilities and infrastructure can help improve and consolidate responsibilities, avoid duplication of tasks, and augment the efficiency and effectiveness of the team. One survey indicated that patients who received care in an interdisciplinary HIV care model had high levels of satisfaction (Vachirasudlekha, 2014).

Ideally, the HIV interdisciplinary care team is colocated (on-site) and fully integrated to allow for open and seamless communication. There are many benefits of the colocalized provision of integrated services. An interdisciplinary coordinated program can simultaneously treat the complexities involved with multiple needs and conditions through minimization of barriers to care, enhanced communication with clinicians, and improved adherence to medical recommendations. However, other models in which team members and various services have been located off-site have had success (Kimmel, 2016). A shared EHR can facilitate communication among team members, especially those located off-site.

ROLES OF TEAM MEMBERS IN DIFFERENT CARE MODELS

In the interdisciplinary HIV care models, both HIV care and primary care may be provided by the same clinician or different clinicians, according to local factors and expertise. In the first model, the infectious diseases (ID) provider handles both the HIV and primary care issues. In the second model the primary care provider (PCP) (or generalist) provides both HIV and primary care. In the third model, the ID physician provides the HIV care, while the PCP handles the issues related to primary care (Rhodes, 2017). While one model may work better in a certain community, it is not the most important factor when quality of care is measured. Studies have consistently found that the most important factor in achieving optimal outcomes across the HIV continuum of care is the HIV provider's volume and experience, regardless of the provider's training (Kitahata, 1996, 2003; Laine, 1998; Landon, 2005; Gallant, 2011; Kimmel, 2016; Rhodes, 2017; O'Neill, 2015).

RECOMMENDED READING

Gardner LI, Giordano TP, Marks G, et al. Enhanced personal contact with HIV patients improves retention in primary care: a randomized trial in six US HIV clinics. *Clin Infect Dis.* 2014;59(5):725–734.

Gopalappa C, Farnham PG, Hutchinson A, et al. Cost effectiveness of the national HIV/AIDS strategy goal of increasing linkage to care for HIV-infected persons. *J AIDS.* 2012;66(1):99–105.

STRATEGIES FOR SUCCESSFUL REFERRAL

LEARNING OBJECTIVE

Describe the steps for obtaining referrals for HIV-infected patients and strategies that can increase the success of referrals.

KEY POINT

- Common types of referrals include specialized medical, dental, mental health, and substance use disorder treatment; home care; child care; peer services; transportation; housing; financial/legal support; spirituality services; and end-of-life care and hospice. The positive impact of effective referrals is demonstrated in data suggesting that supportive services can lead to improvements in adherence, health outcomes, and client satisfaction.

As noted earlier, due to the remarkable advances in ART, for many patients HIV infection has been transformed into a chronic illness. As in the general population, as patients age they often develop additional comorbidities that may require additional medical resources to manage. Numerous factors result in the need for more resources to manage patients with HIV, including the higher rates of homelessness, substance abuse, and mental illness and the fact that patients may be more socioeconomically disadvantaged. Providing comprehensive care for these patients often requires referrals to other healthcare providers, financial counselors, social workers, and ancillary services. Depending on the model and scope of HIV care, the referrals may occur within the same interdisciplinary HIV team, to another provider in the same institution, or to someone outside the system. Effective referrals can be initiated through a structured referral process utilizing established referral sources.

While there is no one approach that will work for all HIV providers or delivery models with regards to appropriate referrals, certain practices may be widely applicable. Initially, an assessment of the patient's referral needs should be performed and objectives for the referral should be clearly defined. Ideally, providers from different disciplines should work together to meet the identified patient healthcare needs. In the interdisciplinary team-based approach, decisions regarding referrals and patient care are shared. In collaborative arrangements, decision-making responsibilities are shared and ownership of changes in care may shift depending on the level of expertise required at a given time. The HIV case manager may be helpful in coordinating appropriate referrals and ensuring that the patient is linked to the needed specialist or services (Gardner, 2005). The case manager can also be helpful in communicating the patient's unique needs to the referring and receiving provider or agency.

It is helpful for team members to become familiar with the various agencies in their community, especially those that maintain a core group of professionals committed to the care of people living with HIV (PLWH). This encourages further support and involvement in the patient's progress. Referral of patients to on-site providers is preferred but referrals off-site may be necessary. This can present with its own set of challenges, especially regarding transportation and communication. There may be a limited number of specialists available who are willing to care for PLWH, and these may have less than adequate methods for reimbursement. The case manager may need to arrange transportation to the off-site specialist or ancillary worker. Communication is a major issue and, if not facilitated, may lead to lack of understanding by the patient and the off-site provider. Thus, the patient's needs may not be adequately addressed. In some cases, if resources allow, the case manager may accompany the patient in order to ensure that the patient attends the appointment and that recommendations are understood by the patient and are carried out. Clear two-way communication between the HIV provider and the specialist is important in order for the goals of care to be met. The specialist should clearly identify the questions and objectives of the referring provider and the patient, and should clearly state the plan of care, which should be readily accessible. A shared EHR can help to alleviate the communication issue. However, direct communication between the referring provider and the specialist, as well as with other team members, is optimal.

Responsibility for the implementation and follow-up of recommended changes in the plan of care should be clearly outlined. Documentation of patient receipt and progress of referral services is critical to ensure the referral services have been provided. Identification of one interdisciplinary team member to be responsible for follow-up on the status of the referral and to assess patient input of referrals is helpful to assess possible future barriers to completion of referrals. Frequent and timely communication between the referring organization and the referral providers can decrease gaps in care and ensure continuity of quality care.

RECOMMENDED READING

Family Health International. Establishing referral networks for comprehensive HIV care in low-resource settings. 2005. Available at http://pdf.usaid.gov/pdf_docs/Pnadf677.pdf. Accessed November 27, 2015.

Gardner LI, Giordano TP, Marks G, et al. Enhanced personal contact with HIV patients improves retention in primary care: a randomized trial in six US HIV clinics. *Clin Infect Dis.* 2014;59(5):725–734.

Gopalappa C, Farnham PG, Hutchinson A, et al. Cost effectiveness of the national HIV/AIDS strategy goal of increasing linkage to care for HIV-infected persons. *J AIDS.* 2012;66(1):99–105.

Kwait J, Valente T, Celentano, D. Interorganizational relationships among HIV/AIDS service organizations in Baltimore: a network analysis. *J Urban Health.* 2001;78(3):468–487.

QUALITY IMPROVEMENT

The goal of the HIV care is to optimize patient health, decrease HIV transmission, and end the AIDS epidemic. A clear vision with focused efforts to improve clinical outcomes and quality can help to develop, improve, and sustain effective patient care practices (Gallant, 2011; Mugavero, 2011). An up-to-date and available patient registry with relevant clinical and retention data can help monitor and measure patient care outcomes. In some clinics, the EHR can be used to create the registry, but in other cases creation of a separate data tool (e.g., an electronic spreadsheet) may be beneficial. Examples of relevant clinical and retention data include adherence, missed appointments, recent contact information and outreach, detectable viral load, status of ART, and evidence of failing or failed primary care (e.g., development of antiretroviral resistance, new opportunistic infections, onset or worsening of comorbid conditions, or clinical decline).

In a resource-limited setting, targeted data collection may be beneficial instead of attempting to obtain all data at once. For example, it may be beneficial to prioritize and focus resources to high-risk and vulnerable patients, such as those who have been out of care for more than 6 months or have a detectable viral load. A patient registry with clinical and laboratory data can also support the measurement of and improve patient outcomes by strategizing quality improvement projects. Examples include annual influenza vaccination among patients with HIV and appropriate sexually transmitted disease screening. Having a registry can facilitate a team member in contacting or collaborating with clinicians to strategize, and in contacting patients by mail, phone call, or during visits to receive these interventions.

In addition to the patient registry, local or state public health, community, or funding organizations may have available patient data, such as detectable viral load, out-of-care patients, involvement with outside services, or other socioeconomic data, which can help in gathering information on why certain patients are not retained in care. Sharing data can help clarify and eliminate duplicating efforts to coordinate care among different healthcare facilities (e.g., a patient engaged in a clinic while still registered as a patient at another facility). Availability of such data may be limited to certain local or state public health, community, or funding organizations. If such data are available, they can also be relevant for both the healthcare facility and the local and state public health, community, and funding organizations to improve services and monitor outcomes along the HIV continuum of care. Moreover, understanding population-based health outcomes can help in the administration, coordination, and improvement of infrastructure and funding of HIV care in the community (CDC, 2014; White House, 2014).

FUNDING FOR HIV CARE

See Chapter __ on funding for a comprehensive discussion on funding in the United States.

Ryan White HIV/AIDS Program

The Ryan White HIV/AIDS Program is an important component of HIV patient care (HRSA HIV/AIDS, 2018; Sood, 2014). This federal program, which began in 1991, funds healthcare and services to PLWH. Program funding is distributed among Parts A–F. Part A provides emergency assistance to eligible areas that are most severely affected by HIV/AIDS. Part B provides grants to all 50 states and US territories or associated jurisdictions. Part C provides outpatient-based comprehensive primary healthcare for PLWH. Part D provides family-centered care for women, infants, children, and youth with HIV/AIDS. Part F provides funds for a variety of programs, such as health information technology, social media, and outreach programs. The program also funds dental care, special projects, training programs, and minority AIDS initiatives.

The Ryan White Program funds cities, states, and local community-based organizations to provide HIV care and treatment services to more than half a million people each year and assists approximately 52% of all people diagnosed with HIV in the United States. In fiscal year 2017, the Ryan White Program provided $2.36 billion in funding (HRSA, 2017). The program is known for its "wrap-around" services to patients with HIV. However, coverage and requirements of Ryan White-funded programs may vary state to state, and grantees of the program should review eligibility and criteria of renewal (including required data collection and conformance with standards of care) (HRSA, 2018). The Ryan White HIV/AIDS Program is always the "payer of last resort."

An important component of the Ryan White Program (under Part B) is ADAP, which provides medications approved by the US Food and Drug Administration (FDA) to low-income people living with HIV who have limited or no health coverage from private insurance, Medicaid, or Medicare. ADAP funds may also be used to purchase health insurance for eligible clients and for services that enhance access to, adherence to, and monitoring of drug treatments. Different states have varied eligibility criteria and renewal processes, including documentation of income status (15 states established income eligibility at 200% or less of the federal poverty level), diagnosis of HIV, opportunistic infections, chronic medical conditions, and/or other service needs (HRSA ADAP, 2018).

Several studies have demonstrated better outcomes for patients receiving care at Ryan White–funded clinics versus nonfunded clinics (Weiser, 2015; Bradley, 2016).

RECOMMENDED READING

Henry Kaiser Family Foundation. Total federal HIV/AIDS grant funding. 2014. Available at http://kff.org/hivaids/state-indicator/total-federal-grant-funding. Accessed August 2, 2018.

Joint United Nations Programme on HIV/AIDS (UNAIDS). 90-90-90 An ambitious treatment target to help end the AIDS epidemic. 2014. Available at http://www.unaids.org/sites/default/files/media_asset/90-90-90_en_0.pdf. Accessed November 29, 2015.

Shah M, Risher K, Berry SA, et al. The epidemiologic and economic impact of improving HIV testing, linkage, and retention in care in the United States. *Clin Infect Dis*. 2016;62(2):220–229.

ACKNOWLEDGMENTS

This Chapter is revised from an earlier edition by Joy H. King and Peter A. Selwyn.

REFERENCES

Bauman LJ, Braunstein S, Calderon Y, et al. Barriers and facilitators of linkage to HIV primary care in New York City. *J AIDS*. 2013;64(1):S20–S26.

Boyd CM, Lucas GM. Patient-centered care for people living with multimorbidity. *Curr Opin HIV AIDS.* 2014;9(4):419–427.

Beane SN, Culyba RJ, DeMayo M, Armstrong W. Exploring the Medical Home in Ryan White HIV care settings: a pilot study. *J Assoc Nurses AIDS Care.* May-June 2014;25(3):191–202.

Bradley H, Viall AH, Wortley PM, et al. Ryan White HIV/AIDS program assistance and HIV treatment outcomes. *Clin Infect Dis.* January 1, 2016;62(1):90–98.

Centers for Disease Control and Prevention (CDC). Revised guidelines for HIV counseling, testing, and referral. *MMWR* 2006b;55(RR14):1–17.

Centers for Disease Control and Prevention (CDC). Revised recommendations for HIV testing of adults, adolescents, and pregnant women in health-care settings. *MMWR Recomm Rep.* 2006a;55(14):1–17.

Centers for Disease Control and Prevention (CDC). HIV surveillance—United States, 1981–2008. *MMWR Recomm Rep.* 2011;60(21):689–693.

Centers for Disease Control and Prevention(CDC), Division of HIV/AIDS Prevention. Understanding the HIV care continuum. 2014. Available at https://stacks.cdc.gov/view/cdc/26481. Accessed November 3, 2015.

Centers for Disease Control and Prevention (CDC). Estimated HIV incidence and prevalence in the United States, 2010–2015. *HIV Surveillance Supplemental Report* 2018;23(No. 1). http://www.cdc.gov/ hiv/library/ reports/hiv-surveillance.html. Published March 2018. Accessed January 7, 2018.

Centers for Disease Control and Prevention (CDC). *HIV Surveillance Report, 2016*; vol. 28. November 2017. http://www.cdc.gov/hiv/library/reports/hiv-surveillance.html. Accessed August 29, 2018.

Chen RY, Accortt NA, Westfall AO, et al. Distribution of health care expenditures for HIV-infected patients. *Clin Infect Dis.* 2006;42:1003–1010.

Chu C, Selwyn PA. An epidemic in evolution: the need for new models of HIV care in the chronic disease era. *J Urban Health.* 2011;88(3):556–566.

Conviser R, Pounds M. The role of ancillary services in client-centered systems of care. *AIDS Care.* 2002;14(1):S119–S131.

Crits-Christoph P, Gallop R, Noll E, et al. Impact of a medical home model on costs and utilization among comorbid HIV-positive Medicaid patients. *Am J Manag Care.* 2018;24:368–375

Dombroski JC, Simoni JM, Katz DA, et al. Barriers to HIV care and treatment among participants in a public health HIV care relinkage program. *AIDS Patient Care STDS.* 2015;29:279–287.

Dykeman M, Sternberg C, Jasek J, et al. A model for the delivery of care for HIV-positive clients. *AIDS Patient Care STDS.* 1996;10:240–245.

Gallant JE, Adimora AA, Carmichael JK, et al. Essential components of effective HIV care: a policy paper of the HIV Medicine Association of the Infectious Diseases Society of America and the Ryan White Medical Providers Coalition. *Clin Infect Dis.* 2011;53:1043–1050.

Gardner EM, McLees MP, Steiner JF, et al. The spectrum of engagement in HIV care and its relevance to test-and-treat strategies for prevention of HIV infection. *Clin Infect Dis.* 2011;52(6):793–800.

Gardner LI, Metsch LR, Anderson-Mahoney P, et al. Efficacy of a brief case management intervention to link recently diagnosed HIV-infected persons to care. *AIDS.* 2005;19:423–431.

Henry Kaiser Family Foundation. Total federal HIV/AIDS grant funding. 2014. Available at http://kff.org/hivaids/state-indicator/total-federal-grant-funding. Accessed August 2, 2018.

Health Resources and Services Administration (HRSA). The Ryan White HIV/AIDS program. Available at http://hab.hrsa.gov/abouthab/aboutprogram.html. Accessed August 8, 2018.

Health Resources and Services Administration (HRSA). Ryan White HIV/AIDS Treatment Extension Act of 2009 (Public Law 111-87) Part B: AIDS drug assistance program. Available at http://hab.hrsa.gov/abouthab/partbdrug.html. Last reviewed October 2017. Accessed August 8, 2018.

Horberg MA, Hurley LB, Towner WJ, et al. Determination of optimized multidisciplinary care team for maximal antiretroviral therapy adherence. *J AIDS.* 2012;60(2):183–190.

Irvine MK, Chamberlin SA, Robbins RS, et al. Improvements in HIV care engagement and viral load suppression following enrollment in a comprehensive HIV care coordination program. *Clin Infect Dis.* 2014;60:298–310.

Kimmel A, Martin E, Galadima H, et al. Clinical outcomes of HIV care delivery models in the US: a systematic review. *AIDS Care.* 2016;28(10):1215–1222.

Kitahata MM, Von Rompaey SE, Dillinghanm PW, et al. Primary care delivery is associated with greater physician experience and improved survival among persons with AIDS. *J Gen Intern Med.* February 2003;18(2):95–103.

Kitahata MM, Koepsell TD, Deyo RA, Maxwell CL, Dodge WT, Wagner EH. Physicians' experience with the acquired immunodeficiency syndrome as a factor in patients' survival. *N Engl J Med.* 1996;334(11):701–706.

Laine C, Markson LE, et al. The relationship of clinic experience with advanced HIV and survival of women with AIDS. *AIDS.* 1998;12:417–424.

Landon BE et al. Physician specialization and the quality of care for Human immunodeficiency virus infection. *Arch Intern Med.* 2005;165:1133–1139.

Magnus M, Schmidt N, Kirkhart N, et al. Association between ancillary services and clinical and behavioral outcomes. *AIDS Patient Care STDS.* 2001;15:137–145.

Mayer K, Chagutur S. Penalizing success: is comprehensive HIV care sustainable? *Clin Infect Dis.* 2006;42:1011–1013.

Mugavero MJ, Norton WE, Saag MS. Health care system and policy factors influencing engagement in HIV medical care: piecing together the fragments of a fractured health care delivery system. *Clin Infect Dis.* 2011;52(Suppl 2):S238–S246.

Nancarrow SA, Booth A, Ariss S, et al. Ten principles of good interdisciplinary team work. *Hum Resour Health.* 2013;11:19.

Ojikutu B, Holman J, Kunches L, et al. Interdisciplinary HIV care in a changing healthcare environment in the USA. *AIDS Care.* 2014;26(6):731–735.

O'Neill M, Karelas GD, Feller DJ, et al. The HIV Workforce in New York State: Does Patient Volume Correlate with Quality? *Clin Infect Dis.* 2015;62:1871–1877.

Rhodes C, Chang Y, Regan S, et al. (2017). Human immunodeficiency virus (HIV) quality indicators are similar across HIV care delivery models. *Open Forum Infect Dis.* Winter 2017;4(1):ofw240.

Samji H, Cescon A, Hogg RS, et al. Closing the gap: increases in life expectancy among treated HIV-positive individuals in the United States and Canada. *PLoS One.* 2014;8(12):e81355.

Scanlon ML, Vreeman RC. Current strategies for improving access and adherence to antiretroviral therapies in resource-limited settings. *HIV AIDS (Auckl).* 2013;5:1–17.

Sood N, Juday T, Vanderpuye-Orgle J, et al. HIV care providers emphasize the importance of the Ryan White program for access to quality of care. *Health Affairs.* 2014;33(3):394–400.

Soto TA, Bell J, Phillen MB. Literature on integrated HIV care: a review. *AIDS Care.* 2004;16(Supplement 1):S43–S55.

US Department of Health and Human Services (USDHHS). Panel on antiretroviral guidelines for adults and adolescents: guidelines for the use of antiretroviral agents in HIV-1-infected adults and adolescents. 2018. Available at https://aidsinfo.nih.gov/contentfiles/lvguidelines/AdultandAdolescentGL.pdf. Accessed July 8, 2018.

US Preventive Services Task Force. Screening for HIV: US Preventive Services Task Force recommendation statement. *Ann Intern Med.* 2013;159(1):51–60.

Wada N, Jacobson LP, Cohen M, et al. Cause-specific mortality among HIV-infected individuals, by CD4[+] cell count at HAART initiation, compared with HIV-uninfected individuals. *AIDS.* 2014;28:257–265.

Weiser J, Beer L, Frazier E, et al. Service delivery and patient outcomes in Ryan White HIV/AIDS program-funded and—nonfunded health care facilities in the United States. *JAMA Intern Med.* 2015;175(10):1650–1659.

White House Office of National AIDS Policy. *National HIV/AIDS strategy: update of 2014 federal actions to achieve national goals and improve outcomes along the HIV care continuum.* Washington, DC: The White House Office of National AIDS Policy; 2014.

Vachirasudlekha B, Cha A, Berkowitz, L, et al. Interdisciplinary HIV care—patient perceptions. *Int J Health Care Qual Assur.* 2014;27(5):405–413.

16.

THE PHARMACIST'S ROLE IN CARING FOR HIV-POSITIVE INDIVIDUALS

Jennifer Cocohoba

CHAPTER GOALS

Upon completion of this chapter, the reader should be able to

- Understand how a pharmacist might be incorporated into a healthcare team that is caring for persons living with HIV

- Discuss medication-related issues for which it would be optimal for an HIV to provide expert consultation on.

INTRODUCTION

HIV, a chronic disease, requires a multidisciplinary approach to ensure that all aspects of a patient's health are addressed. Medications are essential tools used for prevention, treatment, and the management of comorbid conditions. Pharmacists play an important role in all of these because they ensure accurate medication dispensing. Pharmacist specialists have also become essential members of the healthcare team because their expertise extends beyond dispensing. When included on the healthcare team, HIV pharmacist expertise can be channeled into improving the selection, safety, efficacy, and overall quality of medication therapy.

LEARNING OBJECTIVES

- Describe common settings in which HIV pharmacists' practice.

- List three potential ways in which pharmacists can contribute to the care of HIV-positive individuals.

KEY POINTS

- HIV pharmacists are a diverse group of providers who work to improve the health of HIV-positive individuals via medication therapy management, quality assurance practices, research, and other avenues.

- HIV pharmacists may be particularly skilled at managing complex antiretroviral drug–drug interactions, recommending therapies for resistant HIV virus, and providing education and support with regard to adherence.

- If practicing with a physician under a collaborative drug therapy management agreement, an HIV pharmacist may be able to provide more direct disease state management (e.g., prescribing and ordering lab tests) including preexposure prophylaxis, HIV, and associated conditions.

THE HIV CLINICAL PHARMACIST SPECIALIST

Medications for HIV have become more convenient but not less complex. For this reason, having a clinical pharmacist as a part of the healthcare team can greatly enhance the care of HIV-positive patients. HIV-specialized clinical pharmacists typically receive advanced training in HIV during postdoctorate residencies, infectious diseases fellowship programs, or HIV-specific fellowship programs, although some acquire their HIV knowledge through experience and intense self-study. Certification programs such as the American Academy of HIV Medicine's HIV Pharmacist (AAHIVP) certification program and the Introductory HIV Pharmaceutical Care Certificate Program offered through the University of Buffalo can help distinguish pharmacists who are well-versed in aspects of HIV pharmacotherapy (McLaughlin, 2018). Many HIV pharmacists also pursue Board of Pharmacy Specialties certification in infectious diseases (BCIDP) or ambulatory care (BCACP) due to the wide knowledge base, roles, and responsibilities that can be associated with caring for patients living with HIV.

SETTINGS IN WHICH HIV PHARMACISTS PROVIDE PATIENT CARE

People living with HIV/AIDS encounter many different pharmacists who contribute to their care across the spectrum of their disease and medical visits. For patients who are acutely ill, the first setting in which they may interact with an HIV-specialized pharmacist is in the hospital. In many health systems, the infectious diseases (ID) team oversees consultative care for HIV-infected patients. HIV/ID pharmacists on these multidisciplinary teams contribute skills and knowledge to enhance care for HIV-positive patients. The paradigm of test and treat has increased the number of patients initiated on antiretroviral therapy (ART) during a hospital stay, but

HIV pharmacotherapy is riddled with complex drug–drug interactions and requires close monitoring to dose adjust for renal insufficiency or hepatic dysfunction. HIV pharmacists on inpatient clinical services assist the team in selecting ART and appropriate opportunistic infection regimens, screen for complex drug–drug interactions, assist in ordering and interpreting resistance testing or therapeutic drug monitoring assays, provide discharge counseling for patients initiating new ARTs, and can help coordinate benefit coverage for any antiretrovirals prescribed during an inpatient hospital stay.

HIV-specialized pharmacists play an important role in preventing and ameliorating medication errors. Published literature suggests that hospitalized HIV-positive patients are at high risk of incurring medication errors and that these errors—including incorrect antiretroviral regimens, incorrect dosing strategies, incorrect scheduling, or drug–drug interactions—may occur at various points during their hospital stay (Li, 2014).

Pharmacist-led antiretroviral stewardship programs have resulted in reduced ART medication errors in hospitalized HIV patients. One hospital found that 45% of their 334 hospitalized HIV patients had at least one medication error occur during their stay, and 31% of these patients still had uncorrected errors at the time of discharge (Zucker, 2016). After 1 year, a prospective audit and feedback strategy was employed and the proportion of admissions with errors dropped to 31%, although 31% still had uncorrected errors at discharge. During the second year, prospective review plus intervention was implemented. The proportion of medication errors remained stable at 37%, but the rate of uncorrected errors at discharge dropped to 12%. A Texas antiretroviral stewardship program implemented pharmacist education, a pharmacist-led ART checklist, and modifications to the hospital order-entry and verification system to support prospective audit and feedback; this combination of interventions significantly reduced the number of ART-related errors from 208 to 24 (Shea, 2018). Although many studies do not evaluate the financial benefit of preventing errors, one study estimated a cost avoidance of $24,273 per year for less serious HIV medication errors and $124,080 per year for more serious medication errors (Merchen, 2011). Last, errors of omission can greatly impact the health of hospitalized HIV patients. A small study of 139 patients found that hospital pharmacist intervention improved rates of appropriate opportunistic infection prophylaxis from 58% to 93% in patients living with HIV (Schatz, 2016).

Patients in a clinic may interact with HIV-specialized pharmacists who work as part of an interdisciplinary ambulatory care team. These HIV clinical pharmacists have a wide range of duties commensurate with their experience and level of expertise. Responsibilities can include dispensing medications in a clinic-associated pharmacy; reviewing patient charts to ensure optimal pharmacotherapy; providing one-on-one patient education; consulting with patients and medical providers regarding medication-related problems, adherence, or resistance testing results; initiating and managing ART; ordering lab tests; and initiating, adjusting, or discontinuing medications for concomitant disease states.

Clinic-based HIV-specialized pharmacists can have an important impact on patient medication adherence and clinical outcomes. A study of 10,801 HIV-positive individuals conducted at Kaiser Permanente in California compared different clinic team structures to determine the optimal combination of clinicians that would increase adherence (Horberg, 2012). For patients starting a new ART regimen, the largest adherence increases at 12 months were attributable to multidisciplinary teams composed of a clinical pharmacist, a social worker/benefits coordinator, and a non–HIV-specialized primary care provider (8.1% increase in mean adherence; 95% confidence interval [CI], 2.7–13.5%). Kaiser Permanente also conducted an ecological study to assess the effects of its HIV clinical pharmacists on adherence, healthcare utilization, and HIV outcomes (Horberg, 2007). Refill adherence at 24 months was statistically significantly higher for patients seen by an HIV clinical pharmacist (76.7% vs. 68.9%, $p = 0.02$). Odds of having a suppressed viral load or increase in $CD4^+$ cell count were modestly better for patients seen by HIV pharmacists. However, these point estimates did not achieve statistical significance and varied based on other factors, such as provider panel size, and patient factors, such as length of time infected with HIV. The study did find that patients who worked with HIV pharmacists and whose providers had a smaller patient panel had a lower risk for medical office visits (relative risk = 0.81, $p < 0.001$). Rathbun et al. (2005) conducted a small, randomized, controlled clinical trial testing the effect of a pharmacist-run clinic adherence program on adherence and viral load. The intervention consisted of patient education, monitoring, and provision of adherence reminder devices. Patients were counseled at a clinic visit prior to starting ART. After initiation, they were contacted via telephone within 1 week and seen at a clinic visit after 2 weeks. Patients could be followed in additional clinic visits as necessary for the 12-week duration of the study. At week 28, adherence, as recorded by electronic drug monitors (74% vs. 51%), proportion of patients with viral suppression of less than 50 copies/mL (63% vs. 53%), and median $CD4^+$ T cell count increases (142 vs. 97 cells) were all higher in the clinic pharmacist intervention group, although the point estimates did not achieve statistical significance. Apart from this unique randomized controlled trial, most of the published research evaluating impact of HIV pharmacists in clinic settings utilize quasi-experimental before-after study designs. These studies, which examine pharmacist-run adherence programs situated within community clinics, hospital clinics, and academic medical center clinics, found improvements in $CD4^+$ T cell counts, increased rates of viral suppression, fewer acute medical visits, and increased adherence for patients who interact with an HIV clinical pharmacist (Saberi, 2012).

ART is typically dispensed by a community pharmacist. Nearly all HIV-positive patients will interact with one at some point; the community pharmacist may be the healthcare provider with whom a healthy HIV-positive patient interacts most frequently. In larger metropolitan areas, pharmacists and staff who are knowledgeable about HIV disease may frequently be found at pharmacies that specialize in HIV care. These HIV-focused pharmacies may belong to large retail chains or can be independent pharmacies. They may stand alone or be integrated within a larger health system (Gilbert, 2016). They may also undergo an accreditation process to be officially recognized as a specialty pharmacy, although this designation tends to indicate expertise in various other disease states and not HIV alone. Patient education and counseling, provision of reminder devices and adherence aids, managing the practical aspects of synchronizing and coordinating medication refills, and facilitating the procurement of antiretrovirals are just a few of the activities conducted by HIV community pharmacists.

Clinical researchers are beginning to study the impact of HIV-focused community pharmacies on patient-related outcomes. The major challenge of conducting this type of research is that pharmacy records typically do not link to medical and laboratory records, such that pharmacists may more easily evaluate the clinical impact of their interventions. The US Department of Health and Human Services funded a pilot program to support 10 California community pharmacies in providing medication therapy management (MTM) services for 1,353 HIV-positive patients receiving Medicaid (Hirsch, 2009, 2011). Types of services offered in these HIV-focused pharmacies varied greatly; they included adherence enhancements such as automatic refill reminders, reminder packaging, and patient counseling when underuse or overuse of ART was detected (Rosenquist, 2010). After the first year of the program, patients using the pilot pharmacies were more adherent to their ART regimens (defined as having a medication possession ratio between 80% and 120%) compared to patients using nonpilot pharmacies (56.3% vs. 38.1%, $p < 0.001$). This trend continued at 3 years, at which time HIV-positive patients filling their ART at the pilot pharmacies ($n = 2,234$) demonstrated higher medication possession ratios (69.4% vs. 47.3%, $p < 0.001$) and a higher odds of having optimal adherence (odds ratio, 2.74; 95% CI, 2.44–3.10) compared to those filling their ART at traditional pharmacies, after controlling for age, gender, and ethnicity (Hirsch, 2009, 2011). Costs at the end of the first year of the program were approximately $1,014 per pilot pharmacy patient. Although the funding for this program has since concluded, it demonstrates the potential for improvement in pharmacotherapy and adherence associated with patients using HIV-knowledgeable community pharmacies.

A SAMPLE OF PHARMACIST SKILLS

Pharmacists make ideal treatment facilitators due to their extensive training in MTM. The goal of MTM is for a pharmacist to optimize a patient's treatment through identification, resolution, and prevention of medication-related problems (American Pharmacists Association and the National Association of Chain Drug Stores Foundation, 2008). This definition of MTM is intentionally broad so that it may accommodate the wide variety in activities that a pharmacist may perform to optimize a patient's therapy. For example, during a medication therapy review, a pharmacist may discover dangerous drug–drug interactions and poor patient adherence. The pharmacist may work closely with the patient and their medical provider to create an action plan that addresses these issues. This section presents a sample of some of the skills that an HIV pharmacist may exercise when caring for an HIV-positive patient.

IDENTIFICATION AND MANAGEMENT OF DRUG–DRUG INTERACTIONS

Many antiretroviral agents strongly induce or inhibit the cytochrome P450 system, particularly the 3A4 isoform. Because approximately 60% of the most commonly prescribed drugs are also metabolized via cytochrome P450 3A4, pharmacists are trained to carefully review an HIV-positive patient's medication list to identify adverse drug interactions that may result in excess toxicity or subtherapeutic levels of the object drug or that may result in alterations in the HIV drug concentrations. Pharmacists provide management strategies for known interactions. For important theoretical interactions, pharmacists may suggest using therapeutic drug monitoring and can help interpret the levels garnered from these tests.

SUPPORTING ADHERENCE AND PROVIDING PATIENT EDUCATION

In every setting, HIV pharmacists strive to support patient adherence to their antiretroviral regimens. One very basic barrier is that patients may have difficulty adhering to medications that they cannot afford. Pharmacists can provide patients with information and resources regarding pharmaceutical company–run patient assistance programs and state-run AIDS drug assistance programs to help them afford their regimens. Hospital and clinic pharmacists may be knowledgeable regarding the local pharmacies that keep a consistent stock of antiretrovirals. Last, in the era of utilization management, pharmacists and their technicians play a critical role in selecting antiretroviral regimens that adhere to insurance formulary guidelines, providing clinical justification for prior authorizations, and managing those submissions so that patients do not have lapses in therapy.

Pharmacists have access to a wealth of reminder devices that may help improve adherence (Mahtani, 2011; Saberi, 2011). Some pharmacies offer specialized unit-dose packaging in plastic "bubble packs" or on medication cards ("blister packs") to help patients remember to take their doses. Pharmacists can train patients on how to use weekly medication boxes. Some community and clinic pharmacists may offer text messaging or may work with patients to set up cell phone alarms to serve as automated medication reminders. Pharmacies may offer a variety of other adherence-enhancing services, such as online management of medications, automatic prescription refills, telephone refill reminders, and home mailing or courier medication delivery.

Pharmacist services include patient counseling to enhance adherence. HIV clinical pharmacists make ideal treatment advocates because they are knowledgeable about ART and may help bridge the gap between patients and their providers. They offer personalized patient education regarding HIV disease, HIV treatment and opportunistic infection prophylaxis, and management of adverse effects. Using popular counseling techniques such as motivational interviewing, pharmacists may assess a patient's readiness to initiate ART and may help motivate the patient toward that goal (D'Antonio, 2010; Krummenacher, 2011). Although these items may be discussed during the treating clinician's visit rather than during a pharmacist visit, this type of education often takes up more time than allowed in a brief visit focused on acute medical problems. A visit with a pharmacist provides complementary education and serves as an extension of the provider's care. In clinic and community pharmacy settings, pharmacists may package all of these services into structured adherence programs that span the range of patient assessment, education, and counseling; offering reminder devices; dispensing medications; and providing continuity in the refill process. Although no two pharmacist-run adherence programs are exactly alike, many studies have illustrated their benefits with regard to patient outcomes (Dilworth, 2018).

TESTING FOR HIV INFECTION

HIV testing is a service that is emerging predominantly in community pharmacies, although pharmacists in other settings are often included as members of multidisciplinary testing teams (Sherman, 2014). These models of care typically encompass the use of point-of-care rapid HIV tests, counseling, and linkage to confirmatory testing and/or care. In preliminary studies, pharmacy-based testing appears to be acceptable to both patients and pharmacists (Amesty, 2015; Darin, 2015). In one study, 939 HIV tests were provided by 22 pharmacy staff members at six different sites during a 12-month period (Lecher, 2015). Pre- and posttest counseling required an average of 4–12 minutes, and the average cost per person tested ranged from $32.17 to $47.21.

EXPANDING PATIENT CARE VIA COLLABORATIVE PRACTICE AGREEMENTS

In the United States, most states have legislation that allows for pharmacists to engage in collaborative practice; however, the requirements and regulations vary from state to state. In some states, pharmacists may enhance the care of HIV-positive patients via collaborative drug therapy management (CDTM) agreements. The specifics of any CDTM agreement depend on the collaborating physician and the qualifications and experience of the pharmacist.

The American College of Clinical Pharmacy defines a CDTM agreement as

> a collaborative practice agreement between one or more physicians and pharmacists wherein qualified pharmacists working within the context of a defined protocol are permitted to assume professional responsibility for performing patient assessments; ordering drug therapy-related laboratory tests; administering drugs; and selecting, initiating, monitoring, continuing, and adjusting drug regimens (Hammond, 2003, p. 1210).

The American Society of Health Systems Pharmacists recently published an updated statement on pharmacist involvement in HIV care that attempts to summarize the scope of practice for an HIV pharmacist (Schafer, 2016). Collaborative protocols with physicians may allow pharmacists to select and initiate ART or opportunistic infection prophylaxis, draw and interpret pertinent labs that monitor efficacy or toxicity of the regimen, simplify regimens using fixed-dose combination tablets, and manage common antiretroviral-related side effects such as nausea and diarrhea. Knowledgeable pharmacists may order, interpret, and change a patient's ART based on resistance tests. Ma et al. (2010) conducted a before-and-after comparison of clinical outcomes for patients consulting with an HIV clinical pharmacist in a drug optimization clinic. Pharmacists reviewed patient medication histories and resistance tests, simplified or adjusted their ART regimens, and provided adherence training and education. After the pharmacist intervention, refill adherence was improved (89% vs. 81%, $p = 0.003$), a higher proportion of patients achieved undetectable viral loads (96% vs. 63%, $p < 0.001$), and a higher proportion of patients had increased absolute CD4+ T cell counts (491 vs. 423 cells/mm^3 at visit, $p < 0.001$).

In addition to managing ART, some protocols allow pharmacists to assess and adjust medication therapy for HIV-related comorbidities such as depression, diabetes, hypertension, hepatitis C, or dyslipidemia. A retrospective cohort study found that an interdisciplinary primary care team that included an HIV pharmacist produced significantly improved outcomes in lipid management and smoking cessation for patients with HIV and diabetes, hypertension, or hyperlipidemia ($n = 96$) compared to a control group ($n = 50$) that was managed by an individual healthcare provider (Cope, 2015). The interdisciplinary team achieved a cost savings of approximately $3,000 per patient.

An emerging opportunity to utilize CDTM agreements is in the provision of preexposure prophylaxis (PrEP). Recent studies have highlighted gaps in access to PrEP. Some of these gaps may be related to clinician familiarity or time to discuss or manage PrEP, or lack of access to healthcare for certain populations who might benefit from PrEP. Community pharmacies may have unique access to some of these populations. CDTM agreements would allow pharmacists to screen for appropriateness, prescribe PrEP under protocol, draw and review monitoring labs, assess and support adherence, and refill as appropriate. The One-Step-PrEP program in Seattle, Washington, is an example of a pharmacy run PrEP program operating under a CDTA (Tung, 2017). Over a 1-year period from 2015 to 2016, 373 patients sought out this pharmacy-based PrEP service. Of those, 245 persons initiated PrEP and most of these patients (96%) did not have to pay for their PrEP medication. An impressive retention of 75% was achieved over the first year of operation. This study demonstrates that pharmacy-based PrEP services are feasible and desired and remain a promising avenue for pharmacists to contribute to the public health goal of preventing new infections (Okoro, 2018).

A collaborative, interdisciplinary practice coupled with good communication between providers can serve as an excellent model for enhancing the care of HIV-positive patients and extending the provider's ability to reach the greatest number of patients. The roles, responsibilities, and impact of HIV pharmacists in clinical practice are likely to expand in the future as the profession lobbies for all pharmacists to be recognized as healthcare providers under US federal law.

The benefit of having an HIV clinical pharmacist extends beyond direct patient services. Pharmacists are becoming increasingly essential members of HIV hospital or clinic quality improvement teams. Performance measures, such as those for HIVQUAL, often involve chart abstraction to benchmark rates of ART, viral suppression, opportunistic infection prophylaxis, and adherence assessment. HIV clinical pharmacists have the clinical background and skills to assess these items (and others) quickly, accurately, and thoroughly. Pharmacists can also offer valuable insight for plan–do–study–act projects designed to improve any below-target performance measures.

Finally, an increasing number of trained HIV clinical pharmacist scientists are making a strong impact on HIV-related research. Their understanding of study design, drug therapy monitoring, and pharmacotherapy makes HIV clinical pharmacists ideal study coordinators or project managers for research studies being conducted within clinical settings. Advanced training through master's degree programs and complementary PhD programs also places HIV clinical pharmacists in an optimal position to serve as principal investigators on research studies regarding pharmacokinetics, pharmacodynamics, investigational drugs, adherence, drug resistance, or provision of health services. As pharmacists become further trained in clinical research methods, they will continue to contribute valuable information to the body of HIV knowledge.

CONCLUSION

HIV clinical pharmacists are a diverse group of healthcare practitioners with specialized skills and knowledge. Whether they are engaged in patient care, quality assurance, research, or a combination of these, they strive to benefit HIV-positive patients through their efforts. Although not all clinics or hospitals have available resources or grants to house an HIV-specialized pharmacist, collaborations with HIV-focused community pharmacists can ensure that patients have access to this valuable healthcare team member and that they receive the highest quality medication care possible.

RECOMMENDED READING

Durham SH, Badowski ME, Liedtke MD, Rathbun RC, Fulco PP. Acute care management of the HIV-infected patient: a report from the HIV Practice and Research Network of the American College of Clinical Pharmacy. *Pharmacotherapy*. 2017;37:611–629.

Schafer JJ, Cocohoba JM, Sherman EM, Tseng AL, eds. *HIV Pharmacotherapy: The Pharmacist's Role in Care and Treatment*. Bethesda, MD: American Society of Health-System Pharmacists; 2018.

Scott JD, Abernathy KA, Diaz-Linares M, et al. HIV clinical pharmacists: the US perspective. *Farm Hosp*. 2010;34(6):303–308.

REFERENCES

American Pharmacists Association and National Association of Chain Drug Stores Foundation. Medication therapy management in pharmacy practice: Core elements of an MTM service model (version 2.0). *J Am Pharm Assoc (2003)*. 2008;48(3):341–353.

Amesty S, Crawford ND, Nandi V, et al. Evaluation of pharmacy-based HIV testing in a high-risk New York City community. *AIDS Patient Care STDS*. August 2015;29(8):437–444.doi:10.1089/apc.2015.0017.

Cope R, Berkowitz L, Arcebido R, et al. Evaluating the effects of an interdisciplinary practice model with pharmacist collaboration on HIV patient co-morbidities. *AIDS Patient Care STDS*. 2015;29(8):445–453.

D'Antonio, N. Including motivational interviewing skills in the PharmD curriculum. *Am J Pharm Educ*. 2010;74(8):152d.

Darin KM, Scarsi KK, Klepser DG, et al. Consumer interest in community pharmacy HIV screening services. *J Am Pharm Assoc (2003)*. January–February 2015;55(1):67–72.

Dilworth TJ, Klein PW, Mercier RC, et al. Clinical and economic effects of a pharmacist-administered antiretroviral therapy adherence clinic for patients living with HIV. *JMCP*. 2018;24(2):165–172.

Gilbert EM, Gerzenshtein L. Integration of outpatient infectious diseases clinic pharmacy services and specialty pharmacy services for patients with HIV infection. *Am J Health Syst Pharm*. June 1, 2016;73(11):757–763.

Hammond RW, Schwartz AH, Campbell MJ, et al. Collaborative drug therapy management by pharmacists—2003. *Pharmacotherapy*. 2003;23(9):1210–1225.

Hirsch JD, Gonzales M, Rosenquist A, et al. Antiretroviral therapy adherence, medication use, and health care costs during 3 years of a community pharmacy medication therapy management program for Medi-Cal beneficiaries with HIV/AIDS. *J Manag Care Pharm*. 2011;17(3):213–223.

Hirsch JD., Rosenquist A, Best B, et al. Evaluation of the first year of a pilot program in community pharmacy: HIV/AIDS medication therapy management for Medi-Cal beneficiaries. *J Manag Care Pharm*. 2009;15(1):32–41.

Horberg MA, Bartemeier Hurley L, James Towner W, et al. Determination of optimized multidisciplinary care team for maximal antiretroviral therapy adherence. *J Acquir Immune Defic Syndr*. 2012;60(2):183–190.

Horberg MA, Hurley LB, Silverberg MJ, et al. Effect of clinical pharmacists on utilization of and clinical response to antiretroviral therapy. *J AIDS*. 2007;44(5):531–539.

Krummenacher I, Cavassini M, Bugnon O, et al. An interdisciplinary HIV-adherence program combining motivational interviewing and electronic antiretroviral drug monitoring. *AIDS Care*. 2011;23(5):550–561.

Lecher SL, Shrestha RK, Botts LW, et al. Cost analysis of a novel HIV testing strategy in community pharmacies and retail clinics. *J Am Pharm Assoc (2003)*. 2015;55(5):488–492.

Li EH, Foisy MM. Antiretroviral and medication errors in hospitalized HIV-positive patients. *Ann Pharmacother*. May 8, 2014;48(8):998–1010.

Ma A, Chen DM, Chau FM, et al. Improving adherence and clinical outcomes through an HIV pharmacist's interventions. *AIDS Care*. 2010;22(10):1189–1194.

Mahtani KR, Heneghan CJ, Glasziou PP, et al. Reminder packaging for improving adherence to self-administered long-term medications. *Cochrane Database System Rev*. 2011;9:CD005025.

McLaughlin M, Gordon LA, Kleyn TJ, Lamsen M, Scott J. Assessment of the benefits of and barriers to HIV pharmacist credentialing. *J Am Pharm Assoc (2003)*. March–April 2018;58(2):168–173.

Merchen A, Gerzenshtein L, Scarsi K, et al. HIV-specialized pharmacists' impact on prescribing errors in hospitalized patients on antiretroviral therapy. Paper presented at the 51st Interscience Conference on Antimicrobial Agents and Chemotherapy, Chicago, September 17–20, 2011.

Okoro O, Hillman L. HIV pre-exposure prophylaxis: exploring the potential for expanding the role of pharmacists in public health. *J Am Pharm Assoc (2003)*. July-August 2018;58(4):412–420.

Rathbun RC, Farmer KC, Stephens JR, et al. Impact of an adherence clinic on behavioral outcomes and virologic response in the treatment of HIV infection: a prospective, randomized, controlled pilot study. *Clin Ther*. 2005;27(2):199–209.

Rosenquist A, Bes, BM, Miller TA, et al. Medication therapy management services in community pharmacy: a pilot programme in HIV specialty pharmacies. *J Eval Clin Pract*. 2010;16(6):1142–1146.

Saberi P, Dong BJ, Johnson MO, et al. The impact of HIV clinical pharmacists on HIV treatment outcomes: a systematic review. *Patient Prefer Adherence*. 2012;6:297–322.

Saberi P, Johnson MO. Technology-based self-care methods of improving antiretroviral adherence: a systematic review. *PLoS One*. 2011;6(11):e27533.

Schafer JJ, Gill TK, Sherman EM, McNicholl IR. ASHP guidelines on pharmacist involvement in HIV care. *Am J Health-Syst Pharm*. 2016;73:468–494. Available at http://www.ajhp.org/content/73/7/468. Accessed July 7, 2018.

Schatz K, Guffey W, Maccia M, Templin M, Rector K. Pharmacists' impact on opportunistic infection prophylaxis in patients with HIV/AIDS. *J Hosp Infect*. December 2016;94(4):389–392.

Shea KM, Hobbs AL, Shumake JD, Templet DJ, Padilla-Tolentino E, Mondy KE. Impact of an antiretroviral stewardship strategy on medication error rates. *Am J Health Syst Pharm*. June 15, 2018;75(12):876–885.

Sherman EM, Elrod S, Allen D, Eckardt P. Pharmacist testers in multidisciplinary health care team expand HIV point-of-care testing program. *J Pharm Pract*. December 2014;27(6):578–581.

Tung E, Thomas A, Eichner A, Shalit P. Feasibility of a pharmacist-run HIV PreP clinic in a community pharmacy setting. Presented at the Conference on Retroviruses and Opportunistic Infections, Seattle, Washington, February 13–16, 2017. Abstract 961.

Zucker J, Mittal J, Jen SP, Cennimo D. Impact of stewardship interventions on antiretroviral medication errors in an urban medical center: a 3-year, multiphase study. *Pharmacotherapy*. March 2016;36(3):245–251.

17.

THE ROLE OF THE PHYSICIAN ASSISTANT AND THE NURSE PRACTITIONER IN CARING FOR PERSONS LIVING WITH HIV

D. Trew Deckard

CHAPTER GOALS

Upon completion of this chapter, the reader should be able to

- Understand the contributions of Physician Assistants and Nurse Practitioners in HIV/AIDS care since the beginning of the epidemic through today.

- Realize the body of research, clinical applications, and treatment advancements made by Nurse Practitioners and Physician Assistants.

- Recognize the expanding role of the Physician Assistant (PA) and Nurse Practitioner (NP) as the management and treatment of HIV/AIDs continues to evolve.

LEARNING OBJECTIVES

- Review a brief history of nurse practitioner (NP) and physician assistant (PA) professional development.

- Recount outcomes conclusions of NPs and PAs by the HIV Medicine Association (HIVMA) and other organizations.

- Describe multiple areas of HIV/AIDS literature contributions of NPs and PAs.

- Outline the HIV care provider gaps filled by NPs and PAs.

KEY POINTS

- There are currently approximately 115,000 practicing PAs and 248,000 practicing NPs in the United States and around the world.

- NPs and PAs are the providers for more than 1 million HIV/AIDS visits per year.

- Multiple medical reviews support NPs and PAs as HIV/AIDS providers.

- PAs and NPs are responsible for a growing body of research in HIV/AIDS medicine.

Note of clarification of discipline names: Throughout the body of current medical literature, the reader may encounter the professional designations of advanced practice practitioner (APP), advanced practice provider (APP), and non-physician clinician (NPC). Each is referring to NPs and/or PAs.

BACKGROUND OF THE PROFESSIONS OF ADVANCED PRACTICE PROVIDERS: A BRIEF REVIEW

As early as the 1930s and 1940s in the United States, the medical community had begun to see increasing numbers of physicians being trained in specialty fields. More graduating physicians were turning their focus away from primary care and into their respective fields of specialty. This began to leave gaps in primary medical care in many places in the country, especially in rural areas. By the 1960s, it became very clear that new ways of approaching primary care would be needed

In 1965, Duke University established the first physician assistant (PA) program with four ex-Navy corpsmen. This was a natural fit as Navy corpsmen had a level of medical training relevant to their role in the military that couldn't be carried into civilian life. Therefore, the newly developed PA discipline allowed corpsmen to continue their medical training and practice medicine under the supervision of a physician. Since that time, PA students enter their medical training from a wide variety of clinical areas. In 1968, the American Academy of Physician Assistants (AAPA) was established. "AAPA, established in 1968 by students and alumni of the Duke program, extends membership to graduates from programs around the country and becomes the legitimate voice for the profession" (aapa.org, 2018; pahx.org, 2018).

At the same time that the PA profession was being developed, levels of clinical training and expertise were growing in the nursing field. In 1965, the first nurse practitioner (NP) program was established at the University of Colorado by Drs. Loretta Ford and Henry Silver. In 1985, the American Academy of Nurse Practitioners was established (aanp.org, 2018). Since that time, NPs have continued to expand their role and are currently pursuing independent practice authority, which is currently approved in 22 US states (aanp.org, 2018).

THE GROWING ROLE OF PAS AND NPS IN CARING FOR HIV PATIENTS

In the 1980s, when AIDS and its cause, HIV, were identified, its transmission and outcomes were poorly understood. Primary care providers (PCPs) were very frequently the first to identify the patient who was presenting with HIV/AIDS symptoms. This led to a natural relationship between PCPs and the newly diagnosed HIV-positive person. In addition to physicians in infectious diseases caring for people living with HIV (PLWH), so were many in internal medicine, family practice, and general medicine, which often included NPs and PAs.

According to Gilman et al., PAs and NPs were responsible for providing care for 15% of HIV-positive persons in the United States in 2010, with projected rates of 20% by 2015, which represents nearly 1 million visits for that year alone (Gilman, 2016).

Given these statistics it is important to recognize the importance that advanced practice practitioners play in the role of caring for HIV/AIDS patients and the outcomes associated with that care. In order to address the growing need of NPs and PAs to support the medical needs of HIV/AIDS patients in the United States, several studies have reviewed this very important issue. One study from the Health Policy Institute, Medical College of Wisconsin, Milwaukee, even as early as 2001 found that "for many years, non-physician clinicians (NPCs) have participated in the care of patients. However, their numbers were small and their licensed prerogatives were narrow. Over the past decade, these characteristics have changed in three important ways. First, training in many of the NPC disciplines has increased substantially, and the growth of these disciplines is accelerating. Second, state laws and regulations have expanded both the practice prerogatives of NPCs and their autonomy from physician supervision. Third, payers have increased their access to reimbursement. As a consequence, NPCs are undertaking many elements of care that previously were provided by physicians. Their participation is generally cost-effective and is met with a high degree of patient satisfaction" (Cooper, 2001).

Since that time, further data have supported those findings and given more recognition for advanced practice providers as a continued viable choice as PCPs and HIV specialists for PLWH. In 2011, the HIV Medicine Association (HIVMA) came to the following conclusion:

> The availability of effective treatment has transformed HIV disease into a chronic condition requiring a complex hybrid of HIV specialty, primary care and preventive medicine best delivered by a multidisciplinary care team. Advanced Practice Registered Nurses (APRNs) and Physician Assistants (PAs) play a critical role in maximizing the effectiveness of the care team and in providing quality, cost-effective HIV care in the U.S.

Studies indicate that patients with HIV cared for by APRNs and PAs in multi-disciplinary care settings have comparable outcomes to patients managed by physicians. (Gallant, 2011)

Another study released in 2005 in the *Annals of Internal Medicine* (Wilson, 2005) examined patient outcomes for multiple care providers. Comparisons were made between physician HIV experts and NPs or PAs and between physician non–HIV experts and NP or PAs. Their conclusions were as follows: "the quality of HIV care provided by NPs and PAs was similar to that of physician HIV experts and generally better than physician non–HIV experts. Nurse practitioners and PAs can provide high-quality care for persons with HIV."

NUMBERS OF ADVANCED PRACTICE PROVIDERS IN THE UNITED STATES AND AROUND THE WORLD

There were approximately 80,019 certified PAs in the United States at the end of 2010; the profession grew 44.4% over the next 6 years, reaching 115,547 certified PAs at the end of 2016 (Figure 17.1) (National Commission on Certification of Physician Assistants, Inc., 2017). Of this number, 539 were practicing in other countries.

There are more than 248,000 NPs licensed in the United States as of 2018 (Figure 17.2) (NP Fact Sheet, 2018).

In addition, the NP role continues to emerge and evolve around the world. Education, credentialing, and practice for NPs vary by country. The American Association of Nurse Practitioners (AANP) was an active member of the steering committee that led to the development of the ICN Nurse Practitioner/Advanced Practice Nursing Network (ICN NP/APPN) and continues to provide support for the network website. AANP also offers support to those implementing the NP role (aanp.org/international, 2018).

In addition to clinical outcomes of HIV/AIDS patients in the United States under the care of advance practice providers already discussed, there are data to support high-quality outcomes outside of the United States as well. In one African study, the researchers concluded that

> This study of nearly 6000 patients initiating ART during the first 40 months of the Mozambique national ART program found a similar or better quality of HIV care provided by NPC (Non-physician Clinicians) compared with physicians. These results highlight the key role that NPC play in driving ART scale-up, and argue for using all relevant clinical staff to meet the clinical demands in countries with a high HIV burden. The results also underscore the importance of considering NPC training and supervision needs when developing guidelines and regulations for HIV care. (Sherra, 2010)

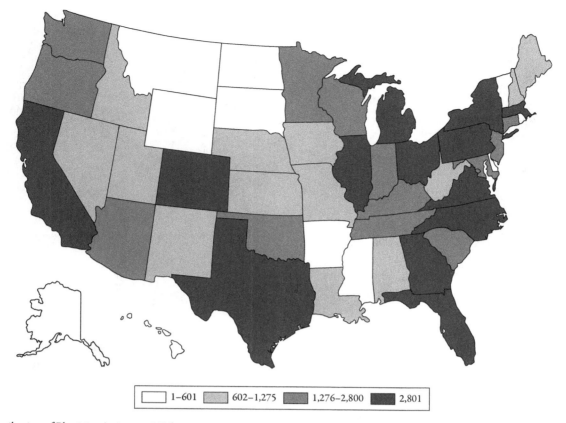

| | 1–601 | | 602–1,275 | | 1,276–2,800 | | 2,801 |

Figure 17.1 Distribution of Physician Assistants: 2016. (National Commission on Certification of Physician Assistants, Inc. (2017, March). 2016 Statistical Profile of Certified Physician Assistants: An Annual Report of the National Commission on Certification of Physician Assistants. Available at: http://www.nccpa.net/research.)

ADVANCE PRACTICE PROVIDERS; PA AND NP CONTRIBUTIONS IN REVIEWING RESEARCH AND ORIGINAL RESEARCH IN HIV LITERATURE

HIV TESTING

NPs and PAs have been involved in virtually all aspects of HIV/AIDS care, as well as in contributing to the medical literature that helps to formulate our approach to that care. Over the past three decades, testing for HIV has taken many permutations, and, as of 2006, the US Centers for Disease Control and Prevention (CDC) recommended routine HIV testing for all persons living in the United States between the ages of 13 and 65. This recommendation has been debated since that time. Different hospitals, organizations, and states have had varying responses to these recommendations.

In 2007, one study revealed that this recommendation was being actively debated. Leonard B. Johnson, MD, and Sharon E. Valenti, NP, were among the investigators whose aggregate conclusions were to "agree with the CDC recommendations to implement rapid HIV screening in the areas of high HIV prevalence. However routine testing of all patients even in areas of high prevalence should be evaluated carefully and weighed against the cost of testing, training residents, and

non–HIV-physicians in HIV 101; and other potential costs of follow-up and the rate of return on successfully identifying patients as HIV positive" (Johnson, 2010).

Other HIV testing studies have focused on how specific populations are affected by access to HIV testing. Gerald Kayingo, PhD, MMSc, PA-C and Robert Douglas Bruce, MD, MA, MSc, researchers at a large community health center in Connecticut found that "Before universal HIV screening, significant sex and racial differences existed among patients visiting this CHC (Community Health Center). Implementation of universal HIV screening has increased the number of people tested, increased the number of minorities tested, and reduced the HIV testing disparities that previously existed between men and women" (Kayingo, 2016).

In 2011, PA Kevin Michael O'Hara, in a study entitled "HIV Exceptionalism and Ethical Concerns Surrounding HIV Testing," concluded that "Clinicians and policy leaders must reflect on the core ethical principles of beneficence, nonmaleficence, and autonomy when evaluating approaches to HIV testing" (O'Hara, 2011).

HIV PREVENTION

In 2013, I had the opportunity to review the data from the CDC's program, "Prevention with Positives" and noted that the declining death rate from HIV and relatively unchanged

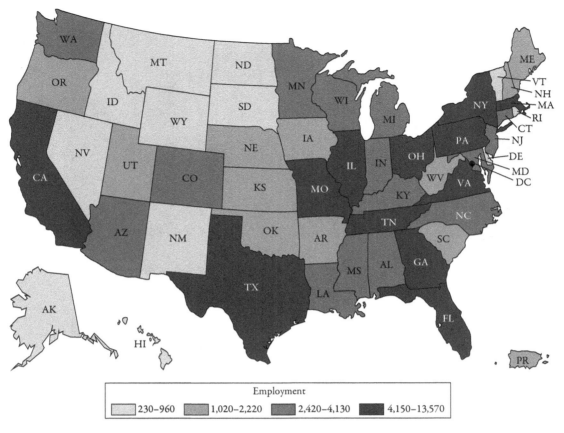

Employment

| 230–960 | 1,020–2,220 | 2,420–4,130 | 4,150–13,570 |

Blank areas indicate data not available.

Figure 17.2 Employment of nurse Practioners, by state, May 2017. (United States Department of Labor, Bureau of Labor Statistics, May 2017. Available at: https://www.bls.gov/oes/2017/may/oes291171.htm.)

annual rate of new infections have contributed to the increasing numbers of PLWH. After reviewing the literature, I concluded "Preventing new HIV infections is a primary goal of the US National HIV/AIDS Strategy. Clinicians should proactively incorporate into their practices the additional tools and interventions provided by new research, continue to search for innovative and interactive ways, and to reach out to communities at high risk for HIV acquisition" (Deckard, 2013).

Also in 2013, Jonathan Baker, MPAS, PA-C, while reviewing conventional behavioral modifications for preventing HIV and their outcomes found that "An understanding of current and emerging HIV prevention options lets patients and their healthcare providers create a patient-centered prevention plan" (Baker, 2013). He noted that this included using prevention plans based on a patient's risk; familiarity with ways to prevent maternal-child HIV transmission; the roles of circumcision, postexposure prophylaxis (PEP), and preexposure prophylaxis (PrEP); familiarity with IV drug use and HIV risk, and the knowledge of emerging biomedical methods such as microbicides and vaccines.

To follow the data presented in 2013, in 2014, Jonathan Baker, MPAS, PA-C, along with Kevin Michael O'Hara, MMSc, MS, PA-C, reported on oral PrEP, finding that "Oral PrEP has recently been demonstrated as an effective

intervention for the prevention of HIV when used with classic prevention strategies including condoms. MSM [men who have sex with men], heterosexual men and women, and IV drug users may benefit from PrEP" (Baker, 2014).

To further this area of work, Gary Spinner, PA, MPH, AAHIVS, in 2015 found that "With extensive data from clinical trials demonstrating that PrEP is highly effective in preventing HIV infections, its use should be encouraged, along with other prevention measures to help further decrease the incidence of new infections in the US and globally" (Spinner, 2015).

In 2017, Barbara Warren, BSN, MPH, PNP, and Lyn Stevens, MS, NP, along with other clinicians reported on a new program called Targeted PrEP Implementation Program (TPIP), which was an 18-month project involving five statewide agencies to assess PrEP implementation in "real-world" settings. They found that "TPIP played a pivotal role in laying the foundation for statewide implementation of PrEP. Throughout the program PrEP was delivered as part of a comprehensive prevention plan that included consistent and correct condom use, safer sex practices, risk reduction counseling, and routine screening for HIV and other STIs that could facilitate HIV transmission" (Parisi, 2018).

As recently as July 2018, Maria Anotonieta Andrews, FNP, and A. J. Dominguez reported on an outreach tool for high-risk populations noting that, as in most parts of the United States, the most recent Arizona HIV/AIDS epidemiology report in 2016 revealed new HIV diagnoses were higher in MSM between the ages of 25 and 29 and second highest were in 20- to 24-year-old MSM. Therefore, on January 2, 2018, the Southwest Center for HIV/AIDS in Phoenix launched a Facebook live broadcast called IGNITE with the "'intention of creating a fun, accessible approach to online education and outreach."

They found that, "Overall by using the evaluation tools built into Facebook Live IGNITE is able to develop best practices and learn valuable lessons about audience engagement and effective outreach. Adopting a social media-based web-broadcast is within reach and has the potential to improve outreach to high risk individuals, thereby addressing the HIV epidemic" (Andrews, 2018).

INITIATING HIV THERAPY

Advanced practice providers are responsible for keeping current with HIV treatment guidelines, as are the physicians who treat this population. In February 2011, Ann Maldonado, MPH, PA-C, reviewed the guidelines in the *Journal of the American Academy of Physician Assistants* (JAAPA) to emphasize the importance of remaining up to date.

As expected with all populations of medical providers who care for PLWH, her conclusion was that "Although this article provides a detailed review of the [US Department of Health and Human Services] DHHS guidelines for the initiation of ARV therapy in the HIV-infected patient, PAs caring for this population are strongly encouraged to obtain, review, and implement the full guidelines in their daily practice in order to follow the current standard of care. (Maldonado, 2011).

ANTIRETROVIRAL THERAPY ADHERENCE

Antiretroviral therapy (ART) adherence has always been a mainstay of HIV treatment by providers, including advanced practice providers. It is understood as the cornerstone for long-term success. There are many approaches to explore determinants of adherence, and the following are two of them.

Cook et al. determined that evaluating motivation is one possible important component. Their study measured PLWH's daily experiences and tested a model to explain the intention–behavior gap. Overall, the proposed model in which adherence results from momentary motivation was partially confirmed, and the researchers concluded that clinicians would be well-advised to assess motivation because of its link to ART adherence based on past and predicted behavior (Cook, 2018).

A controversial but contemporary study by Claborn et al. used emerging data from a large HIV treatment study to explore clinician perspectives on prescribing opioids to incentivize retention in HIV care. Their findings concluded that this study is an important first step toward understanding prescription-based incentives to retain patients in care. Consideration of the ethics and legality of such an approach is important to determine whether additional use of such prescribing practices is justifiable (Claborn, 2018).

HIV AND THE EFFECTS OF CULTURE, SOCIAL DETERMINANTS, ETHNICITY, AND DEMOGRAPHICS

NPs and PAs must make many observations regarding how culture, social environment, and demographics effect outcomes with HIV-impacted patients. Tim Nolan, ANP, AAHIVS, found that, with Latino populations, there are practical tips that have the potential to improve a patient's clinical experience and outcomes. He notes that "As Latino patients present to us with a unique set of challenges, we as HIV specialty providers can work to acquire a distinct set of tools to provide them with integrated care. These tools of course vary from region to region but there are some basics:

a) Speak the language

b) Understand the immigration issue and become involved

c) Read Rafael Diaz's and George Ayala's "Social Discrimination and Health: The Case of Latino Gay Men and HIV"

d) Understand the unique qualities of the varying Latino cultures. (Nolan, 2013)

In addition, Janis Zadel, NP, AAHIVS, also in 2013, reported that "Working with Latinos is the same as anyone working outside of their native population. You must make the effort to get to know the culture. Make the effort to bring out what their health beliefs are and what motivates them so you can relate to them and provide the help and care that they need" (Zadel, 2013).

Intimate partner violence also plays a role in persons at risk for HIV, and this may be exacerbated for Hispanics, as Weidel et al. conclude in their research reported in 2008: "Hispanics have unique cultural and social characteristics and norms that may place them at risk for HIV exposure. An awareness of the distinct cultural differences in gender roles and varying levels of acculturation can assist clinicians in investigating patients' level of risk" (Weidel, 2008).

For the past several years, most of new HIV diagnoses in the United States have been made in persons living in the South. Why this is the case and how to address it have been the subject of many investigations and studies. In 2014, J. Wesley Thompson, PA-C, MHS, DFAAPA, AAHIVS, reported on the Southern HIV/AIDS Strategy Initiative (SASI), finding that "a holistic approach that includes local, state, and federal partnerships and has addressed the multiple factors that contribute to the disproportionate epidemic in the South, such as lack of resources and regional resource inequalities, as well as stigma and high [sexually transmitted infection] STI rates, are needed to adequately address HIV in the region." Last, he notes that "Only through partnership and collaboration can we address the epidemic of HIV in the South" (Thompson, 2014).

HIV AND MSM

Tonia Poteat, PA-C, MPH, AAHIVS, reviewing data from the 2009 American Conference for the Treatment of HIV (ACTHIV) recapped information on risk of HIV acquisition for MSM and most specifically for black MSM, quoting predominantly from a presentation that addressed this specific issue. She reported that "Dr. Millett suggests that annual screening for HIV/STD screening is insufficient to keep up with the rate of infection in this population and suggests more frequent screening." Also that "black MSM must be even more vigilant in engaging in safer sex practices than other groups because of factors that place them at higher risk of infection even when practicing the same behaviors or less risky behaviors as other MSM" (Poteat, 2009).

This article found that "While there are varied and individual reasons that patients drop out of care, the failure to understand the important cultural context from which a patient interacts with the health care system often leads to poor ART adherence and loss of retention in care. How health care providers interact with their patients, attempt to understand their racially and ethnically diverse cultures, and develop a relationship built on trust and free of personal bias is essential to keep patients engaged in and retained in care" ' (Spinner, 2017).

HIV AND ADOLESCENTS

Adolescents are a unique population, and this is especially true with HIV. Advanced practice practitioners play an important role in this area as elsewhere in the care of our HIV/ AIDS population. Nellie Reindeau Lazar, MSN, CRNP-BC, AAHIVS, and Mary Tanney, NP, MSN, MPH, AAHIVS, address this in their current article, "Challenges of Medication Adherence in HIV+ Adolescents."

They note that although the current USDHHS guidelines recommend all HIV-positive persons begin ART as soon as possible, adolescents have unique challenges that may prohibit this. " 'Adhering to medication is a crucial component of living a healthy life with HIV. Youth living with HIV (YLH) are at higher risk for negative outcomes because of higher rate of depression, substance abuse and other risk factors. All of these factors contribute to a youth's ability and drive to adhere to medication. YLH need culturally sensitive, tailored multi-factorial interventions to increase motivation and self-efficacy" (Riendeau Lazar, 2015).

AGING WITH HIV

As HIV providers began to recognize the issues that caregivers faced with an aging population of PLWH, more research began to take place. Jeffrey D. Myers, PA-C, MMSc, MIH, in 2009 reported on this area of research in the article, concluding that "Important epidemiologic and clinical differences exist between younger and older HIV infected persons. Health care providers need to address the issues of sexuality in our older patients and . . . the conditions associated with HIV and those of aging, such as dementia. To address this and other emerging issues, further research is needed on the long-term effects of ARV therapy, HAD, and the many metabolic and hormonal changes that occur in the HIV infected persons." He also suggests that we examine "at-risk behaviors," social trends, public policy, and our own comfort with addressing these issues with our patients (Myers, 2009).

It is estimated that, as of 2015, about 50% of HIV-positive persons in the United States were 50 years and older and that there are increasing clinical needs for this population. An important part of this population are women, who constitute approximately 25% of the total HIV-infected population. Seja Jackson, APRN-BC, AAHIVS reviewed data and current research with this group. She determined that, overall, "Women over 50 living with HIV have unique situations and challenges. Those of us working in the field of HIV need to listen carefully, be sensitive to needs, find answers, and be creative with the solutions for women living and aging with HIV infection. Destigmatizing the HIV diagnosis is particularly important for older women living with HIV in order for them to live comfortable full lives. We must be allies and advocates for this group that is often living the shadows" (Jackson, 2015).

TRANSGENDER HIV PATIENTS

Medical care for transgender patients has been a developing area of medicine for many years and continues to be misunderstood by many. Wesp et al. point out that "Transgender is an umbrella term used to describe individuals who have a gender identify different than the sex they were assigned at birth." They also highlight that trans persons face personal and medical stigma, avoid and/or are turned away from medical care at alarming rates, and have a much higher attempted suicide rate compared to the general population.

The article concludes by acknowledging "Expanding the base of gender-affirming healthcare providers in the U.S. must begin with the adoption of cultural humility on the part of the providers and educators as the foundational component to providing patient-centered care" (Wesp, 2016).

A 2017 article written by Elizabeth Schmidt, MS, PA-C, and Denise Rizzolo PhD, PA-C focuses on how "exogenous use of sex steroids provided as hormone therapy and gender affirming procedures affect screening and prevention." They identify several gaps in our understanding of how to approach medical hormonal therapy and its consequences and note that the US Preventive Service Task Force (USPSTF) is taking steps toward clearer and more expanded recommendations for transgender persons. Currently "the authors recommend integrating the UCSF guidelines, which provide graded evidence with its recommendations to support evidence-based primary care practice" (Schmidt, 2017).

Additional data have been presented with individual case presentations addressing the growing needs of transgender persons (Ferron, 2010).

HIV AND SEXUALLY
TRANSMITTED INFECTIONS

Kristy Goodman, MS, MPH, PA-C, along with Christopher M. Black, MPH, reported on the disconnect between patients being testing for sexually transmitted infections (STIs) and their understanding of which test are begin evaluated. Their findings:

> Most healthcare providers, regardless of practice specialty, will encounter patient infected with STIs. All providers should maintain a working knowledge of current CDC guidelines in order to provide appropriate testing and treatment. . . . Preventing STIs and correctly identifying patients is critical to reducing the prevalence and potentially negative outcomes of these infections. Clear communication between healthcare providers performing STI-testing in all settings is essential to meeting this goal. (Goodman, 2018)

A 2015 American Academy of Physician Assistants (AAPA) Abstract had the stated goal to "increase the number of PA providers capable of providing high quality care to patients with HIV and other STIs." Their study concluded that "Focused training in infectious diseases increased the knowledge, comfort, and skills of PA students and generally improved as the level of training increased" (Swatzell, 2015).

OPPORTUNISTIC INFECTIONS

Opportunistic infections (OIs) were much more frequent and had higher rates of morbidity and mortality in the earlier years of HIV. And although we would like to believe that OIs are a thing of the past, unfortunately they are not.

Carolyn Savini, MSN, FNP, AAHIVS, Beverly Harrington, MSH, FNP-C, and Susan Wilson, ACRN, remind us in a review of Kaposi's sarcoma (KS) in ART-naïve patients that " 'Although recent observational studies report an increase in non–AIDS-defining cancers in HIV patients, clinicians should be reminded that KS continues to occur in the post-HAART era, especially in patients who present later for testing and care" (Savini, 2009), a fact that remains true today.

Another increasingly rare but possible OI is progressive multifocal leukoencephalopathy (PML). In 2007, Meredith Cadorette, MMSc, PA-C, reported on a case of PML and reminds us that "PML is a demyelinating disease that affects immunosuppressed patients. . . . It is a fatal opportunistic infection that occurs in the setting of severe immunosuppression . . . the goal of treatment is restoring immune function. This case demonstrates, however, that even when immune recovery with HAART occurs, unfavorable clinical outcomes and death may still ensue" (Cadorette, 2007).

COMORBIDITIES WITH HIV

Since HAART became the standard of care in 1996, we have been working to decrease the risk of comorbidities with HIV as people now have a near-normal to normal life expectancy. The following researched articles represent both original research and review of the literature by advanced practice practitioners. They represent only a portion of the comorbidities we encounter regularly, but these data continue to emphasize the importance of NPs and PAs working in the field.

Tracy Hicks, MSH, FNP-BC, through her review of the data on major depressive disorder and HIV-positive women reminds us that "MDD is very prevalent in our society and it is imperative that providers adequately assess for symptoms of this condition. Mental illness and chronic disease such as HIV are common in primary care. A collaborative approach is needed to ameliorate segmented patient care and promote a holistic approach to treatment of these conditions" (Hicks, 2015).

In another article on HIV and mental health, Betty D. Morgan, PhD, APRN-BC, and Anne P. Rossi, APRN-BC, CARN, describe the successes and pitfalls of a collaborative approach with psychiatric advanced practice nurses and the ability of this collaboration to manage complex HIV/AIDS patients with psychiatric illness and substance abuse problems (Morgan, 2007).

Another significant comorbid area of HIV care is cardiovascular disease. HIV providers and PCPs have struggled with best practices to treat cardiovascular disease comorbidities in HIV patients for many years. In a retrospective study, Michael J. Kacka, MD, MPH; Sabra Custer DNP, MS, FNP-BC; Crystal Hughley, FNP-BC, and others reviewed atherosclerotic cardiovascular disease (ASCVD) in HIV-positive persons and reported that "ASCVD is a leading cause of death in persons living with HIV (PLWH). These patients likely have a higher risk of heart disease compared to the general population even in the setting of good virological control and have a high prevalence of traditional ASCVD risk factors including smoking, hypertension, dyslipidemia, diabetes, and excess body weight. The need for better ASCVD prevention strategies for this population is being widely recognized and represents new challenges for HIV care providers" (Kacka, 2017). Their findings point to the importance of recognizing rates of hypertension and diabetes, lifestyle factors, statin therapy by 10-year risk, and higher risk categories.

Ocular complaints, especially acute ocular complaints in an HIV-infected patient, are of particular concern. Stephanie D. Kurtz, PA-C, MMSc, and Francois Rollin, MD, MPH, review a case of ocular syphilis and make specific recommendations based on the workup and outcomes: "When evaluating a patient presenting with ocular symptoms and rash, consider syphilis in the differential. Early consultation with the appropriate specialists is key when approaching a patient with a history of HIV and sudden onset of visual complaints, as the differential diagnosis is broad, and the risk of permanent visual compromise is high" (Kurtz, 2014).

When reviewing the overall rate of non-AIDS malignancies, we see that these have increased in the post-HAART era. A report by Erich J. Grant, MMS, PA-C, et al. discusses the current literature around HIV and HPV-associated anal dysplasia. Their findings determined that, although still controversial,

"Early screening and detection of AIN (Anal intraepithelial neoplasia) is critical in preventing anal cancer. Clinician education on high risk populations and appropriate screenings is essential for proper management. Vaccination may also play a role in the prevention of HPV-related anal cancer, but more research and outcome data are needed" (Grant, 2013).

SUPPORTING THE HIV COMMUNITY

There exists several articles and summaries from bodies of work written by APPs who have commented on their support of and contributions directly to their patients and to the HIV community. My own article notes that "the healthiest provider–patient relationship is one where both patient and provider respect each other and are engaged in ongoing, long-term relationship development and sharing of information about the latest developments in HIV care" (Deckard, 2009).

An article written by Susan LeLacheur, DrPH, PA-C, reviews the history of her work with HIV/AIDS patients and the role she has played in increasing the quality of life for her patients. In summarizing her experience, she notes regarding one of her patients "I saw Tommy last week in clinic and as usual each time I see him it was all I could do to hold back tears of joy. For me he is a walking, talking, smiling reminder of what has been accomplished in HIV treatment. . . . There are many reasons patients are lost to follow-up, but I hope that a good PA may sometimes be one reason they come back" (LeLacheur, 2013).

Still another article reminds us that always taking into considerations the patient's needs and desires should be our primary concern, noting that "An HIV positive person's choice may not be ours. His or her life may not be like ours. Developing an educated, professional, empathetic response must be the rule, not the exception when dealing with an HIV positive client." And "in the end a positive difference be made. That is why our work matters" (Myers, 2013).

LEGISLATIVE ISSUES

PAs and NPs have been involved in legislative matters for many years through researching literature involving regulations and laws which impact our patient population, through white coat days, and through working directly with our local, state, and federal legislators. In 2012, I had the opportunity to investigate multiple providers throughout the state of Texas to determine the probable effect on patients of the institution of the Affordable Care Act (ACA). I concluded with "It is clear that, depending upon one's practice setting, payor sources, level of acuity and patient load, perceptions of how the ACA, and more specifically how the Medicaid expansion will effect patient care, are variably interpreted. The constant theme, however, is that no matter what one's practice affiliation, access to care is paramount. Gaining that access is clearly the challenge" (Deckard, 2012).

ORGAN TRANSPLANT IN HIV PATIENTS

In 2018, organ transplantation in the United States is more common and less stigmatized for HIV-positive persons.

R. Patrick Wood, MD, and Schawnte Williams-Taylor, RN, BSN, CCRN, summarize the current state of organ procurement and transplantation availability by stating "Creating awareness of the opportunities for organ donation by individuals living with HIV is vital to saving lives as well as gaining more information through medical research. Individuals with HIV are encouraged to register to be organ donors on the national donor registry, www.donatelife.net or on their state organ donor registry. It is also important to note that once an individual signs up on the donor registry, this serves as first person authorization and their decision to be an organ donor cannot be revoked by their next of kin" (Wood, 2018).

SUMMARY

When we look at the past six decades of clinical service to our patients, both HIV-impacted and non–HIV-impacted, advanced practice providers—both PAs and NPs—have delivered high-level, equitable clinical outcomes to the population served.

Their contributions have been reviewed and acknowledged by multiple medical organizations, and these organizations have consistently shown excellent outcomes for healthcare delivered.

They have made contributions to practice and to the research in virtually every part of HIV/AIDS medicine: comorbidities with HIV; prevention; treatment research; epidemiology; social, cultural, and gender determinants data; legislative issues; and workforce and in additional original research.

NPs and PAs represent a growing percentage of healthcare professionals caring for HIV/AIDS patients, and they also hold growing numbers of positions within medical practices and medical organizations, providing an increasing voice in medical decision-making and advocacy for our patients. PAs and NPs work in most practice settings in collaboration with other healthcare professionals and adjunctive clinicians and with larger clinical care teams to provide best practices outcomes.

The American Academy of HIV Medicine (AAHIVM) which is the only HIV credentialing body in the United States for HIV specialists, recognizes the importance of the advanced practice providers and their level of knowledge, expertise, and clinical outcomes. To that extent, the AAHIVM recognizes that its credentialing exam applies the title of HIV Specialist (AAHIVS) to physicians, PAs, and NPs working in direct clinical care with the HIV population.

REFERENCES

American Academy of Nurse Practitioners. NP fact sheet. Available at https://www.aanp.org/all-about-nps/np-fact-sheet. Accessed August 1, 2018.

American Association of Nurse Practitioners. Historical timeline. Available at https://www.aanp.org/about/about-the-american-association-of-nurse-practitioners-aanp/historical-timeline.

American Academy of Nurse Practitioners. International NP resources. Available at https://www.aanp.org/international.

American Academy of PAs. Website. Available at Aapa.org. Accessed August 1, 2018.

Andrews MA, Dominguez AJ. Social media as a cost-effective outreach tool for high risk populations. HIV awareness in the MSM community. *HIV Specialist.* July 2018;10(2):30–32.

Baker J. Stay current with options for HIV prevention. *JAAPA.* 2013;26(12):14–20.

Baker J, O'Hara KM. Oral preexposure prophylaxis to prevent HIV infection: clinical and public health implications. *JAAPA.* 2014;27(12):10–17.

Cadorette M. A rare, opportunistic disease in a patient with AIDS. *JAAPA.* 2007;20(7):29–32.

Claborn KR, Aston ER, Champion J, et al. Prescribing opioids as an incentive to retain patients in medical care: a qualitative investigation into clinician awareness and perceptions [published online ahead of print June 5, 2018]. *J Assoc Nurses AIDS Care.* September-October 2018;29(5):642–654. doi: 10.1016/j.jana.2018.05.010.

Cook PF, Schmiege SJ, Bradley-Springer L, et al. Motivation as a mechanism for daily experiences' effects on HIV medication adherence. *J Assoc Nurses AIDS Care.* 2018;29(3):383–393.

Cooper RA. Health care workforce for the twenty-first century: the impact of nonphysician clinicians. *Annu Rev Med.* 2001;52:51–61.

Deckard DT. ACA in the state of Texas: perceptions and concerns. *HIV Specialist.* October 2012. Available at https://aahivm.org/wp-content/uploads/2017/03/HIVspecialist_2012_FINAL.pdf. Accessed September 29, 2018.

Deckard DT. Empowerment & encouragement in HIV care. *HIV Specialist.* Winter 2009. Available athttps://aahivm.org.

Deckard DT. Prevention with positives: where we are now. *HIV Specialist.* Fall 2013. Available at https://aahivm.org. Accessed August 15, 2018.

Ferron P, Young S, Boulanger C, et al. Integrated care of an aging HIV-infected male-to-female transgender patient [published online ahead of print March, 19, 2010. *J Assoc Nurses AIDS Care.* 2010;21(3):278–282. doi: 10.1016/j.jana.2009.12.004.

Gallant JE, Adimora AA, et al. Essential components of effective HIV care: a policy paper of the HIV Medicine Association of the Infectious Diseases Society of America and the Ryan White Medical Providers Coalition. *Clin Infect Dis.* 2011;53(11):1043–1050.

Gilman B, Bouchery E, Hogan P, et al. Supply and demand projections from 2010 to 2015. August 2016. *HIV Specialist.* Available at https://wwww.aahivm.org.

Goodman K, Black CM. Patient knowledge of STI testing in an urban clinic. *JAAPA* 2018;31(4):36–41.

Grant EJ, Javier JT, Kelley PA, et al. An approach to managing HPV-associated anal dysplasia. *JAAPA.* August 2013;26(8):62–63.

Hicks T. Major depressive disorder and HIV positive women: how well are we assessing? *HIV Specialist.* July 2015. Available athttps://mydigitalpublication.com/publication/?i=266229 {"issue_id":"266229,""page":26}. Accessed September 29, 2018.

Jackson S. HIV & aging older women. . . living in the shadows. *HIV Specialist.* July 2015. Available at https://mydigitalpublication.com/publication/?i=266229 {"issue_id":"266229,""page":32. Accessed September 29, 2018.

Johnson LB, Valenti SE. Routine testing: not so fast. Spring 2010. *HIV Specialist.* https://www.aahivm.org.

Kacka MJ, Custer S, Gustafson E, et al. Preventing heart disease. how HIV clinics can improve primary prevention. *HIV Specialist.* December 2017. Available athttps://mydigitalpublication.com/publication/?i=464973 {"issue_id":464973,"page":32}.Accessed September 29, 2018.

Kayingo G, Bruce RD. HIV testing at a community health center before and after implementing universal screening. *JAAPA.* 2016;29(8):45–46.

Kurtz SD, Rollin F. Ocular syphilis in a patient with HIV. *JAAPA.* 2014;27(4):32–35.

LeLachur S. Why my work matters. *HIV Specialist.* 2013. Available at https://mydigitalpublication.com/publication/?i=181566 {"issue_id":181566,"page":42}. Accessed September 29, 2018.

Maldonado A. Initiating HIV antiretroviral therapy: criteria, evidence, and controversy based on efficacy data, durability of viral suppression, tolerability and toxicity profiles. *JAAPA.* 2011;24(2):26–30.

Myers J. Growing old with HIV: the AIDS epidemic and an aging population. *JAAPA.* 2009;22(1):20–24.

Morgan BD, Rossi AP. Difficult-to-manage HIV/AIDS clients with psychiatric illness and substance abuse problems: a collaborative practice with psychiatric advanced practice nurses. *J Assoc Nurses AIDS Care.* November-December 2007;18(6):77–84.

National Commission on Certification of Physician Assistants. 2016 Statistical profile of certified physician assistants: an annual report of the National Commission on Certification of Physician Assistants. March 2017. Available at http://www.nccpa.net/research. Accessed August 1, 2018.

Nolan T. Beliefs, borders and barriers. An HIV healthcare provider's guide to helping Latino patients. *HIV Specialist.* April 2013. Available athttps://mydigitalpublication.com/publication/?i=152014 {"issue_id":152014,"page":18}. Accessed September 29, 2018.

O'Hara KM. HIV exceptionalism and ethical concerns surrounding HIV testing. *JAAPA.* 2011;24(4):66–68.

Parisi D, Warren B, Yin S, et al. A multicomponent approach to evaluating a Pre-exposure Prophylaxis (PrEP) implementation program in five agencies in New York [published online ahead of print June 16, 2017]. *J Assoc Nurses AIDS Care.* 2018;29(1):10–19. doi: 10.1016/j.jana.2017.06.006.

Physician Assistant Historical Society. Timeline. Available at https://pahx.org/timeline/. Accessed August 1, 2018.

Poteat T. At the forefront. Risk factors: Black MSM. *HIV Specialist.* Published Fall 2009. Available at https://aahivm.org/wp-content/uploads/2017/03/HIVSpecialistMagazineFall2009.pdf. Accessed September 28, 2018.

Riendeau Lazar N, Tanney M. Challenges of medication adherence in HIV+ adolescents. *HIV Specialist.* October 2015. Available at https://mydigitalpublication.com/publication/?i=279325 {"issue_id":279325,"page":10}. Accessed September 29, 2018.

Savini C, Harrington B, Wilson S. Kaposi's sarcoma in treatment naïve HIV patients. *HIV Specialist.* Published 2009. Available at https://aahivm.org/wp-content/uploads/2017/03/HIVSpecialistMagazine Winter2009.pdf Pages 20–21. Accessed September 29, 2018.

Schmidt E, Rizzolo D. Disease screening and prevention for transgender and gender-diverse adults. *JAAPA.* 2017;30(10):11–16.

Sherra KH, Miceka MA, Gimbel SO, et al. Quality of HIV care provided by non-physician clinicians and physicians in Mozambique: a retrospective cohort study. *AIDS.* January 2010;24(Suppl 1): S59–S66. doi:10.1097/01.aids.0000366083.75945.07.

Spinner GF. The HIV care continuum. *HIV Specialist.* October 2017. Available athttps://mydigitalpublication.com/publication/?i=450299 {"issue_id":450299,"page":14}. Accessed September 29, 2018.

Spinner GF. Potential for PrEP. *HIV Specialist.* April 2015. Available athttps://mydigitalpublication.com/publication/?i=253079 {"issue_id":253079,"page":14}. Accessed September 29, 2018.

Swatzell KE, Caruthers KL, Baddley JW. Increasing the knowledge, comfort, and skills of PA students in the management of patients with HIV and other sexually transmitted infections. Poster session presented at the American Academy of Physician Assistants Annual Meeting, 2015.

Thompson JW. HIV/AIDS—Tale of two souths and the great equalizer. April 2014. Available athttps://mydigitalpublication.com/publication/?i=205250 {"issue_id":205250,"page":18}. Accessed September 29, 2018.

Weidel JJ, Provencio-Vasquez E, Watson SD, et al. Cultural considerations for intimate partner violence and HIV risk in Hispanics. *J Assoc Nurses AIDS Care.* July-August 2008;19(4):247–251.

Wesp L, Dimant O, Cook TE. Excellence in the care of trans patients: expanding the base of gender-affirming healthcare professionals. *HIV Specialist.* July 2016. Available athttps://mydigitalpublication.com/publication/?i=321747 {"issue_id":321747,"page":12}. Accessed September 29, 2018.

Wilson IB, Landon BE, Hirschhorn LR, et al. Quality of HIV care provided by nurse practitioners, physician assistants, and physicians. *Ann Intern Med.* 2005;143:729–736.

Wood RP, Williams-Taylor S. Organ procurement organizations are spreading the word of hope. *HIV Specialist.* 2018. Available at https://aahivm.org/wp-content/uploads/2018/07/FINALHIVspecialist_July2018FINAL-1.pdf. Accessed September 29, 2018.

Zadel J. Outside your native culture. *HIV Specialist.* April 2013. Available athttps://mydigitalpublication.com/publication/?i=152014 {"issue_id":152014,"page":44}. Accessed September 29, 2018.

18.

HOSPICE AND PALLIATIVE CARE IN ADVANCED HIV DISEASE

Paul W. DenOuden

CHAPTER GOALS

Upon completion of this chapter, the reader should be able to

- Demonstrate knowledge about both hospice and palliative care options in the context of end-stage HIV disease.

- Know when each option may be best appropriate.

- Optimally counsel and educate patients and their families in an effective, professional, and sensitive manner.

CARING FOR THE TERMINALLY ILL PATIENT

In the early years of the HIV/AIDS epidemic, caring for the terminally ill patient was a regular and inevitable part of HIV/AIDS care because the disease would progressively advance to end stages in the pretreatment era. Most HIV/AIDS clinicians were dealing with terminal illness on a daily basis, and, in dealing with multiple and recurrent opportunistic infections, there would come a point when the focus changed to palliative/hospice care. Many US cities had multiple AIDS hospices for terminally ill patients. As treatment evolved and became increasingly successful, and especially from the late 1990s onward as death rates plummeted, many hospices closed or changed their focus to skilled nursing, and the daily focus of clinicians became much more geared toward ongoing care of stable patients. However, given the still significant death rates and changing dynamics of causes of mortality in HIV/AIDS patients, it is still important for HIV/AIDS clinicians to be comfortable with and fluent in caring for patients with terminal illnesses. The numbers of end-stage opportunistic infections have decreased, whereas the numbers patients with malignancies, end-stage liver disease, cardiovascular disease, and age-related comorbidities have increased.

It is important to not lose focus on maintaining a close provider–patient relationship in the transition to terminal illness; the provider not only has a responsibility to the patient to journey with him or her through chronic illness to recovery, stabilization, or death but also has a responsibility to him- or herself to do so. By caring for the dying and attempting to provide patients with "good" deaths, physicians may feel a sense of professional satisfaction. Providing good end-of-life care makes physicians better communicators, helping them to better understand and treat suffering while offering them a deeper understanding of the nature of life (Block, 2001; Cherny, 1996).

It is important to reassure patients that they will not be abandoned when hospice care has begun. Patients and their families usually prefer their primary physicians to stay in contact until death, even if the main tasks of palliative care are taken on by another clinician (Han, 2005). Maintaining contact throughout the dying process is most likely the best policy, within reasonable bounds of previous clinical involvement (Quill, 1995).

KEY POINTS

- Palliative care can be accessed at any stage of illness to alleviate ongoing or severe symptoms even in the absence of a terminal illness.

- Hospice care involves an interdisciplinary approach to diagnosing and managing suffering and addressing the physical, psychosocial, and spiritual needs of patients and their families at the end of life.

- Hospice care should be considered when no further interventions or treatments can cure or prolong the life of a terminally ill patient with an estimated life expectancy of 6 months or less.

- Making the decision for hospice care is often challenging for the patient, family, and clinicians alike in the modern antiretroviral therapy (ART) era.

HOSPICE CARE

DEFINITION OF HOSPICE CARE

Hospice care is defined as a comprehensive system of care for patients with limited life expectancy. This system is flexible and can take place either at home or in an inpatient care facility (hospital or nursing home). Hospice care works from a biopsychosocial model rather than a disease model, and it focuses on comfort, dignity, and personal growth at life's end. This encompasses biomedical, psychosocial, and spiritual aspects of the dying experience, emphasizing quality of life and healing or strengthening of interpersonal relationships rather than prolonging the dying process at any cost. A quality hospice program comprises an interdisciplinary team of experts that deals with all aspects of the dying process (Emanuel, 2005).

Often, people may interchange the terms "palliative care" and "hospice care." *Palliative care* is used to address suffering at any stage of illness, from diagnosis to recovery or death. *Hospice* is a formal structured environment for delivering quality palliative care at the end of life.

INDICATIONS FOR HOSPICE CARE

In the early days of the HIV epidemic in the United States, death was common and survival unusual. Advances in ART and treatment of AIDS-related illnesses have resulted in dramatic increases in the life expectancy of HIV-infected people. Unfortunately, several end-stage conditions remain very difficult to treat in patients with extensive antiretroviral resistance or in patients who refuse or cannot tolerate medications. It may be appropriate in these circumstances to discuss end-stage options. In this way, hospice care can focus on comfort and quality of life rather than on treatments with uncomfortable side effects and no further benefit.

One study found that the cause of death of HIV-infected patients in the ART era is increasingly likely to be a chronic medical condition such as hepatic failure or malignancies, with "traditional" opportunistic infections (OIs) declining in importance (Sansone, 2000). Crum and colleagues found that 80% of pre-ART deaths were related to AIDS-defining conditions. This declined to 65% in the early post-ART era and reduced further to 56% in the late post-ART era (Crum, 2006).

Since the advent of ART, the biology of HIV and AIDS has shifted, requiring both patients and healthcare providers to consider the cumulative impact of chronic HIV infection and the long-term side effects of treatment. With longer life spans, people with HIV have become prone to diseases of aging—such as heart disease, diabetes, and osteoporosis—and to progressive conditions such as chronic viral hepatitis (Highleyman, 2005). Chronic viral hepatitis can lead to end-stage liver damage as patients coinfected with HIV and hepatitis B virus and/or hepatitis C virus live longer. Liver problems can also be related to antiretroviral drug toxicity, and ART can increase the risk of cardiovascular disease due to the blood lipid and glucose elevations associated with therapies that include protease inhibitors (Highleyman, 2005).

These changes in end-stage disease have resulted in changes in the approach that caregivers take to their HIV patients and, thus, in how physicians and other clinicians discuss end-of-life options with their patients as they reach the terminal phases of disease. However, it is important to keep in mind that AIDS-defining conditions may still appear, especially toward the end of life, and prevention and treatment of OIs will still have a role in the end-of-life care (Welch, 2002).

ADVANTAGES OF HOSPICE CARE

Hospice and palliative care comprise an interdisciplinary approach to the diagnosis and management of suffering. *Suffering* is a multidimensional disorder of consciousness that includes physical, psychosocial, and spiritual elements. The unit of care in palliative care is the patient–caregiver dyad, with the needs of the family and loved ones being addressed along with the needs of the patient (Emanuel, 2005). Given that there is still stigma associated with HIV/AIDS and that, for many reasons, families are sometimes alienated from HIV/AIDS patients, special care needs to be taken with family dynamics issues that often come to the fore in hospice care with this population. As the usefulness of medical treatments diminishes, the effectiveness of psychosocial and spiritual interventions increases (Peterson, 1996).

When a patient becomes progressively weaker despite treatment, it is time to consider hospice care. Early hospice evaluation can provide great comfort to the patient and his or her loved ones. Palliative care clinicians are experts in pain and symptom management and can usually improve the patient's level of comfort. If symptoms do not respond to conventional medical therapy, addressing psychological and spiritual suffering may benefit the patient. Alternative and complementary therapies may be used, including relaxation, music therapy, meditation, herbal therapy, and acupuncture (Chesney, 1994; O'Neill, 1997).

It takes time to prepare for a good death, and the earlier a hospice referral is made, the more likely the patient will be able to benefit. Unfortunately, the average length of stay in hospice is only 2 weeks, which may be an indication of missed opportunities for referral.

Understanding, reconciliation, acceptance, and, for many, spiritual growth at the end of life may provide great comfort. Table 18.1 lists many of the practical issues involved in the care of dying patients (Cherny, 1996).

Many patients with terminal illnesses prefer to die at home, and patients and their families may want to consider end-of-life care at home using an interdisciplinary care management approach. Home hospice services can be cost-effective and can enhance quality of life for terminally ill patients with HIV (Huba, 1998). Home hospice care usually requires stable housing and willing family, partners, or friends to help with the dying process at home. Sometimes this can be challenging to accomplish for many social reasons, even if a patient is interested in pursuing home hospice.

DIFFICULTIES OF HOSPICE IN THE ART ERA

With the use of ART, death is less common and often less anticipated. Poor outcome is often related to nonadherence, and feelings of guilt and other emotional responses can become a major issue for the patient and the caregiver. People dying of HIV tend to be younger and often suffer from depression and other mental illnesses that need evaluation and treatment.

Several issues can lead to difficult deaths, including the biology of HIV disease, provider and system barriers to accepting hospice care, family issues, and patients' values and choices. Patients can experience dramatic improvement even when close to death; however, deaths from comorbid conditions such as hepatitis and cancer are often more abrupt, unpredictable, and devastating (Karascz, 2003).

Many patients and providers may be very reluctant to abandon research and experimental treatment options even in

Table 18.1 PRACTICAL ISSUES TO BE ADDRESSED
IN THE CARE OF DYING PATIENTS

ISSUE	SPECIFICS TO BE ADDRESSED
Communication	With patient With family With other participating caregivers
Symptom control	Physical Psychological Existential
Evaluation of family well-being	Coping Resources
Evaluation of therapeutic plan	Primary therapies Supportive pharmacotherapies Hydration and nutrition
Contingency planning	Crisis planning Addressing do-not-resuscitate orders
Ongoing care planning	Home/inpatient Home care backup Observation 24-Hour availability of clinician with decision-making authority

SOURCE: Adapted from Cherny et al. (1996) with permission from Elsevier.

the late stages of disease. There is evidence that even patients with severe immunosuppression, very low CD4 cell counts, high viral loads, and/or symptomatic AIDS can still derive significant benefit from ART (Highleyman, 2005). This further complicates the choice to seek hospice care. Many people arrive at the end of life stripped of assets. Although hospice can find community support and provide services not covered by ordinary government and private insurance, most insurance coverage of hospice care, following the lead of Medicare rules, generally prohibits curative options for those seeking coverage for hospice and palliative care at the end of life (Scalia-Foley, 2004).

Patients may face very difficult decisions in choosing to stop ART, both for symptom control and psychological reasons, because so many have been conditioned to stay fully adherent and never stop ART and the complications with hospice coverage make it more difficult to decide how they and their physicians should best face this challenge (Karascz, 2003). Patients with advanced HIV frequently do not fit the cancer model on which hospice often rests. For these patients, an insurance program that requires cessation of ART or will not cover other treatments is often problematic and may result in difficulty in planning and decision-making. Generally, ART is not covered under the Medicare hospice benefit.

PALLIATIVE CARE

Palliative care is often a major part of hospice care, but it can and should be used for any suffering patients even if they are not actively in hospice. Palliative care has been defined by the World Health Organization (WHO, 1990) as

the active total care of patients whose disease is not responsive to curative treatment. Control of pain, of

other symptoms, and of psychological, social, and spiritual problems, is paramount. The goal of palliative care is to achieve the best quality of life for patients and their families.

The subset of palliative care tailored to the terminally ill and associated with hospice care is more accurately termed "end-of-life care." Many end-stage symptoms can be successfully treated in a palliative care setting, making the end of life as comfortable as possible for terminally ill hospice patients. Common and distressing symptoms in terminally ill patients can often be easily managed.

The use of non-oral routes of medication delivery can be helpful in a palliative setting for other symptom management in addition to pain control. Examples of non-oral administration include rectal administration (prochlorperazine suppositories for nausea and diazepam suppositories for agitation), sublingual administration (lorazepam for hiccups or agitation), or subcutaneous/intramuscular administration (clonazepam or haloperidol for acute agitation) (Enck, 2002; Woodruff, 1999).

The following sections describe several common symptoms to be aware of and focus on when providing palliative care to a patient.

Pain

A common fear of patients is that of pain. There are many medication approaches to pain control, and a common treatment model is given by the WHO in its report on cancer pain relief and palliative care (WHO, 1990).

In the terminal phase of disease, oral medications become more difficult for patients, and alternate routes such as the transdermal approach have been shown to be safe and effective in patients with HIV (Newshan, 2001). Another widely used route for effective pain medication delivery is continuous subcutaneous infusion, which is common in the hospice setting and has many potential advantages, including ease of administration/access, decreased infection site complications, less volume overload, and lower cost (Herndon, 2001). Other modalities of pain control in addition to classic opiates are important to remember to optimize effective pain management for patients.

OPIATES	NEUROPATHIC PAIN MEDS	ADJUVANT TREATMENTS
Codeine	Carbamazepine	Acetaminophen
Fentanyl	Duloxetine	Acupuncture
Hydromorphone	Gabapentin	Benzodiazepines
Methadone	Pregabalin	Cannabinoids
Morphine	Tricyclics	Corticosteroids
Oxycodone	Valproic acid	Focal Radiation
Oxymorphone		Lidocaine (topical) Muscle relaxants Nonsteroidal anti-inflammatories (NSAIDs)

Seizures

In patients whose terminal AIDS condition involves intracerebral masses or central nervous system (CNS) infections such as toxoplasmosis or CNS lymphoma, seizures can be a frequent symptom requiring management. There are several common antiepileptic drugs, and because no one drug has shown superiority over the others, they are often used interchangeably, with substitution as needed for lack of effectiveness or side effects (Krouwer, 2000). Adding or increasing corticosteroids to treat related peritumoral edema may be indicated if seizures are occurring with a therapeutic antiepileptic drug level (Krouwer, 2000).

Depression, Fatigue, and Sleep Disturbance

Depression, fatigue, and sleep disturbance are all common and interrelated symptoms that can be addressed effectively in palliative care. Because fatigue and sleep difficulties are common manifestations of depression, effective standard antidepressant treatment (e.g., with a selective serotonin reuptake inhibitor [SSRI] or other appropriate psychopharmacologics) may need to be instituted (see Chapter 39 on psychiatric complications). Psychostimulants (e.g., methylphenidate or dextroamphetamine) have been studied in the palliative care setting and have been found to be effective in treating depression, opioid-induced sedation, and fatigue. Often dosed in the morning and early afternoon, psychostimulants may improve the cognition, neuropsychological function, and energy of terminally ill patients and allow for better quality of life and interaction with loved ones during the final days of life (Dein, 2002).

Delirium

Another related CNS symptom that many hospice patients experience is delirium, which is defined as a transient disorder of cognition and attention, often accompanied by disruption of the normal sleep–wake cycle (Enck, 2002). The causes of delirium are broad and include metabolic disturbances; acute infection and fever; brain metastases; hypoxia; and side effects of drugs frequently used in palliation, such as opiates and corticosteroids (Enck, 2002; Woodruff, 1999).

Management should be directed at the suspected cause; for example, if hypoxia is suspected, empiric oxygen can be administered via cannula/mask, and if a drug side effect is implicated, nonessential medications can be discontinued or the opioid changed (Woodruff, 1999). Sedation may be necessary to alleviate severe agitation, and neuroleptics, most commonly haloperidol (which can be given orally, intravenously, or intramuscularly as needed), are effective and can be titrated individually (Woodruff, 1999). In the last few days of life, an agitated delirium often termed "terminal restlessness" occurs in some patients (Woodruff, 1999). Benzodiazepines are commonly used in this situation because they specifically aid in relieving myoclonus, seizure activity, and restlessness. There are many options with varying half-lives and many possible routes of delivery, such as diazepam rectal suppository, sublingual lorazepam, and subcutaneous clonazepam.

Pruritus

Pruritus is common and may be a symptom of dry skin, underlying organ dysfunction or tumor, or induced by opioid use (Krajnik, 2001; WHO, 1998). Directed treatment often includes topical steroid creams and emollients for dry skin (WHO, 1998). Systemic antihistamines, corticosteroids, and even SSRIs have been found to be of benefit (Krajnik, 2001; WHO, 1998). Nursing care for the skin can include colloidal oatmeal soap baths and warm compresses for comfort.

Dry Mouth

Dry mouth or oral mucosa breakdown has many etiologies, and symptom relief can be quite helpful for patient comfort. Often in advanced HIV, infections contribute to this problem, and treatment is related to the specific cause, for example, antifungals for oral candidiasis or antivirals for herpes simplex ulcers. Mouthwashes, hydration techniques such as use of ice chips or popsicles, and oral hygiene using mouth swabs called toothettes can also lessen discomfort (WHO, 1998). Painful aphthous ulcers can be aided by topical corticosteroid Orabase and local analgesic agents (WHO, 1998), such as viscous lidocaine; use of thalidomide has also been shown to be effective in patients with AIDS (Woodruff, 1999).

Hiccups

Hiccups can be difficult and multifactorial in nature. Promoting gastric emptying with metoclopramide can help (Kinzbrunner, 2002). Treating esophagitis, a common cause of hiccups in advanced HIV (Albrecht, 1994), can be accomplished with antifungals and antacids as appropriate. Symptomatic treatment often includes chlorpromazine or baclofen trials to calm the CNS response (Kinzbrunner, 2002).

Dyspnea

Dyspnea is a common end-of-life symptom and can be an unpleasant sensation causing much anxiety to the patient, which often exacerbates the breathlessness. As with other symptoms, the causes are highly variable, and treatment is always directed to the root cause when known. For example, diuretics may be helpful in cases of congestive heart failure or fluid overload, and significant pleural effusions can be drained for symptom relief. If bronchospasm is noted, inhaled bronchodilators can be used, often in nebulized form with a mask if the patient is unable to use a metered-dose inhaler; systemic corticosteroids can also cause effective bronchodilation. Oxygen therapy is of benefit if the patient is hypoxic (e.g., pulse oximeter saturation <90%) and can be titrated for comfort via either nasal prongs or face mask.

Many patients may remain dyspneic even with oxygen use and other interventions, and the use of morphine may be indicated for the relief of continued respiratory symptoms rather than solely for pain control because morphine has been shown to decrease the respiratory rate and sensation of air hunger. Morphine also has the benefit of administration via the oral, subcutaneous, intravenous, intramuscular, or even the nebulized route. The anxiety that accompanies and often worsens dyspnea can be managed using any of the benzodiazepines via any appropriate route and timing schedule (Enck, 2002; Woodruff, 1999).

The final stages of the dying process are variable but commonly involve irregular or Cheyne–Stokes respirations and difficulty in clearing upper airway secretions. The sounds made by these retained secretions during respiration in this phase, often referred to as "death rattle" or "tracheal secretions," may be quite disturbing to family and caregivers of the terminally ill patient. Standard measures to reduce this potentially disquieting sound include positioning, decreasing parenteral hydration, and gentle suctioning, as well as antisecretory drug therapy. Several anticholinergic drugs have been reported to be successful, including scopolamine, atropine, and hyoscyamine (Wildiers, 2002).

Nausea

Intractable nausea is common in end-stage AIDS (Karus, 2005), and often the source of the nausea is elusive. The many possible causes of discomfort, including both side effects from therapies and direct effects of opportunistic infections, make therapies difficult to generalize (Karus, 2005; Reiter, 1996). The most effective method is to begin with a phenothiazine such as prochlorperazine or trimethobenzamide, increase the dose to the highest tolerable level, and then add another agent of a different class. Many classes of antiemetics are effective, including butyrophenones, benzodiazepines, benzamides, and cannabinoids. However, simultaneous use of three or four agents may be needed to provide adequate relief (Reiter, 1996).

REFERENCES

Block SD. Perspectives on care at the close of life. Psychological considerations, growth, and transcendence at the end of life: the art of the possible. *JAMA*. 2001;285:2898–2905.

Cherny NI, Coyle N, Foley KM. Guidelines in the care of the dying cancer patient. *Hematol Oncol Clin North Am*. 1996;10:261–286.

Chesney MA, Folkman S. Psychological impact of HIV disease and implications for intervention. *Psychiatr Clin North Am*. 1994;17:163–182.

Crum NF, Riffenburgh RH, Wegner S, et al. Comparisons of causes of death and mortality rates among HIV-infected persons: analysis of the pre-, early, and late HAART (highly active antiretroviral therapy) eras. *J AIDS*. 2006;41:194–200.

Dein S, George R. A place for psychostimulants in palliative care? *J Palliat Care*. 2002; 18:196–199.

Emanuel LL, Ferris FD, von Gunten CF, Von Roenn J. *EPEC-O: education in palliative and end-of-life care—oncology*. Chicago: The EPEC Project; 2005.

Enck RE. *The medical care of terminally ill patients*. 2nd ed. Baltimore: Johns Hopkins University Press; 2002.

Han PK, Arnold RM. Palliative care services, patient abandonment, and the scope of physicians' responsibilities in end-of-life care. *J Palliat Med*. 2005;8:1238–1245.

Herndon CM, Fike DS. Continuous subcutaneous infusion practices of United States hospices. *J Pain Symptom Manage*. 2001;22:1027–1034.

Highleyman L. Mortality trends: toward a new definition of AIDS? *BETA*. 2005;17:18–28.

Huba GJ, Cherin DA, Melchior LA. Retention of clients in service under two models of home health care for HIV/AIDS. *Home Health Care Serv Q*. 1998;17:17–26.

Karascz A, Dyche L, Selwyn P. Physicians' experiences of caring for late-stage HIV patients in the post-HAART era: challenges and adaptations. *Soc Sci Med*. 2003;57:1609–1620.

Karus D, Raveis DH, Alexander C, et al. Patient reports of symptoms and their treatment at three palliative care projects servicing individuals with HIV/AIDS. *J Pain Symptom Manage*. 2005;30:408–417.

Kinzbrunner BM, Weinreb NJ, Policzer JS, eds. *Twenty common problems in end-of-life care*. New York: McGraw-Hill; 2002.

Krajnik M, Zylicz Z. Understanding pruritus in systemic disease. *J Pain Symptom Manage*. 2001;21:151–168.

Krouwer HG, Pallagi JL, Graves NM. Management of seizures in brain tumor patients at the end of life. *J Palliat Med*. 2000;3:465–475.

Newshan G, Lefkowitz M. Transdermal fentanyl for chronic pain in AIDS: a pilot study. *J Pain Symptom Manage*. 2001;21:69–77.

O'Neill JF, Alexander CS. Palliative medicine and HIV/AIDS. *Prim Care*. 1997;24:607–615.

Peterson JL, Folkman S, Bakeman R. Stress, coping, HIV status, psychosocial resources, and depressive mood in African American gay, bisexual, and heterosexual men. *Am J Community Psychol*. 1996;24:461–487.

Quill TE, Cassel CK. Nonabandonment: a central obligation for physicians. *Ann Intern Med*. 1995;122:368–374.

Reiter GS, Kudler NR. Palliative care and HIV. Part II: systemic manifestations and late-stage issues. *AIDS Clin Care*. 1996;8:27–30, 33, 36.

Sansone GR, Frengley JD. Impact of HAART on causes of death of persons with late-stage AIDS. *J Urban Health*. 2000;77:166–175.

Scala-Foley MA, Caruso JT, Archer D, Reinhard SC. Medicare's hospice benefits: when cure is no longer the goal, Medicare will cover palliative care. *Am J Nurs*. 2004;104:66–67.

Welch K, Morse A. The clinical profile of end-stage AIDS in the era of highly active antiretroviral therapy. *AIDS Patient Care STDS*. 2002;16:75–81.

Wildiers H, Menten J. Death rattle: prevalence, prevention and treatment. *J Pain Symptom Manage*. 2002;23:310–317.

Woodruff R. *Palliative medicine: symptomatic and supportive care for patients with advanced cancer and AIDS*. Oxford: Oxford University Press; 1999.

World Health Organization (WHO). Cancer pain relief and palliative care. Report of a WHO expert committee. *World Health Organ Tech Rep Ser*. 1990;804:1–75.

World Health Organization (WHO). *Symptom relief in terminal illness*. Geneva: World Health Organization; 1998.

19.

HIV VIROLOGY

Schuyler Livingston, Martin Markowitz, William Wright, Benjamin Young, Poonam Mathur, and Bruce L. Gilliam

---

CHAPTER GOALS

Upon completion of this chapter, the reader should be able to

- Demonstrate and apply knowledge about established and evolving science describing HIV virology, both in the cell and in the host.

- Effectively counsel and educate patients and their communities regarding HIV treatment.

HIV STRUCTURE AND LIFE CYCLE

LEARNING OBJECTIVE

Discuss basic HIV virology and its relevance to current and potential drug targets.

WHAT'S NEW?

Expanded discussion of reverse transcription, viral integration, and viral production is presented.

KEY POINTS

- HIV is a member of the lentivirus subfamily of retroviruses.

- The HIV life cycle can be divided into two phases: (1) virus entry, reverse transcription, entry into the nucleus, and integration of double-stranded DNA (the provirus); and (2) regulation of production of viral proteins and new infectious virions.

- HIV enters the cell via the CD4 receptor and chemokine coreceptors, primarily CCR5 and CXCR4.

- The viral genome is transcribed from RNA to DNA by reverse transcriptase and integrated into the host genome by integrase.

- The HIV genome encodes 15 proteins comprising three categories: structural, regulatory, and accessory.

- After budding from the host cell, the virus matures into its infectious form through cleavage of viral precursor proteins by protease.

VIRAL CLASSIFICATION

Human immunodeficiency virus (HIV) is a member of the lentivirus subfamily of retroviruses; it is distinct from HTLV-1 and HTLV-2, which are members of oncoviruses. Two distinct groups of lentiviruses are pathogenic in humans: HIV-1 and HIV-2. Both are transmitted sexually and known to cause immunodeficiency disease. HIV-2 is less pathogenic and epidemiologically distinct from HIV-1, as it was first isolated from patients in West Africa. Subsequent discussion, therefore, focuses on HIV-1 infection and pathogenesis.

HIV-1 can be subclassified into three groups: M (major), O (outlier), and N (non-M, non-O) (Simon, 1998). The vast majority of HIV-1 infections belong to group M. Group M has at least nine known genetically distinct subtypes (or clades): A, B, C, D, F, G, H, J, and K. Occasionally, genetic material from different clades of HIV-1 may recombine within the same host to form hybrid viruses, called *circulating recombinant forms* (Salminen, 1997).

VIRAL STRUCTURE

HIV-1 is an RNA virus, and its basic genomic structure is typical of other retroviruses. The integrated form of HIV is known as the *provirus*, which is flanked at both ends by a repeated sequence known as the *long terminal repeats* (LTRs). The genes of HIV are located in the central region of the proviral DNA and encode 15 distinct proteins divided into three classes: structural proteins (Gag, Pol, and Env), regulatory proteins (Tat and Rev), and accessory proteins (Vpu, Vpr, Vif, and Nef) (Klimkait, 1990; Willey, 1992). In the mature HIV-1 virion, the inner capsid contains two molecules of single-stranded RNA and key enzymes necessary for infection: reverse transcriptase, integrase, protease, and accessory proteins (Figure 19.1). The capsid is surrounded by structural matrix protein, itself contained within the viral envelope. Composed of a phospholipid bilayer derived from the host cell, the envelope contains trimers of the viral glycoproteins gp120 and gp41. The exposed surfaces of gp120 exhibit a high level of variability, limiting the humoral immune response to circulating virus (Tilton, 2010).

VIRAL ENTRY

The viral envelope contains the necessary proteins for cell fusion and viral entry, initiating infection of the host cell. HIV

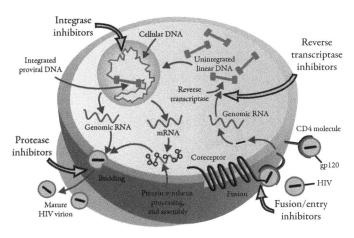

Figure 19.1. HIV life cycle and drug targets. Reproduced from Fauci 2003 with permission from Macmillan Publishers Ltd: Nat Med, copyright 2003.

gains access to its target cells via multiple interactions of viral proteins with receptors on the cell membrane (Figure 19.2). The viral glycoprotein gp120 binds with high affinity to the CD4 receptor, which normally functions as a coreceptor in the activation of helper T cells. CD4 binding induces a conformational change in gp120, exposing its binding sites for coreceptors (either CCR5 or CXCR4) on the host cell surface. Binding of gp120 to the coreceptor exposes the fusion domain of the viral glycoprotein gp41. Then, glycoprotein gp41 inserts its hydrophobic peptide into the target cell membrane, forming a pore

through which the viral capsid enters (Tavasolli, 2011). This process is known as *fusion*. Gp41 is a target of drugs that bind to this glycoprotein and prevent formation of the fusion pore.

Viral strains vary in their coreceptor usage. Those that bind the chemokine receptors CCR5 or CXCR4 are classified as R5-tropic or X4-tropic, respectively. During HIV transmission and early infection, R5-tropic strains predominate. Individuals who do not express CCR5, by virtue of genetic mutation, are highly resistant to HIV infection (Reiche, 2007). Mutant alleles in the CCR5 gene have also been shown to prevent HIV infection by creating a partially nonfunctional coreceptor for HIV entry (Liu, 1996; Samson, 1996).

Drugs that target CCR5 and bind to the coreceptor alter its interaction with gp120. However, these drugs can only be used in patients who are R5-tropic. Through further evolution within the host, some HIV strains become X4-tropic, rendering them resistant to these agents. Deletion of the CCR5 gene through stem cell transplantation or gene therapy has been a proposed mechanism for curing HIV (Deeks, 2012).

REVERSE TRANSCRIPTION AND INTEGRATION

After fusion, viral disassembly (which is distinct from and not merely the reverse of viral assembly) occurs before reverse transcription can take place. In order for HIV-1 to fully establish infection in a susceptible cell, the RNA must undergo reverse transcription into double-stranded DNA and integrate into the host genome (Tekeste, 2015). Reverse transcription

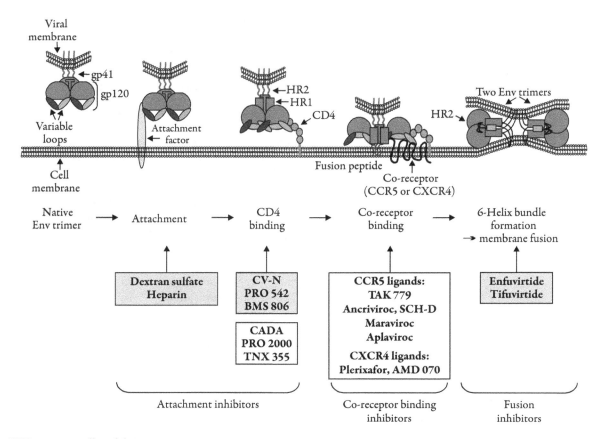

Figure 19.2 HIV entry into cells and drug targets. Reproduced from Reeves and Piefer 2005 with permission from Wolters Kluwer Health.

Table 19.1 VIRAL ACCESSORY AND REGULATORY PROTEIN FUNCTIONS

GENE	FUNCTION
Tat	Transcriptional transactivator
Rev	Allows unspliced viral genomes to leave the nucleus
Nef	Downregulates CD4 receptor and MHC class I, alters T cell activation, aids viral infectivity
Vif	Counters the host restriction factor APOBEC3G
Vpr	Facilitates the nuclear localization of the viral genome
Vpr	Downregulates CD4 receptor, increases viral release

Schwartz O, Marechal V, Le Gall S, et al. Endocytosis of major histocompatibility complex class I molecules is induced by the HIV-1 Nef protein. *Nat Med.* March 1996;2(3):338–342.
Miller MD, Feinberg MB, Greene WC. The HIV-1 nef gene acts as a positive viral infectivity factor. *Trends Microbiol.* August 1994;2(8):294–298.

starts when the viral RNA is released into the host cell cytoplasm, shedding associated proteins in a process known as *uncoating*. The viral enzyme reverse transcriptase (RT) then produces double-stranded DNA from the viral RNA template. RT is a heterodimer composed of a larger, functional subunit (p66) and a smaller, structural subunit (p51). At this stage, the host's natural antiviral immunity is activated, and the enzyme APOBEC3G, found in CD4+ T cells and macrophages, terminates the elongating viral DNA by causing hypermutations. However, HIV has the protein Vif, which binds APOBEC3G and leads to its degradation, overriding the host's natural immunity and allowing propagation of viral DNA (Table 19.1) (Tavasolli, 2011).

The newly synthesized viral DNA then integrates into the host DNA. Integration is catalyzed by integrase (IN), in conjunction with the nuclear localization factor Vpr, to form the preintegration complex. Once in the nucleus, a critical interaction between integrase and the host protein LEDGF/p75 directs this complex to the host DNA (Tavasolli, 2011), and IN mediates strand transfer, linking viral and host DNA through covalent bonds. Coopting host cell proteins, HIV relies on the cell's normal DNA repair mechanism to complete integration. Integration is a vital step in the sustained life of the virus and its progeny; IN-negative HIV mutants do not integrate and therefore do not produce infectious virions (Wiskerchen, 1995).

The newest class of antiretroviral medications are integrase strand transfer inhibitors (INSTIs), which block the penultimate step of integration by preventing strand transfer to the host DNA. Also, since it has been demonstrated in vitro that the RT-IN interaction is biologically significant for reverse transcription (Tekeste, 2015), the interaction between these two enzymes may be a target for new antiretroviral drugs.

VIRUS PRODUCTION

Once integrated into the host DNA, the viral genome can remain latent or undergo active expression. Active expression is dependent on cellular and viral factors that activate viral promotors, including coinfection with other agents, production

of inflammatory cytokines, and cellular activation (Honda, 1998). In active infection, viral DNA is first transcribed into mRNA. Some of the early mRNA produced are 2-kb in size and serve as viral regulatory proteins. These mRNAs can be detected by Northern blot analysis (Kim, 1989) or even polymerase chain reaction (PCR) (Klotman, 1991) within 6 hours of infection. Many of the same transcription factors involved in CD4+ T cell activation also bind to the HIV LTR, promoting expression of the viral genome (Pereira, 2000). The resulting mRNA is spliced, processed, and ultimately translated into viral proteins by the host cell machinery. In a positive feedback loop, the viral protein Tat (trans-activator) promotes further viral transcription by facilitating elongation of nascent viral transcripts (Kao, 1987). The viral protein Gag mediates assembly of progeny virions by packaging genomic RNA within virus particles. Finally, HIV protease catalyzes the cleavage of the gag-pol precursor polyprotein (p55), yielding the structural proteins that form the mature virion. Assembly of mature virus occurs at the cell membrane, and these virus particles exit the cell in a process known as *viral budding*. Budding occurs in areas called *lipid rafts*, located in the cell membrane, composed of high concentrations of cholesterol, sphingolipids, and glycolipids (Liao, 2001). HIV-1 generation time in vivo is 2 days, and the half-life of infected CD4+ T cells is 0.7 days (Markowitz, 2003).

Antiretroviral drugs which target virus production are protease inhibitors (PIs), and they act by preventing viral maturation into infectious particles. These agents have become critical components of antiretroviral medication regimens since they made possible the dual class combination therapy known as highly active antiretroviral therapy (HAART), and second-generation PIs have been shown to have a high genetic barrier to development of viral resistance (Wensing, 2010).

RECOMMENDED READING

Fauci AS. HIV and AIDS: 20 years of science. *Nat Med.* 2003;9(7):834–843.
Greene WC, Peterlin BM. Molecular insights into HIV biology. Available at http://hivinsite.ucsf.edu/InSite?page=kb-02-01-01. Accessed April 20, 2006.
Moore JP, Kitchen SG, Pugach P, et al. The CCR5 and CXCR4 coreceptors: central to understanding the transmission and pathogenesis of human immunodeficiency virus type 1 infection. *AIDS Res Hum Retroviruses.* 2004;20(1):111–126.
Reeves JD, Piefer AJ. Emerging drug targets for antiretroviral therapy. *Drugs.* 2005;65(13):1747–1766.

HIV NATURAL HISTORY

LEARNING OBJECTIVE

Discuss the course of HIV infection and its dynamics in the host over time.

WHAT'S NEW?

Expanded discussion of viral kinetics and latency.

- In mucosal transmission, HIV crosses the epithelial barrier and establishes an expanding infection at the site of entry.

- During acute infection, HIV disseminates to lymphatic tissue throughout the body.

- The rate of fall in plasma viremia with HAART reflects the kinetics of different types of infected host cells.

- HIV exhibits remarkable levels of diversity, both globally and within a single host.

- HIV establishes latent infection in a subset of host cells, allowing it to persist despite HAART.

ESTABLISHMENT OF INFECTION

In sexual transmission, HIV must first breach the epithelial barrier of the genital or rectal mucosa. This may occur via physical breaks in the epithelium related to trauma or sexually transmitted infections, particularly herpes simplex virus. However, HIV can also cross intact mucosa via specialized dendritic cells in the genital tract or transcytosis in the gastrointestinal (GI) tract (Morrow, 2008). Upon crossing the epithelial barrier, the virus encounters multiple potential target cells. The major cellular receptor for fusion and entry of HIV is CD4$^+$ T cells, whose critical role in HIV infection was identified in 1984 (Dalgleish, 1984; Klatzmann, 1984). Initial infection is propagated by dendritic cells (especially the Langerhans cells), components of the innate immune system, which deliver HIV to CD4$^+$ T cells; or, the virus may directly infect local CD4$^+$ T cells without the aid of dendritic cells. The initial proliferation of HIV represents a genetic bottleneck in which a large viral inoculum gives rise to a small founder population of infected cells. In heterosexual transmission, infection results from a single viral genotype in 80% of cases, with preference for the CCR5 coreceptor (Haase, 2010).

The *eclipse phase* refers to the period after mucosal exposure, when the virus remains undetectable in plasma, and lasts approximately 10 days. Once a founder viral population is established at the portal of entry, it must expand locally by rapid migration to regional lymph nodes and dissemination to distant draining lymph nodes via the bloodstream. In a chain reaction of cell-to-cell signaling, termed the *virologic synapse* (Piguet, 2007), dendritic and Langerhans cell-type T cells' exposure to HIV induces the recruitment of more plasmacytoid dendritic cells, and ultimately, more CD4$^+$ T cells (Haase, 2010). Therefore, in addition to the role that lymphoid tissue (in particular dendritic cells) plays in the initiation of HIV infection, it also is responsible for the dissemination of HIV infection. These early events may be altered to prevent infection, and they figure prominently in research on microbicides, preexposure prophylaxis, and preventative vaccines.

ACUTE INFECTION

Once infection is established in draining lymph nodes, activated CD4$^+$ T lymphocytes become the predominant source of viral replication. Immune activation increases the pool of susceptible activated CD4$^+$ T cells, creating a positive feedback loop. An exponential increase in plasma viremia ensues, and patients may develop symptoms of the acute retroviral syndrome. HIV disseminates and infects other lymphatic tissues throughout the body. The CD4$^+$ T cell count in peripheral blood declines markedly, thought to occur through several proposed mechanisms: increased destruction of cells by direct infection by HIV, activation of apoptosis, increased lymphocyte turnover, and decreased production by reduced thymic output and redistribution of cells from peripheral blood to lymphoid tissue. A profound depletion of CD4$^+$ T cells also occurs in the gut-associated lymphatic tissue (GALT), causing permanent damage.

The events in acute infection have long-term consequences for the patient. Activation of CD4$^+$ T cells and HIV RNA replication causes fibrosis to occur in the lymphoid architecture, leading to incomplete immune reconstitution after initiation of HAART (Brenchley, 2004). Damage to the GI epithelium and mucosal immune response allows an increase in microbial translocation (Haase, 2011), which may serve as a stimulus to systemic immune activation, magnifying the positive feedback loop for the virus. Over time, microbial translocation likely contributes to chronic immune activation and progression to AIDS. Finally, a reservoir of latently infected cells is established, which later prevents viral eradication with HAART. Important reservoir sites include GALT and peripheral lymphoid tissues. In the rare cases in which HIV is diagnosed during primary infection, immediate ART may have potential to attenuate, although not reverse, these changes.

VIRAL KINETICS AND LATENCY

Plasma HIV RNA levels reflect a dynamic interplay between the infection of susceptible cells and the destruction of infected cells. With initiation of ART, susceptible host cells are protected from infection. Consequently, the rate of decline in the viral load following initiation of HAART reflects the kinetics of the death of HIV-infected cells (Figure 19.3) (Palmer, 2011).

Viral decay occurs in four distinct phases. The viral load declines dramatically in the first phase of 7–10 days, reflecting clearance of activated CD4$^+$ T cells ($t_{1/2}$ = 1 or 2 days), with roughly 90% of the decrease in plasma HIV occurring in these first weeks of therapy (Markowitz, 2003). The second phase, characterized by a more gradual decline in viral load and average half-life of 14 days (Andrade, 2013), correlates with the intermediate half-lives of partially activated CD4$^+$ T cells, macrophages, and possibly dendritic cells. In the third phase (the slowest), plasma HIV continues to decline, although at levels detectable only by ultrasensitive assays. This phase may represent decay of latently infected resting CD4$^+$ T cells that are producing HIV, but HIV RNA levels are unobserved since they have fallen below the limit of detection (Andrade, 2013). The fourth phase occurs 4–5 years after ART initiation and finally stabilizes at very low levels (<1–5 copies/mL) (Siliciano, 2003). Research has focused on the resting memory CD4$^+$ T cell as the source of viral replication during these latter stages.

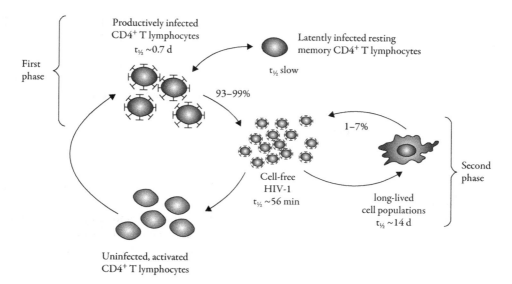

Figure 19.3 Rates of clearance of different cell populations and viral turnover. Reproduced from Simon and Ho 2003, with permission from Macmillan Publishers Ltd: Nat Rev Microbiol, copyright 2003.

Despite fully suppressive HAART, the proportion of resting CD4+ T cells that are latently infected shows minimal decline over time, yielding an estimated half-life of 44 months (Siliciano, 2003). By this estimate, HIV eradication would require approximately 60 years of uninterrupted HAART.

Since HIV latency is the chief obstacle to eradicating HIV, increasing attention has turned to the mechanisms that maintain latent infection. In latent infection, proviral DNA is integrated into the host genome but remains in a transcriptionally silent, but inducible, state. Latently infected cells serve as a reservoir for virus that can reactivate and drive HIV viral loads to pretreatment levels if ART is interrupted (Rouzine, 2015). In rhesus macaque models, simian immunodeficiency virus (SIV) established latency in reservoir cells as early as 3 days after infection, before viremia was detected (Whitney, 2014). Different biological processes, such as host transcription factors, histone deacetylase-mediated epigenetic silencing, and cytokines, have been shown to play a role in HIV latency. The host transcription factors (NF-κB, NFAT, and P-TEFβ) and the viral protein tat promote expression of proviral DNA, but they are present at low levels in resting CD4+ T cells. Histone deacetylation and DNA methylation at the HIV LTR alter the local chromatin environment, denying access to the machinery of transcription (Palmer, 2011). Cytokines promote the activation of resting CD4+ T cells. Therapies that promote expression of the proviral genome or activate resting CD4+ T cells have the potential to speed decay of the latent reservoir, leading to eradication of HIV from patients receiving HAART. In addition, drugs that prevent histone deacetylation (HDAC inhibitors) are under active investigation as a therapy to eradicate latent infection. Last, ongoing studies are measuring the ability of interleukin-7 to deplete the latent reservoir in patients receiving HAART. Though HIV latency reactivation has been extensively studied, the kinetics of viral mRNA and viral protein production following reactivation at the single-cell level are still being investigated, which

may serve to determine sites of action for potential HIV cures (Martrus, 2016).

VIRAL DIVERSITY

During untreated infection, HIV replicates at a very high rate, with roughly 10 billion new virions produced each day in a given patient. Reverse transcriptase, in contrast to DNA polymerases, lacks proofreading activity (Taylor, 2008). As a result, frequent mutations occur in the daughter viral genome, potentially altering the structure and function of viral proteins. HIV recombination is another means of viral diversity and occurs when one person is coinfected with two strains of the virus which replicate within the cell (Taylor, 2008). The rapid rate of production, combined with frequent mutations and recombination, leads to the production of diverse quasispecies. Strikingly, the genetic diversity observed in a single individual after 6 years of HIV infection is roughly equivalent to that observed worldwide in influenza A virus within a given year (Korber, 2001). However, the genetic diversity that occurs in acute infection occurs at a much higher rate than in chronic infection. The high number of replication cycles also allows for selection of resistant variants, either due to drug pressure or the immune system. Emergence of drug resistance mutations is governed by selection forces and drift (Maldarelli, 2013).

Viral diversity presents a unique challenge for producing an HIV vaccine. Historically, vaccines have prevented infection by stimulating antibody or cell-mediated immunity in susceptible patients. Both HIV and SIV have been shown to escape from these host immune responses by virtue of their extreme diversity. An effective HIV vaccine may need to elicit broad immune responses that protect against multiple quasi-species and possibly other HIV subtypes. The impact of viral diversity is well known to clinicians engaged in the treatment of HIV. The administration of multiple agents, so-called *drug cocktails*, is required to suppress viral replication to levels at which drug-resistant strains are unlikely to emerge. Likewise, viral diversity underpins the importance of strict adherence to HIV therapy. More broadly, the continued evolution of HIV has necessitated the increased use of resistance testing and the development of antiretrovirals with novel therapeutic mechanisms.

RECOMMENDED READING

Finzi D, Blankson J, Siliciano JD, et al. Latent infection of CD4⁺ T cells provides a mechanism for lifelong persistence of HIV-1, even in patients on effective combination therapy. *Nat Med.* 1999;5(5):512–517.

Harris RS, Liddament MT. Retroviral restriction by APOBEC proteins. *Nat Rev Immunol.* 2004;4(11):868–877.

Mehandru S, Tenner-Racz K, Racz P, et al. The gastrointestinal tract is critical to the pathogenesis of acute HIV infection. *J Allergy Clin Immunol.* 2005;116(2):419–422.

Persaud D, Zhou Y, Siliciano JM, et al. Latency in human immunodeficiency virus type 1 infection: no easy answers. *J Virol.* 2003;77(3):1659–1665.

Simon V, Ho DD. HIV-1 dynamics in vivo: Implications for therapy. *Nat Rev Microbiol.* 2003;1(3):181–190.

OVERVIEW OF ANTIRETROVIRAL THERAPY

LEARNING OBJECTIVES

- Discuss the goals of antiretroviral treatment.

- Discuss the rationale for initiating ART in all HIV-infected persons.

- Discuss the principles for antiretroviral regimen selection in HIV-infected, treatment-naïve patients.

- Discuss the principles of switching, or simplifying, ART.

WHAT'S NEW?

- HAART is associated with the potential to decrease both viral-related and non–viral-related comorbidities, as well as reduce levels of population-based HIV transmission.

- Guidelines for treatment now recommend starting HAART in all who are ready for treatment, regardless of CD4⁺ cell count, to prevent comorbidities and transmission.

- Newer antiretroviral agents and regimens can improve tolerability and durable viral suppression in HIV-infected treatment-naïve patients.

- The recommended initial regimens in the most recent guidelines by the US Department of Health and Human Services (USDHHS) have moved away from starting PIs and instead focus on using integrase inhibitors.

KEY POINTS

- Untreated and uncontrolled HIV replication is associated with HIV-related inflammation, accelerated aging, and a higher rate of comorbid illnesses that has been shown to be reduced by earlier initiation of HAART.

- Studies have indicated improved clinical outcomes with treatment initiation at CD4⁺ cell counts greater than 500/mm³. Based on these studies, treatment is now recommended for all HIV-infected patients regardless of CD4⁺ cell count.

- Treatment of HIV with HAART can reduce/prevent HIV-1 transmission.

- Choice of regimen is now focused on what is best suited for the patient and his or her comorbidities to ensure adherence and long-term durability. The factors considered include medication tolerability and toxicities, resistance, and patient comorbidities.

INTRODUCTION

Great strides have been made in ART since the introduction of zidovudine in 1987 and combination of therapy in 1996. ART has reduced HIV-associated morbidity and mortality, making HIV a chronic disease that can be managed with potent and simple medication regimens. In addition, treatment with HAART has been shown to reduce HIV transmission. With these advances, many HIV-infected patients can now expect to live a near-normal lifetime. However, only 55% of people with HIV in the United States have suppressed viral loads (USDHHS, 2018) due to undiagnosed infections or difficulty linking patients to care.

Paramount to the success of HAART is the patient's willingness and commitment to adhere to life-long therapy. In the past, acute and long-term adverse effects associated with HAART limited adherence to therapy, leading to treatment failure. However, with the advent of newer agents and better understanding of antiretroviral treatment management, current therapy combinations are now associated with less toxicity, reduced pill burden, and improved potency, allowing many patients to achieve greater than 95% adherence. However, as alluded to earlier, concerns remain which have a significant impact on antiretroviral treatment success, including access to and the cost of long-term HAART (particularly in resource-limited areas); social and economic factors; drug–drug interactions; and comorbid medical conditions such as hepatitis B (HBV) and C (HBC), liver disease, tuberculosis, cardiovascular disease, diabetes, osteoporosis or osteopenia, hyperlipidemia, renal disease, psychological disorders, and chemical dependency. Recognizing and addressing the individual barriers to adherence for each patient prior to initiation of ART has had a dramatic effect on long-term treatment outcomes.

WHEN TO START ANTIRETROVIRAL THERAPY

Similar to the options for ART, the decision of when to start therapy in HIV-infected patients has evolved over time. Early studies demonstrated a clear benefit of combination ART in patients with AIDS (defined as a CD4⁺ cell count <200 cells/mm³ and/or an AIDS-defining illness) and symptomatic

HIV-infection (Cameron, 1998; Hammer, 1997). Subsequent studies demonstrated decreased mortality or reduced risk of disease progression in treated patients with CD4$^+$ cell counts of 201–350 cells/mm^3 (Egger, 2002; Opravil, 2002; Palella, 2003). Although the baseline CD4$^+$ cell count was the predominant marker that significantly predicted the probability of progression to AIDS and/or death, a plasma HIV viral load greater than 100,000 copies/mL was also associated with a higher probability of these risk events (Egger, 2002; Philips, 2004). These and other studies balanced the costs and toxicities of antiretroviral agents and eventually led to recommending initiation of antiretroviral treatment at CD4$^+$ cell counts of less than 350 cells/mm^3.

An analysis of 18 cohort studies in 2009 involving 21,247 patients reported a higher rate of progression to AIDS and death among patients who deferred therapy initiation until their CD4$^+$ cell count dropped below 350 cells/mm^3 compared to those who started HAART with a CD4$^+$ cell count of 351–450 cells/mm^3 (Sterne, 2009). This study advocated for initiation of HAART prior to the minimal threshold of 350 cells/mm^3 but found no significant rate of progression to AIDS and/or death among the two groups starting therapy with a CD4$^+$ cell count threshold of 450 cells/mm^3. Meanwhile, the investigators of a large North American Cohort (NA-ACCORD) analyzed data from 17,517 patients with asymptomatic HIV infection and reported a higher risk of death among patients starting therapy with a CD4$^+$ cell count less than 350 cells/mm^3 compared to those who started therapy with a count greater than this threshold (Kitahata, 2009). In addition, these investigators reported a significant reduction in mortality among patients starting HAART with a CD4$^+$ cell count of 351–500 cells/mm^3 compared to patients with a count above this threshold. Although these investigators also found a mortality difference among patients starting HAART with a CD4$^+$ cell count greater than 500 cells/mm^3 (compared to a CD4$^+$ cell count less than this threshold), there were not enough risk events to demonstrate a significant difference between the two groups. Both of these studies demonstrated the benefit of earlier initiation of antiretroviral treatment; however, the interpretation of the results varied among different groups globally.

The discordance in study results and international guideline recommendations changed in August 2015, with the publication of the Strategic Timing of Antiretroviral Treatment (START) trial results. In this prospective, randomized controlled trial, asymptomatic HIV-positive adults were randomized to receive HAART at CD4$^+$ T cell levels greater than 500/mm^3 (the immediate initiation group) or were started on HAART only after CD4$^+$ T cell levels decreased below 350/mm^3 (the deferred initiation group/delayed HAART). A total of 4,685 patients in 35 countries were followed for a mean of 3 years and assessed for a composite end point of serious AIDS-related events and serious non–AIDS-related events, including death from causes other than AIDS, only after CD4$^+$ T cell levels decreased below 350/mm^3. The study was stopped at an interim analysis because a significant benefit was demonstrated in the immediate initiation group,

and all patients in the deferred initiation group were offered ART. Importantly, no increased rate of adverse effects from HAART was observed in the immediate initiation group (INSIGHT START Initiation Group, 2015).

Due to the results of the START trial, the British HIV Association, the European AIDS Clinical Society (EACS), and the World Health Organization (WHO) joined the USDHHS and the International Antiviral Society–USA in recommending starting all patients with HIV on HAART (with caution in cases of TB or cryptococcal meningitis), prompting a cohesive global recommendation regarding initiation of ART for all patients with HIV/AIDS and eliminating the variability previously present for providers in different nations.

In addition to findings from the START trial, arguments for initiating earlier HAART include reduction of the risks associated with HIV-mediated chronic immune activation leading to end-organ damage, non–AIDS-related infections, malignancies, liver disease, and viral transmission (Cohen, 2011; Donnell, 2010; Ferry, 2009; Granich, 2009; Marin, 2009). The benefits of HAART in preventing or reducing the incidence of the aforementioned HIV-associated comorbidities were demonstrated in studies that predated the START trial. In a multicenter cohort study involving 9,858 patients (aged 16 years or older), investigators suggested that non–AIDS-defining conditions (e.g., cardiovascular disease, non–AIDS-related infections and malignancies, and liver disease) were increased in association with advancing immunodeficiency (defined as a prolonged period below a CD4$^+$ T cell count of 350 cells/mm^3). This study noted that only an increased risk of cardiovascular disease and death were associated with an elevated plasma HIV viral load (>200 copies/mL), regardless of receiving HAART (the plasma viral load is considered a surrogate marker for HIV-related endothelial inflammation). Although there was also an association with liver disease–related deaths and an elevated plasma HIV viral load, patients receiving HAART appeared to have a protective effect. Another cohort of 1,281 patients treated with a PI–based regimen and followed over a median period of 7.3 years demonstrated that non–AIDS-defining conditions occurred at a higher frequency than HAART toxicities or AIDS-defining conditions (Ferry, 2009). The earlier implementation of HAART has also reduced sexual transmission of HIV and clinical end points such as tuberculosis, bacterial infections, and death in a large cohort of serodiscordant couples in Africa (Cohen, 2011). "Treatment at prevention" was demonstrated in a study by Donnell et al., in which 3,400 HIV-infected patients were treated with HAART. There was a 92% decrease in HIV transmission rates to those patients' heterosexual, serodiscordant partners (Donnell, 2010). A randomized control trial of either immediate or delayed ART for HIV-infected partners of heterosexual serodiscordant couples found a 96% reduction in HIV transmission when immediate ART was initiated, as well as increased CD4$^+$ T cell counts and decreased rates of extrapulmonary tuberculosis (Cohen, 2011).

In addition to the data promoting earlier initiation of ART, the armamentarium of antiretroviral agent options has expanded with many new drugs that have improved toxicity and side effect profiles, lower pill burdens, and easier dosing schedules. At the same time, our understanding of many aspects of HIV has also dramatically increased, including the impact of HIV on comorbid conditions and their effect on HIV progression, the role of mutation threshold of drugs and resistance, the importance of pharmacokinetics and drug–drug interactions, the knowledge of side effects/toxicities and how to manage them, and the impact of medication adherence.

CURRENT TREATMENT GUIDELINES

In the United States, the guidelines published by the USDHHS (2018) and the International Antiviral Society–USA (IAS-USA; Saag, 2018) are similar and constantly updated to reflect the release of new medications, new data on timing of HAART association, new drug regimens, and HIV treatment in special populations. The guidelines also address patients' readiness for therapy, barriers to adherence, and comorbid conditions. More importantly, the most recent version of the guidelines reflects the release and use of the INSTIs dolutegravir and bictegravir, and regimen switching. The USDHHS and IAS-USA guidelines reflect the data from the START trial and recommend treatment in all patients with HIV, regardless of CD4+ T cell lymphocyte count, in order to reduce the morbidity and mortality associated with HIV infection and prevent HIV transmission. In some cases, ART may be deferred due to psychosocial factors, but medication should be started as soon as the patient is ready and psychosocial factors have stabilized. The following conditions should be considered urgent and discourage deferring treatment initiation:

1. Pregnancy
2. AIDS-defining conditions, including HIV-associated dementia and AIDS-defining malignancies
3. Opportunistic infections
4. CD4+ T cell counts below 200 cells/mm³
5. HIV-associated nephropathy
6. HBV or HCV coinfection

SELECTION OF AN INITIAL ANTIRETROVIRAL REGIMEN

Currently, there are more than 25 different antiretroviral agents that consist of six different mechanisms of action aimed at providing maximal viral suppression when used in combination (USDHHS, 2018; Saag, 2018). The available classes of agents include nucleoside and non-nucleoside reverse transcriptase inhibitors (NRTIs and NNRTIs), PIs, fusion inhibitors, CCR5 receptor antagonists, and INSTIs. Ritonavir and cobicistat are pharmacokinetic (PK) enhancers to improve the PK profiles of PIs and the INSTI elvitegravir. Regimens that do not require boosting are favored (Saag, 2018).

When considering which treatment combination to start, providers should tailor the regimen based on the following factors:

1. Patient readiness and barriers to adherence
2. Cost, convenience (e.g., pill burden), dosing frequency, potential drug toxicities, and potential drug–drug interactions
3. Pregnancy state or potential among women of childbearing age
4. Comorbid conditions (e.g., cardiovascular disease, liver disease, kidney disease, co-infection with HBV and HCV, psychiatric disorders, and chemical dependency)
5. Viral resistance testing results (if available)

The USDHHS and IAS-USA recommend the following as initial regimens for most people with HIV (in alphabetical order; references to tenofovir are either tenofovir alafenamide or tenofovir disoproxil fumarate)

- Bictegravir/tenofovir/emtricitabine
- Dolutegravir/abacavir/lamivudine (if HLA B*5701 is negative)
- Dolutegravir plus tenofovir/emtricitabine

In addition, the USDHHS lists these as options for initial regimens:

- Elvitegravir/cobicistat/tenofovir/emtricitabine
- Raltegravir plus tenofovir/emtricitabine

The USDHHS recommends that the following ART drugs no longer be used due to suboptimal potency, unacceptable toxicities, high pill burden, or pharmacologic concerns: delavirdine, didanosine, indinavir, nelfinavir, and stavudine.

Historically, treatment regimens evolved from the use of one or two NRTIs to a combination of two NRTIs and a third antiretroviral agent, since most clinical trial data have been based on the use of two NRTIs. Combination therapy with three or four NRTIs has demonstrated antiviral activity but either lacks comparable data with other regimens or has been shown to be inferior to other combination regimens (DART, 2006; Gulick, 2004). In the past, initial recommended regimens included two NRTIs with a boosted PI, but the DHHS has moved away from PIs as part of initial regimen recommendations (as noted earlier) and now includes use of INSTIs. The PI darunavir used to be a recommended initial regimen, but now it is recommended in certain clinical situations since INSTI-based regimens have shown improved outcomes with fewer side effects compared to darunavir. Darunavir may be used, for example, in a situation where there is concern for ART-resistance and a medication with a high genetic barrier to resistance is needed.

Some research has investigated different approaches to regimens, including trials with class-sparing regimens. In particular, there has been an interest in nucleoside-sparing regimens to avoid metabolic toxicities and viral resistance while maintaining maximal viral suppression (Riddler, 2008). As suggested earlier, studies with INSTI-based regimens have been shown to achieve high rates of viral suppression without the tolerability issues of PI- or NNRTI-based regimens (Eron, 2010; Messiaen, 2013; Squires, 2016). Also, tenofovir alafenamide has been shown to have less bone and kidney toxicity and may be advantageous for patients who have bone or kidney disease or for those who are at risk for these conditions (Flamm, 2017; Grant, 2016; Rijnders, 2016; Wang, 2016).

Other research has focused on the use of two-drug regimens, even as options for initiation of therapy. The regimens that are under investigation include dolutegravir and lamivudine, as well as darunavir/ritonavir and lamivudine (Saag, 2018). These regimens would have the advantage of avoiding the toxicity of three drugs, however, the efficacy of two-drug regimens is still under investigation.

Dual NRTI fixed-dose combinations available are abacavir/lamivudine, tenofovir alafenamide/emtricitabine, and tenofovir disoproxil/emtricitabine. The ACTG 5202 study (Sax, 2009) and the HEAT study (Smith, 2009) demonstrated equal efficacy between the abacavir/lamivudine and tenofovir disoproxil/emtricitabine combinations; however, an association between abacavir and myocardial infarction was first reported in the D:A:D study (Worm, 2010; Sabin, 2008), and there have been several subsequent studies that have found an association. Other studies, however, including a meta-analysis done by the US Food and Drug Administration (FDA) of 26 randomized clinical trials (Ding, 2012), have not found an association between abacavir and cardiovascular disease. There is no consensus in the USDHHS guidelines regarding this association.

On March 27, 2018, the USDHHS issued a statement regarding the use of a fixed-dose combination of bictegravir/tenofovir alafenamide/emtricitabine as one of the recommended initial regimens (USDDHS, 2018). Bictegravir (BIC) is a new INSTI that, in clinical trials, is noninferior to TAF/FTC plus DTG or ABC/3TC/DTG for up to 48 weeks (Sax, 2017; Gallant, 2017). In vitro, BIC has been shown to have at least as high of a resistance barrier as DTG (Tsiang, 2016), but there are no data available on the use of BIC in patients with prior INSTI failure or those with INSTI-associated resistance mutations. BIC/TAF/FTC has also been shown to be efficacious as a switch regimen for patients virally suppressed on other regimens, with no resistance mutations noted to the components of the combination regimen (Daar, 2017).

Recommendations for antiretroviral regimens are similar among the USDHHS (2018) and IAS-USA (Saag, 2018) guidelines as well as the British HIV Association guidelines (Ahmed, 2016) and European AIDS Clinical Society (EACS, 2017) guidelines; however the British HIV Association and EACS guidelines include PIs (boosted atazanavir and/or boosted darunavir) in recommended initial regimens. The differences in the recommended agents are based on differing interpretations of clinical data. All of these combination regimens have been demonstrated to be efficacious. All individual antiretroviral agents and regimens have different pharmacokinetic profiles, drug–drug interactions, side effects, and toxicities. The optimal choice of agents for a regimen is dependent on the specific needs, situation, and comorbidities of the individual being treated. The critical issues to consider are adherence barriers and lifestyle (e.g., once- vs. twice-daily regimens, need for coadministration with food, and coformulated agents), comorbidities (e.g., hepatitis B, pregnancy, and kidney disease), and tolerability (side effects that the patient can tolerate). The successful regimen will be that which is well-tolerated and well-suited for the individual's lifestyle.

The guidelines have been drafted with the average patient and provider in mind. However, alternative regimens and strategies may also be effective for specific individuals. One of the important issues in the current treatment of HIV is the management of comorbidities and medication toxicities. Combinations listed as alternative or acceptable in the guidelines may be particularly well-suited for specific situations and should not be discouraged for the individual patient with those characteristics. Other treatment regimens may not currently have adequate data to allow them to be recommended as preferred or alternative regimens. Because our knowledge of antiretroviral agents is constantly changing, when new data are available, some agents or combinations may well be recommended or removed from the list of acceptable alternatives. The addition of new classes to our armamentarium also means that we do not yet know about many possible treatment combinations including agents such as the CCR5 antagonists and integrase inhibitors or the best combinations of these and other classes. A phase IIb randomized controlled trial with antiretroviral-naïve adults showed that the investigational INSTI, cabotegravir, plus NRTIs had potent antiviral activity during 24 weeks of initial treatment compared to treatment with efavirenz. When these patients switched to cabotegravir plus rilpivirine (an NNRTI), antiviral activity was found to be the same as that of dual NRTIs and efavirenz at the end of a 96-week follow-up period. This study adds to the data that suggest that certain two-drug regimens, without NRTIs, might be acceptable for ART-naïve patients (Margolis, 2015).

The initial recommended regimens by the IAS-USA and USDHHS have evolved to reflect new data revealing efficacious combinations with the least toxicities (including metabolic, cardiovascular, and renal) and best long-term durability in formulations that facilitate adherence.

WHEN TO SWITCH OR SIMPLIFY ANTIRETROVIRAL THERAPY

Side effects or toxicities due to antiretroviral medications are often encountered in clinical practice. Because patients may have to take antiretroviral medications for a lifetime, side effects and toxicities must be addressed to avoid metabolic complications and decreased adherence leading to virologic failure. With the advent of newer agents with improved toxicity profiles, easier dosing schedules, and fewer pills, providers are often confronted with the question of whether to change individual agents or whole regimens. Although the optimal time for changing therapy remains undetermined, most studies have investigated changes in therapy for patients who have been controlled on a HAART regimen for at least 6 months. The main goal of switching therapy is to maintain viral suppression without jeopardizing the availability of future treatment options. According to the IAS-USA and USDHHS, these are some reasons to consider changing therapy (USDHHS, 2018; Saag, 2018):

1. Reduce pill burden or dosing frequency

2. Reduce short- or long-term toxicity and enhance tolerability

3. Change food or fluid requirements

4. Minimize drug–drug interactions

5. Optimize ART regimen for pregnancy or in case of pregnancy

Switching to a simplified, less toxic regimen in patients with an extensive treatment history remains complex. Simply changing one agent may not be possible, and a complete review of the patient's treatment history, resistance testing, treatment tolerance, and drug–drug interactions should be conducted prior to designing a new regimen.

In general, two approaches to changing therapy in virally suppressed patients have been changing one agent to another agent within the same class (within-class simplification) or changing one agent to an alternate class (out-of-class simplification) (USDHHS, 2018). Within-class simplification can decrease toxicity, dosing frequency, and pill burden, especially when coformulated agents are used. For example, a regimen that includes the NRTI zidovudine could be changed to a regimen that includes tenofovir or abacavir, reducing immediate side effects and dosing frequency (USDHHS, 2018). Another example of a within-class change is switching from tenofovir disoproxil to tenofovir alafenamide for decreased long-term bone and renal effects (Gallant, 2016). However, the long-term adverse effects of the NRTIs tenofovoir, abacavir, and lamivudine must be noted. In a 2013 population-based study of approximately 100 patients, these NRTIs (stavudine and didanosine were not studied) were shown to inhibit telomerase activity, leading to accelerated shortening of telomere length in mononuclear cells (tenofovir was found to be the most potent inhibitor). This study suggests that NRTIs are a potential factor in contributing to HIV-associated accelerated aging, and switching patients off NRTI-based regimens may become a higher priority in the future (Leeansyah, 2013).

Similar to NRTIs, within-class simplification of NNRTIs can reduce toxicities and adverse side effects. In a randomized trial involving 38 men switching from efavirenz to etravirine

due to central nervous system toxicity, researchers reported a significant reduction in adverse events in patients whose regimen was changed to etravirine, with all participants maintaining a suppressed viral load at 24 weeks (Waters, 2011). In addition, in an analysis of four randomized clinical trials, researchers found that patients on efavirenz were twice as likely to experience suicidal thoughts or attempt to or actually commit suicide compared to those not receiving efavirenz (Mollan, 2014).

The majority of studies investigating class switches have evaluated the replacement of a PI agent with an alternative class, such as an NRTI, NNRTI, or INSTI. This can be done to reduce the toxicities experienced by the patient or to change to a simple, once-daily coformulated agent. Although this is generally successful in patients without resistance, it can lead to virologic failure in patients with previous underlying resistance. This was seen in the SWITCHMRK study, when patients who were randomized to change from boosted lopinavir to raltegravir had improved serum lipid concentrations, but they also had a higher failure rate than those who remained on lopinavir/ritonavir, leading to study termination at 24 weeks (Eron, 2010).

In most of the aforementioned studies, ART regimen changes occurred in patients who were virologically suppressed. If regimen switching is done in patients with virologic failure (HIV RNA > 1,000 copies/mL) or suboptimal viral load reduction, HIV drug-resistance testing should be performed to assist with the selection of active ART drugs. For patients who have virologic failure while on an INSTI, genotype testing specifically for INSTI resistance should be performed (some resistance testing profiles do not include INSTI in the standard lab order). The drug resistance testing should be done while the patient is on ART or within 4 weeks of discontinuation. The addition of phenotypic testing to genotypic testing is recommended for patients with complex resistance patterns. In addition, if switching to an abacavir-based regimen, HLA-B*5701 allele testing should be done to reduce the risk of a hypersensitivity reaction. When switching regimens for someone with hepatitis B coinfection, a drug regimen effective for both HIV and HBV should be used.

After switching regimens, patients should be evaluated closely to ensure that no new side effects have emerged, and a repeat viral load 4–8 weeks after a regimen switch should be obtained to ensure the patient is virally suppressed. If preexisting laboratory abnormalities were attributed to the previous ART regimen (i.e., hyperlipidemia assumed to be from PIs), these laboratory values should be rechecked 3 months after switching regimens.

SUMMARY

The USDHHS, IAS-USA, WHO, EACS, and British HIV Association guidelines now recommend treatment of all HIV-infected individuals, regardless of the CD4$^+$ count. Currently, the critical issues in antiretroviral treatment are focused on optimizing regimens for the individual patient. Barriers to adherence and addressing those factors remain paramount; resolution prior to treatment initiation is important to achieve treatment success. Once the patient is "ready" for therapy, the key issues in the future will be tailoring medication regimens for patient's medical comorbidities, medication toxicities, and lifestyle. Switching to newer agents must be done prudently, with careful consideration of the patient's resistance history and comorbidities. Just as there has been enormous progress in the past, we will continue to witness significant change in the future as we seek to find the optimal treatments for our patients.

RECOMMENDED READING

Günthard HF, Aberg JA, Eron JJ, et al.; International Antiviral Society–USA Panel. Antiretroviral treatment of adult HIV infection: 2014 recommendations of the International Antiviral Society–USA Panel. *JAMA.* 2014;312(4):410–425.

Johnson JA, Sax PE. Beginning antiretroviral therapy for patients with HIV. *Infect Dis Clin North Am.* 2014;28(3):421–438.

Sellers CJ, Wohl DA. Antiretroviral therapy: when to start. *Infect Dis Clin North Am.* 2014;28(3):403–420.

US Department of Health and Human Services (USDHHS), Panel on Antiretroviral Guidelines for Adults and Adolescents. Guidelines for the use of antiretroviral agents in HIV-1-infected adults and adolescents. Available at https://www.aidsinfo.nih.gov/ContentFiles/AdultandAdolescentGL.pdf. Accessed July 17, 2018.

Volberding PA, Deeks SG. Antiretroviral therapy and management of HIV infection. *Lancet.* 2010;376(9734):49–62.

ACKNOWLEDGMENTS

Dr. Gilliam's contribution was made while on faculty at the University of Maryland School of Medicine.

REFERENCES

Ahmed N, Angus B, Boffito M, et al. British HIV Association guidelines for the treatment of HIV-1 positive adults with antiretroviral therapy (Interim update) 2016. Available at http://www.bhiva.org/guidelines.aspx. Accessed July 17, 2018.

Andrade A, Rosenkranz S, Cillo A, et al. Three distinct phases of HIV-1 RNA decay in treatment-naïve patients receiving raltegravir-based antiretroviral therapy: ACTG A5248. *J Inf Dis.* 2013;208(6):884–891.

Brenchley JM, Schacker TW, Ruff LE, et al. CD4+ T cell depletion during all stages of HIV disease occurs predominantly in the gastrointestinal tract. *J Exp Med.* September 20, 2004;200(6):749–759.

Cameron DW, Heath-Chiozzi M, Danner S, et al. Randomized placebo-controlled trial of ritonavir in advanced HIV-1 disease. *Lancet.* 1998;351:543–549.

Cohen MS, Chen YQ, McCauley M, et al. Prevention of HIV-1 infection with early antiretroviral therapy. *N Engl J Med.* 2011;365:493–505.

Daar E, DeJesus E, Ruane P, et al. Phase 3 randomized, controlled trial of switching to fixed-dose bictegravir/emtricitabine/tenofovir alafenamide (B/F/TAF) from boosted protease inhibitor-based regimens in virologically suppressed adults: week 48 results. Presented at ID Week, San Diego, CA, 2017.

Dalgleish AG, Beverly PC, Clapham PR, et al. The CD4(T4) antigen is an essential component of the receptor for the AIDS retrovirus. *Nature.* 1984;312:763–767.

DART Virology Group and Trial Team. Virological response to a triple nucleoside/nucleotide analogue regimen over 48 weeks in HIV-1-infected adults in Africa. *AIDS.* 2006;20:1391–1399.

Deeks SG, Autran B, et al.; International AIDS Society Scientific Working Group on HIV Cure. Towards an HIV cure: a global scientific strategy. *Nat Rev Immunol.* 2012;12:607–614.

Ding X, Andraca-Carrera E, Cooper C, et al. No association of abacavir use with myocardial infarction: findings of an FDA meta-analysis. *J AIDS.* 2012;61(4):441–447.

Donnell D, Baeten JM, Kiarie J, et al. Heterosexual HIV-1 transmission after initiation of antiretroviral therapy: a prospective cohort analysis. *Lancet.* 2010;375:2092–2098.

Egger M, May M, Chene G, et al.;the ART Cohort Collaboration. Prognosis of HIV-1 infected patients starting highly active antiretroviral therapy: a collaborative analysis of prospective studies. *Lancet.* 2002;360:119–129.

Eron JJ, Young B, Cooper DA, et al.;the SWITCHMRK 1 and 2 investigators. Switch to a raltegravir-based regimen versus continuation of a lopinavir–ritonavir-based regimen in stable HIV-infected patients with suppressed viremia (SWITCHMRK 1 and 2): two multicentre, double-blind, randomized controlled trials. *Lancet.* 2010;375:396–407.

European AIDS Clinical Society (EACS). Guidelines. Version 9.0. October 2017. Available at Accessed July 17, 2018.

Ferry T, Raffi F, Collin-Filleul F, et al.; the ANRS CO8 (APROCO-COPILOTE) Study Group. Uncontrolled viral replication as a risk factor for non-AIDS severe clinical events in HIV-infected patients on long-term antiretroviral therapy: APROCO/COPILOTE (ANRS CO8) cohort study. *J AIDS.* 2009;23:1743–1753.

Flamm J, Vanig T, Gathe J. Efficacy and safety of tenofovir alafenamide vs. tenofovir disoproxil fumarate in HIV-infected, virologically suppressed black and non-blacks adults through week 96: subgroup analysis of a randomized switch study. *Curr Opin HIV AIDS.* 2016;11(3):326–332.

Gallant J, Lazzarin A, Mills A, et al. Bictegravir, emtricitabine, and tenofovir alafenamide versus dolutegravir, abacavir, and lamivudine for initial treatment of HIV-1 infection (GS-US-380-1489): a double-blind, multicentre, phase 3, randomised controlled non-inferiority trial. *Lancet.* 2017;390(10107):2063–2072.

Gallant JE, Daar ES, Raffi F, et al. Efficacy and safety of tenofovir alafenamide versus tenofovir disoproxil fumarate given as fixed-dose combinations containing emtricitabine as backbones for treatment of HIV-1 infection in virologically suppressed adults: a randomised, double-blind, active-controlled phase 3 trial. *The Lancet HIV.* 2016;3(4):e158–165.

Granich RM, Gilks GF, Dye C, et al. Universal voluntary HIV testing with immediate antiretroviral therapy as a strategy for elimination of HIV transmission: a mathematical model. *Lancet.* 2009;373:48–57.

Grant PM, Cotter AG. Tenofovir and bone health. *Curr Opin HIV AIDS.* 2016;11(3):326–332.

Gulick RM, Ribaudo HJ, Shikuma CM, et al.;the AIDS Clinical Trials Group Study A5095 Team. Triple-nucleoside regimens versus efavirenz-containing regimens for the initial treatment of HIV-1 infection. *N Engl J Med.* 2004;350:1850–1861.

Haase A. Targeting early infection to prevent HIV-1 mucosal transmission. *Nature.* 2010;464:217–223.

Hammer SM, Squires KE, Hughes MD, et al. A controlled trial of two nucleoside analogues plus indinavir in persons with human immunodeficiency virus infection and CD4$^+$ cell counts of 200 per cubic millimeter or less. *N Engl J Med.* 1997;337:725–733.

Heinzinger NK, Bukrinsky MI, Haggerty SA, et al. The Vpr protein of human immunodeficiency virus type 1 influences nuclear localization of viral nucleic acids in nondividing host cells. *Proc Natl Acad Sci USA.* July 19, 1994;91(15):7311–7315.

Honda Y, Rogers L, Nakata K, et al. Type I interferon induces inhibitory 16-kD CCAAT/enhancer binding protein (C/EBP) beta, repressing the HIV-1 long terminal repeat in macrophages: pulmonary tuberculosis alters C/EBP expression, enhancing HIV-1 replication. *J Exp Med.* 1998;188:1255–1265.

INSIGHT START Study Group. Initiation of antiretroviral therapy in early asymptomatic HIV infection. *N Engl J Med*. 2015;373(9):795–807.

Kao SY, Calman AF, Luciw PA, et al. Anti-termination of transcription within the long terminal repeat of HIV-1 by tat gene product. *Nature*. December 3, 1987;330(6147):489–493.

Kim SY, Byrn R, Groopman J, et al. Temporal aspects of DNA and RNA synthesis during human immunodeficiency virus infection: evidence for differential gene expression. *J Virol*. 1989;63:3708–3713.

Kitahata MM, Gange SJ, Abraham AG, et al.; the NA-ACCORD Investigators. Effect of early versus deferred antiretroviral therapy for HIV on survival. *N Engl J Med*. 2009;360:1815–1826.

Klatzmann D, Champagne E, Chamaret S, et al. T-lymphocyte T4 molecule behaves as receptor for human retrovirus LAV. *Nature*.1984;312:767–768.

Klimkait T, Strebel K, Hoggan MD, et al. The human immunodeficiency virus type 1-specific protein vpu is required for efficient virus maturation and release. *J Virol*. February 1990;64(2):621–629.

Klotman ME, Kim S, Buchbinder A, et al. Kinetics of expression of multiply spliced RNA in early human immunodeficiency virus type 1 infection of lymphocytes and monocytes. *Proc Natl Acad Sci U S A*. 1991;88:5011–5015.

Korber B, Gaschen B, Yusim K, et al. Evolutionary and immunological implications of contemporary HIV-1 variation. *Br Med Bull*. 2001;58:19–42.

Leeansyah E, Cameron P, Solomon A, et al. Inhibition of telomerase activity by human immunodeficiency virus (HIV) nucleos(t)ide reverse transcriptase inhibitors: a potential factor contributing to HIV-associated accelerated aging. *J Infect Dis*. 2013;207:1157–1165.

Liao Z, Cimakasky LM, Hampton R, et al. Lipid rafts and HIV pathogenesis: host membrane cholesterol is required for infection by HIV type 1. *AIDS Res Hum Retroviruses*. 2001;17:1009–1019.

Liu R, Paxton W, Choe S, et al. Homozygous defect in HIV-1 coreceptor accounts for resistance of some multiply-exposed individuals to HIV-1 infection. *Cell*. 1996;86:367–377.

Luria S, Chambers I, Berg P. Expression of the type 1 human immunodeficiency virus Nef protein in T cells prevents antigen receptor-mediated induction of interleukin 2 mRNA. *Proc Natl Acad Sci USA*. June 15, 1991;88(12):5326–5330.

Maldarelli F, Kearney M, Palmer S, et al. HIV populations are large and accumulate high genetic diversity in a nonlinear fashion. *J Virol*. 2013;87(18):10313–10323.

Margolis D, Brinson C, Smith G, et al. Cabotegravir plus rilpivirine, once a day, after induction with cabotegravir plus nucleoside reverse transcriptase inhibitors in antiretroviral-naive adults with HIV-1 infection (LATTE): a randomised, phase 2b, dose-ranging trial. *Lancet Inf Dis*. 2015;15:1145–1155.

Marin B, Thiebaut R, Bucher HC, et al. Non-AIDS-defining deaths and immunodeficiency in the era of combination antiretroviral therapy. *AIDS*. 2009; 23:1743–1753.

Markowitz M, Louie M, Hurley A, et al. A novel antiviral intervention results in more accurate assessment of human immunodeficiency virus type 1 replication dynamics and T-cell decay in vivo. *J Virol*. 2003;77:5037–5038.

Martrus G, Niehrs A, Cornelis R, et al. Kinetics of HIV-1 latency reversal quantified on the single-cell level using a novel flow-based technique. *J Virol*. 2016;90(20):9018–9028.

Messiaen P, Wensing AMJ, Fun A, et al. Clinical use of HIV integrase inhibitors: a systematic review and meta analysis. *PLoS ONE*. 2013;8(1): e52562.

Miller MD, Feinberg MB, Greene WC. The HIV-1 nef gene acts as a positive viral infectivity factor. *Trends Microbiol*. August 1994;2(8):294–298.

Mollan KR, Smurzynski M, Eron JJ, et al. Association between efavirenz as initial therapy for HIV-1 infection and increased risk for suicidal ideation or attempted or completed suicide: an analysis of trial data. *Ann Int Med*. 2014;161:1–10.

Morrow G, Vachot L, Vagenas P, et al. Current concepts of HIV transmission. *Curr Infect Dis Rep*. May 2008;10(2):133–139.

Opravil M, Ledergerber B, Furrer H, et al.;the Swiss HIV Cohort Study. Clinical efficacy of early initiation of HAART in patients with asymptomatic HIV infection and CD4+ cell count >350 × 10(6)/1. *AIDS*. 2002;16:1371–1381.

Palella FJ Jr, Deloria-Knoll M, Chmiel JS, et al.; the HIV Outpatient Study Investigators. Survival benefit of initiating antiretroviral therapy in HIV infected persons in different CD4+ cell strata. *Ann Intern Med*. 2003;138:620–626.

Palmer S, Josefsson L, Coffin JM. HIV reservoirs and the possibility of a cure for HIV infection [published online ahead of print October 27, 2011. *J Intern Med*. 2011;270(6):550–560. doi: 10.1111/j.1365-2796.2011.02457.x.

Pereira LA, Bentley K, Peeters A, et al. A compilation of cellular transcription factor interactions with the HIV-1 LTV promoter. *Nucleic Acids Res*. 2000;28(3):663–668.

Phillips A, Pezzotti P, and the CASCADE Collaboration. Short-term risk of AIDS according to current CD4+ cell count and viral load in antiretroviral drug-naive individuals and those treated in the monotherapy era. *AIDS*. 2004;18:51–58.

Piguet V, Steinman RM. The interaction of HIV with dendritic cells: outcomes and pathways. *Trends Immunol*. 2007;28:503–510.

Reiche EM, Bonametti AM, Voltarelli JC, et al. Genetic polymorphisms in the chemokine and chemokine receptors: impact on clinical course and therapy of the human immunodeficiency virus type 1 infection (HIV-1). *Curr Med Chem*. 2007;14:1325–1334.

Riddler SA, Haubrich R, DiRienzo AG, et al.; the AIDS Clinical Trials Group Study A5142 Team. Class-sparing regimens for initial treatment of HIV-1 infection. *N Engl J Med*. 2008;258:2095–2106.

Rijnders BJ, Post FA, Rieger A, et al. Longer-term renal safety of tenofovir alafenamide vs tenofovir disoproxil fumarate. Presented at the Conference on Retroviruses and Opportunistic Infections, Boston, 2016. Available at http://www. croiconference.org/sessions/longer-term-renal-safety-tenofovir-alafenamide-vs-tenofovir-disoproxil-fumarate. Accessed July 9, 2018.

Rouzine I, Weinberger A, Weinberger L. An evolutionary role for HIV latency in enhancing viral transmission. *Cell*. 2015;160(5):1002–1012.

Saag M, Benson C, Gandhi R, et al. Antiretroviral drugs for treatment and prevention of HIV infection in adults: 2018 recommendations of the International Antiviral Society-USA Panel. *JAMA*. 2018;320(4):379–396.

Sabin CA, Worm SW, Weber R, et al. Use of nucleoside reverse transcriptase inhibitors and risk of myocardial infarction in HIV-infected patients enrolled in the D:A:D study: a multi-cohort collaboration. *Lancet*. 2008;371(9622):1417–1426.

Salminen MO, Carr JK, Robertson DL, et al. Evolution and probably transmission of intersubtype recombinant human immunodeficiency virus type 1 in a Zambian couple. *J Virol*. April 1997;71(4)2647–2655.

Samson M, Libert F, Doranz B, et al. Resistance to HIV-1 infection in caucasian individuals bearing mutant alleles of the CCR-5 chemokine receptor gene. *Nature*. 1996;382:722–725.

Sax PE, Tierney C, Collier A, et al. Abacavir-lamivudine versus tenofovir-emtricitaibine for initial HIV-1 therapy. *N Engl J Med*. 2009;361:2230–2240.

Sax PE, Pozniak A, Montes ML, et al. Coformulated bictegravir, emtricitabine, and tenofovir alafenamide versus dolutegravir with emtricitabine and tenofovir alafenamide, for initial treatment of HIV-1 infection (GS-US-380-1490): a randomised, double-blind, multicentre, phase 3, non-inferiority trial. *Lancet*.2017;390(10107):2073–2082.

Schwartz O, Marechal V, Le Gall S, et al. Endocytosis of major histocompatibility complex class I molecules is induced by the HIV-1 Nef protein. *Nat Med*. March 1996;2(3):338–342.

Siliciano JD, Kaidas J, Finzi D, et al. Long-term follow-up studies confirm the stability of the latent reservoir for HIV-1 in resting CD4+ T cells [published online ahead of print May 18, 2003]. *Nat Med*. June 2003;9(6):727–728. doi: 10.1038/nm880.

Simon F, Mauclere P, Roques P, et al. Identification of a new human immunodeficiency virus type 1 distinct from group M and group O. *Nat Med*. 1998;4(9):1032–1037.

Smith KY, Patel, Fine D. Randomized, double-blind, placebo-matched, multicenter trial of abacavir/lamivudine or tenofovir/emtricitabine with lopinavir/ritonavir for initial HIV treatment. *AIDS.* 2009;23(12):1547–1556.

Squires K, Kityo C, Hodder S. Integrase inhibitor versus protease inhibitor based regimen for HIV-1 infected women (WAVES): a randomised, controlled double-blind, phase 3 study. *Lancet HIV.* 2016;3(9):e410–e420.

Sterne JA, May M, Costagliola D, et al.; the When to Start Consortium. Timing of initiation of antiretroviral therapy in AIDS-free HIV-1-infected patients: a collaborative analysis of 18 HIV cohort studies. *Lancet.* 2009;373:1352–1363.

Tavasolli A. Targeting the protein-protein interactions of the HIV lifecycle. *Chem Soc Rev.* 2011;40(3):1337–1346.

Taylor B, Sobieszczyk M, McCutchan F, et al. The challenge of HIV-1 subtype diversity. *N Engl J Med.* 2008;358(15):1590–1602.

Tekeste SS, Wilkonson TA, Weiner EM, et al. Interaction between reverse transcriptase and integrase is required for reverse transcription during HIV-1 replication. *J Virology.* 2015;89(23):12058–12069.

Tilton JC, Doms RW. Entry inhibitors in the treatment of HIV-1 infection [published online ahead of print August 14, 2009. *Antiviral Res.* January 2010;85(1):91–100. doi: 10.1016/j.antiviral.2009.07.022.

Tsiang M, Jones G, Goldsmith J. Antiviral activity of Bictegravir (GS-9883), a novel potent HIV-1 integrase strand transfer inhibitor with an improved resistance profile. *Antimicrob Agents Chemother.* 2016;60(12):7086–7097.

US Department of Health and Human Services (USDHHS), Panel on Antiretroviral Guidelines for Adults and Adolescents. Guidelines for the use of antiretroviral agents in HIV-1-infected adults and adolescents. May 30, 2018. Available at https://www.aidsinfo.nih.gov/ContentFiles/AdultandAdolescentGL.pdf. Accessed July 9, 2018.

Wang H, Lu X, Yang X. The efficacy and safety of tenofovir alafenamide versus tenofovir disoproxil fumarate in antiretroviral regimens or HIV-1 therapy. *Medicine (Batimore).* 2016;95(41):e5146.

Waters L, Fisher M, Winston A, et al. A phase IV, double-blind, multicentre, randomized, placebo-controlled, pilot study to assess the feasibility of switching individuals receiving efavirenz with continuing central nervous system adverse events to etravirine. *AIDS.* 2011;25:65–71.

Wensing A, van Maarseveen N, Nijhuis M. Fifteen years of HIV protease inhibitors: raising the barrier to resistance. *Antiviral Res.* 2010;85(1):59–74.

Whitney JB, Hill AL, Sanisetty S, et al. Rapid seeding of the viral reservoir prior to SIV viraemia in rhesus monkeys. *Nature.* 2014;512:74–77.

Willey RL, Maldarelli F, Martin MA, et al. Human immunodeficiency virus type 1 Vpu protein regulates the formation of intracellular gp160-CD4 complexes. *J Virol.* January 1992;66(1):226–234.

Wiskerchen M, Muesing MA. Human immunodeficiency virus type 1 integrase: effects of mutations on viral ability to integrate, direct viral gene expression from unintegrated viral DNA templates, and sustain viral propagation in primary cells. *J Virol.* 1995;69:376–386.

World Health Organization. Guideline on when to start antiretroviral therapy and on pre-exposure prophylaxis for HIV. September 2015. Available at http://www.who.int/hiv/pub/guidelines/earlyrelease-arv/en. Accessed November 5, 2015.

Worm SW, Sabin C, Weber R, et al. Risk of myocardial infarction in patients with HIV infection exposed to specific individual antiretroviral drugs from the 3 major drug classes: the data collection on adverse events of anti-HIV drugs (D:A:D) study. *J Infect Dis.* 2010;201(3):318–330.

20.

PRINCIPLES OF APPLIED CLINICAL PHARMACOKINETICS AND PHARMACODYNAMICS IN ANTIRETROVIRAL THERAPY

Neha Sheth Pandit and Emily L. Heil

CHAPTER GOALS

Upon completion of this chapter, the reader should be able to

- Understand the basic principles of applied pharmacokinetics and pharmacodynamics of antiretroviral agents, and apply this knowledge to improve individual patient treatment regimens.

INTRODUCTION

Understanding the basic principles of applied clinical pharmacokinetics and pharmacodynamics can help the clinician gain insight into contemporary HIV pharmacotherapy and improve therapeutic responses. This information can be used to improve antiretroviral (ARV) treatment for the individual patient by gaining a fundamental working knowledge of concepts that contribute to the occurrence of drug–drug interactions (DDIs), adverse drug reactions, poor adherence, decreased efficacy, and the selection of viral resistance. These factors, alone or in combination, can lead to treatment failure of antiretroviral therapy (ART) and subsequent progression of HIV disease. This chapter discusses some of the applied clinical pharmacokinetic and pharmacodynamic principles that relate to the treatment of HIV.

LEARNING OBJECTIVES

- Describe the basic pharmacokinetic properties of classes of antiretroviral (ARV) medications.

- Explain the benefits and shortcomings of using ritonavir or cobicistat for pharmacokinetic enhancement of protease inhibitors (PIs) and/or integrase inhibitors.

- Review the potential role for therapeutic drug monitoring for ARV medications.

WHAT'S NEW?

- The pharmacokinetics of ARV drugs in anatomical sanctuary sites or reservoirs such as the central nervous system (CNS) and genital tract has been extensively studied for the treatment of HIV-associated neurocognitive disorders (HAND) as well as for insights for disease prevention.

- There is continued interest in individualizing ARV dosing based on the genetic polymorphisms that affect metabolism and drug transport, such as cytochrome P450 (CYP) enzymes and P-glycoprotein (P-gp).

- Ongoing development of co-formulated fixed-dose combinations with drugs that share similar half-lives and long-acting formulations to decrease overall medication administration frequency will continue to offer convenient and well-tolerated treatment options ensuring adequate drug exposure and maximizing treatment outcomes.

KEY POINTS

- Systemic concentrations of ARV drugs are influenced by the pharmacokinetic properties of absorption, distribution, metabolism, and excretion (ADME).

- Pharmacokinetics and local drug exposure can differ significantly within anatomical sanctuary sites compared with the systemic compartment.

- High variability in interpatient ARV concentrations is common, which makes population ARV pharmacokinetics very difficult to interpret. HIV replication is dynamic and requires combination ARV therapy with multiple active agents in order to achieve durable virologic suppression.

- Direct and indirect relationships between drug exposure, efficacy, and/or toxicity are common for most ARVs and can be used to improve overall treatment success.

- Suboptimal adherence can result in inadequate concentrations, drug resistance, and virologic failure.

- Therapeutic drug monitoring can be considered in certain scenarios that should be evaluated on a case-by-case basis.

The science of *pharmacokinetics* studies the amount of drug in various locations or compartments of the body and attempts to explain the effect that the body has on the drug through the assessment of multiple factors, such as (1) absorption or bioavailability of the drug, (2) distribution of the drug throughout body compartments, (3) metabolism of the drug, and (4) elimination or excretion of the drug from the body. Clinical pharmacokinetics is the application of these pharmacokinetic principles to the therapeutic management of a drug in a patient with the goal of enhancing efficacy while minimizing toxicity.

In contrast, *pharmacodynamics* examines the relationship between the drug concentration and response or the impact that the drug has on the body, which may have an intended or unintended pharmacologic effect. It also attempts to describe how drugs may interact with each other and display an additive effect (1 + 1 = 2), a synergistic effect (1 + 1 = 3), or an antagonistic effect (1 + 1 = 0). An example is the combination of zidovudine and ganciclovir causing additive bone marrow toxicity resulting in neutropenia. The combination of zidovudine and stavudine has also been shown to be antagonistic because these drugs compete for the same site of action on the viral reverse transcriptase target (US Department of Health and Human Services [USDHHS], 2018).

PHARMACOKINETICS

ABSORPTION

Absorption of medications highly depends on the route of administration. Oral formulations of ARV medications have varying degrees of bioavailability that affect a patient's serum ARV concentration. Currently, only zidovudine and ibalizumab are available in an intravenous formulation, and enfuvirtide is the only ARV available for subcutaneous injection. Ibalizumab, a humanized monoclonal antibody, was approved as an intravenous infusion given every 14 days for heavily treatment-experienced patients (Emu, 2017). Long-acting injectable formulations of rilpivirine (RPV) and an investigational integrase strand transfer inhibitor (INSTI), cabotegravir, are being evaluated for intramuscular administration (Margolis, 2015). For the solid dosage forms, tablets or capsules, absorption first requires the dissolution of the tablet or capsule, allowing the drug to be absorbed through the gastrointestinal (GI) tract and then into the systemic circulation from which it will be distributed to its site of action.

Drug absorption is a function of ionization and aqueous solubility, and this can be impacted by factors such as gastric pH, gastric mobility (emptying), absorptive capacity, biliary function, GI enzymes, splanchnic blood flow, CYP enzyme expression in the gut, and transporters, such as P-gp. Absorption can be further affected under different patient conditions, such as use of nasogastric or percutaneous endoscopic gastrostomy tubes for medication administration, or when liquid formulations of medications are required, such as for pediatric patients or patients who have difficulty swallowing solid dosage forms. Many ARVs are available in oral solutions or suspensions to facilitate administration in these circumstances. The bioavailability of many ARV medications can be significantly compromised by manipulation of the dosage form, such as crushing tablets or opening up the contents of capsules (Bastiaans, 2014). For example, administration of crushed lopinavir/ritonavir tablets significantly decreased the exposure of both components, with a decrease in area under the plasma drug concentration–time curve (AUC) of 45% and 47%, respectively, compared to swallowing the tablets whole (Best, 2011).

Food can impact the bioavailability and rates of absorption for certain medications because food increases the pH in the stomach and delays gastric emptying to the small intestine, which serves as the site of absorption for many medications. For example, the relative bioavailability and maximum plasma drug concentration (C_{max}) of efavirenz (EFV) are increased after a high-fat meal, and it is recommended that the drug be taken on an empty stomach (Sustiva package insert, Bristol-Myers Squibb, 2017). The solubility of a drug and surface area for absorption can be affected by gastric bypass procedures, which may impact the absorption of ART (Smith, 2011). In addition, the AUC and trough concentrations of INSTIs can be significantly reduced when coadministered with polyvalent cation products such as iron and calcium supplements or antacids containing aluminum, magnesium, or calcium. INSTIs should be given at least 2 hours before or 6 hours after products containing polyvalent cations (USDHHS, 2018).

Some ARVs require an acidic environment for solubility to occur, and acid-reducing agents may impact the dissolution of these drugs. Atazanavir (ATV) is a protease inhibitor (PI) whose absorption is dependent on a highly acidic environment (Falcon, 2008). Up to 40 mg by mouth twice daily of famotidine with boosted and unboosted ATV was found to decrease ATV AUC by approximately 20% (Wang, 2009). A pharmacokinetic study of boosted ATV and omeprazole 40 mg reported a 76% reduction in ATV AUC and a 79% reduction in ATV trough concentration (C_{trough}) compared with boosted ATV alone (Agarwala, 2005). Increased gastric pH by acid-reducing agents such as proton pump inhibitors (PPIs) do not cause changes in absorption with other PIs such as lopinavir/ritonavir or darunavir/ritonavir (DHHS, 2018). Increased gastric pH will also decrease RPV absorption, leading to suboptimal concentrations. RPV 150 mg was given with omeprazole 20 mg to 16 HIV-negative patients. RPV AUC and C_{max} decreased by 40%. Based on this study, PPIs are contraindicated with RPV use, and H_2 antagonists should be taken 12 hours before or 4 hours after RPV ingestion (Crauwels, 2008).

DISTRIBUTION

After ARVs are absorbed into the bloodstream, they distribute into the interstitial and intracellular fluids depending on the individual physiochemical properties (pK, molecular weight/size, and lipophilicity) of each drug (Minuesa, 2011). Many of the ARVs circulate in the bloodstream reversibly bound to plasma proteins. Albumin primarily binds acidic drugs, and α_1 acid glycoprotein primarily binds basic drugs. Only free, or unbound, drug is pharmacologically active, and the greater the free fraction of the drug, the better it distributes into tissues or compartments. A decrease in plasma protein binding may be seen in patients with cirrhosis or cancer (Morse, 2006).

Unbound drug can enter cells or tissues primarily through carrier-mediated transport mechanisms, although some drugs can pass through via transcellular diffusion (Griffin, 2011).

The individual distribution characteristics of ARV compounds are under extensive investigation because each ARV drug may differ in the ability to penetrate into "sanctuary sites" throughout the body. These are areas where HIV can undergo compartmentalized viral replication with the potential to select resistant viral mutations due to suboptimal ARV drug concentrations within these sites. For example, HIV can reside within these anatomical sanctuary sites or reservoirs such as the male and female genital tract and/or the CNS (Pomerantz, 2002; Tseng, 2014). In addition, understanding drug distribution in the genital tract is essential for selecting agents for preexposure prophylaxis. Drug distribution to the male and female genital tracts is influenced by many patient factors, including hormonal changes, inflammation, concomitant sexually transmitted infections, and drug factors such as protein binding and lipophilicity (Trezza, 2014).

METABOLISM

Many ARV drugs, including C-C chemokine receptor type 5 (CCR5) inhibitors, non-nucleoside reverse transcriptase inhibitors (NNRTIs), and PIs, are metabolized by CYP enzymes, which are located in the smooth endoplasmic reticulum in cells throughout the body, primarily the liver and intestines. Inhibition of gut CYP3A4 enzymes leads to increased bioavailability, whereas inhibition of liver CYP3A4 metabolism results in delayed elimination and a prolonged elimination half-life. Ritonavir is a highly potent inhibitor of the CYP3A4 enzyme, and coadministration of a subtherapeutic dose (~100 mg) of ritonavir is sufficient to enhance (or "boost") the pharmacokinetic profile of most of the currently licensed PIs (Larson, 2014). Cobicistat, an inhibitor of CYP3A enzymes, is approved by the US Food and Drug Administration (FDA) to provide pharmacokinetic enhancement to the PIs ATV and darunavir, and the INSTI elvitegravir (EVG). Due to its selective inhibition of CYP3A enzymes, cobicistat has less potential for off-target DDIs. Cobicistat has no anti-HIV activity and is also more soluble than ritonavir, facilitating the development of coformulated products (Larson, 2014; Shah, 2013).

Pharmacokinetic enhancement of PI concentrations with ritonavir or cobicistat may have a number of benefits, including the following:

- Higher C_{trough} levels, reducing the risk of selection for drug-resistant viral quasispecies
- Higher plasma levels throughout the 24-hour day, minimizing the need for food requirements, reducing or eliminating the significance of interactions with other agents that induce the metabolism of PIs, and potentially lessening the effects of interpatient variations in drug levels due to factors such as gender, smoking, alcohol consumption, or liver disease

- Increased plasma half-life, resulting in reduced dosing frequency and pill burden
- Increased levels of "forgiveness" with missed or late doses, potentially delaying/preventing the development of viral mutations

P-gp is a cellular protein pump involved in transporting molecules in and out of the cell. P-gp is found extensively in the intestine, and its action is important in drug exposure and bioavailability. PIs are known to be substrates for P-gp. Overexpression of P-gp by certain individuals may result in lower intracellular concentrations of some PIs and thus decreased overall drug exposure (Sankatsing, 2004). Ritonavir is a potent inhibitor of P-gp, whereas cobicistat is a weak P-gp substrate and inhibitor that does not lead to clinically relevant interactions (Larson, 2014; Shah, 2013).

EXCRETION

Antiretroviral drugs are eliminated from the body either unchanged by the process of excretion or converted to metabolites that may be more readily excreted. The kidney is the most important organ for the elimination of drugs and their metabolites, whereas the liver is the principal organ responsible for drug metabolism and biliary excretion (Verbeeck, 2009).

Renal and hepatic diseases are progressive illnesses that may occur as comorbidities in the HIV population. Chronic kidney disease is a condition marked by deteriorating kidney function and subsequent decreases in medication elimination. Nucleoside/nucleotide reverse transcriptase inhibitors (NRTIs) are primarily eliminated via the kidney, with the exception of abacavir. If there is a decrease in the glomerular filtration rate (GFR) in chronic kidney disease, it may be necessary to decrease the NRTI dose or increase the dosing frequency interval to prevent high systemic drug concentrations that may lead to adverse drug reactions. It is important for the clinician to routinely check kidney function at least every 6 months (USDHHS, 2018). The National Kidney Foundation Kidney Disease Outcomes Quality Initiative recommends the use of kidney function estimating equations of either Cockroft–Gault or the Modification of Diet in Renal Disease (MDRD) for the routine estimation of GFR. Note that most FDA medication package insert dosage guidelines for renal impairment are based on only the Cockcroft–Gault estimating equation. Guidelines for renal dosage adjustments of ARV agents are provided in the USDHHS guidelines (2018).

PHARMACODYNAMICS

The need to maintain adequate drug concentrations that are effective in controlling HIV replication and preventing resistance has resulted in considerable interest in the relationship between ARV drug exposure and virologic response or drug-related toxicity. This relationship is better known as therapeutic drug monitoring (TDM) and is often used to optimize medication dosing to ensure efficacy and prevent toxicities. TDM has been well established with certain medications, such as digoxin, vancomycin, aminoglycosides, and immunosuppressants (Pretorius, 2011). However, the use of TDM for the routine management of ART is not without limitations. Specifically, there is a lack of large prospective studies showing improved outcomes, a lack of established therapeutic concentration ranges for ARV agents, intrapatient variability in concentrations, a lack of availability of Clinical Laboratory Improvement Amendments-compliant clinical laboratories that reliably perform ARV concentrations, and a shortage of experts to assist with analysis and application of ARV concentrations (USDHHS, 2018; Pretorius, 2011).

The current strategy for using TDM for ARVs includes patients who may have compromised ADME. For example, absorption may be disrupted in patients with DDIs or impairment of GI, hepatic, and renal function. Distribution may be affected due to age, weight, and pregnancy. Metabolism may be affected in those who are on concurrent CYP P450-interacting ARVs, and excretion may be compromised, leading to toxicities for patients with hepatic or renal impairment (USDHHS, 2018; Pretorius, 2011). For patients who are experiencing virologic rebound, adherence to their treatment regimen should be thoroughly evaluated prior to TDM as noncompliance is the most common cause for treatment failure.

PROTEASE INHIBITORS

All PIs are CYP3A4 substrates and most are inhibitors of CYP3A; thus, there is a risk of DDIs with commonly used concurrent medications for other disease states that may be substrates of, induce or inhibit the same CYP enzymes. The most common example of this type of interaction is the boosting effect of ritonavir or cobicistat with other PIs or the INSTI, EVG.

A retrospective analysis of 240 HIV-infected patients on boosted and unboosted ATV found a direct correlation between ATV plasma concentrations and the incidence and severity of hyperbilirubinemia, percentage increase in triglycerides, and incidence of nephrolithiasis. These toxicities and increased plasma concentrations were seen mostly in the boosted ATV group, and the study suggests that concentrations greater than 800 ng/mL were likely the cause (Gervasoni, 2015).

NON-NUCLEOSIDE REVERSE TRANSCRIPTASE INHIBITORS

Similar to PIs, NNRTIs are also substrates of the CYP3A4 enzyme; however, unlike PIs, most NNRTIs act as inducers as opposed to inhibitors of CYP enzymes. This still places the NNRTIs at high risk for DDIs and therefore potential candidates for TDM. Unlike the PIs, NNRTIs have a low barrier to resistance. Single-point mutations such as the K103N can cause resistance to first-generation NNRTIs. Second-generation NNRTIs, including RPV, have a higher genetic barrier to resistance (Usach, 2013). The risk of virologic failure with EFV-based ART was associated with low EFV plasma levels in one small study (Marzolini, 2001). In a larger study,

trough levels and AUC_{24} of nevirapine and EFV were not predictive of virologic failure, although for EFV there was an association between these parameters and virologic failure (Leth, 2006). An analysis of etravirine from the DUET trials failed to show any relationship between etravirine pharmacokinetics and efficacy or toxicities (Kakuda, 2010). RPV is currently being studied as a long-acting subcutaneous injection that could be given at least every 4 weeks. The plasma RPV concentrations seen in the long-acting studies have been similar to those seen with oral RPV use (Williams, 2015).

EFV-induced CNS toxicities have been correlated with elevated plasma concentrations (Marzolini, 2001). Through the use of TDM, elevated plasma EFV concentrations were reduced to the recommended therapeutic range while maintaining undetectable viral loads (Mello, 2011). Although subjects in this trial were stable on long-term EFV, a significant improvement in anxiety scores and a trend toward lower stress scores were noted with the reduction in concentrations. EFV 400 mg was also compared to the standard 600 mg dose, and it was found that the lower 400 mg dose was noninferior to the standard 600 mg dose for virologic suppression but was associated with fewer EFV-related adverse events (ENCORE1 Study Group, 2015). A fixed-dose combination tablet including EFV 400 mg is FDA-approved to help minimize toxicities (Symfi Lo, Mylan, 2018).

INTEGRASE STRAND TRANSFER INHIBITORS

INSTIs are the newest class of ARVs, with the first agent, raltegravir (RAL), being approved in 2007. RAL, dolutegravir (DTG), and bictegravir (BIC) are metabolized by UGT1A1, whereas EVG acts similarly to a PI because it is a substrate of CYP3A4 requiring pharmacokinetic enhancing, with the potential for many DDIs. BIC is a minor substrate of CYP3A4 so concomitant administration of potent inducers of CYP3A, P-gp, or UGT1A1 should be avoided (Biktarvy, Gilead, 2018). A study that evaluated RAL 800 mg once daily compared to 400 mg twice daily, both given with emtricitabine/tenofovir disoproxil fumarate (TDF), in treatment-naïve individuals found that although patients in both groups had similar AUCs, a sixfold decrease was seen in C_{trough} in the 800 mg group (Rizk, 2012). Even with the decrease in C_{trough}, similar response rates were seen in both groups, with a baseline viral load of 100,000 copies/mL or less. The once-daily dosing arm was statistically inferior to the standard twice-daily dosing arm in those patients with a baseline viral load of more than 100,000 copies/mL and a CD4$^+$ T cell count 200 mm^3 or less (Eron, 2011). Another study comparing RAL 1200 mg once daily to 400 mg twice daily both in combination with TDF in ART-naïve patients found that the once-daily option was noninferior to twice-daily dosing. RAL HD 600 mg tablets are now available and FDA approved for a total 1,200 mg dosage taken orally once daily (Deeks, 2017). DTG 50 mg/d has been shown to achieve a 2.5 log decrease in HIV RNA after 10 days of DTG therapy (Lalezari, 2009). Similar results were seen with the use of EVG, which resulted in a greater than 1 log decrease in HIV RNA after once- and twice-daily dosing (DeJesus, 2006).

APPLIED PHARMACOKINETICS AND PHARMACODYNAMICS

CENTRAL NERVOUS SYSTEM EFFECTIVENESS OF ANTIRETROVIRAL DRUGS

The CNS is reached by considerable blood flow, but two anatomical barriers—the blood–brain barrier and the blood–cerebrospinal fluid (CSF) barrier—prevent the free passage of drugs into the brain (Calcagno, 2014). The CNS HIV Antiretroviral Therapy Effects Research (CHARTER) study group developed the CNS penetration-effectiveness (CPE) ranking scheme of CNS effectiveness of ARVs based partly on the physiochemical properties of the drug, such as lipophilicity, protein binding, and efflux substrate, that affect penetration into the CNS (Letendre, 2008). Regimens with higher CPE scores may have greater effectiveness in controlling HIV replication in the CSF. However, the use of CPE rankings to affect the course and severity of HAND has not been demonstrated consistently (Caniglia, 2014; Ellis, 2014).

THERAPEUTIC DRUG MONITORING

The combined use of didanosine (ddI) and tenofovir results in tenofovir-induced increases in ddI concentrations as well as a poor $CD4^+$ T cell count response with early virologic failure and rapid selection of resistant mutations (Negredo, 2008). Minimal data exist on the relationship between concentrations of new ARV agents such as DTG, maraviroc, and darunavir and their potential for toxicities. A retrospective study of 1,807 samples found that the majority of concentrations for ARVs are above the upper therapeutic threshold and could likely benefit from dose optimization using TDM (Cattaneo, 2014). The current dosing strategy for ARVs is to dose to ensure the highest probability of success despite lower doses with equivalent efficacy. Currently, the only ARV dosed to the lowest efficacious dose is RPV. This dosing strategy has led to post-approval dose reduction in ARVs such as zidovudine, didanosine, stavudine, and EFV. Other medications that are efficacious at lower doses include lopinavir, ATV, darunavir, and RAL (Crawford, 2012).

SUMMARY

The pharmacokinetic drug properties of ADME will determine the amount of systemic drug concentration that is available for the inhibition of viral synthesis. Other factors, such as drug–drug interactions, drug–food interactions, and concomitant comorbidities contributing to altered GI, renal, and hepatic function, may cause variations in the systemic drug exposure of the ARV agent. Pregnancy, sex differences, and genetic differences can also contribute to pharmacokinetic variability. It is important to note that due to these variables, the same dose of drug does not produce the same drug concentration among patients because of interpatient differences in ADME. Studies are currently under way regarding the use of pharmacogenomics to individualize dosing of ARVs to improve drug therapy outcomes while minimizing the risk of toxicities (Aceti, 2015; Bonora, 2015). Due to the high interpatient variability of ARV concentrations, it is also important to understand that drug toxicities and efficacy can occur at different plasma concentrations for all patients, and future studies may focus on individualizing treatment strategies.

SCENARIO

Consider the management of a HIV-1 infected patient who is experiencing severe depression on EFV 600 mg/tenofovir disoproxil fumarate 300 mg/emtricitabine 200 mg once daily. This patient has been on treatment for 3 months, takes the fixed-dose combination at night on an empty stomach, and is virologically suppressed. Although historically the standard dosing for EFV has been 600 mg/d, in patients who are persistently experiencing CNS toxicities due to high concentrations of EFV, decreasing the dose to 400 mg may improve the pharmacodynamics outcomes of CNS toxicities while maintaining viral suppression. This would be a practical way to use pharmacokinetic and pharmacodynamic principles to help achieve and/or maintain viral suppression.

REFERENCES

Aceti A, Gianserra L, Lambiase L, et al. Pharmacogenetics as a tool to tailor antiretroviral therapy: a review. *World J Virol.* 2015;4:198–208.

Agarwala S, Gray K, Wang Y, et al. Pharmacokinetic effect of omeprazole on atazanavir co-administered with ritonavir in healthy subjects [Abstract 658]. Presented at the 12th Conference on Retroviruses and Opportunistic Infections; Boston, MA February 22–25, 2005.

Bastiaans D, Cressey T, Vromans H, et al. The role of formulation on the pharmacokinetics of antiretroviral drugs. *Expert Opin Drug Metab Toxicity.* 2014; 10:1019–1037.

Best GM, Capparelli EV, Diep H, et al. Pharmacokinetics of lopinavir/ritonavir crushed versus whole tablets in children. *J AIDS.* 2011;58:385–391.

Biktarvy [Package Insert]. Foster City, CA. Gilead, 2018.

Bonora S, Rusconi S, Calcagno A, et al. Successful pharmacogenetics-based optimization of unboosted atazanavir plasma exposure in HIV-positive patients: a randomized, controlled, pilot study (the REYAGEN study). *J Antimicrob Chemother.* 2015;70:3096–3099.

Calcagno A, Di Perri G, Bonora S. Pharmacokinetics and pharmacodynamics of antiretrovirals in the central nervous system. *Clin Pharmacokinet.* 2014;53:891–906.

Caniglia EC, Cain LE, Justice A, et al. Antiretroviral penetration into the CNS and incidence of AIDS-defining neurologic conditions. *Neurology.* 2014;83:134–141.

Cattaneo D, Baldelli S, Castoldi S, et al. Is it time to revise antiretrovirals dosing? A pharmacokinetic viewpoint. *AIDS.* 2014;28:2477–2479.

Crauwels HM, van Heeswijk RP, Kestens D, et al. The pharmacokinetic interaction between omeprazole and TMC 278, an investigational NNRTI [Abstract P239]. Presented at the 9th International Congress on Drug Therapy in HIV Infection, Glasgow, Scotland, November 2008.

Crawford KW, Ripin DHB, Levin AD, et al. Optimising the manufacture, formulation, and dose of antiretroviral drugs for more cost-effective delivery in resource-limited settings: a consensus statement. *Lancet Infect Dis.* 2012;12:550–560.

Deeks ED. Raltegravir once-daily tablet: a review in HIV-1 infection. *Drugs*. 2017;77: 1789–1795.

DeJesus E, Berger D, Markowitz M, et al. Antiviral activity, pharmacokinetics, and dose response of the HIV-1 integrase inhibitor GS-9137 (JTK-303) in treatment-naïve and treatment-experienced patients. *J AIDS*. 2006;43:1–5.

Ellis RJ, Letendre S, Vaida F, et al. Randomized trial of central nervous system-targeted antiretrovirals for HIV-associated neurocognitive disorder. *Clin Infect Dis*. 2014;58:1015–1022.

Emu B, Fessel WJ, Schrader s, et al. Forty-eight week safety and efficacy on-treatment analysis of ibalizumab in patients with multi-drug resistant HIV-1. *Open Forum Infect Dis*. 2017;4(Suppl 1):S38–S39.

ENCORE1 Study Group. Efficacy and safety of efavirenz 400 mg daily versus 600 mg daily: 96-week data from the randomized, double-blind, placebo-controlled, non-inferiority ENCORE1 study. *Lancet Infect Dis*. 2015;15:793–802.

Eron JJ, Rockstroh JK, Reynes J, et al. Raltegravir once daily or twice daily in previously untreated patients with HIV-1: a randomised, active-controlled, phase 3 non-inferiority trial. *Lancet Infect Dis*. 2011;11:907–915.

Falcon RW, Kakuda TN. Drug interactions between HIV protease inhibitors and acid-reducing agents. *Clin Pharmacokinet*. 2008;47:75–89.

Gervasoni C, Meraviglia P, Minisci D, et al. Metabolic and kidney disorders correlate with high atazanavir concentrations in HIV-infected patients: is it time to revise atazanavir dosage? *PLoS One*. 2015;10:1–12.

Griffin L, Annaert P, Brouwer KL. Influence of drug transport proteins on the pharmacokinetics and drug interactions of HIV protease inhibitors. *J Pharm Sci*. 2011;100:3636–3654.

Kakuda TN, Wade JR, Snoeck E, et al. Pharmacokinetics and pharmacodynamics of the non-nucleoside reverse-transcriptase inhibitor etravirine in treatment-experienced HIV-1-infected patients. *Clin Pharmacol Ther*. 2010;88:695–703.

Lalezari J, Sloan L, DeJesus E, et al. Potent antiviral activity of S/GSK1349572, a next generation integrase inhibitor (INI) in INI-naïve HIV-1-infected patients: ING111521 protocol [Abstract TUAB105]. Presented at the 5th Conference on HIV Pathogenesis, Treatment and Prevention; Cape Town, South Africa, July 19–22, 2009.

Larson KB, Wang K, Delille C, et al. Pharmacokinetic enhancers in HIV therapeutics. *Clin Pharmacokinet*. 2014;53:865–872.

Letendre S, Marquie-Beck J, Capparelli E, et al. Validation of the CNS penetration-effectiveness rank for quantifying antiretroviral penetration into the central nervous system. *Arch Neurol*. 2008;65:65–70.

Leth FV, Kappelhoff BS, Johnson D, et al. Pharmacokinetic parameters of nevirapine and efavirenz in relation to antiretroviral efficacy. *AIDS Res Hum Retroviruses*. 2006;22:232–239.

Margolis DA, Boffito M. Long-acting antiviral agents for HIV treatment. *Curr Opin HIV AIDS*. 2015;10:246–283.

Marzolini C, Telenti A, Decosterd LA, et al. Efavirenz plasma levels can predict treatment failure and central nervous system side effects in HIV-1-infected patients. *AIDS*. 2001;15:71–75.

Mello AF, Buclin T, Decosterd LA, et al. Successful efavirenz dose-reduction guided by therapeutic drug monitoring. *Antivir Ther*. 2011;16:189–197.

Minuesa G, Huber-Ruano I, Pastor-Anglada M, et al. Drug uptake transporters in antiretroviral therapy. *Pharmacol Ther*. 2011;132:268–279.

Morse GD, Catanzaro LM, Acosta EP. Clinical pharmacodynamics of HIV-1 protease inhibitors: use of inhibitory quotients to optimise pharmacotherapy. *Lancet Infect Dis*. 2006;6:215–225.

Negredo E, Garrabou G, Puig J, et al. Partial immunological and mitochondrial recovery after reducing didanosine doses in patients on didanosine and tenofovir-based regimens. *Antivir Ther*. 2008;13:231–240.

Pomerantz RJ. Reservoirs of human immunodeficiency virus type 1: the main obstacles to viral eradication. *Clin Infect Dis*. 2002;34:91–97.

Pretorius E, Klinker H, Rosenkranz B. The role of therapeutic drug monitoring in the management of patients with human immunodeficiency virus infection. *Ther Drug Monit*. 2011;33:265–274.

Rizk ML, Hang Y, Luo WL, et al. Pharmacokinetics and pharmacodynamics of once-daily versus twice-daily raltegravir in treatment-naïve HIV-infected patients. *Antimicrob Agents Chemother*. 2012;56:3101–3106.

Sankatsing SUC, Beijnen JH, Schinkel AH, et al. P glycoprotein in human immunodeficiency virus type 1 infection and therapy. *Antimicrob Agents Chemother*. 2004;48:1073–1081.

Shah BM, Schafer JJ, Priano J, et al. Cobicistat: a new boost for the treatment of human immunodeficiency virus infection. *Pharmacotherapy*. 2013;33:1107–1116.

Smith A, Henrisksen B, Cohen A. Pharmacokinetic considerations in Roux-en-Y gastric bypass patients. *Am J Health Syst Pharm*. 2011;68:2241–2247.

Sustiva [package insert] Princeton, NJ: Bristol-Myers Squibb; 2017.

Symfi Lo [package insert] Morgantown, WV: Mylan; 2018.

Trezza CR, Kashuba AD. Pharmacokinetics of antiretrovirals in genital secretions and anatomic sites of HIV transmission: implications for HIV prevention. *Clin Pharmacokinet*. 2014;53:611–624.

Tseng A, Seet J, Phillips EJ. The evolution of three decades of antiretroviral therapy: challenges, triumphs and the promise of the future. *Br J Clin Pharmacol*. 2014;79:182–194.

US Department of Health and Human Services (USDHHS), Panel on Antiretroviral Guidelines for Adults and Adolescents. Guidelines for the use of antiretroviral agents in adults and adolescents living with HIV. Available at http://www.aidsinfo.nih.gov/contentfiles/lvguidelines/AdultandAdolescentGL.pdf. 2018. Accessed July 20, 2018.

Usach I, Melis V, Peris JE. Non-nucleoside reverse transcriptase inhibitors: a review on pharmacokinetics, pharmacodynamics, safety and tolerability. *J Int AIDS Soc*. 2013;16:1–14.

Verbeeck RK, Musuamba FT. Pharmacokinetics and dosage adjustment in patients with renal dysfunction. *Eur J Clin Pharmacol*. 2009;65:757–773.

Wang X, Chung E, Mahnke L, et al. Effects of famotidine on the pharmacokinetics of atazanavir when given with ritonavir with or without tenofovir in HIV-infected subjects [Abstract P30]. Presented at the 10th International Workshop on Clinical Pharmacology of HIV Therapy, Amsterdam, April 2009.

Williams PE, Crauwels HM, Basstanie ED. Formulation and pharmacology of long-acting rilpivirine. *Curr Opin HIV AIDS*. 2015;10:239–245.

21.

CLASSES OF ANTIRETROVIRALS

David E. Koren

CHAPTER GOALS

Upon completion of this chapter, the reader should be able to

- Describe the classes of antiretroviral (ARV) medications and the factors influencing treatment dosing.

- Understand the US Department of Health and Human Services panel's recommended initial HIV treatments and relevant clinical trials.

- Recognize recently approved co-formulated medications, pharmacogenomics, and clinical trials design.

MECHANISMS OF ANTIRETROVIRAL AGENTS

LEARNING OBJECTIVE

Describe the mechanisms of action of the antiretroviral (ARV) classes.

WHAT'S NEW?

Ibalizumab, a monoclonal antibody, is characterized as a post-attachment inhibitor and adds to the diverse class of medications that inhibit initial viral entry into the $CD4^+$ cell.

KEY POINTS

- There are five major categories of ARV agents: inhibitors of viral entry, two types of reverse transcriptase inhibitors, inhibitors of HIV protease, and inhibitors of HIV integrase.

- Combination ARV therapy (ART) is recommended for all people living with HIV.

As recommended by the US Department of Health and Human Services (USDHHS) since 2012 and as further validated by the more recent START (INSIGHT START GROUP, 2015) and TEMPRANO (TEMPRANO ANRS 12136 STUDY GROUP, 2015) trials, ART is indicated for all patients living with HIV without regards to $CD4^+$ T cell count. There are currently 32 unique US Food and Drug Administration (FDA)-approved agents to treat HIV by targeting five major steps in the HIV replication cycle (Figure 21.1). Classes of ARVs can be divided into nucleoside/nucleotide reverse transcriptase inhibitors (NRTIs/NtRTIs), non-nucleoside reverse transcriptase inhibitors (NNRTIs), protease inhibitors (PIs), entry inhibitors (comprising a fusion inhibitor [FI], a CCR5 coreceptor antagonist, and a post-attachment inhibitor [PAI]), and integrase strand transfer inhibitors (INSTIs). The primary goal of combination ART is to achieve viral suppression (USDHHS, 2018).

NUCLEOSIDE REVERSE TRANSCRIPTASE INHIBITORS

NRTIs inhibit the HIV-encoded reverse transcriptase enzyme in the host cell cytoplasm. This blocks the conversion of single-stranded RNA viral chromosome to double-stranded DNA, ultimately preventing incorporation of HIV genetic material into the host chromosome. NRTIs are nucleoside analogs; when reverse transcriptase incorporates them into the growing DNA, chain elongation is terminated. NRTIs must first be activated in the cell through three phosphorylation steps before they can become active chain terminators. NRTIs are poor substrates for human nuclear DNA polymerases, but some NRTIs can be utilized by human mitochondrial DNA polymerases and can cause toxicity. This class of ARVs approved by the FDA include abacavir (ABC), emtricitabine (FTC), lamivudine (3TC), and zidovudine (ZDV).

NUCLEOTIDE REVERSE TRANSCRIPTASE INHIBITORS

NtRTIs and NRTIs act by the same mechanism; however, parent NtRTI compounds are monophosphorylated and therefore require only two enzymatic reactions to become active triphosphorylated moieties. Tenofovir DF (TDF) and tenofovir alafenamide (TAF) are the only NtRTIs approved by the FDA for HIV treatment.

NON-NUCLEOSIDE REVERSE TRANSCRIPTASE INHIBITORS

NNRTIs also inhibit reverse transcriptase in the cytoplasm of the host cell. They act at the same point in the HIV-1

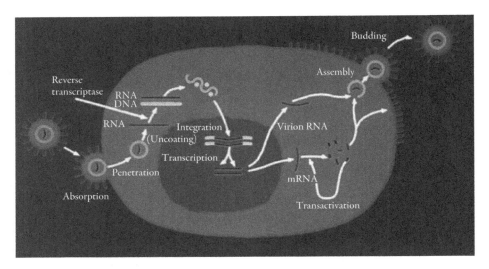

Figure 21.1 HIV replication cycle.

replication cycle as do the NRTIs, but NNRTIs bind the reverse transcriptase adjacent to the active site, causing structural alterations in the enzyme that sterically prevent it from adding any new nucleosides to the growing DNA chain. Because of this different mechanism of action, the viral mutations that encode for resistance to NNRTIs are different from those that encode for resistance to NRTIs. Doravirine (DOR), efavirenz (EFV), etravirine (ETR), nevirapine (NVP), and rilpivirine (RPV) are currently FDA-approved NNRTIs.

PROTEASE INHIBITORS

PIs act when a nearly mature virion is budding from the surface of the infected host cell. These compounds bind HIV-1 protease, preventing it from cleaving the gag precursor polyprotein, an essential process for HIV core maturation. Thus, the viruses that bud from the cell have immature cores, rendering them defective and unable to infect further host cells. First-line PI regimens that include a pharmacologically boosted PI characteristically are associated with no to very low rates of treatment-emergent drug resistance at the time of virologic failure.

While there are six currently FDA-approved PIs, only three, atazanavir (ATV), darunavir (DRV), and ritonavir-boosted lopinavir (LPV/r), are noted in the USDHHS Guidelines (2018) for use in certain clinical situations. The remaining three include fosamprenavir (FPV), saquinavir (SQV), and tipranavir (TPV), but these are no longer recommended by the USDHHS guidelines.

ENTRY INHIBITORS

HIV entry inhibitors are a diverse class with different mechanisms of action. Enfuvirtide (T-20), the only FDA-approved fusion inhibitor, binds the HIV envelope protein gp41, preventing virus–cell fusion. Coreceptor inhibitors act by binding to the coreceptors CCR5 or CXCR4, resulting in allosteric changes that prevent HIV binding, attachment, and subsequent fusion. The only FDA-approved entry inhibitor is maraviroc (MVC), a CCR5 coreceptor antagonist. Use of MVC requires the testing

of viral coreceptor utilization. Patients who harbor virus using CXCR4 or mixed coreceptors receive significantly less virological benefit from maraviroc. Ibalizumab (IBA), a monoclonal antibody characterized as a post-attachment inhibitor, sterically inhibits post-CD4 binding events through attachment to domain 2 of the $CD4^+$ receptor.

INTEGRASE STRAND TRANSFER INHIBITORS

Integrase inhibitors inhibit the viral enzyme integrase, which is responsible for inserting HIV proviral DNA into the host cell's chromosomes. There are four FDA-approved integrase inhibitors: raltegravir (RAL), elvitegravir (EVG), dolutegravir (DTG), and bictegravir (BIC). Regimens that include an INSTI are associated with more rapid viral load declines and greater $CD4^+$ T cell increases than NNRTI- or PI-based regimens.

RECOMMENDED READING

Coffey S. Antiretroviral drug profiles. In: Peiperl L, Coffey S, Bacon O, et al., eds. *HIV InSite Knowledge Base*. San Francisco: University of California at San Francisco. Available at http://hivinsite.ucsf.edu/InSite?page=kb-00&doc=ar-drugs. Accessed August 20, 2018.

ANTIRETROVIRAL DOSING

LEARNING OBJECTIVE

Describe the usual dosing, dose modifications for weight or impaired renal or hepatic clearance, and food requirements for currently FDA-approved ARV therapies.

KEY POINTS

- The selection of an ARV dose should take into consideration the drug concentration that inhibits viral replication and the drug concentration that causes toxicity.

- ARV dosing does not require precise timing; rather, current ARVs are dosed either once or twice daily without need for exact 24- or 12-hour dosing.

- Multiple factors affect drug exposures, including renal and/or hepatic insufficiency, ARV food requirements, and drug–drug interactions.

The selection of an appropriate dosage of an ARV is based on the amount of drug needed to inhibit viral replication and the ability to physiologically obtain these concentrations without causing significant toxicities. Ideally, the maximum concentration should not cause adverse events, and the minimum drug concentrations at the end of a dosing interval should be in excess of the target concentration needed to inhibit viral replication.

Many ARV agents are metabolized by the liver and/or eliminated by the kidney; thus, changes in hepatic or renal function can cause drug accumulation. This increases the potential for adverse drug events and might necessitate dosing changes. Food requirements are important to ensure optimal drug absorption or minimize adverse drug effects. Appendix B of the USDHHS Guidelines (Adults and Adolescents) lists the standard dose, food requirements, and dosage adjustments in renal and/or hepatic impairment for the FDA-approved ARVs. In those situations in which renal and/or hepatic impairment requires dosage modifications, the use of certain fixed-dose, single-tablet regimens (e.g., Atripla, Biktarvy, Complera, Delstrigo, Genvoya, Odefsey, Stribild, and Triumeq) may not be possible; these situations may require the use of individual agents, when available, with the proper dosage adjustment for each agent.

Counseling patients on optimal dosing and adherence is critical to the success of ARV treatment. Evidence-based guidelines for improving adherence are available and include recommendations for the routine collection of self-reported adherence data and the use of pharmacy refill data adherence monitoring (International Advisory Panel on HIV Care Continuum Optimization, 2015). Nearly all ARV medications currently prescribed are dosed either once or twice daily. Note that this does not imply, nor require, that patients take their medications exactly every 24 or 12 hours but, rather, aim to take their medications within a more generous time window.

Many ARV medications should be taken with food for optimal absorption. Some medications require an acidic stomach environment and may have negative drug–drug interactions with acid-lowering agents such as proton pump inhibitors (e.g., ATV and RPV). Others require dietary fat for optimal absorption (e.g., RPV). Counseling and patient adherence to dietary restrictions are important elements for optimal response to ART.

RECOMMENDED READING

International Advisory Panel on HIV Care Continuum Optimization. IAPAC guidelines for optimizing the HIV care continuum for adults and adolescents. *J Int Assoc Provid AIDS Care.* 2015; 14(Suppl. 1):S3–S34. doi:10.1177/2325957415613442

US Department of Health and Human Services, Panel on Antiretroviral Guidelines for Adults and Adolescents. Guidelines for the use of antiretroviral agents in HIV-1-infected adults and adolescents. Available at https://aidsinfo.nih.gov/contentfiles/lvguidelines/adultandadolescentgl.pdf. Accessed August 31, 2018.

RECOMMENDED AND RECENTLY APPROVED ANTIRETROVIRAL AGENTS

LEARNING OBJECTIVE

Describe the USDHHS-recommended initial ART regimens and recently FDA-approved ARV agents in terms of their class, dosing requirements, adverse effects, and resistance profile.

WHAT'S NEW?

- HIV integrase inhibitors are the standard of care for initial therapy. The USDHHS HIV treatment guidelines now recommend five ARV regimens (combining both forms of tenofovir) for most people with HIV. Additional recommendations for certain clinical situations exist, including PI- or NNRTI-based regimens.

- BIC is a new INSTI and is the first to be formulated in a nonboosted, single-tablet regimen containing tenofovir alafenamide.

- Doravirine is a new NNRTI with a unique resistance profile. It is available both as a single agent and as a single-tablet regimen combined with lamivudine and tenofovir disoproxil fumarate

- Ibalizumab is the first monoclonal antibody to be approved for HIV treatment and comprises a new mechanism of action (post-attachment inhibitor).

KEY POINTS

- The USDHHS recommends five regimens for initial treatment of HIV.

- All USDHHS-recommended initial regimens for most people with HIV include an HIV INSTI with two NRTIs.

- Additional USDHHS-recommended initial regimens containing PIs and NNRTIs exist for certain clinical situations that may arise.

This section reviews and summarizes currently recommended initial ARV regimens and newly FDA-approved ARVs. Today's HIV treatments have revolutionized the prognosis for people living with HIV. Once a typically fatal disease, with care and modern treatment, patients can expect near-normal life expectancy, with low risk of AIDS-related complications and few, if any, significant side effects from medications. HIV treatment is prevention, and US and global HIV treatment guidelines now recommend treatment for all people living with HIV, independent of CD4+ T cell count or clinical stage. Viral transmission, HIV-related morbidity/mortality, and non-HIV morbidity/mortality decrease with successful viral suppression. The obstacles to achieving these goals, however, are improving access to HIV testing and medications and engagement and retention in care.

The selection of ARV agents for the treatment of HIV is typically aided by evidence-based guidelines, among the most rigorous are the "Guidelines for the Use of Antiretroviral Agents in HIV-1-Infected Adults and Adolescents" issued by the Panel on Antiretroviral Guidelines for Adults and Adolescents of the USDHHS (2018). The USDHHS guidelines underwent a significant revision in 2017, no longer identifying preferred/alternative regimens for treatment initiation, but rather reclassifying regimens into recommended initial regimens for most people with HIV and designating those regimens as having "demonstrated virologic efficacy, favorable tolerability and toxicity profiles, and ease of use." An additional category was created for recommended initial regimens in certain clinical situations, designating those regimens as "effective and tolerable, but have some disadvantages . . . or have less supporting data from randomized clinical trials." All five recommended initial regimens for most people with HIV (combining tenofovir formulations) include two nucleoside/tide reverse transcriptase inhibitors with an integrase inhibitor (USDHHS, 2018).

These regimens are as follows (in alphabetical order, based on "third" agent):

- Bictegravir/tenofovir alafenamide/emtricitabine (BIC/TAF/FTC; Biktarvy)

- Dolutegravir/abacavir/lamivudine (DTG/ABC/3TC; Triumeq) only for patients who are HLA-B*5701 negative

- Dolutegravir (DTG; Tivicay) plus tenofovir disoproxil fumarate/emtricitabine (TDF/FTC; Truvada) or tenofovir alafenamide/emtricitabine (TAF/FTC; Descovy)

- Elvitegravir/cobicistat/TDF/FTC (EVG/cobi/TDF/FTC; Stribild) or elvitegravir/cobicistat/FTC/tenofovir alafenamide (EVG/c/FTC/TAF; Genvoya)

- Raltegravir (RAL; Isentress) plus TDF/FTC or TAF/FTC

Previously recommended darunavir-, atazanavir-, efavirenz-, and rilpivirine-containing regimens remain recommended but must be taken into account with certain clinical scenarios (e.g., pretreatment viral loads <100,000 copies/mL for rilpivirine regimens) summarized in table 7 of the USDHHS guidelines (2018).

The USDHHS panel recommends taking into consideration pretreatment conditions in selecting initial ART. For example, tenofovir alafenamide has been associated with fewer bone and kidney markers of toxicity than the disoproxil fumarate formulation; however, TDF is associated with lower lipid levels than tenofovir alafenamide. Additionally, patients with high cardiac risk may avoid the use of ABC, although the data to support this remains controversial (USDHHS, 2018).

Recent ARV approvals for the treatment of HIV are summarized in Table 21.1.

KEY CHARACTERISTICS AND FINDINGS OF RECENT CLINICAL TRIALS OF USDHHS-RECOMMENDED REGIMENS

BICTEGRAVIR-BASED REGIMENS

BIC is the fourth FDA-approved INSTI available only in a fixed-dose single-tablet regimen with the NtRTI tenofovir alafenamide and the NRTI emtricitabine. BIC/TAF/FTC is a regimen recommended by the USDHHS for most people living with HIV. BIC is generally very well-tolerated, and adverse drug reactions are uncommon. Characteristic adverse effects are diarrhea, nausea, and headache.

BIC is dosed once daily and has no dietary requirements. As with all INSTIs, oral absorption of these agents is affected by divalent cations, and so dose separation between BIC and divalent cation (aluminum, magnesium, iron, and calcium)-containing products is recommended. Alternatively, iron- and calcium-containing supplements can be taken with BIC together with food (as with DTG). BIC causes reversible inhibition of renal tubular transporters, resulting in decreased tubular excretion of creatinine. This has the effect of increasing serum creatinine levels without impairment of glomerular filtration, also as seen with DTG. Increases were seen in clinical trials after 4 weeks and remained stable through week 48.

Two phase 3 clinical trials evaluated BIC-containing treatments (with either TAF/FTC or ABC/3TC) for initial therapy in adults. GS-380-1489 was a multicenter, randomized, double-blind noninferiority study comparing once daily BIC/TAF/FTC versus DTG/ABC/3TC in 631 patients. The primary endpoint at week 48 demonstrated noninferiority between the two regimens with regard to viral suppression (<50 copies/mL) (Gallant, 2017).

GS-380-1490 was a similarly designed multicenter, randomized, double-blind noninferiority study comparing once daily BIC/TAF/FTC versus DTG + TAF/FTC in 657 treatment-naïve adults. Overall, the two regimens performed

Table 21.1 ANTIRETROVIRAL MEDICATIONS APPROVED BY THE FOOD AND DRUG ADMINISTRATION (FDA) SINCE 2017

TRADE NAME	DRUG/DOSE	ARV CLASS(ES)	DOSE	FOOD REQUIREMENT
Isentress HD (2017)	RAL (600mg)	1 INSTI	2 tablets q.d.	No
Juluca (2017)	RPV (25 mg) DTG (50 mg)	1 NNRTI + 1 INSTI	1 tablet q.d.	Yes
Biktarvy (2018)	TAF (25 mg) FTC (200 mg) BIC (50 mg)	1 NtRTI + 1 NRTI + 1 INSTI	1 tablet q.d.	No
Cimduo (2018)	TDF (300 mg) 3TC (300 mg)	1 NtRTI + 1 NRTI	1 tablet q.d.	No
Symfi (2018)	TDF (300 mg) 3TC (300 mg) EFV (600 mg)	1 NtRTI + 1 NRTI + 1 NNRTI	1 tablet q.d.	No
Symfi Lo (2018)	TDF (300 mg) 3TC (300 mg) EFV (400 mg)	1 NtRTI + 1 NRTI + 1 NNRTI	1 tablet q.d.	No
Symtuza (2018)	TAF (10 mg) FTC (200 mg) DRV (800 mg) COB (150mg)	1 NtRTI + 1 NRTI + 1 PI + 1 PKE	1 tablet q.d	Yes
Trogarzo (2018)	IBA (150 mg/mL)	PAI	2000mg IV load followed by 800mg IV every 2 weeks	No
Pilfeltro (2018)	DOR (100mg)	1 NNRTI	1 tablet q.d.	
Delstrigo (2018)	DOR (100mg) TDF (300mg) 3TC (300mg)	1 NtRTI + 1 NRTI + 1 NNRTI	1 tablet q.d.	

ARV, antiretroviral; BIC, bictegravir; COB, cobicistat; DOR, doravirine; DRV, darunavir; DTG, dolutegravir; EFV, efavirenz; FTC, emtricitabine; IBA, ibalizumab-uiyk; INSTI, integrase strand transfer inhibitor; NRTI, nucleoside reverse transcriptase inhibitor; NNRTI, non-nucleoside reverse transcriptase inhibitor; NtRTI, nucleotide reverse transcriptase inhibitor; PAI, post-attachment inhibitor; PI, protease inhibitor; PKE, pharmacokinetic enhancer; RPV, rilpivirine; TAF, tenofovir alafenamide; TDF, tenofovir disoproxil fumarate; 3TC, lamivudine.

very similarly at week 48 demonstrating noninferiority between the two regimens with regard to viral suppression (<50 copies/mL) (Sax, 2017). These studies suggest that BIC, dosed as part of a single-tablet regimen, is a potent available treatment option for persons initiating therapy.

No treatment-emergent resistance mutations resulted in either clinical trial. BIC retains in vitro activity against some viral strains resistant to other INSTIs, although cross-resistance is possible in isolates harboring a resistance mutation at integrase gene codon 118 or with multiple integrase resistance mutations in combination.

DOLUTEGRAVIR-BASED REGIMENS

DTG is an INSTI commercially available as a stand-alone product (Tivicay), as a fixed-dose combination with NRTIs ABC and 3TC (Triumeq), and as a fixed-dose combination with the NNRTI RPV (Juluca). DTG + TDF/FTC or TAF/FTC and DTG/ABC/3TC are both DHHS-recommended initial treatment regimens. DTG is generally very well-tolerated, and adverse drug reactions are uncommon. Characteristic adverse effects are diarrhea, nausea, and headache. In 2018, an unplanned analysis of the Tsepamo trial was released as an ongoing surveillance study for birth outcomes in Botswana. In this analysis, four cases of neural tube defects were seen in infants from HIV-positive mothers who had received DTG prior to and through conception and pregnancy (Zash, 2018). This study is still ongoing, with final readout expected in April 2019. It is now recommended to check current USDHHS or WHO guidance when starting DTG in women of child-bearing age.

DTG has multiple dosing recommendations in adults: once daily in INSTI-naïve patients or in those who are INSTI-experienced without associated resistance substitutions, and twice daily in patients receiving concurrent cytochrome P450-3A4 inducers (e.g., carbamazepine or rifampin) or who are INSTI-experienced with associated INSTI-resistance substitutions. DTG has no dietary requirements. Oral absorption of INSTIs is affected by divalent cations. Dose separation between DTG and divalent cation (aluminum, magnesium, iron, and calcium)-containing products is recommended. Alternatively, iron- and calcium-containing supplements can be taken with DTG together with food. In order to reduce the risk of abacavir hypersensitivity reaction, DTG/ABC/3TC should be administered only to individuals who test negative for the HLA B-5701 allele. DTG causes reversible inhibition of the renal tubular transporter, resulting in decreased tubular excretion of creatinine. This has the effect of increasing serum creatinine levels without impairment of glomerular filtration.

Four phase 3 clinical trials evaluated DTG-containing treatments (with either TDF/FTC or ABC/3TC) for initial therapy in adults. The SINGLE study was a randomized, double-blind, 144-week study that compared DTG + TDF/FTC to single-tablet EFV/TDF/FTC in approximately 800 treatment-naïve adults (Pappa, 2014; Walmsley, 2013). The primary end point demonstrated the statistical superiority of DTG + TDF/FTC, with the difference driven by discontinuations due to side effects related to EFV. There was no significant difference in the rates of viral suppression between treatment groups. The superiority of the DTG study arm was maintained through 144 weeks of follow-up.

SPRING-2 was a randomized, double-blind study that compared DTG to RAL (dosed twice daily) with NRTI backbone, ABC/3TC, or TDF/FTC in approximately 800 treatment-naïve patients (Raffi, 2013). Overall, the two study arms performed very similarly, with approximately 3% discontinuation due to treatment-related adverse effects and rare treatment-emergent drug resistance (none in the DTG arm), demonstrating noninferiority between the two INSTIs.

FLAMINGO was an open-label clinical trial comparing DTG to DRV/r (with TDF/FTC or ABC/3TC) in treatment-naïve adults (Clotet, 2014; Molina, 2014). The 48- and 96-week results demonstrated the superiority of DTG to DRV/r. The difference between the two study arms was driven by a combination of more frequent virologic and tolerability discontinuations in the DRV/r arm. Changes in fasting lipids were lower among subjects in the DTG arm.

ARIA was the first fully powered all-women's phase 3 clinical trial comparing DTG/ABC/3TC to ritonavir-boosted atazanavir + TDF/FTC in 499 women (Orrell, 2017). After 48 weeks, DTG/ABC/3TC met a predetermined statistical noninferiority endpoint of viral suppression of less than 50 copies/mL compared to the ritonavir-boosted protease inhibitor arm. Fewer patients receiving DTG reported drug-related adverse effects than with ATV (83 [33%] vs. 121 [41%]). Additionally, fewer patients receiving the INSTI-based regimen experienced adverse effects that led to discontinuation (10 [4%] vs. 17 [7%]).

Treatment-emergent resistance to DTG in clinical trials of initial ART is exceptionally rare, with only one case reported with no corresponding decrease in DTG susceptibility (Tivicay package insert, ViiV Healthcare, 2018). Moreover, resistance to NRTI components to initial therapy has not been reported in phase 3 clinical trials. DTG retains activity against some viral strains resistant to other INSTIs, although cross-resistance is possible in isolates harboring resistance mutations at integrase gene codon 148 (in combination with at least two other integrase inhibitor-resistance mutations).

ELVITEGRAVIR-BASED REGIMENS

EVG was the second INSTI approved for treatment of HIV. EVG requires pharmacologic boosting, typically with coformulated cobicistat. EVG/cobi is generally well-tolerated, and adverse drug reactions are uncommon. The characteristic adverse effects of EVG/cobi are gastrointestinal. Two fixed-dose combinations of EVG/cobi are FDA-approved: EVG/cobi/TDF/FTC (Stribild) and in combination with tenofovir alafenamide (TAF), EVG/cobi/FTC/TAF (Genvoya). Both fixed-dose combinations are recommended by the USDHHS guidelines among most patients living with HIV. EVG/cobi is usually well-tolerated; its characteristic adverse effects are nausea, diarrhea, and rash.

Cobicistat is a potent CYP3A4 inhibitor and used to boost EVG levels. EVG/cobi can cause a wide range of drug–drug interactions with CYP3A4 substrates. Cobicistat causes inhibition of the renal tubular transporter, resulting in decreased tubular excretion of creatinine. This has the effect of increasing serum creatinine levels without impairment of glomerular filtration.

EVG/cobi is dosed once daily and should be taken with food. Oral absorption of INSTIs is affected by divalent cations. Dose separation between EVG and divalent cation (aluminum, magnesium, iron, and calcium)-containing products is recommended. EVG/cobi/TDF/FTC is only recommended for patients with baseline creatinine clearance (CrCl) of 70 mL/min or more and should be discontinued if CrCl decreases to less than 50 mL/min. EVG/cobi/FTC/TAF is approved for use in individuals with an estimated glomerular filtration rate (eGFR) 30 mL/min or greater (Gupta, 2015).

EVG/COBI/TDF/FTC

EVG/cobi/TDF/FTC was the first single-tablet INSTI-containing regimen approved in 2012. This fixed-dose combination was studied in three large randomized clinical trials in treatment-naïve individuals. In a 144-week, randomized, double-blind study of 700 ART-naïve individuals comparing two single-tablet regimens, EVG/cobi/TDF/FTC was shown to be statistically noninferior to EFV/TDF/3TC, with similar virologic effectiveness and rates of treatment discontinuation for adverse events (DeJesus, 2012; Wohl, 2015).

The GS 236-0103 clinical trial randomized 708 ART-naïve individuals to receive either EVG/cobi/TDF/FTC or ritonavir-boosted atazanavir + TDF/FTC (Sax, 2015). After 144 weeks, the two study groups showed similar overall results, supporting the finding of noninferiority of EVG/cobi/TDF/FTC.

WAVES was the first fully powered all-women's phase 3 clinical trial comparing EVG/cobi/TDF/FTC to ritonavir-boosted atazanavir + TDF/FTC in 575 women (Kityo, 2015). After 48 weeks, EVG/cobi/TDF/FTC demonstrated statistical superiority to the ritonavir-boosted protease inhibitor arm, with differences driven by less frequent discontinuations due to adverse events (1.7% vs. 6.6%). Declines in bone mineral density were similar in both treatment arms. No treatment-emergent drug resistance was detected among the EVG/cobi/TDF/FTC-treated patients.

EVG/COBI/FTC/TAF

In two large phase 3 clinical trials, EVG/cobi/FTC/TAF was noninferior to EVG/cobi/TDF/FTC in approximately 1,700 treatment-naïve adults (with pretreatment eGFR ≥50 mL/min) at 48 and 96 weeks (Sax, 2015). The study subjects who received TAF had lower declines in eGFR and loss of bone mineral density, suggesting a favorable renal and bone toxicity profile. Lipid parameters were slightly less favorable in the TAF compared with the TDF study arm.

EVG/cobi/FTC/TAF was also studied in an open-label, single-arm study of virologically suppressed patients with mild to moderate renal insufficiency (eGFR, 30–69 mL/min), supporting the FDA indication for the use of EVG/c/FTC/TAF in adults with eGFR of 30 mL/min or more (Gupta, 2015).

Resistance to EVG is characterized by mutations at codons T66I/A/K, E92Q/G, T97A, S147G, Q148R/H/K, and N155H in the viral integrase gene. Resistance to EVG commonly confers cross-resistance to RAL and occasionally to DTG.

RALTEGRAVIR-BASED REGIMEN

RAL was the first FDA-approved INSTI (2007). The combination of RAL with TDF/FTC is a USDHHS-recommended initial regimen. RAL is generally very well-tolerated, and adverse drug reactions are uncommon. Characteristic adverse effects are diarrhea, nausea, and headache.

Depending on formulation, RAL can be dosed once or twice daily and has no dietary restrictions. RAL is metabolized by glucuronidation and has no interaction with CYP3A4 substrates. Oral absorption RAL is decreased by divalent cations; coadministration with aluminum- or magnesium-containing antacids is not recommended.

STARTMRK was a 240-week, randomized, double-blind, placebo-controlled study comparing RAL + TDF/FTC compared to EFV/TDF/FTC in 566 ART-naïve individuals (DeJesus, 2012). At the primary end point of 48 weeks, RAL + TDF/FTC was noninferior to EFV/TDF/FTC. The 4- and 5-year analysis showed virologic and immunologic superiority of RAL, with the virologic differences driven by EFV/TDF/FTC discontinuations due to adverse effects (Rockstroh, 2013).

ACTG A5257 was a large randomized open-label trial of more than 1,800 treatment-naïve subjects that compared twice-daily RAL with once-daily ATV/r or once-daily DRV/r, each administered with TDF/FTC (Lennox, 2014). At week 96, the RAL group was statistically superior to both once-daily PI regimens. Although the regimens had similar virologic suppression rates, there were differences in discontinuations due to side effects and toxicity. Of note, participants receiving RAL had less change in fasting lipids and less decrease in bone mineral density compared to both boosted PI arms.

The SPRING-2 was a double-blind study that randomized treatment-naïve subjects to receive RAL or DTG and was discussed previously (Raffi, 2013). Over 96 weeks of follow-up, the two study arms performed nearly identically, demonstrating noninferiority of the two INSTIs.

The phase 3 ONCEMRK trial was a randomized, double-blind, active controlled trial comparing RAL 400 mg twice daily versus RAL 1,200 mg daily, dosed as two 600 mg tablets (plus TDF+FTC) in approximately 800 treatment-naïve patients. Noninferiority was met at week 48 using a snapshot analysis, including in patients with pretreatment viral loads greater than 100,000 copies/mL.

Resistance to RAL is characterized by mutations at codons 143, 148, and 155 in the viral integrase gene. Resistance to RAL typically confers cross-resistance to EVG and sometimes to DTG. Treatment-emergent resistance to RAL is uncommon. In the STARTMRK and SPRING-2 studies, in individuals initiating ART with RAL + TDF/3TC, INSTI resistance was detected after virologic failure in 4 of 281 (STARTMRK; 240-week data) and 1 of 411 treated individuals (SPRING-2; 96-week data). No INSTI resistance emerged after the first 48 weeks of treatment.

OTHER RECENTLY FDA-APPROVED ANTIRETROVIRAL AGENTS

Non-Nucleoside Reverse Transcriptase Inhibitor

Doravirine (DOR, Pifeltro, Delstrigo) is an NNRTI approved in 2018. Its development presents two unique advantages over other agents in the class: the lack of a food requirement for absorption and a resistance profile not seen among failures with currently available NNRTIs (V106A, Y188L, and F227L). DOR is available as an individual 100 mg tablet (Pifeltro) and as part of a single-tablet regimen containing DOR/TDF/3TC (100 mg/300 mg/300 mg, Delstrigo) and approved for use in adults with no prior ARV experience. As with other regimens containing TDF, the single-tablet regimen should not be given to patients with an estimated CrCl of less than 50 mL/min.

Post Attachment Inhibitor

Ibalizumab-uiyk (IBA, Trogarzo) was approved in 2018. As part of the TMB-301 clinical trial, IBA was developed for usage in patients with multidrug-resistant virus in conjunction with other active ARVs. It possesses a unique mechanism of action (described earlier in this chapter) and has both minimal adverse effects and drug–drug interactions (Emu, 2018). Resistance to IBA is possible if given as monotherapy, demonstrating a patient mandate to take the entire regimen and not to rely on IBA alone.

RECOMMENDED READING

US Department of Health and Human Services, Panel on Antiretroviral Guidelines for Adults and Adolescents. Guidelines for the use of antiretroviral agents in HIV-1-infected adults and adolescents. Available at https://aidsinfo.nih.gov/contentfiles/lvguidelines/adultandadolescentgl.pdf. Accessed August 7, 2018.

COFORMULATIONS

LEARNING OBJECTIVE

Describe current coformulations utilized in HIV therapy.

WHAT'S NEW?

Since 2017, eight new coformulated products have been licensed for the treatment of HIV. Notable are the first single-tablet regimen containing a non-boosted INSTI (Biktarvy), the first single-tablet regimen containing a protease inhibitor (Symtuza), and the first dual-agent single-tablet regimen (Juluca).

KEY POINTS

- Coformulated medications reduce pill burden and improve adherence to ART.

- There are currently four USDHHS panel-recommended single-tablet regimens for initial HIV treatment.

- A two-drug regimen of DTG and rilpivirine has been proved to treat HIV as well as three drugs in selected populations.

Co-formulated ARV medications have been used for the treatment of HIV since 1997. The rationale for coformulation is to decrease pill burden, thereby facilitating treatment adherence while decreasing risk of selective nonadherence or supply chain gaps. A meta-analysis comparing single-tablet regimens (STRs) to multitablet ARV regimens (MTRs) concluded that STRs were associated with statistically significantly more adherence compared to patients on MTRs of any frequency (odds ratio [OR], 2.37; 95% confidence interval [CI], 1.68–3.35; $p < 0.001$; four studies), twice-daily MTR (OR, 2.53; 95% CI, 1.13–5.66; $p = 0.02$; two studies), and once-daily MTR (OR, 1.81; 95% CI, 1.15–2.84; $p = 0.01$; two studies) (Clay, 2015). The relative risk (RR) for 48-week viral load suppression was improved with STRs (RR, 1.09; 95% CI, 1.04–1.15; $p = 0.0003$; three studies), whereas RR of grade 3 to 4 laboratory abnormalities was lower among patients on STRs (RR, 0.68; 95% CI, 0.49–0.94; $p = 0.02$; two studies).

As of 2018, there are 23 coformulations licensed for use in HIV therapy in the United States (Table 21.2).

NON-NUCLEOSIDE REVERSE TRANSCRIPTASE INHIBITORS

Delstrigo, an STR of DOR/TDF/3TC was approved in 2018. This approval was based on two phase 3 clinical studies, DRIVE AHEAD and DRIVE FORWARD, in treatment-naïve adults. In DRIVE AHEAD DOR/TDF/3TC demonstrated noninferiority compared to EFV/FTC/TDF through 48 weeks (Orkin, submitted). In DRIVE FORWARD DOR once daily was compared to DRV/r (800 mg/100 mg) once daily, each in combination with FTC/TDF

or ABC/3TC. DOR + 2 NRTIs demonstrated noninferiority compared to DRV/r + 2 NRTIs through 48 weeks (Molina, 2018). Across both studies 7/747 (0.9%) developed genotypic and phenotypic resistance to DOR. In the DRIVE-AHEAD EFV treatment group, 12/364 (3.3%) developed genotypic and phenotypic resistance to EFV. DOR has a unique resistance pathway; selected viruses from phase 3 studies had V106 or F227 substitutions (Lai, 2018).

Protease Inhibitors

A single-tablet regimen containing darunavir/cobicistat/tenofovir alafenamide/emtricitabine (DRV/COB/TAF/FTC, Symtuza) was approved in 2018. This combination product represents the first STR containing a protease inhibitor. FDA approval was based on the AMBER and EMERALD phase 3 clinical trials in treatment-naïve and -experienced patients, respectively, demonstrating noninferiority from its individual components (Eron, 2018; Orkin, 2018). This regimen retains a high genetic barrier to resistance, but possesses the similar gastrointestinal side effects seen with other agents within the class.

Dual-Agent Treatment Regimens

Recent research in HIV treatment has attempted to simplify treatment regimens in order to prevent lifetime exposure to ARVs. Reducing exposure to certain ARVs may, in turn, reduce long-term side effects of the medications while maintaining viral suppression. The similarly designed SWORD 1 and 2 trials determined the efficacy of two-drug therapy versus three-drug among patients already suppressed on ARVs and who did not have baseline resistance-associated mutations. The studied regimen of DTG and rilpivirine has shown to be similarly efficacious through 100 weeks of follow-up and has been approved as a complete regimen for HIV treatment among patients already virally suppressed and who do not have associated resistance substitutions to either agent: Juluca (DTG/RPV, 2017) (Aboud, 2018; Llibre, 2018). It is noted that when using this regimen that rilpivirine has a dietary fat/acid requirement for absorption and thus cannot be coadministered with many acid-suppressing agents. Further study of other dual-agent regimens is currently under way.

RECOMMENDED READING

Clay PG, Nag S, Graham CM, et al. Meta-analysis of studies comparing single and multi-tablet fixed dose combination HIV treatment regimens. *Medicine*. 2015; 94(42):e1677.

Libre, JM, Hung CC, Brinson C, Castelli F, et al. Efficacy, safety, and tolerability of dolutegravir-rilpivirine for the maintenance of virologic suppression in adults with HIV-1: phase 3 randomised, noninferiority SWORD-1 and SWORD-2 studies. *Lancet HIV*. 2018; 391(10123):839–849.

Table 21.2 US FOOD AND DRUG ADMINISTRATION (FDA)-APPROVED COFORMULATED ANTIRETROVIRAL MEDICATIONS

TRADE NAME	DOSE	CLASSES	DOSE
Combivir (1997)	AZT (300 mg) 3TC (150 mg)	2 NRTIs	1 tablet b.i.d.
Trizivir (2000)	AZT (300 mg) 3TC (150 mg) ABC (300mg) ABC (300 mg)	3 NRTIs	1 tablet b.i.d.
Kaletra (2000)	LPV (200 mg) RTV (50 mg)	2 PIs	2 tablets b.i.d. For treatment-naïve patients only: 4 tablets q.d.
Truvada (2004)	FTC (200 mg) TDF (300 mg)	1 NRTI + 1 NtRTI	1 tablet q.d.
Epzicom (2004)	ABC (600 mg) 3TC (300 mg)	2 NRTI	1 tablet q.d.
Atripla (2006)	FTC (200 mg) TDF (300 mg) EFV (600 mg)	2 NRTI + 1 NNRTI	1 tablet q.d.
Complera (2011)	FTC (200 mg TDF (300 mg) RPV (25 mg)	2 NRTI + 1 NNRTI	1 tablet q.d.
Stribild (2012)	EVG (150 mg) COB (150mg) FTC (200 mg) TDF (300 mg)	1 NRTI + 1 NtRTI + 1 INSTI + 1 PK booster	1 tablet q.d.
Triumeq (2014)	ABC (600 mg) 3TC (300 mg) DTG (50 mg)	2 NRTI + 1 INSTI	1 tablet q.d.
Prezcobix (2015)	DRV (800 mg) COB (150 mg)	1 PI + 1 PK booster	1 tablet q.d.
Evotaz (2015)	ATV (300 mg) COB (150 mg)	1 PI + 1 PK booster	1 tablet q.d.
Genvoya (2015)	EVG (150 mg) COB (150mg) FTC (200 mg) TAF (25 mg)	1 NRTI + 1 NtRTI + 1 INSTI + 1 PK booster	1 tablet q.d.
Dutrebis (2015)	3TC (150 mg) RAL (300 mg)	1 NRTI + 1 INSTI	1 tablet b.i.d.
Odefsey (2016)	RPV (25 mg) TAF (25 mg) FTC (200 mg)	NRTI + NtRTI + NNRTI	1 tablet q.d.
Descovy (2016)	TAF (25 mg) FTC (200 mg)	NRTI + NtRTI	1 tablet q.d.
Juluca (2017)	RPV (25 mg) DTG (50 mg)	1 NNRTI + 1 INSTI	1 tablet q.d.
Biktarvy (2018)	TAF (25 mg) FTC (200 mg) BIC (50 mg)	1 NtRTI + 1 NRTI + 1 INSTI	1 tablet q.d.
Cimduo (2018)	TDF (300 mg) 3TC (300 mg)	1 NtRTI + 1 NRTI	1 tablet q.d.

(continued)

Table 21.2 CONTINUED

TRADE NAME	DOSE	CLASSES	DOSE
Symfi (2018)	TDF (300 mg) 3TC (300 mg) EFV (600 mg)	1 NtRTI + 1 NRTI + 1 NNRTI	1 tablet q.d.
Symfi Lo (2018)	TDF (300 mg) 3TC (300 mg) EFV (400 mg)	1 NtRTI + 1 NRTI + 1 NNRTI	1 tablet q.d.
Symtuza (2018)	TAF (10 mg) FTC (200 mg) DRV (800 mg) COB (150mg)	1 NtRTI + 1 NRTI + 1 PI + 1 PKE	1 tablet q.d
Delstrigo (2018)	DOR (100mg) TDF (300mg) 3TC (300mg)	1 NtRTI + 1 NRTI + 1 NNRTI	1 tablet q.d.

ABC, abacavir; ARV, antiretroviral; ATV, atazanavir; AZT, zidovudine; BIC, bictegravir; COB, cobicistat; DOR, Doravirine; DRV, darunavir; DTG, dolutegravir; EFV, efavirenz; EVG, elvitegravir; FTC, emtricitabine; INSTI, integrase strand transfer inhibitor; LPV, lopinavir; NRTI, nucleoside reverse transcriptase inhibitor; NNRTI, non-nucleoside reverse transcriptase inhibitor; NtRTI, nucleotide reverse transcriptase inhibitor; PI, protease inhibitor; PK, pharmacokinetic; RAL, raltegravir; RPV, rilpivirine; RTV, ritonavir; 3TC, lamivudine; TAF, tenofovir alafenamide; TDF, tenofovir disoproxil fumarate.

CLINICAL TRIALS DESIGN AND ACCESS PROGRAMS

LEARNING OBJECTIVE

Describe the differences between phase 1, 2, 3, and 4 research clinical trials and expanded access programs.

KEY POINTS

- Phase 1 studies are the earliest clinical trials, focusing mainly on safety and pharmacokinetics.

- Phase 2 studies further evaluate safety and begin to evaluate efficacy and dosing. Dose selection is done in early phase 2.

- Phase 3 studies focus on safety and efficacy in the target population.

- Phase 4 studies, sometimes referred to as *post-marketing trials*, occur after FDA approval and study the use of the drug in different patient populations and long-term safety.

- Expanded-access programs make a drug available to patients who are in particular need prior to the drug being available commercially. These programs are generally not established until after phase 3 studies have been fully enrolled.

PHASES OF CLINICAL TRIALS

In general, there are four phases to drug development, which are guided by procedures described in the US Code of Federal Regulations 21 CFR 314.126 (FDA, 2001b):

- Phase 1 is the most preliminary clinical work in small numbers of human subjects and helps to determine safety/toxicity (FDA, 2001a). Phase 1 studies usually start as single-dose studies and then progress to multiple-dose studies (mainly using healthy volunteers). They evaluate a range of aspects, such as pharmacokinetics (including drug bioavailability), dosing interval, food effects, tolerability, and toxicity (to define maximum tolerated dose, sentinel adverse effects, and target organ toxicity).

- Phase 2 studies further evaluate toxicity and the effectiveness of the drug for a particular indication in a larger number of patients who have the disease or condition under study, and they potentially establish dosage (FDA, 2001a). This is usually the initial assessment of activity or proof-of-concept study. It includes several doses and a short course of monotherapy or functional monotherapy. It may include randomized dosing and control or may be dose escalating. Phase 2 studies also collect data on pharmacokinetics, dose response, tolerability, and toxicity. In HIV, these studies are usually divided into phase 2a and phase 2b. Phase 2a trials are generally conducted in a small number of HIV-infected patients and usually are of short duration. Phase 2b trials usually involve longer term dosing, are almost always in combination with other agents, and have a control arm. Longer term tolerability, toxicity, and effectiveness are important outcomes.

- Phase 3 studies are primarily geared toward large cohort efficacy and (along with the accumulated weight of safety and toxicity studies) form the basis for submission to and approval by the FDA (FDA, 2001a). Phase 3 studies are typically large randomized studies that can provide the main core information for submission and regulatory approval. They frequently include blinded therapy. For ARVs, the end point for the most part has traditionally been some measurement of HIV-1 RNA response.

- Phase 4 studies are post-marketing or post-approval trials and may be mandated by the FDA to further determine long-term toxicities or may serve as vehicles for expanded indications or dosing changes (USDHHS, 2005).

Expanded-access programs are often created for patients in particular need to make a drug available before it is licensed. These programs are an outgrowth of the expedited review process for HIV drugs and are usually limited in the number of patients enrolled and the duration of availability. Typically, expanded-access programs are established after phase 3 studies have been fully enrolled and before drug approval. They are subject to FDA oversight (FDA, 2001a; USC, 2002), although considerably less so than are registrational trials. Due to the number of treatment options available today, expanded-access programs are much less common than in the past.

MECHANISMS FOR EXPANDED ACCESS

There are five mechanisms for expanded access.

Emergency Investigational New Drug

For an emergency investigational new drug (E-IND), a physician, on behalf of the patient, contacts the FDA and/or pharmaceutical manufacturer. In this type of emergency situation, a written submission is not needed; however, the FDA expects the physician to submit an IND application as soon as possible (FDA, 1998).

Open-Label Protocol

Open-label protocol is designed to account for the time between the completion of a clinical trial and the FDA approval of an investigational drug. This allows for the continuation of treatment and the end of a phase 3 study. Compliance with the patient safeguard processes must also be demonstrated (FDA, 1998).

Treatment Investigational New Drug

The treatment investigational new drug (T-IND) allows patients, most of whom are very ill, access to investigational drugs when there are no alternative therapies. These are sometimes referred to as "compassionate use" studies and are used to collect safety data in very ill patients who use the new therapy (FDA, 1998).

Parallel Track

This mechanism has been developed to expand availability of INDs to patients with AIDS or other related diseases. Patients in a parallel track study, or a study that is being run in parallel with controlled clinical studies for a particular investigational agent, are those who would not otherwise have access to the treatment because of geographical location or because they do not meet the specific entry criteria for the original study. Only patients who cannot enroll in the available original trial and who are not eligible for marketing standard treatment may enroll in these studies (FDA, 1998).

In 2009, the FDA issued two new rules related to expanded access. The first rule, titled "Expanded Access to Investigational Drugs for Treatment Use," clarifies the criteria for access to investigational drugs, enumerates the requirements for access submissions, establishes safeguards to protect patients from adverse side effects, and implements mechanisms for maintaining meaningful data about treatment use and results. Per the rule, those who may be granted access to investigational drugs include individuals with a serious or immediately life-threatening disease and for whom there is no comparable satisfactory alternative therapy, intermediate-size patient populations comprising individuals who are ineligible to participate in clinical trials or whose disease is so rare that a drug is not being developed, and larger populations under a treatment protocol or in a trial conducted as part of an IND application.

The expanded-access rule specifies that pharmaceutical companies are responsible for submitting IND safety reports (and annual reports when the protocol continues for 1 year or more) and for providing treating physicians with necessary information to maximize the benefits and minimize the risks of treatment. Physicians who administer the treatments, who are considered "investigators" for purposes of this rule, must report adverse drug events to the sponsor, ensure that informed consent requirements are met, and maintain accurate case histories and drug disposition records. In support of the effort to help seriously ill patients gain access to these therapies, the FDA has a website that provides information for patients and their physicians about options for access to investigational drugs (see http://www.fda.gov/ForConsumers/ByAudience/ForPatientAdvocates/AccesstoInvestigationalDrugs/ucm176098.htm).

The second rule, titled "Charging for Investigational Drugs Under an Investigational New Drug Application," amends the existing rules concerning when drug manufacturers may charge patients for investigational drugs. This rule specifies that a company that wishes to charge a clinical trial participant for a drug must show that the drug may provide a significant advantage over other available treatments (as demonstrated by the trial), that the data from the trial are essential to demonstrating the drug's safety and efficacy, and that charging participants is essential because the cost of the drug is "extraordinary to the sponsor" (FDA, 2009).

Right to Try

In 2018, President Trump signed into law the Trickett Wendler, Frank Mongiello, Jordan McLinn, and Matthew Bellina Right to Try Act of 2017 (Right to Try Act). This law amends the Federal Food, Drug, and Cosmetic Act to establish a new pathway for access of post-phase 1 trial medications in patients who have life-threatening illnesses or who have exhausted approved treatment options and are unable to enter a clinical trial. It is unknown what process this will be at this time.

RECOMMENDED READING

US Food and Drug Administration. Expanded access to investigational drugs for treatment use. Title 21 CFR Parts 312 and 316. 2009 ed. Available at https://www.gpo.gov/fdsys/pkg/FR-2009-08-13/pdf/E9-19005.pdf. Accessed November 30, 2015.

US Food and Drug Administration. Expanded access to investigational drugs for treatment use—Questions and answers: Guidance for industry. May 2013 ed. Available at http://www.fda.gov/downloads/drugs/guidancecomplianceregulatoryinformation/guidances/ucm351261.pdf. Accessed November 30, 2015.

PHARMACOGENOMICS

LEARNING OBJECTIVE

Demonstrate how pharmacogenomics are applied in the clinical management of HIV-infected patients.

KEY POINTS

- Pharmacogenomics uses genetic information to guide treatment decision-making.

- Drug resistance testing is an example of viral pharmacogenomic testing.

- Patient pharmacogenomic testing for the HLA B5701 haplotype reduces the risk of abacavir hypersensitivity reaction and is recommended prior to the initiation of abacavir-containing therapy.

Pharmacogenomics refers to the concept of using information about genetic variation to individualize therapeutic decision-making. With regard to HIV therapy, pharmacogenomics could be exploited to identify the most effective or tolerated ARV medications for an individual virus or patient. Possible applications of pharmacogenomics can be broadly categorized into the following areas: (1) ARV susceptibility, (2) explaining pharmacokinetic or pharmacodynamic variability, and (3) predicting adverse drug reaction.

The use of genotypic drug resistance testing is well established and recommended prior to the initiation of treatment and after treatment failure. Such viral testing is a well-established example of the use of pharmacogenomics, albeit using genetic markers to predict susceptibility to ARV medications. Management of HIV drug resistance is detailed in Chapter 21.

Efavirenz is associated with characteristic neuropsychological side effects. These side effects correlate with plasma levels of efavirenz. The metabolism of efavirenz is subject to variable metabolism, with higher efavirenz levels associated with genetic polymorphisms of cytochrome CYP2B6 (Rotger, 2007). In one clinical trial from Japan, individuals harboring the CYP2B6*6 or -*26 allele had successful maintenance of plasma efavirenz levels with dose reduction (Gatanaga, 2007).

Atazanavir is occasionally associated with severe hyperbilirubinemia. Genetic polymorphisms in the UGT1A1 gene appear to influence plasma levels of atazanavir (Rotger, 2005) and are weakly associated with the risk of discontinuation of atazanavir among Hispanic recipients (Ribaudo, 2012).

One of the best characterized examples of pharmacogenomic biomarkers is the association between the HLA-B*5701 allele and abacavir hypersensitivity. Without genetic screening, approximately 5–8% of individuals exposed to abacavir develop the hypersensitivity reaction (HSR). Genetic screening identified the HLA-B*5701 allele as a predictor of HSR. The PREDICT study (Mallal, 2008) was a randomized study of HLA screening of 1,956 predominantly white individuals who were treated with abacavir-containing ART. The use of genetic screening dramatically reduced clinically suspected HSR from 7.8% to 3.4%. Skin patch test immunologically confirmed HSR was reduced from 2.7% to 0%. In a large, racially diverse group of North American patients, HLA-B*5701 screening resulted in 0.8% of individuals having clinically suspected HSR and no immunologically confirmed cases (Young, 2008). HLA-B*5701 allele screening is now recommended prior to the use of abacavir by multiple national treatment guidelines, including USDHHS guidelines (DHHS, 2018).

ACKNOWLEDGMENTS

I thank the authors of previous editions of this chapter, Benjamin Young, MD, Nicholas Bellos, MD, and Amy Keller.

RECOMMENDED READING

Gatanaga H, Hayashida T, Tsuchiya K, et al. Successful efavirenz dose reduction in HIV type 1-infected individuals with cytochrome P450 2B6*6 and *26. *Clin Infect Dis.* 2007; 45(9):1230–1237.

Haas DW, Tarr PE. Perspectives on pharmacogenomics of antiretroviral medications and HIV-associated comorbidities. *Curr Opin HIV AIDS.* 2015; 10(2):116–122.

Phillips E, Mallal S. Successful translation of pharmacogenetics into the clinic: the abacavir example. *Mol Diagn Ther.* 2009; 13(1):1–9.

Ribaudo HJ, Daar ES, Tierney C, et al. Impact of UGT1A1 Gilbert variant on discontinuation of ritonavir-boosted atazanavir in AIDS Clinical Trials Group Study A5202. *J Infect Dis.* 2013; 207(3):420–425.

Young B, Squires K, Patel P, et al. First large, multicenter, open-label study utilizing HLA-B*5701 screening for abacavir hypersensitivity in North America. *AIDS.* 2008; 22:1673–1681.

REFERENCES

Aboud M, Orkin C, Podzamczer D, et al. Durable suppression 2 years after switch to DTG+RPV 2-drug regimen: Sword 1&2 studies. Program and abstracts of the 22nd International AIDS conference; July 23–28, 2018; Amsterdam, The Netherlands. Abstract THPEB047.

Cahn P, Kaplan R, Sax PE, et al. Raltegravir 1200mg once daily versus raltegarvir 400 mg twice daily, with tenofovir disoproxil fumarate and emtricitabine, for previously untreated HIV-1 infection: a randomized, double-blind, parallel-group, phase 3, noninferiority trial. *Lancet HIV.* 2017; 4(11):e486–e494.

Clay PG, Nag S, Graham CM, et al. Meta-analysis of studies comparing single and multi-tablet fixed dose combination HIV treatment regimens. *Medicine.* 2015; 94(42):e1677.

Clotet B, Feinberg J, van Lunzen J, et al.; the ING114915 Study Team. Once-daily dolutegravir versus darunavir plus ritonavir in antiretroviral-naïve adults with HIV-1 infection (FLAMINGO): 48 week results from the randomised open-label phase 3b study. *Lancet.* 2014 Jun 28; 383(9936):2222–2231. [Erratum in: *Lancet.* 2015 Jun 27; 385(9987):2576]

DeJesus E, Rockstroh JK, Henry K, et al. Co-formulated elvitegravir, cobicistat, emtricitabine, and tenofovir disoproxil fumarate versus ritonavir-boosted atazanavir plus co-formulated emtricitabine and tenofovir disoproxil fumarate for initial treatment of HIV-1 infection: A randomised, double-blind, phase 3, noninferiority trial. *Lancet.* 2012; 379(9835):2429–2438.

DeJesus E, Rockstroh JK, Lennox JL, et al. Efficacy of raltegravir versus efavirenz when combined with tenofovir/emtricitabine in treatment-naïve HIV-1-infected patients: Week-192 overall and subgroup analyses from STARTMRK. *HIV Clin Trials.* 2012; 13(4):228–232.

Department of Health and Human Services (DHHS). Information on clinical trials and human research studies: glossary. 2005. Available at: http://www.clinicaltrials.gov/ct/gui/info/glossary#phasel.

Emu B, Fessel J, Schrader S, et al. Phase 3 Study of Ibalizumab for Multidrug-Resistant HIV-1. *N Eng J Med.* 2018; 379:645–654.

Eron JJ, Orkin C, Gallant J, et al. A week-48 randomized phase-3 trial of darunavir/cobicistat/emtricitabine/tenofovir alafenamide in treatment-naïve HIV-patients. *AIDS.* 2018; 32(11):1431–1442.

Food and Drug Administration (FDA). Information sheets: 1998 Guidance for Institutional Review Boards and Investigators. 1998. Available at: http://www.fda.gov/oc/ohrt/irbs/drugsbiologics.html.

Food and Drug Administration (FDA). 21 CFR 312.21. Investigational new drug application. In: Food and Drugs. April 1, 2001a. Available at: http://www.access.gpo.gov/nara/cfr/waisidx_01/21cfr312_01.html.

Food and Drug Administration (FDA). 21 CFR 314.126. Applications for FDA approval to market a new drug. In: Food and Drugs. April 1, 2001b. Available at: http://www.access.gpo.gov/nara/cfr/waisidx_01/21cfr314_01.html.

Gallant J, Lazzarin A, Mills A, et al. Bictegravir, emtricitabine, and tenofovir alafenamide versus dolutegravir, abacavir, and lamivudine for initial treatment of HIV-1 infection (GS-US-380–1489): a double-blind, multicenter, phase 3, randomized controlled noninferiority trial. *Lancet.* 2017; 390(10107):2063–2072.

Gatanaga H, Hayashida T, Tsuchiya K, et al. Successful efavirenz dose reduction in HIV type 1-infected individuals with cytochrome P450 2B6*6 and *26. *Clin Infect Dis.* 2007; 45(9):1230–1237.

Gupta S, Pozniak A, Arribas J, et al. Subjects with renal impairment switching from tenofovir disoproxil fumarate to tenofovir alafenamide have improved renal and bone safety through 48 weeks [Abstract TUAB0103]. 8th International AIDS Society Conference on HIV Pathogenesis, Treatment, and Prevention, July 19–22, 2015, Vancouver.

INSIGHT START Study Group. Initiation of Antiretroviral Therapy in Early Asymptomatic HIV Infection. *N Eng J Med.* 2015; 373:795–807.

International Advisory Panel on HIV Care Continuum Optimization. IAPAC guidelines for optimizing the HIV care continuum for adults and adolescents. *J Int Assoc Provid AIDS Care.* 2015; 14(Suppl. 1):S3–S34. doi:10.1177/2325957415613442

Kityo C, Squires K, Johnson M, et al. The efficacy and safety of elvitegravir/cobicistat/emtricitabine/tenofovir disoproxil fumarate and ritonavir-boosted atazanavir plus emtricitabine/tenofovir disoproxil fumarate in treatment-naïve women with HIV-1 infection: Week 48 analysis of the phase 3, randomized, double-blind study. EACS 2015 Oct 21–24, Barcelona, Spain—15th European AIDS Conference.

Orkin C, Squires KE, Molina JM, et al. Doravirine/lamivudine/TDF is noninferior to efavirenz/emtricitabine/TDF in treatment naïve adults with HIV-1 infection; week 48 results of the phase 3 DRIVE-AHEAD study. *Clinical Infect Dis.* 2019;68(4):535–544.

Orkin C, Molina JM, Negredo E, Arribas JR, et al. Efficacy and safety of switching from boosted protease inhibitors plus emtricitabine and tenofovir disoproxil fumarate regimens to single-tablet darunavir, cobicistat, emtricitabine, and tenofovir alafenamide at 48 weeks in adults with virologically suppressed HIV-1 (EMERALD): a phase 3, randomized, noninferiority trial. *Lancet HIV.* 2018; 5(1):e23–e34.

Orrell C, Hagins DP, Belonosova E, et al. Fixed-dose combination dolutegravir, abacavir, and lamivudine versus ritonavir-boosted atazanavir plus tenofovir disoproxil fumarate and emtricitabine in previously untreated women with HIV-1 infection (ARIA): week 48 results from a randomized, open-label, noninferiority, phase 3b study. *Lancet HIV.* 2017; 4(12):e536–e546.

Lai MT, Xu M, Ngo W, et al. Characterization of doravirine-selected resistance patterns from participants in treatment-naïve phase 3 clinical trials. 22nd International AIDS Conference. Amsterdam, The Netherlands. July 23–27, 2018. Abstract THBDB01.

Lennox JL, Landovitz RJ, Ribaudo HJ, et al. Efficacy and tolerability of 3 nonnucleoside reverse transcriptase inhibitor-sparing antiretroviral regimens for treatment-naïve volunteers infected with HIV-1: A randomized, controlled equivalence trial. *Ann Intern Med.* 2014; 161(7):461–471.

Libre, JM, Hung CC, Brinson C, Castelli F, et al. Efficacy, safety, and tolerability of dolutegravir-rilpivirine for the maintenance of virologic suppression in adults with HIV-1: phase 3 randomised, noninferiority SWORD-1 and SWORD-2 studies. *Lancet HIV.* 2018; 391(10123):839–849.

Mallal S, Phillips E, Carosi G, et al. HLA-B*5701 screening for hypersensitivity to abacavir. *N Engl J Med.* 2008 Feb 7; 358(6):568–579.

Mills A, Arribas JR, Andrade-Villanueva J, et al. Switching from tenofovir disoproxil fumarate to tenofovir alafenamide in antiretroviral regimens for virologically suppressed adults with HIV-1 infection: A randomised, active-controlled, multicentre, open-label, phase 3, noninferiority study. *Lancet Infect Dis.* 2016; 16(1):43–52.

Molina JM, Clotet B, van Lunzen J, et al. Once-daily dolutegravir is superior to once-daily darunavir/ritonavir in treatment-naïve HIV-1-positive individuals: 96 week results from FLAMINGO. *J Int AIDS Soc.* 2014; 17(4 Suppl. 3):19490.

Molina JM, Squires K, Sax P, et al. Doravirine versus ritonavir-boosted darunavir in antiretroviral naïve adults with HIV-1 infection (DRIVE-FORWARD); 48-week results from a randomized, double-blinded, phase 3 noninferiority trial. *Lancet HIV.* 2018;5(5):e211–e220.

Pappa K, Baumgarten A, Felizarta F, et al. Dolutegravir (DTG) plus abacavir/lamivudine once daily superior to tenofovir/emtricitabine/efavirenz in treatment-naïve HIV subjects: 144-week results from SINGLE (ING114467). Paper presented at the Interscience Conference on Antimicrobial Agents and Chemotherapy (ICAAC), 2014, Washington, DC.

Raffi F, Jaeger H, Quiros-Roldan E, et al. Once-daily dolutegravir versus twice-daily raltegravir in antiretroviral-naïve adults with HIV-1 infection (SPRING-2 study): 96 week results from a randomised, double-blind, noninferiority trial. *Lancet Infect Dis.* 2013; 13(11):927–935.

Ribaudo HG, Daar ES, Tierney C, et al. Impact of UGT1A1 Gilbert variant on discontinuation of ritonavir-boosted atazanavir in AIDS Clinical Trials Group Study A5202. *J Infect Dis.* 2013 Feb 1; 207(3):420–425.

Rockstroh JK, DeJesus E, Lennox JL, et al. Durable efficacy and safety of raltegravir versus efavirenz when combined with tenofovir/emtricitabine in treatment-naïve HIV-1-infected patients: Final 5-year results from STARTMRK. *J Acquir Immune Defic Syndr.* 2013; 63(1):77–85.

Rotger M, Tegude H, Colombo S, et al. Predictive value of known and novel alleles of CYP2B6 for efavirenz plasma concentrations in HIV-infected individuals. *Clin Pharmacol Ther.* 2007 Apr; 81(4):557–566.

Sax PE, Wohl D, Yin MT, et al. Tenofovir alafenamide versus tenofovir disoproxil fumarate, coformulated with elvitegravir, cobicistat, and emtricitabine, for initial treatment of HIV-1 infection: Two randomised, double-blind, phase 3, noninferiority trials. *Lancet.* 2015; 385(9987):2606–2615.

Sax PE, Pozniak A, Montes ML, et al. Coformulated bictegravir, emtricitabine, and tenofovir alafenamide versus dolutegravir with emtricitabine and tenofovir alafenamide, for initial treatment of HIV-1 infection (GS-US-380-1490): a randomized, double-blind, multicenter, phase 3, noninferiority trial. *Lancet*. 2017; 390(10107):2073–2082.

TEMPRANO ANRS 12136 Study Group. A Trial of Early Antiretrovirals and Isoniazid Preventive Therapy in Africa. *N Engl J Med*. 2015; 373:808–822.

US Code. 21 USC 360bbb. General provisions relating to drugs and devices: expanded access tounapproved therapies and diagnostics. In: Food and Drugs: Drugs and Devices. January 24, 2002. Available at: http://frwebgate.access.gpo.gov/cgi-bin/getdoc.cgi?dbname=browse_usc&docid=Cite:+21USC360bbb.

US Department of Health and Human Services, Panel on Antiretroviral Guidelines for Adults and Adolescents. Guidelines for the use of antiretroviral agents in HIV-1-infected adults. Available at http://aidsinfo.nih.gov/contentfiles/lvguidelines/AdultandAdolescentGL.pdf.and adolescents. Available at https://aidsinfo.nih.gov/contentfiles/lvguidelines/adultandadolescentgl.pdf.

US Food and Drug Administration. Expanded access to investigational drugs for treatment use. Title 21 CFR Parts 312 and 316. 2009 ed. Available at https://www.gpo.gov/fdsys/pkg/FR-2009-08-13/pdf/E9-19005.pdf. Accessed November 30, 2015.

ViiV Healthcare. Tivicay Package Insert. September, 2018. Available at: https://www.gsksource.com/pharma/content/dam/GlaxoSmithKline/US/en/Prescribing_Information/Tivicay/pdf/TIVICAY-PI-PIL.PDF#page=1. Accessed September 19, 2018.

Walmsley SL, Antela A, Clumeck N, et al. Dolutegravir plus abacavir–lamivudine for the treatment of HIV-1 infection. *N Engl J Med*. 2013; 369(19):1807–1818.

Wohl DA, Cohen C, Gallant JE, et al. A randomized, double-blind comparison of single-tablet regimen elvitegravir/cobicistat/emtricitabine/tenofovir DF versus single-tablet regimen efavirenz/emtricitabine/tenofovir DF for initial treatment of HIV-1 infection: Analysis of week 144 results. *J Acquir Immune Defic Syndr*. 2014; 65(3):e118–e120.

Wohl D, Oka S, Clumeck N, et al. A randomized, double-blind comparison of tenofovir alafenamide vs. tenofovir disoproxil fumarate, each coformulated with elvitegravir, cobicistat, and emtricitabine, for initial HIV-1 treatment: Week 96 results. 15th European AIDS Conference, 2015, Barcelona, Spain.

Young B, Squires K, Patel P, et al. First large, multicenter, open-label study utilizing HLA-B*5701 screening for abacavir hypersensitivity in North America. *AIDS*. 2008; 22:1673–1681.

Zash R, Jacobson D, et al. Dolutegravir/tenofovir/emtricitabine (DTG/TDF/FTC) started in pregnancy is as safe as efavirenz/tenofovir/emtricitabine (EFV/TDF/FTC) in nationwide birth outcomes surveillance in Botswana. 9th IAS 2017 Paris, France.

22.

INITIATION OF ANTIRETROVIRAL THERAPY

WHAT TO START WITH

Saira Ajmal and Zelalem Temesgen

CHAPTER GOALS

Upon completion of this chapter, the reader should be able to

- Discuss categories of regimens for first-line antiretroviral therapy.

- Recognize the basis for the US Department of Health and Human Services (USDHHS) guidelines for initial antiretroviral therapy.

- Recognize and apply recommended regimens for initiation of antiretroviral therapy.

INTRODUCTION

The benefits of antiretroviral therapy (ART) are becoming increasingly appreciated. The primary goal of therapy is to prevent HIV-associated morbidity and mortality. In addition to the dramatic decline in HIV-related illness and death that has been observed as a result of the introduction and expansion of combination ART, evidence is emerging that uncontrolled HIV replication also has a deleterious impact on conditions that are not conventionally associated with immune deficiency, including cardiovascular disease, kidney disease, liver disease, neurologic complications, and malignancy (Deeks, 2011). Other studies have found an independent association between cumulative exposure to replicating virus over time and mortality (Mugavero, 2011). Emerging data also increasingly support the earlier use of ART (INSIGHT START Study Group, 2015). Although it may still be true that ART is beneficial even when started later in the course of HIV disease, it is becoming clear that the damage by unchecked replication done earlier in the course of HIV disease may be irreparable. It has also been shown that the extent of CD4$^+$ recovery is directly associated with the CD4$^+$ T cell count at initiation of ART. The landmark study, HPTN 052, demonstrated the benefit of ART in preventing HIV transmission to uninfected sexual partners of HIV-infected persons on treatment (Cohen, 2011). Effective ART can reduce viremia and transmission of HIV to sexual partners by more than 96%, making reducing the risk of HIV transmission a secondary goal of ART (Cohen, 2015).

The recommendation to start ART in all HIV-infected patients regardless of pretreatment CD4$^+$ T cell counts has recently been changed to class A1 (strong recommendation based on data from randomized controlled trials) based on the START and TEMPRANO trial results. Both of these randomized controlled trials demonstrated that the clinical benefits of ART were greater when started early with CD4$^+$ T cell counts greater than 500 cells/mm^3 than when initiated at a lower CD4$^+$ threshold (INSIGHT START Study Group, 2015; TEMPRANO ANRS 12136 Study Group, 2015).

Currently, there are 29 US Food and Drug Administration (FDA)-approved individual antiretroviral (ARV) drugs classified in seven categories based on their mechanism of action: nucleoside/nucleotide analogue reverse transcriptase inhibitors (NRTIs), non-nucleoside analogue reverse transcriptase inhibitors (NNRTIs), protease inhibitors (PIs), entry inhibitors (fusion inhibitor, CCR5 antagonist, integrase strand transfer inhibitors [INSTIs]), and post-attachment inhibitors. In addition, two drugs (pharmacokinetic boosters [PK]) are used to improve the pharmacokinetic profiles of some ARV drugs.

A panel of leading HIV specialists, convened by the US Department of Health and Human Services (USDHHS), has been developing and updating recommendations for use of ARV agents in HIV-infected individuals since the early days of the highly active antiretroviral therapy (HAART) era. The most recent revised guidelines were released on May 30, 2018, and included key updates to several sections, including changes in recommendations for initial combination regimens for the ARV-naïve patient (USDHHS, May 30, 2018).

FIRST-LINE ANTIRETROVIRAL REGIMENS

In general, an ART regimen has been defined as a three- or four-drug combination consisting of two NRTIs (NRTI backbone) with an INSTI with or without a PK enhancer, NNRTI, or PI with or without a PK enhancer as the third drug. Such regimens have resulted in favorable virologic and immunologic outcomes in most patients in clinical trials as well as in clinical practice. The specific regimen should be selected based on each patient's individual requirements,

Table 22.1 FACTORS FOR CONSIDERATION IN ANTIRETROVIRAL THERAPY (ART) REGIMEN SELECTION

PATIENT CHARACTERISTICS	COMORBIDITIES	REGIMEN-SPECIFIC CONSIDERATIONS
Pretreatment HIV RNA level	Cardiovascular disease, hyperlipidemia, renal disease, osteoporosis, psychiatric illness, neurologic disease, drug abuse requiring narcotic replacement therapy	Regimen's genetic barrier to resistance
Pretreatment CD4$^+$ T cells	Pregnancy or pregnancy potential	Potential adverse effects of medications
HIV genotypic drug resistance	Coinfections: hepatitis C, hepatitis B, tuberculosis	Drug interactions
HLA-B*5701 status		Convenience—pill burden, dosing frequency, availability of fixed-dose combination products, food requirement
Patient's anticipated compliance		Cost
Patient's preference		

taking into account any concerns for virologic efficacy, potential adverse effects, pill burden, dosing frequency, drug–drug interaction, patient's resistance profile, comorbid conditions, and cost. A summary of factors to consider when selecting an ARV regimen is provided in Table 22.1.

According to the latest ARV treatment guidelines, INSTI-based regimens are recommended as initial therapy for most people with HIV. The recommendations by the USDHHS guidelines panel are based primarily on a regimen's efficacy, potency, durability of efficacy, and toxicity profile, as evidenced from published reports of a randomized, prospective clinical trial with an adequate sample size and adequate duration. Darunavir-based (DRV) regimens, which had previously been one of the preferred regimens for initial therapy are now relegated to the category of "Recommended Initial Regimens in Certain Clinical Situations." This decision was based on evidence from clinical trials that showed better outcomes with INSTI-based regimens, in part because of more adverse drug events with DRV-based regimens. Providers should further individualize selection of an ARV regimen on the basis of other considerations, including potential for drug–drug interactions, comorbid conditions, and resistance test results.

RECOMMENDED NRTI BACKBONES

The NRTI combinations of tenofovir DF or tenofovir alafenamide (TAF)/emtricitabine (TDF/FTC or TAF/FTC) or abacavir/lamivudine (ABC/3TC) comprise the nucleoside backbone in each of the recommended and alternative regimens. All of these NRTI combinations are available as coformulated, fixed-dose tablets and as components of coformulated single-tablet regimens. Choosing between the NRTI pairs is directed mainly by differences between TDF, TAF, and ABC. TAF, an oral prodrug of tenofovir (TFV), is available in several coformulated preparations (TAF/FTC, elvitegravir/cobicistat/TAF/FTC (EVG/c/TAF/FTC), and rilpivirine (RPV/TAF/FTC).

In two clinical studies, ACTG 5202 and ASSERT, regimens with ABC/3TC were shown to have an inferior virologic response compared with regimens containing TDF/

FTC (Sax, 2009; Post, 2010). ACTG 5202 compared the efficacy and safety of ABC/3TC to that of TDF/FTC when each was used in combination with either efavirenz (EFV) or ritonavir-boosted atazanavir (ATV/r); differences in virologic efficacy were noted in those with baseline HIV RNA level greater than 100,000 copies/mL (Sax, 2009). The ASSERT study compared ABC/3TC to TDF/FTC, with each also receiving EFV. The proportion of participants with HIV RNA less than 50 copies/mL was lower among ABC/3TC-treated participants (Post, 2010). However, other studies have documented virologic equivalence between ABC/3TC and TDF/FTC. The HEAT study compared ABC/3TC to TDF/FTC, each in combination with ritonavir-boosted lopinavir (LPV/r); there was no difference in virologic efficacy, including in patients with baseline HIV RNA greater than 100,000 copies/mL (Smith, 2009). Similarly, ABC/3TC has shown comparable virologic efficacy to TDF/FTC when used in combination with dolutegravir (DTG) (Walmsley, 2013).

ABC has been associated with a hypersensitivity reaction—a systemic illness with fever, rash, constitutional symptoms, and multiorgan involvement—in 5–8% of individuals. Testing for HLA-B*5701 should precede ABC's clinical uses because the risk of an ABC-related hypersensitivity reaction is highly associated with the presence of this allele; ABC is contraindicated in patients who are HLA-B*5701 positive (ViiV Healthcare, 2013).

ABC has also been associated with myocardial infarction (MI) in some observational studies but not in others. No consensus has been reached on the association between ABC use and MI risk or the mechanism for such an association (Monforte, 2013; Palella, 2015; Sabin, 2014; Worm, 2010; Young, 2015).

Tenofovir disoproxil fumarate (TDF) has been associated with renal impairment. The risk for this adverse event may be greater when TDF is used in regimens containing PIs or elvitegravir boosted with ritonavir or cobicistat (Mocroft, 2015). The use of TDF has also been associated with a decrease in bone mineral density (McComsey, 2011).

Tenofovir alafenamide fumerate (TAF) is an oral prodrug of TFV that has been designed to achieve higher active metabolite concentrations inside peripheral blood mononuclear cells and lower plasma TFV exposures than TDF. This results in comparable antiviral efficacy but less renal and bone mineral adverse effects. The approval of TAF and the two TAF-containing regimens—elvitegravir 150 mg/cobicistat 150 mg/emtricitabine 200 mg/TAF 10 mg (EVG/c/TAF/FTC) and rilpivirine 25 mg/TAF 25mg/FTC 200 mg (RPV/TAF/FTC)—was supported by 48-week data from two pivotal phase 3 studies in which EVG/c/TAF/FTC was found to be noninferior to elvitegravir 150 mg/cobicistat 150 mg/emtricitabine 200 mg/TDF 300 mg (EVG/c/TDF/FTC) among treatment-naïve adult patients. The safety and efficacy of TAF/FTC were also demonstrated in one switch study of virologically suppressed patients who were randomized to continue TDF/FTC or switch to TAF/FTC (Gallant, 2016; Pozniak, 2016). Bioequivalence studies have demonstrated that stand-alone TAF/FTC achieved the same drug levels of TAF/FTC in the blood as EVG/c/TDF/FTC. Bioequivalence studies have also demonstrated that RPV/TAF/FTC achieved similar drug levels of emtricitabine and TAF in the blood as EVG/c/TAF/FTC and similar drug levels of RPV as stand-alone RPV. Based on these results, EVG/c/FTC/TAF is considered as a recommended initial regimen for ART-naïve patients with an estimated creatinine clearance 30 mL/min or more. TAF/FTC is now included as a component of several recommended regimens and offers clinicians an additional NRTI backbone option. Two doses of TAF have been approved: 25 and 10 mg. The 10-mg dose is intended for use in combination with ritonavir or cobicistat; otherwise, the 25-mg dose of TAF is recommended.

CHOOSING BETWEEN INSTIS

The choice of the third drug in an initial ARV regimen lies between an INSTI, NNRTI, or PI is based on consideration of the regimen's efficacy, genetic barrier to resistance, adverse effects, convenience, comorbidities, and drug–drug interactions. Based on these considerations, the following observations have been noted:

- The efficacy and safety of DTG-based regimens (with either ABC/3TC or TDF/FTC) have been evaluated in three clinical trials (SPRING-2, SINGLE, and FLAMINGO). DTG-based regimens were found to be noninferior or superior to other INSTI-, NNRTI-, or PI-based regimens. Thus, DTG/ABC/3TC and DTG + TDF/FTC are among recommended first-line ART regimens (Clotet, 2014; Raffi, 2013; Walmsley, 2013).

- The efficacy and safety of RAL (with either TDF/FTC or ABC/3TC) have been evaluated in a number of clinical trials, in which it was shown to be superior to EFV-, ATV/r-, and DRV/r-based regimens and noninferior to DTG-based regimens (Lennox, 2009, 2014; Raffi, 2013).

- The four-drug, fixed-dose combination product, EVG/c/TDF/FTC, has been evaluated in two randomized clinical trials, in which it was found to be noninferior to EFV/TDF/FTC or ATV/r plus TDF/FTC (Rockstroh, 2013; Zolopa, 2013).

- Bictegravir (BIC) is a new FDA-approved INSTI that is available as part of a single-tablet, once-daily regimen that includes TAF and FTC (BIC/TAF/FTC). The efficacy of BIC in ART-naïve adults was compared to DTG plus two NRTIs in two large, phase 3, randomized, double-blinded clinical trials (Sax, 2017; Gallant, 2017). The proportion of participants with plasma HIV RNA less than 50 copies/mL at week 48 in the BIC arms was noninferior to that noted in the DTG arms in both trials (89% vs. 93% and 92.4% vs. 93%, respectively).

- Clinical studies of DRV/r + TDF/FTC have shown it to be noninferior to RAL and superior to LPV/r. Compared to DTG-based regimens in the FLAMINGO study, DRV/r was inferior to DTG, with adverse events being the primary driver for this difference (Clotet, 2014).

- Historically, EFV, particularly the single-tablet regimen EFV/TDF/FTC, has played a central role in the preferred first-line ARV regimen category. This was based on its demonstrated superiority or noninferiority to all the regimens against which it was compared. However, recent studies have shown superiority of DTG, RAL, and RPV (in patients with baseline HIV RNA <100,000 copies/mL and CD4 cell count >200 cells/mm^3) to EFV; these results were primarily driven by differences in adverse events. Concern regarding EFV-related adverse events was further enhanced by a possible association with suicidality observed in one analysis of four clinical trials (Mollan, 2014). Thus, EFV/TDF/FTC has been relegated to the alternative "Recommended Initial Regimens in Certain Clinical Situations" category.

- Until recently, ATV/r + TDF/FTC was among the preferred first-line ARV regimens based on its virologic efficacy, which is equivalent to that of a number of comparator regimens, including EFV/TDF/FTC, EFV + ABC/3TC, LPV/r + TDF/FTC, and EVG/c/TDF/FTC. However, a recent study, ACTG 5257, compared ATV/r with DRV/r or RAL, each in combination with TDF/FTC. Virologic efficacy was comparable among the three groups; however, more adverse events and treatment discontinuations were noted among patients on ATV/r compared to the other two groups (Lennox, 2015). Thus, ATV/r has been relegated to the "Recommended Initial Regimens in Certain Clinical Situations" category.

RECOMMENDED INITIAL REGIMENS FOR MOST PEOPLE WITH HIV

Regimens classified as recommended by the USDHHS guidelines are those that have shown optimal and durable virologic efficacy in randomized controlled trials, are easy to use, and have favorable tolerability and toxicity profiles. The regimens recommended as initial regimens for most people with HIV are all INSTI-based regimens and are listed in Table 22.2.

RECOMMENDED INITIAL REGIMENS IN CERTAIN CLINICAL SITUATIONS

These regimens are effective but have some potential disadvantages (e.g., pill burden, dosing, schedule, toxicity

Table 22.2 RECOMMENDED INITIAL ANTIRETROVIRAL THERAPY (ART) REGIMENS

INSTI-BASED REGIMENS

Bictegravir/tenofovir alafenamide/emtricitabine[b]

Dolutegravir/abacavir/lamivudine (DTG/ABC/3TC)[a,b]—if HLA-B*5701 negative

Dolutegravir plus tenofovir/emtricitabine (DTG + TDF/FTC or TAF/FTC)[a,c]

Elvitegravir/cobisistat/tenofovir/emtricitabine ((EVG/c/TDF/FTC or TAF/FTC)[d]—

Raltegravir plus tenofovir/emtricitabine (RAL + TDF/FTC or TAF/FTC)[a,c]

ml/min[b]

---

[a] Lamivudine (3TC) may be interchanged with emtricitabine (FTC) or vice versa.

INSTI, integrase strand transfer inhibitors

[b] Single-pill, once-daily regimen.

[c] Fixed-dose co-formulated product for nucleoside backbone.

[d] TAF and TDF are two forms of tenofovir approved by the Food and Drug Administration. TAF has fewer bone and kidney toxicities than TDF, while TDF is associated with lower lipid levels. Safety, cost and access are among the factors to consider when choosing between these drugs.

---

profile, baseline HIV RNA levels, and CD4 cell count) compared to preferred regimens for most people, or they may have less supporting data from randomized clinical trials. However, there may be situations in which these regimens

Table 22.3 ALTERNATIVE ANTIRETROVIRAL THERAPY (ART) REGIMENS

NNRTI-BASED REGIMENS	PI-BASED REGIMENS
Efavirenz/tenofovir/emtricitabine (EFV/TDF/FTC)[b,c]	Cobicistat-boosted atazanavir (ATV/c) plus tenofovir/emtricitabine (TDF/FTC)[a,c]—only if pretreatment estimated CrCl ≥70 mL/min
Rilpivirine/tenofovir/emtricitabine (RPV/TDF/FTC)[a,b]—if pretreatment HIV RNA <100000 copies/mL and CD4+ T cell count >200 cells/mm³	Ritonavir-boosted atazanavir (ATV/r) plus tenofovir/emtricitabine (TDF/FTC)[a,c]
	Cobicistat-boosted darunavir (DRV/c) or ritonavir-boosted Darunavir (DRV/r) plus abacavir/lamivudine (ABC/3TC)[a,c]—if HLA-B*5701 negative
	Cobicistat-boosted darunavir (DRV/c) plus tenofovir/emtricitabine (TDF/FTC)[a,c]—if pretreatment estimated CrCl ≥70 mL/min

NNRTI, non-nucleoside analogue reverse transcriptase inhibitors; PI, protease inhibitor.

[a] Lamivudine (3TC) may be interchanged with emtricitabine (FTC) or vice versa.

[b] Single-pill, once-daily regimen.

[c] Fixed-dose co-formulated product for nucleoside backbone.

Table 22.4 BASELINE CHARACTERISTICS

SCENARIO	RECOMMENDED ACTION
Low CD4+ T cell count (<200 cells/mm³)	Do not use RPV or DRV/r plus RAL
Pre-treatment HIV RNA >100,000 copies/mL	Do not use RPV, ABC/3TC with EFV or ATV/r, or DRV/r plus RAL

might be preferred in an individual patient (e.g., treatment of a pregnant woman). These alternative regimens are categorized as NNRTI-based regimens and PI-based regimens (Table 22.3).

Table 22.5 CONCOMITANT MEDICAL CONDITIONS

SCENARIO	RECOMMENDED ACTION
Cardiac disease	Consider avoiding ABC, LPV/r and DRV/r
Chronic kidney disease	Avoid TDF with a PK enhancer, in particular[a] EVG/c/TDF/FTC ATV/c with TDF DRV/c with TDF
HIV-associated dementia	Avoid EFV because its psychiatric effects may cloud the clinical picture. Favor use of DRV- or DTG-based regimens due to the possibility of increased central nervous system penetration.
Osteoporosis	Consider avoiding TDF.
Hyperlipidemia	EFV, ABC, PI/r, and EVG/c have been associated with increases in lipids.
Psychiatric illness	Consider avoiding EFV. It can exacerbate psychiatric symptoms. It may be associated with suicidality.
Hepatitis B virus co-infection	Use TDF/FTC or TDF/3TC. If TDF use is contraindicated, recommend use of FTC or 3TC with entecavir.
Tuberculosis	If rifampin is used, EFV/TDF/FTC is the recommended regimen, however DTG 50mg BID has been shown to be effective If a PI/r-based ART regimen is used, rifabutin is the rifamycin of choice in the tuberculosis regimen.
Gastroesophageal reflux disease requiring the use of proton pump inhibitors	Avoid ATV or RPV.
Situations when neither tenofovir nor abacavir can be used	DRV/r plus RAL (treatment-naïve) LPV/r plus 3TC (treatment-naïve) DTG plus 3TC (treatment-naïve) DTG/RPV (virally suppressed with no previous virologic failure)

[a] Lamivudine (3TC) may be interchanged with emtricitabine (FTC) or vice versa.

INCORPORATING USDHHS RECOMMENDATIONS FOR FIRST-LINE ANTIRETROVIRAL REGIMEN INTO CLINICAL PRACTICE: SELECT CLINICAL SCENARIOS

The USDHHS guidelines provide an evidence-based menu for selecting an initial ARV regimen. However, it remains the responsibility of clinicians to select the regimen most suited to the clinical scenario at hand. Tables 22.3, 22.4 and 22.5 present select clinical scenarios to illustrate this point.

RECOMMENDED READING

US Department of Health and Human Services (USDHHS), Panel on Antiretroviral Guidelines for Adults and Adolescents. Guidelines for the use of antiretroviral agents in HIV-1-infected adults and adolescents. Available at https://aidsinfo.nih.gov/guidelines/html/1/adult-and-adolescent-treatment-guidelines/0. Accessed April 20, 2016.

US Department of Health and Human Services (USDHHS), Panel on Antiretroviral Guidelines for Adults and Adolescents. Panel on Antiretroviral Guidelines for Adults and Adolescents includes a fixed-dose combination of elvitegravir/cobicistat/emtricitabine/tenofovir alafenamide among the recommended regimens for antiretroviral treatment-naïve individuals with HIV-1 infection. Available at https://aidsinfo.nih.gov/news/1621/evg-c-ftc-taf-statement-from-adult-arv-guideline-panel. Accessed November 22, 2015.

REFERENCES

Cohen MS, Chen YQ, McCauley M, et al. Prevention of HIV-1 infection with early antiretroviral therapy. *N Engl J Med.* 2011;365:493–505.

Cohen MS, Chen Y, McCauley M, et al. Final results of the HPTN 052 randomized controlled trial: antiretroviral therapy prevents HIV transmission [Abstract MOAC0101LB]. Presented at the 8th IAS Conference on HIV Pathogenesis, Treatment & Prevention, Vancouver, British Columbia, July 19–22, 2015.

Clotet B, Feinberg J, van Lunzen J, et al. Once-daily dolutegravir versus darunavir plus ritonavir in antiretroviral-naive adults with HIV-1 infection (FLAMINGO): 48 week results from the randomised open-label phase 3b study. *Lancet.* 2014;383(9936):2222–2231.

Deeks SG. HIV infection, inflammation, immunosenescence, and aging. *Annu Rev Med.* 2011;62:141–155.

Gallant JE, Daar ES, Raffi F, et al. Efficacy and safety of tenofovir alafenamide versus tenofovir disoproxil fumarate given as fixed-dose combinations containing emtricitabine as backbones for treatment of HIV-1 infection in virologically suppressed adults: a randomised, double-blind, active-controlled phase 3 trial. *Lancet HIV.* 2016;3(4):e158–e165.

Gallant J, Lazzarin A, Mills A, et al. Bictegravir, emtricitabine, and tenofovir alafenamide versus dolutegravir, abacavir, and lamivudine for initial treatment of HIV-1 infection (GS-US-380-1489): a double-blind, multicentre, phase 3, randomised controlled non-inferiority trial. *Lancet.* 2017;390(10107):2063–2072.

INSIGHT START Study Group. Initiation of antiretroviral therapy in early asymptomatic HIV infection. *N Engl J Med.* 2015;373:795–807.

Lennox JL, DeJesus E, Lazzarin A, et al. Safety and efficacy of raltegravir-based versus efavirenz-based combination therapy in treatment-naïve patients with HIV-1 infection: a multicentre, double-blind randomised controlled trial. *Lancet.* September 5, 2009;374(9692):796–806.

Lennox JF, Landovitz RJ, Ribaudo HJ. Three nonnucleoside reverse transcriptase inhibitor-sparing antiretroviral regimens for treatment-naïve volunteers infected with HIV-1. *Ann Intern Med.* March 17, 2015;162(6):461–462.

Lennox JL, Landovitz RJ, Ribaudo HJ, et al. Efficacy and tolerability of 3 nonnucleoside reverse transcriptase inhibitor-sparing antiretroviral regimens for treatment-naive volunteers infected with HIV-1: a randomized, controlled equivalence trial. *Ann Intern Med.* October 7, 2014;161(7):461–471.

McComsey GA, Kitch D, Daar ES, et al. Bone mineral density and fractures in antiretroviral-naive persons randomized to receive abacavir-lamivudine or tenofovir disoproxil fumarate-emtricitabine along with efavirenz or atazanavir-ritonavir: AIDS Clinical Trials Group A5224s, a substudy of ACTG A5202. *J Infect Dis.* 2011;203(12):1791–1801.

Mocroft A, Lundgren JD, Ross M, et al. Exposure to antiretrovirals (ARVs) and development of chronic kidney disease (CKD) [Abstract 142]. Presented at the 2015 Conference on Retroviruses and Opportunistic Infections, Seattle, Washington, February 23–24, 2015.

Mollan KR, Smurzynski M, Eron JJ, et al. Association between efavirenz as initial therapy for HIV-1 infection and increased risk for suicidal ideation or attempted or completed suicide: an analysis of trial data. *Ann Intern Med.* July 1, 2014;161(1):1–10.

Monforte Ad, Reiss P, Ryom L, et al. Atazanavir is not associated with an increased risk of cardio- or cerebrovascular disease events. *AIDS.* January 28, 2013;27(3):407–415.

Mugavero MJ, Napravnik S, Cole SR, et al. Viremia copy-years predicts mortality among treatment-naïve HIV-infected patients initiating antiretroviral therapy. *Clin Infect Dis.* November 1, 2011;53(9):927–935.

Palella F, Althoff KN, Moore R, et al. NA-ACCORD: recent abacavir use and risk of MI [Abstract 749 LB]. Presented at the 2015 Conference on Retroviruses and Opportunistic Infections, Seattle, Washington, February 23–26, 2015.

Post FA, Moyle GJ, Stellbrink HJ, et al. Randomized comparison of renal effects, efficacy, and safety with once-daily abacavir/lamivudine versus tenofovir/emtricitabine, administered with efavirenz, in antiretroviral-naive, HIV-1-infected adults: 48-week results from the ASSERT study. *J AIDS.* 2010;55(1):49–45.

Pozniak A, Arribas JR, Gathe J, et al. Switching to tenofovir alafenamide, coformulated with elvitegravir, cobicistat, and emtricitabine, in HIV-infected patients with renal impairment: 48-week results from a single-arm, multicenter, open-label phase 3 study. *J AIDS.* April 15, 2016;71(5):530–537.

Raffi F, Jaeger H, Quiros-Roldan E, et al. Once-daily dolutegravir versus twice-daily raltegravir in antiretroviral-naive adults with HIV-1 infection (SPRING-2 study): 96 week results from a randomised, double-blind, non-inferiority trial. *Lancet Infect Dis.* 2013;13(11):927–935.

Rockstroh J, DeJesus E, Henry K, et al. A randomized, double-blind comparison of coformulated elvitegravir/cobicistat/emtricitabine/tenofovir DF vs. ritonavir-boosted atazanavir plus coformulated emtricitabine and tenofovir DF for initial treatment of HIV-1 infection: analysis of week 96 results. *J AIDS.* 2013;62(5):483–486.

Sabin C, Reiss P, Ryom L, et al. Is there continued evidence for an association between abacavir and myocardial infarction risk? [Abstract 747]. Presented at the 21st Conference on Retroviruses and Opportunistic Infections, Boston, 2014.

Sax P, Tierney C, Collier A, et al. Abacavir–lamivudine versus tenofovir–emtricitabine for initial HIV-1 therapy. *N Engl J Med.* December 3, 2009;361(23):2230–2240.

Sax PE, Pozniak A, Montes ML, et al. Coformulated bictegravir, emtricitabine, and tenofovir alafenamide versus dolutegravir with emtricitabine and tenofovir alafenamide, for initial treatment of HIV-1 infection (GS-US-380-1490): a randomised, double-blind, multicentre, phase 3, non-inferiority trial. *Lancet.* 2017;390(10107):2073–2082.

Smith KY, Patel P, Fine D, et al. Randomized, double-blind, placebo-matched, multicenter trial of abacavir/lamivudine or tenofovir/emtricitabine with lopinavir/ritonavir for initial HIV treatment. *AIDS.* July 31, 2009;23(12):1547–1556.

TEMPRANO ANRS 12136 Study Group. A trial of early antiretrovirals and isoniazid preventive therapy in Africa. *N Engl J Med.* 2015;373:808–822.

US Department of Health and Human Services (USDHHS), Panel on Antiretroviral Guidelines for Adults and Adolescents. Guidelines for the use of antiretroviral agents in adults and adolescents living with HIV. Available at http://aidsinfo.nih.gov/contentfiles/lvguidelines/AdultandAdolescentGL.pdf. Accessed July 26, 2018.

ViiV Healthcare. Ziagen (abacavir) US prescribing information. 2013. Available at http://www.accessdata.fda.gov/drugsatfda_docs/label/2012/020977s025,020978s029lbl.pdf. Accessed April 30, 2016.

Walmsley SL, Antela A, Clumeck N, et al. Dolutegravir plus abacavir-lamivudine for the treatment of HIV-1 infection. *N Engl J Med.* 2013;369(19):1807–1818.

Worm SW, Sabin C, Weber R, et al.;DAD Study Group. Risk of myocardial infarction in patients with HIV infection exposed to specific individual antiretroviral drugs from 3 major drug classes. *J Infect Dis.* 2010;201:318–330.

Young J, Xiao Y, Moodier EE, et al. Effect of cumulating exposure to abacavir on the risk of cardiovascular disease events in patients from the Swiss HIV cohort study. *J AIDS.* 2015;69(4):413–421.

Zolopa A, Sax P, DeJesus E, et al. A randomized double-blind comparison of coformulated elvitegravir/cobicistat/emtricitabine/tenofovir disoproxil fumarate versus favirenz/emtricitabine/tenofovir disoproxil fumarate for initial treatment of HIV-1 infection: analysis of week 96 results. *J AIDS.* 2013;63:96–100.

23.

HIV-1 RESISTANCE TO ANTIRETROVIRAL DRUGS

Tamara Bininashvili, Quentin Doperalski, and Naiel Nassar

LEARNING OBJECTIVE

Discuss the different HIV drug resistance mutations and cross-resistance patterns in each class of HIV medication.

WHAT'S NEW?

In recent years, newer HIV medications have been introduced, and several studies have identified resistance mutations associated with the newer medications.

KEY POINTS

- Previous exposure to antiretroviral (ARV) medications has a significant role in the development of drug resistance, especially in patients who are noncompliant with medications.

- Drug resistance testing should be done in the setting of treatment failure because it can help achieve better virologic response.

- There is extensive cross-resistance with first-generation non-nucleoside reverse transcriptase inhibitors (NNRTIs) and first-generation integrase strand inhibitors (INSTIs).

EPIDEMIOLOGY OF DRUG RESISTANCE

Numerous epidemiologic studies of ARV resistance in both treatment-experienced and treatment-naïve individuals have been performed in the potent combination antiretroviral therapy (ART) era. The development of ARV resistance depends on previous ARV exposure, compliance with the medication, and availability of a fully active ARV regimen for the individual patient. A patient's historical ARV usage will have a major effect on the rate of resistance. For instance, in populations in whom a large percentage of patients were previously treated with mono- and dual-nucleoside therapy, there will be higher rates of ARV resistance.

In the developed world, current rates of ARV resistance in treatment-experienced individuals are declining as the rates of virologic failure decrease with the availability of more potent and better tolerated regimens. Also, patients who were previously exposed to suboptimal therapy are becoming a smaller proportion of the total HIV-infected population. According to the Swiss HIV cohort study from 1998 to 2012, the rate of ARV resistance in treatment-experienced patients is declining over time but that in treatment-naïve patients is not (Yang, 2015).

In treatment-naïve individuals, the rate of transmitted drug resistance (TDR) is related to the prevalence of drug resistance in individuals practicing high-risk behaviors in a community. Thus, rates of TDR can vary widely between locales. Recent studies include a cohort comprising all ART-naïve adults in Kaiser Permanente Northern California (KPNC) undergoing genotypic resistance testing between January 2003 and December 2016 at the Stanford University Healthcare Diagnostic Virology Laboratory. Between 2012 and 2016, TDR rates to any drug class ranged from 15.7% to 19.2% and class specific rates from 10% to 12.8% for NNTRIs, 4.1% to 8.1% for nucleoside reverse transcriptase inhibitors (NRTIs), and 3.6% to 5.2% for protease inhibitors (PIs). Thymidine analogue mutations M184V/I and the tenofovir-associated K65R and K70E/Q/G/N/T accounted for 82.9% (Soo-Yon Rhee, 2018).

With expanding worldwide use of ART, low- and middle-income countries have also seen an increase in acquired and transmitted drug resistance. The prevalence of TDR is highest for NRTIs and NNRTIs, lower for PIs, and, so far, rare for INSTIs. Surveillance conducted by the World Health Organization (WHO) between 2015 and 2016 in 11 countries estimated annual increases of resistance for NNRTIs of 23% (95% confidence interval [CI], 16–29) in southern Africa, 17% (95% CI, 5–30) in eastern Africa, 17% (95% CI, 6–29) in western and central Africa, 11% (95% CI, 5–18) in Latin America and the Caribbean, and 11% (95% CI, 2–20) in Asia. In the United Kingdom, TDR prevalence peaked in 2002 at 14% and dropped to 8–9% in 2009 and to 6.6% in 2013. Data on the transmission of INSTI resistance are scant. The larger studies, to date from the Swiss HIV Cohort Study and the United Kingdom, did not find any transmitted major integrase inhibitor resistance mutations since the class was introduced in 2007, despite the fact that thousands of patients are being treated with these drugs. Thus, as seen for all drugs used at high frequency, INSTI TDR will likely increase over time (Günthard, 2018).

GUIDELINES FOR THE USE OF RESISTANCE TESTING

Several expert panels have issued guidelines for the optimal use of resistance testing, including the British HIV association, the International Antiviral Society, and the US Department of Health and Human Services (Angus, 2016; Günthard, 2018; USDHHS, 2018). All the panels recommend the use of resistance testing in the setting of treatment failure. Several randomized studies have demonstrated that this strategy (regardless of whether genotypic or phenotypic testing is used) leads to superior virologic responses (Baxter, 2000; Cohen, 2002; Durant, 1999). With treatment failure, either genotypic or phenotypic resistance testing is appropriate. In patients with a complex treatment history, the combination of genotypic and phenotypic resistance testing may be helpful. Ideally, resistance testing should be performed while the patient is still on the failing regimen. With removal of drug selection pressure, wild-type virus would be expected to quickly replace the resistant virus as the dominant population circulating in the plasma.

For treatment-naïve adults, earlier versions of treatment recommendations only supported resistance testing in early HIV infection. However, studies have shown that TDR can be detected many years after initial infection (Little, 2008). Because patients infected with resistant virus do not have a reservoir of drug-susceptible virus, TDR is only replaced by drug-susceptible virus by back mutation, a process that can take months to years. Furthermore, abundant evidence indicates that TDR, particularly to NNRTIs, leads to suboptimal virologic response (Kuritzkes, 2008; Little, 2002). A cost-effectiveness analysis found baseline genotyping to be cost-effective when the background rate of TDR is 5% or greater (a situation that is likely in most locales in the developed world) (Sax, 2005). Consequently, resistance testing in chronically infected treatment-naïve patients is now recommended by all three leading agencies. Resistance testing should be performed when the patient enters clinical care, regardless of whether ART is planned in the near term, because the sensitivity of resistance testing declines with time due to the fact that there is some back mutation to wild-type virus. Due to cost considerations and its improved sensitivity for detecting viral mixtures, genotypic testing is preferred in this setting. Resistance testing is also recommended for treatment-naïve pregnant and pediatric patients.

RESISTANCE TESTING

GENOTYPIC RESISTANCE TESTING: THE TEST AND ITS INTERPRETATION

Genotype testing involves the detection of specific genetic mutations in a patient's dominant viral isolate that are known to be associated with ARV resistance. To perform a genotypic resistance test, polymerase chain reaction (PCR) is used to amplify reverse transcriptase and protease. Many labs can now amplify integrase if requested. Direct PCR dideoxynucleotide sequencing is performed. Overlapping sequencing reactions are performed in both directions and resolved electrophoretically in a sequencer. The amino acid sequence is then compared to the standard HIV subtype B consensus sequence. Differences in amino acids at positions that have been found to be associated with resistance are reported. It should be noted that there is some variability in labs' ability to perform genotypic resistance testing at low viral loads (e.g., <1,000 copies/mL).

Numerous genotypic interpretation systems (GIS) are available (Table 23.1). In addition, many scores for individual drugs have been created (Pellegrin, 2008; Vingerhoets, 2008). Until 2013, Virco offered a virtual phenotype (the "Vircotype"), which used available genotype–phenotype pairs within the company's database to predict the phenotype based on the detected genotype. However, there is little evidence that the virtual phenotype outperforms rules-based GIS when predicting virologic response (Torti, 2003), and, due to declining demand, the test is no longer available for clinical use.

Although the outputs of the most commonly used GIS are relatively straightforward, there is still a significant role for the expert clinician in deciding on the optimal salvage regimen. The benefit of additional expert advice compared with provider-only interpretation of genotype testing results was clearly demonstrated by the Havana trial (Tural, 2002). Using a factorial design, the investigators randomized subjects with virologic failure to receive a combination of genotype resistance testing and/or expert advice prior to the choice of the salvage regimen. The study demonstrated that a salvage regimen selected based on both resistance testing as well as expert advice improved virologic outcomes with increased likelihood of undetectable viral load. The combination of genotype resistance testing with expert advice was superior to either strategy alone.

A newer test, GenoSure Archive (Monogram Biosciences), is now available for use when standard resistance testing cannot be performed due to low levels of plasma viral load. This test interrogates the viral archive from mononuclear cells in the peripheral blood and analyzes the proviral DNA with next generation sequencing (NGS) methods to assign drug

Table 23.1 EXAMPLES OF WIDELY USED WEB-BASED GENOTYPIC INTERPRETATION SYSTEMS

French ANRS (National Agency for AIDS Research)	http://www.hivfrenchresistance.org
International AIDS Society USA Mutation List	http://www.iasusa.org/content/ drug-resistance-mutations-in-HIV
Rega Institute	https://rega.kuleuven.be
Stanford University HIV Resistance Database	http://hivdb.stanford.edu

resistance or susceptibility predictions. Testing is available for NRTIs, NNRTIs, INSTIs, and PIs. Clinical utility is highest when prior genotype testing is not available, and a medication switch is being considered.

GIS are similar in their ability to predict the activity of a drug based on a set of mutations (Grant, 2008). Multiple clinical studies have shown that a genotypic susceptibility score (GSS) created from a GIS is a strong predictor of virologic response (Cooper, 2008; Fätkenheuer, 2008). A GSS that weighs the activity of the boosted PI in the salvage regimen may have the capacity to improve the predictive value of a GSS derived from a GIS (Fox, 2007).

PHENOTYPIC RESISTANCE TESTING: THE TEST AND ITS INTERPRETATION

Phenotypic resistance testing measures in vitro susceptibility to specific drugs and may complement genotypic testing in complex cases in which there are multiple resistance mutations, especially in protease, that may make it difficult to predict the outcome of mutational interactions.

Phenotypic resistance testing is available as commercial tests from Monogram Biosciences and Virco (Hertogs, 1998; Monogram Biosciences, 2016), both of which use similar methods and require a viral load 500 copies/mL or greater to be performed successfully. However, due to declining demand, since April 2010, the phenotype test from Virco has not been available for routine clinical use. Initially, PCR is used to amplify the reverse transcriptase (RT) and protease (PR) sequences of the patient's virus (and integrase, if requested). This sequence is then transfected into a lab strain of HIV (which has its RT and PR sequences deleted). The chimeric virus is then cultured with CD4 cell lines in the presence of different concentrations of drugs. In the Monogram assay, a reporter gene (luciferase) indicates infection of cells. Both assays report a fold change for each drug that is determined by the ratio of the IC_{50} (the concentration of a drug that is required for 50% viral inhibition) from the patient's chimeric virus divided by the IC_{50} of a wild-type virus. The interpretation of the phenotype is based on defined clinical cutoffs for each drug. There are potentially two important cutoffs for each drug. The lower cutoff would define when the susceptibility begins to decline but the drug still has partial activity, and the upper cutoff would be the fold change at which all drug activity is lost. If these clinical cutoffs have not been defined for a given drug, the clinician is provided a biological cutoff, which is based on the normal variation in fold changes in wild-type virus. If the fold change is above the upper cutoff, it will be reported as decreased susceptibility. However, if the fold change is below the lower cutoff, it will be reported as increased susceptibility.

The PhenoSense assay also reports replication capacity (RC), an attempt to provide a surrogate for in vivo fitness of a virus. Reduced RC measured by this methodology has been associated with slower disease progression in treatment-naïve individuals (Goetz, 2007). However, currently, RC plays a relatively limited role in the clinical management of patients.

RESISTANCE TESTING IN RESOURCE-LIMITED SETTINGS

Because of the limited availability of resistance testing in resource-limited settings, it is not generally used to guide therapy choices. The World Health Organization (WHO) does use a sentinel monitoring system to assess the levels of TDR in various sites in the developing world.

ANTIRETROVIRAL CROSS-RESISTANCE

DEFINITION OF CROSS-RESISTANCE AND FACTORS AFFECTING LIKELIHOOD OF OCCURRENCE

When HIV replicates in the presence of an incompletely suppressive regimen, the viral mutations that are selected by a specific drug may confer resistance to that drug, as well as to other drugs in the same therapeutic class. This phenomenon has been recognized for NRTIs, NNRTIs, PIs, and INSTIs. The rate at which cross-resistance develops and the extent to which it affects other drugs in the class vary for the different ARV agents. For the first-generation NNRTIs and INSTIs, there is a high level of cross-resistance. Among NRTIs, the potential for cross-resistance varies, although there is complete cross-resistance between lamivudine and emtricitabine. Among PIs and second-generation NNRTIs, as more resistance mutations accumulate during virologic failure to drugs in their class, there is an increasing degree of resistance. There is also extensive cross-resistance between integrase inhibitors dolutegravir, bictegravir, and cabotegravir with accumulation of G140S/Q148H mutations (Zhang, 2018).

CROSS-RESISTANCE PATTERNS IN NRTIS

Nucleoside analogue-associated mutations (NAMs) are a set of RT mutations that confer some degree of resistance to NRTIs and are selected when HIV is exposed to drugs in the NRTI class. These include M41L, E44D, K65R, D67N, 69 insertions, L74V/I, K70R, V118I, Q151M, M184V/I, L210W, T215Y/F, and K219Q/E.

A subset of NAMs that are associated with resistance to zidovudine and stavudine are known as thymidine analogue mutations (TAMs) and occur at positions 41, 67, 70, 210, 215, and 219. An accumulation of TAMs causes loss of susceptibility to the broad NRTI class, independent of the specific mutations associated with resistance to other NRTIs (Whitcomb, 2003).

Two other resistance profiles are also associated with broad NRTI cross-resistance. Q151M usually appears after HIV is exposed to didanosine plus either stavudine or zidovudine. Four other supporting mutations arise afterward (A62V, V75I, F77L, and F116Y), with resulting loss of susceptibility to all NRTIs except tenofovir.

The codon 69 insertion is less common than the Q151M complex. It is composed of a T69S mutation followed by the addition of two amino acids, including serine and usually a second serine, alanine, or glycine. It always arises on a background of TAMs and a few other mutations to create resistance to all currently approved NRTIs.

Most other drug-specific resistance mutations act like the Q151M complex by improving RT's ability to discriminate between NRTIs and the natural nucleoside substrates. For these non-thymidine mutations, the implications of cross-resistance increase when drugs with similar resistance profiles are used together.

K65R confers resistance to the non-thymidine NRTI drugs, including abacavir, didanosine, emtricitabine, lamivudine, and tenofovir. Although uncommon with currently used therapies, K65R developed at high rates in individuals prescribed NRTI-only regimens that lacked a thymidine analogue (e.g., abacavir/lamivudine/tenofovir). The use of thymidine analogues in a regimen appears to decrease the risk of the emergence of K65R because K65R antagonizes the ability of TAMs to facilitate NRTI removal (White, 2006).

The L74V and M184V mutations can also cause cross-resistance. L74V alone causes some decreased susceptibility to abacavir and didanosine. M184V causes resistance to lamivudine and emtricitabine, decreased susceptibility to abacavir and didanosine, and increased susceptibility to tenofovir and zidovudine.

CROSS-RESISTANCE PATTERNS IN NNRTIS

There is extensive cross-resistance between the first-generation NNRTIs (e.g., delavirdine, efavirenz, and nevirapine). Etravirine is unique among currently available NNRTIs in that both in vitro and clinical evidence suggest that it retains antiviral activity in the presence of resistance to first-generation NNRTIs (Madruga, 2007; Vingerhoets, 2008). Rilpivirine has an in vitro profile similar to that of etravirine (Rimsky, 2009). Rilpivirine may also retain antiviral activity in patients with resistance failing treatment with efavirenz and nevirapine (Theys, 2015). Rilpivirine-based regimens are well-tolerated and associated with fewer virologic failures in full virally suppressed treatment-experienced patients upon switching from other ART regimens for different reasons (Gazaignes, 2014).

Mutations at RT codons 103 or 188 lead to high-level resistance to the first-generation NNRTIs. K103N does not reduce the activity of etravirine, whereas Y188L leads to low-level etravirine resistance. Mutations at position 181 lead to high-level resistance to nevirapine and subsequent rapid development of high-level resistance to efavirenz. The Y181C/I/V mutation also is an important mutation for etravirine and is among the mutations given the greatest weighting within Tibotec's scoring system for etravirine (the others being L100I, K101P, and M230L) (Vingerhoets, 2008).

CROSS-RESISTANCE PATTERNS IN PROTEASE INHIBITORS

Several protease mutations emerge during exposure to a variety of PIs, especially unboosted PIs. The accumulation of four or more mutations at codons 10, 32, 46, 54, 82, 84, and 90 is associated with resistance to most agents in the class. However, darunavir and tipranavir both frequently maintain activity against viruses resistant to older PIs and have shown clinical benefit in patients with extensive drug resistance.

CROSS-RESISTANCE PATTERNS IN INSTIS

There is extensive cross-resistance between the first-generation INSTIs raltegravir and elvitegravir. Raltegravir resistance occurs by three main, occasionally overlapping, mutational pathways: N155H followed by E92Q and other accessory mutations, Q148H/R/K + G140S/A and other accessory mutations, and Y143C/R + T97A and other accessory mutations. With the exception of Y143C/R, most raltegravir-resistance mutations confer cross-resistance to elvitegravir. Likewise, it appears that most elvitegravir-resistance mutations are likely to confer cross-resistance to raltegravir.

Dolutegravir, a second-generation INSTI, has a higher barrier to resistance than raltegravir and elvitegravir. Dolutegravir has good activity against most of the viral strains resistant to raltegravir and elvitegravir. However, the virologic response of dolutegravir is significantly reduced when the Q148 mutation is associated with two or more secondary mutations (G140A/C/S, E138A/K/T, or L74I) compared to no Q148 mutation (Castagna, 2014).

New second-generation integrase inhibitors bictegravir and cabotegravir have thus far shown good efficacy and tolerability. They have also shown to be much more proficient at inhibiting mutants than their earlier counterparts. However, the potency of the second-generation INSTI, including dolutegravir, can be affected by triple mutants, which arise when polymorphic mutations are combined (Smith, 2018). There was a substantial decrease in susceptibility to dolutegravir, bictegravir, and cabotegravir when T97A and L74M substitutions were combined with G140S/Q148H (Zhang, 2018).

CONSIDERATIONS FOR RESOURCE-LIMITED SETTINGS

In many resource-limited settings, access to resistance testing is limited or unavailable. However, it is still important to understand the implications of resistance when attempting to sequence therapies in these settings. In the absence of resistance testing, a patient who is experiencing virologic failure on an NNRTI-based regimen despite good adherence should be assumed to harbor NNRTI-associated resistance and switched to boosted PI-based regimen if available.

ANTIRETROVIRAL RESISTANCE MUTATIONS

Figures 23.1 through 23.4 detail the mutations that are associated with resistance to RT, protease, entry, and integrase inhibitors.

Drugs for which a single mutation results in a major change in susceptibility are said to have a low "genetic barrier"

Nucleoside and Nucleotide Analogue Reverse Transcriptase Inhibitors (nRTIs)

69 Insertion Complex (affects all nRTIs currently approved by the US FDA)

Multi-nRTI Resistance

	M 41	A 62	▼ 69	K 70		L 210	T 215	K 219
	L	V	Insert	R		W	Y	Q
							F	E

151 Complex (affects all nRTIs currently approved by the US FDA except tenofovir)

Multi-nRTI Resistance

	A 62	V 75	F 77	F 116	Q 151
	V	I	L	Y	M

Thymidine Analogue-Associated Mutations (TAMs; affect all nRTIs currently approved by the US FDA other than emtricitabine and lamivudine)

Multi-nRTI Resistance

	M 41	D 67	K 70		L 210	T 215	K 219
	L	N	R		W	Y	Q
						F	E

Abacavir

	K 65	L 74	Y 115	M 184
	R	V	F	V
	E			
	N			

Didanosine

	K 65	L 74
	R	V
	E	
	N	

Emtricitabine

	K 65	M 184
	R	V
	E	I
	N	

Lamivudine

	K 65	M 184
	R	V
	E	I
	N	

Stavudine

	M 41	K 65	D 67	K 70		L 210	T 215	K 219
	L	R	N	R		W	Y	Q
		E					F	E
		N						

Tenofovir

	K 65	K 70
	R	E
	E	
	N	

Zidovudine

	M 41	D 67	K 70		L 210	T 215	K 219
	L	N	R		W	Y	Q
						F	E

Nonnucleoside Analogue Reverse Transcriptase Inhibitors (NNRTIs)

Efavirenz

	L 100	K 101	K 103	V 106	V 108	Y 181	Y 188	G 190	P 225	M 230
	I	P	N	M	I	C	L	S	H	L
			S			I		A		

Etravirine

	V 90	A 98	L 100	K 101	V 106	F 138	V 179	Y 181	G 190	M 230
	I	G	I	E	I	A	D	C	S	L
				H		G	F	I	A	
				P		K	T	V		
						Q				

Nevirapine

	L 101	K 101	K 103	V 106	V 108	Y 181	Y 188	G 190	M 230
	I	P	N	A	I	C	C	A	L
			S	M		I	L		
							H		

Rilpivirine

	L 100	K 101	E 138	V 179	Y 181	Y 188	H 221	F 227	M 230
	I	E	A	L	C	L	Y	C	L
		P	G		I				
			K		V				
			Q						
			R						

Figure 23.1 Mutations in the reverse transcriptase gene associated with resistance to reverse transcriptase inhibitors. NRTIs, nucleoside and nucleotide analogue reverse transcriptase inhibitors.   From Wensing et al. (2017).

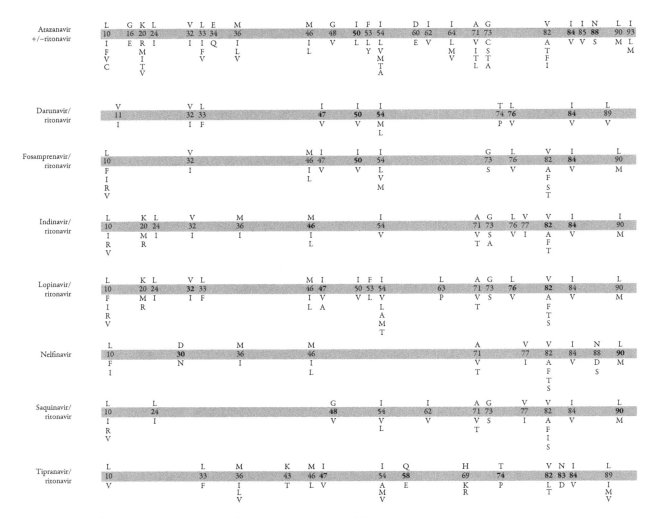

Figure 23.2 Mutations in the protease gene associated with resistance to protease inhibitors. From Wensing et al. (2017).

to resistance. Examples of such drugs include lamivudine, emtricitabine, enfuvirtide, delavirdine, efavirenz, nevirapine, raltegravir, and elvitegravir. Boosted PIs, etravirine and dolutegravir, have higher genetic barriers to resistance and require multiple mutations that occur in a stepwise manner to confer substantially reduced drug susceptibility.

RESISTANCE ASSOCIATED WITH NRTIS

Mechanisms

As with all enzymatic reactions, reverse transcription exists as an equilibrium between a forward and a reverse reaction.

The forward reaction is characterized by attack of the 3′-hyroxyl group of the primer on the α-phosphate of the incoming deoxynucleoside triphosphate (dNTP) to form a phosphodiester bond, releasing pyrophosphate. This extends the length of the primer chain by one base. This process continues to extend the primer until natural completion or until an incoming dNTP is a nucleoside analogue, which lacks the 3′-hydroxyl group and therefore prematurely terminates the chain. The reverse reaction removes the terminal nucleoside monophosphate from the primer by coupling with free pyrophosphate or adenosine triphosphate. This is termed *pyrophosphorolysis*. If the terminal base is a nucleoside analogue, its removal from the terminated primer

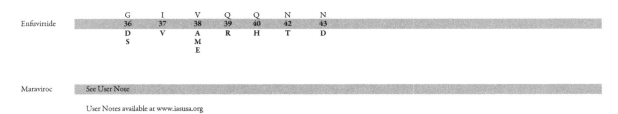

User Notes available at www.iasusa.org

Figure 23.3 Mutations in the envelope gene associated with resistance to entry inhibitors.

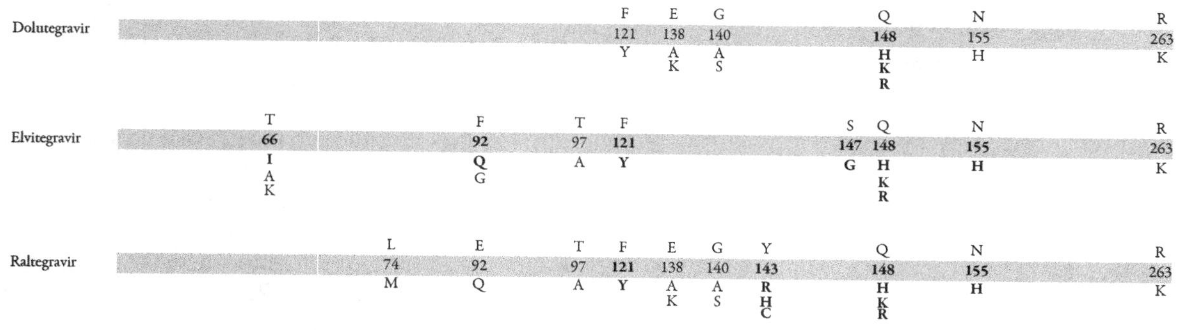

Figure 23.4 Mutations in the integrase gene associated with resistance to integrase strand transfer inhibitors. From Wensing et al. (2017).

	66	74	92	97	121	138	140	143	147	148	155	263
Dolutegravir					F / Y	E / A K	G / A S			Q / H K R	N / H	R / K
Elvitegravir	T / I A K		F / Q	T / A	F / Y				S / G	Q / H K R	N / H	R / K
Raltegravir		L / M	E / Q	T / A	F / Y	E / A K	G / A S	Y / R H C		Q / H K R	N / H	R / K

will unblock the chain so it can continue extension. This is referred to as *primer unblocking.*

In general, NRTI-associated resistance mutations cause resistance by either increasing the rate of primer unblocking or decreasing the incorporation of nucleoside analogues compared with the natural dNTPs. Allosteric interference with the incorporation of the nucleoside analogue is the major mechanism by which the mutations M184V, Y115F, Q151M, L74V, V118I, and K65R cause resistance. The TAMs M41L, D67N, K70R, L210W, T215Y/F, and K219Q/E/N enhance primer unblocking. An increase in the number of TAMs proportionally increases the degree of primer unblocking. Insertions at position 69 also enhance primer unblocking, especially in the presence of the TAMs.

Thymidine Analogue Mutations

Zidovudine and stavudine select for mutations at RT positions 41, 67, 70, 210, 215, and 219. Although these TAMs are selected by the thymidine analogues, either alone or in combination with other drugs, increasing numbers of TAMs decrease the in vivo activity of all NRTIs. There are generally two different clusters of evolution among these mutations. The first and most common pathway is M41L, L210W, and T215Y. The second pathway includes D67N, K70R, T215F, and K219Q/E/N. The second pathway results in less phenotypic cross-resistance to other NRTIs compared to the first pathway.

M184V/I

Lamivudine and emtricitabine select for the M184I and V mutations. M184I develops first and then is generally replaced by the M184V mutation due to a fitness advantage. However, in an unusual example of "cross-talk" between the NRTI- and NNRTI-associated mutations, patients with failure to rilpivirine/tenofovir/emtricitabine are more likely to develop M184I (rather than M184V) in combination with E138K (Kulkarni, 2012; Rimsky, 2012). M184V/I is also selected by abacavir and didanosine, and it confers some degree of cross-resistance to these drugs, although this mutation alone is not enough to significantly decrease the response to either. M184V/I reverses TAM-associated resistance to zidovudine, stavudine, and tenofovir.

K65R

K65R is selected by tenofovir and, to a lesser extent, abacavir and didanosine. Interestingly, it also appears more commonly in subtype C virus during failure with stavudine-containing regimens (Doualla-Bell, 2006). K65R confers partial resistance to didanosine, abacavir, tenofovir, lamivudine, emtricitabine, and possibly stavudine. K65R results in in vitro hypersusceptibility to zidovudine, although the clinical relevance of this finding is unclear (Grant, 2010).

L74V

L74V was the most common mutation that arose in patients receiving didanosine monotherapy but also was seen in patients receiving abacavir monotherapy. L74V is rarely selected in combination therapies that include thymidine analogues and didanosine or abacavir; however, it can occur with combination therapies that include didanosine/lamivudine or abacavir/lamivudine. L74V confers resistance or partial resistance to didanosine, lamivudine, emtricitabine, and abacavir. Like M184V and K65R, L74V reduces TAM-associated resistance to zidovudine.

Q151M Complex

Q151M develops in 5–10% of patients treated with thymidine analogue/didanosine combinations and causes moderate resistance to all NRTIs. The Q151M mutation is generally associated with mutations at positions A62V, V75I/F, F77L, and F116Y. Each of these mutations substantially increases the degree of resistance and the fitness of isolates containing Q151M. Tenofovir retains some activity against HIV with this mutational complex, and lamivudine may also have activity.

Position 69 Insertions

Insertions at the fingers region between codons 67 and 70, most commonly two amino acids at position 69, occur in 1% or 2% of patients treated extensively with NRTIs. These inserts are typically found in strains that also contain TAMs. Isolates with insertions at codon 69 and TAMs are highly cross-resistant to all the currently available NRTIs.

E44D/A and V118I

Mutations E44D/A and V118I both occur in untreated patients, but their prevalence increases in subjects who have had extensive exposure to NRTIs. These mutations cause low-level resistance to lamivudine and emtricitabine and probably to each of the other NRTIs.

RESISTANCE ASSOCIATED WITH NNRTIS

Mechanisms

The catalytic domain for reverse transcription has a three-dimensional structure often compared to a right hand. Despite their diverse chemical structure, NNRTIs all bind to a similar location within a hydrophobic pocket in HIV-1 RT outside the active domain of the enzyme. The binding of an NNRTI results in a conformational change in RT, thus resulting in the displacement of the catalytic aspartate residues in relation to the polymerase binding site. Nearly all the NNRTI resistance mutations are within or adjacent to this NNRTI-binding pocket and alter the shape of the NNRTI pocket to exclude the NNRTI. The second-generation NNRTI, etravirine, has a more flexible chemical structure that allows it to bind within the pocket despite the presence of mutations.

K103N

K103N occurs in more than 50% of patients failing efavirenz and also leads to high-level resistance to nevirapine and delavirdine. However, K103N does not affect antiviral response to etravirine and in vitro does not affect susceptibility to rilpivirine.

Y181C

Y181C is often selected for by nevirapine and confers only minimal resistance to efavirenz. However, attempts to sequence drugs using nevirapine followed by efavirenz have resulted in rapid development of resistance to efavirenz, likely due to an emergence of preexisting minority-resistant quasispecies (Lecossier, 2005).

Y188 C/L/H and G190A/S

Mutations at positions 188 and 190 in RT confer resistance to nevirapine and efavirenz but remain susceptible to delavirdine, although no studies have shown the utility of delavirdine in this setting. Etravirine also maintains activity in the presence of these mutations.

E138K

E138K is the most common mutation selected for by rilpivirine. It is selected less frequently by etravirine and reduces its susceptibility by approximately fivefold. E138K reduces the susceptibility of nevirapine and efavirenz approximately two- to fivefold.

RESISTANCE ASSOCIATED WITH PROTEASE INHIBITORS

Mechanisms

Protease processes the gag and gag/pol polyprotein precursors necessary for viral maturation. The visualization of protease using X-ray crystallography allowed for the development of the PI drug class. Protease exists as a homodimer, with each subunit consisting of 99 amino acids, creating a cleft that is the active site of protease. PIs act as competitive inhibitors, binding within this cleft and disabling the enzyme. Mutations within the cleft can exclude PIs, leading to resistance. Most PI-resistant viruses also require at least one ag cleavage site mutation to compensate for the altered substrate cleft caused by resistance mutations within protease.

Major Mutations

PI resistance mutations are generally categorized as major mutations (ones that confer significant resistance) and accessory mutations (ones that enhance resistance or viral fitness when a primary resistance mutation is present). Most major mutations lead to some degree of cross-class resistance, but a few signature mutations are not associated with cross-class resistance. The I50L mutation to atazanavir and the D30N mutation to nelfinavir are the best examples of signature mutations that do not lead to class-wide resistance.

The presence of signature mutations in protease that do not lead to cross-resistance led some to advocate for the sequencing of PIs. However, because primary resistance to boosted PIs is very rare in treatment-naïve individuals failing boosted PI-based regimens, the argument for the sequencing of boosted PIs is not strong.

The major protease mutations that lead to some degree of cross-class resistance are V32I, M46I/L, G48V/M, I50V, I54V/T/A/L/M, L76V, V82A/T/F/S, I84V, N88S, and L90M. PI cross-resistance is complex as a result of the large number of PI-resistance mutations and the fact that different mutations at the same position can have markedly different effects on PI susceptibility. This is particularly the case for mutations at positions 50, 54, and 82.

Darunavir, however, usually retains activity even in the presence of multiple major PI-associated mutations (Talbot, 2010) and has supplanted lopinavir/ritonavir as first-line treatment in patients harboring extensive PI-associated resistance. In clinical trials, the presence of three or more of the following mutations was associated with a diminished response to darunavir: V11I, V32I, L33F, I47V, I50V, I54L/M, G73S, L76V, I84V, and L89V (De Meyer, 2008).

Tipranavir also has activity against virus with high-level protease resistance. Although genotypic scores have been developed for tipranavir (Scherer, 2007), none of the scores performs well in predicting susceptibility to tipranavir (Talbot, 2010), and a phenotype may be particularly useful when tipranavir is being considered for use. However, tipranavir is rarely used in clinical practice given the preserved activity of darunavir in most cases and tipranavir's multiple drug–drug interactions and concerning side-effect profile (US Food and Drug Administration, 2005).

RESISTANCE ASSOCIATED WITH INSTIS

Mechanisms

HIV integrase catalyzes a multistep process that allows the double-stranded HIV cDNA to be incorporated irreversibly within the host DNA. INSTIs inhibit the final step of integration ("strand transfer"), the covalent bonding of the primed viral ends to the cleaved host DNA. INSTIs bind only to integrase bound to viral DNA, attaching closely to the enzyme's active site and disrupting the correct positioning of the viral DNA relative to the active site and the interaction of integrase with the two essential magnesium ions. Although the multiple mutations associated with resistance against INSTIs have been identified, the full-length crystal structure of HIV integrase is still not developed.

N155H

The N155H mutation develops early in the course of virologic failure to raltegravir and is accompanied by E92Q and other accessory mutations. N155H is associated with high-level raltegravir and elvitegravir resistance. However, dolutegravir, a second-generation INSTI, appears to retain activity in the presence of N155H.

Q148H/R/K

Mutations at codon 148 in integrase often develop later in individuals failing raltegravir-based therapy. Mutations at codon 148 are accompanied by mutations at codon 140 and lead to high-level resistance to raltegravir and elvitegravir. Dolutegravir dosed at 50 mg twice daily provides a good response in patients with resistance to raltegravir/elvitegravir (Eron, 2011). However, mutations at codon 148 together with two or more secondary mutations (G140A/C/S, E138A/K/T, or L74I) are also associated with low response to dolutegravir (Castagna, 2014). There was a substantial decrease in susceptibility to dolutegravir, bictegravir, and cabotegravir when T97A and L74M substitutions were combined with G140S/Q148H (Zhang, 2018).

Y143C/R

Mutations at codon 143 in integrase develop relatively uncommonly with failure to a raltegravir-containing regimen. Site-directed mutagenesis experiments suggest that mutations at codon 143 do not lead to cross-resistance to elvitegravir (Métifiot, 2011), but clinical data are lacking to support elvitegravir's use for this indication.

E92Q

E92Q is the most common integrase mutation that develops during virologic failure to elvitegravir. The mutation leads to cross-resistance with raltegravir, but dolutegravir is expected to maintain activity.

R263K

According to an in vitro study, R263K mutation can lead to low resistance to dolutegravir (Quashie, 2012).

MUTATIONS ASSOCIATED WITH ENTRY INHIBITORS

CCR5 Antagonists

Maraviroc binds to the CCR5 receptor and antagonizes the gp120–CCR5 interaction. Resistance to maraviroc can develop through two distinct mechanisms. Most commonly, the virus can begin using the CXCR4 coreceptor for entry; less commonly, mutations can occur that allow gp120 to bind the bound CCR5 receptor.

When a virus appears to switch from CCR5-tropic to dual/mixed-tropic or CXCR4-tropic, this is more frequently due to outgrowth of a minority variant than a de novo switch. Monogram's second-generation enhanced-sensitivity Trofile assay is more sensitive in detecting these minority variants compared to the first-generation assay. Due to clinicians' experience with the Trofile assay and its use for the evaluation of tropism in clinical trials for maraviroc, this assay remains the gold standard in assessing tropism (Gulick, 2008). However, genotypic interpretation of tropism has been shown to have a high degree of concordance with the Trofile and had a similar ability compared to the first-generation Trofile to predict short-term virologic response to maraviroc (Harrigan, 2009; Raymond, 2008).

When CCR5-tropic viruses become resistant to CCR5 antagonists, they generally show changes in the V3 loop stem in gp120, although changes in gp41 have also been associated with resistance to CCR5 antagonists (Anastassopoulou, 2009). There appears to be a wide variety of mutational patterns in the env gene, and no predictive rules based on genotypic changes have been developed.

Fusion Inhibitors

Currently, enfuvirtide is rarely used given the frequent injection site reactions that develop with its use. Several mutations in the gp41 envelope gene have been associated with resistance or reduced susceptibility to enfuvirtide, primarily at codons 36–45 of the first heptad repeat (HR1) region.

Post-Attachment Inhibitors

In 2018, the FDA approved ibalizumab (TaiMed), the first CD4-directed post-attachment inhibitor for the treatment of multidrug-resistant HIV-1. To date, there is no evidence of any cross-resistance between ibalizumab and other classes of ARV medications.

ACKNOWLEDGMENTS

We thank the authors of previous editions of this chapter, Philip M. Grant, Andrew R. Zolopa, and Ye Thu.

REFERENCES

Anastassopoulou CG, Ketas TJ, Klasse PJ, et al. Resistance to CCR5 inhibitors caused by sequence changes in the fusion peptide of HIV-1 gp41. *Proc Natl Acad Sci USA*. 2009;106:5318–5323.

Angus B, Brook G, Awosusi F, et al. BHIVA guidelines for the routine investigation and monitoring of adult HIV-1-positive individuals. Available at http://www.bhiva.org/monitoring-guidelines.aspx.

Baxter JD, Mayers DL, Wentworth DN, et al. A randomized study of antiretroviral management based on plasma genotypic antiretroviral resistance testing in patients failing therapy. *AIDS*. 2000;14:F83–F93.

Cane P, Chrystie I, Dunn D, et al. Time trends in primary resistance to HIV drugs in the United kingdom: multicentre observational study. *Br Med J*. 2005;331:1368.

Castagna A, Maggiolo F, Penco G, et al. Dolutegravir in antiretroviral-experienced patients with raltegravir- and/or elvitegravir-resistant HIV-1: 24-week results of the phase III VIKING-3 study. *J Infect Dis*. 2014;210(3):354–362.

Cohen CJ, Hunt S, Sension M, et al. A randomized trial assessing the impact of phenotypic resistance testing on antiretroviral therapy. *AIDS*. 2002;16:579–588.

Cooper DA, Steigbigel RT, Gatell JM, et al. Subgroup and resistance analyses of raltegravir for resistant HIV-1 infection. *N Engl J Med*. 2008;359:355–365.

De Meyer S, Dierynck I, Lathouwers E, et al. Identification of mutations predictive of a diminished response to darunavir/ritonavir: analysis of data from treatment-experienced patients in POWER 1, 2, 3 and Duet-1 and Duet-2 [Abstract 54]. Paper presented at the 6th European HIV Drug Resistance Workshop, Budapest, 2008.

Doualla-Bell FA, Avalos B, Brenner T, et al. High prevalence of the K65R mutation in human immunodeficiency virus type 1 subtype C isolates from infected patients in Botswana treated with didanosine-based regimens. *Antimicrob Agents Chemother*. 2006;50:4182–4185.

Durant J, Clevenbergh P, Halfon P, et al. Drug-resistance genotyping in HIV-1 therapy: the VIRADAPT randomised controlled trial. *Lancet*. 1999;353:2195–2199.

Eron J, Kumar P, Lazzari A, et al. DTG in subjects with HIV exhibiting RAL resistance: functional monotherapy results of VIKING study cohort II [Abstract 151LB]. Paper presented at the 18th Conference on Retroviruses and Opportunistic Infections, Boston, February 27–March 2, 2011.

Fätkenheuer G, Nelson M, Lazzarin A, et al. Subgroup analyses of maraviroc in previously treated R5 HIV-1 infection. *N Engl J Med*. 2008;359:1442–1455.

Fox ZV, Geretti AM, Kjaer J, et al. The ability of four genotypic interpretation systems to predict virological response to ritonavir-boosted protease inhibitors. *AIDS*. 2007;21:2033–2042.

Gazaignes S, Resche-Rigon M, Yang C, et al. Efficacy and safety of rilpivirine-based regimens in treatment-experienced HIV-1 infected patients: a prospective cohort study. *J Int AIDS Soc*. 2014;17(4 Suppl 3):19796.

Goetz M, Leduc R, Kostman J, et al. HIV replicative capacity is an independent predictor of disease progression in persons with untreated chronic HIV infection [Abstract WEPDB07]. Paper presented at the 4th IAS Conference on HIV Pathogenesis, Treatment and Prevention, Sydney, Australia, July 22–25, 2007.

Grant P, Taylor J, Nevins A, et al. Antiviral activity of zidovudine and tenofovir in the presence of the K65R mutation in reverse transcriptase: an international cohort analysis. *Antimicrob Agents Chemother*. 2010;54:1520–1525.

Grant P, Wong EC, Rode R, et al. Virologic response to lopinavir-ritonavir-based antiretroviral regimens in a multicenter international clinical cohort: comparison of genotypic interpretation scores. *Antimicrob Agents Chemother*. 2008;52:4050–4056.

Gulick RM, Lalezari J, Goodrich J, et al. Maraviroc for previously treated patients with R5 HIV-1 infection. *N Engl J Med*. 2008;359:1429–1441.

Günthard HF, Calvez V, Paredes R, et al. Human immunodeficiency virus drug resistance: 2018 recommendations of the International Antiviral Society–USA Panel. *Clin Infect Dis*. July 20, 2018. ciy463, https://doi.org/10.1093/cid/ciy463.

Harrigan PR, McGover R, Dong W, et al. Screening for HIV tropism using population based V3 genotypic analysis: a retrospective virological outcome analysis using stored plasma screening samples from MOTIVATE-1 [Abstract 15]. Paper presented at the XVIII International HIV Drug Resistance Workshop, Fort Myers, FL, June 9–13, 2009.

Hertogs K, de Bethune MP, Miller V, et al. A rapid method for simultaneous detection of phenotypic resistance to inhibitors of protease and reverse transcriptase in recombinant human immunodeficiency type 1 isolates from patients treated with antiretroviral drugs. *Antimicrob Agents Chemother*. 1998;42:269–276.

Kulkarni R, Babaoglu K, Lansdon EB, et al. The HIV-1 reverse transcriptase M184I mutation enhances the E138K-associated resistance to rilpivirine and decreases viral fitness. *J AIDS*. 2012;59:47–54.

Kuritzkes DR, Lalama CM, Ribaudo HJ, et al. Preexisting resistance to nonnucleoside reverse-transcriptase inhibitors predicts virologic failure of an efavirenz-based regimen in treatment-naive HIV-1-infected subjects. *J Infect Dis*. 2008;197:867–870.

Lecossier D, Shulman NS, Morand-Joubert L, et al. Detection of minority populations of HIV-1 expressing the K103N resistance mutation in patients failing nevirapine. *J AIDS*. 2005;38:37–42.

Little SJ, Frost SD, Wong JK, et al. Persistence of transmitted drug resistance among subjects with primary human immunodeficiency virus infection. *J Virol*. 2008;82:5510–5518.

Little SJ, Holte S, Routy JP, et al. Antiretroviral-drug resistance among patients recently infected with HIV. *N Engl J Med*. 2002;347:385–394.

Madruga JV, Cahn P, Grinsztejn B, et al. Efficacy and safety of TMC125 (etravirine) in treatment-experienced HIV-1 infected patients in Duet-1: 24-week results from a randomized, double-blind placebo-controlled trial. *Lancet*. 2007;37:29–38.

Métifiot M, Vandegraaff N, Maddali K, et al. Elvitegravir overcomes resistance to raltegravir induced by integrase mutation Y143. *AIDS*. 2011;25:1175–1178.

Monogram Biosciences. Available at http://www.monogramvirology.com/hiv-tests/resistance-testing/phenotype. Accessed April 29, 2016.

Ocfemia CB, Kim D, Ziebell R, et al. Prevalence and trends of transmitted drug resistance-associated mutations by duration of infection among persons newly diagnosed with HIV-1 infection: 5 states and 3 municipalities, US, 2006 to 2009 [Abstract 730]. Paper presented at the 19th Conference on Retroviruses and Opportunistic Infections, Seattle, WA, March 5–8, 2012.

Pellegrin I, Wittkop L, Joubert LM, et al. Virological response to darunavir/ritonavir-based regimens in antiretroviral-experienced patients (PREDIZISTA study). *Antiviral Ther*. 2008;13:271–279.

Quashie P, Mesplède T, Han Y, et al. Characterization of the R263K mutation in HIV-1 integrase that confers low-level resistance to the second-generation integrase strand transfer inhibitor dolutegravir. *J Virol*. 2012;86(5):2696–2705.

Raymond S, Delobel P, Mavigner M, et al. Correlation between genotypic predictions based on V3 sequences and phenotypic determination of HIV-1 tropism. *AIDS*. 2008;22:F11–F16.

Rimsky L, Vingerhoets J, Van Eygen V, et al. Genotypic and phenotypic characterization of HIV-1 isolates obtained from patients on rilpivirine therapy experiencing virologic failure in the phase 3 ECHO and THRIVE studies: 48-week analysis. *J AIDS*. 2012;59:39–46.

Rimsky LT, Azijn H, Tirry I, et al. In vitro resistance profile of TMC278, a next-generation NNRTI: evidence of a higher genetic barrier and a more robust resistance profile than first generation NNRTIs [Abstract 120]. Paper presented at the XVIII International Drug Resistance Workshop, Fort Myers, FL, June 9–13, 2009.

Sax PE, Islam R, Walensky RP, et al. Should resistance testing be performed for treatment-naive HIV-infected patients? A cost-effectiveness analysis. *Clin Infect Dis*. 2005;41:1316–1323.

Scherer J, Boucher C, Baxter JD, et al. Improving the prediction of virologic response to tipranavir: the development of a tipranavir weighted score [Abstract P3.4/07]. Paper presented at the 11th European AIDS Conference, Madrid, 2007.

Shafer RW, Hertogs K, Zolopa AR, et al. High degree of interlaboratory reproducibility of human immunodeficiency virus type 1 protease and reverse transcriptase sequencing of plasma samples from heavily treated patients. *J Clin Microbiol*. 2001;39:1522–1529.

Smith S, Zhao X, Burke T, et.al. Efficacies of Cabotegravir and Bictegravir against drug-resistant HIV-1 integrase mutants. *Retrovirology*. 2018;15:37.

Soo-Yon R, Clutter D, Fessel WJ, Klein D, et al. Trends in the molecular epidemiology and genetic mechanisms of transmitted human immunodeficiency virus Type 1 drug resistance in a large US clinic population. *Clin Infect Dis*. ciy453, https://doi.org/10.1093/cid/ciy453.

Talbot A, Grant P, Taylor J, et al. Predicting tipranavir and darunavir resistance using genotypic, phenotypic and virtual phenotypic resistance patterns: an independent cohort analysis of clinical isolates highly resistant to all other protease inhibitors. *Antimicrob Agents Chemother*. 2010;54:2473–2479.

Theys K, Camacho R, Gomes P, et al. Predicted residual activity of rilpivirine in HIV-1 infected patients failing therapy including NNRTIs efavirenz or nevirapine. *Clin Microbiol Infect*. 2015;21(6):607.e1–e8.

Torti C, Quiros-Roldan E, Keulen W, et al. Comparison between rules-based human immunodeficiency virus type 1 genotype interpretations and real or virtual phenotype: concordance analysis and correlation with clinical outcome in heavily treated patients. *J Infect Dis*. 2003;188:194–201.

Tural C, Ruiz L, Holtzer C, et al. Clinical utility of HIV-1 genotyping and expert advice: the Havana trial. *AIDS*. 2002;16:209–218.

US Department of Health and Human Services (USDHHS), Panel on Antiretroviral Guidelines for Adults and Adolescents. Guidelines for the use of antiretroviral agents in HIV-1-infected adults and adolescents. January 28, 2016. Available at https://aidsinfo.nih.gov/contentfiles/lvguidelines/AdultandAdolescentGL.pdf. Accessed April 29, 2016.

US Food and Drug Administration. New therapy for HIV patients with advanced disease. *FDA Patient Safety News*, Show 44. October 2005.

Vingerhoets J, Peeters M, Azijn H, et al. An update of the list of NNRTI mutations associated with decreased virologic response to etravirine (ETR): multivariate analyses on the pooled DUET-1 and DUET-2 clinical trial data. Paper presented at the XVII HIV Drug Resistance Workshop, Sitges, Spain, June 10–14, 2008.

Weinstock HS, Zaidi I, Heneine W, et al. The epidemiology of antiretroviral drug resistance among drug-naive HIV-1-infected persons in 10 US cities. *J Infect Dis*. 2004;189:2174–2180.

Wensing AM, Calvez V, Günthard HF, et al. 2015 update of the drug resistance mutations in HIV-1. *Top Antivir Med*. October-November 2015;23(4):132–141.

Wheeler W, Mahle K, Bodnar U, et al. Antiretroviral drug-resistance mutations and subtypes in drug-naïve persons newly diagnosed with HIV-1 infection, US, March 2003 to October 2006 [Abstract 648]. Paper presented at the 14th Conference on Retroviruses and Opportunistic Infections, Los Angeles, CA, February 25–28, 2007.

Whitcomb JM, Parkin NT, Chappey C, et al. Broad nucleoside reverse-transcriptase inhibitor cross-resistance in human immunodeficiency virus type 1 clinical isolates. *J Infect Dis*. 2003;188:992–1000.

White KL, Chen JM, Feng JY, et al. The K65R reverse transcriptase mutation in HIV-1 reverses the excision phenotype of zidovudine resistance mutations. *Antivir Ther*. 2006;11:155–163.

Yang W, Kouyos R, Scherrer A, et al. Assessing the paradox between transmitted and acquired HIV type 1 drug resistance mutations in the Swiss HIV cohort study from 1998 to 2012. *J Infect Dis*. 2015;212(1):28–38.

Zhang J, Rhee SY, Taylor J, et al. Comparison of the precision and sensitivity of the Antivirogram and PhenoSense HIV drug susceptibility assays. *J AIDS*. 2005;38:439–344.

Zhang W, Cheung P, Oliveira N, et al. Accumulation of multiple mutations in vivo confers cross-resistance to new and existing integrase inhibitors. *J Infect Dis*. jiy428, https://doi.org/10.1093/infdis/jiy428.

24.

MANAGING THE PATIENT WITH MULTIDRUG-RESISTANT HIV

Quentin Doperalski, Tamara Bininashvili, and Naiel Nassar

INTRODUCTION

During the past 15 years, HIV infection has been transformed into a chronic, manageable disease primarily due to the effectiveness of antiretroviral therapy (ART). Well-tolerated, potent combination ART with simpler dosing schedules has led to a reduction in the rates of virologic failure and the proportion of patients harboring multidrug-resistant HIV.

Treatment guidelines emphasize achieving maximal virologic suppression. Given the newer integrase strand inhibitors (e.g., bictegravir and dolutegravir) and existing classes with extended spectra of antiretroviral (ARV) activity (e.g., darunavir, etravirine) and with the potential promise fewer long-term side effects (e.g., tenofovir alafenamide), it is now possible to achieve maximal virologic suppression in virtually all adherent patients, even those harboring viruses with extensive drug resistance. This chapter outlines strategies for managing patients with multidrug-resistant virus, including treatment simplification in virologically suppressed patients.

LEARNING OBJECTIVE

Explain how to construct ARV regimens for patients with multidrug-resistant HIV.

WHAT'S NEW?

- Ibalizumab is a post-attachment inhibitor and the first monoclonal antibody to be approved for HIV treatment. It is approved for usage in highly treatment-experienced patients.

- Although it has been general practice to include nucleoside/nucleotide reverse transcriptase inhibitors in salvage regimens, there is not a significant difference in virologic failure rates between regimens containing them versus those that do not.

- Fostemsavir, an oral attachment inhibitor, has demonstrated acceptable safety and efficacy in treating patients with multidrug-resistant HIV and will most likely be approved by the US Food and Drug Administration (FDA) soon.

KEY POINTS

- Treatment guidelines emphasize the need for at least two or preferably three fully active medications in any ART regimen of patients experiencing virologic failure.

- The new regimen should be started with as little interruption as possible because the structured interruption of treatment in patients with multidrug-resistant HIV infection is associated with greater progression of the disease.

- The pharmacokinetic enhancer, cobicistat, is available as a fixed-dose combination product with ARV medication, which allows the treatment to be simplified and reduces the pill burden.

CONSTRUCTING AN ANTIRETROVIRAL DRUG REGIMEN IN PATIENTS EXPERIENCING VIROLOGIC FAILURE

In patients experiencing virologic failure, multiple studies have demonstrated that resistance testing (either genotypic or phenotypic) leads to improved virologic outcomes (Baxter, 2000; Cohen, 2002). Treatment guidelines emphasize the need for at least two or preferably three fully active medications in the ART regimens of patients experiencing virologic failure (US Department of Health and Human Services [USDHHS], 2018). In treatment-experienced patients, multiple clinical studies demonstrate higher rates of virologic suppression with an increasing number of active drugs in a salvage regimen (Cooper, 2008; Fätkenheuer, 2008). However, rates of virologic response plateau when three active drugs are included in an ART regimen; regimens including four or five active drugs do not outperform those with three (Cooper,

2008; Staszewski, 1999; Markowitz, 2014). In addition, multiple studies have shown higher baseline CD4$^+$ T cell count, and lower HIV RNA levels predict good virologic response (Cooper, 2008; Fätkenheuer, 2008).

OPTIMAL THERAPY FOR "EARLY" SALVAGE

According to the current USDHHS guidelines, ARV regimens for most treatment-naïve patients should preferentially include an integrase strand inhibitor (INSTI) plus two nucleoside/nucleotide reverse transcriptase inhibitors (NRTIs). Because resistance to INSTIs in treatment-naïve patients is relatively rare, 85–90% of these patients have a good virologic response to these regimens. However, if a patient who is already on NRTIs plus non-nucleoside reverse transcriptase inhibitors (NNRTIs) develops virologic failure, switching to a regimen containing a boosted protease inhibitor (PI) plus two NRTIs is associated with a better response compared to boosted PI alone (Bunupuradah, 2012). Also, based on another study, a regimen containing a boosted PI plus an INSTI is not inferior to a boosted PI plus two NRTIs (Boyd, 2013). Therefore, a boosted PI plus an INSTI-containing regimen can be another reasonable option (Huhn, 2017). This can also significantly simplify the patient's regimen, especially in number of pills and frequency of dosing.

OPTIMAL THERAPY FOR PATIENTS HARBORING VIRUS WITH MORE EXTENSIVE RESISTANCE

As per USDHHS guidelines, drug resistance testing should be done for patients with virologic failure. To increase the chance of detecting selected mutations, the test should be done while the patient is taking the failing ARV regimen or within 4 weeks after discontinuation of the treatment. The basic principle is to construct a new regimen containing at least two or, if possible, three fully active agents. The new treatment regimen should be formulated based on the drug resistance testing and previous drug experience. The new regimen should be started with as little interruption as possible. It has been shown that the structured interruption of treatment in patients with multidrug-resistant HIV infection is associated with greater progression of the disease and does not provide any immunologic or virologic benefit (Lawrence, 2003).

With the availability of medications such as dolutegravir, etravirine, and darunavir that have a higher barrier of resistance, it is now easier than in the past to formulate the treatment regimen to achieve the maximum virologic response even for patients with multidrug-resistance HIV. According to one study, dual therapy with darunavir/ritonavir and etravirine is effective in patients with virologic failure (Bernardino, 2014).

Resistance to INSTI is very rare in patients who are naïve to this class of therapy (Doyle, 2015). However, for INSTI-experienced patients with resistance to raltegravir and elvitegravir, a good virologic response has been achieved with dolutegravir administered as 50 mg twice daily (Castagna, 2014).

For entry inhibitors, maraviroc can be considered fully active in patients with CCR5-tropic virus by the second-generation enhanced-sensitivity Trofile assay (ESTA) or a genotypic tropism assay (Harrigan, 2009). With dual/mixed or CXCR4-tropic viruses, maraviroc should not be used. Enfuvirtide is rarely required in salvage regimens because usually three other active drugs can be found, but for enfuvirtide-naïve patients, it should be considered a fully active drug. For patients with prior ongoing viremia on enfuvirtide, resistance has likely developed, and enfuvirtide cannot be expected to provide residual activity. Ibalizumab (IBA), a monoclonal antibody characterized as a post-attachment inhibitor, sterically inhibits post-CD4 virus binding events through attachment to domain 2 of the CD4$^+$ receptor. IBA was approved in 2018 for usage in patients with multidrug-resistant virus in conjunction with other active ARVs. It has both minimal adverse effects and drug–drug interactions (Emu, 2018). Resistance to IBA is possible if given as monotherapy, demonstrating a basic ARV tenet strongly discouraging monotherapy and a patient mandate to take his or her entire regimen and not to rely on IBA alone.

The BRIGHTE study is an ongoing phase 3 randomized clinical trial evaluating fostemsavir in heavily treatment-experienced patients infected with multidrug-resistant HIV-1 for whom a viable ART regimen was not possible to construct. Fostemsavir is an investigational, first-in-class prodrug of the active moiety temsavir, which binds to HIV-1 gp120 and prevents attachment to CD4 receptor on T cells, and other immune cells, thereby blocking virus infection. Week 48 rates of virologic suppression (HIV-1 RNA <40 copies/mL, mITT; Snapshot analysis) were 54% (146/272). Sixty-nine percent of participants achieved viral loads of less than 200 copies/mL at week 48. CD4$^+$ T cell counts increased, and mean change from baseline was an increase of 139 cells/µL (Aberg, 2018). It is expected that, based on these data, fostemsavir will be FDA-approved at some time in 2019.

With the availability of these newer and soon-to-approved drugs, some may question the need for NRTIs in salvage therapy. Previously, general practice was to routinely include NRTIs in salvage regimens, but there is no significant difference in virologic failure rate for salvage regimens without NRTIs compared to regimens containing NRTIs (Tashima, 2015). Examples of these regimens include boosted PIs plus INSTI or boosted PI plus NNRTI (Bernardino, 2014; Boyd, 2013).

SIMPLIFICATION OF ANTIRETROVIRAL THERAPY IN VIROLOGICALLY SUPPRESSED PATIENTS HARBORING MULTIDRUG-RESISTANT HIV

Given the efficacy of modern ARV regimens, fewer patients are now experiencing virologic failure. However, many patients maintain virologic suppression on overly complex or poorly tolerated regimens or on regimens with increased rates of long-term toxicities.

According to USDHHS (2018) guidelines, regimen switching in the setting of viral suppression can be considered "to simplify the regimen by reducing pill burden and dosing frequency to improve adherence, to enhance tolerability and decrease short- or long-term toxicity, to change food or fluid requirements, to avoid parenteral administration, to minimize or address drug interaction concerns, to reduce costs." Treatment simplification requires the clinician to be aware of the patient's ARV treatment history and results of previous resistance testing. If CCR5 coreceptor antagonists are being considered during a regimen switch in a patient with undetectable viral load, a proviral DNA tropism assay can be used. If CXCR4 or D/M tropic virus is detected, maraviroc should not be used.

In altering established therapy in virologically suppressed patients with a history of virologic failure, regimens should be chosen that would be predicted to be highly active based on the individual's past treatment history and resistance profile (USDHHS, 2018). In general, substitutions of medications within the same ARV drug class (generally with coformulated medications or with newer, better-tolerated or potent agents) are straightforward with a low risk of virologic failure (Mallolas, 2009; Martin, 2009).

Many patients with multidrug-resistant HIV are taking regimens with boosted PIs because they have a higher barrier of resistance. Prior to the introduction of cobicistat, ritonavir was the only available pharmacokinetic enhancer for protease or integrase (elvitegravir) inhibitors. However, the pharmacokinetic enhancer cobicistat was introduced to the market in 2015 and 2016 as part of coformulated regimens and later as a single agent (Tyboost). The major advantage of cobicistat compared to ritonavir is cobicistat's solubility and dissolution rate, which allow cobicistat as a fixed-dose combination product with ARV medication. This allows the treatment regimen to be simplified and also reduces pill burden. In one study, darunavir/cobicistat was generally well tolerated and had a similar virologic and immunologic response as that of darunavir/ritonavir (Tashima, 2014).

Cobicistat was also studied as a pharmacokinetic enhancer for integrase inhibitors. It has been demonstrated that coformulated elvitegravir, cobicistat, emtricitabine (FTC), and tenofovir disoproxil fumarate (TDF) are not inferior to the ritonavir-boosted PI/FTC/TDF regimen (Arribas, 2014; Huhn, 2015). It should be noted that cobicistat typically increases the serum creatinine level by 0.1–0.15 mg/dL and decreases the estimated glomerular filtration rate (GFR) by 10–15 mL/min. This is due to its effect of blocking cellular transporters within proximal renal tubular cells' secretion of creatinine; thus, the physiologic GFR is not changed with use of cobicistat (German, 2012). However, cobicistat is not recommended for administration with TDF in patients with estimated GFR of less than 70 mL/min because dosage adjustment for TDF has not been established for this regimen.

Out-of-class substitutions potentially hold greater risk if not carefully considered. This is especially true when switching a patient off of a PI to another class of medication with a lower barrier to resistance (e.g., a NNRTI or integrase inhibitor). A number of regimen switch studies have shown increased rates of virologic failure when patients with previous histories of virologic failure on PI-based regimens were switched off the PI to a medication class with a lower barrier to resistance (Eron, 2010; Martinez, 2007). Although there are valid reasons to switch patients off PIs, this must be done cautiously in patients with histories of virologic failure and drug resistance.

REFERENCES

Aberg J, Molina J-M, Kozal M et al. Week 48 safety and efficacy of the HIV-1 attachment inhibitor prodrug fostemsavir in heavily treatment-experienced participants (BRIGHTE study) [Abstract O344A]. Glasgow, 2018.

Arribas JR, Pialoux G, Gathe J, et al. Simplification to coformulated elvitegravir, cobicistat, emtricitabine, and tenofovir versus continuation of ritonavir-boosted protease inhibitor with emtricitabine and tenofovir in adults with virologically suppressed HIV (STRATEGY-PI): 48 week results of a randomised, open-label, phase 3b, non-inferiority trial. *Lancet Infect Dis.* 2014;14(7):581–589.

Baxter JD, Mayers DL, Wentworth DN, et al. A randomized study of antiretroviral management based on plasma genotypic antiretroviral resistance testing in patients failing therapy. *AIDS.* 2000;14:F83–F93.

Bernardino JI, Zamora FX, Valencia E, et al. Efficacy of a dual therapy based on darunavir/ritonavir and etravirine in ART-experienced patients. *J Int AIDS Soc.* 2014;17(4 Suppl 3):19787.

Boyd MA, Kumarasamy N, Moore CL, et al. Ritonavir-boosted lopinavir plus nucleoside or nucleotide reverse transcriptase inhibitors versus ritonavir-boosted lopinavir plus raltegravir for treatment of HIV-1 infection in adults with virological failure of a standard first-line ART regimen (SECOND-LINE): a randomised, open-label, non-inferiority study. *Lancet.* 2013;381(9883):2091–2099.

Bunupuradah T, Chetchotisakd P, Ananworanich J, et al. A randomized comparison of second-line lopinavir/ritonavir monotherapy versus tenofovir/lamivudine/lopinavir/ritonavir in patients failing NNRTI regimens: the HIV STAR study. *Antivir Ther.* 2012;17(7):1351–1361.

Castagna A, Maggiolo F, Penco G, et al. Dolutegravir in antiretroviral-experienced patients with raltegravir- and/or elvitegravir-resistant HIV-1: 24-week results of the phase III VIKING-3 study. *J Infect Dis.* 2014;210(3):354–362.

Cohen CJ, Hunt S, Sension M, et al. A randomized trial assessing the impact of phenotypic resistance testing on antiretroviral therapy. *AIDS.* 2002;16:579–588.

Cooper DA, Steigbigel RT, Gatell JM, et al. Subgroup and resistance analyses of raltegravir for resistant HIV-1 infection. *N Engl J Med.* 2008;359:355–365.

Doyle T, Dunn D, Ceccherini-Silberstein F, et al. Integrase inhibitor (INI) genotypic resistance in treatment-naive and raltegravir-experienced patients infected with diverse HIV-1 clades. *J Antimicrob Chemother.* 2015;70(11):3080–3086.

Emu B, Fessel J, Schrader S et al. Phase 3 study of ibalizumab for multidrug-resistant HIV-1. *N Engl J Med.* 2018;379:645–654.

Eron JJ, Young B, Cooper DA, et al. Switch to a raltegravir-based regimen versus continuation of a lopinavir–ritonavir-based regimen in stable HIV-infected patients with suppressed viremia (SWITCHMRK 1 and 2): two multicentre, double-blind, randomised controlled trials. *Lancet.* 2010;375:396–407.

Fätkenheuer G, Nelson M, Lazzarin A, et al. Subgroup analyses of maraviroc in previously treated R5 HIV-1 infection. *N Engl J Med.* 2008;359:1442–1455.

German P, Liu H, Szwarcberg J, et al. Effect of cobicistat on glomerular filtration rate in subjects with normal and impaired renal function. *J AIDS.* 2012;61(1):32–40.

Swenson LC, Mo T, Dong WW. Deep sequencing to infer HIV-1 co-receptor usage: application to three clinical trials of maraviroc in treatment-experienced patients. *J Infect Dis.* 2011;203(2):237–245.

Harrigan PR, McGover R, Dong W, et al. Screening for HIV tropism using population based V3 genotypic analysis: a retrospective virological outcome analysis using stored plasma screening samples from MOTIVATE-1 [Abstract 15]. Paper presented at the XVIII International HIV Drug Resistance Workshop, Fort Myers, FL, June 9–13, 2009.

Huhn G, Tebas P, Gallant J, et al. Strategic simplification: the efficacy and safety of switching to elvitegravir/cobicistat/emtricitabine/tenofovir alafenamide (E/C/F/TAF) plus darunavir (DRV) in treatment-experienced HIV-1 infected adults (NCT01968551). *J AIDS.* 2017;74(2):193–200.

Lawrence J, Mayers D, Hullsiek KH, et al. Structured treatment interruption in patients with multidrug-resistant human immunodeficiency virus. *N Engl J Med.* 2003;349:837–846.

Mallolas J, Podzamczer D, Milinkovic A, et al. Efficacy and safety of switching from boosted lopinavir to boosted atazanavir in patients with virological suppression receiving a LPV/r-containing HAART: the ATAZIP study. *J AIDS.* 2009;51:29–36.

Markowitz M, Evering TH, Garmon D, Caskey, M. Randomized open-label study of three- versus five-drug combination antiretroviral therapy in newly HIV-1 infected individuals. *J AIDS.* 2014;66(2):140–147.

Martin A, Bloch M, Amin J, et al. Simplification of antiretroviral therapy with tenofovir–emtricitabine or abacavir–lamivudine: a randomized, 96-week trial. *Clin Infect Dis.* 2009;49:1591–1601.

Martinez E. The NEFA study: results at three years. *AIDS Rev.* 2007;9:62.

Staszewski S, Morales-Ramirez J, Tashima KT, et al. Efavirenz plus zidovudine and lamivudine, efavirenz plus indinavir, and indinavir plus zidovudine and lamivudine in the treatment of HIV-1 infection in adults. Study 006 Team. *N Engl J Med.* 1999;341:1865–1873.

Tashima K, Crofoot G, Tomaka FL, et al. Cobicistat-boosted darunavir in HIV-1-infected adults: week 48 results of a phase IIIb, open-label single-arm trial. *AIDS Res Ther.* 2014;11:39.

Tashima K, Smeaton L, Fichtenbaum C, et al. HIV salvage therapy does not require nucleoside reverse transcriptase inhibitors: a randomized, controlled trial. *Ann Intern Med.* 2015;163(12):908–917.

US Department of Health and Human Services (USDHHS), Panel on Antiretroviral Guidelines for Adults and Adolescents. Guidelines for the use of antiretroviral agents in HIV-1-infected adults and adolescents. Available at https://aidsinfo.nih.gov/guidelines/html/1/adult-and-adolescent-treatment-guidelines/0. Accessed November 11, 2018.

25.

FUTURE ANTIRETROVIRALS, IMMUNE-BASED STRATEGIES, AND THERAPEUTIC VACCINES

Niyati Jakharia, Adrian Majid, Bruce L. Gilliam, and Rohit Talwani

CHAPTER GOALS

Upon completion of this chapter, the reader should be able to to gain knowledge about new antiretroviral drugs in development, different strategies to restore the immune system and eliminate the latent HIV reservoir, and also discuss the role and current research of preventive and therapeutic vaccines.

INTRODUCTION

Currently available antiretroviral medications consistently achieve durable suppression of HIV, however are not able to eliminate the latent reservoir of infection or significantly modulate host immune responses in a manner that improves clinical outcomes. In this chapter, we will discuss new antiretroviral drugs in development and various strategies targeting immune dysregulation and T cell homeostasis. We also update the status of clinical research evaluating immunomodulators and vaccines in late stage clinical development.

LEARNING OBJECTIVES

- Discuss new antiretroviral (ARV) drugs from traditional drug classes in development.

- Describe novel pharmaceuticals that will change HIV treatment in the future.

WHAT'S NEW?

New medications within existing classes of ARV agents are in clinical trials and will likely offer activity against resistant HIV-1 strains and provide alternatives for combination pill therapy. Novel therapeutics including oral attachment inhibitors and monoclonal antibody (mAb) treatments continue to show efficacy against HIV-1 and progress in clinical trials.

KEY POINTS

- Among traditional classes of HIV treatment, cabotegravir, an integrase strand inhibitor, is a newer agent with activity against resistant virus.

- A nucleoside reverse transcriptase translocation inhibitor (MK-8591) with a novel mechanism of action with a high potency and a long half-life has entered into phase 2 studies.

- Early phase 3 study results of a new type of oral HIV entry inhibitor with good oral bioavailability (fostemsavir) has demonstrated efficacy in heavily pretreated HIV-infected patients with limited treatment options.

- mAbs directed against CCR5 (PRO 140) and the CD4 receptor (TNX-355) have shown potency in early clinical trials.

FUTURE DIRECTIONS IN ANTIRETROVIRAL TREATMENT

ANTIRETROVIRAL DRUGS IN DEVELOPMENT

Highly active antiretroviral therapy (HAART) remains the mainstay of treatment for patients chronically infected with HIV. Novel drugs, both within existing classes and new ones, are in various stages of development and testing (Table 25.1).

New types of entry inhibitors are also being investigated. Fostemsavir, an oral attachment inhibitor, binds to HIV-1 gp120, blocking viral attachment to host CD4$^+$ T cells. In phase 2a trials of monotherapy in both treatment-naïve and treatment-experienced patients over 8 days, it has been shown to decrease viral load and increase CD4$^+$ T cell count (Nettles, 2012). In other recent trials, fostemsavir, when combined with tenofovir (TDF) and raltegravir, led to comparable rates of viral suppression as a similar regimen with atazanavir (ATV) and ritonavir (RTV) (Lalezari, 2015). Because the drug attaches to a viral target, HIV subtype-specific polymorphisms at the gp120 site may contribute to variable efficacy of the drug, an area of further research with this agent. The ongoing phase 3 BRIGHTE study evaluated fostemsavir in two cohorts of heavily treatment-experienced participants. In the randomized cohort, 272 participants were randomized 3:1 to receive 7 days of blinded therapy with either fostemsavir or placebo in addition to their failing background regimen. The primary endpoint of this study was the reduction in HIV RNA at day 8 at which time the

Table 25.1 ANTIRETROVIRAL DRUGS IN CLINICAL TRIALS

AGENT	DESCRIPTION	STAGE OF DEVELOPMENT
	NRTIs	
Elvucitabine	Cytosine nucleoside analogue that can be used in cases of resistance to FTC or 3TC	Phase 2 trials completed Drug out licensed for further development in China, Taiwan, and Hong Kong
MK 8591 Nucleoside reverse transcriptase translocation inhibitor Phase II	MK 8591 Nucleoside reverse transcriptase translocation inhibitor Phase II	MK 8591 Phase II
	INSTIs	
Cabotegravir (GSK1265744 or GSK744)	Available in both an oral and a long-acting intramuscular formulation; intramuscular formulation being investigated for role in treatment and pre-exposure prophylaxis	Phase 3
	Entry and Fusion Inhibitors	
Fostemsavir	Attaches to HIV gp120 to prevent HIV attachment to the host CD4 cell	Phase 3
Cenicriviroc	Once-daily CCR5 antagonist that also has CCR2 activity (anti-inflammatory effect)	Phase 2 trial demonstrated improvement in neurocognition among participants with AIDS demential complex. Phase 3 trials in HIV planned, currently undergoing phase 3 clinical trials in participants with NASH
	Inhibitors of Rev-Mediated Viral RNA Biogenesis	
ABX464	Enhances viral mRNA splicing by interfering with these Rev-mediated functions (Campos, 2015)	Phase 2 trials

ATV, atazanavir; Cobi, cobicistat; ELV, elvucitabine; FTC, emtricitabine; INSTIs, integrase strand inhibitors; NNRTIs, non-nucleoside reverse transcriptase inhibitors; NRTIs, nucleoside reverse transcriptase inhibitors; RPV, rilpivirine; 3TC, lamivudine.

mean reduction in HIV RNA was 0.79 $\log_{10}$ copies/mL in the fostemsavir group and .17 $\log_{10}$ copies/mL in the placebo group. All participants then went on to receive open-label fostemsavir and an optimized background regimen for a planned 96 weeks. A second nonrandomized cohort included in this study evaluated open-label fostemsavir and optimized background therapy in 99 participants with limited treatment options (no fully active approved agents) with a planned treatment duration of 96 weeks. Interim data were recently presented and demonstrated that 54% of those in the randomized cohort and 36% of those in the nonrandomized cohort had HIV RNA levels of less than 40 copies/mL after 24 weeks of treatment (Kozal, 2017).

Cabotegravir, an investigational integrase strand inhibitor and structural analogue of dolutegravir, is available as both a short-acting daily tablet and a long-acting intramuscular formulation. Cabotegravir has shown similar efficacy at viral suppression to efavirenz as part of an induction regimen with a nucleoside reverse transcriptase inhibitor (NRTI) backbone for ARV-naïve patients (Margolis, 2015). When used as part of a dual maintenance regimen with rilpivirine once the HIV-1 RNA is less than 50 copies/mL, it had similar antiviral efficacy as efavirenz with an NRTI backbone. The phase 2b LATTE-2 study showed that the long-acting intramuscular cabotegravir plus rilpivirine given every 4 or 8 weeks was as effective as three-drug oral therapy of cabotegravir, abacavir, and lamivudine in patients with HIV RNA of less than 50 copies/mL (Margolis,

2017). After 96 weeks of treatment, 87% of participants who received the injection every 4 weeks, 94% of those who received the injection every 8 weeks, and 84% of those who received the daily oral regimen had an HIV RNA of less than 50 copies/mL. Because of its long-acting duration of activity, cabotegravir LA is also being studied in phase 3 trials for use as preexposure prophylaxis (PrEP) and HIV treatment maintenance.

MK-8591 is a nucleoside reverse transcriptase translocation inhibitor in clinical development. MK-8591 triphosphate (MK-8591 TP) is the active phosphorylated form which has a half–life of 78-128 hours in human peripheral blood mononuclear cells. In an open label study, a single dose of MK-8591 in HIV-1 treatment-naïve subjects showed a greater than 1 $\log_{10}$ viral load decline after 7–10 days. (Matthews, 2017) A phase 2 randomized trial to evaluate the safety, tolerability, and ARV activity of MK-8591 in combination with doravirine and lamivudine is ongoing. Primate studies have demonstrated clinically relevant drug exposures for more than 6 months after single a single dose of parenterally administered MK-8591, supporting evaluation of extended dosing formulations which may have utility as PrEP or treatment maintenance (Barrett AAC, 2018).

Other interesting ARV agents in early stage development include a capsid inhibitor (GS-6207; Zheng, 2018), a maturation inhibitor (GSK3640254; Krystal, 2016), an entry inhibitor(combinectin-GSK3732394) which works through 3 independent modes of action using adnectin, and an NRTI active against resistant virus (GS-9131; White, 2017).

Monoclonal Antibody Therapy

During the past decade, multiple mAbs have been developed against various viral targets, including viral membrane targets (e.g., gp120 and gp41), the CD4 receptor, and the CCR5 coreceptor (Chen, 2012). Very few of these mAbs have shown clinical benefit despite efficacy in nonhuman primate models due, in part, to the challenge of generating broadly neutralizing antibodies against genetically diverse HIV-1 isolates and the virus's ability to rapidly develop resistant variants. Nonetheless, several promising compounds and treatment approaches have evolved recently and are discussed here.

PRO 140, a humanized CCR5 mAb, has been shown to have potent and prolonged ARV activity when given in both intravenous and subcutaneous (SQ) formulations in early clinical trials (Jacobson, 2008, 2010). One of these studies was a randomized, controlled trial of 44 R5-tropic patients with CD4 cell counts of more than 300 cells/μL and HIV-1 RNA of more than 5,000 copies/mL off antiretroviral therapy (ART) for 12 months or longer (Jacobson, 2010). It showed that SQ PRO 140 administered weekly or biweekly produced a dose-dependent and statistically significant reduction in HIV-1 viral load— a more potent effect that was seen even with some of the initial trials of FTC/TDF. PRO 140 is being investigated in clinical trials to determine if weekly subcutaneous dosing can replace oral ART in patients with HIV-1 who are virologically suppressed. The use of CCR5 mAbs that recognize different epitopes has also been shown to be synergistic with small-molecule CCR5 antagonists such as maraviroc and fusion inhibitors such as enfuvirtide (Murga, 2006; Safarian, 2006).

Clinically relevant mAbs to host cellular receptors have also shown efficacy in clinical trials. Ibalizumab is a humanized mouse mAb directed against the extracellular domains of human CD4 cells aimed at preventing HIV entry into the cell. It has activity against both CCR5- and CXCR4-tropic viruses. Two phase 2 trials have shown that, in treatment-experienced patients, TNX-355 in addition to HAART led to statistically significant reductions in HIV-1 viral load up to 1 year after drug initiation without any significant safety concerns noted to date (Bruno, 2010; Khanlou, 2011). A phase 3 trial evaluated the safety and efficacy of ibalizumab in 40 participants with multidrug-resistant HIV infection in combination with an optimized background regiment (including 17 who also received fostemsavir). After 25 weeks of treatment, 43% of participants had an HIV RNA of less than 50 copies/mL (Emu, 2018). Ibalizumab was approved by the US Food and Drug Administration (FDA) for heavily treatment-experienced patients with multiple resistance mutations in March 2018. It is administered intravenously every 2 weeks.

BROADLY NEUTRALIZING MONOCLONAL ANTIBODIES

HIV-1 immunotherapy with first-generation mAb in the preclinical and clinical settings was largely ineffective. A new generation of potent mAb has shown increased potency and breadth of activity, and there has been increased interest in the administration of these antibodies for prevention and immunotherapy. In chronically simian/human immunodeficiency virus (SHIV)-infected rhesus macaques, a cocktail of mAb against the CD4 binding site (3BNC117) and a single N332 glycan-dependent mAb (PGT121) led to a rapid decline in plasma viremia (3.1 log decline in 7 days) in addition to reduced proviral DNA in peripheral blood, gastrointestinal mucosa, and lymph nodes (Barouch, 2013). Another SHIV primate model showed viral suppression for 3–5 weeks in macaques infused with a single infusion of antibodies directed against the CD4 binding site and V3 region, with a second infusion helping to control virus rebound (Shingai, 2013). In phase 1 human trials, a single infusion of 3BNC17 led to a 0.8–2.5 $\log_{10}$ reduction in viral load sustained for 28 days (Caskey, 2015). Another study evaluated early administration of combination bNAb (10-1074 and 3BNC117), which targets nonoverlapping envelope peptide, in macaques challenged with mucosal or parenteral SHIV and demonstrated sustained viral suppression (up to 177 days) (Nishimura, 2017). The combination of bNAb 10-1074 and 3BNC117 was evaluated in a phase 1b study of 7 HIV-infected volunteers of whom 4 had dual antibody sensitive viruses and had a 2.05 $\log_{10}$ reduction in HIV RNA which was maintained for 90 days after last antibody infusion (Bar-Om, 2018).

A phase 2 open-label study showed that 3BNC117 infusions were able to suppress viral rebound up to 19 weeks in HIV-infected humans with treatment interruptions. They also observed that most of the rebound viruses had high resistance to 3BNC117, suggesting that it exerts strong selective pressure on the latent reservoir during treatment interruption (Scheid, 2016). These results will need to be studied further, especially with regard to impact on the latent reservoir and immune dysregulation because chronic antigen stimulation should be reduced by these antibodies.

VRC01 is a bNAb that targets the CD4-binding site of the HIV envelope glycoprotein. In two open-label trials on HIV patients with treatment interruptions, VRC01 slightly delayed viral rebound but did not maintain viral suppression by week 8, and many patients had preexisting resistance to VRC01 (Bar, 2016). VCR01 is undergoing phase 2b studies. A phase 1 study evaluating a long-acting form of VRC01 (VRC01LS) was recently completed in healthy volunteers. Results from this study demonstrated that VRC01LS was safe, well-tolerated, had a fourfold greater half-life than VRC01, and elicited HIV-1 neutralizing activity in serum (Gaudinski, 2018).

$\alpha_4\beta_7$ Antibody

Early HIV infection of lymphocytes within gut-associated lymphoid tissue (GALT) and subsequent depletion of gut CD4+ T cells appears to significantly contribute to dysfunction observed in chronic HIV infection. Durable suppression of HIV replication with HAART does not significantly reverse the damage caused to GALT during early infection. Accordingly, therapies aimed at attenuating HIV-mediated destruction of GALT may serve as an effective strategy to treat and/or prevent HIV infection. One such approach involves disruption of the interaction between gut homing receptors on immune effector cells and the gut endothelial cell adhesion molecules to which these receptors home to. Specifically, $\alpha_4\beta_7$ is a gut homing receptor expressed on CD4 and CD8 T cell subsets which mediates trafficking to

GALT via interaction with mucosal addressing cell adhesion molecules (MAdCAM) expressed on gut endothelial cells. Furthermore, HIV has been shown to interact with $\alpha_4\beta_7$ via the V2 domain of the gp120 subunit, and CD4$^+$ T cells with high expression of $\alpha_4\beta_7$ appear to be preferentially infected during acute HIV or SIV infection. A commercially available humanized anti-$\alpha_4\beta_7$ mAb vedolizumab (Act-1) is currently approved for use in inflammatory bowel disease. This antibody blocks binding to MAdCAM via binding to the b7 chain of $\alpha_4\beta_7$, which thereby inhibits the migration of lymphocytes into the gastrointestinal tract and reduces localized inflammatory responses. Blocking this antibody may attenuate HIV-mediated damage to GALT by putatively reducing the number of target cells in GALT that can be infected by HIV. Initial studies evaluating this approach have been conducted in primate models. A primatized version of Act-1 was evaluated when administered prior to SIV infection in macaques and resulted in lower peak viral RNA levels, lower set points, and reduction in the amount of SIV in GALT (Ansari, 2011). Another study evaluated the effect of coadministration of ART and $\alpha_4\beta_7$ in rhesus macaques (Byareddy, 2016). In this study, initiation of ART 5 weeks after SIV infection followed by a rhesus mAb against $\alpha_4\beta_7$ started 4 weeks after ART led to durable viral control in both peripheral blood and gut tissue for more than 9 months after ARV treatment cessation. A phase 1 study evaluating vedolizumab in participants with HIV infection undergoing analytical treatment interruption is under way.

RECOMMENDED READING

Arthos JA, Cicala C, Nawaz F, et al. The role of integrin $\alpha_4\beta_7$ in HIV pathogenesis and treatment. *Curr Opin HIV AIDS*. 2018;15:127–135.

Olender SA, Taylor BS, Wong M, et al. CROI 2015: Advances in antiretroviral therapy. *Top Antivir Med*. 2015;23(1):28–45.

Pace P, Markowitz M. Monoclonal antibodies to host cellular receptors for the treatment and prevention of HIV-1 infection. *Curr Opin HIV AIDS*. 2015;10(3):144–150.

Richman DD, Margolis DM, Delaney M., et al. The challenge of finding a cure for HIV infection. *Science*. 2009;323(5919):1304–1307.

IMMUNOMODULATORY AGENTS AND GENE THERAPY

LEARNING OBJECTIVES

- Describe different strategies to help restore the immune system in patients chronically infected with HIV-1 and potentially eliminate the latent reservoir.

- Discuss the different gene therapy modalities currently being tested and their potential benefits and limitations to clinical use.

WHAT'S NEW?

A new generation of broadly neutralizing antibodies has demonstrated potency at suppressing HIV-1 viremia in clinical trials and may play a role in immunotherapy and prevention. Latency reversing agents (e.g., histone deacetylase inhibitors) and gene therapy strategies using autologous CD4 T cells and hematopoietic stem cells continue to be evaluated in trials.

KEY POINTS

- Interleukin-7 (IL-7) and IL-21 are cytokines being studied as immunomodulatory agents.

- It has been demonstrated in the "Berlin patient" that CCR5 null cells can be engrafted, curing this patient and renewing interest in gene therapy strategies.

- Histone deacetylase inhibitors are being studied as agents targeting the HIV-1 latent reservoir and immune dysregulation in HIV-1.

- A new generation of broadly neutralizing mAbs has demonstrated more potency and breadth than prior generations.

- Ribozymes, RNA interference aptamers, and zinc finger nucleases (ZFNs) are gene therapy strategies being studied as immunotherapy for HIV-1.

- Currently, the potential implementation of immune-based strategies is limited, most notably by cost and patient access.

ARV drugs are currently the mainstay of treatment for HIV-1, but these medications do not achieve cure, have potential side effects, and require life-long adherence. Many HIV-infected patients treated with ART alone also do not achieve immune restoration despite viral suppression. The importance of immune restoration was highlighted by a large trial of HIV-infected adults achieving virologic suppression for 3 years with CD4 counts 200 cells/μL or less (Engsig, 2014). These patients had significantly greater mortality compared to those with CD4 counts of more than 200 cells/μL (adjusted hazard ratio, 2.6). Given significant evidence that CD4 counts have been correlated with normal life expectancy (ART Collaboration Cohort, 2008; Lewden, 2007), attention has turned to strategies to control chronic immune activation and loss of normal T cell homeostasis seen in HIV. This section discusses some of these strategies in further detail, as well as the feasibility for future implementation.

CYTOKINES

IL-2, an autocrine T cell growth factor, is produced by CD4$^+$ T cells and is therefore deficient and dysfunctional in HIV-infected patients. Based on promising phase 2 trials showing increased CD4$^+$ T cell counts in patients receiving recombinant IL-2 (rIL-2) (Pett, 2010), two phase 3 trials were performed. In the ESPRIT study, 4,111 HIV-infected patients with CD4 counts of 300 cells/μL or more were randomized to receive SQ IL-2 (three 5-day cycles 8 weeks apart) with HAART or HAART alone (Abrams, 2009). Although the rIL-2 group had a significantly higher CD4 count, this difference seemed to decline with time, and clinical outcomes, including opportunistic infection/death and all-cause mortality, did not significantly differ between the two groups. In addition, there were more grade 4 adverse events in the group receiving IL-2, most notably deep venous thrombosis. Subsequent analysis also raised concern for an increased incidence of pneumonia in patients receiving rIL-2 less than 180 days previously (Pett, 2011).

The SILCAAT study, another phase 3 trial, randomized 1,695 patients with CD4 counts of 50–299 cells/mm^3 to similar treatment arms, except the IL-2 group received six cycles at a lower dose (Abrams, 2009). CD4 cell counts were again higher in the IL-2 group, but statistically significant differences in opportunistic infection/death, all-cause mortality, and grade 4 clinical events were not seen. Both studies do not support an additional clinical benefit to rIL-2 with HAART.

IL-2 has also been studied as a means to eradicate HIV from latently infected CD4 cells and, therefore, reduce the viral reservoir. One randomized trial did not show an impact of rIL-2 with HAART on proviral DNA in blood, lymph nodes, and cerebrospinal fluid compared to HAART alone (Stellbrink, 2002). Other potential uses of rIL-2, such as a means to delay HAART initiation or facilitate HAART treatment interruption or as a vaccine adjunct (discussed later), have been challenged by clinical studies. In the STALWART study, a phase 2 trial in patients not on HAART with CD4 counts greater than 300 cells/µl, rIL-2 use was associated with more opportunistic disease and death and a statistically significant increase in grade 3 or grade 4 events (Tavel, 2010).

Other cytokines currently being studied for use in HIV include IL-7, IL-15, and IL-21. IL-7 plays a key role in T cell homeostasis, leading to expansion and survival of naïve and memory T cells and preventing apoptosis of CD4 and CD8 cells in HIV-infected patients in vitro. In early clinical trials, human recombinant IL-7 therapy was well-tolerated and induced a significant and dose-dependent increase in functional naïve and memory CD4 and CD8 cells in lymphopenic patients with HIV on HAART (Levy, 2009; Sereti, 2009). In a randomized, placebo-controlled trial of recombinant IL-7 in ARV-treated HIV-infected persons, there were brisk CD4 increases of naïve and central memory T cells (averaging 323 cells/µL at 12 weeks) with a durable response seen up to 1 year (Levy, 2012).

In macaque models, IL-21 has improved beneficial immune responses, such as natural killer (NK) and T cell cytotoxicity, with reduced levels of intestinal T cell proliferation and microbial translocation. With this novel profile, it may become a useful treatment for augmenting immune response while ameliorating intestinal immune activation (Pallikkuth, 2011, 2013).

IL-15, like IL-2, has lymphocyte stimulatory activity and is significantly increased in HIV patients with a virologic and immunologic response to HAART compared to ARV-naïve patients (Forcina, 2004), which has prompted theoretical interest in its role in immune therapy.

OTHER IMMUNOMODULATORY TREATMENTS

Several new classes of medications are being studied for their role in altering immune dysregulation in HIV. Histone deacetylase inhibitors (HDACs), a class of anticancer drugs, have been proposed as latency-reversing agents. There are conflicting data on the ability to HDACs to induce T cell activation and substantial increases in HIV-1 mRNA in latently infected cells. A study that examined panobinostat, vorinostat, and romidepsin did not find any significant increase in HIV-1 production (Bullen, 2014). However, romidepsin has been shown in a single trial to induce a sixfold increase in intracellular RNA levels in latently infected cells, which persisted for 48 hours and correlated with inhibition of cell-associated HDAC activity (Wei, 2014). A recent phase 1b/2a trial showed that romidepsin, administered intravenously once weekly for 3 weeks to six aviremic HIV-1–infected patients on ART, significantly increased HIV-1 transcription and plasma HIV-1 RNA levels in five of the six patients without decreasing the number of HIV-1–specific T cells or inhibiting T cell cytokine production (Sogaard, 2015). Many of these compounds have entered into pilot phase 2 single-center studies, and results are forthcoming.

In combination with protein C agonists, HDACs have also been shown to induce HIV-1 transcription and virus production in ex vivo analysis, contributing to latency reversal without the release of proinflammatory cytokines by resting CD4$^+$ T cells (Laird, 2015). Phase 1/2 clinical trials of romidepsin are ongoing, as are trials examining its use in conjunction with the therapeutic vaccine Vacc-4x.

Another molecular target is PD-1, a signaling molecule on the surface of CD4 T cells that can be transiently expressed with T cell activation and persistently expressed in a type of cellular dysfunction called *T cell exhaustion*. This molecule is of specific interest with regard to HIV because it is preferentially expressed by latently infected CD4 T cells, and anti–PD-1 antibodies may be able to restore the function of CD4 and CD8 T cells that have become exhausted (Porichis, 2012). A significant proportion of the HIV reservoir in patients receiving HAART appears to reside in PD-1–positive T cells. It is speculated that blocking this receptor could facilitate restoration of host cell pathways needed for T cell activation and subsequent transcription of latently infected HIV. BMS-936559, a human antibody against PD ligand 1, has been shown in a trial of rhesus macaques to delay viral load rebound after ARV cessation and to significantly lower viral load setpoint (Mason, 2014). In a phase 1 randomized clinical trial in 8 HIV-1 patients on ART with CD4 counts of greater than 350 cells/µL and detectable viral load who received a single infusion of BMS-936559, 2 patients showed an increase in the mean percentage of HIV-1 Gag-specific CD8$^+$ T cells expressing interferon-γ (INF-γ; Gay, 2017). While this drug is no longer in clinical development, these studies did demonstrate, as a proof of concept, the potential utility of immune checkpoint inhibitors in targeting the HIV reservoir. Other immune checkpoint inhibitors have been approved as cancer therapies, including nivolumab, an anti–PD-1 antibody, which, as described in a case report, appeared to decrease the HIV reservoir (as suggested by a decrease in cell-associated HIV-DNA, increase in HIV-RT and Nef-specific CD8 cells, and increase in T cell activation) in a 51-year-old man with non–small cell carcinoma and well-controlled HIV infection who was treated with nivolumab (Guihot, 2018). Several phase 1 and 2 studies evaluating PD-1 antibodies in HIV-infected participants have started enrollment and are ongoing.

Because T cell activation is controlled by a number of signaling pathways, inhibitors of these pathways may also play a role in reducing the size of the latent viral reservoir. Early preclinical research has shown that mTOR inhibitors (e.g., sirolimus, temsirolimus, and everolimus) may play a role in reducing T cell activation and inflammation (Heredia, 2015; Martin, 2015; Palmer, 2015), although clinical trial data are lacking. A phase 4 study evaluating impact of everolimus on HIV persistence post kidney or liver transplant recently completed enrollment, and results are forthcoming.

BROADLY NEUTRALIZING MONOCLONAL ANTIBODIES

HIV-1 immunotherapy with first-generation mAbs in the preclinical and clinical settings was largely ineffective. A new generation of potent mAbs has shown increased potency and breadth of activity, and there has been increased interest in the administration of these antibodies for prevention and immunotherapy. In chronically SHIV-infected rhesus macaques, a cocktail of mAbs against the CD4 binding site (3BNC117) and a single N332 glycan-dependent mAb (PGT121) led to a rapid decline in plasma viremia (3.1 log decline in 7 days) in addition to reduced proviral DNA in peripheral blood, gastrointestinal mucosa, and lymph nodes (Barouch, 2013). Another SHIV primate model showed viral suppression for 3–5 weeks in macaques infused with a single infusion of antibodies directed against the CD4 binding site and V3 region, with a second infusion helping to control virus rebound (Shingai, 2013). In phase 1 human trials, a single infusion of 3BNC17 led to a 0.8–2.5 $\log_{10}$ reduction in viral load sustained for 28 days (Caskey, 2015). Another study in evaluated early administration of combination bNAb (10-1074 and 3BNC117), which target non-overlapping envelope peptide, in macaques challenged with mucosal or parenteral SHIV and demonstrated sustained viral suppression (up to 177 days) (Nishimura, 2017).

GENE THERAPY

Gene therapy, also referred to as "intracellular immunization," involves the insertion of protective genes either mechanically or by viral vectors. The goal of gene therapy in HIV is to have the target cells produce gene products that protect them and their progeny from HIV infection. There has been increasing interest in gene therapy after reports of the "Berlin patient," an HIV-positive male with acute myelogenous leukemia who received an allogeneic stem cell transplant from a donor homozygous for the CCR5-delta 32 mutation, known to naturally confer resistance to HIV infection (Hutter, 2009). He successfully engrafted with CCR5 null cells and has remained free of detectable virus for more than 6 years without ART.

Gene therapy research has focused on two areas: the disruption of cellular genes involved in HIV entry, such as the CCR5 coreceptor, and the introduction of genes to disrupt HIV replication. The use of various technologies including ribozymes, aptamers, RNA-based interference strategies, and ZFNs is currently being investigated.

RIBOZYMES, APTAMERS, AND RNA-BASED INTERFERENCE

Ribozymes are small, catalytically active RNA molecules that can be engineered to target specific RNA sequences. In HIV, they can target viral RNA during uncoating and after transcription, leading to RNA degradation. Although in vitro studies of ribozyme gene therapy have been promising, retroviral vectors delivering ribozymes targeting viral targets (e.g., tat and rev) have been plagued by problems with low transduction efficiency.

The first phase 2 randomized, controlled trial of an anti-HIV ribozyme was conducted in 74 HIV-1-infected individuals on HAART receiving either autologous stem cells transduced with a ribozyme targeting the overlapping tat and vpr reading frames of HIV-1 (OZ1) or placebo (Mitsuyasu, 2009). No significant adverse events were reported with the infusion, but the subjects also had low engraftment levels and short persistence of the ribozyme. There was a trend, but no statistically significant difference, in HIV-1 viral load at the primary end point; however, after treatment interruption at 40 weeks, patients continuing to express OZ1 RNA had a statistically significant decrease in HIV-1 viral load.

RNA interference utilizes short RNAs that mediate the degradation of mRNAs in a sequence-specific manner. Theoretically, multiple short hairpin RNAs (shRNA) in a single vector are thought to prevent HIV-1 escape. With this strategy, antisense oligonucleotides can bind mRNA and trigger degradation through an RNase H-dependent pathway or block ribosome binding, thus preventing gene expression. Clinical research in this field is evolving, but it has been limited by difficulty delivering the RNAs to the correct target cells, poor cellular uptake and stability, and viral escape (Zhou, 2011). VRX496 (Lexgenleucel-T), antisense env in a lentiviral vector, has progressed to phase 2 trials, in which it has been delivered via autologous CD4+ T cell infusion to both patients on failing regimens and patients on a fully suppressive ART regimen. In one trial, 17 patients received Lexgenleucel-T over 16 weeks, with HAART interruption 1 month later in 13 of these patients (Tebas, 2013). Six of 8 patients analyzed were noted to have a decrease in viral load set point. The use of a short-interfering RNA targeting a unique triple repeat of NF-κB has also been shown to achieve long-term suppression of HIV-1 subtype C (Singh, 2014).

Aptamers are single-stranded RNA or DNA molecules that can bind viral proteins, preventing them from carrying out their function in the viral life cycle (Figure 25.1). In clinical trials, when used alone, they have not been shown to be effective. However, strategies combining aptamers, ribozymes, and RNA interference, based on in vitro efficacy, require further investigation because they have been shown to exhibit potent inhibition of HIV-1 in vitro (Centlivre, 2013; ter Brake, 2008).

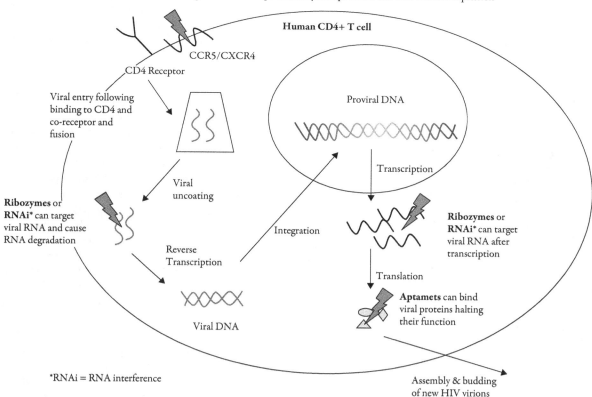

Zinc finger nucleases can permanently disrupt CCR5 and even CXCR4 expression

Figure 25.1 Schematic diagram of the HIV viral life cycle in host cell and gene therapy targets. From Zeller et al. (2011).

Theoretically, gene therapy can also be used to inhibit viral fusion. C46, a structurally similar peptide to enfuvirtide, has been engineered to be expressed on autologous T cells and seems to be well-tolerated in clinical trials, although clinical efficacy has not yet been demonstrated (van Lundzen, 2007). Calimmune, a small, public-/private-funded biotech company based in Pasadena, California, has developed Cal-1, an anti-HIV-1 lentiviral vector containing CCR5 shRNA and C46 that has been shown in preclinical studies to be nontoxic and to protect gene-modified cells from both CXCR4- and CCR5-tropic HIV-1 strains (Wolstein, 2014). A phase 1/2 clinical trial has recently been completed using autologous, Cal-1–modified CD4+ cells and hematopoietic progenitor/stem cells with and without bone marrow condition in HIV-positive patients to test the Cal-1 construct for the treatment of HIV-1, and results are forthcoming.

ZINC FINGER NUCLEASES

ZFNs are engineered proteins with two functional domains—one that recognizes DNA, and one that cleaves it. ZFNs can bind specific DNA sequences, produce a double-stranded break, and then lead to permanent gene disruption when cellular repair pathways lead to the addition or deletion of nucleotides at the break site. ZFNs have been shown to disrupt CCR5 expression in human stem cells administered in a mouse model of HIV and to be associated with lower HIV viral loads after HIV challenge (Holt, 2010).

SB-728T, an infusion of ZFN-modified autologous CD4 T cells with the ability to knock out CCR5 expression, has been shown to increase CD4 cell over time, decrease proviral DNA, and restore the CD4-depleted population of the gut mucosa in chronically infected patients with CD4 counts of more than 200 cells/µL (June, 2012; Lalezari, 2012). One subject with the highest level of CCR5 modification had an undetectable viral load when HAART treatment interruption occurred. In a well-publicized clinical trial, SB-728T was demonstrated to be safe in 12 patients who received the treatment, with one serious infusion reaction noted (Tebas, 2014). These subjects had significantly increased CD4+ T cell counts, and the gene-modified CD4 T cells persisted at low levels during long-term follow-up. Six of these patients underwent 12-week ART interruption, but in only 1 patient (heterozygous for the CCR5-delta 32 mutation) did the viral load decline to an undetectable level prior to ART reinitiation.

Additional studies of SB-728T are under way, with one examining CCR5-delta 32 heterozygotes and another examining the use of cytoxan prior to CD4+ T cell infusion to decrease the number of existing CD4+ T cells. Early data from the latter trial have demonstrated that cytoxan treatment is well-tolerated with a dose-related increase in total CD4+ T cell count and engraftment of CCR5-modified cells (Blick, 2014).

One novel gene therapy approach currently in phase 1 trials is the use of MazF-T, autologous CD4+ T cells modified with the MAZF endoribonuclease gene, which can render T cells resistant to HIV replication (Saito, 2014). Additional trials using modified stem cells are also in early clinical stages for AIDS patients with hematologic malignancies. Although promising, it will be difficult to develop the previously discussed gene strategies for widespread use. Cost of the agents/technology, the development of an infrastructure for delivery, lack of availability of this technology in areas most affected by HIV-1, and patient insurance limitations all pose significant barriers to implementation.

RECOMMENDED READING

Ahlensteil CL, Suzuki K, Marks K, et al. Controlling HIV-1: non-coding RNA gene therapy approaches a functional cure. *Front Immunol.* 2015;6:474.

Barouch DH, Deeks SG. Immunologic strategies for HIV-1 remission and eradication. *Science.* 2014; 45(6193):169–174.

Chomont N, El-Far M, Ancuta P, et al. HIV reservoir size and persistence are driven by T cell survival and homeostatic proliferation. *Nat Med.* 2009;15(8):893–900.

Frater J. New approaches in HIV eradication research. *Curr Opin Infect Dis.* 2011;24(6):593–598.

Kitchen SG, Shimizu S, An DS. Stem cell-based anti-HIV gene therapy. *Virology.* 2011;411:260–272.

Levy J. Not an HIV cure but encouraging new directions. *N Engl J Med.* 2009;360:724–725.

Lewin S, Rouzioux C. HIV cure and eradication: how will we get from the laboratory to effective clinical trials? *AIDS.* 2011;25:885–897.

THERAPEUTIC VACCINES

LEARNING OBJECTIVE

Discuss the progression and current status of research in HIV therapeutic vaccines.

WHAT'S NEW?

HIV therapeutic vaccine research has seen a resurgence in recent years with different classes of vaccines showing promise in clinical trials.

KEY POINTS

- Therapeutic immunization is a strategy for boosting anti–HIV-1 immunity in chronically infected patients.

- Recent studies of therapeutic vaccines have provided more durable and diverse immune responses and lowering of viral load set points.

- Many different types of vaccines have progressed to phase 2 trials, including DNA, subunit, and dendritic cell vaccines.

Therapeutic immunization aims to induce a cellular immune response through vaccination with components of HIV-1 that will help contain viral replication through reconstitution of anti–HIV-1 immune responses. Data support the observation that the cellular immune response is critical in controlling HIV-1 replication, as reported in patients with primary HIV-1 infection and long-term nonprogressors (Borrow, 1994; Cao, 1995; Kroup, 1994; Rosenberg, 1997). Therapeutic vaccines can potentially be of benefit to ART-naïve patients by potentially delaying progression to AIDS and time to initiation of ART. Among patients on ART, development of a durable vaccine can potentially intensify the effects of ART (accelerate response time to therapy, decrease risk of transmission, and potentiate the immune effects of ART including reduction of proviral DNA), simplify ART regimens, and support regimens with treatment interruption (Ensoli, 2014).

Clinical therapeutic vaccine research for HIV started prior to the introduction of HAART, first with a gp120-depleted inactivated HIV-1 preparation and then with vectors expressing viral proteins (e.g., gag p17 and p24). Clinical trials of these agents largely failed to show efficacy and a sustained HIV-1–specific response (Hardy, 2007). Subsequent vaccines with recombinant HIV-1 glycoproteins (e.g., gp120 and gp160) also fared poorly, not altering the decline in CD4 count or halting disease progression in HIV-1–infected individuals in phase 2 trials (Eron, 1996; Pontesilli, 1998; Sandstrom, 1999; Tsoukas, 1998). In one of the largest of these trials, 608 HIV-1–infected individuals with CD4$^+$ T cell counts of greater than 400 cells/mm^3 were repeatedly immunized with a recombinant gp160 vaccine (VaxSyn HIV-1) or placebo and followed for 3–5 years. Although the vaccine had excellent immunogenicity (~70%), it failed to show a difference in reaching the primary clinical end points: a 50% decline in CD4$^+$ T cell count or disease progression to Walter Reed stages 4, 5, and 6 (Birx, 2000).

ANRS 093, a study of 70 HIV-1–infected patients, compared HAART to immunization with recombinant canarypox vector expressing several HIV genes (env, gag, pol, and nef) and lipo-6T (HIV-1 lipopeptides) followed by SQ IL-2. The vaccine elicited a statistically significant INF-γ–producing CD8$^+$ T cell response that correlated with virologic control (Levy, 2005). The vaccine group was able to have a lower viral set point and, therefore, a significantly greater number of days off HAART (Levy, 2006), but the results of this study await validation in larger trials. In ACTG 5197, administration of a replication-defective adenovirus type 5 HIV-1 gag vaccine to HIV-infected patients with CD4$^+$ T cell counts of more than 500 cells/mm^3 failed to be sufficiently immunogenic and lacked statistically significant efficacy (Schooley, 2010). The finding that the plasma viral load was 0.5 log$_{10}$ lower in the vaccine arm at 16 weeks post-HAART interruption prompted further analysis of the HLA class I alleles in all 110 participants because HLA classes have previously been shown to influence viral evolution and disease progression. Vaccinated patients with neutral HLA alleles in this cohort had a lower plasma viral load than those of both patients vaccinated with protective alleles and placebo participants with neutral alleles (Li, 2011).

One novel therapeutic vaccine strategy with promising results has targeted Tat, a transactivator of HIV gene expression essential for viral replication that is relatively conserved among HIV-1 subtypes. This vaccine is aimed at patients on ART with the hope of decreasing viral reservoirs and restoring immune homeostasis. In phase 2 trials, 168 patients controlled on ART and anti-Tat antibody negative at baseline administered the vaccine three or five times monthly showed specific and durable immune responses when followed for up to 144 weeks (Ensoli, 2015). Most patients (79%) developed anti-Tat antibodies, which was associated with significant reduction of proviral DNA seen after week 72. The vaccine was also associated with a restoration of T, B, and NK cells and CD4$^+$ and CD8$^+$ central memory subsets.

A multinational phase 2 trial examined the safety and immunogenicity of Vacc-4x, a peptide-based HIV-1 therapeutic vaccine targeting the conserved domains of p24Gag (Pollard, 2014). In chronically infected HIV-1 patients who were virologically suppressed on ART, the Vacc-4x vaccine did not alter time to ART resumption and did not lead to significant changes in CD4 count at week 28 during treatment interruption. However, there was a statistically significant difference in HIV viral load at both week 48 (23,000 vs. 71,800 copies/mL) and week 52 (19,500 vs. 51,000 copies/mL).

The DNA plasmid vaccine GTU-multiHIV B, aimed at inducing immune responses to HIV-1 regulatory genes, has shown efficacy in HIV-1 subtype C chronically infected patients not on ART. In a population of 63 patients, the vaccine was deemed safe and was associated with a statistically significant decline in log pHIV-RNA with an increase in CD4$^+$ T cell counts nearing significance compared to placebo, especially after intramuscular injections (Vardas, 2012). The efficacy of GTU-multi-HIV B DNA vaccine and LIPO-5 vaccine in a prime-boost strategy for lowering viral set point after treatment interruption for patients virologically suppressed on ART is currently being studied in phase 2 trials.

Significant attention has also focused on dendritic cells as cellular adjuvants for therapeutic HIV-1 vaccines because they have been shown to elicit strong CD4 and CD8 T cell responses in vivo. One uncontrolled study of immunization of 18 HIV-1–infected treatment-naïve patients with dendritic cells pulsed with inactivated autologous virus reported a 90% decrease in viral load during the course of a year (Lu, 2004). A subsequent randomized control trial of 24 treatment-naïve subjects with a similar vaccine, however, showed a weak HIV-1–specific response and a modest decrease in viral load compared to placebo (Garcia, 2011). In a trial of chronically infected patients on ART with CD4$^+$ T cell counts of more than 450 cells/mm^3, the use of a monocyte-derived dendritic cell pulse with heat-inactivated whole HIV helped lower plasma viral load set point after treatment interruption, with an associated increased in HIV-1–specific T cell responses compared to placebo (Garcia, 2013). Recent trials have continued to demonstrate better vaccine responses and control of viral replication (Levy, 2014). Dendritic cells expressing the HIV proteins Gag, Tat, Rev, and Nef administered as a vaccine have been shown to elicit potent antiviral T cell responses in HIV-1 patients on HAART, including a Gag-specific IFN-γ response that correlated with HIV-1 inhibitory activity (van Gulck, 2012).

Although no therapeutic vaccine is currently FDA approved, the future of therapeutic vaccine research for both naïve and ART-treated patients remains promising. Some of the key vaccines in development are highlighted in Table 25.2.

Recent data have been encouraging, but the results of therapeutic vaccine trials have not yielded a therapeutic vaccine strategy that can be implemented. In addition to further clinical trials of the vaccines discussed previously, additional studies investigating the heterogeneity of response to vaccines (e.g., genetic determinants) and the immunologic correlates of vaccine efficacy are needed for the field to advance.

PREVENTIVE VACCINES

Although a preventive HIV-1 vaccine would help control the worldwide AIDS pandemic, there have been many obstacles to its development. HIV-1 itself has significant genetic and antigenic diversity that is difficult to target with a vaccine. The failure to induce broadly neutralizing antibodies against the virus and the lack of clear immune correlates of protection have also been challenges. Additionally, SIV/SHIV nonhuman primate models on which preclinical testing of the vaccines is typically done have often showed promising results not reproduced in clinical trials.

Multiple phase 1 and 2 trials of vaccines have occurred dating back to 1987, but very few trials have reached phase 2b/3. Initial vaccine trials involved using recombinant proteins to induce neutralizing antibodies. In two large randomized controlled trials, VAX003 and VAX004, involving vaccination with recombinant gp120 subunits, there were no statistically significant reductions in HIV infection in the vaccinated groups (Flynn, 2005; Pitisuttithum, 2006). In subsequent analysis, these vaccines seemed to fail due to a lack of a broad neutralizing antibody response.

Vaccine development subsequently shifted toward the use of live viral or bacterial vectors engineered to carry genes encoding the HIV antigens. These antigens are expressed in the cytoplasm of the target cell, broken down, and then presented on the surface of the cell, priming a CD8$^+$ response. In the STEP trial, HIV-negative subjects received immunization with three shots of a replication-incompetent recombinant adenovirus vector expressing HIV-1 Gag, Pol, and Nef (Buchbinder, 2008). The vaccine did not show any benefit in preventing transmission or reducing early viral load after infection.

Surprisingly, however, patients vaccinated who were seropositive for AD-5 or uncircumcised had higher rates of HIV-1 infection than placebo for unclear reasons, a finding prompting discontinuation of another clinical trial with the same vaccine at the time. Subsequent genetic sequencing of the HIV-1 strains from the vaccine and placebo groups revealed that the virus infecting the vaccine group had different epitopes from those in the placebo group (Rolland, 2011). The divergence was confined to the vaccine components of the virus, supporting the notion of selective pressure from vaccine-induced T cell responses.

More recent vaccine strategies have used a heterologous prime-boost strategy to activate both cellular and humoral immune arms by priming with a certain vaccine (e.g., DNA

Table 25.2 SELECT THERAPEUTIC VACCINE TRIALS

VACCINE	DESCRIPTION	STAGE OF DEVELOPMENT	RESULTS
DNA Vaccines			
Dermavir	Topically applied DNA vaccine	Phase 2	Safe and immunogenic in ART-treated patients with GAG-specific T cell responses (Rodriguez, 2013)
GTU-multiHIV B	DNA plasmid vaccine, contains complete sequences of HIV-1 Rev, Nef, Tat, and Gag (p17/p24) and a number of T cell epitopes from Pol and Env	Phase 2	Statistically significant decrease in log pHIV RNA in ART-naïve patients compared to placebo; currently being studied with LIPO-5 as a prime boost strategy for patients on ART
Subunit Vaccines			
Tat protein vaccine	Recombinant biologically active HIV-1 B Clade Tat protein	Phase 2	Induction of anti-Tat antibodies in most patients on ART restoring T, B, and NK cells and CD4[+] and CD8[+] central memory subsets (Ensoli, 2015); significant reduction in proviral DNA seen at week 72
Vac-3S	Peptide-based vaccine aimed at eliciting a humoral response against the highly conserved region of gp41	Phase 2	An increase in CD4 count was observed in patients with higher antibody levels.
Vacc-4x	Peptide-based vaccine with four synthetic peptides based on the HIV-1 p24 protein	Phase 2	Statistically significant lower HIV viral set point at week 48 compared to placebo in patients on ART; no change to time in treatment interruption and Cd4 count (primary endpoints)
HIV-v	T cell epitope HIV vaccine with synthetic peptides from conserved regions of Vpr, Vif, Rev, and Nef	Phase 1b/2	Safe, IgG responses in up to 75% of volunteers with 1 log reduction in viral load in ART-naïve males with this response compared to placebo and non-responders (Boffito, 2013)
Dendritic Cell Vaccines			
AGS-004	Patient-derived dendritic cells and loaded ex vivo with RNA encoding four (Gag, Nef, Rev, and Vpr) antigens plus CD40L	Phase 2	Delay in continuous ART resumption in 24 treated subjects, but no improvement in CD4[+] T cell counts (DeBenedette, 2014). Greater effect on HIV-specific effector/memory CD8 T-cell responses but no effect on viral load after treatment interruption. (Jacobson, 2016)
THV-01 (THV01-1 and THV01-2)	Live lentiviral vector vaccines, carries transgene that induces cellular response and eliminated HIV infected cells	Phase 2	Able to elicit vaccine specific CD4[+] and CD8[+] responses in patients on suppressive ART Trials ongoing.

ART, antiretroviral therapy; NK, natural killer.

vaccine) and then boosting the immune response with another type of vaccine (e.g., live vector vaccine) (Girard, 2011). The RV144 trial, a phase 3 randomized controlled trial, involved priming subjects with two successive doses of a canarypox vector (ALVAC) encoding Gag/Pro and Env antigens followed by two additional immunizations with this vector and AIDSVAX B/E, a bivalent HIV gp120 envelope glycoprotein derived from a subtype B and subtype E envelope (Rerks-Ngarm, 2009). The trial showed that 74 of 7,325 in the placebo group and 51 of 7,347 in the vaccine group developed HIV-1 infection at 96 weeks, offering a mildly statistically significant 31% efficacy. These results have been encouraging, but there was not a significant broadly neutralizing antibody response, and the vaccine efficacy peaked in the first 6–12 months (50–60%) only to decrease thereafter. Recently presented analysis of the RV144 trial, however, has shown two immune correlates of infection risk after vaccination (Haynes, 2012). Binding of IgG antibodies to the variable regions of Env inversely correlated with infection rates, while plasma IgA binding to Env was directly correlated.

Building on the RV144 data, The HIV Vaccine Trials Network implemented HVTN 100, a phase 1/2, randomized controlled, double-blind trial in South Africa that compared a canarypox vector, ALVAC-HIV[vCP2438], in combination with an envelope (env) glycoprotein (gp120), both adapted to circulating strains in South Africa and paired with a more potent adjuvant to placebo. This combination induced strong humoral and cellular responses (Bekker, 2018). These encouraging results led to the development of HVTN 702, a phase 2b/3 efficacy trial which is currently being implemented in South Africa.

Another strategy was evaluated in the APPROACH trial, a multicenter, randomized, double-blind, placebo-controlled phase 1/2a trial in Africa, South Africa, Thailand, and the United States. The participants received Ad26.Mos.HIV expressing mosaic HIV-1 envelope (Env)/Gag/Pol antigens and aluminium-adjuvanted clade C Env gp140 protein or placebo. Researchers evaluated the vaccine safety, tolerability, and antibody responses at weeks 28 and 52. A parallel study was also conducted in rhesus monkeys. It elicited Env-specific binding antibody responses (100%) and antibody-dependent cellular phagocytosis responses (80%) at week 52 and T cell responses at week 50 (83%) in humans. The most common adverse reaction was injection site (69–88%). A phase 2 clinical efficacy trial is ongoing in sub-Saharan Africa (Barouch, 2018).

Recently progress has been made toward the development of a preventive HIV vaccine. Key issues in development remain the identification of the correlates of immunity, induction of broadly neutralizing antibody responses, and the durability of these responses. Trials building on the results of RV144 are in progress and further development, and it is hoped that they will provide insight into the correlates of immunity and eventually lead to an effective preventive vaccine strategy.

RECOMMENDED READING

Ensoli B, Cafaro A, Monini P, et al. Challenges in HIV vaccine research for treatment and prevention. *Front Immunol.* 2014;5:417.

Gilliam BL, Redfield RR. Therapeutic HIV vaccines. *Curr Top Med Chem.* 2003;3(13):2536–1553.

Gotch FM, Imami N, Hardy G. Candidate vaccines for immunotherapy in HIV. *HIV Med.* 2001;2:260–265.

Levy Y. Therapeutic HIV vaccines: an update. *Curr HIV/AIDS Rep.* 2005;2(1):5–9.

Van Gulck E, Van Tendeloo VF, Berneman ZN, et al. Role of dendritic cells in HIV immunotherapy. *Curr HIV Res.* 2010;8(4):310–322.

REFERENCES

Abrams D, Levy Y, Losso MH, et al.; INSIGHT-ESPRIT Study Group;SILCAAT Scientific Committee. Interleukin 2 therapy in patients with HIV infection. *N Engl J Med.* 2009;361(16):1548–1559.

ART Collaboration Cohort. Life expectancy of individuals on combination antiretroviral therapy in high-income countries: a collaborative analysis of 14 cohort studies. *Lancet.* 2008;372:293–299.

Bar KJ, Sneller MC, Harrison LJ, et al. Effect of HIV antibody VRC01 on viral rebound after treatment interruption. *N Engl J Med.* 2016;375(21):2037–2050.

Barouch DH, Tomaka FL, Wegmann F, et al. Evaluation of a mosaic HIV-1 vaccine in a multicentre, randomised, double-blind, placebo-controlled, phase 1/2a clinical trial (APPROACH) and in rhesus monkeys (NHP 13–19). *Lancet.* 2018;392 (10143):232–243.

Barouch DH, Whitney JB, Moldt B, et al. Therapeutic efficacy of potent neutralizing HIV-1-specific monoclonal antibodies in SHIV-infected rhesus monkeys. *Nature.* 2013;503:224–229.

Bekker L-G, Moodie Z, Grunenberg N, et al. Subtype C ALVAC-HIV and bivalent subtype C gp120/MF59 HIV-1 vaccine in low-risk, HIV-uninfected, South African adults: a phase 1/2 trial. *Lancet HIV.* 2018;5(7):PE366–E378.

Birx D, Loomis-Price LD, Aronson N, et al. Efficacy of recombinant human immunodeficiency virus (HIV) gp160 as a therapeutic vaccine in early-stage HIV-1-infected volunteers. *J Infect Dis.* 2000;181:881–889.

Blick G, Lalezari J, Hsu R, et al. Cyclophosphamide enhances SB-728T engraftment to levels associated with HIV-RNA control [Abstract 141]. Paper presented at the 21st Conference on Retroviruses and Opportunistic Infections, Boston, March 2014.

Boffito M, Folx J, Bowman C, et al. Safety, immunogenicity and efficacy assessment of HIV immunotherapy in a multi-centre, double blind randomized placebo-controlled phase Ib human trial. *Vaccine.* 2013;31(48):5680–5686.

Borrow P, Lewicki H, Hahn BH, et al. Virus specific CD8 cytotoxic T-lymphocyte activity associated with control of viremia in primary human immunodeficiency virus type 1 infection. *J Virol.* 1994;68:6103–6110.

Bruno JB, Jacobson JM. Ibalizumab: an anti-CD4 monoclonal antibody for the treatment of HIV-1 infection. *J Antimicrob Chemother.* 2010;65:1839–1841.

Bullen CK, Laird GM, Durand CM, et al. New ex vivo approached distinguish effective and ineffective single agents for reversing HIV-1 latency in vivo. *Nat Med.* 2014; 20(4):425–429.

Callebaut C, Stepan G, Tian Y, et al. In vitro virology profile of tenofovir alafenamide, a novel oral prodrug of tenofovir with improves antiviral activity compared to that of tenofovir disoproxil fumarate. *Antimicrob Agents Chemother.* 2015;59(10):5909–5916.

Campos N, Myburgh R, Garcel A, et al. Long lasting control of viral rebound with a new drug ABX 464 targeting Rev-mediated viral RNA biogenesis. *Retrovirology.* 2015;12:64–66.

Cao Y, Qin L, Zhang L, et al. Virologic and immunologic characterization of long-term survivors of human immunodeficiency virus type 1 infection. *N Engl J Med.* 1995;332:201–208.

Caskey M, Klein F, Lorenzi JC, et al. Viraemia suppressed in HIV-1 infected humans by broadly neutralizing antibody 3BNC117. *Nature.* 2015;522:487–493.

Centlivre M, Legrand N, Klamer S, et al. Preclinical in vivo evaluation of the safety of a multi-shRNA-based gene therapy against HIV-1. *Mol Ther Nucleic Acids.* 2013; 2:e120.

Chen W, Dmitrov D. Monoclonal antibody-based candidate therapeutics against HIV type 1. *AIDS Res Hum Retroviruses.* May 2012;28(5):425–434.

Daar ES, DeJesus E, Ruane P, et al. Efficacy and safety of switching to fixed-dose bictegravir, emtricitabine, and tenofovir alafenamide from boosted protease inhibitor-based regimens in virologically suppressed adults with HIV-1: 48 week results of a randomised, open-label, multicentre, phase 3, non-inferiority trial. *Lancet HIV.* 2018;5(7):e347-e356.

DeBenedette M, Tcherepanova I, Gamble A, et al. Immune function and viral load post AGS-004 administration to chronic HIV subjects undergoing STI [Abstract 343]. Paper presented at the 21st Conferences on Retroviruses and Opportunistic Infections (CROI), Boston, March 2014.

Emsig FN, Zangerle R, Katsarou O, et al. Long-term mortality in HIV-positive individuals virally suppressed for >3 years with incomplete CD4 recovery. *Clin Infect Dis.* 2014;58(9):1312–1321.

Ensoli B, Cafaro A, Monini P, et al. Challenges in HIV vaccine research for treatment and prevention. *Front Immunol.* 2014;5:417.

Ensoli F, Cafaro A, Casabianco A, et al. HIV-1 Tat immunization restores immune homeostasis and attacks the HAART-resistant blood HIV DNA: results of a randomized phase II clinical exploratory clinical trial. *Retrovirology.* 2015;12:33.

Eron JJ Jr, Ashby MA, Giordano MF, et al. Randomized trial of MNrgp120 HIV-1 vaccine in symptomless HIV-1 infection. *Lancet.* 1996;348:1547–1551.

Forcina G, d'Ettorre G, Mastroianni C, et al. Interleukin-15 modulated interferon-γ and β-chemokine production in patients with HIV infection: implications for immune-based therapy. *Cytokine.* 2004;25:283–290.

Gallant J, Lazzarin A, Mills A, et al. Bictegravir, emtricitabine, and tenofovir alafenamide versus dolutegravir, abacavir, and lamivudine for initial treatment of HIV-1 infection (GS-US-380-1489): a double-blind, multicentre, phase 3, randomised controlled non-inferiority trial. *Lancet*. 2017;390:2063–2072.

Garcia F, Climent N, Assoumou L, et al. A therapeutic dendritic cell-based vaccine for HIV-1 infection. *J Infect Dis*. 2011;203:473–478.

Garcia F, Climent N, Guardo AC, et al. A dendritic cell- based vaccine elicits T cell responses associated with control of HIV- 1 replication. *Sci Transl Med*. 2013;5:166ra62.

Gatell J, Raffi F, Plettenber A, et al. Efficacy and safety of doravirine 100 mg QD vs. efavirenz 600 mg QD with TDF/ FTC in ART- naïve HIV- infected patients: week 24 results [Abstract TUAB0104]. Paper presented at the 8th International AIDS Society Conference on HIV Pathogenesis, Treatment and Prevention, Vancouver, British Columbia, July 2015.

Gatell JM, Morales- Ramirex JO, Hagens DP, et al. Forty- eight week efficacy and safety and early CNS tolerability of doravirine (MK-1439), a novel NNRTI, with TDF/ FTC in ART-naïve HIV-positive patients. *J Int AIDS Soc*. 2014;17(4 Suppl 3):19532.

Gaudinski MR, Coates EE, Houser K, et al. Safety and pharmacokinetics of the Fc-modified HIV-1 human monoclonal antibody VRC01LS: a Phase 1 open-label clinical trial in healthy adults. *PLoS Med*. January 24, 2018;15(1):e1002493. doi: 10.1371/journal.pmed.1002493. eCollection January 2018.

Gay CL, Bosch RJ, Ritz J, et al. Clinical trial of the anti-PD-L1 antibody BMS-936559 in HIV-1 infected participants on suppressive antiretroviral therapy. *J Infect Dis*. 2017;215(11):1725–1733.

Guihot A, Marcelin AG, Massiani AM, et al. Drastic decrease of the HIV reservoir in a patient treated with nivolumab for lung cancer. *Ann Oncol*. 2018;29(2):517–518.

Hardy GA, Imami N, Nelson MR. A phase I, randomized study of combined IL- 2 and therapeutic immunization with antiretroviral therapy. *J Immune Based Therapies Vaccines*. 2007;5:6.

Heredia A, Le N, Gartenhaus RB, et al. Targeting of mTOR catalytic site inhibits multiple steps of the HIV- 1 lifecycle and suppresses HIV- 1 viremia in humanized mice. *Proc Natl Acad Sci USA*. 2015;112(30):9412–9417.

Holt N, Wang J, Kim K, et al. Human hematopoietic stem/ progenitor cells modified by zinc- finger nucleases targeted to CCR5 control HIV- 1 in vivo. *Nat Biotechnol*. 2010;28(8);839–847.

Hutter G, Nowak D, Mossner M, et al. Long-term control of HIV by CCR5 delta 32/ delta 32 stem cell transplantation. *N Engl J Med*. 2009;360:692–698.

Hwang C, Schurmann D, Sobotha C, et al. Second generation HIV- 1 maturation inhibitor BMS- 955176: overall antiviral activity and safety results from the phase IIa proof- of- concept study [Abstract AI468002]. Paper presented at the 15th European AIDS Conference, Barcelona, Spain, October 2015.

Jacobson JM, Routy J-P, Welles S, et al. Dendritic cell immunotherapy for HIV-1 infection using autologous HIV-1 RNA: a randomized, double-blind, placebo-controlled clinical trial. *J AIDS (1999)*. 2016;72(1):31–38.

Jacobson JM, Saag MS, Thompson MA, et al. Antiviral activity of a single dose PRO 140, a CCR5 monoclonal antibody in HIV- infected adults. *J Infect Dis*. 2008;198:1345–1352.

Jacobson JM, Thompson M, Lalezari J, et al. Anti- HIV- 1 activity of weekly or biweekly treatment with subcutaneous PRO 140, a CCR5 monoclonal antibody. *J Infect Dis*. 2010;201(10):1481–1487.

June C, Tebas P, Stein D, et al. Induction of acquired CCR5 deficiency with zinc finger nuclease-modified autologous CD4 T cells (SB-728-T) correlates with increases in CD4 count and effects on viral load in HIV-infected subjects [Abstract 155]. Paper presented at the 19th Conference on Retroviruses and Opportunistic Infection, Seattle, WA, February 2012.

Khanlou H, Devente J, Fessel J, et al. Durable efficacy and continued safety of ibalizumab in treatment- experienced patients. Abstracts of the IDSA Annual Meeting, Boston, MA, 2011. Abstract LB9.

Kroup RA, Safrit JT, Cao Y, et al. Temporal association of cellular immune responses with the initial control of viremia in primary human immunodeficiency virus type 1 syndrome. *J Virol*. 1994;68:4650–4655.

Krystal M, et al. HIV-1 Combinectin BMS-986197: a long-acting inhibitor with multiple modes of action [Abstract 97]. Presented at the 23rd Conference on Retroviruses and Opportunistic Infection, Boston, February 22–25, 2016.

Laird GM, Bullen CK, Rosenbloom DI, et al. Ex vivo analysis identifies effective HIV- 1 latency reversing drug combinations. *J Clin Invest*. 2015;125(5):1901–1902.

Lalezari J, Mitsuyasu R, Wang S, et al. A single infusion of zinc finger nuclease CCR5 modified autologous CD4 T cells (SB-728T) increased CD4 counts and leads to decrease in HIV proviral load in an aviremic HIV-infect subject [Abstract 433]. Paper presented at the 19th Conference on Retroviruses and Opportunistic Infection, Seattle, WA, February 2012.

Lalezari JP, Latiff GH, Brinson C, et al. Safety and efficacy of the HIV-1 attachment inhibitor prodrug BMS-663068 in treatment-experienced individuals: 24 week results of AI438011, a phase 2b randomized controlled trial. *Lancet HIV*. 2015;2(10):e427–e437.

Levy Y, Durier C, Lascaux AS, et al. Sustained control of viremia following therapeutic immunization in chronically HIV-1 infected individuals. *AIDS*. 2006;20:405–413.

Levy Y, Gahery-Segard H, Durier C, et al. Immunologic and virologic efficacy of therapeutic immunization combined with interleukin-2 in chronically HIV-1 infected patients. *AIDS*. 2005;19:279–286.

Levy Y, Lacabaratz C, Weiss L, et al. Enhanced T cell recovery in HIV-1 infected adults through IL-7 treatment. *J Clin Invest*. 2009;119(4)997–1007.

Levy Y, Sereti I, Tambussi G, et al. Effects of recombinant human interleukin 7 on T-cell recovery and thymic output in HIV- infected patients receiving antiretroviral therapy: results of a phase I/ IIa randomized, placebo-controlled multicenter study. *Clin Infect Dis*. 2012;55(2):291–300.

Levy Y, Thiebaut R, Montes M, et al. Dendritic cell-based therapeutic vaccine elicits polyfunctional HIV-specific T-cell immunity associated with control of viral load. *Eur J Immunol*. 2014;44:2802–2810.

Lewden C, Chene G, Morlat P, et al. HIV- infected adults with a CD4 cell count greater than 500 cells/ µl on long-term combination antiretroviral therapy reach same mortality rates as the general population. *J AIDS*. 2007;46(1):72–77.

Li J, Brumme Z, Brumme C, et al. Factors associated with viral rebound in HIV-1 infected individuals enrolled in a therapeutic HIV-1 gag vaccine trial. *J Infect Dis*. 2011;203:976–983.

Lu W, Arraes C, Ferreira WT, et al. Therapeutic dendritic cell vaccination for chronic HIV-1 infection. *Nat Med*. 2004;10:1359–1365.

Margolis DA, Brinson CC, Smith G, et al. Cabotegravir plus rilpivirine, once a day, after induction with cabotegravir plus nucleoside reverse transcriptase inhibitors in antiretroviral-naïve adults with HIV-1 infection (LATTE): a randomised, phase 2b, dose-ranging trial. *Lancet Infect Dis*. 2015;15:1145–1155.

Margolis DA, Gonzalez-Garcia J, Stellbrink H-J, et al. Long-acting intramuscular cabotegravir and rilpivirine in adults with HIV-1 infection (LATTE-2): 96-week results of a randomised, open-label, phase 2b, non-inferiority trial. *Lancet*. 2017;390:1499–1510.

Martin AR, Siciliano RF. Immune modulation with rapamycin as a potential strategy for HIV-1 eradication [Abstract 415]. Paper presented at the 22nd Conference on Retroviruses and Opportunistic Infections, Seattle, WA, February 2015.

Mason SW, Sanisetty S, Osuna Gutierrez C, et al. Viral suppression was induced by anti-PD-L1 following ARV-interruption in SIV-infected monkeys [Abstract 318LB]. Paper presented at the 21st Conference on Retroviruses and Opportunistic Infections, Boston, March 2014.

Matthews RP, Schurmann D, Rudd DJ, et al. Single doses as low as 0.5 mg of the novel NRTTI MK-8591 suppress HIV for at least seven days. Presented at the 9th International AIDS Society Conference on HIV Science, Paris, July 2017.

Mitsuyasu RT, Merigan TC, Carr A, et al. Phase 2 gene therapy trial of anti-HIV ribozyme in autologous CD34[+] cells. *Nat Med.* 2009;15(3):285–292.

Molina J-M, Ward D, Brar I, et al. Switching to fixed-dose bictegravir, emtricitabine, and tenofovir alafenamide from dolutegravir plus abacavir and lamivudine in virologically suppressed adults with HIV-1: 48 week results of a randomised, double-blind, multicentre, active-controlled, Phase 3, non-inferiority trial. *Lancet HIV.* 2018;5(7):e357–e365

Murga JD, Franti M, Pevear DC, et al. Potent antiviral synergy between monoclonal antibody and small molecule CCR5 antagonists of human immunodeficiency virus type 1. *Antimicrob Agents Chemother.* 2006;50(10):3289–3296.

Nettles R, Schurmann D, Zhu L, et al. Pharmacodynamics, safety, and pharmacokinetics of BMS- 663068: an oral HIV attachment inhibitor in HIV-1-infected patients. *J Infect Dis.* 2012;206(7):1002–1011.

Nowicka-Sans B, Protack T, Lin Z, et al. Characterization of a second-generation HIV-1 maturation inhibitor [Poster TUPEAO78]. Presented at the 8th International AIDS Society Conference on HIV Pathogenesis, Treatment and Prevention, Vancouver, British Columbia, July 2015.

Pallikkuth S, Micci L, Ende ZS, et al. Maintenance of intestinal Th17 cells and reduced microbial translocation in SIV-infected rhesus macaques treated with interleukin (IL)-21. *PLoS Pathog.* 2013;9:e1003471.

Pallikkuth, S, Rogers K, Villinger F, et al. Interleukin-21 administration to rhesus macaques chronically infected with simian immunodeficiency viruses increases cytotoxic effector molecules in T cells and NK cells and enhances B cell function without increasing immune activation or viral replication. *Vaccine.* 2011;29:9929–9938.

Palmer CS, Ostrowski M, Zhou J, et al. The mTORC1 inhibitors, temsirolimus and everolimus, suppress HIV-patient-derived CD4[+] T-cell death and activation in vitro [Abstract 320]. Paper presented at the 22nd Conference on Retroviruses and Opportunistic Infections, Seattle, WA, February 2015.

Pett SL, Carey C, Lin E, et al. Predictors of bacterial pneumonia in Evaluation of Subcutaneous Interleukin-2 in Randomized International TRIAL (ESPRIT). *HIV Med.* 2011;12(4):219–227.

Pett SL, Kelleher AD, Emery S. Role of interleukin-2 in patients with HIV infection. *Drugs.* 2010;70(9):1115–1130.

Pollard RB, Rockstroh JK, Pantaleo G, et al. Safety and efficacy of the peptide-based therapeutic vaccine for HIV-1, Vacc-4x: a phase 2 randomised double-blind, placebo-controlled trial. *Lancet Infect Dis.* 2014;14(4):291–300.

Pontesilli I, Guerra ES, Ammassari A, et al. Phase II controlled trial of post-exposure immunization with recombinant gp160 versus anti-retroviral therapy in asymptomatic HIV-1 infected adults. *AIDS.* 1998;12:473–480.

Porichis F, Kaufmann DE. Role of PD-1 in HIV pathogenesis and as a target for therapy. *Curr HIV/AID Rep.* 2012;9(1):81–90.

Rerks-Ngarm S, Pitisuttithum P, Nitayaphan S, et al. Vaccination with ALVAC and AIDSVAX to prevent HIV-1 infection in Thailand. *N Engl J Med.* 2009;361(23):2209–2220.

Rodriguez B, Asmuth DM, Matining RM, et al. Safety, tolerability and immunogenicity of repeated doses of dermavir, a candidate therapeutic HIV vaccine, in HIV-infected patients receiving combination antiretroviral therapy. *J AIDS.* 2013;64(4):351–359.

Rosenberg ES, Billingsley JM, Caliendo AM, et al. Vigorous HIV-1-specific CD4R T cell responses associated with control of viremia. *Science.* 1997;278:1447–1450.

Safarian D, Carnec X, Tsamis F, et al. An anti-CCR5 monoclonal antibody and small molecular CCR5 antagonists synergize by inhibiting different stages of human immunodeficiency virus type 1 entry. *Virology.* 2006;352(2):477–484.

Saito N, Chono H, Shibata H, et al. CD4[+] T cells modified by endoribonuclease MazF are safe and can persist in SHIV-infected rhesus macaques. *Mol Ther Nucleic Acids.* 2014;3(6):e168.

Sandstrom E, Wahren B; Nordic Vac-04 Study Group. Therapeutic immunization with recombinant gp160 in HIV-1 infection: a randomized double blind placebo- controlled trial. *Lancet.* 1999;353:1735–1742.

Sax PE, Saag MS, Yin MT, et al. Renal and bone safety tenofovir alafenamide vs. tenofovir disoproxil fumarate [Abstract 143LB]. Paper presented at the 22nd Conference on Retroviruses and Opportunistic Infection, Seattle, WA, February 2015.

Scheid JF, Horwitz JA, Bar-On Y, et al. HIV-1 antibody 3BNC117 suppresses viral rebound in humans during treatment interruption. *Nature.* 2016;535(7613):556–560.

Schooley RT, Spritzler J; Wang H, et al.; AIDS Clinical Trials Group 5197. A placebo-controlled trial of immunization of HIV-1-infected persons with a replication-deficient adenovirus type 5 vaccine expressing the HIV-1 core protein. *J Infect Dis.* 2010;202(5):705–716.

Sereti I, Dunham RM, Spritzler J, et al. IL-7 administration drives T cell entry and expansion in HIV-1 infection. *Blood.* 2009;113(25):6304–6314.

Shingai M, Nishumura Y, Klein F, et al. Antibody-mediated immunotherapy of macaques chronically infected with SHIV suppresses viraemia. *Nature.* 2013;503:277–281.

Singh A, Palanichamy JK, Ramalingam P, et al. Long-term suppression of HIV-1 C virus production in human peripheral blood mononuclear cells by LTR heterochromatization with a short double-stranded RNA. *J Antimicrob Chemother.* 2014;69:405–415.

Sogaard OS, Graversen ME, Leth S, et al. The depsipeptide romdiepsin reverses HIV-1 latency in vivo. *PLoS Pathog.* 2015;11(9):e1005142.

Stellbrink HJ, van Lundzen J, Westby M, et al. Effects of interleukin-2 plus highly active antiretroviral therapy on HIV-1 replication and proviral DNA (COSMIC trial). *AIDS.* 2002;16:1479–1487.

Tavel JA; INSIGHT STALWART Study Group. Effect of intermittent IL-2 alone or with peri-cycle antiretroviral therapy in early HIV-1 infection: the STALWART study. *PloS One.* 2010;5(2):e9334.

Tebas P, Stein D, Binder-Scholl G, et al. Antiviral effects of autologous CD4 T cells genetically modified with a conditionally replicating lentiviral vector expressing long antisense to HIV. *Blood.* 2013;121(9):1524–1533.

Tebas P, Stein D, Tang WW, et al. Gene editing of CCR5 in autologous CD4 T cells of persons infected with HIV. *N Engl J Med.* 2014;370(10):901–910.

ter Brake O, 't Hooft K, Liu YP, et al. Lentiviral vector design for multiple shRNA expression and durable HIV-1 inhibition. *Mol Ther.* 2008;16:557–564.

Tsoukas CM, Raboud J, Bernard NF, et al. Active immunization of patients with HIV infection: a study of VaxSyn, a recombinant HIV envelope subunit vaccine, on progression of immunodeficiency. *AIDS Res Hum Retroviruses.* 1998;14:483–490.

Van Gulck E, Vlieghe E, Vekemans M, et al. mRNA-based dendritic cell vaccination induced potent antiviral responses in HIV-1 infected patients. *AIDS.* 2012;26:F1–F12.

Van Lundzen J, Glausinger T, Stahmer I, et al. Transfer of autologous gene-modified T cells in HIV-infected patients with advanced immunodeficiency and drug-resistant virus. *Mol Ther.* 2007;15:1024–1033.

Vardas E, Stanescu I, Leinonen M, et al. Indicators of a therapeutic effect in FIT-06, a phase II trial of a DNA vaccine, GTU-Multi-HIVB, in untreated HIV-1 infected subjects. *Vaccine.* 2012;30(27):4046–4054.

Wei DG, Chaiang V, Fyne E, et al. Histone deacetylase inhibitor romidepsin induces HIV expression in CD4 T cells from patients on suppressive antiretroviral therapy at concentrations induced by clinical dosing. *PLoS Pathog.* 2014;10(4):e1004071.

White, et al. GS-9131 is a novel NRTI with activity against NRTI-resistant HIV-1 [Abstract 436]. Presented at the 24th Conference on Retroviruses and Opportunistic Infection, Seattle, WA, February 13–16, 2017.

Wohl D, Pozniack DA, Thompson M, et al. Tenofovir alafenamide (TAF) in a single tablet regimen in initial HIV-therapy [Abstract 113LB]. Paper presented at the 22nd Conference on Retroviruses and Opportunistic Infection, Seattle, WA, February 2015.

Wolstein O, Boyd M, Millington M, et al. Preclinical safety and efficacy of an anti-HIV-1 lentiviral vector containing a short hairpin RNA to CCR5 and the C46 fusion inhibitor. *Mol Ther Methods Clin Dev.* 2014;1:11.

Zeller S, Kumar P. RNA-based gene therapy for the treatment and prevention of HIV: from bench to bedside. *Yale J Biol Med.* 2011;84(3):301–309.

Zheng, et al. GS-CA2: a novel, potent and selective first-in-class inhibitor of HIV-1 capsid function displays nonclinical pharmacokinetics supporting long-acting potential in humans [Abstract 539]. Presented at ID Week 2018, San Francisco, October 3–7, 2018

Zhou J, Rossi JJ. Current progress in the development of RNAi based therapeutics for HIV-1. *Gene Ther.* 2011;18:1134–1138.

26.

SOLID ORGAN TRANSPLANTATION IN PERSONS LIVING WITH HIV

Eurides Lopes and Jennifer Husson

INTRODUCTION

The arrival of combination antiretroviral therapy (ART) in 1996 resulted in increased life expectancy for HIV-positive patients. Consequently, end-organ failure and associated disease has become a major cause of morbidity and mortality in this population. Up to 30% of HIV-positive individuals have end-stage renal disease (ESRD) as a direct consequence of HIV infection (HIV-associated nephropathy [HIVAN]), drug toxicities, or other comorbidities (Ahuja, 2002), accounting for 12.2% of HIV-related deaths (Locke, 2014). Because HIV-positive individuals with ESRD have a 5-year survival of only 65% compared to 94% for HIV-uninfected individuals with ESRD, and given the fact that coinfection with hepatitis C virus (HCV) is prevalent in this population and contributes an additional risk factor for chronic kidney disease (CKD) and progressive liver disease, there is a growing need for renal and liver transplantation in these patients (Rodriguez, 2003; Lucas, 2013; Peters, 2012).

LEARNING OBJECTIVE

Discuss the evaluation and management of the HIV-positive transplant candidate and current clinical outcomes for HIV-positive solid organ transplant recipients.

WHAT'S NEW?

- Studies have found that patient and graft survival rates in HIV-positive transplant recipients can be as good as those in noninfected recipients.

- The HIV Organ Policy Equity (HOPE) Act, which was signed into law in the United States in November 2013, allows the use of HIV-positive donor organs for transplantation into HIV-positive recipients under research protocols.

KEY POINTS

- End-organ disease has become a major cause of morbidity and mortality in HIV-positive patients due to increased life expectancy, thus increasing the demand for organ transplantation in these patients.

- The care of HIV-positive transplant recipients warrants a multidisciplinary team approach, including the specific organ transplant team, pharmacists, infectious disease specialists, nurses, and patients and their families.

- The immunosuppression of HIV-positive recipients post-transplant does not appear to further advance HIV disease.

- The post-transplant risk of opportunistic infections (OIs) for HIV-positive recipients does not appear to be increased by immunosuppression. However, the overall rate of infections is high, especially in HCV coinfected transplant recipients.

- HIV/HCV coinfected recipients generally have worse outcomes than both liver and kidney HIV-positive recipients, although this may be changing with increased use of curative treatment for HCV prior to or following transplant.

PRETRANSPLANT EVALUATION

CRITERIA FOR TRANSPLANTATION

- Any OIs or malignancies should be completely treated prior to transplant. Patients with histories of OIs or malignancies with suboptimal or noncurative therapies (e.g., progressive multifocal leukoencephalopathy [PML], visceral Kaposi's sarcoma, chronic cryptosporidiosis, or primary central nervous system lymphoma) are generally not good candidates for transplantation (Stock, 2010).

- Recipients must meet standard criteria for transplantation.

- Recipients must be on a stable antiretroviral therapy (ART) regimen.

Renal Transplant

- CD4$^+$ T cell count should be 200 cells/μL or higher prior to transplantation.

- HIV RNA should be below the limit of detection for *at least* 6 months prior to transplantation (Harbell, 2013; Stock, 2010).

Liver Transplant

- CD4$^+$ T cell count must be 100 cells/μL or higher, or they must be 200 cell/μL or higher for recipients who have a history of previous OIs or malignancy. The CD4$^+$ T cell count threshold is lower for liver transplant recipients due to presumed splenic sequestration secondary to portal hypertension.

- Ideally, HIV RNA should be suppressed to below the level of detection at the time of transplant.

- For recipients who are not able to tolerate ART or who have recently started ART, an infectious diseases (ID) physician must be able to predict full HIV suppression on a tolerable and effective ART regimen (Harbell, 2013). This situation is increasingly less common due to new antiretroviral (ARV) agents such as INSTIs.

PRETRANSPLANT INFECTION SCREENING AND VACCINATIONS

Tuberculin Skin Test or Quantiferon Gold

- All candidates must be screened for latent tuberculosis (TB) prior to transplantation. Patients should be treated if they have a positive Quantiferon TB test, a tuberculin skin test of greater than 5 mm, or recent contact with a person with active TB. The preferred regimen is isoniazid (INH) $^+$ vitamin B$_6$ for 9 months, completing at least 6 of the 9 months prior to transplantation. For liver transplantation, when prophylactic treatment cannot be completed prior to or the risk of toxicity is too high, treatment should be completed as soon as possible after transplant.

Syphilis

- Test for and treat syphilis prior to transplant.

Serologies

- Test for cytomegalovirus (CMV), Epstein–Barr virus, herpes simplex virus, varicella zoster virus, and viral hepatitis serologies in all candidates. In addition, coccidioides and strongyloides serologies should be tested if the recipient has prolonged exposure to endemic areas.

Vaccinations

- All candidates should be vaccinated against hepatitis A and B if not already immune.

- Inactivated influenza vaccine should be given yearly. The high-dose vaccine has been shown to have better immunogenicity and to be safe in solid organ transplant recipients (Mombelli, 2018).

- Pneumococcal/Prevnar vaccine should be given if not given in the past 5 years.

- TDaP vaccine should be given if not given in the past 10 years.

- The HPV vaccine should be given for ages 15–26 years.

- The meningococcal vaccine should be given in appropriate context.

- Varicella vaccine should be given to those who are VZV seronegative prior to transplant.

- The shingles, varicella, and mumps/measles/rubella (MMR) vaccines are contraindicated if CD4$^+$ T cell count is less than 300 cells/μL (Miro, 2014). Trials of a recombinant, adjuvant herpes zoster vaccine approved in 2017 have shown safety and immunogenicity in immunocompromised populations (Berkowitz, 2015; Stadtmauer, 2014).

- Live, attenuated vaccines are contraindicated after transplant.

WHEN TO REFER

Renal Transplant

- All HIV-positive patients on hemodialysis or with a glomerular filtration rate 25 mL/min or less should be referred to a renal transplant center as long they meet the HIV inclusion criteria.

Liver Transplant

- All HIV-positive patients with decompensated cirrhosis, symptomatic disease, or hepatocellular carcinoma who meet the inclusion criteria should be referred for liver transplant evaluation. Patients with an albumin of less than 3 g/dL, a prolonged prothrombin time, or a modified Child–Turcotte–Pugh score of 7 or higher should also be considered.

POSTTRANSPLANT MANAGEMENT AND CARE

All pre-, peri-, and posttransplant care should be coordinated among a multidisciplinary team consisting of the transplant surgeon, an ID or HIV specialist, a nephrologist or hepatologist, a primary care provider, a transplant coordinator, a transplant pharmacist, a social worker, and nursing staff.

IMMUNOSUPPRESSION THERAPY

Induction

The multicenter HIVTR study suggested that the use of anti-thymocyte globulin (ATG) was associated with a higher risk of graft loss with renal transplantation (Stock, 2010). However, subsequent studies found a 2.6-fold lower risk of acute rejection with ATG induction, with graft survival rates equivalent to those of a non–HIV-positive cohort (Locke, 2014). A subsequent study of 830 HIV-positive renal transplant recipients found a 40% lower rate of rejection among those who received ATG for induction compared to either no induction or anti–IL-2R induction (Kucirka, 2016). The choice of induction therapy should be patient-specific, accounting for the individual's risk of rejection, although recent evidence suggests ATG is generally safe in people living with HIV (PLWH) undergoing renal transplantation.

Maintenance

Maintenance immunosuppression generally consists of triple therapy including calcineurin inhibitors (CNIs) (e.g., cyclosporine and tacrolimus) with an antimetabolite (e.g., mycophenolate mofetil) and corticosteroids. An mTOR inhibitor (e.g., sirolimus and everolimus) may be substituted if a patient is not able to tolerate CNIs or antimetabolites. The HIVTR study found an increased risk of rejection with the use of cyclosporine compared to tacrolimus (Stock, 2010), and sirolimus was found to be associated with a higher rate of rejection (Locke, 2014). However, given the uncertainty with drug interactions and small numbers of patients, the optimal regimen remains unclear.

ANTIRETROVIRAL THERAPY

ART should be reinitiated posttransplant as soon as oral medications can be tolerated (Roland, 2006). The regimen varies based on the individual patient's viral resistance pattern and prior ARV exposure. There are also drug–drug interactions between CNIs, mTOR inhibitors, protease inhibitors (PIs), and non-nucleoside reverse transcriptase inhibitors (NNRTIs) due to their inducing or inhibiting effects on cytochrome P450 (CYP) 3A4 drug metabolism and P-glycoprotein (Frasetto, 2007; Trullas, 2011). This is significant because changes in antiretroviral medications (as well as other medications) can lead to altered metabolism of the immunosuppressants, thus leading to organ rejection or drug toxicity (van Maarseveen, 2012). However, there are no absolute contraindications because dosing modifications based on therapeutic drug monitoring of the

immunosuppressants can compensate for the altered metabolism of these drugs.

Nucleoside Reverse Transcriptase Inhibitors

When possible, nucleoside reverse transcriptase inhibitors (NRTIs) with significant mitochondrial toxicity should *not* be used with mycophenolate. Zidovudine and stavudine may have some antagonism when used with mycophenolate, and zidovudine may exacerbate bone marrow suppression. Abacavir, on the other hand, may have synergistic activity against HIV when used with mycophenolate (Chapuis, 2000; Margolis, 1999). Tenofovir should be avoided when possible due to the associated increase in creatinine, though its newer formulation (tenofovir alafenamide) may be a safe alternative.

Non-Nucleoside Reverse Transcriptase Inhibitors

NNRTIs are strong CYP3A4 inducers, thus increasing the metabolism of CNIs and decreasing their serum levels. The dose of these immunosuppressive agents frequently needs to be increased with close monitoring of drug levels.

Protease Inhibitors

Boosted PIs are both strong CYP3A4 inhibitors (and sometimes also weak inducers) that decrease the metabolism of CNIs and mTOR inhibitors resulting in higher levels of these agents. Thus, it is imperative that if boosted PIs must be used in the ART regimen, the dosages of both CNIs and mTOR inhibitors commonly must be decreased and the dosing interval increased with close monitoring of drug levels. The use of boosted PIs in post-kidney transplant has been linked to an increased risk of graft loss and death in one recent study, while in another study it was found to actually be associated with reduced graft failure rates (Sawinski, 2017; Sparkes, 2018). This suggests that PIs should be used sparingly and with careful monitoring.

Boosted PIs also decrease the clearance of glucocorticoids, which may cause a Cushing-like syndrome. In addition, they may exacerbate hyperlipidemia posttransplant and potentiate CNI-induced impaired glucose tolerance.

Integrase Inhibitors

Integrase inhibitors (INSTIs) have no or only minimal effects on CYP3A metabolism; thus, there are few potential drug interactions with immunosuppressants, making this class of ARVs well-suited for use in PLWH during solid organ transplantation.

CCR5 Antagonists

Sirolimus reduces the expression of CCR5 receptors and may enhance the antiviral activity of CCR5 antagonists such as maraviroc (Gilliam, 2007; Heredia, 2008).

POSTTRANSPLANT INFECTION PROPHYLAXIS

In addition to standard posttransplant CMV prophylaxis, HIV solid-organ transplant (SOT) recipients should receive the following prophylaxis:

- *Pneumocystis jiroveci*
  - Prophylaxis with trimethoprim/sulfamethoxazole (TMP/SMX) or dapsone (if sulfa allergic or bone marrow suppression is an issue) as long as glucose-6-phosphate dehydrogenase (G-6PD) levels are normal Atovaquone can also be used as a secondary alternative to TMP/SMX.
  - The duration of prophylaxis is generally recommended life-long (Blumberg, 2013), though it may be reasonable to end prophylaxis when patients are on stable immunosuppression and maintain CD4$^+$ T cell counts higher than 200 cells/μL for more than 3 months (Masur, 2014).
- *Mycobacterium avium* complex (MAC)
  - 1,200 mg of azithromycin dosed weekly with food should be used if CD4$^+$ T cell count is less than 75 cells/μL.
- Toxoplasmosis
  - TMP/SMX should be used if CD4$^+$ T cell count is less than 200 cells/μL and if either the recipient or the donor carries IgG antibodies against *Toxoplasma gondii*. Atovaquone can be used if a patient cannot tolerate TMP/SMX or dapsone.
- Prior OIs
  - Continue secondary prophylaxis for OIs such as cryptococcus or coccidioidomycosis until CD4$^+$ T cell counts are above the threshold (i.e., CD4$^+$ >200 cells/μL) for approximately 3–6 months, although many may prefer life-long secondary prophylaxis (Harbell, 2013).

OUTCOMES

PATIENT AND GRAFT SURVIVAL AND REJECTION

Renal Transplant

The overall patient and graft survival rates of HIV-positive renal transplant recipients in the HIVTR study were between the rates observed in HIV-uninfected, older recipients and all recipients, with rates of 94.6% ± 2% and 90.4% at 1 year and 88.2% ± 3.8% and 73.7% at 3 years, respectively. Living donor grafts were also found to be protective, and the use of ATG, HCV coinfection, and older age were associated with decreased survival (Stock, 2010). Subsequently, the use of ATG induction was found to be associated with patient and graft survival rates equivalent to those of an HIV-uninfected cohort (Locke, 2014).

In the HIVTR study, the rate of acute rejection was found to be two- to threefold higher, and acute rejection was more aggressive, with a rate of 31% at 1 year and 41% at 3 years in HIV-positive recipients compared to the national rates (Stock, 2010). Further studies have also found higher rates of rejection, with a rate of 55% at 12 months and notably 28% at 1 month (Malat, 2012). ATG induction was associated with a 2.6-fold decrease in the rate of acute rejection compared to that of patients who did not receive any induction (Locke, 2014) and a 40% lower rate of rejection compared to those who received either no induction or anti–IL-2R induction (Kucirka, 2016).

Liver Transplant

Studies have shown that dual-organ (liver and kidney) transplantation, a lower pretransplant body mass index, older age, and HCV coinfection were associated with decreased patient survival, although there was a survival benefit for liver recipients with a pretransplant Model for End-Stage Liver Disease (MELD) score of 15 or higher (Stock, 2010). Recent data suggest that outcomes for mono-infected, HIV-positive recipients have improved, with outcomes superior to those for HCV mono-infected or HIV/HCV coinfected recipients (Sawinski, 2015). However, there remains a 1.68-fold increased risk for death and 1.70-fold increased risk for graft loss compared to those risks for HIV noninfected recipients independent of HCV status (Locke, 2016). In addition, the 3-year rejection rate was 1.6-fold higher in HIV/HCV coinfected liver recipients compared to HCV mono-infected recipients (Terrault, 2012).

HIV/HCV COINFECTION

Renal Transplant

HIV/HCV coinfected renal transplant recipients have the lowest 3-year patient survival and graft survival rates (73% and 60%, respectively) compared to non–coinfected recipients (90% and 86%, respectively), HIV mono-infected recipients (89% and 81%, respectively), and HCV mono-infected recipients (84% and 78%, respectively) (Sawinski, 2015). Coinfected recipients are also at a higher risk of acute rejection at 1 year, and the use of induction in this population confers a survival benefit (Vivanco, 2013). These findings are consistent with those of other studies, suggesting that HCV coinfection has a negative impact on renal transplantation outcomes and emphasizing the need to cure HCV infection with direct acting anti-HCV agents (DAAs) either pre- or posttransplant (Sawinski, 2015).

Liver Transplant

In general, HIV/HCV coinfected recipients tend to have poorer outcomes. Initial studies of liver transplantation in HIV-positive recipients showed that the 3-year patient and graft survival rates for the HIV/HCV coinfected patients were lower (53% and 74%, respectively) than those for HCV mono-infected recipients (60% and 79%, respectively) (Terrault, 2012). One explanation is that many of these patients will have recurrent HCV infection that can be very aggressive, leading to graft loss and death. Previously reported 5-year survival of approximately 50–55% may increase to 80% in coinfected liver recipients in whom the HCV viral infection has been cleared (Miro, 2015). With the increasing use of DAAs, the negative patient and graft survival effects of coinfection with HCV are predicted to decline.

HIV/HEPATITIS B VIRUS COINFECTION

Renal Transplant

Kidney recipients with hepatitis B virus (HBV) infection have overall lower survival rates compared to noninfected recipients. The 10-year patient survival rate was 51.4% in HBV-infected recipients compared to 82.8% in noninfected recipients, and graft survival rates were 44% for HBV-infected recipients compared to 74.2% for noninfected recipients (Lee, 2001).

Liver Transplant

The overall outcomes for HIV/HBV coinfected recipients appear to be equivalent to those of HBV mono-infected recipients. A small study found that no patients developed clinical evidence of HBV recurrence despite low-grade viremia in 54% of coinfected recipients when treated with HBV immunoglobulin (HBIg) with or without anti-HBV antiviral therapy (Coffin, 2010). The recommended management for HBV-infected liver recipients includes two NRTIs with anti-HBV activity (lamivudine, tenofovir, and entecavir) and HBIg, with HBV DNA monitoring every 6 months (Harbell, 2013); this should be incorporated into or added to HIV/HBV coinfected recipients' ARV therapy.

PROGRESSION OF HIV DISEASE

The HIVTR study reported five cases of new opportunistic infections, including two cases of cutaneous Kaposi's sarcoma, one case of cryptosporidiosis, one presumed case of *P. jiroveci*, and one case of candidal esophagitis. Despite an initial decline in CD4+ T cell count posttransplant, which was more pronounced with ATG induction, there was no increase in complications associated with HIV disease or progression of HIV (Stock, 2010).

RISK OF INFECTION, IMMUNE RECOVERY, AND MALIGNANCY

Overall, 38% of kidney recipients had infections posttransplant in the HIVTR study, which is higher than historical rates previously seen in non-HIV recipients. The infections consisted of predominantly genitourinary infections (26%), respiratory tract infections (20%), and bacteremias (19%). This study also found that HCV coinfected recipients had an even higher rate of serious infections compared to HCV-uninfected recipients (Stock, 2010).

Patients with pre-transplant CD4+ T cell counts of less than 350 cells/μL had a lower CD4+ T cell nadir 4-weeks posttransplant and were associated with prolonged CD4+ T cell lymphopenia, which was associated with an increased risk for serious infections (Suarez, 2016). Induction with ATG is associated with a more significant CD4+ T cell nadir posttransplant; however, more recent studies suggest that there is no significant increase in infectious risk (Kucirka, 2016).

Based on available data, the incidence of new or recurrent after SOT in HIV-positive patients is low and not significantly different from that of HIV-uninfected patients. In the HIVTR study, 9% of patients (11.2% of liver recipients and 8.7% of kidney recipients) developed posttransplant malignancies (including skin cancer, cutaneous Kaposi's sarcoma, penile squamous cell cancer, head and neck cancer, renal cell cancer, lymphoma, recurrence of pretransplant hepatocellular carcinoma, and cholangiocarcinoma), and 3% of patients died from a cancer-related cause (Stock, 2010). The same study showed an increased risk of developing high-grade squamous intraepithelial lesions after transplantation in 89 patients followed for anal cytology, which requires further study (Nissen, 2012).

FUTURE DIRECTIONS

With the increasing numbers of HIV-positive patients with ESRD and end-stage liver disease and the increased mortality associated with these conditions, the demand for organ transplantation is increasing. However, the organ pool does not currently meet demand. The use of HIV-positive donor organs may help to narrow this gap. Until recently, HIV-positive individuals were not allowed to be included in the transplant donor pool. There are still many concerns regarding the use of HIV-positive donor organs—namely the risk of superinfection with a new, possibly resistant HIV strain; the risk of transmitting donor-derived opportunistic infections; and the increased risk of acute rejection. Despite these concerns, in 2013, the HOPE Act, which allows the use of HIV-positive donor organs for transplantation into HIV-positive recipients, was signed into law in the United States. In addition, preliminary data from South Africa show patient survival rates among HIV-positive recipients of HIV-positive donor kidneys to be 84% at 1 year, 84% at 3 years, and 74% at 5 years, with graft survival rates of 93% at 1 year and 84% at both 3 and 5 years and rejection rates of 8% at 1 year and 22% at 3 years (Muller, 2015). The availability of these organs has increased and HIV-positive to HIV-positive transplantation research is ongoing to evaluate the safety and efficacy of these transplants.

CONCLUSION

HIV-positive patients have good survival benefit from transplantation, especially renal transplantation and some selected liver transplantation. Posttransplant immunosuppression does not appear to advance HIV disease or have an increased risk of opportunistic infection. HIV/HCV coinfected recipients continue to appear to have worse outcomes, partially due to a more aggressive posttransplant HCV recurrence, which emphasizes the importance of HCV cure with DAAs prior to or immediately posttransplant now that newer, less toxic therapies are available. The management of drug–drug interactions remains a crucial part of this process that cannot be ignored. This is a task that should include a large, integrated group of providers, including the transplant team, pharmacists, infectious disease specialists, and nurses, in addition to the patients.

REFERENCES

Ahuja TS, Grady J, Khan S. Changing trends in the survival of dialysis patients with human immunodeficiency virus in the United States. *J Am Soc Nephrol.* 2002;13(7):1889–1893.

Berkowitz EM, Moyle G, Stellbrink H-J, et al. Safety and immunogenicity of an adjuvanted herpes zoster subunit candidate vaccine in HIV-positive adults: a phase 1/2a randomized, placebo-controlled study. *J Infect Dis.* 2015;211(8):1279–1287.

Blumberg EA, Rogers CC. Human immunodeficiency virus in solid organ transplantation. *Am J Transplant.* 2013;13(s4):169–178.

Chapuis AG, Paolo Rizzardi G, D'Agostino C, et al. Effects of mycophenolic acid on human immunodeficiency virus infection in vitro and in vivo. *Nat Med.* 2000;6:762–768.

Coffin CS, Stock PG, Dove LM, et al. Virologic and clinical outcomes of hepatitis B virus infection in HIV–HBV co-infected transplant recipients. *Am J Transp.* 2010;10:1268–1275.

Frasetto LA, Browne M, Cheng A, et al. Immunosuppressant pharmacokinetics and dosing modifications in HIV-1 infected liver and kidney transplant recipients. *Am J Transplant.* December 2007;7(12):2816–2820. https://www.ncbi.nlm.nih.gov/pubmed/17949460

Gilliam B, Heredia A, Devico A, et al. Rapamycin reduces CCR5 mRNA levels in macaques: potential applications in HIV-1 prevention and treatment. *AIDS.* 2007;21(15):2108–2110.

Harbell J, Terrault NA, Stock P. Solid organ transplants in HIV-positive patients. *Curr HIV/AIDS Rep.* 2013;10:217–225.

Heredia A, Latinovic O, Gallo RC, et al. Reduction of CCR5 with low-dose rapamycin enhances the antiviral activity of vicriviroc against both sensitive and drug-resistant HIV-1. *Proc Natl Acad Sci USA.* 2008;105(51):20476–20481.

Kucirka LM, Durand CM, Bae S, et al. Induction immunosuppression and clinical outcomes in kidney transplant recipients infected with human immunodeficiency virus. *Am J Transplant.* 2016;16(8):2368–2376.

Lee WC, Shu KH, Cheng CH, et al. Long-term impact of hepatitis B, C virus infection on renal transplantation. *Am J Nephrol.* 2001;21:300–306.

Locke JE, Durand C, Reed RD, et al. Long-term outcomes after liver transplantation among human immunodeficiency virus-infected recipients. *Transplantation.* 2016;100(1):141–146.

Locke JE, James NT, Mannon RB, et al. Immunosuppression regimen and the risk of acute rejection in HIV-positive kidney transplant recipients. *Transplantation.* 2014;97(4):446–450.

Lucas GM, Jing Y, Sulkowski M, et al. Hepatitis C viremia and the risk of chronic kidney disease in HIV-positive individuals. *J Infect Dis.* 2013;208(8):1240–1249.

Malat GE, Ranganna KM, Sikalas N, et al. High frequency of rejections in HIV-positive recipients of kidney transplantation: a single center prospective trial. *Transplantation.* 2012;94:1020–1024.

Margolis D, Heredia A, Gaywee J, et al. Abacavir and mycophenolic acid, an inhibitor of inosine monophosphate dehydrogenase, have profound and synergistic anti-HIV activity. *J AIDS.* 1999;21:362–370.

Masur H, Brooks JT, Benson CA, et al. Prevention and treatment of opportunistic infections in HIV-positive adults and adolescents: updated guidelines from the Centers for Disease Control and Prevention, National Institutes of Health, and HIV Medicine Association of the Infectious Diseases Society of America. *Clin Infect Dis.* 2014;58(9):1308–1311.

Miro JM, Agüero F, Duclos-Vallée JC, et al. Infections in solid organ transplant HIV-positive patients. *Clin Microbiol Infect.* 2014;20:119–130.

Miro JM, Stock P, Teicher E, et al. Outcome and management of HCV/HIV coinfection pre- and post-liver transplantation: a 2015 update. *J Hepatol.* 2015;62:701–711.

Mombelli M, Rettby N, Perreau M, et al. Immunogenicity and safety of double versus standard dose of the seasonal influenza vaccine in solid-organ transplant recipients: a randomized controlled trial. *Vaccine.* 2018;36(41):6163–6169.

Muller E, Barday Z, Kahn D. HIV-positive-to-HIV-positive kidney transplantation: results at 3 and 5 years. *N Engl J Med.* 2015;372:613–620.

Nissen NN, Barin B, Stock PG. Malignancy in the HIV-positive patients undergoing liver and kidney transplantation. *Curr Opin Oncol.* 2012;24:517–521.

Peters L, Grint D, Lundgren JD, et al. Hepatitis C virus viremia increases the incidence of chronic kidney disease in HIV-positive patients. *AIDS Lond Engl.* 2012;26(15):1917–1926.

Richterman A, Blumberg E. The challenges and promise of HIV-positive donors for solid organ transplantation. *Curr Infect Dis Rep.* 2015;17:17.

Rodriguez RA, Mendelson M, O'Hare AM, et al. Determinants of survival among HIV-positive chronic dialysis patients. *J Am Soc Nephrol.* 2003;14(5):1307–1313.

Roland ME, Barin B, Huprikar S, et al; HIVTR Study Team. Survival in HIV-positive transplant recipients compared with transplant candidates and with HIV-negative controls. *AIDS.* 2016;30(3):435–444.

Roland ME, Stock PG. Liver transplantation in HIV-positive recipients. *Semin Liver Dis.* 2006;26(3):273–284.

Sawinski D, Forde KA, Eddinger K, et al. Superior outcomes in HIV-positive kidney transplant patients compared with HCV-infected or HIV/HCV co-infected recipients. *Kidney Int.* 2015;88:341–349.

Sawinski D, Goldberg DS, Blumberg E, et al. Beyond the NIH multicenter HIV transplant trial experience: outcomes of HIV+ liver transplant recipients compared to HCV+ or HIV+/HCV+ co-infected recipients in the United States. *Clin Infect Dis.* 2015;61(7):1054–1062.

Sawinski D, Shelton BA, Mehta S, et al. Impact of protease inhibitor-based anti-retroviral therapy on outcomes for HIV+ kidney transplant recipients. *Am J Transplant.* 2017;17(12):3114–3122.

Sparkes T, Manitpisitkul W, Masters B, et al. Impact of antiretroviral regimen on renal transplant outcomes in HIV-positive recipients. *Transpl Infect Dis.* 2018;e12992.

Stadtmauer EA, Sullivan KM, Marty FM, et al. A phase 1/2 study of an adjuvanted varicella-zoster virus subunit vaccine in autologous hematopoietic cell transplant recipients. *Blood.* 2014;124(19):2921–2929.

Stock P, Barin B, Murphy B, et al. Outcomes of kidney transplantation in HIV-positive recipients. *N Engl J Med.* 2010;363:2001–2014.

Suarez JF, Rosa R, Lorio MA, et al. Pretranspalnt CD4 count influences immune reconstitution and risk of infectious complications in Human Immunodeficiency Virus-infected kidney allograft recipients. *Am J Transpl.* 2016;16(8):2463–2472.

Terrault N, Roland ME, Schiano T, et al. Outcomes of liver transplant recipients with hepatitis C and human immunodeficiency virus coinfection. *Liver Transpl.* 2012;18(6):716–726.

Trullas JC, Cofan F, Tuset M, et al. Renal transplantation in HIV-positive patients: 2010 update. *Kidney Int.* April 2011;79(8):825–842. https://www.ncbi.nlm.nih.gov/pubmed/21248716

van Maarseveen EM, Rogers CC, Trofe-Clark J, et al. Drug–drug interactions between antiretroviral and immunosuppressive agents in HIV-positive patients after solid organ transplantation: a review. *AIDS Patient Care STDs.* 2012;26(10):568–581.

Vivanco M, Friedmann P, Zia Y, et al. Campath induction in HCV and HCV/HIV-seropositive kidney transplant recipients. *Transpl Int.* 2013;26(10):1016–1026.

27.

ANTIRETROVIRAL THERAPY IN PREGNANT WOMEN

William R. Short and Jason J. Schafer

CHAPTER GOAL

Upon completion of this chapter, the reader should be able to describe the appropriate management of antiretrovirals for pregnant women living with HIV.

INTRODUCTION

Over time, research has demonstrated that proper prevention strategies and interventions during pregnancy, labor, and delivery can significantly reduce the rate of mother-to-child transmission (MTCT) of HIV. In 1994, a pivotal study in the field of HIV medicine, the Pediatric AIDS Clinical Trials Group 076, demonstrated that the use of zidovudine (ZDV) monotherapy during pregnancy substantially reduced the risk of HIV transmission to infants by 67% (Connor, 1994). The protocol is summarized in Table 27.1. It consisted of oral administration of ZDV initiated between 14 and 34 weeks of gestation and continued throughout pregnancy, followed by intrapartum administration of intravenous ZDV and oral administration of ZDV to the newborn for 6 weeks after delivery. Additional studies have demonstrated the effectiveness of the use of combination antiretroviral therapy (ART), further decreasing the risk of HIV transmission to 1–2% (Cooper, 2002). Based on recent data, there have been modifications to the original protocol, including a more selective use of intravenous ZDV based on maternal viral load and changes to postpartum administration of ART to the newborn.

LEARNING OBJECTIVE

Review the clinical management of HIV-positive pregnant women including recommendations for use of antiretrovirals (ARVs) and drug disposition.

WHAT'S NEW?

- Initial results from an ongoing study in Botswana noted an increased risk of neural tube defects in infants whose mother became pregnant while receiving a dolutegravir-based regimen as compared to an efavirenz-based regimen (0.94% vs. 0.05%), prompting the US Department of Health and Human Services (USDHHS) to issue a statement with new recommendations for dolutegravir use in women of childbearing age.

- When a pregnant woman presents on an elvitegravir/cobicistat regimen, providers should consider switching to a more effective regimen. If an elvitegravir/cobicistat regimen is continued, the viral load should be monitored more frequently, and therapeutic drug monitoring may be helpful.

- There are inadequate data to determine whether administration of ZDV intravenously to women with a HIV viral load between 50 and 999 copies/mL provides any additional protection against perinatal transmission, but some experts would administer intravenous ZDV to women with RNA levels in this range, as the transmission risk is slightly higher when HIV RNA is in the range of 50–999 copies/mL compared to less than 50 copies/mL.

KEY POINTS

- ARVs should be initiated in all HIV-positive pregnant women regardless of CD4 count or HIV-1 RNA level. ARVs should be given in combination therapy, similar to nonpregnant patients, with the goal of complete virologic suppression.

- Treatment changes during pregnancy have been associated with the loss of virologic control and independently associated with MTCT.

- All cases of prenatal antiretroviral exposure should be reported to the antiretroviral pregnancy registry (www.apregistry.com).

PHYSIOLOGIC CHANGES DURING PREGNANCY

There are physiologic changes that occur during pregnancy which may alter drug disposition and lead to decreased drug exposure. These changes may be associated with incomplete virologic suppression, virologic failure, and/or the development of drug resistance (Mirochnick, 2004). An understanding of the pharmacokinetic changes that can occur with ARVs during pregnancy is essential for making proper dose modifications to maintain efficacy and minimize toxicity. Summarized in Table 27.2 are some of the physiologic

Table 27.1 THREE-PART ZIDOVUDINE (ZDV) CHEMOPROPHYLAXIS REGIMEN BASED ON PEDIATRIC AIDS CLINICAL TRIALS GROUP (PACTG) 076

TIME OF ZDV ADMINISTRATION	REGIMEN
Antepartum	Oral administration of 100 mg ZDV 5 times daily,[a] initiated at 14–34 weeks gestation and continued throughout pregnancy.
Intrapartum	During labor, intravenous administration of ZDV in a 1-hour initial dose of 2 mg/kg body weight, followed by a continuous infusion of 1 mg/kg body weight/hour until delivery.
Postpartum	Oral administration of ZDV to the newborn (ZDV syrup at 2 mg/kg body weight/dose every 6 hours) for the first 6 weeks of life, beginning at 8–12 hours after birth[b]

[a]Oral ZDV administered as 200 mg three times daily or 300 mg twice daily is currently used in general clinical practice and is an acceptable alternative regimen to 100 mg five times daily.
[b]Intravenous dosage for full-term infants who cannot tolerate oral intake is 1.5 mg/kg body weight intravenously every 6 hours. ZDV dosing for infants of less than 35 weeks' gestation at birth is 1.5 mg/kg/dose intravenously, or 2.0 mg/kg/dose orally, every 12 hours, advancing to every 8 hours at 2 weeks of age if greater than 30 weeks' gestation at birth or at 4 weeks of age if less than 30 weeks gestation at birth.

changes that occur during pregnancy which could affect drug disposition.

TRANSPLACENTAL TRANSFER OF ANTIRETROVIRAL DRUGS

The placenta functions to transfer nutrients and oxygen to the fetus and assist in the removal of waste products (Syme, 2004). In general, nucleoside reverse transcriptase inhibitors (NRTIs), non-nucleoside reverse transcriptase inhibitors (NNRTIs), and integrase inhibitors (INSTIs) readily cross

Table 27.2 EFFECT OF PREGNANCY ON DRUG DISPOSITION

COMPONENTS OF DRUG DISPOSITION

Absorption
Decrease intestinal motility resulting in increased gastric emptying
Reduced gastric acid secretion with gastric pH increase affecting absorption of weak acids and bases
Nausea and vomiting
Distribution
Total body water increases
Protein binding to albumin and α-1 acid glycoprotein decreases
Metabolism
Induction of hepatic metabolic pathways
Estrogen and progesterone may compete for metabolic binding sites
Excretion
Increased clearance of drugs eliminated by renal clearance

the placenta. Protease inhibitors (PIs), such as darunavir/ritonavir (DRV/r), are highly protein bound and therefore only the small percentage of drug that is unbound is free to transfer (Panel on Treatment of HIV-positive Pregnant Women and Prevention of Perinatal Transmission, 2018).

BASIC PRINCIPLES OF USE OF ANTIRETROVIRALS IN PREGNANCY

- ARVs should be initiated in all HIV-positive pregnant women regardless of CD4+ T cell count or HIV-1 viral load.

- The regimen should have good efficacy and should be safe and well-tolerated.

    o The regimen should have one or more NRTI with good placental passage.
- The provider should consider multiple factors when selecting a regimen, including baseline ARV resistance (determined by HIV genotype and treatment history), comorbidities, convenience, adverse effects, drug interactions, pharmacokinetics, and experience in pregnancy.

- Women entering pregnancy on ARVs should continue their regimen if it is effective, well-tolerated, and does not contain agents that are teratogenic.

RECOMMENDATIONS

ARV-Naïve Patients

All HIV-positive women should receive a potent ARV regimen to reduce the risk of perinatal transmission. Table 27.3 lists the updated current USDHHS *preferred* and *alternate* regimens for women who have never received ART and are pregnant. There is also a section on drug regimens that are no longer recommended and the rationale for the discontinuation of their use.

HIV-POSITIVE PREGNANT WOMEN ON ANTIRETROVIRAL THERAPY

HIV-positive pregnant women who present for care in the first trimester should be counseled about the risks and benefits of ART. If possible, they should be maintained on their current ART regimen as discontinuations may lead to the loss of virologic control. This could adversely affect the health of the fetus, including HIV infection. In a prospective cohort of 937 mother–infant pairs, interruption of ART during the first and third trimesters was independently associated with MTCT. The overall rate of MTCT was 1.3%, compared to the rate associated with first- and third-trimester interruptions of ART, which were 4.9% and 18.2%, respectively (Galli, 2009).

In the past, there has been concern over the teratogenic effects of efavirenz use in the first trimester of pregnancy. Preclinical primate data and retrospective reports raised

Table 27.3 RECOMMENDATIONS FOR USE OF ANTIRETROVIRAL DRUGS IN PREGNANT WOMEN

DRUG	COMMENT
Preferred Regimens Regimens with clinical trial data in adults demonstrating optimal efficacy and durability with acceptable toxicity and ease of use, PK data available in pregnancy, and no evidence to date of teratogenic effects or established adverse outcomes for mother/fetus/newborn. To minimize the risk of resistance, a PI regimen is preferred for women who may stop ART during the postpartum period.	
Preferred Two-NRTI backbone	
ABC/3TC	Available as FDC. Can be administered once daily. ABC *should not be used* in patients who test positive for HLA-B*5701 because of the risk of hypersensitivity reaction. ABC/3TC with ATV/r or with efavirenz is not recommended if pretreatment HIV RNA >100,000 copies/mL.
TDF/FTC or 3TC	TDF/FTC available as FDC. Either TDF/FTC or TDF and 3TC can be administered once daily. TDF has potential renal toxicity, thus TDF-based dual NRTI combinations should be used with caution in patients with renal insufficiency.
Preferred PI Regimens	
ATV/r + a preferred 2-NRTI backbone	Once-daily administration. Extensive experience in pregnancy. Maternal hyperbilirubinemia. No clinically significant neonatal hyperbilirubinemia or kernicterus reported, but neonatal bilirubin monitoring recommended. Cannot be administered with proton-pump inhibitors; specific timing recommended for H_2 blockers.
DRV/r + a preferred 2-NRTI backbone	Better tolerated than LPV/r. PK data available. Increasing experience with use in pregnancy. DRV/r must be used twice daily in pregnancy.
Preferred Integrase inhibitor Regimen	
RAL plus a preferred two-NRTI backbone	PK data available and increasing experience in pregnancy. Rapid viral load reduction (potential role for women who present for initial therapy late in pregnancy). Useful when drug interactions with PI regimens are a concern. Twice-daily dosing required.
Preferred Integrase Inhibitor Regimen	
RAL plus a Preferred Two-NRTI Backbone	PK data available and increasing experience in pregnancy. Rapid viral load reduction. Useful when drug interactions with PI regimens are a concern. Twice-daily dosing required.
Alternative Regimens Regimens with clinical trial data demonstrating efficacy in adults, but one or more of the following apply: experience in pregnancy is limited, data are lacking or incomplete on teratogenicity, or regimen is associated with dosing, formulation, toxicity, or interaction issue.	
Alternative Two-NRTI backbone	
ZDV/3TC	Available as FDC. NRTI combination with most experience for use in pregnancy but has disadvantages of requirement for twice-daily administration and increased potential for hematologic toxicity.
Alternative PI Regimens	
LPV/r + a preferred 2-NRTI backbone	Abundant experience and established PK in pregnancy. More nausea than preferred agents. Twice-daily administration. Once-daily LPV/r is not recommended for use in pregnant women.
Alternative NNRTI Regimen	
Efavirenz plus a preferred two-NRTI backbone	Concern because of birth defects seen in primate studies, but data not borne out in human studies and extensive experience in pregnancy; cautionary text remains in package insert.
RPV/TDF/FTC (or RPV plus a preferred two-NRTI backbone)	RPV not recommended with pretreatment HIV RNA >100,000 copies/ml or CD4+ T cell count <200 cells/mm³. Do not use with PPIs. PK data available in pregnancy but relatively little experience with use in pregnancy. Available in co-formulated single-pill once-daily regimen.

(continued)

Table 27.3 CONTINUED

DRUG	COMMENT
Insufficient Data in Pregnancy to Recommend Routine Use in ART-Naïve Women Drugs that are approved for use in adults but lack adequate pregnancy-specific PK or safety data	
TAF/FTC Fixed dose combination	No data on use of TAF in pregnancy
RPV/TAF/FTC Fixed Drug Combination	No data on use of TAF in pregnancy
Not Recommended Drugs whose use is not recommended because of toxicity, lower rate of viral suppression, pharmacologic data suggesting insufficient serum drug levels in pregnancy, or because not recommended in ART-naïve populations.	
EVG/COBI/TDF/FTC Fixed dose combination	Limited data on the use of EVG/COBI component in pregnancy. Inadequate levels of both EVG and COBI in first and third trimesters, as well as viral breakthroughs have been reported. Specific timing and/or fasting recommendations especially if taken with calcium or iron (prenatal vitamins).
EVG/COBI/TAF/FTC	Limited data on the use of EVG/COBI component in pregnancy as above; additionally, no data on use of TAF in pregnancy. Inadequate levels of both EVG and COBI in second and third trimesters, as well as viral breakthroughs have been reported. Specific timing and/or fasting recommendations especially if taken with calcium or iron (prenatal vitamins).
ABC/3TC/ZDV	Generally not recommended due to inferior virologic efficacy.
COBI	Limited data on use of COBI (including coformulations with ATV or DRV) in pregnancy.
d4T	Not recommended due to toxicity
ddI	Not recommended due to toxicity
FPV	Limited data on use in pregnancy. Not recommended in ART-naïve population.
IDV/r	Nephrolithiasis, maternal hyperbilirubinemia.
MVC	MVC requires tropism testing before use. Few case reports of use in pregnancy. Not recommended in ART-naïve populations.
NFV	Lower rate of viral suppression with NFV compared to LPV/r or efavirenz in adult trials
RTV	RTV as a single PI is not recommended because of inferior efficacy and increased toxicity
SQV/r	Not recommended based on potential toxicity and dosing disadvantages. Baseline ECG is recommended before initiation of SQV/r because of potential PR and QT prolongation; contraindicated with preexisting cardiac conduction system disease. Limited data in pregnancy. Large pill burden. Twice daily dosing required.
ETR	Not recommended in ART-naïve populations
NVP	Not recommended because of greater potential for adverse events, complex lead-in dosing, and low barrier to resistance. NVP should be sued in caution when initiating ART in women with CD4 count > 250 cells/mm^3. Use NVP and ABC together with caution; both can cause hypersensitivity reactions within the first few weeks after initiation.
T20	Not recommended in ART- naïve populations
TPV	Not recommended in ART- naïve populations

3TC, lamivudine; ABC, abacavir; ART, antiretroviral therapy; ARV, antiretroviral; ATV/r, atazanavir/ritonavir; CD4, CD4 T lymphocyte; COBI, cobicistat; d4T, stavudine; ddI, didanosine; DTG, dolutegravir; DRV/r, darunavir/ritonavir; ECG, electrocardiogram; efavirenz, efavirenz; ETR, etravirine; EVG, elvitegravir; FDC, fixed drug combination; FPV/r, fosamprenavir/ritonavir; FTC, emtricitabine; HSR, hypersensitivity reaction; IDV/r, indinavir/ritonavir; LPV/r, lopinavir/ritonavir; MVC, maraviroc; NFV, nelfinavir; NRTI, nucleoside reverse transcriptase inhibitor; NNRTI, non-nucleoside reverse transcriptase inhibitor; NVP, nevirapine; PI, protease inhibitor; PK, pharmacokinetic; PPI, proton pump inhibitor; RAL, raltegravir; RPV, rilpivirine; RTV, ritonavir; SQV/r, saquinavir/ritonavir; T20, enfuvirtide; TAF + tenofovir alafenamide; TDF, tenofovir disoproxil fumarate; TPV, tipranavir; TPV/r, tipranavir/ritonavir; ZDV, zidovudine.

SOURCE: Panel on Treatment of HIV-positive Pregnant Women and Prevention of Perinatal Transmission. Recommendations for use of antiretroviral drugs in pregnant HIV-1-infected women for maternal health and interventions to reduce perinatal HIV transmission in the United States. Available at: http://aidsinfo.nih.gov/contentfiles/PerinatalGL.pdf. Accessed July 31, 2018.

Table 27.4 DOLUTEGRAVIR USE IN PREGNANCY OR IN ADULTS OR ADOLESCENTS OF CHILDBEARING POTENTIAL

CLINICAL SCENARIO	RECOMMENDATIONS
ARV-naïve or receiving non-dolutegravir ART and Considering switch to dolutegravir-based regimen	
Pregnant, < 8 wks from last menstrual period	- Do not initiate dolutegravir
Pregnant, > 8 wks from last menstrual period	- If ARV naïve, initiate dolutegravir or another ARV drug - If currently receiving non-dolutegravir regimen, continue current regimen or switch to dolutegravir or another option
Wanting to become pregnant or not using effective contraception	- Do not initiate dolutegravir
Not wanting to become pregnant and using effective contraception	- Dolutegravir-based ART can be considered - Pregnancy testing is recommended before dolutegravir initiation - Discuss potential impact of dolutegravir on fetus and importance of effective contraception use
Currently receiving dolutegravir	
Pregnant, <8 wks from last menstrual period	- Switch dolutegravir to an alternative option or continue dolutegravir after weighing the risks and benefits of both approaches - Do not stop dolutegravir without replacing it with another effective ARV drug - Discuss potential risk of dolutegravir to the fetus and explain that switching after neural tube has formed is unlikely to confer benefit - ARV history, current and previous resistance profiles, patient and fetus safety, tolerance, and drug interaction potential should be considered when determining an optimal alternative to dolutegravir
Pregnant, >8 wks from last menstrual period	- Dolutegravir can be continued - Neural tube defects occur in first 4 weeks following conception or 6 weeks from last menstrual period
Wanting to become pregnant or not using effective contraception and have effective treatment options other than dolutegravir	- Switch dolutegravir to an alternative option - Do not stop dolutegravir without replacing it with another effective ARV drug - Discuss potential risk of dolutegravir to the fetus - ARV history, current and previous resistance profiles, patient and fetus safety, tolerance, and drug interaction potential should be considered when determining an optimal alternative to dolutegravir
Wanting to become pregnant or not using effective contraception and with drug-resistant HIV using dolutegravir as part of salvage regimen, with no other effective ART options	- Continue dolutegravir - Discuss potential risk of dolutegravir to the fetus and risk of viral rebound if dolutegravir is discontinued, including potential for HIV transmission to the fetus
Not wanting to become pregnant and using effective contraception	- Dolutegravir-based ART can be continued - Discuss potential impact of dolutegravir on fetus and importance of effective contraception use

concern about an increased risk of neural tube defects with efavirenz use in pregnancy. It is important to note that the neural tube closes at 36–39 days after the last menstrual period. Thus, the risk of neural tube defects is restricted to the first 5–6 weeks of pregnancy. Finally, a meta-analysis that included data on 1,437 first-trimester efavirenz exposures showed *no* overall increased risk of birth defects compared to women on other ARV drugs. There was one neural tube defect, giving an incidence of 0.07% (Ford, 2011). The panel on treatment of HIV-positive pregnant women has recently updated its recommendation, noting that efavirenz is an alternative NNRTI regimen due to extensive experience in pregnancy. Atripla is the preferred regimen in women who require coadministration of drugs with significant interactions with

preferred agents or those who need the convenience of a single tablet and are not eligible for RPV. It is important to screen for antenatal and postpartum depression (USDHHS, 2018).

DOLUTEGRAVIR USE IN PREGNANCY

The Tsepamo birth outcome study is an ongoing observational study funded by the US National Institutes of Health (NIH) in Botswana comparing birth outcomes among pregnant women taking efavirenz- versus dolutegravir-based regimens. An analysis done on women who were taking dolutegravir-containing regimen before or during conception revealed 4 out of 429 (0.94%) had neural tube defects. In comparison, neural tube defects occurred in 14 out of 11,3000 (0.0012%) of infants born to women receiving any non–dolutegravir-based regimen from conception and 3 out of 5787 (0,05%) of women on an efavirenz-containing regimen (Zash, 2018a). In an updated analysis, the prevalence was noted to be 4/596 (0.67%) which is still above all other exposure groups (Zash, 2018b). The next updated analysis will be in March 2019.

The Panel on Antiretroviral Guidelines for Adults and Adolescents, the Panel on Antiretroviral Therapy and Medical Management of Children Living with HIV, and the Panel on Treatment of Pregnant Women Living with HIV and Prevention of Perinatal Transmission issued recommendations regarding the use of dolutegravir in adults and adolescents with HIV who are pregnant or of childbearing potential (https://aidsinfo.nih.gov/news/2094/statement). See Table 27.4.

HIV-POSITIVE PREGNANT WOMEN WITH LACK OF VIRAL SUPPRESSION

In late pregnancy, lack of virologic suppression could be due to either inadequate time on ART, poor adherence, or virologic failure. Providers must consider several things when evaluating a pregnant woman with lack of viral suppression including adherence, tolerability, correct dosing, drug interactions, and resistance. If there is a concern for resistance, ARV resistance studies should be sent and consultation with an expert is advised.

There have been case reports on the use of raltegravir-containing regimens in late pregnancy due to the rapid viral decay that has been demonstrated with integrase inhibitors (INSTIs). There are no comparative data available in pregnancy (USDHHS, 2018).

INTRAPARTUM ZIDOVUDINE DURING LABOR

HIV-infected women with HIV-1 RNA counts of greater than 1,000 copies/mL or an unknown viral load near delivery should receive intravenous ZDV (Briand, 2013). In the past, all HIV-positive women were given intravenous ZDV during pregnancy regardless of viral load, as this was part of the PACTG 076 protocol noted earlier (Table 27.1).

The French Perinatal Cohort evaluated perinatal transmission in more than 11,000 HIV-positive pregnant women receiving ARV. The overall rate of perinatal transmission was 0.9% in those who received intravenous ZDV and 1.8% without intravenous ZDV. Among women with HIV RNA counts of more than 1,000 copies/mL, the risk of transmission was increased without ZDV (10.2%) compared to 2.5% with intravenous ZDV if neonates received only ZDV for prophylaxis but was no different without or with intrapartum ZDV if the neonate received intensified prophylaxis with two or more ARV drugs. Among women with HIV RNA counts of less than 1,000 copies/mL at delivery, no (zero) transmissions occurred among 369 women who did not receive intravenous ZDV, compared to 0.6% of those receiving intravenous ZDV (Briand, 2013). A few additional studies were reported; based on these studies, intravenous ZDV should continue to be administered to women with HIV RNA counts of greater than 1,000 copies/mL near delivery regardless of intrapartum regimen. The panel recommends intrapartum ZDV administration to women with HIV RNA levels in the range of 50 to 999 copies/mL as the risk of transmission is slightly higher (1–2% vs. 1% or less).

ANTIRETROVIRAL PREGNANCY REGISTRY

Established in 1989, the Antiretroviral Pregnancy Registry (APR) collects data on HIV- infected pregnant women taking ARVs with the goal of detecting any major teratogenic effects. Registration is voluntary and confidential; however, providers are strongly encouraged to enroll pregnant patients in the registry at the time of the initial evaluation of the pregnant woman. This is an observational, exposure registration and follow-up study. The APR is an international registry that has received reports from 67 countries, with the reports predominantly coming from the United States. More information can be obtained by visiting the registry website at www.APRegistry.com.

REFERENCES

Briand N, Warszawski J, Mandelbrot L, et al. Is intrapartum intravenous zidovudine for prevention of mother-to-child HIV-1 transmission still useful in the combination antiretroviral therapy era? *Clin Inf Dis*. 2013;57(6):903–914.

Connor EM, Sperling RS, Gelber R, et al. Reduction of maternal-infant transmission of human immunodeficiency virus type 1 with zidovudine treatment. *N Engl J Med*. 1994;331(18):1173–1180.

Cooper ER, Charurat M, Mofenson L, et al; Combination Antiretroviral strategies for the treatment of pregnant women HIV-1 infected women and prevention of perinatal HIV-1 transmission. Women and Infants' Transmission Study Group. *J AIDS*. 2002;29(5):489–494.

Ford N, Calmy A, Mofenson L. Safety of efavirenz in the first trimester of pregnancy: an updated systematic review and meta-analysis. *AIDS*. 2011;25(18):2301–2304.

Galli L, Puliti D, Chiappini E, Gabiano C, Ferraris G, Mignone F, et al. Is the interruption of antiretroviral treatment during pregnancy an additional major risk factor for mother-to-child transmission of HIV type 1? *Clin Infect Dis*. 2009;48:1310–1317. https://aidsinfo.nih.gov/news/2094/statement-on-potential-safety-signal-in-infants-born-to-women-taking-dolutegravir-from-the-hhs-antiretroviral-guideline-panels.

Mirochnick M, Capparelli E. Pharmacokinetic of antiretrovirals in pregnant women. *Clin Pharmacokinetics*. 2004;43(15):1071–1087.

Panel on Treatment of HIV-positive Pregnant Women and Prevention of Perinatal Transmission. Recommendations for use of antiretroviral drugs in pregnant HIV-1-infected women for maternal United States. Available at http://aidsinfo.nih.gov/contentfiles/PerinatalGL.pdf. Accessed August 30, 2018.

Syme MR, Paxton JW, Keelan JA. Drug transfer and metabolism by the human placenta. *Clin Pharmacokinetics*. 2004;43(8):487–514.

Zash R, Holmes L, Makhema J, et al. Surveillance for neural-tube defects following antiretroviral exposure from conception [Abstract MOAX0202LB]. Presented at the 9th IAS Conference, Amsterdam, 2018a.

Zash R, Makhema J, Shapiro RL. Neural-tube defects with Dolutegravir treatment from the time of conception. *N Engl J Med*. 2018b;379:979–981.

28.

ANTIRETROVIRAL THERAPY FOR CHILDREN AND NEWBORNS

Karin Nielsen-Saines

CHAPTER GOALS

Upon completion of this chapter, the reader should be able to

- Understand the basics regarding pathogenesis of mother to child HIV transmission (MTCT) and be aware of landmark studies targeting prevention of HIV mother to child transmission (PMTCT).

- Understand the concept of HIV-exposure versus HIV-infection.

- Comprehend the specific challenges of early HIV diagnosis of infants and understand the importance of timing of transmission for diagnosis and pathogenesis.

- Be aware of the concept of HIV remission in early treated infants.

- Have a general idea of HIV disease course in children and surrogate markers of disease.

- Be aware of specific caveats guiding antiretroviral use in children.

INTRODUCTION

In the absence of interventions to curtail mother-to-child HIV-1 transmission, HIV-1 infection in children parallels that of women of childbearing age. Perinatal transmission of HIV-1 accounts for nearly all worldwide cases of pediatric HIV-1 infection today, with the exception of adolescent acquisition of HIV-1 via adult risk behaviors. HIV-1 transmission from mother-to-child occurs in 25–30% of cases when there is no maternal ARV treatment (Newell, 1991; Scott, 1989); if breastfeeding until 12 months of age is included, transmission risk can be as high as 40%. Infection may be transmitted during pregnancy, at the time of labor and delivery, and via breastfeeding. Worldwide, approximately 2,000 HIV-infected infants are born daily, with 90% of cases occurring in sub-Saharan Africa (Marston, 2011). Breastfeeding transmission contributes another 300,000 infant infections per year (Marston, 2011). Although cART can reduce MTCT transmission to less than 1% in developed countries (Dorenbaum, 2002), failure to recognize HIV-1 infection in women and/or unavailability of treatment still contributes to continuing

mother-to-child HIV transmission worldwide. Management of HIV-1 infection in children has to take into consideration several factors. These include early diagnosis of infection, the natural history of HIV-1 infection in children and surrogate markers of disease, suitable pediatric drug formulations for children, drug metabolism and pharmacokinetics of ARVs in children, and the general paucity of pediatric treatment data as compared to adults.

LEARNING OBJECTIVES

- Discuss advances in antiretroviral therapy (ART) for the prevention of mother-to-child HIV transmission, particularly for postexposure infant prophylaxis.

- Review pediatric-specific issues of early HIV diagnosis, timing and pathogenesis of HIV disease, and use of surrogate markers of HIV infection in this population.

- Discuss current guidelines for management of antiretrovirals (ARVs) in children within the context of what drugs to use, when to start, and when to change ART.

WHAT'S NEW?

- The US Department of Health and Human Services (USDHHS) ARV treatment guidelines for children were recently updated and now offer more options for ARV postexposure prophylaxis for children. Guidelines continue to recommend that definitive exclusion or confirmation of HIV infection in children between the ages of 18 and 24 months who are HIV antibody-positive should be based on a nucleic acid test (NAT) rather than on maternal antibody results because there could be residual maternal antibody in this age group.

- Pharmacokinetic and safety data on select ARV agents for HIV-infected preterm infants and term infants younger than 15 days have been updated. There are dosing guidelines for the use of raltegravir in infants with suspected or confirmed HIV infection. Nevertheless, USDHHS guidelines continue to recommend that neonatal care providers who are considering a three-drug ARV treatment regimen for term infants younger than 2 weeks or premature infants contact a pediatric HIV expert for guidance and individual case assessment of the risk-benefit ratio of treatment and for the latest information on neonatal drug doses. The National Perinatal HIV Hotline (1-888-448-8765) provides free clinical consultation on perinatal HIV care.

- Early diagnosis of HIV infection in the United States was largely made through the use of DNA polymerase chain reaction (PCR) testing via the Amplicor HIV-1 DNA test, which is no longer commercially available. In its absence, measurement of HIV RNA PCR for diagnosis is an acceptable alternative. It is important to note that the sensitivity and specificity of noncommercial HIV-1 DNA tests which are now being used may differ from the sensitivity and specificity of the previously US Food and Drug Administration (FDA)-approved Amplicor HIV-1 DNA test, and false-positive or false-negative results may occur. It is important to confirm HIV DNA results with FDA-approved HIV RNA assays.

- Studies have continued to demonstrate a significant benefit of early ARV treatment to infants less than 12 months of age in the prevention of HIV mortality and morbidity, and treatment is recommended to all HIV-infected infants in this age group in all geographic settings, regardless of clinical findings, CD4+ T cell counts, or viral load. The updated recommendation is that treatment of infants under 12 months of age who are diagnosed with HIV should be expedited and characterizes an urgent situation. HIV diagnosis is an emergency, and infants identified as HIV-exposed should be tested as soon as possible. Treatment should not be delayed and can be started as early as the first day of life if HIV diagnosis is confirmed. ARV agents that can be used from birth for which there is PK data include zidovudine, nevirapine, lamivudine, and raltegravir. Lopinavir/ritonavir can be used as early as 2 weeks of age, and abacavir as early as 3 months. Tenofovir disoproxil fumarate is not recommended for use in children less than 2 years of age and tenofovir alafenamide (TAF) has not been studied in young children.

- Infant postexposure prophylaxis with 2 or 3 ARV agents initiated within 48 hours of life continues to be preferred to standard zidovudine prophylaxis in situations where mothers did not receive ARVs during pregnancy until the time of labor and delivery. This strategy has been shown to further reduce the risk of intrapartum HIV acquisition in non-breastfeeding populations.

- World Health Organization (WHO) guidelines for resource-limited settings recommend combined ART (cART) in all pregnant women with HIV-infection regardless of CD4+ T cell count or virus load throughout pregnancy, for the duration of breastfeeding, and continuing thereafter for life (WHO Option B+).

- Initial combination therapy for ARV treatment-naïve children includes the use of integrase strand transfer inhibitor (INSTI)-based regimens as agents to be used in combination with two nucleoside analogue reverse transcriptase inhibitors (NRTIs). Dolutegravir is licensed for children aged 12 years and older. Raltegravir is licensed for infants as young as 4 weeks of age but can be used in the neonatal period when necessary. The protease inhibitor (PI) atazanavir boosted with ritonavir is now considered an alternative PI in children aged 3 months through 5 years and remains a preferred drug for children 6 years and older. The two-NRTI combination of zidovudine and lamivudine or emtricitabine is now considered an alternative combination for adolescents older than 13 years.

- Perinatal studies such as IMPAACT P1115 are under way to determine the extent and duration of HIV remission following prompt initiation of combination ARV treatment in HIV-infected infants who are treated shortly after birth (i.e., during the acute infection process).

KEY POINTS

- HIV-infected infants and children have a different, more progressive disease course as compared to adults given that early infection leads to sustained, high-magnitude viremia with significant seeding of reservoirs in the first months of life, prior to full maturation of the immune system.

- Early diagnosis of HIV infection is pivotal in the management of infants and in the prevention of HIV-associated morbidity and mortality.

- The availability of potent pediatric ARV formulations encompassing different classes of drugs for infected infants and young children is still limited and needs further development.

- Infant postexposure HIV prophylaxis varies according to the risk scenario.

- Early ARV treatment (i.e., at the time of diagnosis) is still the mainstay of pediatric HIV infection, particularly for infants less than 12 months of age, but is also highly recommended for older children.

- Early treatment of young infants diagnosed shortly after birth appears to be the best approach to reduce the seeding of viral reservoirs and to potentially attain prolonged periods of HIV remission off ARVs, a strategy evaluated in prospective clinical trials.

ANTIRETROVIRALS TO THE HIV-EXPOSED INFANT

Advances in perinatal primary ART and antepartum, peripartum, and postpartum delivery of zidovudine in non–breast-feeding, HIV-infected women without severe immuno-suppression in the United States led to a decrease in perinatal transmission rates. The US Centers for Disease Control and Prevention (CDC) estimates that the number of infants born annually with HIV in the United States decreased from 1,650 in 1991 to 100–200 in 2004, which is approximately the number observed in the United States in 2018. The provision of ARVs to infants born to HIV-infected mothers as prophylaxis has been standard of care in the Unites States since 1994, when results of Pediatric AIDS Clinical Trials Group study 076 were published (Connor, 1994). The study demonstrated that zidovudine monotherapy given to the mother starting at 16 weeks' gestation, accompanied by an intravenous zidovudine infusion during labor and delivery and followed by four times per day dosing of zidovudine to the infant from birth to 6 weeks of age was highly efficacious in preventing mother-to-child HIV transmission as compared to placebo (8% vs. 25% respectively, $p < 0.001$). In the developed country setting, 4–6 weeks of zidovudine to the infant initiated at birth, given at 2 mg/kg per dose four times a day or 4 mg/kg per dose twice a day is standard of care (Ruane, 2013). The major toxicities of zidovudine used as infant prophylaxis include anemia and neutropenia; however, these are dose-dependent and self-limiting, tend to occur toward the end of the course of treatment, and rarely require interruption of prophylaxis (Lahoz, 2010). In resource limited-settings, single-dose nevirapine to the infant (2 mg/kg) shortly after birth was used for many years as standard of care, following publication of HIVNET 012 (Guay, 1999), which documented the efficacy of this approach in reducing MTCT when associated with single-dose nevirapine given to the mother at the time of labor. Nevertheless, this approach induced a large wave of ARV resistance in infants who ultimately became infected, rendering nevirapine use problematic for early infant treatment strategies in the developing world. Among HIV-infected infants whose mothers were not treated with ARVs throughout the course of pregnancy and are therefore at higher risk of HIV acquisition, double ARV prophylaxis initiated within 48 hours of birth with three doses of nevirapine in the first week of life concurrently with 6 weeks of zidovudine has been shown to be more efficacious for the prevention of HIV intrapartum infection than zidovudine alone (Nielsen-Saines, 2011). An alternative, equally efficacious regimen was the use of lamivudine and nelfinavir in the first 2 weeks of life concurrent with 6 weeks of zidovudine (Nielsen-Saines, 2011). Due to the current lack of availability of pediatric formulations of nelfinavir, however, the nevirapine/zidovudine combination is preferable. Lopinavir/ritonavir suspension is currently not recommended by the FDA for use in infants younger than 2 weeks of age. In resource-limited settings, the use of daily nevirapine prophylaxis to the HIV-exposed infant for prevention of MTCT has been evaluated up to 6 months of age and has been shown to be effective and safe in the prevention of postpartum HIV acquisition (Coovadia, 2012). Presently however, most settings in sub-Saharan Africa have transitioned to WHO Options B+, which recommend treatment with cART to all HIV-infected women during pregnancy, lactation, and onward with no further treatment interruption (WHO, 2014).

The selection of ART to reduce perinatal HIV transmission must include consideration of optimal treatment for the infected pregnant women and balance potential for fetal harm. Maternal factors that should be considered include the mother's viral load, degree of immunosuppression, medications for use in treatment of comorbid conditions (e.g., tuberculosis, hepatitis C virus), and the potential for inducing viral resistance. Transmission of resistant HIV to infants has been described in the literature, but it is an infrequent event (De Lourdes Teixeira, 2015; Yeganeh, 2018). Other considerations to prevent perinatal transmission of HIV include scheduled delivery to minimize prolonged rupture of membranes, including a recommendation from the American College of Obstetrics for scheduled cesarean section for women with viral loads exceeding HIV RNA levels of 1,000 copies/mL (Committee on Obstetric Practice ACOG, 2001). In a meta-analysis of 15 North American and European cohorts of HIV-infected pregnant women ($n = 100$ women), vertical transmission rates differed by 5% for those with scheduled delivery by cesarean section (transmission rate, 2%) as compared with those with other delivery modes (transmission rate, 7.3%; International Perinatal HIV Group, 1999). Evaluation of the morbidity and mortality related to such scheduled cesarean sections suggests that HIV-infected pregnant women may have a higher incidence of postpartum hemorrhage with resultant transfusion, sepsis, pneumonia, and death than do their noninfected pregnant peers undergoing the same scheduled procedure (odds ratio, 1.6) (Louis, 2007). HIV-infected pregnant women without detectable viral loads should be informed preoperatively of their risk for having morbidity related to cesarean section performed to prevent perinatal HIV transmission. Although intravenous zidovudine was recommended in the past for use throughout labor and delivery, for women with an undetectable viral load during pregnancy, the current recommendation is to continue the current oral ARV regimen throughout labor delivery without the need for intravenous zidovudine.

DIAGNOSIS

Early diagnosis of HIV-1 infection is crucial for identification of at-risk infants and consequent initiation of treatment. All HIV-1 exposed infants carry maternal HIV-1 antibodies until approximately 15–18 months of age. Thus, early pediatric diagnosis relies on identification of the virus, usually via HIV-1 DNA or RNA PCR techniques. The former measures integrated virus in the host genome, and the latter measures circulating plasma virus. HIV-1 co-culture is not routinely performed because of cost and time, although it is also a reliable diagnostic method. Infants infected in utero usually have positive PCR results within the first 48 hours of birth, while infants infected at the time of labor and delivery may have a negative HIV DNA or RNA PCR result at birth, followed by a positive result 1 week to 2 months following birth (Bryson, 1992). Breastfed infants have continuing HIV exposure and thus can develop a positive HIV DNA or RNA PCR result at any time. The risk of transmission by breastfeeding from an HIV-positive mother is approximately 16% (Fowler, 2002). Therefore, repeat PCR testing in the first few months of life is critical for determination of the timing of infection, with sensitivity of a PCR result reaching 96% by 4 weeks of life in the absence of breastfeeding (Dunn, 1992; Nielsen, 2000).

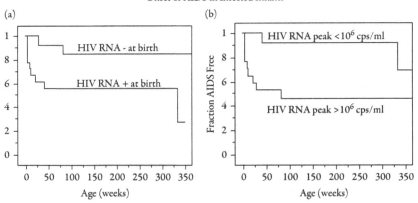

Onset of AIDS in Infected Infants

Figure 28.1 In utero acquisition of HIV infection and sustained peak viremia greater than 10^6 copies/mL of plasma in the first year of life are predictive of HIV disease progression.　From Dickover (1998).

TIMING OF INFECTION

Acquisition of HIV infection may occur in utero, intrapartum, or through breastfeeding. Even before ARV treatment was recommended to pregnant women, two-thirds of HIV-exposed infants escaped HIV infection. Perinatal HIV infection rates have declined substantially in the developed world since 1994, following publication of the landmark PACTG 076 study which demonstrated reduction of perinatal HIV transmission in women who used zidovudine in pregnancy as compared to placebo (Connor, 1994). Approximately 30–50% of infants who contract HIV infection will acquire it in utero, and 50–70% will acquire the infection during the intrapartum period (Cao, 1997; Dickover, 1996; Mayaux, 1997). In order to characterize the timing of HIV infection, a working definition was created for acquisition of infection in utero and intrapartum (Bryson, 1992). An infant is considered to have in utero infection if virologic tests (HIV DNA or RNA PCR) are positive within 48 hours of life. Due to the risk of contamination with maternal blood, cord blood samples should not be used for diagnostic evaluations. Infants are considered to have intrapartum HIV infection if diagnostic tests within the first 48 hours of life are negative but further virologic testing after 1 week of life is positive. There is evidence that most cases of HIV transmission occur late in pregnancy or at delivery.

Postpartum transmission of HIV via breastfeeding has been a continuing problem for the prevention of MTCT of HIV efforts worldwide. HIV can be transmitted as cell-associated or cell-free virus in breast milk (Lyimo, 2012). Mastitis, which triggers migration of inflammatory cells, is also a known risk factor for HIV breastmilk transmission (Semrau, 2013), as is nonexclusive breastfeeding (Coutsoudis, 1999) or the presence of oral thrush in the infant (Read, 2009). Longer duration of breastfeeding is also a well-known risk factor for transmission (Becquet, 2005), as is maternal primary infection during lactation (Morrison, 2015). In areas where safe alternatives to breastfeeding are not available, however, formula feeding is associated with higher morbidity and mortality. Provision of combination ART to lactating HIV-infected mothers has been demonstrated to significantly increase HIV-free survival

in infants with improved infant outcomes in terms of growth and reduced infections (Marazzi, 2007, 2009, 2010; Interagency Task Team on the Prevention and Treatment of HIV Infection in Pregnant Women Mothers and Children (IATT) CDC WHO and UNICEF, 2015). Successful screening of pregnant women with availability of ARV treatment for HIV-positive pregnant and lactating women through the WHO B+ program (CDC, 2015) has decreased early and late postpartum HIV transmission via breastfeeding over time. In women with $CD4^+$ T cell counts higher than $350/\mu L$ in sub-Saharan Africa, the Promise Study observed a mother-to-child in utero transmission rate of HIV at 1 week of age of 0.5% when women received cART during pregnancy (Fowler, 2016). Further follow-up of the same infants revealed very low breastfeeding transmission rates when mothers received cART during lactation (HIV transmission 0.57%) or infants received prophylactic infant nevirapine (HIV transmission 0/58%) during the first 18 months of life or following cessation of breastfeeding, whichever occurred first (Flynn, 2018).

The timing of HIV-1 infection (in utero vs. intrapartum) is somewhat predictive of the patient's subsequent clinical course (Dickover, 1994). Early onset of AIDS-defining conditions is more frequently observed in in utero infected infants who sustain early, prolonged elevated HIV RNA levels.

As in adults, prolonged periods of elevated HIV RNA levels are predictive of disease progression. HIV-infected infants undergo primary infection, either in utero or shortly after birth. Therefore, they tend to have very elevated virus loads in the first months of life (Figure 28.2).

MATERNAL RISK FACTORS FOR HIV TRANSMISSION

Maternal risk factors associated with enhanced perinatal HIV transmission identified through national surveillance in reported AIDS cases include untreated HIV disease, seroconversion during pregnancy or breastfeeding, drug abuse, heterosexual infection by sexual partners with risk factors for acquiring HIV disease, and maternal transfusion before 1985. Prospective and retrospective evaluations of maternal

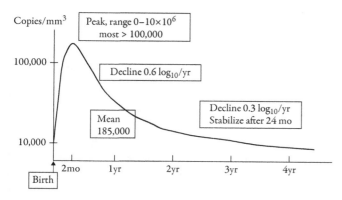

Dynamics of HIV-RNA in Infants

Copies/mm³

Peak, range 0–10×10⁶ most > 100,000

Decline 0.6 log₁₀/yr

Decline 0.3 log₁₀/yr Stabilize after 24 mo

Mean 185,000

100,000

10,000

Birth   2mo   1yr   2yr   3yr   4yr

Figure 28.2 Natural course of HIV RNA viremia in children. From Palumbo et al. (1998).

predictors for perinatal HIV transmission have been the focus of multiple studies. Maternal transmission predictors identified to date include maternal viremia (measured as quantitative HIV RNA PCR or viral load; Gabiano, 1992; Magder, 2005) maternal immunosuppression, or an inadequate immune response (measured by the CD4⁺ T cell count, neutralizing antibody production; Magder, 2005) and viral characteristics (chemokine receptor tropism, resistance patterns of maternal virus at delivery or infant virus at birth; Scarlatti, 2004). Pregnancy and placental variables (delivery mode, duration of rupture of membranes, chorioamnionitis) also may influence the risk for perinatal transmission of HIV (Mwanyumba, 2002, St Louis, 1993, International Perinatal HIV Group, 1999). Infant variables evaluated as predictors of transmission of HIV include specific human leukocyte antigen (HLA) markers and the infant cellular immune response (cytokine production, activated T cell function; European Collaborative Study, 1991; Luzuriaga, 1991; Magder, 2005; Polycarpou, 2002). In addition, immunogenetic factors (chemokine coreceptor expression) have been suggested to confer protection against progression of disease (Sei, 2001).

EARLY TREATMENT INITIATION AND HIV REMISSION IN HIV-EXPOSED INFANTS

ART to infants and children suppresses viremia, reduces the high infant mortality, and improves clinical outcome; however, children must continue life-long ARV treatment. The major barrier to achieving HIV remission in children, as in adults, is the early establishment of long-lived latent cellular reservoirs in CD4⁺ T cells and other sites, with continued low-level replication and rebound viremia once taken off ARTs (Persaud, 2012). It is postulated that, through treatment of very early HIV infection, the establishment, quantity, or even elimination of latent reservoirs could be achieved by reducing viral spread into memory CD4⁺ T cell reservoirs, which would potentially allow patients to thrive off of ARTs without viral rebound, as evidenced by the "Mississippi baby" who remained in ARV-free viral remission

for 27 months post early cART (Persaud, 2013; Siliciano, 2014; Luzuriaga, 2015). Importantly, there are emerging data that very early therapy during acute HIV infection in both adult and children quantitatively modifies HIV persistence and may influence the rate of reservoir decay. This approach is presently being further evaluated in ongoing clinical trials.

DISEASE COURSE

The natural history of pediatric HIV-1 infection is bimodal (Scott, 1991). Studies conducted in developed countries prior to the availability of ARVs demonstrate that approximately 20% of children exhibit very rapid disease progression, with rapid loss of CD4⁺ T cell counts and development of AIDS-defining conditions before 2 years of age (Nielsen, 1997). The majority of HIV-infected children, however (approximately 60–65%) will have intermediate disease progression, with the presence of AIDS-defining events by 7–8 years of age. There is a small subset of children (as there is in adults), approximately 15–20% of patients, who have very slow to no disease progression by age 8 years, and an even smaller set of elite controllers (<5%). These children enter adolescence with minimal to no symptoms of HIV disease. Studies conducted in Africa have demonstrated an even faster pace of disease progression, with the majority of pediatric patients having AIDS-defining conditions by age 5 years (Newell, 2004). This might be due to the higher overall burden of disease and presence of multiple coinfections. cART makes it possible to alter the natural history of HIV disease and transform disease progressors into nonprogressors. This translates into improvements in the quality of life and reduction in HIV-associated disease morbidity and mortality.

Infants with in utero infection appear to have a more rapid disease course when compared to infants who acquire HIV infection intrapartum (Dickover, 1996). In utero infected infants still have normal CD4⁺ T cell values at birth and are usually born with a low virus load (as measured by DNA or RNA PCR) (Mayaux, 1996). In addition, even in utero HIV-infected infants are asymptomatic at birth. In utero HIV appears to result from transplacental passage of virus or ascending viral infection in patients with prolonged rupture of membranes (Minkoff, 1995). In the animal model, researchers have demonstrated that viral infection of the amniotic fluid with simian immunodeficiency virus (SIV) resulted in infection of all the offspring (Van Rompay, 1995). Intrapartum transmission of HIV infection is responsible for the majority of perinatal cases. In a prospective study of 271 HIV-infected infants using HIV DNA PCR, 38% of children were found to be positive within 48 hours of life, 93% were positive by 14 days of age, and 96% of the total number of infected children were positive by 4 weeks of age (Dunn, 1992). There are infants who might not have detectable virus as late as 3 months following delivery in selected cases. Untreated infants tend to maintain a very high virus burden throughout their first year of life, and immunologic patterns of primary viremia in infants have long been described (Luzuriaga, 1997). High-level viremia might persist for a longer period of time in infants than in adults undergoing primary infection; untreated early infection is associated with a high mortality risk (Violari, 2008). Many years prior to the advent of cART, discordant twin infections were reported, with the first-born twin having a higher risk of infection (Duliege, 1995).

SURROGATE MARKERS OF DISEASE

The goal of ART is to reduce the HIV-1 viral load as much as possible while restoring or preserving immune function. Viral load is generally measured via plasma HIV-1 RNA reverse transcriptase (RT) PCR (Roche Molecular Systems), HIV RNA quantitation by branched (b) DNA (Chiron Corporation), or nucleic acid sequence-based amplification (NASBA) HIV-1 RNA quantitative (QT) assay (Organon Teknika). All three methods are reliable parameters for the measurement of free virus in plasma, with new-generation assays being able to identify virus isolates of different subtypes. Immune function in HIV disease is measured primarily by evaluating T cell subsets, particularly $CD4^+$ T cell absolute numbers and percentages. Three-color flow cytometry is generally the methodology employed for this purpose. Declining counts parallel disease progression, with declines in $CD4^+$ T cells usually following peak HIV RNA viremia. One important caveat in the management of HIV-infected children is that $CD4^+$ T cell numbers, particularly in infants, differ significantly from adults and do not achieve similar levels until after 5 years. Therefore, an infant with a $CD4^+$ T cell count of 750 cells/mm^3 or less is at significant risk for development of AIDS-defining conditions because normal values are generally greater than 2,000 cells/mm^3.

ANTIRETROVIRALS IN CHILDREN

One general principle in the use of ARV therapy is that continued viral replication in the presence of ARV drugs promotes development of drug resistance. Resistance to one specific ARV agent may in turn confer resistance to other drugs within the same class. Current standard of practice is that, once therapy is started, long-term or life-long treatment is warranted. In children, the efficacy of ARV therapy often is extrapolated from data obtained from adult clinical trials because of lack of pediatric data. There are, however, significant age-related differences between children and adults. These encompass body composition, renal excretion, liver metabolism, and gastrointestinal function. This leads to differences in drug distribution and metabolism, drug clearance, drug dosing, and different toxicities between children and adults. In addition, protein binding and drug clearance of some specific ARVs may differ by race due to the presence of genetic polymorphisms. Nevertheless, often therapeutic doses for infants and children are not available. Liquid or palatable formulations for children do not exist for many ARVs, and adherence depends on adult caretakers. It is crucial when initiating ARV therapy to take into consideration the presence of comorbidities and concomitant medications in order to avoid overlapping drug toxicities. It is also important to consider cross-resistance and later therapeutic options.

GUIDELINES

Treatment guidelines have been developed over the years in order to address critical concerns about the use of ARV therapy in children. Major concerns have always included the optimal timing of initiation of ARV therapy, the preferred choice of ARVs, best ways to monitor efficacy and toxicities, and when to change therapy. There are decreased variations in guidelines between developed and developing countries. In the United States, traditionally, most children have been treated when identified as having HIV-1 infection, regardless of symptomatology. Given multiple therapeutic options and the general availability of viral load monitoring, guidelines in developed countries over the years have relied on virus load measures for predicting early switches in therapy (Panel on Antiretroviral Therapy and Medical Management of HIV-Infected Children, 2018). Randomized clinical trials, such as the CHER trial in South Africa, demonstrated that early ARV treatment to infants diagnosed before 12 months of age is clearly beneficial in reducing morbidity and mortality (Violari, 2008).

The current US pediatric ARV treatment guidelines Panel has increased the strength of its recommendations for initiating ART in children aged 1 year or older who are asymptomatic or who have mild symptoms and those who have $CD4^+$ T cell counts of 1,000 cells/mm^3 or greater (for those aged 1–6 years) or $CD4^+$ T cell counts of 500 cells/mm^3 or greater (for those aged $\geq$6 years); recommendations ratings have been changed from Moderate (BI*) to Strong (AI*) (Panel on Antiretroviral Therapy and Medical Management, 2011, 2015, 2018). Thus, the Panel now recommends that all children receive ART, regardless of symptoms or $CD4^+$ T cell count. WHO treatment guidelines, however, recommend treatment for all children under the age of 12 months regardless of clinical findings and otherwise for children who have WHO clinical stage 3 or 4 (i.e., more symptomatic patients). WHO guidelines also use T cell subset measures as the main laboratory surrogate markers of disease (when available), as opposed to virus load measures for dictating initiation or switches in ARV therapy (Violari, 2008). Regardless of the specific guidelines in use, however, the decision to initiate therapy is based on disease severity and the risk of disease progression.

TIMING OF INITIATION OF THERAPY

Early versus deferred initiation of ARV treatment in HIV-infected children was a controversial matter, but this is no longer a subject of debate. It is currently universally accepted in both the developed and developing world that ART should be started at the time of HIV diagnosis in all children, regardless of age. Starting therapy early in asymptomatic children controls viral replication before genetic mutations develop, leading to fewer number of circulating viral strains. It also prevents immune system destruction and avoids disease progression. With this strategy, viral seeding of latent cells or $CD4^+$ T cell reservoirs can often be circumvented. Given the significant repercussions to cognitive development when treatment is delayed, there is no justification at the present time to delay treatment to HIV-infected children.

CHANGE IN THERAPY

The decision to change ARVs varies slightly according to the pediatric guidelines employed. The variability is mostly due to the surrogate markers used. Nevertheless, most experts would agree that indicators of treatment failure include progression of HIV disease, growth failure, development of opportunistic infections while on established therapy, decline in CD4+ percentiles, development or worsening HIV encephalopathy, and significant increases in virus load. Tolerability, palatability, and drug toxicities are also reasons why ARV regimens are switched in children, as in adults. Simplification of treatment regimens are recommended whenever possible, as the greatest predictor of achieving an undetectable plasma virus load is adherence.

SPECIFIC ANTIRETROVIRAL AGENTS

ARVs currently available for use in the United States are listed in Table 28.1. Optimal ARV combinations for children may differ slightly from that of adults. In infants, particularly those under 1 year of age, there is often a need to use very potent ARV regimens for reduction of persistently elevated viral loads (Luzuriaga, 2004; Palumbo, 2010). Therefore, in this scenario, four-drug combinations including a PI, two nucleoside analogs, and a non-nucleoside analog such as nevirapine may be indicated. The use of many ARVs is also limited in younger children (especially those under 4 years) because of the lack of liquid formulations, as depicted in Table 28.1. Prevalent ART regimens in pediatrics include one PI such as ritonavir/lopinavir, or atazanavir or darunavir (in older children) in combination with a double NRTI backbone such as ZDV + 3TC, D4T + 3TC, ZDV + DDI, D4T + ABC, ABC + 3TC, or FTC/TDFC (in older children). The PIs may be substituted with NNRTIs such as nevirapine or efavirenz (the latter in older children). In special circumstances, it may be necessary to boost the main PI with additional PIs such as ritonavir or the pharmaco-enhancer cobicistat in order to achieve higher blood concentrations. This is, for instance, the case of atazanavir when used with tenofovir; additional boosting with 100 mg of ritonavir in the treatment of older children is often warranted. Specific ARV regimens to be avoided include any type of mono or dual therapy, atazanavir with tenofovir without ritonavir boosting, combinations of ZDV+ D4T, DDC with 3TC, D4T or DDI, or D4T and DDI in pregnant patients. Clinical trials in the United States are currently evaluating the pharmacokinetics of integrase inhibitors in children, as well as the pharmacokinetics of CCR5 chemokine receptor blockers. Newer generation NNRTI drugs, such as etravirine or rilpivirine, have not yet been evaluated in children nor are there dosing recommendations for multiple ARVs in children under 4 years of age. TAF has not been studied in young children (Ruane, 2013). In resource-limited settings, treatment studies have demonstrated greater durability of viral load suppression in children treated with ritonavir/lopinavir-based regimens as opposed to nevirapine-based regimens, although, interestingly, nevirapine has been shown to be associated with improved growth in this population (Chadwick, 2011).

TOXICITIES AND ADVERSE EFFECTS

The complications and side effects of specific ARV are multiple. The most frequent toxicities of zidovudine are hematologic, particularly anemia, and neutropenia. These may resolve with dose reduction. All NRTIs may cause some degree of mitochondrial toxicity. Zidovudine may cause myopathy, and peripheral neuropathy is seen with this drug as well as with DDI, DDC, D4T, and rarely with 3TC. DDI is associated with pancreatitis. D4T is associated with lipoatrophy and, in combination with DDI, may induce liver fatty acid syndrome, particularly during pregnancy. Abacavir is famous for a fatal hypersensitivity reaction, which occurs in 1% of pediatric patients. It presents as flu-like symptoms with or without a rash, abdominal pain, sore throat, and myalgias. If the drug has been interrupted in this scenario, shock will ensue when restarted. The NNRTIs most commonly cause skin rashes (about 40%) and have rarely been associated with Steven-Johnsons syndrome. Efavirenz is teratogenic, and central nervous system findings such as dizziness, insomnia, and nightmares have been reported shortly after initiation of treatment with this drug. There is some concern about the use of nevirapine during pregnancy in women with CD4+ T cell counts greater than 250/mm³ due to an increased risk of hepatic failure (Hitti, 2004), but there is still controversy on the subject since additional studies have failed to demonstrate an association (De Lazzari, 2008).

Table 28.1 ANTIRETROVIRALS AVAILABLE FOR TREATMENT IN THE UNITED STATES USED IN PEDIATRICS

Nucleoside reverse transcriptase inhibitors (NRTIs)	**Protease inhibitors (PIs)**
Zidovudine (ZDV/AZT) [a]	Saquinavir soft gel
Lamivudine (3TC) [a]	Ritonavir[a]
Abacavir (ABC) [a]	Nelfinavir
Tenofovir disoproxil fumarate (TDF)	Lopinavir/ritonavir[a]
Tenofovir alafenamide (TAF)	Atazanavir
Emtricitabine (FTC)	Darunavir
Non-nucleoside reverse transcriptase inhibitors (NNRTIs)	**Fusion inhibitors**
Nevirapine[a]	
Efavirenz	
Rilpivirine	
Doravirine	
Combination antiretrovirals[b]:	**Other classes**
AZT/3TC	R-5 receptor inhibitors: Maraviroc
AZT/3TC/ABC	Integrase inhibitors:
TDF/FTC or TAF/FTC	Raltegravir
ABC/3TC	Dolutegravir
EFV/TDF/FTC	*Elvitegravir/cobicistat/ TAF/FTC*
FTC/RPV/TDF (or TAF)	

[a] Pediatric formulations available

[b] Additional formulations such as NVP/ZDV/3TC and NVP/D4T/3TC are available to children in pediatric formulations as generic drugs in resource-limited settings

PIs have multiple drug–drug interactions because of their cytochrome P450 metabolism in the liver. Their most common side effects are gastrointestinal symptoms. Hepatitis and hyperbilirubinemia are not uncommon. In adults, they have been shown to induce lipodystrophy, diabetes, and increased atherosclerosis because of lipid abnormalities. These findings are now being recognized in children, although complications are to a lesser extent. There are also recent concerns about the potential for osteopenia and osteoporosis in children, either induced by ART (notably TDF) or HIV disease itself (Mora, 2004).

IMMUNE RECONSTITUTION INFLAMMATORY SYNDROME

One recognized potential complication of potent ARV therapy is the immune reconstitution inflammatory syndrome (IRIS). It is most frequently observed in patients who initiate ART with low $CD4^+$ T cell counts. It is associated with a wide range of reactivation of previously latent pathogens, with tuberculosis being a common underlying condition. The underlying pathogenesis appears to start with unrecognized, low-level colonization of opportunistic pathogens in patients who have moderate to severe immunosuppression. With the initiation of ART and subsequent recovery of immunity to the organism, there is a paradoxical clinical deterioration due to a dysregulated, overly exuberant immune response. This syndrome usually presents in the first 6 weeks of ART and may resolve either with the use of steroids or temporary discontinuation of ART. It is infrequently seen in pediatric HIV practiced in developed countries, particularly because children are generally treated earlier. However, it is very prevalent in the developing world and may carry high morbidity and mortality.

BENEFITS OF THERAPY

Despite the complications and controversies, the benefits of ART in children with HIV are overwhelming. In the United States, the annual mortality in pediatric HIV patients decreased to less than 1% as of 1999 due to the availability of treatment (Gortmaker, 2001; Jeremy, 2005). ART decreases the virus load, preserves and restores the immune function, decreases the risk of comorbidities, decreases hospitalizations, improves survival, improves quality of life, and restores hope to children and their families. Many perinatally infected children who initiated treatment early in life are now adults who have families and children of their own. ART has also changed the AIDS paradigm. As one patient once said, HIV is no longer a disease you die from, but a disease you live with.

REFERENCES

Becquet R, Ekouevi DK, Viho I, et al. Acceptability of exclusive breast-feeding with early cessation to prevent HIV transmission through breast milk, ANRS 1201/1202 Ditrame Plus, Abidjan, Cote d'Ivoire. *J AIDS*. 2005;40(5):600–608.

Bryson YJ, Luzuriaga K, Sullivan JL, et al. Proposed definitions for in utero versus intrapartum transmission of HIV-1. *N Engl J Med*. 1992;327:1246–1247.

Cao Y, Krogstad P, Korber BT, et al. Maternal HIV-1 viral load and vertical transmission of infection: the Ariel Project for the prevention of HIV transmission from mother to infant. *Nat Med*. 1997;3(5):549–552.

Chadwick EG, Yogev R, Alvero CG, et al.; International Pediatric Adolescent Clinical Trials Group (IMPAACT) P1030 Team. Long-term outcomes for HIV-infected infants less than 6 months of age at initiation of lopinavir/ritonavir combination antiretroviral therapy. *AIDS*. 2011;25:643–649.

Committee on Obstetric Practice. ACOG committee opinion scheduled cesarean delivery and the prevention of vertical transmission of HIV infection: number 234, May 2000 (replaces number 219, August 1999). *Int J Gynaecol Obstet*. 2001;73:279–281.

Connor EM, Sperling RS, Gelber R, et al. Reduction of maternal-infant transmission of human immunodeficiency virus type 1 with zidovudine treatment. Pediatric AIDS Clinical Trials Group Protocol 076 Study Group. *N Engl J Med*. 1994;331(18):1173–1180.

Coovadia HM, Brown ER, Fowler MG, et al.; HPTN 046 PRotocol Team. Efficacy and safety of an extended nevirapine regimen in infant children of breastfeeding mothers with HIV-1 infection for prevention of postnatal HIV-1 transmission (HPTN 046): a randomised, double-blind, placebo-controlled trial. *Lancet* 2012; 379(9812):221–228.

Coutsoudis A, Pillay K, Spooner E, et al. Influence of infant-feeding patterns on early mother-to-child transmission of HIV-1 in Durban, South Africa: a prospective cohort study. South African Vitamin A Study Group. *Lancet*. 1999;354(9177):471–476.

De Lazzari E, León A, Arnaiz JA, et al. Hepatotoxicity of nevirapine in virologically suppressed patients according to gender and CD4 cell counts. *HIV Med*. 2008;9:221–226.

de Lourdes Teixeira M, Nafea S, Yeganeh N, et al. High rates of baseline antiretroviral resistance among HIV-infected pregnant women in an HIV referral centre in Rio de Janeiro, Brazil. *Int J STD AIDS*. November 2015;26(13):922–928.

Dickover RE, Dillon M, Gillette SG, et al. Rapid increases in load of human immunodeficiency virus correlate with early disease progression and loss of CD4 cells in vertically infected infants. *J Infect Dis*. 1994;170:1279–1284.

Dickover RE, Dillon M, Leung KM, et al. Early prognostic indicators in primary perinatal human immunodeficiency virus type 1 infection: importance of viral RNA and the timing of transmission on long-term outcome. *J Infect Dis*. 1998;178:375–387.

Dickover RE, Garratty EM, Herman SA, et al. Identification of levels of maternal HIV-1 RNA associated with risk of perinatal transmission. Effect of maternal zidovudine treatment on viral load. *JAMA*. 1996;275(8):599–605.

Dorenbaum A, Cunningham CK, Gelber RD, et al. Two-dose intrapartum/newborn nevirapine and standard antiretroviral therapy to reduce perinatal HIV transmission: a randomized trial. *JAMA*. 2002;288:189–198.

Duliege AM, Amos CI, Felton S, et al. Birth order, delivery route, and concordance in the transmission of human immunodeficiency virus type 1 from mothers to twins. International Registry of HIV-Exposed Twins. *J Pediatr*. 1995;126:625–632.

Dunn DT, Newell ML, Ades AE, et al. Risk of human immunodeficiency virus type 1 transmission through breastfeeding. *Lancet*. 1992;340:585–588.

European Collaborative Study. Children born to women with HIV-1 infection: natural history and risk of transmission. *Lancet*. 1991;337:253–260.

Flynn PM, Taha TE, Cababasay M, et al. Prevention of HIV-1 transmission through breastfeeding: efficacy and safety of maternal antiretroviral therapy versus infant nevirapine prophylaxis for duration of breastfeeding in HIV-1-infected women with high CD4 cell count (IMPAACT PROMISE): a randomized, open-label, clinical trial. *J AIDS*. April 1, 2018;77(4):383–392.

Fowler MG, Newell ML. Breastfeeding and HIV-1 transmission in resource-limited settings. *J AIDS*. 2002;30:230–239.

Fowler MG, Qin M, Fiscus SA, et al. Benefits and risks of antiretroviral therapy for perinatal HIV prevention. *N Engl J Med*. 2016;375(18):1726–1737.

Gabiano C, Tovo PA, de Martino M, et al. Mother-to-child transmission of human immunodeficiency virus type 1: risk of infection and correlates of transmission. *Pediatrics*. 1992;90:369–374.

Gortmaker SL, Hughes M, Cervia J, et al.; Pediatric AIDS Clinical Trials Group Protocol 219 Team. Effect of combination therapy including protease inhibitors on mortality among children and adolescents infected with HIV-1. *N Engl J Med*. 2001;345(21):1522–1528.

Guay LA, Musoke P, Fleming T, et al. Intrapartum and neonatal single-dose nevirapine compared with zidovudine for prevention of mother-to-child transmission of HIV-1 in Kampala, Uganda: HIVNET 012 randomised trial. *Lancet*. 1999;354(9181):795–802.

Hitti J, Frenkel LM, Stek AM, et al.; PACTG 1022 Study Team. Maternal toxicity with continuous nevirapine in pregnancy: results from PACTG 1022. *J AIDS*. 2004;36:772–776.

Inter-agency Task Team on the Prevention and Treatment of HIV Infection in Pregnant Women Mothers and Children (IATT) CDC WHO and UNICEF. Monitoring & evaluation framework for antiretroviral treatment for pregnant and breastfeeding women living with HIV and their infants. 2015. Available at http://www.who.int/hiv/mtct/iatt-me-framework/en/. Accessed October 14, 2018.

International Perinatal HIV Group. The mode of delivery and the risk of vertical transmission of human immunodeficiency virus type 1—a meta-analysis of 15 prospective cohort studies. *N Engl J Med*. 1999;340(13):977–987.

Jeremy RJ, Kim S, Nozyce M, et al.; Pediatric AIDS Clinical Trials Group (PACTG) 338 & 377 Study Teams. Neuropsychological functioning and viral load in stable antiretroviral therapy-experienced HIV-infected children. *Pediatrics*. 2005;115:380–387.

Lahoz R, Noguera A, Rovira N, et al. Antiretroviral-related hematologic short-term toxicity in healthy infants: implications of the new neonatal 4-week zidovudine regimen. *Ped Inf Dis J*. 2010;29(4):376–379.

Louis J, Landon MB, Gersnoviez RJ, et al. Perioperative morbidity and mortality among human immunodeficiency virus infected women undergoing cesarean delivery. *Obstet Gynecol* 2007;110(2 Pt 1):385–390.

Luzuriaga K, Bryson Y, Krogstad P, et al. Combination treatment with zidovudine, didanosine, and nevirapine in infants with human immunodeficiency virus type 1 infection. *N Engl J Med*. 1997;336:1343–1349.

Luzuriaga K, Gay H, Ziemniak C, et al. Viremic relapse after HIV-1 remission in a perinatally infected child. *N Engl J Med*. 2015;372:786–788.

Luzuriaga K, Koup RA, Pikora CA, et al. Deficient human immunodeficiency virus type 1-specific cytotoxic T cell responses in vertically infected children. *J Pediatr*. 1991;119:230–236.

Luzuriaga K, McManus M, Mofenson L, et al.; PACTG 356 Investigators. A trial of three antiretroviral regimens in HIV-1-infected children. *N Engl J Med*. 2004; 350(24):2471–2480.

Lyimo MA, Mosi MN, Housman ML, et al. Breast milk from Tanzanian women has divergent effects on cell-free and cell-associated HIV-1 infection in vitro. *PLoS One*. 2012;7(8):e43815.

Magder LS, Mofenson L, Paul ME, et al. Risk factors for in utero and intrapartum transmission of HIV. *J AIDS*. 2005;38:87–95.

Marazzi CM, Germano P, Liotta G, et al. Implementing anti-retroviral triple therapy to prevent HIV mother-to-child transmission: a public health approach in resource-limited settings. *Eur J Pediatr*. 2007;166(12):1305–1307.

Marazzi MC, Liotta G, Nielsen-Saines K, et al. Extended antenatal antiretroviral use correlates with improved infant outcomes throughout the first year of life. *AIDS*. 2010;24(18):2819–2826.

Marazzi MC, Nielsen-Saines K, Buonomo E, et al. Increased infant human immunodeficiency virus-type one free survival at one year of age in sub-Saharan Africa with maternal use of highly active antiretroviral therapy during breast-feeding. *Ped Inf Dis J*. 2009;28(6):483–487.

Marston M, Becquet R, Zaba B, et al. Net survival of perinatally and postnatally HIV-infected children: a pooled analysis of individual data from sub-Saharan Africa. *Int J Epidemiol*. 2011;40:385–396.

Mayaux MJ, Burgard M, Teglas JP, et al. Neonatal characteristics in rapidly progressive perinatally acquired HIV-1 disease. The French Pediatric HIV Infection Study Group. *JAMA*. 1996;275:606–610.

Mayaux MJ, Dussaix E, Isopet J, et al. Maternal virus load during pregnancy and mother-to-child transmission of human immunodeficiency virus type 1: the French perinatal cohort studies. SEROGEST Cohort Group. *J Infect Dis*. 1997;175(1):172–175.

Minkoff H, Burns DN, Landesman S, et al. The relationship of the duration of ruptured membranes to vertical transmission of human immunodeficiency virus. *Am J Obstet Gynecol*. 1995;173:585–589.

Mora S, Zamproni I, Beccio S, et al. Longitudinal changes of bone mineral density and metabolism in antiretroviral-treated human immunodeficiency virus-infected children. *J Clin Endocrinol Metab*. 2004;89:24–28.

Morrison S, John-Stewart G, Egessa JJ, et al. Rapid antiretroviral therapy initiation for women in an HIV-1 prevention clinical trial experiencing primary HIV-1 infection during pregnancy or breastfeeding. *PLoS One*. 2015;10(10):e0140773.

Mwanyumba F, Gaillard P, Inion I, et al. Placental inflammation and perinatal transmission of HIV-1. *J AIDS*. 2002;29:262–269.

Newell ML. The natural history of vertically acquired HIV infection. The European Collaborative Study. *J Perinat Med*. 1991;19(Suppl 1):257–262.

Newell ML, Coovadia H, Cortina-Borja M, et al.; Ghent International AIDS Society (IAS) Working Group on HIV Infection in Women and Children. Mortality of infected and uninfected infants born to HIV-infected mothers in Africa: a pooled analysis. *Lancet*. 2004;364:1236–1243.

Nielsen K, Bryson YJ. Diagnosis of HIV infection in children. *Pediatr Clin N Am*. 2000;47:39–63.

Nielsen K, McSherry G, Petru A, et al. A descriptive survey of pediatric human immunodeficiency virus-infected long-term survivors. *Pediatrics*. 1997;99:pe4.

Nielsen-Saines K, Watts DH, Veloso VG, et al.; for the NICHD HPTN 040/ PACTG 1043 Protocol Team. Phase III randomized trial of the safety and efficacy of three neonatal antiretroviral regimens for prevention of intrapartum HIV-1 transmission (NICHD HPTN 040/ PACTG 1043) [Late Breaker Abstract 124LB]. Presented at the 18th Conference on Retroviruses and Opportunistic Infections, Boston, February 27–March 2, 2011.

Palumbo P, Lindsey JC, Hughes MD, et al. Antiretroviral treatment for children with peripartum nevirapine exposure. *N Engl J Med*. 2010;363:1510–1520.

Palumbo PE, Raskino C, Fiscus S, et al. Predictive value of quantitative plasma HIV RNA and CD4+ lymphocyte count in HIV-infected infants and children. *JAMA*. 1998;279:756–761.

Panel on Antiretroviral Therapy and Medical Management of HIV-Infected Children. Guidelines for the use of antiretroviral agents in pediatric HIV infection. Updated May 22, 2018. Available at https://aidsinfo.nih.gov/contentfiles/lvguidelines/pediatricguidelines.pdf. Accessed October 14, 2018.

Panel on Antiretroviral Therapy and Medical Management of HIV-Infected Children. Guidelines for the use of antiretroviral agents in pediatric HIV infection. August 11, 2011. Available at http://aidsinfo.nih.gov/contentfiles/lvguidelines/pediatricguidelines.pdf. Accessed March 25, 2011.

Panel on Antiretroviral Therapy and Medical Management of HIV-Infected Children. Guidelines for the use of antiretroviral agents in pediatric HIV infection. March 5, 2015. Available at https://aidsinfo.nih.gov/guidelines/html/2/pediatric-arv-guidelines/45/whats-new-in-the-guidelines. Accessed December 23, 2015.

Persaud D, Gay G, Ziemniak C, et al. Absence of detectable HIV-1 viremia after treatment cessation in an infant. *N Engl J Med*. 2013;369:1828–1835.

Persaud D, Palumbo PE, Ziemniak C, et al. Dynamics of the resting CD4+ T cell latent HIV reservoir in infants initiating highly active antiretroviral therapy less than six months of age. *AIDS*. July 31, 2012;26(12):1483–1490.

Polycarpou A, Ntais C, Korber BT, et al. Association between maternal and infant class I and II HLA alleles and of their concordance with the risk of perinatal HIV type 1 transmission. *AIDS. Res Hum Retroviruses*. 2002;18:741–746.

Read JS, Mwatha A, Richardson B, et al. Primary HIV-1 infection among infants in sub-Saharan Africa: HPTN 024. *J AIDS*. 2009;51(3):317–322.

Ruane PJ, DeJesus E, Berger D, et al. Antiviral activity, safety, and pharmacokinetics/pharmacodynamics of tenofovir alafenamide as 10-day monotherapy in HIV-1-positive adults. *J AIDS*. 2013;63(4):449–455.

Scarlatti G. Mother-to-child transmission of HIV-1: advances and controversies of the twentieth centuries. *AIDS Rev.* 2004;6:67–78.

Scott GB. HIV infection in children: clinical features and management. *J AIDS*. 1991;4:109–115.

Scott GB, Hutto C, Makuch RW, et al. Survival in children with perinatally acquired human immunodeficiency virus type 1 infection. *N Engl J Med*.1989;321:1791–1796.

Sei S, Boler AM, Nguyen GT, et al. Protective effect of CCR5 delta 32 heterozygosity is restricted by SDF-1 genotype in children with HIV-1 infection. *AIDS*. 2001;15:1343–1352.

Semrau K, Kuhn L, Brooks DR, et al. Dynamics of breast milk HIV-1 RNA with unilateral mastitis or abscess. *J AIDS*. 2013;62(3):348–355.

Siliciano JD, Siliciano RF. Recent developments in the search for a cure for HIV-1 infections: targeting the latent reservoir for HIV-1. *J Allergy Clin Immunol*. 2014;134:12–19.

St Louis ME, Kamenga M, Brown C, et al. Risk for perinatal HIV-1 transmission according to maternal immunologic, virologic, and placental factors. *JAMA*. 1993;269:2853–2859.

Van Rompay KK, Otsyula MG, Marthas ML, et al. Immediate zidovudine treatment protects simian immunodeficiency virus-infected newborn macaques against rapid onset of AIDS. *Antimicrob Agents Chemother*. 1995;39:125–131.

Violari A, Cotton MF, Gibb DM, et al.; CHER Study Team. Early antiretroviral therapy and mortality among HIV-infected infants. *N Engl J Med*. 2008;359:2233–2244.

World Health Organization (WHO). March 2014 Supplement to the 2013 Consolidated guidelines on the use of antiretroviral drugs for treating and preventing HIV infection recommendations for a public health approach. March 2014. Available at http://apps.who.int/iris/bitstream/10665/104264/1/9789241506830_eng.pdf?ua=1 Accessed December 29, 2015.

Yeganeh N, Kerin T, Ank B, et al. HIV antiretroviral resistance and transmission in mother-infant pairs enrolled in a large perinatal study. *Clin Inf Dis*. 2018;66(11):1770–1777.

29.

IMMUNOSUPPRESSANTS AND ANTIRETROVIRAL THERAPY IN HIV-POSITIVE TRANSPLANT PATIENTS

Carolyn Kramer and Emily Blumberg

CHAPTER GOALS

Upon completion of this chapter, the reader should be able to

- Explain the key drug-drug interactions between immunosuppressive agents and HIV antiretroviral therapy.

- Describe the expected effect of administration of protease inhibitors on drug levels and need for monitoring of immunosuppressive agents.

- Describe the expected effect of administration of non-nucleoside reverse transcriptase inhibitors on drug levels and need for monitoring of immunosuppressive agents.

- Explain the rationale behind the preferred choice of antiretroviral therapy in in HIV-positive solid organ transplant recipients.

INTRODUCTION

As survival for HIV-positive individuals improves and advances in antiretroviral therapy (ART) allow more patients to remain suppressed on more tolerable combination therapies, the focus of HIV care has shifted to management of chronic comorbidities. End-stage renal disease (ESRD) and cirrhosis occur frequently among this population due to shared comorbidities. Solid organ transplant, once considered contraindicated among HIV-positive individuals, has been increasingly successful. A retrospective review of 1,431 HIV-positive patients listed for renal transplant showed a relative risk of mortality at 5 years of 0.21 for patients who underwent transplant compared with those who remained on dialysis (Locke, 2017). Several studies have shown patient and graft survival rates for HIV-positive renal transplant recipients that are largely comparable to the transplant population as a whole. A prospective, nonrandomized US National Institutes of Health (NIH) study of 150 patients with well-controlled HIV who underwent renal transplant demonstrated 1- and 3-year patient and graft survival rates that fell below national survival rates for all renal transplant recipients but were above the rates for recipients over the age of 65 (Stock, 2010). In the absence of hepatitis C virus (HCV) coinfection, survival

rates may be even closer to that of HIV-negative recipients. A review of the Scientific Registry of Transplant Recipients which included 510 HIV-positive renal transplant recipients showed similar 5- and 10-year graft survival for HIV-negative recipients and HIV-monoinfected recipients (Locke, 2015). A similar review of national registry data evaluated more than 148,000 patients who underwent renal transplant between 1996 and 2013. Among patients who were HCV-negative, graft survival and overall survival were similar for HIV-positive and HIV-negative recipients (Sawinski, 2015). There are promising data as well for liver transplantation in HIV-positive patients. Liver transplantation confers a survival benefit in HIV-positive patients with end-stage liver disease (ESLD) and Model for End-Stage Liver Disease (MELD) score of greater than 15 (Roland, 2016). In the absence of HCV coinfection, HIV-positive liver transplant recipients have a risk of death and graft loss similar to that of uninfected recipients (Sawinski, 2015). Cardiac transplant in HIV-positive patients is infrequent, and data on outcomes are limited. However, recent case reports describe successful heart transplant in HIV-positive patients who maintained viral suppression with a 5-year survival rate similar to that of HIV-negative heart transplant recipients (Aguero, 2016).

Managing interactions between immunosuppressive agents and ART can be a particularly challenging aspect of caring for the HIV-positive transplant recipient. In the outpatient setting, clinicians will most frequently encounter maintenance immunosuppressive regimens consisting of a combination of a calcineurin inhibitor (tacrolimus or cyclosporine), corticosteroids, and potentially an antiproliferative agent (mycophenolate mofetil or azathioprine). In some cases, a mammalian target of rapamycin (mTOR) inhibitor (sirolimus or everolimus) will be used in place of one of these agents or as adjunctive therapy. Understanding the pharmacokinetics of each of these drug classes is crucial to safely managing ART. Calcineurin inhibitors are substrates as well as weak inhibitors of cytochrome P450 3A4 (CYP3A4) and therefore have potential for significant interaction with antiretroviral agents that are inhibitors or inducers of CYP3A4. mTOR inhibitors are substrates of CYP3A4, and dosing must be adjusted in the presence of inhibitors or inducers of CYP3A4. The antimetabolites mycophenolate mofetil and azathioprine are not substrates for CYP3A4, and they have no expected or documented interactions with ART.

Explain the key drug–drug interactions between immunosuppressive agents and ART in HIV-positive solid organ transplant recipients.

WHAT'S NEW?

With the increase in number and availability of integrase inhibitors, clinicians and patients can frequently choose an antiretroviral regimen that minimizes the risk of drug interactions while limiting side effects, maintaining ease of administration, and preserving a high barrier to resistance.

KEY POINTS

- Protease inhibitors (PIs), especially ritonavir, are potent inhibitors of CYP3A4. They can significantly increase levels of calcineurin inhibitors (tacrolimus or cyclosporine) and mTOR inhibitors (sirolimus or everolimus). Whenever possible PI-free regimens are preferred.

- Cobicistat is an inhibitor of CYP3A4, and its effect on levels of calcineurin inhibitors and mTOR inhibitors is likely to be similar to that of ritonavir.

- Some non-nucleoside reverse transcriptase inhibitors (NNRTIs) are clinically significant inducers of CYP3A4. Efavirenz in particular may result in lower concentrations of calcineurin inhibitors and mTOR inhibitors.

- Dose reduction and careful attention to monitoring drug levels are critical to avoid toxicity and maintain therapeutic immunosuppressive concentrations when PIs or cobicistat are coadministered with calcineurin inhibitors or mTOR inhibitors. If NNRTIs are used, calcineurin inhibitor and mTOR inhibitor doses may need to be increased; careful monitoring is required.

- Nucleoside/nucleotide reverse transcriptase inhibitors (NRTIs) are not metabolized by CYP3A4, nor are they inducers or inhibitors of CYP3A4. These classes are not expected to significantly alter dosing or levels of immunosuppressants.

- Some integrase inhibitors are metabolized in part by CYP3A4; however, none is a significant inducer or inhibitor of CYP3A4. As a class, integrase inhibitors would not be expected to alter levels of calcineurin inhibitors or mTOR inhibitors. Mycophenolate mofetil and azathioprine are not substrates for CYP3A4 and have no expected or documented interactions with ART.

- Although there is no formalized recommendation for the ideal ART regimen in HIV-positive transplant recipients, a regimen consisting of two NRTIs and an integrase inhibitor minimizes the risk of drug–drug interactions and simplifies dosing of immunosuppressive agents while maintaining a high barrier to resistance.

KEY DRUG–DRUG INTERACTIONS

PROTEASE INHIBITORS

PIs are both substrates and inhibitors of CYP3A4. Both boosted (i.e., coadministered with ritonavir or cobicistat) and unboosted PIs can significantly alter metabolism of calcineurin inhibitors and mTOR inhibitors, resulting in increased levels of these immunosuppressive agents. Case reports of coadministration of calcineurin inhibitors and PIs suggest that significant dose reductions in tacrolimus or cyclosporine and frequent monitoring of drug levels are critical to minimize toxicity related to overexposure and to avoid subtherapeutic trough levels. An observational study of patients undergoing orthotopic liver transplantation found that those who initiated therapy with lopinavir/ritonavir required a dose reduction of tacrolimus of 99% to maintain therapeutic levels (Teicher, 2007). A similar dose reduction is necessary to maintain appropriate trough levels of cyclosporine when coadministered with PIs. Liver transplant recipients receiving a ritonavir-boosted PI showed an increase in half-life of cyclosporine of up to 38 hours, requiring reductions to 5–20% of standard doses (Vogel, 2004). Even with awareness of the need for drastic dose reduction, achieving stable target levels can be difficult. A 2017 case report of a renal transplant patient receiving an antiretroviral regimen of darunavir, ritonavir, and dolutegravir showed an increase in tacrolimus level to well above the desired target level despite initial dose reduction and close monitoring (Yilmaz, 2017). Modeling pharmacokinetic curves of pretransplant test doses of tacrolimus in patients on a ritonavir-boosted regimen may allow for more targeted posttransplant dosing (van Maarseveen, 2013). mTOR inhibitors have shown similar pharmacokinetic alterations when coadministered with PIs. A case study of an HIV-positive liver transplant recipient who initiated nelfinavir showed that the 24-hour trough level of sirolimus was increased by fivefold, peak concentration was increased by 3.2 times, and half-life was extended by 60% (Jain, 2002). While some adjustments can be made to immunosuppressant dosing in the setting of PI use, there is evidence that graft and overall survival are reduced for patients who remain on these regimens. In a review of 332 HIV-positive kidney transplant recipients, risk of graft loss was 1.8 times higher and risk of death was 1.9 times higher compared with HIV-positive renal transplant recipients receiving non-PI based regimens (Sawinski, 2017). Given the difficulties managing immunosuppressive regimens in patients receiving PIs, their avoidance is recommended whenever possible.

Cobicistat (which is structurally very similar to ritonavir but lacks direct activity against HIV) is an inhibitor of CYP3A4, and similar caution should be used when coadministered with an immunosuppressive regimen. In a 2016 case report, a renal transplant recipient who began a cobicistat-containing HIV regimen demonstrated elevated tacrolimus levels and acute kidney injury (Han, 2016). Consequently, cobisistat-based regimens should be avoided whenever possible.

NON-NUCLEOSIDE REVERSE TRANSCRIPTASE INHIBITORS

The most commonly administered NNRTIs are substrates of CYP3A4. In addition, efavirenz, nevirapine, and etravirine are inducers of CYP3A4. Although published data are sparse, the effect of NNRTIs on immunosuppressant metabolism may be greatest for efavirenz. In a study of 35 liver or kidney transplant patients, those taking efavirenz required significantly increased doses of cyclosporine (Frassetto, 2007). A case report of a heart transplant recipient taking efavirenz demonstrated a need for an increased dose of everolimus to maintain therapeutic levels (Durante-Mangoni, 2014). Available data suggest that the effect may be less pronounced for concomitant administration of nevirapine and immunosuppressants. In a 2013 pharmacokinetic analysis, a significantly higher dose of cyclosporine was required for patients taking efavirenz than for those taking nevirapine. The same study showed no clinically significant effect on pharmacokinetics of tacrolimus for patients taking concomitant nevirapine (Frasetto, 2013). There is limited information regarding rilpivirine interactions; therapeutic dose monitoring is recommended for all patients on calcineurin inhibitors or mTOR inhibitors and rilpivirine. Transplant recipients on an antiretroviral regimen that includes an NNRTI, particularly efavirenz, should have immunosuppressant levels monitored closely, with the expectation that they may require higher doses of calcineurin and mTOR inhibitors than typically administered.

NUCLEOSIDE REVERSE TRANSCRIPTASE INHIBITORS

NRTIs are not metabolized via the CYP pathway, and there is no expected interaction between immunosuppressant agents and NRTIs. A pharmacokinetic study of tacrolimus coadministered with tenofovir/emtricitabine to healthy volunteers demonstrated no clinically relevant interaction between these drugs (Chittick, 2008). Case reports among HIV-positive transplant recipients are consistent with this expectation. A 2007 study of tacrolimus pharmacokinetics in HIV-positive liver transplant recipients reported little change in the tacrolimus dose required to maintain therapeutic levels in a patient who initiated therapy with an NRTI-based regimen (Teicher, 2007). The current standard dual-NRTI backbone of ART appears to be appropriate and safe in transplant recipients and does not require alterations to standard doses of immunosuppressive agents.

INTEGRASE INHIBITORS

Integrase inhibitors, which are metabolized by glucuronidation and, to varying degrees, via CYP3A4, are neither inducers nor inhibitors of CYP3A4. As a class, they have been shown to have negligible effect on levels of calcineurin inhibitors and mTOR inhibitors. Although experience is greatest with raltegravir, the absence of interaction and stability of immunosuppressant dosing are likely to be similar for other integrase inhibitors, including bictegravir. A pharmacokinetic study among four HIV-positive liver transplant recipients showed no interaction between raltegravir and cyclosporine (Barau, 2014), and case reports have demonstrated successful coadministration of these agents (Di Biagio, 2009). Case reports and a small retrospective study have shown similar stability without dose adjustment of tacrolimus when administered with raltegravir (Bickel, 2010; Miro, 2010). An observational study of 13 HIV-positive liver and kidney transplant recipients maintained on a combination of two NRTIs and raltegravir found that target levels of tacrolimus and cyclosporine were stable and easily achieved with no adjustment to standard immunosuppressant doses. Among these 13 patients, HIV viral suppression was maintained, and there were no cases of acute rejection (Tricot, 2009). Data for sirolimus, although limited, suggest a similar safety profile without need for dose adjustment. A case report of a liver transplant recipient with tacrolimus-induced renal toxicity in the setting of PI coadministration demonstrated safety of raltegravir and sirolimus with no adjustment to standard dosing of sirolimus (Moreno, 2008). Because dolutegravir interferes with tubular secretion of creatinine, mild elevations of creatinine may occur that do not represent a decline in glomerular filtration rate (Lee, 2016).

Integrase inhibitors provide a safe option for ART that, when combined with dual NRTIs, avoids clinically relevant drug interactions with immunosuppressive agents.

SUMMARY

In caring for HIV-positive organ transplant recipients, understanding interactions between immunosuppressive agents and ART is critical to maintaining viral suppression and promoting longevity of the transplant organ. PIs, as inhibitors of CYP3A4, can drastically increase levels of calcineurin inhibitors and mTOR inhibitors, resulting in overexposure and potential toxicity if doses are not adjusted and levels monitored carefully. Some NNRTIs, particularly efavirenz, are inducers of CYP3A4 and can decrease levels of calcineurin inhibitors and mTOR inhibitors, resulting in subtherapeutic trough levels and ultimately increasing the risk of rejection. The ideal ART regimen, although not formally defined, may be a combination of NRTIs and an integrase inhibitor; neither of these classes has significant interactions with calcineurin inhibitors or mTOR inhibitors. Clinicians caring for HIV-positive transplant recipients should be aware of the key interactions between ART and immunosuppressive agents and take these interactions into consideration when initiating or adjusting antiretroviral regimens.

ACKNOWLEDGMENTS

This chapter is an extension of the work by the authors of previous editions of this chapter, Ian R. McNicholl and Joan J. McNicholl.

RECOMMENDED READING

Blumberg EA, Rogers CC; AST Infectious Diseases Community of Practice. Human immunodeficiency virus in solid organ transplantation. *Am J Transplant*. 2013;13(Suppl 4):169–178.

Conte AH, Kittleson, MM, Dilibero D, et al. Successful orthotopic heart transplantation and immunosuppressive management in 2 human immunodeficiency virus-seropositive patients. *Tex Heart Inst J*. 2016;43(1):69–74.

Locke JE, James NT, Mannon RB, et al. Immunosuppression regimen and the risk of acute rejection in HIV-infected kidney transplant recipients. *Transplantation*. 2014;97(4):446–450.

REFERENCES

Aguero F, Castel MA, Cocchi S, et al. An update on heart transplantation in human immunodeficiency virus-infected patients. *Am J Transplant*. 2016;16(1):21–28.

Barau C, Braun J, Vincent C, et al. Pharmacokinetic study of raltegravir in HIV-infected patients with end-stage liver disease: the LIVERAL-ANRS 148 study. *Clin Infect Dis*. 2014;59(8):1177–1184.

Bickel M, Anadol E, Vogel M, et al. Daily dosing of tacrolimus in patients treated with HIV-1 therapy containing a ritonavir-boosted protease inhibitor or raltegravir. *J Antimicrob Chemother*. 2010;65(5):999–1004.

Chittick GE, Zong J, Begley JA, et al. Pharmacokinetics of emtricitabine/tenofovir disoproxil fumarate and tacrolimus at steady state when administered alone or in combination. *Int J Clin Pharmacol Ther*. 2008;46(12):627–636.

Di Biagio A, Rosso R, Siccardi M, et al. Lack of interaction between raltegravir and cyclosporine in an HIV-infected liver transplant recipient. *J Antimicrob Chemother*. 2009;64(4):874–875.

Durante-Mangoni E, Maiello C, Limongelli G, et al. Management of immunosuppression and antiretroviral treatment before and after heart transplant for HIV-associated dilated cardiomyopathy. *Int J Immunopathol Pharmacol*. 2014;27(1):113–120.

Frasetto L, Floren L, Barin B, et al. Changes in clearance, volume, and bioavailability of immunosuppressants when given with HAART in HIV-1 infected liver and kidney transplant recipients. *Biopharm Drug Dispos*. 2013;34(8):442–451.

Frassetto LA, Browne M, Cheng A, et al. Immunosuppressant pharmacokinetics and dosing modifications in HIV-1 infected liver and kidney transplant recipients. *Am J Transplant*. 2007;7(12):2816–2820.

Han Z, Kane BM, Petty LA, et al. Cobicistat significantly increases tacrolimus serum concentrations in a renal transplant recipient with human immunodeficiency virus infection. *Pharmacotherapy*. 2016;36(6):e50–53.

Jain AK, Venkataramanan R, Fridell JA, et al. Nelfinavir, a protease inhibitor, increases sirolimus levels in a liver transplantation patient: a case report. *Liver Transpl*. 2002;8(9):838–840.

Lee DH, Malat GE, Bias TE, et al. Serum creatinine elevation after switch to dolutegravir in a human immunodeficiency virus-positive kidney transplant recipient. *Trans Inf Disease*. 2016;18(4):625–627.

Locke JE, Gustafson MD, Mehta S, et al. Survival benefit of kidney transplantation in HIV-infected patients. *Ann Surg*. 2017;265(3):604–608.

Locke JE, Mehta S, Reed RD, et al. A national study of outcomes among HIV-infected kidney transplant recipients. *J Am Soc Nephrol*. 2015;265:2222–2229.

Moreno A, Barcena R, Quereda C, et al. Safe use of raltegravir and sirolimus in an HIV-infected patient with renal impairment after orthotopic liver transplantation. *AIDS*. 2008;22(4):547–548.

Miro JM, Ricart MJ, Trullas JC, et al. Simultaneous pancreas–kidney transplantation in HIV-infected patients: a case report and literature review. *Transplant Proc*. 2010; 42(9):3887–3891.

Roland ME, Barin B, Huprikar S, et al.; HIVTR Study Team. Survival in HIV-positive transplant recipients compared with transplant candidates and with HIV-negative controls. *AIDS*. January 28, 2016;30(3):435–444.

Sawinski D, Forde KA, Eddinger K, Troxel AB, et al. Superior outcomes in HIV-positive kidney transplant patients compared with HCV-infected or HIV/HCV coinfected recipients. *Kidney International*. 2015;88:341–349.

Sawinski D, Goldberg DS, Blumberg E, et al. Beyond the NIH multicenter HIV transplant trial experience: outcomes of HIV+ liver transplant recipients compared to HCV+ or HIV+/HCV+ coinfected recipients in the United States. *Clin Infect Dis*. 2015;61(7):1054–1062.

Sawinski D, Shelton B, Mehta S, et al. Impact of protease inhibitor-based anti-retroviral therapy on outcomes for HIV kidney transplant recipients. *Am J Transpl*. 2017;17(12):3114–3122.

Stock PG, Barin B, Murphy B, et al. Outcomes of kidney transplantation in HIV-infected recipients. *N Engl J Med*. 2010;363(21):2004–2014.

Teicher E, Vincent I, Bonhomme-Faivre L, et al. Effect of highly active antiretroviral therapy on tacrolimus pharmacokinetics in hepatitis C and HIV co-infected liver transplant recipients in the ANRS HC-80 study. *Clin Pharmacokinet*. 2007;46(11):941–952.

Tricot L, Teicher E, Peytavin G, et al. Safety and efficacy of raltegravir in HIV-infected transplant patients cotreated with immunosuppressive drugs. *Am J Transplant*. 2009;9(8):1946–1952.

van Maarseveen EM, Crommelin HA, Mudrikova T, et al. Pretransplant pharmacokinetic curves of tacrolimus in HIV-infected patients on ritonavir-containing cART: a pilot study. *Transplantation*. 2013;95(2):397–402.

Vogel M, Voigt E, Michaelis HC, et al. Management of drug-to-drug interactions between cyclosporine A and the protease-inhibitor lopinavir/ritonavir in liver-transplanted HIV-infected patients. *Liver Transpl*. 2004;10(7):939–944.

Yilmaz, Gokengin D, Bozbiyik O, et al. Kidney transplant in a Human Immunodeficiency Virus positive patient: case report of drug interactions. *Exp Clin Transplant*. 2017; epub.

30.

UNDERSTANDING AND MANAGING ANTINEOPLASTIC AND ANTIRETROVIRAL THERAPY

Jason J. Schafer, Elizabeth M. Sherman, Taylor K. Gill, and Jatandra Birney

---

CHAPTER GOAL

Upon completion of this chapter, the reader should be able to

- Identify contemporary challenges and describe strategies in managing antineoplastic and antiretroviral therapy in patients with cancer and HIV infection.

INTRODUCTION TO CANCER IN HIV

In 2010, more than 7,500 of the estimated 1.1 million people living with HIV (PLWH) in the United States were diagnosed with cancer (National Comprehensive Cancer Network [NCCN] Guidelines, 2018). The incidence is approximately 50% greater than the incidence of cancer expected in the general population. The elevated risk of cancer in PLWH is likely multifactorial and due to underlying immune deficiency, coinfection with oncogenic viruses, and a higher prevalence of other cancer-related risk factors such as the use of tobacco products.

LEARNING OBJECTIVE

To review both general and specific concepts regarding the safe and effective use of antineoplastic and antiretroviral therapy (ART) in patients living with HIV and cancer.

WHAT'S NEW?

To address the challenges of complicated interactions and toxicities associated with antiretroviral and antineoplastic therapies, patients living with HIV and cancer should receive multidisciplinary care that includes primary care providers, infectious disease clinicians, hematologists/oncologists, and clinical pharmacists.

KEY POINTS

- The use of combination ART in patients with malignancies is associated with improved HIV- and cancer-related outcomes.

- Combining antiretroviral and antineoplastic therapy is often complicated by significant drug–drug interactions, drug–disease state monitoring interactions, and overlapping toxicities.

- Definitive pharmacokinetic studies evaluating drug interactions between antineoplastics and antiretrovirals are uncommon, and clinical judgment must often be used to determine the potential for significant interactions.

- Adjusting ART in response to significant drug interactions or overlapping toxicities is often more feasible than modifying antineoplastic protocols.

Before the widespread use of ART, AIDS-defining malignancies (ADMs) such as Kaposi's sarcoma, non-Hodgkin's lymphoma, and invasive cervical cancer accounted for the largest burden of cancer in PLWH (Rubinstein, 2014). These malignancies occur most commonly in patients with severe immune suppression characterized by advanced HIV, and all are associated with oncogenic viruses.

Following the widespread use of combination ART in the mid-1990s, a substantial decline in the number of new AIDS diagnoses and AIDS-related deaths was observed (Rubinstein, 2014). The ability to reconstitute the immune system with ART also led to a decrease in ADMs. During the same time period, however, the occurrence of non–AIDS-defining malignancies (NADMs) increased. These malignancies include Hodgkin's lymphoma, leukemia, and cancers of the head, neck, lung, kidney, liver, gastrointestinal tract, anus, and skin. Currently, NADMs cause more cancer-related morbidity and mortality than ADMs and will remain common among PLWH, with lung and prostate cancer expected to emerge as the most prevalent cancer types in the next decade (Shiels, 2018).

Although ADMs most commonly occur in patients with severe immune suppression, low $CD4^+$ T cell counts (<500 cells/mm^3) have been identified as a risk factor for both ADMs and NADMs (Torres, 2014). This suggests that initiating ART to suppress HIV replication and reconstituting $CD4^+$ T cell counts may reduce the overall risk of malignancies in patients living with HIV. Recently, viral suppression, particularly long-term suppression with ART, has been linked with ADM and

NADM prevention. Despite this, cancer risk can remain elevated even in virally suppressed PLWH in comparison to persons without HIV infection (Park, 2018).

In patients with cancer, the use of ART alongside chemotherapy is now routinely recommended to improve overall survival. The administration of chemotherapy and ART concurrently can be complicated by a number of factors (Rudek, 2011), including limited data regarding safe and effective therapy combinations; significant drug–drug interactions among ART, antineoplastics, and supportive care medications; drug–disease state monitoring interactions; and overlapping drug toxicities (Table 30.1). This chapter reviews contemporary information regarding the use of chemotherapy and ART in combination, including strategies for managing potential and established drug–drug interactions and considerations for preventing and/or monitoring for toxicity.

GENERAL CONSIDERATIONS FOR COMBINING ANTINEOPLASTIC AND ANTIRETROVIRAL THERAPY

DRUG INTERACTIONS: CYP450

Drug interactions between ART and antineoplastic agents may occur via several different mechanisms. The most common are the interactions that occur during metabolism of medications from active to inactive substances via the hepatic cytochrome P450 system (CYP450). Medications may be substrates of the CYP450 system, meaning that they use this system for metabolism, and their concentrations may be altered by concurrent administration with other agents. In addition, medications may be inducers or inhibitors of individual CYP450 isoenzymes, such as 3A4. CYP450 inducers will increase the metabolism of CYP450 substrates, thus decreasing the concentration of medication, which may lead to subtherapeutic medication levels. Conversely, CYP450 inhibitors will decrease the metabolism of CYP450 substrates, thus increasing the medication concentration, which may lead to toxicity. The timing of the CYP450 interactions may also vary as enzyme inhibition occurs rapidly, with maximum effect occurring when a medication is at steady state and enzyme induction occurring more slowly due to the need for enzyme synthesis (Di Francia, 2014). Many antiretroviral, antineoplastic, and supportive care medications utilize the CYP450 system for metabolism, and drug interactions are expected to be a challenge in this setting.

DRUG INTERACTIONS: P-GLYCOPROTEIN

To add to the complexity of interactions that occur with medication metabolism, there may also be absorption interactions with the p-glycoprotein efflux pump in the gastrointestinal tract. Similar to the CYP450 interactions, medications may be p-glycoprotein substrates, inducers, or inhibitors. P-glycoprotein inducers stimulate the efflux of medications back into the gastrointestinal lumen thus decreasing the absorption and plasma concentrations of these medications. Likewise, p-glycoprotein inhibitors will increase the absorption of medication and increase plasma concentrations of substrates, which could lead to toxicities. Literature has shown that p-glycoprotein is highly expressed in HIV-associated malignancies such as non-Hodgkin's lymphoma and plays a significant role in the effectiveness of both antiretroviral and antineoplastic therapy (Klibanov, 2007). Clinicians should be aware of antiretroviral, antineoplastic, and supportive care agents that affect p-glycoprotein and should realize the potential for drug interactions with medications that influence, or are influenced by, this mechanism.

MEDICATION TOXICITIES

Clinicians will also need to consider overlapping toxicities of medication classes. Some ART and antineoplastic agents are known for causing severe adverse effects that may become additive when used in combination. It is vitally important when devising medication regimens that serious adverse effects of all agents be identified and overlapping toxicities minimized when possible.

DRUG–DISEASE INTERACTIONS

The presence of drug–disease interactions will need to be recognized when combining antiretroviral and antineoplastic agents. Disease monitoring interactions are a concern because there are certain antiretroviral medications that increase oncologic disease markers such as bilirubin. Conversely, there are also concerns that antineoplastic agents may affect the level of CD4+ T cells, rendering the monitoring parameters of both disease states inaccurate (Klibanov, 2007). To supplement these monitoring parameter concerns, there may also be medication absorption concerns due to the presence of disease complications such as gastrointestinal tumors, mucositis, and graft-versus-host disease (Torres, 2014). Clinicians may need to be creative in these situations, such as selecting medication regimens available in liquid formulations or alternative routes of administration.

The key concepts of drug interactions, overlapping toxicities, and drug–disease interactions are just a few examples of the complexity in utilizing combination antiretroviral and antineoplastic therapy. Specific literature and guideline recommendations to assist in the selection, dosing, and monitoring of these agents when used in combination are scarce. Thus, these concepts should be considered on a case-by-case basis and explored when crafting a medication regimen in the treatment of both HIV and oncologic diseases.

Table 30.1 POTENTIAL DRUG INTERACTIONS AND OVERLAPPING TOXICITIES IN A SAMPLE OF COMMONLY USED ANTINEOPLASTIC AND ANTIRETROVIRAL AGENTS

ANTINEOPLASTIC	SOME CANCERS TREATED	INFLUENCES OR INFLUENCED BY CYP450	OTHER METABOLISM	INFLUENCES OR INFLUENCED BY P-GLYCOPROTEIN	DOCUMENTATION OF INTERACTIONS WITH ANTIRETROVIRAL THERAPY	OVERLAPPING TOXICITY	COMMENT
Folate Antagonists							
Methotrexate	Most cancers	No	Renal (80% unchanged drug)	No	No	Renal, BMS	Caution when used with sulfamethoxazole–trimethoprim
Pyrimidine/Purine Antagonists							
5-Fluorouracil	A, C, Br, L, Pan, H&N	Yes	DPD metabolism	No	No	Mucositis, diarrhea, rash	
Cytarabine	Leuk, HD, NHL	Yes	Cytidine deaminase	No	No	Renal, BMS	
Gemcitabine	Br, HD, NHL, L, Pan, S	No	Cytidine deaminase	No	No	BMS, hepatic	
Platinums							
Cisplatin	Most solid tumors	No	Possibly spontaneous degradation	Yes	No	Renal, PN	May need to renally adjust ART due to cisplatin toxicity
Carboplatin	B, Br, H&N, L	No	Spontaneous hydrolysis	No	No data available	N	Active study pending results with ART and carboplatin
Oxaliplatin	C, HD, NHI, Br, Pan	No	Extensive biotransformation in blood	No	No	N	
Alkylating Agents							
Cyclophosphamide/iphosphamide	Most cancers	Yes	Renal excretion	No	No	BMS, renal	
Dacarbazine	B, HD, Pan, S	Yes	Hepatic activation	No	Yes	Hepatic	Regimen ABVD with ritonavir-boosted regimen had documented increased toxicities
Procarbazine	B, HD, L, MM, NHL	Yes	Renal excretion	No	No	BMS, rash	

(continued)

Table 30.1 CONTINUED

ANTINEOPLASTIC	SOME CANCERS TREATED	INFLUENCES OR INFLUENCED BY CYP450	OTHER METABOLISM	INFLUENCES OR INFLUENCED BY P-GLYCOPROTEIN	DOCUMENTATION OF INTERACTIONS WITH ANTIRETROVIRAL THERAPY	OVERLAPPING TOXICITY	COMMENT
Antitumor Antibiotics							
Dactinomycin	Leuk, Br, KS, S	Unknown	Hepatic	Yes	No data available	BMS, hepatic, rash	
Doxorubicin	Leuk, Br, H&N, KS, HD, NHL, L, MM, S	Yes	Hepatic	Yes	No	BMS, hepatic	Regimen ABVD with ritonavir-boosted regimen had documented increased toxicities
Idarubicin	Leuk	Yes	Plasma	No	No	BMS	
Bleomycin	H&D, HD, NHL, KS, S	Unknown	Intracellular hydrolysis	No	Yes	Renal, rash	Regimen ABVD with ritonavir-boosted regimen had documented increased toxicities
Mitomycin	A, C, L, Br, Pan, H&N	Unknown	Hepatic	Yes	No data available	BMS	No data published about interactions with ART in anal cancer studies
Microtubules							
Vinblastine	Br, Leuk, H&N, HD, NHL, KS, L	Yes	Hepatic	Yes	Yes	N	Caution when used with ritonavir-boosted regimens
Vincristine	Leuk, B, Br, CRC, S, H&N, KS, L, MM, P, HD, NHL	Yes	Hepatic	Yes	No	N	
Taxanes							
Docetaxel	L, H&N, Br, KS, Pan, S	Yes	Hepatic	Yes	Yes	N, BMS	Caution when used with ritonavir-boosted regimens
Paclitaxel	Br, H&N, L, KS	Yes	Hepatic	Yes	Yes	BMS, mucositis	Conflicting reports of interactions in published data

A, anal; ART, antiretroviral therapy; ABVD, doxorubicin, bleomycin, vinblastine, dacarbazine; B, brain; BMS, bone marrow suppression; Br, breast; C, ; CRC, colorectal; DPD, dihydropyrimidine dehydrogenase; G, gastric; HD, Hodgkin's lymphoma; H&N, head and neck; KS, Kaposi's sarcoma; L, lung; Leuk, leukemia; MM, Multiple myeloma; N, neck; NHL, non-Hodgkin lymphoma; Pan, pancreas; S, sarcoma; UGT, uridine 5'-diphosphoglucuronosyltransferase.

SOURCE: Gold Standard, Inc. Clinical pharmacology [database online]. Available at http://www.clinicalpharmacology.com. Accessed December 3, 2015.

SPECIFIC CONSIDERATIONS FOR COMBINING ANTINEOPLASTIC AND ANTIRETROVIRAL THERAPIES BY ANTIRETROVIRAL DRUG CLASS

ENTRY/FUSION INHIBITORS

There are limited data on the use of HIV entry/fusion inhibitors (maraviroc, enfuvirtide, and ibalizumab) with chemotherapy agents. Maraviroc, a CCR5 antagonist entry inhibitor, is a substrate of CYP3A4 but does not induce or inhibit this enzyme. It is also a substrate of p-glycoprotein. Therefore, maraviroc is unlikely to affect levels of antineoplastic drugs, although levels of maraviroc may be altered by drug interactions with antineoplastic and supportive care medications. The prescribing information for maraviroc contains a warning of hepatotoxicity associated with allergic features including rash and fever approximately 4 weeks after starting treatment (Selzentry package insert, GlaxoSmithKline). Such an adverse effect should be considered when combining maraviroc with chemotherapy agents with a high risk of hepatotoxicity due to the potential for overlapping toxicity.

Ibalizumab, a novel entry inhibitor, is a monoclonal antibody that binds the CD4 receptor and blocks HIV entry into cells. It is administered via intravenous infusion and has no significant liver or kidney metabolism. To date, no drug interaction studies have been conducted with ibalizumab. However, based on ibalizumab's mechanism of action and target-mediated drug disposition, drug–drug interactions are not expected. Use of ibalizumab in antiretroviral regimens is limited by its paucity of data, requirement for intravenous infusion every 14 days, and approval specifically for use in persons with extensive HIV drug resistance to existing ART classes.

Enfuvirtide, an HIV fusion inhibitor, is not metabolized by nor an inhibitor or inducer of CYP450 enzymes. Rather, it undergoes catabolism to its constituent amino acids. Enfuvirtide is not expected to have drug interactions with any antineoplastic agent or supportive therapy agent. However, the use of enfuvirtide is limited by its tolerability, which includes injection site reactions.

NUCLEOSIDE/NUCLEOTIDE REVERSE TRANSCRIPTASE INHIBITORS

The nucleoside/nucleotide reverse transcriptase inhibitors (NRTIs) were the first available class of antiretrovirals and are still commonly used today. The class consists of eight individual agents and is the backbone of many current HIV treatment regimens. Therefore, it should be expected that at least one and probably two agents in this class will be used concurrently with antineoplastic agents. In analyzing the concurrent usage of this class and oncologic treatments, fewer drug interactions are expected but concern regarding additive and overlapping adverse effects remains.

Regarding drug interactions, NRTIs are excreted unchanged in the urine or metabolized outside of the hepatic CYP450 system. In addition, NRTIs do not induce or inhibit any of the CYP450 enzymes. The majority of NRTIs are also completely absorbed without involvement of the p-glycoprotein system, with the exception of tenofovir disoproxil fumarate and tenofovir alafenamide, which are p-glycoprotein substrates (Torres, 2014). Due to these pharmacokinetic properties, the NRTIs have minimal drug interactions with other medications. When devising complex antineoplastic medication regimens, the NRTIs will be easy to utilize concurrently, and drug interactions should not be a major concern.

Although NRTIs have the benefits of being efficacious and easily utilized in combination regimens due to lack of drug interactions, their tolerability and adverse effects have historically been limitations. While many early NRTIs had severe adverse effect profiles (i.e., zidovudine, stavudine, and didanosine) subsequent agents in this medication class have better tolerability (i.e., lamivudine, abacavir, tenofovir, and emtricitabine). There are specific overlapping toxicities that should be considered when NRTIs and antineoplastic agents are utilized in combination:

- *Neutropenia*: The most severe and troublesome is the occurrence of neutropenia when zidovudine is used with any cytotoxic class of chemotherapy. Due to both medications causing a decrease in the white blood cell count (WBC), it is recommended to avoid the use of zidovudine and use other NRTI agents (NCCN Guidelines, 2018). If this is not possible, then it is recommended to use less toxic chemotherapy (Rudek, 2011).

- *Peripheral neuropathy*: Two specific NRTI agents, didanosine and stavudine, may cause severe and potentially nonreversible peripheral neuropathy. There are also certain classes of chemotherapy agents, such as taxanes, platinums, vinca alkaloids, and the individual agent bortezomib, that may cause peripheral neuropathy. The development of peripheral neuropathy is often dose-related and cumulative with ongoing therapy. Also, peripheral neuropathy may be expected when utilizing these agents in combination. The literature suggests using different NRTI medications or changing to an alternative chemotherapy regimen (Rudek, 2011).

- *Hepatotoxicity*: Many medications have the potential to cause hepatotoxicity, but some NRTIs have a higher propensity than others. As previously mentioned, the older NRTIs of zidovudine, didanosine, and stavudine have more adverse effects and also have the potential for hepatotoxicity. Therefore, it is recommended that these agents not be used in combination with cytotoxic chemotherapy agents that undergo hepatic metabolism. The newer NRTIs, such as abacavir, lamivudine, emtricitabine, and tenofovir, may be preferred in combination with such chemotherapy, or a reduced antineoplastic dose may be considered (Rudek, 2011).

- *Nephrotoxicity*: Tenofovir disoproxil fumarate (TDF), a commonly used NRTI, has been associated with the occurrence of nephrotoxicity. When used in combination with nephrotoxic chemotherapy such as cisplatin or carboplatin, an additive toxic effect may occur, and rigorous monitoring of serum creatinine is recommended (Rubinstein, 2014). A new formulation of tenofovir, tenofovir alafenamide (TAF), was approved by the US Food and Drug Administration (FDA) in 2015 with the aim of decreasing the adverse effect profile seen with the TDF formulation. TAF achieves higher intracellular concentrations allowing for 90% lower systemic exposure with reduced nephrotoxicity and bone mineral density abnormalities. Due to these properties, TAF may also have less overlapping renal toxicity with chemotherapy and is therefore theoretically preferable in patients receiving nephrotoxic chemotherapy (Welz, 2017).

NON-NUCLEOSIDE REVERSE TRANSCRIPTASE INHIBITORS

There are four commonly used non-nucleoside reverse transcriptase inhibitors (NNRTIs): efavirenz, nevirapine, etravirine, and rilpivirine. The potential for drug interactions with these agents is high because they are extensively metabolized by and induce or inhibit the CYP450 system. In addition, NNRTI-mediated modulation of p-glycoprotein may provide another mechanism whereby the pharmacokinetics of antineoplastic drugs are altered.

Both efavirenz and nevirapine are metabolized by CYP3A4 and CYP2B6 enzymes and induce CYP3A4. In addition, efavirenz inhibits CYP2B6, CYP3A4, and CYP2C9/19, whereas nevirapine induces CYP3A4, CYP2B6, and p-glycoprotein. The use of these NNRTIs in combination with chemotherapy agents is limited by their drug interactions and prolonged half-life. Theoretically, either efavirenz or nevirapine could lower therapeutic levels of chemotherapeutic agents that are metabolized by CYP3A4 due to strong enzyme induction. Interacting agents include vinblastine, vincristine, paclitaxel, docetaxel, iphosphamide, cyclophosphamide, tyrosine kinase inhibitors, and corticosteroids that are metabolized by CYP3A4 (Rubinstein, 2014).

Etravirine is a substrate of CYP3A4, CYP2C9, and CYP2C19, and it can both induce and inhibit P450 enzymes. Etravirine acts as an inhibitor of CYP2C9/19 and an inducer of CYP3A4 and p-glycoprotein. There is limited experience in using this NNRTI in patients with cancer, which has unpredictable drug interactions with both chemotherapeutic agents and immunosuppressants (Torres, 2014).

Rilpivirine is a substrate of CYP450 3A4 but does not induce or inhibit the CYP450 system and theoretically should not affect chemotherapeutic or immunosuppressant drug levels. Rilpivirine may cause QT-interval prolongation. Many anti-cancer agents including anthracyclines, tamoxifen, tyrosine kinase inhibitors, and arsenic trioxide may also prolong the QT interval (Welz, 2017). Coadministration of rilpivirine with these antineoplastic agents should be closely monitored. Additionally, rilpivirine may cause benign increases in serum creatinine due to inhibition of tubular creatinine secretion without effects on actual glomerular filtration. This elevation normally occurs in the first few weeks of treatment and then stabilizes. Patients receiving rilpivirine-containing ART regimens should have serum creatinine monitored routinely. If serum creatinine elevations higher than 0.1–0.4 mg/dL occur, particularly outside of this time window, other causes should be considered.

Various NNRTI-based regimens are associated with rash and hepatic transaminase elevations, and overlapping toxicities with antineoplastic agents should be considered. Hepatotoxicity is also common with most chemotherapeutic classes. The literature supports chemotherapeutic agents that can be administered without any dose reductions in the setting of liver toxicity, including cisplatin, gemcitabine, and bleomycin (Rubinstein, 2014).

INTEGRASE INHIBITORS

The integrase inhibitor class of antiretroviral medications is the newest and perhaps most diverse HIV medication class. This class includes raltegravir, elvitegravir, dolutegravir, and bictegravir. Although all have the same mechanism of action, the agents differ dramatically in terms of their pharmacokinetic profiles. Therefore, it is important to assess each agent individually in terms of drug interactions and additive adverse effect potential.

Regarding drug interactions, the first-generation integrase inhibitor raltegravir is metabolized by uridine 5-diphosphate–glucuronosyltransferase (UGT) 1A1 and is unlikely to have any major drug interactions with antineoplastic therapy (Beumer, 2014). Conversely, elvitegravir is a CYP450 3A4 substrate and modest 2C9 inducer and must be boosted by the potent CYP3A4 and 2D6 inhibitor cobicistat. Therefore, when boosted, or given as the once-daily single-tablet regimen of Stribild or Genvoya, elvitegravir can be expected to cause drug interaction concerns. Antineoplastic therapy that utilizes or influences CYP450 3A4, 2D6, or 2C9 will need to be monitored closely when used with elvitegravir boosted with cobicistat because this agent may lead to heightened chemotherapy concentrations. The second-generation integrase inhibitors dolutegravir and bictegravir are primarily metabolized by UGT and, to a lesser extent, CYP450 3A4. Specifically, dolutegravir and bictegravir are substrates but are neither inducers nor inhibitors of the CYP450 3A4 isoenzyme. Caution should be used when these second-generation integrase inhibitors are used with chemotherapy agents that are inhibitors or inducers of CYP450 3A4 as alterations in dolutegravir or bictegravir concentrations may occur.

In addition to CYP450 interactions, p-glycoprotein effects are also agent-specific. Raltegravir has no p-glycoprotein involvement and is not expected to cause drug interactions via this mechanism. When boosted with cobicistat, elvitegravir is a p-glycoprotein inducer and may decrease the concentration of antineoplastic agents that utilize p-glycoprotein for absorption. Dolutegravir and bictegravir are p-glycoprotein substrates, and absorption may be altered by antineoplastic therapies that are p-glycoprotein inhibitors or inducers. Thus, within the integrase inhibitor class, raltegravir is considered the cleanest agent in terms of drug interactions and has been specifically studied in combination with chemotherapy. Literature has shown raltegravir-based ART is safe and effective when combined with antineoplastic chemotherapy, regardless of the tumor type and the type and duration of chemotherapy (Banon, 2014).

Although the metabolism of the individual integrase inhibitors differs, a benefit of the class as a whole is that these inhibitors have minimal adverse effects. Integrase inhibitors are well-tolerated, and overlapping toxicities with antineoplastic agents are not projected to be a major concern. Therefore, due to the lack of drug interactions and minimal adverse effects, the integrase inhibitor raltegravir is an attractive option within a complete ART regimen when antiretroviral and antineoplastic therapy must be given concurrently.

PROTEASE INHIBITORS

The HIV protease inhibitors (PIs) remain commonly used antiretroviral drugs, although their use as initial therapy is decreasing as initial INSTI-based ART increases as per current treatment guidelines. They are potent antiretrovirals that are often effective in both treatment-naïve and -experienced patients, and they have a high barrier to HIV resistance. In addition, newer PIs have a more favorable dosing schedule than previous agents as a result of pharmacologic boosting. All PIs (aside from nelfinavir) can be pharmacologically boosted when coadministered with cobicistat or low-dose ritonavir.

The boosting process begins in the gastrointestinal tract, where low doses of ritonavir or cobicistat inhibit intestinal p-glycoprotein and CYP3A4. Because nearly all PIs are substrates of both p-glycoprotein and CYP3A4, the inhibition of these proteins allows the companion PI to achieve better bioavailability. The process continues in the liver, where ritonavir and cobicistat inhibit CYP3A4-mediated PI metabolism. This step prolongs therapeutic PI concentrations, reducing the need for frequent dosing.

Boosting improves the administration of PIs but also results in a higher likelihood of significant drug–drug interactions with other medications. Several antineoplastic agents are substrates, inducers, or inhibitors of CYP3A4 and/or p-glycoprotein (Rubinstein, 2014). For example, alkylating agents, taxanes, tyrosine kinase inhibitors, and vinca alkaloids can be substrates and inhibitors or inducers of CYP isoenzymes. The result is complex bidirectional interactions with ART (Rudek, 2011). Furthermore, although pharmacologic boosting improves the pharmacokinetic profile of PIs through CYP3A4 inhibition, both ritonavir and cobicistat can cause collateral drug interactions with other metabolic and drug elimination pathways. For example, ritonavir and cobicistat also inhibit CYP2D6, whereas ritonavir can induce CYP2B6, CYP2C9, and certain enzymes involved in glucuronidation. Again, the result is complex interactions with antineoplastic agents that could limit efficacy or introduce the possibility of toxicity.

With regard to toxicity, PIs have been found to potentiate the myelosuppressive effects of certain chemotherapy (Torres, 2014). They may also lead to greater gastrointestinal upset, including nausea, vomiting, and diarrhea. Specific PIs, such as atazanavir and lopinavir/ritonavir, have been associated with QT prolongation (Rudek, 2014). Because of the potential for arrhythmias and sudden death, these PIs should be avoided when antineoplastic agents also known to cause QT prolongation are administered. These include anthracyclines, arsenic trioxide, dasatinib, lapatinib, and tamoxifen.

In addition to some overlapping toxicities, some PIs may also complicate the dosing and monitoring of certain chemotherapy (Beumer, 2014). For example, bilirubin is often used as a means for determining dosage adjustments for a number of chemotherapeutic agents, such as docetaxel, paclitaxel, doxorubicin, etoposide, irinotecan, imatinib, and vincristine. Atazanavir may cause unconjugated hyperbilirubinemia secondary to UGT1A1 inhibition, leading to possible inaccuracies in chemotherapy dosage calculations.

STRATEGIES FOR CLINICAL MANAGEMENT OF PATIENTS WITH CANCER AND HIV

Treatment of patients with HIV-related malignancies is complex. The administration of ART with chemotherapy improves clinical response and prolongs survival, but concerns often arise regarding pharmacokinetic drug interactions and additive toxicity. The data regarding pharmacokinetic and pharmacodynamic interactions between antiretrovirals and chemotherapy agents are limited. To address the challenges of these complicated interactions and toxicities, PLWH and cancer should be treated using a multidisciplinary approach including primary care providers, infectious disease clinicians, hematologists/ oncologists, and clinical pharmacists. Communication among these professions is essential.

In combining ART and anticancer drug therapy, overlapping toxicity profiles can be avoided by altering either the ART regimen or the chemotherapy regimen. Interruption of ART is not recommended because it has been associated with an increase in mortality. In many instances, one or more components of a patient's ART regimen may be substituted in order to avoid risk of drug interactions or additive toxicity. ART regimen changes should always be carried out in conjunction with an HIV specialist utilizing the patient's complete antiretroviral treatment history, past adverse events, and resistance test results. More intensive monitoring of tolerability, viral suppression, adherence, and laboratory changes is recommended during the first 3 months after a regimen switch. In addition, modifications to the drugs in an antineoplastic regimen may also be considered due to concerns regarding drug interactions and/or overlapping toxicities. Dose adjustments of anticancer therapy, based on patient tolerance and response, can also be considered. Regardless, both ART and chemotherapy should be individualized according to patient characteristics.

For the majority of antiretroviral drugs that are CYP450 substrates, inducers, or inhibitors, coadministration with other metabolized drugs could result in drug accumulation and possible toxicity or in decreased efficacy of one or both drugs. Because standardized dosing algorithms do not exist for managing such interactions, increased monitoring for efficacy and toxicity is recommended when coadministering any ART regimen with chemotherapy. When determining interaction potential, drug interaction resources such as the following should be consulted: the Toronto General Hospital Immunodeficiency Clinic (https://hivclinic.ca/drug-information/antiretroviral-interactions-with-chemotherapy-regimens/) and the University of Liverpool HIV drug interaction website (http://www.hiv-druginteractions.org). Due to the paucity of relevant literature and the variability in the quality of evidence, clinical management should be assessed individually for each patient.

Last, in PLWH and cancer, opportunistic infection prophylaxis should be tailored and expanded with antimicrobials required for specific chemotherapy regimens or hematopoietic stem cell transplantation. The need for opportunistic infection prophylaxis should be re-evaluated on a regular basis and adjusted as needed via coordination among both the infectious disease team and the oncology team. Prophylaxis may need to be modified as the patient's CD4+ T cell count decreases with some chemotherapy regimens or increases after completion of therapy.

FUTURE DIRECTIONS

As PLWH live longer and develop ADMs or NADMs, more information on how to treat patients with anticancer treatment and supportive therapies will be needed. The AIDS Malignancy Consortium, a National Cancer Institute clinical trials group, aims to meet these needs by conducting prospective clinical trials with molecularly targeted agents in HIV-infected patients receiving ART. As anticancer therapy moves from cytotoxics to molecularly targeted agents, there may be fewer concerns about drug interactions and overlapping toxicities with ART. Due to the rapidly evolving nature of both HIV and cancer treatments, clinicians should be cognizant of the potential for interactions and toxicities and remain current on the latest clinical information.

REFERENCES

Banon S, Machuca I, Araujo S, et al. Efficacy, safety and lack of interactions with the use of raltegravir in HIV-infected patients undergoing antineoplastic chemotherapy. *J Intern AIDS*. 2014;17(Suppl 3):19590.

Beumer JH, Venkataramanan R, Rudek MA. Pharmacotherapy in cancer patients with HIV/AIDS. *Clin Pharmcol Ther*. 2014;95(4):370–372.

Di Francia R, Di Paolo M, Valente D, et al. Pharmacogenetic based drug–drug interactions between highly active antiretroviral therapy (HAART) and antiblastic chemotherapy. *WCRJ*. 2014;1(2):e386.

Gold Standard. Clinical pharmacology [database online]. Available at http://www.clinicalpharmacology.com. Accessed December 3, 2015.

Klibanov OM, Clark-Vetril R. Oncologic complications of human immunodeficiency virus infection: changing epidemiology, treatments, and special considerations in the era of highly active antiretroviral therapy. *Pharmacotherapy*. 2007;27(1):122–136.

National Comprehensive Cancer Network (NCCN). Clinical Practice Guidelines in Oncology. Cancer in people living with HIV. Version 1.2018. https://www.nccn.org/professionals/physician_gls/. Accessed May 24, 2018.

Park LS, Tate JP, Sigel K, et al. Association of viral suppression with lower AIDS-defining and non-AIDS-defining cancer incidence in HIV-infected veterans: a prospective cohort study. *Ann Intern Med*. 2018;169(2):87–96.

Rubinstein PG, Aboulafia DM, Zloza A. Malignancies in HIV/AIDS: from epidemiology to therapeutic challenges. *AIDS*. 2014;28(4):453–465.

Rudek MA, Chang CY, Steadman K, et al. *Cancer Chemother Pharmacol*. 2014;73(4):729–736.

Rudek MA, Flexner C, Ambinder RF. Use of antineoplastic agents in patients with cancer who have HIV/AIDS. *Lancet Oncol*. 2011;12(9):905–912.

Selzentry [package insert]. Available at https://www.accessdata.fda.gov/drugsatfda_docs/label/2007/022128lbl.pdf. Accessed December 1, 2015.

Shiels MS, Islam JY, Rosengerg PS, et al. Projected cancer incidence rates and burden of incident cancer cases in HIV-infected adults in the United States through 2030. *Ann Intern Med*. 2018;168(12):866–873.

Torres HA, Mulanovich V. Management of HIV infection in patients with cancer receiving chemotherapy. *Clin Infect Dis*. 2014;59(1):106–114.

Welz T, Wyen C, Hensel M. Drug interactions in the treatment of malignancy in HIV-Infected patients. *Oncol Res Treat*. 2017;40:120–127.

31.

SUBSTANCE ABUSE IN HIV POPULATIONS

Elizabeth David, John P. Casas, and Rakel Beall Wilkins

CHAPTER GOAL

Upon completion of this chapter, the reader should be able to

- Discuss issues, implications, diagnosis, and treatment of substance abuse in HIV-positive individuals.

INTRODUCTION

The prevalence of substance use in HIV-positive individuals is high, with rates of abuse/dependence much greater than those in the normal population. These substances include alcohol, opioids, cocaine/crack, methamphetamine, MDMA ("ecstasy" or "molly"), benzodiazepines, marijuana, ketamine, γ-hydroxybutyrate (GHB), anabolic steroids, nitrite inhalants, barbiturates, nicotine, and newer synthetic compounds ("bath salts," "kush," etc.)—all of which can have long- and short-term physiological, psychological, social, and neurocognitive effects when used in excess.

The relationship between substance use and HIV illness, illness progression, and treatment is complex. Whereas early in the course of the epidemic it was theorized that substance abuse was a causative factor or cofactor in HIV disease (Friedman, 1988; Goedert, 1984; Newell, 1985), it has become increasingly obvious that the interaction is behavioral as much as biological. Many behaviors associated with substance use result in increased risk of exposure to the virus, both directly through routes such as needle sharing and more indirectly through mechanisms relating to impaired judgment (unprotected sex, sex with multiple partners, trading sex for drugs, and "adventurous" sex including anal penetration) (Hillfors, 2007; Mackesy-Amiti, 2010; Semples, 2009) and sociocultural issues (homelessness and being embedded in a community with a high incidence of HIV disease) (Millett, 2007). In addition, low adherence to HIV treatment in this population with poor impulse control, unstructured and unhealthy lifestyles, multiple barriers to treatment (including fear of legal reprisals), and patterns of immediate wish gratification lead to increased morbidity and mortality (Cofrancesco, 2008; DeLorenze, 2011).

Mental illness and substance abuse are separate and additive risk factors for HIV infection. One study of HIV-positive patients revealed that those who have the dual diagnosis of mental illness and substance use have an HIV prevalence of 4.7% as opposed to 2.4% for those with substance use disorder diagnosis alone—almost double the rate. This highlights the importance of a comprehensive approach in the treatment of those with dual diagnoses, which inherently place them at a higher risk of contracting or transmitting sexually transmitted diseases (STDs) including HIV. Problems with adherence to medical treatment seem to be additive in this group (Moore, 2008; Sullivan, 2011). Finally, substance abuse is associated with a host of medical sequelae (liver disease, infection, diabetes, cardiovascular disease, and neurocognitive changes), complicating treatment of the virus in a population already at risk for these problems and leading to increased disease progression. Despite this known connection between substance abuse and HIV, and despite the knowledge that successful treatment of substance abuse can increase adherence to combination antiretroviral therapy (ART) regimens to levels comparable to those of non–substance abusers (Catz, 2000; Palepu, 2011; Vallecillo, 2010), a study revealed that fewer than half of all US substance abuse treatment facilities conduct on-site infectious disease screening (Substance Abuse and Mental Health Services Administration [SAMHSA], 2010).

LEARNING OBJECTIVES

- Describe the bidirectional interactions between HIV and unhealthy substance use.

- Recognize unhealthy substance use in their patients.

- Provide an initial outline of potential approaches to the treatment of substance use disorders in this population.

WHAT'S NEW?

The chapter has been updated to reflect the terminology of the fifth edition of the *Diagnostic and Statistical Manual of Mental Disorders* (American Psychiatric Association, 2013). More thorough and specific treatment modalities and recommendations are included.

DIAGNOSIS AND GENERAL ISSUES IN THE TREATMENT OF SUBSTANCE USE DISORDERS

Although there are precise criteria for the diagnosis of abuse and dependence (American Psychiatric Association, 2013), delineating the degree of severity of use is difficult and may ultimately be relatively insignificant. Some drugs are extremely destructive with almost any use, whereas some people manage to adapt and function despite ongoing and heavy abuse. Practically speaking, substance use disorders represent maladaptive patterns of substance use that interfere with a person's ability to function on a day-to-day basis. Generally, when use reaches these levels, there is disturbance of employment, disruption of relationships, possible medical consequences, and the substance use becomes central to the person's daily life, requiring increasingly more of the substance to feel "normal" or get the same high/sense of relief as previously experienced. Despite these obvious costs, the patient frequently does not view his or her use as a problem ("denial") or, perceiving a problem, cannot cut down. Despite traditional views of this as a condition of character weakness or poor choice, addiction is recognized as a disease process by the medical community.

These patients are often difficult to treat. Their frequent relapses—the norm rather than an exception—tend to demoralize them and those treating them. In addition, their patterns of denial and of using and abusing often extend to the people and systems around them, leaving treaters (as well as family, friends, and sometimes strangers) feeling angry, drained, frustrated, manipulated, and overwhelmed. When possible, the use of a treatment team (primary care physician, substance abuse counselor, psychiatrist when necessary, nursing staff, and social services/case manager) and a very clear treatment contract can mitigate these difficulties.

Screening for substance abuse can be done quickly and easily. Numerous specific screening questionnaires are available through the National Institute on Alcohol Abuse and Alcoholism, the Center for Substance Abuse Treatment, and other governmental agencies. However, the validity of simple one-question ("How often in the past year have you had 4 (for women)/5 (for men) or more drinks?" [Smith, 2009]), two-question ("Have you ever had a substance use problem? When was your last use of that substance?" [Cyr, 1988]), or the CAGE/CAGE-AID (cut down, annoyed, guilty, eye-opener) (Brown, 1995; Willenbring, 2009) instrument is well-established, including the modifications made for various other substances. Even for those not currently using, ongoing monitoring of substance use is important in this population known for frequent relapse, and questions at each visit as well as periodic urine drug screens, liver function tests, and complete blood count (to check mean corpuscular volume) can be helpful.

There are several stages in the treatment of substance abuse. When denial and continued use are unquestioned by the abuser, he or she is said to be in a "precontemplative" phase—a term suggesting that everyone has a hope for treatment. Prior to initiation of treatment ("contemplative" phase), there must be acknowledgment by the individual that there is a problem and the beginnings of readiness to consider stopping use. This is followed by detoxification—abstaining from active use of the drug until it is no longer present in the body and the immediate effects of intoxication are gone, usually within 4–10 days, depending on the drug of abuse. Only at this point is the individual physically and cognitively prepared to move on to the tasks of sobriety. Rehabilitation, the next phase, usually lasts approximately 30 days and involves reorganizing one's life patterns to exclude abuse and finding more healthy and adaptive ways of coping. For those with a lengthy history of substance use and/or early onset of use, the rehabilitation portion of treatment is likely to be longer and much more complex. This process may be augmented by participation in a therapeutic community, which is a less structured but still supportive transitional living arrangement, typically lasting 6 months to 1 year. During the rehabilitation phase, active and aggressive treatment of any comorbid psychiatric illness should be initiated (see Chapter 38). The fifth phase is relapse prevention. Finally, because relapse is very common in this population, rapid response to relapse must be considered as yet another part of treatment.

Traditional outpatient treatment involves the use of frequent diagnosis-specific psychosocial groups—12-step programs such as Alcoholics Anonymous, Narcotics Anonymous, and Cocaine Anonymous—accompanied by more individualized interaction with a personal sponsor. These groups are readily available to patients in almost every community, and they are organized and led by individuals with similar problems who have achieved some period of sobriety. Individuals utilizing this approach ("working the program") have access to a strong support network but remain within their own community (family, employment, and neighborhood). Thus, they often encounter problems when habit patterns have formed around the circumstances and stressors that exist within their home environment—potentially a positive situation if they continue to utilize the resources and skills they are building in the treatment process. These programs often incorporate spiritual beliefs into their techniques, and, in Western culture, that often involves a Judeo-Christian outlook, which some might find problematic; but, unlike organized religions, 12-step programs allow each participant to formulate his or her own sense of a "higher power" which can have no religious connection at all.

There are other treatment approaches that rely on totally different mechanisms. Acupuncture is a less traditional outpatient adjunct to reduce cravings and is recognized by the National Institutes of Health (1997), although questions about efficacy have been raised (Margolin, 2002). Cognitive-behavioral therapy (group or individual) has also been used with some success (Roll, 2006). Use of various medications to reduce cravings, block effects of intoxication, and negatively reinforce use is discussed later.

Individuals with long-standing abuse, with physiological dependence (particularly with benzodiazepines, barbiturates, or alcohol, withdrawal from which can be life-threatening), with a history of frequent relapses, or with other significant risk factors (including medical illness and pregnancy) may require an inpatient rehab program. Both medical and nonmedical programs are available, with the nonmedical facilities traditionally prohibiting all psychoactive substances, including medications for mental health issues and pain management as well as those to assist in detox. These medications include tapered doses of benzodiazepines, usually long-acting, to safely withdraw from benzodiazepines or alcohol, sometimes with the addition of carbamazepine or gabapentin to prevent seizures; tapering doses of long-acting narcotics along with symptomatic treatment with clonidine and nonsteroidal anti-inflammatory drugs for comfortable detox from narcotic drugs; and antidepressants or clonidine for comfortable withdrawal from cocaine or methamphetamine.

Traditionally, the goal of treatment is sustained abstinence from all drugs of abuse. This involves strategies for relapse prevention, including avoiding prescribing medications that could lead to increased cravings (e.g., judicious use of benzodiazepines), appropriate treatment of pain (a frequent trigger for relapse), careful observation during periods of increased stress, and prompt treatment of mental health issues (New York State Department of Health AIDS Institute, 2009). Even short-term abstinence, however, can be helpful in stabilizing the individual's life and support network, allowing the body a chance to heal what it can and decreasing the degree of physiological tolerance to a given agent. Psychopharmacological strategies to assist in maintenance of sobriety and relapse prevention include aversive therapy (disulfiram for alcohol abuse), blockade of reinforcement (naltrexone for opioid abuse), drive suppression (bupropion, varenicline, or naltrexone for tobacco abuse; buprenorphine for opiate abuse; and bupropion, modafinil, or baclofen for methamphetamine abuse), substituted addiction (methadone, levo-α-acetylmethadol [LAAM], or buprenorphine for opioid abuse), and tapered addiction (nicotine patch, spray, gum, inhaler for smoking cessation). The treatment regimens for withdrawal and sustained sobriety for specific drugs of abuse are discussed later.

An alternative approach to substance abuse treatment involves establishing a hierarchy of harm reduction. The highest level of harm reduction is, of course, abstinence. In the case of intravenous drug use, if the patient is not yet ready for total cessation of use, will he or she consider stopping injection use? If not stopping injection, will the patient use new needles and syringes? Will the patient clean needles/syringes with bleach? Will he or she avoid sharing injection equipment with others? Will the patient inject in social environments in which consequences of intoxication are lower (i.e., less risk of unsafe sex while intoxicated)?

SPECIFIC DRUGS OF ABUSE

ALCOHOL

As previously noted, alcohol use/misuse is closely linked to risk behaviors exposing individuals to HIV and other STDs. These risk factors have been shown to increase proportionally with higher consumption of alcohol and decrease with abstinence. The impact of alcohol on these risk factors has been shown to be independent of other drug use (Ruiz, 2007). Treatment strategies for alcohol abuse relate to achievement of sobriety/abstinence.

Medications for achieving and maintaining abstinence have utilized two mechanisms of action, one through blocking the reinforcing effects of intoxication by interfering with reward systems and the other focusing on stabilizing systems that have become deregulated by chronic alcohol use.

Disulfiram (Antabuse)

Originally studied as a possible antiparasitic treatment, this medication was discovered to have aversive effects when used with alcohol. In 1954, the US Food and Drug Administration (FDA) approved disulfiram for the treatment of alcohol dependence in the United States. Disulfiram causes irreversible inhibition of acetaldehyde dehydrogenase, a key enzyme in the metabolism of alcohol that leads to buildup of acetaldehyde, resulting in very unpleasant symptoms, including nausea, vomiting, tachycardia, headaches, hypertension (HTN)/hypotension, diaphoresis, flushing, vertigo, dysphoria, and dyspnea—thus the aversive reaction. Disulfiram works best in individuals who are motivated or where abstinence is strictly supervised. Adherence to disulfiram increases with behavioral couples' therapy (BCT), which provides contingency for sobriety and increased psychosocial support for positive change. In BCT, couples provide a caring and supportive positive, nonjudgmental environment. Meta-analysis of randomized studies of BCT has shown superior results in reducing alcohol use, consequence of use, and integrity relationships with others (O'Farrell, 2000). Disulfiram should be avoided in patients with a history of cardiovascular disease, myocardial infarction (MI), congestive heart failure, and end-stage liver disease. Caution should also be used in patients with a history of psychosis (inhibition of dopamine dehydroxylase results in increased dopamine levels, potentially increasing psychotic symptoms), those with peripheral neuropathy (can be exacerbated), and those taking metronidazole (will trigger aversive side effects). Aversive reactions can occur up to 2 weeks after the last dose and can be precipitated by alcohol-containing foods and alcohol in over-the-counter medicines and toiletries. Patients must wait at least 12 hours after a last drink before starting disulfiram.

Naltrexone

Naltrexone is a μ-opioid receptor antagonist originally marketed for opioid dependence. In 1994, it was approved by the FDA for prevention of heavy alcohol bingeing in those with alcohol dependence. It acts through blockade of naturally occurring opiates (i.e., endorphins and encephalins) released during alcohol consumption, minimizing release of dopamine in the nucleus accumbens and thus blocking the effects of pleasure and reinforcement. This results in decreased craving as well as disruption of the euphoric feelings associated with alcohol intoxication. Naltrexone use is contraindicated in patients with significant liver disease (hepatitis and liver failure), and all patients should have liver function tested prior to initiation of this drug because it may cause liver damage, especially in HIV patients, in whom certain antiviral medications can also impair liver function. Naltrexone should also be avoided in those who are currently going through acute opioid withdrawal. Patients should be opioid free for a minimum of 7–10 days prior to starting naltrexone because it can precipitate severe opioid withdrawal. Patients should be started first on the short-acting oral formulation, and if tolerable, they may be switched to monthly injections. The medication may initially cause symptoms of dysphoria, which patients often describe as "feeling weird, odd, not right." These symptoms are due to naltrexone's indirect effect on dopamine levels in the nucleus accumbens. Symptoms will eventually subside as neurochemical systems stabilize. Some patients may try to overcome naltrexone μ-receptor blockade by taking large amounts of exogenous opioids, which may lead to life-threatening opioid intoxication.

Acamprosate (Campral)

Acamprosate is an N-methyl-D-aspartic acid (NMDA) receptor antagonist that modulates γ-aminobutyric acid (GABA) and glutamate activity, resulting in alleviation of negative dysphoric symptoms associated with alcohol abstinence while also decreasing cravings. It is recommended that it be started as soon as possible after alcohol withdrawal and establishment of sobriety and that it should be continued even when relapse occurs. Common side effects include nausea, vomiting, diarrhea, gas, stomach pain, loss of appetite, headache, drowsiness, dizziness, constipation, fatigue, weight gain/loss, muscle/joint pain, change in sexual desire, and decreased sexual ability. Acamprosate carries a warning for possible increase in suicidal behavior. Although many of these events occurred in the context of alcohol relapse, no consistent pattern of relationship between the clinical course of recovery from alcoholism and the emergence of suicidality was identified (Campral/acamprosate product information, Forest Pharmaceuticals, 2004). The interrelationship between alcohol dependence, depression, and suicidality is well-recognized and complex. All alcohol-dependent patients, including those being treated with this medication, should be monitored for the development of symptoms of depression or suicidal thinking. Families and caregivers of patients being treated with acamprosate should be advised to monitor patients for the emergence of symptoms of depression. This drug is eliminated by kidney and is contraindicated in patients with severe renal impairment. Dosage must be adjusted for patients with less severe renal impairment.

OPIOIDS

Use of opioid-based drugs, particularly intravenous drug abuse, has long been associated with HIV infection and transmission. The risk has been shown to be even higher in those who also have psychiatric illness. Depression in intravenous drug users has been linked to increased rates of sharing of needles and other paraphernalia, resulting in a greater risk for HIV infection. It is therefore crucial to treat both the psychological disorders and the behavioral risk factors in intravenous drug use (Ruiz, 2007).

The degree to which opioids are abused depends on the interaction between each opioid and its receptor (full agonist, partial agonist, or antagonist). Drugs that act as a full agonist (heroin, morphine, codeine, oxycodone, hydrocodone, meperidine, methadone, propoxyphene, fentanyl, and LAAM) have a high likelihood of being abused. They produce positive mood effects (euphoria) as well as physical signs such as myosis, nausea, vomiting, constipation, mental clouding, and decreased libido. Abrupt cessation after sustained use results in withdrawal, with specific symptoms depending on when opioids were last used: Early symptoms (24 hours to 2 weeks) include rhinorrhea, lacrimation, gastrointestinal disturbance, piloerection, insomnia, and irritability; late symptoms (2 weeks to 2 years—" late abstinence syndrome") include depressed mood, anhedonia, decreased libido, bone pain, and muscle aches. Overdoses and death are common with intravenous opioid use because the purity of street drugs is notoriously uneven. Overdoses result in respiratory depression, pinpoint pupils, coma, hypotension, bradycardia, and pulmonary edema.

Initial treatment of opioid dependence consists of a period of detoxification, which can be assisted by use of methadone, buprenorphine, clonidine, and lofexidine, as well as supportive/symptomatic treatments for specific complaints. If rapid detox is necessary, clonidine and naltrexone are generally used. There is also the possibility for "ultra-detoxification," which would involve inpatient care and sedation/anesthesia. Because partial agonist and antagonist agents cause less euphoria, are generally less rewarding, and are generally less abused, they have become a staple of longer term medication treatment for opiate abuse. With the exception of methadone, most of the medications used to treat opioid dependence are from these classes of receptor action.

MEDICATION-ASSISTED TREATMENT (MAT) FOR OPIOID DEPENDENCE

METHADONE

Developed in the 1960s, methadone is a μ-receptor agonist as well as a weak NMDA receptor antagonist, and it has proved to be a very effective treatment for opiate addiction. The use of methadone has been shown to decrease the use of intravenous opioid drugs and the spread of communicable diseases such as HIV, hepatitis B virus, and hepatitis C virus by modifying behaviors such as intravenous drug use (Lollis, 2000). Methadone treatment for opioid dependence is provided in specialized opioid treatment programs (OTPs), which require federal licensing and certification. In addition to supplying methadone to its patients, OTP clinics also give counseling, drug testing, and vocational training/assistance. It is illegal for noncertified healthcare entities to provide methadone maintenance treatment. Doses are carefully titrated to the needs of the patient. Studies have shown that methadone doses in the range of 20–40 mg/d are effective in suppressing symptoms of withdrawal, but they may not be effective in reducing or stopping symptoms of craving (Strain, 1993a, 1993b).

Unfortunately, there are many issues with the use of methadone in HIV-positive individuals because this medication has many side effects and drug–drug interactions. Methadone prolongs QT/QTc intervals; therefore, close monitoring is required in patients who are taking other QT interval-prolonging drugs. Antiretrovirals known to significantly interfere with methadone serum levels include lopinavir/

ritonavir, efavirenz, and nevirapine. Other medications that have been shown to have drug–drug interaction with methadone include the anticonvulsants carbamazepine and phenytoin as well as some antibiotics, such as rifampin. In general, use of these medications should be avoided in patients who are being treated or plan to be treated with methadone. If such medication combinations are required, then methadone doses should be titrated upward to avoid withdrawal symptoms and continue maximized treatment. Methadone has been shown to be safe during pregnancy (especially relative to opioid use or withdrawal) and safe with breastfeeding. Some newborns may experience neonatal abstinence syndrome, which consists of blotchy skin coloring (mottling), diarrhea, high-pitched crying, excessive sucking, fever, hyperactive reflexes, increased muscle tone, irritability, poor feeding, and, in rare cases, seizures.

Buprenorphine (Subutex) and Buprenorphine Plus Naloxone (Suboxone)

Buprenorphine is a partial agonist to the μ-opioid receptor and antagonist at the κ-opioid receptor. When patients are not taking opioids, buprenorphine acts as an agonist, whereas it acts as an antagonist when patients attempt to take opioids. Naloxone is added to reduce the abuse potential of the drug. These medications require special certification for prescription, but they can be prescribed in an office setting. Initial doses are low (regardless of the patient's wish to start at higher dose) to avoid potential side effects—2 or 4 mg is standard, and ideally patients should be in some form of opioid withdrawal. If well-tolerated and there are still signs of withdrawal, this dosage can be repeated 1 or 2 hours later. Titration to the target dose (generally 8–16 mg/d, although up to 24 mg/d can be used) is done quickly to minimize patient dropout and withdrawal symptoms. If a patient requires doses greater than 24 mg/d, issues of diversion or misuse must be considered. Suboxone has ceiling effects: Unlike other opioid treatment drugs, it plateaus at a certain dose (32 mg/d), and a higher dose has no therapeutic benefit. Overdose can still occur, resulting in respiratory distress that may require airway management. Other potential side effects include central nervous system depression and hepatitis. Those with a history of traumatic brain injury should be monitored for increased intracranial pressure because all potent opioids may elevate cerebrospinal fluid pressure. Buprenorphine is metabolized by CYP450 3A4 enzyme, and there are several clinically significant drug–drug interactions. Those taking CYP450 3A4 inhibitors such as nefazodone, fluvoxamine, fluoxetine, ketoconazole, itraconazole, erythromycin, clarithromycin, grapefruit juice, and most protease inhibitors (especially ritonavir) should take reduced doses of buprenorphine.

Naltrexone

See the section on alcohol.

In recent years, opioid addiction has emerged as one of America's most pressing public health concerns, prompting greater consideration of how this growing epidemic could be impacting the transmission and treatment of HIV and other blood-borne infections, such as hepatitis C (HCV). In 2016, 2.1 million Americans were estimated to have an opioid use disorder, with nearly 12 million Americans estimated to have misused opioids during the preceding year (SAMHSA, 2016). Apart from the heightened morbidity and mortality associated with opioid overdose, this epidemic also places affected individuals at additional risk of contracting and transmitting infectious diseases during the course of their addiction. Research shows that people who misuse and abuse opioids commonly move from oral use to inhalation to injection use as they build tolerance to the drug's effects and require more potent concentrations to achieve their desired level of intoxication (Peters, 2016). Moreover, it is estimated that 10–20% of people who abuse prescription opioids move on to inject either opioids or heroin (Van Handle, 2016). Given the long-standing association between injection drug use and transmission of HIV and HCV via needle sharing, public health providers must necessarily remain vigilant in hopes of identifying co-occurring trends in these epidemics. One such instance was documented in 2015, in Scott County, Indiana, where opioid use was implicated in an HIV outbreak that resulted in 181 individuals being diagnosed with HIV, most of whom were coinfected with HCV (Van Handle, 2016). As individuals engaged in escalating drug use, they became more susceptible to transmission of HIV and HCV by way of high-risk sexual activity and injection drug use behaviors. This incident was integral in prompting the US Centers for Disease Control and Prevention (CDC) to identify 220 jurisdictions that might be equally vulnerable to similar co-occurring outbreaks due to the preponderance of opioid addiction and high-risk needle sharing, as well as limited access to care in those geographic areas (Van Handle, 2016). Targeted interventions such as these must be undertaken not only in hopes of preventing and rapidly identifying subsequent epidemics, but also as a means of ensuring that individuals with comorbid opioid dependence and HIV have adequate access to both MAT for opioid use disorder and ART. In 2016, a systematic review and meta-analysis of 4,685 articles and 32 studies revealed that MAT for opioid use disorder was associated with a 69% increase in recruitment into ART, a 54% increase in ART coverage, a twofold increase in ART adherence, a 23% decrease in the odds of attrition, and a 45% increase in odds of viral suppression (Low, 2016). Taken together, these striking statistics illustrate the importance of substance abuse recovery in both preventing the spread of HIV and improving the overall quality of life and treatment for persons living with HIV and opioid use disorder. It is imperative that individuals with opioid dependence are screened early for HIV/HCV, then promptly referred for MAT to reduce morbidity and mortality and mitigate the impact of these epidemics across the general population.

COCAINE/CRACK

In addition to the increased incidence of risk behaviors in cocaine abusers, recent studies have shown that cocaine abuse may have broad-ranging effects on human immunity. With regard to HIV infection, in vitro studies have shown that cocaine enhances infection of stimulated lymphocytes. Moreover, cohort studies in the pre- and post-highly active ART (HAART) era have linked stimulant abuse with increased HIV pathogenesis (Baum, 2009). It is therefore crucial to treat HIV-positive patients with cocaine dependence.

Cocaine blocks dopamine (DA) reuptake at the presynaptic site, thus increasing levels of DA at the nucleus accumbens, resulting in its addictive properties. Cocaine effects depend on the mode of use, with smoked (crack) and intravenous administration having the quickest effects (seconds to 30 minutes; peak, 15–30 minutes) and intranasal administration having slightly more delayed effects (5–90 minutes; peak, 30 minutes). Mild to moderate intoxication gives sympathomimetic symptoms—generally increased heart rate and blood pressure, decreased appetite, insomnia, euphoria, hyperalertness, and irritability. With severe intoxication, there is dilation of the pupils, and severe HTN, hyperthermia, cardiac arrhythmias/MIs, stroke, seizures, coma, and death may occur. At any level of intoxication, there may also be psychiatric symptoms—auditory/visual/tactile hallucinations, delusions, paranoia, and aggression/violence. For patients with severe cocaine intoxication (i.e., malignant HTN, hyperthermia, and seizure), the goal is stabilization of vital signs and the elimination of seizure activities. Patients should be given phentolamine, cooling, and other supportive measures for HTN crisis and hyperthermia; benzodiazepine should be given to prevent seizures and agitation. Antipsychotics may be useful for severe agitation/aggression/psychosis but should be avoided in patient with seizures because neuroleptics may further decrease the seizure threshold.

Research into medications for treating cocaine addiction has failed to show conclusive evidence of effectiveness, but efforts are ongoing. Recent ongoing research has been focused on creating a cocaine vaccine that uses modified cold virus attached to cocaine-like molecules to trigger the body to produce cocaine antibodies. Other promising agents include modafinil, topiramate, and desipramine, which may decrease cocaine craving.

METHAMPHETAMINE

Unlike many of the other drugs of abuse, which tend to be predominate in urban areas, methamphetamine use has grown exponentially in both rural and urban areas during the past few decades. It is an extremely addictive drug that heightens sexual arousal with reduced inhibition and judgment, placing its users at risk of contracting STDs such as HIV. It can be smoked, eaten, snorted, injected, or rectally inserted. It is a fairly inexpensive drug with rapid onset and long-lasting high (half-life of 11–12 hours). Use increases the release of newly synthesized dopamine, norepinephrine, and serotonin. It is also an indirect catecholamine and serotonin (5-HT) agonist. Like cocaine, methamphetamine can deplete dopamine stores and lead to significant symptoms of depression and, in some cases, suicide. Other symptoms that may be experienced include psychosis (that may last weeks to months), aggression, thought disorders, and gum disease with long-term use. Acute intoxication of methamphetamine is treated similar to cocaine with phentolamine, cooling, and other supportive measure for HTN crisis and hyperthermia; benzodiazepine is used to prevent seizures and agitation. Antipsychotics may also be required to control severe aggression/agitation. Addiction is more difficult to treat because there are no current approved FDA medications. Some medications have shown promise, including naltrexone, mirtazapine, and topiramate. Unlike other drugs of its kind, methamphetamine may induce sensitization, which results in enhanced response to the drug because of prior exposure and thus a higher likelihood of overdosing.

ECSTASY OR MOLLY (MDMA)

Dubbed the "intimacy drug," ecstasy use has been shown to produce profound feelings of closeness, which may lead to high-risk sexual behavior and HIV exposure. Some studies have shown that those using ecstasy may perceive less danger of contracting HIV and other STDs compared to nonusers of ecstasy (Theall, 2006). It is therefore critical that those with HIV and those at higher risk of contracting HIV be educated about the dangers of ecstasy use in addition to the other known heath issues that may result from ecstasy use. Currently, there is no FDA-approved medication for treatment of ecstasy abuse, and acute management is geared toward treating life-threatening conditions such as serotonin syndrome and hyperthermia that are commonly seen in rave parties.

SPECIAL CONSIDERATIONS IN HIV POPULATIONS

Interactions between substances of abuse and antiretroviral (ARV) agents have been reported. The toxicity of amphetamines, MDMA, meperidine, and GHB is dangerously increased by ritonavir. Barbiturates induce the cytochrome systems responsible for metabolism of protease inhibitors (PI), non-nucleoside reverse transcriptase inhibitors (NNRTIs), maraviroc, elvitegravir, and dolutegravir, significantly decreasing their effectiveness. Oral midazolam and triazolam are contraindicated with PIs, NNRTIs, and efavirenz. The toxicity of ketamine and phencyclidine (PCP) is dangerously increased by PIs and etravirine.

All the agents listed for use in detox and maintenance of sobriety have utility in the HIV population, but there are special considerations:

- Buprenorphine administration is office-based but requires special training and certification. Also, clinically significant interactions occur with ARVs, including atazanavir, darunavir, and ritonavir (increased buprenorphine activity and sedation—especially with atazanavir) and etravirine, nevirapine, and tipranavir (decreased buprenorphine activity, with tipranavir levels also significantly decreased). Fluconazole can increase the activity of buprenorphine, whereas phenobarbital, phenytoin, rifabutin, and rifampin decrease the effective amounts, sometimes causing withdrawal symptoms.

- Bupropion (used for smoking cessation) decreases the seizure threshold, particularly in patients with weight loss or electrolyte instability.

- Disulfiram (Antabuse) has a high risk of hepatotoxicity and cannot be used with tipranavir/ritonavir capsules (they contain alcohol). Use in individuals with heart disease is also problematic.

- Methadone maintenance cannot be done outside a registered clinic, and this agent has several clinically significant adverse interactions with ARVs (blood levels of abacavir are decreased; blood level of zidovudine is increased; abacavir increase blood levels of methadone and dose adjustment may be required to avoid sedation; efavirenz, nevirapine, darunavir, lopinavir, ritonavir (even in boosting doses), and tipranavir all decrease methadone availability, with withdrawal symptoms reported in some cases). Drug interactions with other medications frequently used in the HIV population are also reported (carbamazepine, phenobarbital, phenytoin, and rifampin sharply decrease methadone levels, and fluconazole significantly increases methadone blood levels).

- Naltrexone cannot be used in individuals requiring narcotic pain control but does not seem to interact with ARVs.

SUMMARY

Substance use or misuse is common in the HIV population and requires early and aggressive diagnosis and treatment, both to minimize further spread of the disease through ungoverned risk behaviors and to maximize the ability of the individual to fully participate in HIV treatment. Both of these will obviously decrease morbidity and mortality from both conditions. Adequate treatment with decreased substance use can improve adherence to HIV regimens (clinic visits and ARV use) to levels comparable to those seen in nonaddicted HIV populations. These principles apply even more stringently in those with "triple diagnosis"—substance abuse, mental illness, and HIV. As with any treatment process, success involves establishing a collaborative alliance—a therapeutic relationship between treatment staff and patient. This sets the stage for honest communication, mutual respect of boundaries, and continued participation in treatment (on both sides) despite temporary setbacks and failures. Integrated treatment of substance abuse and HIV (or substance abuse, HIV, and mental illness in the case of triple diagnosis) offers distinct advantages for these complex cases with multiple barriers to participation. Factors in a decision to start antiretroviral treatment in

individuals with active substance abuse are obviously complex, but substance use alone should not be an absolute contraindication to HAART.

RECOMMENDED READING

Ruiz P, Strain EC. Alcohol abstinence pharmacotherapy treatment. In *The Substance Abuse Handbook*. Philadelphia: Lippincott Williams & Wilkins; 2014.

Ruiz P, Strain EC. Amphetamines and other stimulants. In *The Substance Abuse Handbook*. Philadelphia: Lippincott Williams & Wilkins; 2014.

Ruiz P, Strain EC. Buprenorphine treatment. In *The Substance Abuse Handbook*. Philadelphia: Lippincott Williams & Wilkins; 2014.

Ruiz P, Strain EC. Cocaine and crack. In *The Substance Abuse Handbook*. Philadelphia: Lippincott Williams & Wilkins; 2014.

Ruiz P, Strain EC. Methadone maintenance treatment. In *The Substance Abuse Handbook*. Philadelphia: Lippincott Williams & Wilkins; 2014.

Ruiz P, Strain EC. Naltrexone and other pharmacotherapies for opioid dependence. In *The Substance Abuse Handbook*. Philadelphia: Lippincott Williams & Wilkins; 2014.

REFERENCES

American Psychiatric Association. *Diagnostic and statistical manual of mental disorders*. 5th ed. Washington, DC: APA Press; 2013.

Baum MK, Rafie C, Lai S, et al. Crack-cocaine use accelerates HIV disease progression in a cohort of HIV-positive drug users. *J AIDS*. 2009;50(1):93–99.

Brown RL, Rounds LA. Conjoint screening questionnaires for alcohol and other drug abuse: criterion validity in primary practice. *Wisc Med J*. 1995;94:135–140.

Campral (Acamprosate calcium) delayed release tablets [product information]. St. Louis, MO: Forest Pharmaceuticals; 2004.

Catz SL, Kelly JA, Bogart LM, et al. Patterns, correlates, and barriers to medication adherence among persons prescribed new treatments for HIV disease. *Health Psychol*. 2000;19:124–133.

Cofrancesco J Jr, Scherzer R, Tien PC, et al. Illicit drug use and HIV treatment outcomes in a US cohort. *AIDS*. 2008;22:237–245.

Cyr MG, Wartman SA. The effectiveness of routine screening in the detection of alcoholism. *JAMA*. 1988;259:51–54.

DeLorenze GN, Weisner C, Tsai AL, et al. Excess mortality among HIV-positive patients diagnosed with substance use dependence or abuse receiving care in a fully-integrated medical care program. *Alcohol Clin Exp Res*. 2011;35:203–210.

Friedman H, Klein T, Sperter S, et al. Drugs of abuse and virus susceptibility. *Adv Biochem Psychopharmacol*. 1988;44:125–137.

Goedert JJ. Recreational drugs: relationship to AIDS. *Ann N Y Acad Sci*. 1984;437:192–199.

Hillfors DD, Iritani BJ, Miller WC, et al. Sexual and drug behavior patterns and HIV and STD racial disparities: the need for new directions. *Am J Public Health*. 2007;97(1):125–132.

Lollis CM, Strothers HS, et al. Sex, drugs and HIV: does methadone maintenance reduce drug use and risky sexual behavior? *J Behav Med*. 2000;23(;6):545–557.

Low AJ, Mburu G, Welton NJ, et al. Impact of opioid substitution therapy on antiretroviral therapy outcomes: a systematic review and meta-analysis. *Clin Infect Dis*. 2016;63(8):1094–1104.

Mackesy-Amiti ME, Fendrich M, Johnson TP. Symptoms of substance dependence and risky sexual behavior in a probability sample of HIV negative men who have sex with men in Chicago. *Drug Alcohol Dependence*. 2010;110(1–2):38–43.

Margolin A, Avants SK, Holford TR. Interpreting conflicting findings from clinical trials of auricular acupuncture for cocaine addiction: does treatment context influence outcome? *J Altern Complement Med.* 2002;8:111–121.

Millett GA, Flores SA, Bakeman R. Explaining disparities in HIV infection among Black and White men who have sex with men: a meta-analysis of HIV risk behaviors. *AIDS.* 2007;21(15):2083–2091.

Moore RM, Gebo KA, Lucas GM, et al. Rate of co-morbidities not related to HIV infection or AIDS among HIV-positive patients by CD4 count and HAART use status. *Clin Infect Dis.* 2008;47(8):1102–1104.

National Institutes of Health. Acupuncture. *NIH Consensus Statement.* 1997;15:1–34.

New York State Department of Health AIDS Institute. *Substance use in patients with HIV/AIDS.* Albany, NY: New York State Department of Health; 2009.

Newell GR, Mansell PW, Spitz MR, et al. Volatile nitrites: use and adverse effects related to the current epidemic of the acquired immune deficiency syndrome. *Am J Med.* 1985;78(5):811–816.

O'Farrell TJ, William-Fals S. Behavioral couples therapy for alcoholism and drug abuse. *J Substance Abuse Treatment.* 2000;18:51–54.

Palepu A, Milloy MJ, Derr T, et al. Homelessness and adherence to antiretroviral therapy among a cohort of HIV-positive injection drug users. *J Urban Health.* 2011;88(3):545–555.

Peters P, et al. HIV infection linked to injection use of oxymorphone in Indiana, 2014–2015. *N Engl J Med.* 2016;375:229–239.

Roll JM, Petry NM, Stitzer ML, et al. Contingency management for the treatment of methamphetamine use disorders. *Am J Psychiatry.* 2006;163:1993–1999.

Ruiz P, Strain EC. Psychiatric complications of HIV-1 infection and drug abuse. In: *The substance abuse handbook.* Philadelphia: Lippincott Williams & Wilkins; 2014.

Semples SJ, Strathdee SA, Zians J, et al. Sexual risk behavior associated with co-administration of methamphetamine and other drugs in a sample of HIV-positive men who have sex with men. *Am J Addict.* 2009;18:65–72.

Smith PC, Schmidt SM, Allensworth-Davies D, et al. Primary care validation of a single-question alcohol screening test. *J Gen Intern Med.* 2009;24:783–788.

Strain EC, Stitzer ML, Lisbon IA, et al. Dose–response effects of methadone in the treatment of opioid dependence. *Ann Intern Med.* 1993a;119:23–27.

Strain EC, Stitzer ML, Lisbon IA, et al. Methadone dose and treatment outcome. *Drug Alcohol Depend* 1993b;33:105–117.

Substance Abuse and Mental Health Services Administration (SAMHSA). National survey of substance abuse treatment services: the N-SSATS report. February 25, 2010.

Substance Abuse and Mental Health Services Administration (SAMHSA). 2016 National survey on drug use and health. https://www.samhsa.gov/data/sites/default/files/NSDUH-FFR1-2016/NSDUH-FFR1-2016.pdf.

Sullivan LE, Goulet JL, Justice AC, et al. Alcohol consumption and depressive symptoms over time: a longitudinal study of patients with and without HIV infection. *Drug Alcohol Depend.* 2011;117:158–163.

Theall KP, Elifson KW, Sterk CE. Sex, touch, and HIV risk among ecstasy users. *AIDS Behav.* 2006;10(2):169–178.

Vallecillo G, Sanvisens A, Martinez E, et al. Use of highly active antiretroviral therapy is increasing in HIV-positive severe drug users. *Curr HIV Res.* 2010;8(8):641–648.

Van Handle M, et al. County-level vulnerability assessment for rapid dissemination of HIV or HCV infections among persons who inject drugs, United States. *J AIDS.* 2016;73(3):323–331.

Willenbring ML, Gardner MB. Helping patients who drink too much: an evidence-based guide for primary care clinicians. *Am Fam Phys.* 2009;80:44–50.

32.

UNDERSTANDING THE USE OF ANTIRETROVIRALS IN THE AGING PATIENT

Brandon H. Samson and James D. Scott

CHAPTER GOALS

Upon completion of this chapter, the reader should be able to

- Discuss the course of HIV disease in people >50 years of age.

- List treatment concerns that are of greater concern in older people with HIV.

- Discuss the outcomes of clinical trials focused on older people with HIV.

- Discuss the factors that make drug–drug interactions more complicated in older people with HIV.

INTRODUCTION

More than half of HIV-positive individuals in the United States are now over the age of 50, with HIV care intersecting further into management considerations for geriatric care (Guaraldi, 2017). Often, healthcare providers and older people mistake the presence/progression of HIV with the normal aging process, especially since both involve chronic inflammation and activation of the immune system (Nasi, 2014). This presents a unique challenge to healthcare providers since they must balance optimal antiretroviral therapy (ART) selection with additional noncommunicable diseases/comorbidities, drug–drug interactions (DDIs), renal and/or hepatic function, and the increased likelihood of ART-associated events. There is currently a paucity of clinical trials, systematic reviews, and guidelines available to assist healthcare providers in safe and appropriate decision- making for the geriatric HIV population. Currently, outcome measures essential to aging HIV-positive patients have only been included in a small number of studies (Guaraldi, 2017). Nevertheless, the significance of patients living longer while on ART cannot be ignored.

While the association between long-term antiretroviral (ARV) exposure and increased toxicity is less apparent, there is evidence that older age is significantly associated with higher viral load at diagnosis and, consequently, faster CD4$^+$ T cell count decline (Winston, 2015; Grabar, 2004).

With ART associated with both beneficial and deleterious effects, healthcare providers should weigh negative effects against the positive effects of viral suppression (Guaraldi, 2014). There is unfortunately a lack of data on the long-term safety of specific ARV drugs in older patients, with recommendations for older patients based on the adverse effects of therapy based on renal, hepatic, cardiovascular, metabolic, and bone health (US Department of Health and Human Services [USDHHS], 2016). In addition, the majority of existing guidelines for geriatric conditions remain organ-based (Guaraldi, 2017). In the absence of information about the pharmacokinetic effects of long-term ARV use in HIV-positive individuals older than 60 years, what follows are important practice-related considerations regarding ARV use in geriatric populations (Schoen, 2013).

LEARNING OBJECTIVE

Identify the growing relevance of long-term ARV use in geriatric populations and be able to apply treatment strategies involving ARV use for this population.

WHAT'S NEW?

HIV studies pertaining to the geriatric population have been updated with additional studies conducted since the previous publication date of the chapter. Information on a recent drug therapy approved by the US Food and Drug Administration (FDA) and its implications on the geriatric population is also included.

KEY POINTS

- Treatment of HIV in aging patients is based on the consideration of adverse effects associated with ART with regard to renal, hepatic, cardiovascular, metabolic, and bone health as well as the potential for increased DDIs.

- The effect of ART on cardiovascular disease (CVD) risk is mediated by the underlying cardiovascular risk associated with HIV infection itself; hence, ART is not guaranteed to reduce the risk of CVD.

- Certain ARV agents (notably tenofovir disoproxil fumarate) are associated with nephrotoxicity, so monitoring of renal function is crucial, especially in patients also receiving additional nephrotoxic agents.

- Multiple classes of ARV agents are associated with hepatotoxicity, and certain agents have such a severe risk of liver injury that they are no longer recommended as preferred agents by guidelines.

- ART is associated with decreased bone mineral density, with a variable amount of bone loss being a consistent feature of agents used for initial treatment.

- Healthcare providers should routinely review patients' medication lists to look for significant DDIs and perform drug interaction checks using available resources.

METABOLIC COMPLICATIONS ASSOCIATED WITH ANTIRETROVIRAL THERAPY

ART approved prior to 2009 that was associated with lipodystrophy was predictive of atherosclerotic lesions in HIV patients. While newer drugs have a more lipid-friendly profile from a metabolic standpoint, this benefit does not necessarily translate into a guaranteed CVD risk reduction in HIV-positive patients since the effect of ART on CVD risk is mediated by the underlying cardiovascular risk associated with HIV infection itself. As an additional consideration, an initial ritonavir-boosted protease inhibitor–based regimen should be avoided in individuals with diabetes mellitus or hyperinsulinemia if possible (Abrass, 2012).

RENAL COMPLICATIONS ASSOCIATED WITH ANTIRETROVIRAL THERAPY

Optimal ART can prevent the development or stop the progression of HIV-associated nephropathy based on studies showing preservation of renal function associated with ART, possible improvement in renal function, and declining renal function during treatment interruption. However, certain ARV agents (notably tenofovir disoproxil fumarate [TDF]) are associated with nephrotoxicity, so monitoring of renal function is crucial, especially in patients also receiving additional nephrotoxic agents (Hall, 2011). For additional information on effective renal dosing, the US DHHS guidelines provide a valuable reference for medication dosing in settings involving renal or hepatic dysfunction. A newer formulation of tenofovir (tenofovir alafenamide [TAF], currently available as a component of the combination products marketed as Genvoya, Odefsey, Descovy, and Symtuza) has clinical data showing smaller increases in serum creatinine and smaller decreases in estimated glomerular filtration rate compared to tenofovir disoproxil fumarate and, accordingly, lower creatinine clearance cutoffs for treatment initiation (Sax, 2015; Genvoya insert, 2015). In a randomized, noninferiority trial evaluating 1,436 virologically suppressed adults to either a TAF group or one of four TDF-containing regimens, there were significant improvements in urine protein and albumin-to-creatinine ratios in the TAF group compared to TDF (p <0.001) (DeJesus, 2018).

HEPATOTOXICITY ASSOCIATED WITH ANTIRETROVIRAL THERAPY

Multiple classes of ARV agents are associated with hepatotoxicity, and certain agents have such an increased risk of liver injury that they are no longer recommended as preferred agents by guidelines (e.g., didanosine associated with noncirrhotic portal hypertension and stavudine associated with increased frequency of acute liver injury) (Chang, 2012; Clark, 2002). The 2012 World Health Organization (WHO) guidelines on the use of ARV drugs for treating and preventing HIV infection included recommendations to progressively reduce the use of stavudine due to well-recognized toxicities including lipoatrophy, peripheral neuropathy, and lactic acidosis (WHO, 2013). With regard to currently relevant ARV agents in use (most notably protease inhibitors), hepatotoxicity may occur some months after commencing treatment. Further hepatic deterioration may also result in impaired drug elimination and drug accumulation.

EFFECTS ON BONE AND VITAMIN D ASSOCIATED WITH ANTIRETROVIRAL THERAPY

ART is associated with decreased bone mineral density, with varying amounts of bone loss a consistent feature of all agents used for initial treatment. This is believed to be caused by a decrease in bone turnover as ART reduces viral load and increases inflammatory cytokines. In addition, certain agents (efavirenz, zidovudine) can also affect vitamin D levels. For those patients with known risk factors for osteoporosis, long-term concurrent use of proton pump inhibitors (PPIs) or corticosteroids should be avoided if possible. Consistent with the previous study evaluating TAF and TDF in virologically suppressed adults, there were improvements noted in hip and spine bone mineral density for TAF-assigned patients compared to TDF (p <0.001) (DeJesus, 2018).

CENTRAL NERVOUS SYSTEM TOXICITY ASSOCIATED WITH ANTIRETROVIRAL THERAPY

ART, most notably efavirenz, may be associated with neurocognitive/psychiatric complications. Peripheral neuropathy can also be associated with combination ART, but less so with current regimens. In the absence of further available recommendations, caution should be exercised in individual clinical situations. Sleep disturbances have been reported with some integrase strand transfer inhibitors, mainly dolutegravir (DeBoer, 2016; Hoffman, 2017).

CARDIOVASCULAR DISEASE COMPLICATIONS ASSOCIATED WITH ANTIRETROVIRAL THERAPY

HIV-positive patients, regardless of geriatric stature, are known to have an increased risk of chronic CVD (e.g., coronary artery disease, myocardial fibrosis, congestive heart failure, and ischemic stroke). Certain ARV medications (e.g., protease inhibitors and the aforementioned risk of hyperlipidemia) are associated with adverse event profiles that could potentially increase risk of cardiovascular events. Studies have noted the association between abacavir and CVD, although this has not been confirmed in all studies (Wing, 2016). Additional studies have shown that boosted protease inhibitors are also associated with an increased risk of cardiovascular events (Ryom, 2018).

DRUG-DRUG INTERACTIONS/ MEDICATION FATIGUE ASSOCIATED WITH ANTIRETROVIRAL THERAPY

While healthcare providers should communicate the critical need for adherence to ART, they must also be aware of common DDIs among older patients. Although there are many drug interaction studies documenting significant DDIs between ARV drugs and medications that are commonly prescribed in older patients, the majority of these pharmacokinetic studies were conducted in young, healthy volunteers who are not HIV-positive. As a result, these studies may not be generalizable to older HIV-positive patients. Healthcare providers should routinely review patients' medication lists to look for significant DDIs and perform drug interaction checks using available online resources (e.g., http://www.hiv-druginteractions.org), the US DHHS Guidelines for the Use of Antiretroviral Agents, or the Guidelines for the Prevention and Treatment of Opportunistic Infections published by the US Centers for Disease Control and Prevention (CDC)/National Institutes of Health (NIH) (Nachega, 2012).

RECENTLY APPROVED DRUGS AND INFORMATION RELATING TO GERIATRIC POPULATIONS

In 2018, ibalizumab (marketed under the brand name Trogarzo) was approved by the FDA for heavily treatment-experienced adults with multidrug-resistant HIV-1 infection. Ibalizumab, a CD4 cell surface marker-directed, post-attachment HIV-1 inhibitor, interferes with binding and attachment of the infecting virus to the susceptible $CD4^+$ T lymphocyte, a critical step required for the entry of the HIV-1 virus into host cells. Of note, ibalizumab does not impact $CD4^+$ T cell function. To date, ibalizumab has not been evaluated in geriatric patients or in drug interaction studies (Trogarzo insert, 2018).

STUDIES INVESTIGATING ANTIRETROVIRAL MEDICATION RESPONSE IN OLDER HIV-POSITIVE PATIENTS

- A post-hoc analysis evaluating potential differences in efficacy and safety in older (≥50 years) versus younger (<50 years) patients from the ECHO and THRIVE trials revealed similar virologic response rates between older (77%) and younger (76%) patients on rilpivirine. In fact, virologic response was numerically higher in older (84%) versus younger (76%) patients on efavirenz (Ryan, 2013). No clinically relevant age-related differences were observed in immunologic responses. Small differences were noted in older versus younger patients in adverse events (higher rates of depression, insomnia, and rash in older EFV-treated patients), laboratory abnormalities (increased low-density lipoprotein cholesterol and hyperglycemia in older EFV-treated patients and increased amylase in older patients across treatments), bone mineral density (larger decreases in older patients across treatments), and progression to severe vitamin D deficiency (greater in older versus younger EFV-treated patients).

- In a national, retrospective cohort analysis of 161 patients 50 years old or older when they began first combination ART (112 starting with FTC/TDF and 49 with other nucleotide reverse transcriptase inhibitors [NRTIs]), use of FTC/TDF was generally safe and effective without any statistically significant differences between FTC/TDF and non-FTC/TDF users for any output except for persistence (log rank 0.001; adjusted hazard odds ratio [aHOR], 2.10; 95% CI, 1.34–3.29) (Blanco, 2013). They defined persistence as the duration during which a patient remains on a prescribed therapy.

- In a study that enrolled 12,196 eligible patients, immunologic response decreased with increasing age (age groups: 18 to <30: reference; 30 to <40: aHOR, 0.92 [0.85, 1.00]; 40 to <50: aHOR, 0.85 [0.78, 0.92]; 50 to <60: aHOR, 0.82 [0.74, 0.90]; >60: aHOR, 0.74 [0.65, 0.85]), and this relationship was independent of the ARV regimen (Althoff, 2010).

- The COHERE study enrolled 49,921 ARV-naïve patients who started ART from 1998 to 2006 with the objective of measuring virological and immunological response by age (Collaboration of Observational HIV Epidemiological Research Europe, 2008). The probability of virologic response was higher in those aged 50–54 (aHOR, 1.24), 55–59 (1.24), and at least 60 (1.18) years, but the probability of immunologic response in participants aged 60 years or older was 7% less [0.93 (0.87–0.98)]. After adjusting for the latest $CD4^+$ T cell count as a time-updated covariate, the risk of AIDS remained higher in those aged 55–59 and 60 years or older [55–59 years: 1.18 (1.05–1.34); 60 years or older 1.32 (1.17–1.48)].

- Additional supporting data are available from a retrospective cohort analysis of HIV-positive patients being treated throughout Kaiser Permanente California where virologic and immunologic outcomes were measured and stratified by age group in a retrospective analysis of 5,090 patients (Silverberg, 2007). Patients older than 50 were more likely to achieve an undetectable viral load than younger patients, but this age effect disappeared when ARV adherence was controlled for. In contrast, younger patients had a higher probability of achieving a greater increase in CD4$^+$ cells (131.8 cells/μL/year) than patients older than 50 years (111.8 cells/μL/year, $p = 0.046$). This effect was most pronounced during the first year of ART. A greater risk for increased serum creatinine and lower hemoglobin concentrations was also noted for patients older than 50 years.

- The mean time to undetectable viral loads was shorter in older patients (>50 years) than younger (<40 years), with a mean time to undetectable viral load of 3.2 months versus 4.4 months ($p = 0.001$) (Greenbaum, 2008). In this study, no differences were noted in either age group with regard to immunologic response. Unfortunately, older patients also had a shorter survival time and an overall higher mortality than younger patients, with both of these outcomes being statistically significant.

- The GEPPO study was a cross-sectional study aimed at describing ARV regimens in a geriatric HIV population. A total of 1,222 HIV-positive patients were evaluated based on the presence of multidrug or less drug regimens, multiple morbidities, and polypharmacy. Multivariate logistic regression showed that multiple morbidities and polypharmacy were predictive of patients receiving mono/dual, NRTI-sparing, and TDF-sparing combinations while female sex and age were predictors of boosted-free ARV regimens (Nozza, 2017).

- The immunologic and clinical responses to ART in patients 50 years old and older receiving care for HIV was measured in a retrospective analysis conducted in sub-Saharan Africa. A total of 728 patients were evaluated and showed a late median absolute increase in CD4$^+$ at 48 months significantly higher in younger patients than in elderly patients (+241.5 cells/mm^3 vs. +146 cells/mm^3, $P = 0.007$). The proportion of patients with a CD4$^+$ count of 350 cells/μL or more was higher in younger groups at a follow-up time of 48 months (33.9% vs. 30.1%, $P = 0.2$) (Mpondo, 2016).

RECOMMENDED READING

Nachega JB, Hsu AJ, Uthman OA, et al. Antiretroviral therapy adherence and drug–drug interactions in the aging HIV population. *AIDS* July 31, 2012;26 Suppl 1:S39–53.

United States Department of Health and Human Services (USDHHS). HIV and the older patient. January 28, 2016. Available at https://aidsinfo.nih.gov/guidelines/html/1/adult-and-adolescent-arv-guidelines/277/hiv-and-the-older-patient. Accessed August 5, 2018.

REFERENCES

Abrass CK, Appelbaum JS, Boyd CM, et al. Summary report from the Human Immunodeficiency Virus and Aging Consensus Project: treatment strategies for clinicians managing older individuals with the human immunodeficiency virus. *J Am Geriatr Soc.* May 2012;60(5):974–979.

Althoff KN, Justice AC, Gange SJ, et al. Virologic and immunologic response to HAART, by age and regimen class. *AIDS.* 2010;24(16):2469–2479.

Blanco JR, Caro-Murillo AM, Castano MA, et al. Safety, efficacy, and persistence of emtricitabine/tenofovir versus other nucleoside analogues in naive subjects aged 50 years or older in Spain: the TRIP study. *HIV Clin Trials.* 2013;14(5):204–215.

Chang HM, Tsai HC, Lee SS, et al. Noncirrhotic portal hypertension associated with didanosine: a case report and literature review. *Jpn J Infect Dis.* 2012;65(1):61–65.

Clark SJ, Creighton S, Portmann B, et al. Acute liver failure associated with antiretroviral treatment for HIV: a report of six cases. *J Hepatol.* February 2002;36(2):295–301.

DeBoer MGJ, van den Berk GEL, van Holten N, et al. Intolerance of dolutegravir-containing combination antiretroviral therapy regimens in real-life clinical practice. *AIDS.* 2016;30(18):2831–2834.

DeJesus E, Haas B, Segal-Maurer S, et al. Superior efficacy and improved renal and bone safety after switching from a tenofovir disoproxil fumarate- to a tenofovir alafenamide-based regimen through 96 weeks of treatment. *AIDS Res Hum Retroviruses.* 2018;34(4):337–342.

Collaboration of Observational HIV Epidemiological Research Europe (COHERE) Study Group, Sabin CA, Smith CJ, et al. Response to combination antiretroviral therapy: variation by age. *AIDS.* 2008;22(12):1463–1473.

Genvoya [package insert]. Redwood City, CA: Gilead Sciences; 2015.

Grabar S, Kousignian I, Sobel A, et al. Immunologic and clinical responses to highly active antiretroviral therapy over 50 years of age. Results from the French Hospital Database on HIV. *AIDS.* 2004;18(15):2029–2038.

Greenbaum AH, Wilson LE, Keruly JC, et al. Effect of age and HAART regimen on clinical response in an urban cohort of HIV-positive individuals. *AIDS.* 2008;22(17):2331–2339.

Guaraldi G, Palella FJ, Jr. Clinical implications of aging with HIV infection: perspectives and the future medical care agenda. *AIDS.* 2017;31(Suppl 2):S129–S135.

Guaraldi G, Prakash M, Moecklinghoff C, et al. Morbidity in older HIV-positive patients: impact of long-term antiretroviral use. *AIDS Rev.* April–June 2014;16(2):75–89.

Hall A, Hendry B, Nitsch D, et al. Tenofovir-associated kidney toxicity in HIV-positive patients: a review of the evidence. *Am J Kidney Dis.* 2011;57:773–780.

Hoffman C, Welz T, Sabranski M, et al. Higher rates of neuropsychiatric adverse events leading to dolutegravir discontinuation in women and older patients. *HIV Med.* 2017;18:56–63.

Mpondo BC, Gunda DW, Kilonzo SB, et al. Immunological and clinical responses following the use of antiretroviral therapy among elderly HIV-positive individuals attending care and treatment clinic in Northwestern Tanzania: a retrospective cohort study. *J Sex Transm Dis.* 2016;2016:5235269.

Nachega JB, Hsu AJ, Uthman OA, et al. Antiretroviral therapy adherence and drug–drug interactions in the aging HIV population. *AIDS.* July 31, 2012;26(Suppl 1):S39–S53.

Nasi M, Pinti M, De Biasi S, et al. Aging with HIV infection: a journey to the center of inflammAIDS, immunosenescence and neuroHIV. *Immunol Lett.* November 2014;162(1 Pt B):329–333.

Nozza S, Malagoli A, Maia L, et al. Antiretroviral therapy in geriatric HIV patients: the GEPPO cohort study. *J Antimicrob Chemother.* 2017;72(10):2961.

Ryan R, Dayaram YK, Schaible D, et al. Outcomes in older versus younger patients over 96 weeks in HIV-1- infected patients treated with rilpivirine or efavirenz in ECHO and THRIVE. *Curr HIV Res.* 2013;11(7):570–575.

Ryom L, Lundgren JD, El-Sadr W, et al. Cardiovascular disease and use of contemporary protease inhibitors: the D:A:D international prospective multicohort study [published online ahead of print May 3, 2018]. *Lancet HIV*. 2018;5(6):e291–e300. doi: 10.1016/S2352-3018(18)30043-2.

Sax PE, Wohl D, Yin MT, et al. Tenofovir alafenamide versus tenofovir disoproxil fumarate, coformulated with elvitegravir, cobicistat, and emtricitabine, for initial treatment of HIV-1 infection: two randomised, double-blind, phase 3, non-inferiority trials. *Lancet*. June 27, 2015;385(9987):2606–2615.

Schoen JC, Erlandson KM, Anderson PL. Clinical pharmacokinetics of antiretroviral drugs in older persons. *Expert Opin Drug Metab Toxicol*. May 2013;9(5):573–588.

Silverberg MJ, Leyden W, Horberg MA, et al. Older age and the response to and tolerability of antiretroviral therapy. *Arch Intern Med*. 2007;167(7):684–691.

Trogarzo [package insert]. Quebec, Canada: Theratechnologies; 2018.

US Department of Health and Social Services (USDHHS). Considerations for antiretroviral use in special populations: HIV and the older patient. January 28, 2016. Available at https://aidsinfo.nih.gov/guidelines/html/1/adult-and-adolescent-arv-guidelines/277/hiv-and-the-older-patient. Accessed August 5, 2018.

Wing EJ. HIV and aging. *Int J Infect Dis*. 2016;53:61–68.

Winston A, Underwood J. Emerging concepts on the use of antiretroviral therapy in older adults living with HIV infection. *Curr Opin Infect Dis*. February 2015;28(1):17–22.

World Health Organization (WHO). Phasing out stavudine: progress and challenges. Available at http://www.who.int/hiv/pub/guidelines/arv2013/arv2013supplement_to_chapter09.pdf. Accessed August 8, 2018.

33.

OPPORTUNISTIC INFECTIONS

Lisa Armitige and Karen J. Vigil

> **CHAPTER GOAL**
>
> Upon completion of this chapter, the reader should be able to
> - Recognize and manage the most common opportunistic infections found in persons infected with HIV.

TIMING OF ANTIRETROVIRAL THERAPY INITIATION AND IMPACT ON OPPORTUNISTIC INFECTIONS

LEARNING OBJECTIVES

- Describe the issues concerning starting ART in the setting of an opportunistic infection.

- Summarize the recommendations for starting ART in the setting of an opportunistic infection.

WHAT'S NEW?

Data and guidelines on starting ART in patients with cryptococcal meningitis have been updated.

KEY POINTS

- Early initiation of ART was associated with a decrease in AIDS progression and death in ACTG A5164.

- Early initiation of ART near the time of starting treatment for an OI should be considered for most patients, with the possible exception of patients with cryptococcal or tuberculous meningitis.

The question of when to initiate antiretroviral therapy (ART) in the setting of an acute or ongoing opportunistic infection (OI) has been controversial. On the one hand, the immediate initiation of ART in the presence of an OI may provide better clinical outcomes as the immune system improves. On the other hand, rapidly decreasing viral load has been associated with the immune reconstitution inflammatory syndrome (IRIS), which may lead to further complications in the setting of an OI. There are also questions of increasing pill burden, potential drug–drug interactions, additive toxicity and adverse events, and the more practical problem of continuity of care

if ART is started in a hospital setting for a newly diagnosed patient with HIV, without established outpatient care already in place. This problem could be particularly troublesome for patients who do not have health insurance or otherwise do not have affordable access to ART in the outpatient setting.

Some OIs associated with severe immunosuppression, such as cryptosporidiosis, microsporidiosis, progressive multifocal leukoencephalopathy (PML), do not have adequate specific treatment other than ART. For these patients, the only way to improve the condition is by starting ART, so it makes sense to start ART immediately. Similarly, patients with mild to moderate Kaposi's sarcoma may improve this condition after the initiation of ART even without chemotherapy. However, for OIs such as *Pneumocystis jirovecii* pneumonia (PCP), *Cryptococcus neoformans* meningitis, or *Mycobacterium tuberculosis* meningitis, targeted antimicrobial treatment is available to stabilize the condition, and the patient can improve in the absence of ART. It is for these patients that controversy has existed about the optimal time to start ART.

CLINICAL TRIAL RESULTS

AIDS Clinical Trials Group (ACTG) A5164 was designed to address the question of the optimal timing of ART initiation for individuals presenting with AIDS-defining OIs or serious bacterial infections (BIs), other than tuberculosis, for which effective antimicrobial therapies were available. This was a randomized, open-label strategy trial to evaluate early (defined as within 14 days of starting acute OI treatment) versus deferred (given after OI treatment is completed) initiation of ART in patients starting treatment of acute OIs or BIs, using clinical and virologic end points at 48 weeks (Zolopa, 2009). A total of 282 patients were evaluable, with 141 in each arm. Most study participants were from racial/ethnic minority groups (73%) and male (85%), with a median age of 38 years, median CD4$^+$ T cell count of 29 cells/mm^3, and a median HIV RNA of 5.07 log$_{10}$ copies/mL. The most common entry OIs included PCP (63%), cryptococcal meningitis (12%), and BIs (12%). ART was initiated a mean of 12 days after starting OI treatment in the "early" arm and a mean of 45 days after OI treatment in the "deferred" arm.

The study found a statistically significant decrease in the proportion of study patients experiencing progression to a new AIDS-defining disease and death (composite endpoint) in the early treatment arm (14.2%) compared to the deferred arm (24.1%) (odds ratio [OR], 0.51; 95% confidence interval [CI], 0.27–0.94). The time to AIDS progression and death was also longer in the early treatment arm compared to the deferred group (hazard ratio, 0.53; 95% CI, 0.30–0.92). The impact of these differences was seen most prominently in the first 6 months after diagnosis of the OI. The number of adverse events was not different in the two arms, and IRIS was reported in 8 participants in the early arm and 12 participants in the deferred arm. Based on these data, it is clear that early initiation of ART during treatment for an acute OI or serious BI is life-saving or at least serious morbidity–reducing if there are no major contraindications to starting ART. A cost-effectiveness analysis, supportive of this early treatment strategy, has also been published (Sax, 2010).

The overall rates of IRIS in A5164 were lower than rates observed in previous retrospective trials. This was possibly because of the types of the OIs in this study (largely PCP) and because patients with *M. tuberculosis* infection were excluded from entry due to the fact that it was the subject of separate trials. Factors that were found to be associated with IRIS in A5164 were the presence of fungal infections (*Cryptococcus* or *Histoplasma*), lower baseline CD4$^+$ T cell counts, and higher baseline HIV RNA levels. IRIS was also associated with higher CD4$^+$ T cell counts and lower HIV RNA levels while on ART. Early initiation of ART did not increase the incidence of IRIS in this study.

However, recommendations regarding the timing of starting ART specifically in the setting of meningitis due to *C. neoformans* or *M. tuberculosis* have been more complex. A study on IRIS related to meningitis caused by *C. neoformans* was published in 2009 (Sungkanuparph, 2009). Although this study of 101 patients employed a different methodology than ACTG 5164, it also found no association between the timing of ART initiation and the diagnosis of IRIS. Rather, it found that an increased baseline serum cryptococcal antigen titer was a risk factor for IRIS. In contrast, a study of 54 patients in Zimbabwe showed early initiation of ART (within 72 hours of diagnosis) in patients with cryptococcal meningitis versus delayed initiation (after 10 weeks of treatment with fluconazole alone) was associated with increased mortality in that setting, in which the optimal management of increased intracranial pressure (decreasing cerebrospinal fluid (CSF) volume by lumbar puncture or other sterile procedure) may not be available (Makadzange, 2010). Furthermore, a 2014 study of 177 patients from Uganda and South Africa who had cryptococcal meningitis reported increased mortality (hazard ratio, 1.73) at 26 weeks for patients who started ART within 1 or 2 weeks compared to those who had deferral of ART for 5 weeks (Boulware, 2014). Patients in the early group started ART a median of 8 days after antifungal therapy, and patients in the deferred group started ART at a median of 36 days. Most of the increase in mortality was observed within the first 8–30 days of the study. The differences in mortality were especially pronounced in patients who had CSF white blood cell (WBC) counts of less than 5 cells/µL, although it was unclear if the increase in mortality in this study was due to progression of cryptococcal disease or IRIS. Current US Department of Health and Human Services (USDHHS) guidelines recommend a short delay in initiating ART in the presence of cryptococcal meningitis (discussed later).

There are limited data on the optimal timing for the initiation of ART in patients with tuberculous meningitis. A study conducted in Vietnam randomized 253 participants with advanced AIDS and tuberculous meningitis to initiate ART within 7 days or 2 months after starting TB treatment (Török, 2011) Early initiation of ART did not translate in improvement of the 9-month mortality (hazard ratio, 1.12; 95% CI 0.81–1.55; $p = 0.50$) or the time to new AIDS event (hazard ratio, 1.16; 95% CI 0.87–1.55; $p = 0.31$). However, more grade 4 adverse events were reported by participants in the early treatment arm than in the deferred arm (102 vs. 87, respectively; $p = 0.04$).

Implementation of the findings of A5164 and similar studies may prove difficult in practice, particularly in settings in which patients may not have existing linkage to primary care and limited access to ongoing treatment with ART after the resolution of the acute OI. However, effective implementation of early ART was accomplished and published by an academic medical center, and this may be a model for bringing early ART to a "real-world" population (Geng, 2011).

RECOMMENDATIONS OF GUIDELINES

The guidelines for prevention and treatment of OIs in HIV-positive adults and adolescents were updated in May 2018 and are available in the latest form online (https://aidsinfo.nih.gov/guidelines/html/4/adult-and-adolescent-opportunistic-infection/0, accessed August 29, 2018). These guidelines provide recommendations regarding the timing of initiation of ART in the setting of specific opportunistic conditions, and they should be referenced for guidance in the treatment of patients with those conditions. These guidelines generally reiterate the findings of A5164, suggesting that, unless contraindications are present, early initiation of ART near the time of treatment of an OI should be considered for most patients with an acute OI. Other elements that should be considered are degree of immunosuppression, availability of treatment for the OI, drug–drug interactions and overlapping toxicities, and the risk and potential consequences of IRIS.

In many instances, it is recommended that ART should be started as soon as possible. These conditions include PML, which is caused by the John Cunningham (JC) virus; cryptosporidiosis; microsporidiosis; and fungal infections other than meningitis caused by *C. neoformans*. For PCP and invasive BIs, the guidelines recommend starting ART within 2 weeks of diagnosis, although the panel notes that no patients with respiratory failure requiring mechanical ventilation were enrolled in study A5164. For *Toxoplasma gondii* encephalitis, the panel cites expert opinion to start ART within 2 or 3 weeks after diagnosis and initiation of specific treatment for toxoplasmosis based on the data from A5164, which studied only 5% of participants diagnosed with toxoplasmosis. For disseminated *Mycobacterium avium* complex, the panel cites expert opinion to consider starting ART after the first 2 weeks of antimycobacterial therapy in order to decrease the overall initial pill burden and also to decrease the possibility for IRIS. For cytomegalovirus (CMV) retinitis, the panel notes that many experts would not delay ART for more than 2 weeks after the start of CMV-specific treatment.

Regarding cryptococcal meningitis, the panel notes that it would be prudent to defer ART at least until the initial 2-week antifungal induction is complete and possibly until the completion of the consolidation phase at 10 weeks, especially if the patient has increased intracranial pressure or a low CSF WBC count. The panel also notes that if ART is started prior to 10 weeks of antifungal treatment, then the clinician should be prepared to promptly investigate and treat manifestations of IRIS, including increased intracranial pressure. Last, there is very limited randomized clinical trial evidence to guide the optimal time for initiation of ART in the setting of concomitant tuberculous meningitis. Expert opinion remains relevant in managing these patients.

SUMMARY

Although substantial barriers to early initiation of ART in the setting of an acute OI exist, the weight of the available evidence falls on the side of starting ART as soon as possible for most patients with acute OIs and invasive BIs, with the notable exception of meningitis due to *C. neoformans* or *M. tuberculosis*.

RECOMMENDED READING

Abdool Karim SS, Naidoo K, Grobler A, et al. Timing of initiation of antiretroviral drugs during tuberculosis therapy. *N Engl J Med*. February 25, 2010;362(8):697–706. Available at http://www.ncbi.nlm.nih.gov/pubmed/20181971.

Blanc FX, Sok T, Laureillard D, et al. Earlier versus later start of antiretroviral therapy in HIV-positive adults with tuberculosis. *N Engl J Med*. October 20, 2011;365(16):1471–1481. Available at http://www.ncbi.nlm.nih.gov/pubmed/22010913.

Boulware DR, Meya DB, Muzoora C, et al. Timing of antiretroviral therapy after diagnosis of cryptococcal meningitis. *N Engl J Med* June 26, 2014;370(26):2487–2498.

Havlir DV, Kendall MA, Ive P, et al. Timing of antiretroviral therapy for HIV-1 infection and tuberculosis. *N Engl J Med*. October 20, 2011;365(16):1482–1491. Available at http://www.ncbi.nlm.nih.gov/pubmed/22010914.

Mfinanga SG, Kirenga BJ, Chanda DM, et al. Early versus delayed initiation of highly active antiretroviral therapy for HIV-positive adults with newly diagnosed pulmonary tuberculosis (TB-HAART): a prospective, international, randomised, placebo-controlled trial. *Lancet Infect Dis*. July 2014;14(7):563–571. Available at http://www.ncbi.nlm.nih.gov/pubmed/24810491.

Temprano ANRS Study Group, Danel C, Moh R, et al. A trial of early antiretrovirals and isoniazid preventive therapy in Africa. *N Engl J Med*. August 27, 2015;373(9):808–822. Available at http://www.ncbi.nlm.nih.gov/pubmed/26193126.

Zolopa A, Andersen J, Powderly W, et al. Early antiretroviral therapy reduces AIDS progression/death in individuals with acute opportunistic infections: a multicenter randomized strategy trial. *PLoS One*. 2009;4(5):e5575.

MYCOBACTERIAL INFECTIONS

LEARNING OBJECTIVE

Discuss the available tests and treatment modalities to appropriately manage patients with HIV and infection with *M. tuberculosis, M. avium* complex, and *M. kansasii*, the most common mycobacterial diseases associated with HIV infection.

KEY POINTS

- HIV infection markedly increases the likelihood of a patient progressing from latent tuberculosis infection (LTBI) to active TB disease.

- Interferon-γ release assays (IGRAs) increase specificity but not sensitivity over tuberculin skin testing in the diagnosis of TB in HIV-positive patients.

- Rifamycins are a critical component of effective TB therapy in HIV patients but have many drug–drug interactions.

- *M. avium* complex (MAC) disease most commonly presents as disseminated disease with fever, night sweats, weight loss, and gastrointestinal symptoms.

- Optimal treatment of MAC disease should include medications for both MAC and HIV (to reconstitute the immune system).

- MAC should be treated with multidrug therapy, including clarithromycin (or azithromycin) and ethambutol optimally.

- Individuals with a CD4$^+$ T cell count of less than 75 cells/mm^3 should receive chemoprophylaxis for MAC with azithromycin or clarithromycin once they have been ruled out for active disease.

- *M. kansasii* infection closely resembles TB, with more frequent pulmonary presentation than MAC.

- First-line antituberculosis drugs (except for pyrazinamide) are highly effective against *M. kansasii*.

- Diagnosis and treatment of *M. kansasii* as outlined in the American Thoracic Society guidelines are the same for HIV-positive and -uninfected individuals.

MYCOBACTERIUM TUBERCULOSIS

Epidemiology

There were 9.6 million cases of TB worldwide in 2014; 1.2 million of these cases (~12%) were in HIV-positive individuals (World Health Organization, 2015a). Recognition of the vulnerability of the HIV population to TB and increased awareness of the need to rapidly diagnose and treat TB/HIV-coinfected individuals have led to a steady decrease in HIV-associated TB deaths since the numbers peaked globally in 2004. Deaths from TB in HIV-positive individuals declined from 540,000 in 2004 to 360,000 in 2013. Despite these gains, TB still kills an estimated 1 in 5 persons with AIDS annually worldwide (World Health Organization, 2015b).

Rates of TB in the United States are declining, with 3.0 new cases of TB disease per 100,000 population (a total of 9,105 cases) reported in 2017, a decrease from 2016 and the lowest case count on record in the United States (CDC, 2018). The prevalence of LTBI in the general population of the United States is 4.7% (Miramontes, 2015), which has remained unchanged since the last survey in 1999–2000. The incidence of HIV-related TB has declined more rapidly than the rate of active TB in the general population, in part due to the widespread use of ART. For all ages, the estimated percentage of HIV coinfection in persons who reported HIV testing (positive, negative, or indeterminate test results) with TB decreased from 48% to 6% overall from 1993–2017, and from 63% to 9% among persons 25 to 44 years of age during this period (CDC, 2018). Like TB disease in the general population of the United States, HIV-related TB is increasingly a disease of persons born outside of the United States. Notably, TB disease has not decreased significantly in recent years among foreign-born persons with HIV disease in the United States (USDHHS OI Guidelines, May 2018).

Unlike other HIV-related opportunistic infections, CD4+ T cell count does not predict risk of TB infection. Rates of TB in HIV-positive patients are higher than those in non–HIV-positive individuals at all CD4 counts.

Clinical Presentation

Infection with *M. tuberculosis* generally occurs after inhalation of infectious particles coughed into the air by a person with active pulmonary TB disease. A less common route of infection involves ingestion of unpasteurized dairy products produced from the milk of *M. bovis*-infected cows (bovine TB). Once infected, individuals will either progress to active disease (progressive primary disease) or their immune system will contain growth of the organism but not kill it (LTBI). Host immune factors play a major role in which route initial infection will take. Host factors also play a role in whether patients with LTBI will progress to active TB disease (post-primary or reactivation disease).

Tuberculosis in individuals who are not infected with HIV typically presents as pulmonary disease. Often, the upper lobes of the lung are involved, and cavitary lesions are characteristic. Pulmonary disease is frequently accompanied by constitutional symptoms such as fever, night sweats, and weight loss. These findings are more typical of reactivation disease rather than progressive primary infection found when there is poor containment of the infecting organism by the immune system.

CD4+ T cells play a pivotal role in the containment of *M. tuberculosis*. As HIV infection progresses and there is a decline in the number of these cells, there is less containment of infecting organisms. The clinical presentation of TB in HIV-positive individuals differs based on the CD4+ T cell count. Patients with counts of greater than 350 cells/mm³ often present with the classic pulmonary presentation described. As the CD4+ T cell count decreases, the clinical presentation can look more like progressive primary disease. In patients with CD4+ T cell counts of less than 200 cells/mm³, pulmonary lesions may involve any lobe of the lungs and range from infiltrates to pneumonia. Cavitary lesions become less common with advanced HIV disease, and HIV–TB coinfected patients may have no abnormalities on chest X-ray.

Another feature of HIV-associated TB is extrapulmonary disease. Extrapulmonary disease is found in up to 50% of individuals in some series. Lymph node disease is the most common extrapulmonary site. Disseminated (military) disease and mycobacteremia are far more common in patients with low CD4+ T cell counts.

Diagnosis

Diagnosis of TB infection in an HIV-positive patient requires a high index of suspicion. Recent advances in diagnostic tests for TB, such as IGRAs, have not translated into a major improvement in the diagnosis of TB in patients with HIV. Diagnosis requires the HIV physician to remain vigilant.

Traditionally, screening for TB infection has been via the tuberculin skin test (TST). The assay involves injection of 0.1 mL (comprising 5 tuberculin units) of purified protein derivative subcutaneously into the volar surface of the forearm. Individuals who have been previously infected with *M. tuberculosis* develop a delayed-type hypersensitivity reaction to the injected proteins. Induration caused by this reaction is measured after 48–72 hours. A TST measurement of 5 mm of induration or greater is considered positive in a person infected with HIV. Sensitivity of this test has always been poor in HIV-positive individuals, and it can be as low as 30% in TB patients with CD4+ counts of less than 200 cells/mm³. It is also important to note that the TST will not distinguish between patients with latent TB infection and those with active TB, and it may be falsely positive in patients vaccinated with Bacillus Calmette–Guérin (BCG) due to cross-reaction with the antigens found in the BCG vaccine.

IGRAs are newer diagnostic tests developed in the past 10 years for detection of *M. tuberculosis* infection. These tests are based on immune responses to antigens unique to *M. tuberculosis*. IGRAs have the benefits of negating the false positives seen with BCG vaccination and offering a blood draw that requires a single visit. There are two commercially available IGRAs approved by the US Food and Drug Administration (FDA)—the QuantiFERON-TB Gold In-Tube (QFT-GIT) and the T.SPOT.*TB* (T-spot). Meta-analyses (Cattamanchin, 2011; Santin, 2012) show the sensitivity of these tests to be approximately 60% for the QFT-GIT and 70% for the T-spot. Although this appears to be an improvement over the TST, there was not a significant difference in head-to-head sensitivity with either test compared to the TST. The T-spot seems to be less affected by the level of immunosuppression than either the QFT-GIT or TST in HIV-positive patients. The studies highlight the fact that there are still a large number of cases of LTBI or active disease that may be missed by these tests, and a high index of suspicion is still warranted. As highlighted in the recommendations on IGRAs outlined by the US Centers for Disease Control (CDC) (2010), these tests are most useful in BCG-vaccinated populations (adding greater specificity) and in populations with poor rates of return (negating the need for a return visit for reading). These same guidelines state clearly that routine testing with both the TST and an IGRA is not recommended.

HIV-positive individuals should be screened for TB infection by a TST or IGRA at the time of HIV diagnosis and regularly thereafter. Individuals who travel to countries with a high TB burden or who reside in areas with high rates of TB should be tested annually. All others should be tested when there is suspicion of exposure to an active case after their initial testing. Individuals with CD4$^+$ counts of less than 200 cells/mm^3 at HIV diagnosis should have a repeat diagnostic test after CD4$^+$ count recovery to greater than 200 cells/mm^3.

An individual with a positive diagnostic test (TST or IGRA) without evidence of active TB disease should be given a diagnosis of LTBI. HIV patients with LTBI are at very high risk for advancing to active TB. Individuals with LTBI without HIV have a 5–10% lifetime risk of developing active TB, whereas individuals with HIV and LTBI have a 10% annual risk. Generally, persons with HIV and LTBI are 29.6 (27.1–32.1) times more likely to progress to active disease than persons without HIV (World Health Organization, 2015 factsheet). LTBI treatment in this population is paramount and has formed the cornerstone of progress in reducing global TB cases.

Diagnosis of active TB disease requires utilization of many pieces of data. A thorough history is useful in most cases. Important information to note includes exposure to an active TB case, residence in high-risk settings such as jail or homeless shelters, and prior diagnosis of untreated LTBI. Signs and symptoms of active disease may include cough lasting longer than 3 weeks, unexplained weight loss, fevers, and/or night sweats. There are no physical exam findings specific for TB, but a thorough physical exam may reveal suspicious lymphadenopathy, draining fistulas, respiratory sounds, or signs of meningitis.

Diagnostic tests such as the TST and IGRA can add to available data but cannot be relied on entirely. One may also consider performing more than one of these tests to increase sensitivity, especially when the patient has a low CD4 count. In general, a positive TST or IGRA result should be taken as evidence of infection.

All patients suspected of having active TB should receive a chest X-ray because the lungs are the most common entry point and a frequent site of infection. As previously noted, the chest X-ray can be normal in patients with culture-positive pulmonary TB. Any patient with respiratory symptoms, regardless of chest X-ray findings, should have sputum (three specimens) collected 8–24 hours apart with at least one sputum being an early morning specimen.

Patients with lower CD4$^+$ counts are more likely to have extrapulmonary TB with infection in tissues that are more difficult to access and that have fewer organisms. It may be necessary to obtain biopsy specimens such as lymph nodes, bone marrow, or lung tissue to make the diagnosis. Cerebrospinal, ascitic, or abscess fluid may also be diagnostic. All tissue from suspected sites of infection should be submitted for smear and culture analysis for acid-fast bacilli and, if indicated, histopathologic analysis searching for characteristic granulomas on pathology.

Treatment

Treatment of latent TB in HIV-positive patients is essentially the same as that in patients without HIV. The preferred regimen for treatment of LTBI in HIV-positive patients is 9 months of isoniazid (INH) dosed daily or intermittently (twice weekly) by directly observed therapy (DOT).

In individuals without HIV, 6 months of INH is an acceptable alternative, but this regimen has a lower rating for HIV-positive individuals.

Rifampin taken for 4 months is an acceptable LTBI treatment in patients who are intolerant of INH or who are exposed to an INH-resistant case. Rifampin interacts with all antiretrovirals except the nucleoside analogues (excluding zidovudine) and enfuvirtide. In many cases, rifabutin can be substituted for rifampin. When a rifamycin is used in the treatment of a patient on ART, drug–drug interactions must be carefully considered. Guidance is available in a regularly updated document at https://aidsinfo.nih.gov.

The most recently approved treatment regimen for LTBI is INH–rifapentine dosed weekly for 12 weeks by DOT. Although this regimen is appropriate for patients with HIV, it is contraindicated in patients receiving any form of antiretroviral treatment.

Treatment of active TB in HIV-positive patients is also essentially the same as that for HIV-negative patients. All patients diagnosed in the United States with active TB should be started on a four-drug regimen consisting of isoniazid, rifampin, ethambutol, and pyrazinamide unless there is known resistance or baseline severe impairment of hepatic or renal function. After 2 months of this four-drug therapy (initial phase) and if the patient's organism is not resistant, the regimen can be reduced to INH and rifampin for the duration of treatment (continuation phase). Length of treatment will depend on the site and extent of disease. Most cases can be treated with 6–9 months of total therapy, whereas infections involving the bones or meninges should be treated for a total of 9–12 months. Infections of the pericardium or meninges should be treated with steroids in addition to anti-TB medications.

The most significant differences between treatment of HIV-positive patients and that of HIV-negative patients involve use of the rifamycins and frequency of dosing. As previously noted, there is significant interaction between rifampin and most antiretrovirals, so care must be taken in introducing this class of medications into the regimen. Treatment regimens for active TB that do not contain a rifamycin require up to 18 months of therapy and have very high rates of relapse. Every effort should be made to include a rifamycin in the treatment of patients coinfected with HIV and TB. Regularly updated guidance on how to manage drug interactions can be found at https://aidsinfo.nih.gov.

DOT is highly recommended for all cases of active TB treated in the United States. Patients can receive intermittent dosing but only if receiving DOT. Highly intermittent dosing of TB therapy (once- or twice-weekly dosing) is associated with an increased risk of relapse with rifampin-resistant disease and should be avoided in patients infected with HIV (CDC, 2003). This is especially noted in patients with CD4$^+$ counts of less than 100 cells/mm^3.

The question of when to initiate antiretroviral treatment in a patient coinfected with HIV and TB is not a trivial one. Treatment for both diseases simultaneously can result in a large pill burden, potential for multiple drug interactions, and potential for multiple drug toxicities. Although it is clear that patients who are diagnosed with TB should be started immediately on anti-TB medications, until recently, the timing of adding ART was less clear. Several studies (Blanc, 2011; Karim, 2011; Martinson, 2011) conducted at multiple sites have shown a survival benefit (reduced mortality) when starting ART within 2 weeks of starting TB medications in patients with CD4$^+$ counts of less than 50 cells/mm^3. At CD4 counts higher than 50 cells/mm^3, the incidence of IRIS events increased. In patients with severe disease who have CD4$^+$ counts of 50 cells/mm^3 or higher, the current recommendation is to start treatment for HIV within 2–4 weeks of starting TB therapy and within 8–12 weeks in patients with CD4$^+$ counts 50 cells/mm^3 or higher who do not have severe disease.

If IRIS does occur in the course of treatment, it is important that both antiretroviral and TB treatment be continued. Mild cases of IRIS can be observed or treated with nonsteroidal anti-inflammatory agents, or, if more severe, a short course of steroids may be necessary.

Special consideration should be given to patients with HIV and TB meningitis. IRIS involving central nervous system disease leads to worse outcomes. Patients with HIV and TB meningitis must be monitored carefully and treated with steroid therapy to reduce the inflammatory effects associated with disease. Treatment with antiretroviral medication should be added, with careful monitoring of the patient for any evidence of IRIS.

Drug-resistant disease in an HIV-positive patient requires individualized therapy and should be approached with an expert in drug-resistant TB. Patients with multidrug-resistant or extensively drug-resistant TB should have ART initiated within 2–4 weeks after initiation of second-line TB drug therapy.

Prevention

Individuals with HIV should be screened for TB by a TST or IGRA at the time of diagnosis and periodically thereafter. Individuals with HIV who are found to have a positive TST or IGRA without evidence of active disease should be treated for LTBI to prevent progression to active disease.

HIV-positive individuals who are contacts to an infectious pulmonary case of TB and have no evidence of active disease should be treated with a full course of therapy for LTBI, even with a negative diagnostic test. As outlined previously, available diagnostic tests are not sensitive enough to rule out TB infection, and patients exposed to an infectious case are highly susceptible. Active disease should be ruled out in all patients prior to initiation of treatment for LTBI.

Patients who have a history of untreated or inadequately treated TB who do not have evidence of currently active disease should receive treatment for LTBI. This may be manifest as old fibrotic lesions on chest X-ray noted during routine screening.

MYCOBACTERIUM AVIUM COMPLEX

Epidemiology

MAC, also known as MAI, consists of *M. avium* and *M. intracellulare*, two organisms so similar that they can only be differentiated using DNA probes. MAC infections are the most common nontuberculous mycobacteria (NTM) infections in both HIV-positive and HIV-negative patients (Griffith, 2007).

These organisms are ubiquitous and are found environmentally in water, soil, and animal sources. Despite the many places from which the organisms can be isolated, the actual route of infection in HIV-positive patients is unclear. There is no evidence for human-to-human or animal-to-human transmission.

Disseminated disease is the most common presentation of MAC infection associated with HIV and occurs almost exclusively in patients with profound immunosuppression who are not yet receiving ART. Disseminated disease is most commonly found in patient with CD4$^+$ counts of less than 50 cells/mm^3. Having a high HIV viral load (>100,000 copies/mm^3) has also been identified as a risk factor. The incidence of disseminated MAC has declined steadily since the introduction of effective antiretroviral treatment, with most cases occurring in individuals who have not accessed care.

Clinical Presentation

As stated previously, the most common presentation of MAC infection in HIV patients is disseminated disease. Symptoms tend to be nonspecific and typically include fever, night sweats, anorexia, weight loss, and gastrointestinal symptoms such as nausea, vomiting, diarrhea, and abdominal pain. It is important to remember that these same symptoms can be associated with other opportunistic infections, such as TB and fungal disease.

Disseminated MAC infection tends to involve the reticuloendothelial system and, subsequently, physical exam findings may include hepatomegaly, splenomegaly, and lymphadenopathy. Pulmonary disease is rare, even with disseminated disease, but occasionally can manifest as nodules, infiltrates, cavities, or mediastinal/hilar adenopathy. Pulmonary findings are more likely to be associated with infection due to *M. tuberculosis* or *M. kansasii*.

Immune reconstitution in patients newly started on ART may "unmask" preexisting, previously undetected disease. The presentation in this case may manifest as disseminated disease or perhaps localized disease.

Diagnosis

Isolation of MAC from a normally sterile site, such as the blood, should be considered diagnostic for disseminated disease. In the absence of a positive blood culture, other more invasive approaches, such as lymph node, liver, or bone marrow biopsy, may be necessary to obtain an adequate specimen for diagnosis.

Isolation of MAC from nonsterile sites such as the respiratory or gastrointestinal tracts may represent true pathology but can also represent colonization. In these cases, it is important to make an effort to determine if other pathogens may be at play.

Treatment

Optimally, the approach to treatment of disseminated MAC disease should include treatment of both MAC and HIV. Like treatment of TB and other NTM infections, treatment of MAC infection should include multidrug therapy.

Clarithromycin should be the first drug added to a MAC treatment regimen. In the event of clarithromycin intolerance or unacceptable drug interaction with other medications, azithromycin may be substituted. Studies have shown treatment with clarithromycin to be associated with faster clearance of bacteremia than treatment with azithromycin (CDC, 2015).

The second drug added should be ethambutol. Addition of ethambutol to a macrolide is associated with decreased relapse in the treatment of MAC. Rifabutin can also be added to the MAC treatment regimen but has not been shown to improve outcomes over the combination of a macrolide and ethambutol alone. Addition of rifabutin also adds the potential for significant interaction with many antiretrovirals and can lower serum drug levels of clarithromycin when used in combination. Prior to addition of rifabutin to the treatment of a mycobacterial infection, TB must be ruled out to prevent the emergence of rifampin-resistant TB disease.

Based on data from non-HIV-positive patients, agents such as amikacin and streptomycin can be utilized if there is a need for additional medication options due to resistance or toxicity.

IRIS has been documented with treatment of MAC disease, as it has with TB. The presentation generally manifests as a return of fever and worsening lymphadenitis with negative blood cultures. Mild cases can be simply monitored or treated with a nonsteroidal anti-inflammatory agent or, in severe cases, a short course of steroids. Treatment for both MAC and HIV should be continued during management of IRIS reactions.

Treatment of disseminated disease should continue until there is a response to ART. Patients who complete a 12-month course of therapy, who remain free of signs or symptoms of disease, and who show a sustained increase in CD4+ count to more than 100 cells/mm³ for at least 6 months have a low risk of relapse. If a previously treated patient experiences a decrease in CD4+ count to less than 100 cells/mm³, the patient should be placed back on preventive prophylaxis treatment.

Prevention/Prophylaxis

No direct route for infection with MAC has been identified and, thus, there is no specific action known to prevent exposure to MAC. Patients with a CD4+ T cell count of less than 50 cells/mm³ are at high risk for disseminated MAC and should receive chemoprophylaxis to prevent development of disease.

Azithromycin dosed at 1,200 mg weekly is the preferred prophylactic regimen. Clarithromycin dosed at 500 mg twice daily is effective, but due to the increased pill burden, it is considered an alternative to azithromycin. Before starting prophylaxis, disseminated MAC should be ruled out.

Rifabutin is an alternative when there is evidence of macrolide-resistant disease or macrolide intolerance, but rifabutin is less effective in this capacity and adds increased risk of drug interactions with many of the antiretrovirals. Before use of rifabutin, every effort should be made to rule out active TB.

MYCOBACTERIUM KANSASII

Epidemiology

M. kansasii infection is the second most common NTM infection in HIV-positive patients (after MAC infection). Tap water appears to be the most likely environmental reservoir for strains causing human disease (Griffith, 2002; Jones, 2002). Lung disease caused by M. kansasii closely resembles disease caused by M. tuberculosis in both HIV-positive and –negative patients. Despite its similarities to TB, there is no evidence of human-to-human transmission of M. kansasii. Similar to MAC, infection with M. kansasii is most commonly found in patients with CD4+ T cell counts of less than 50 cells/mm³.

Clinical Presentation

Unlike MAC disease, which is most commonly disseminated and rarely pulmonary, M. kansasii can be disseminated but is more commonly pulmonary. Radiographically, M. kansasii infection closely resembles infection with M. tuberculosis, with symptoms that include cough, fever, night sweats, weight loss, and hemoptysis.

Diagnosis

Diagnosis requires isolation of the organism from a sterile site or meeting the criterion outlined in the guidelines set forth by the American Thoracic Society (ATS, 2000). Briefly, the ATS criteria for both HIV-positive and noninfected individuals require that the individual in question have pulmonary symptoms with suggestive radiography, exclusion of other diagnoses, positive culture results from two separate expectorated sputa, or at least one bronchoalveolar lavage specimen or bronchial biopsy with suggestive histopathology.

M. kansasii isolated from the sputum of a patient with pulmonary lesions can trigger an unnecessary public health investigation for TB. Testing with a nucleic acid amplification test can rule out TB in these cases.

Treatment

M. kansasii responds well to anti-TB medications with the exception that the organism is widely resistant to pyrazinamide. Treatment with isoniazid, ethambutol and rifampin or rifabutin is recommended for 18 months, with at least 12 months of culture-negative sputum. Rifamycins in the treatment regimen of M. kansasii patients (unlike those with MAC disease) provide clear benefit and prevent relapse. The choice and dose of rifamycin should be guided by the patient's antiretroviral treatment, with special attention to potential drug interactions.

As with infections caused by other mycobacteria, IRIS has been documented with treatment of *M. kansasii*. Mild cases can be simply monitored or treated with a nonsteroidal anti-inflammatory agent or, in severe cases, a short course of steroids. It is important that treatment for both *M. kansasii* and HIV be continued during management of IRIS reactions.

OPPORTUNISTIC INFECTIONS: VIRAL INFECTIONS

LEARNING OBJECTIVE

Discuss the established and evolving science regarding diagnosis, treatment, and prophylaxis of opportunistic viral infections associated with HIV infection in order to improve quality of life and length of survival.

WHAT'S NEW?

A new recombinant zoster vaccine was approved in October 2017. The Advisory Committee for Immunization Practices (ACIP) is still evaluating recommendations for people living with HIV (PLWH).

KEY POINTS

Herpes Simplex Virus

- Herpes simplex virus (HSV) is a very common disease in PLWH, typically presenting with orolabial, genital, and/or anorectal ulcers that may be very severe in the setting of advance immunosuppression. HSV could also manifest as proctitis (particularly in men who have sex with men), esophagitis, keratitis, meningitis, encephalitis, radiculitis, and retinitis (presenting as acute retinal necrosis).

- Treatment is generally with acyclovir or one of its derivatives. Acyclovir resistance is more common among PLWH. HSV suppression should be considered for individuals with frequent or severe recurrent episodes.

Varicella Zoster Virus

- Varicella zoster reactivation disease in PLWH is often more severe, multidermatomal, or disseminated. Severe complications such as progressive outer retinal necrosis must be treated quickly to prevent permanent sequelae. For mild disease, oral therapy with acyclovir or one of its derivatives is appropriate; in severe cases, however, intravenous therapy is required.

Cytomegalovirus

- Cytomegalovirus may cause a variety of clinical manifestations in PLWH with CD4+ T cell counts of less than 50 cells/mm³. Retinitis and colitis are the most common manifestations. Ganciclovir (or the oral prodrug valganciclovir) or foscarnet are the most common therapies, but they carry significant risk of toxicity. Primary prophylaxis is not recommended.

JC Virus

- JC virus causes progressive multifocal leukoencephalopathy, a progressive, demyelinating disease of the central nervous system that leads to relatively rapid accumulation of neurologic deficits with dementia, coma, and death. Diagnosis is generally made clinically with the support of typical magnetic resonance imaging (MRI) findings and polymerase chain reaction (PCR) testing for JC virus in the CSF. Definitive diagnosis is made by brain biopsy. No specific antiviral therapy exists for JC virus. ART often results in stabilization or regression of disease.

HERPESVIRUS

Herpes Simplex Virus

Herpes simplex virus types 1 and 2 (HSV-1 and HSV-2) are highly prevalent in PLWH. Classically, HSV-1 caused oral ulcers, whereas HSV-2 caused genital ulcers; currently, however, both are recognized as a cause of genital infection, especially in young women and men who have sex with men.

HSV-2 is one of the most common sexually transmitted infections worldwide and the primary cause of genital ulcer disease. The overall national HSV-2 prevalence was reported as 16.2% in 2010 (Xu, 2006); however, seroprevalence rates near 70% have been reported in PLWH (Corey, 2004). The primary mode of transmission is through direct contact with oral secretions or genital secretions. Clinical HSV disease is common in the absence of HIV infection, but manifestations are more common, more severe, or atypical in the setting of HIV infection.

Clinical Presentation

The classical presentation of herpes infection is large, painful, grouped vesicles with an erythematous base typically in the orolabial, genital, and anorectal regions; however, they may involve any areas of the body. In patients with advanced HIV-associated immunosuppression, anogenital lesions may be severe, and they may be refractory to treatment or secondary to acyclovir-resistant virus (Safrin, 1994). Dissemination is possible, but it is rarely seen in PLWH. Proctitis, particularly in men who have sex with men (MSM), keratitis, meningitis, encephalitis, radiculitis, and retinitis (presenting as acute retinal necrosis) are possible complications. HSV esophagitis may occur in people with CD4+ T cell counts of less than 50 cells/mm³ and typically presents with retrosternal chest pain and odynophagia.

Reactivation of HSV is more common in PLWH. Recurrent lesions are often more frequent, more extensive, and of longer duration in this population. In addition, there is prolonged shedding of the virus even in the absence of lesions, especially in patients with lower CD4$^+$ T cell counts and higher plasma HIV-1 RNA levels.

Diagnosis

Diagnosis is made clinically. However, laboratory confirmation should be done, when possible, with viral culture, examination of lesion scrapings using immunofluorescent staining, Tzanck preparation (multinucleated giant cells), or PCR amplification techniques. Culture specimens can also be tested for antiviral drug susceptibility.

Treatment

Table 33.1 shows the current treatment recommendations from the 2018 Panel on Opportunistic Infections in HIV-Positive Adults and Adolescents (Guidelines for the Prevention and Treatment of Opportunistic Infections in HIV-positive adults and adolescents: Recommendations from the CDC, the National Institutes of Health, and the HIV Medicine Association of the Infectious Diseases Society of America). Oral acyclovir, valacyclovir, and famciclovir are comparable alternatives. In patients with extensive mucocutaneous lesions, it is recommended to use intravenous acyclovir.

Resistance to acyclovir has been reported in up to 5% of PLWH with HSV-2 infection and is more frequent in patients with prolonged acyclovir use. Acyclovir inhibits HSV-specific DNA polymerase after incorporation into the growing DNA, resulting in a chain termination due to the absence of the 3' hydroxyl group. It requires phosphorylation by a virally encoded thymidine kinase in order to be active. Altered, reduced, or absent thymidine kinase or altered viral DNA polymerase confers resistance to acyclovir and all the class including

ganciclovir. In these cases, foscarnet or cidofovir are the only alternate options.

Prophylaxis

Condoms are recommended to prevent transmission of HSV-2. The use of 1% tenofovir vaginal gel has been shown to be associated with a 50% risk reduction of HSV-2 acquisition in women at high risk of HIV infection. However, this has not been confirmed in other studies. In addition, in patients taking oral tenofovir, the rates of vaginal shedding of HSV-1 and HSV-2 are similar. Suppressive therapy with oral acyclovir, valacyclovir, or famciclovir is effective in preventing genital herpes recurrences, and it should be discussed with all HSV-2-infected patients (Table 33.2). Immune reconstitution improves the frequency and severity of clinical episodes of genital herpes, but it does not decrease shedding.

In individuals with CD4$^+$ T cell count of less than 250 cells/mm^3 who will start ART, there is an increased risk of HSV-2 shedding and genital ulcer diseases in the first 6 months. It is recommended to give suppressive antiviral therapy because it decreases the risk of genital ulcer diseases by 60%.

VARICELLA ZOSTER VIRUS

Varicella zoster virus (VZV), the third herpesvirus, causes initial infection in childhood (chickenpox) and later reactivates, causing herpes zoster. The prevalence of herpes zoster is 3–5% in the general population, but it is 15–25 times higher in PLWH (Buchbinder, 1992). Lower CD4$^+$ T cell counts have been associated with more atypical presentations of the disease but not with increased incidence.

Table 33.1 HERPES SIMPLEX VIRUS TREATMENT RECOMMENDATIONS

CONDITION	FIRST CHOICE TREATMENT	ALTERNATIVE TREATMENT
Orolabial lesions	Valacyclovir 1 g PO b.i.d. or Famciclovir 500 mg PO b.i.d. or Acyclovir 400 mg PO t.i.d. for 5–10 days	
Initial or recurrent genital lesions	Valacyclovir 1 g PO b.i.d. or Famciclovir 500 mg PO b.i.d. or Acyclovir 400 mg PO t.i.d. for 5–10 days	
Severe mucocutaneous lesions	Acyclovir 5 mg/kg IV every 8 hours until lesions regress, then switch to acyclovir 400 mg PO t.i.d. until lesions are healed	
Esophagitis	Valacyclovir 1 g PO t.i.d. or Famciclovir 500 mg PO t.i.d. or Acyclovir 400 mg PO five times daily for 14–21 days	
Encephalitis and hepatitis	Acyclovir 10–15 mg/kg IV every 8 hours for 21 days	
Acyclovir-resistant herpes	Foscarnet 80–120 mg/kg/day IV 2–3 times daily until clinical response	Topical trifluridine, or Cidofovir 1% gel, or Topical imiquimod 5% three times weekly for 21–28 days or longer based on clinical response

Table 33.2 HERPES SIMPLEX VIRUS SUPPRESSIVE THERAPY RECOMMENDATIONS

CONDITION	FIRST CHOICE TREATMENT
Genital lesions	Valacyclovir 500 mg PO b.i.d. or
	Famciclovir 500 mg PO b.i.d. or
	Acyclovir 400–800 mg PO b.i.d. or t.i.d.

Clinical Presentation

The initial clinical presentation is similar to that of immunocompetent patients. It manifests as a prodrome of cutaneous burning or pain, followed by a cutaneous eruption of grouped vesicles on an erythematous base along a dermatome. However, PLWH are at increased risk for multidermatomal or disseminated zoster, including neurologic and ophthalmologic complications. Approximately 20–30% of PLWH will experience subsequent episodes of herpes zoster, either in the same or in different dermatomes. The probability of a recurrence of herpes zoster within 1 year of the index episode is 10% (Gebo, 2005). Postherpetic neuralgia is reported in 10–15% of PLWH (Gebo, 2005; Harrison, 1999).

Atypical VZV presentations such as chronic hyperkeratotic lesions or chronic disseminated ecthyma have also been reported. Meningitis, multifocal leukoencephalitis, ventriculitis, myelitis, cranial nerve palsies, and focal brainstem lesions are possible neurological complications.

Involvement of the ophthalmic division of the trigeminal nerve causes anterior uveitis, corneal scarring, and vision loss. Ocular involvement with acute retinal necrosis and progressive outer retinal necrosis are syndromes similar to CMV retinitis but of faster progression that typically occurs at $CD4^+$ T cell counts of less than 100 cells/mm^3 and may result in retinal blindness (Engstromm, 1994).

Diagnosis

The diagnosis is made clinically. Laboratory confirmation could be done by viral culture, direct immunofluorescence testing, and the PCR assay, which is the most sensitive test.

Treatment

VZV treatment is summarized in Table 33.3.

Prevention

Long-term prophylaxis or suppressive treatment is not recommended. VZV vaccine is recommended for PLWH with $CD4^+$ T cell counts 200 cells/mm^3 or higher who have no documented history of vaccination or laboratory confirmation of disease. Primary varicella vaccination (Varivax) requires 2 doses administered 3 months apart. In the event that vaccination results in disease, acyclovir is recommended.

Postexposure prophylaxis is recommended for PLWH susceptible to VZV and close contact with a person who has active varicella or herpes zoster. The preferred regimen is a single

Table 33.3 VARICELLA ZOSTER VIRUS TREATMENT RECOMMENDATIONS

CONDITION	FIRST CHOICE TREATMENT
Varicella zoster virus infection, immunocompromised patients	SEVERE: Acyclovir 10–15 mg/kg IV every 8 hours for 7–10 days. May switch to PO if no evidence of visceral involvement. UNCOMPLICATED: Valacyclovir (1 g PO 3 times daily), or famciclovir (500 mg PO 3 times daily) for 5 to 7 days.
Herpes zoster, acute localized dermatomal	Valacyclovir 1 g t.i.d. or famciclovir 500 mg t.i.d. or Acyclovir 800 mg PO 5 times daily Each administered for 7–10 days. Consider longer duration if lesions slow to resolve.
Herpes zoster, extensive cutaneous lesion or visceral involvement	Acyclovir 10–15 mg/kg IV every 8 hours After clinical improvement is evident, switch to oral therapy: Valacyclovir 1 g t.i.d. or Famciclovir 500 mg t.i.d. or Acyclovir 800 mg 5 times daily Each administered for 10–14 days
Acute retinal necrosis	Acyclovir 10 mg/kg IV every 8 hours for 10–14 days; followed by oral valacyclovir 1 g t.i.d. for 6 weeks PLUS ganciclovir 2 mg/0.05mL intravitreal twice weekly × 1–2 doses
Progressive outer retinal necrosis	Ganciclovir 5 mg/kg IV and/or Foscarnet 90 mg/kg IV every 12 hours plus Ganciclovir 2 mg/0.05 ml intravitreal twice weekly × 1–2 doses
Acyclovir-resistant varicella zoster virus infection	Foscarnet 90 mg/kg IV every 12 hours

intramuscular dose of VariZIG dosed on body weight (maximum of 625 IU) administered as soon as possible and within 10 days after exposure. Alternatively, acyclovir or valacyclovir could be given starting 7–10 days after exposure.

There are two vaccines available for the prevention of zoster: a live attenuated virus zoster vaccine (ZVL) and a nonlive recombinant vaccine (RZV). ZVL was studied in a phase II, randomized, double-blind, placebo-controlled clinical trial designed to evaluate its safety, tolerability, and immunogenicity in PLWH on ART with $CD4^+$ T cell counts of 200 cells/mm^3 or higher and virologic suppression (Benson, 2018). A total of 295 participants received the vaccine. ZVL was safe and immunogenic. Those with $CD4^+$ T cell counts of 350 cells/mm^3 or higher developed the highest zoster antibody levels post-vaccination. A small phase 1/2a, randomized, observer-masked, placebo-controlled study evaluated the safety and immunogenicity of RZV in 123 PLWH. The vaccine was found to have a clinically acceptable safety profile and elicited strong gE-specific cell-mediated and humoral immune responses that persisted at least 1 year after the last vaccination. (Berkowitz, 2015). However, recommendations of RZL for PLWH have not been released yet.

CYTOMEGALOVIRUS

CMV is a DNA herpesvirus and the largest virus that infects humans. It is typically acquired from close contact during youth or adolescence. In the general population, the percentage of people with evidence of previous CMV infection ranges from 40% to 100% and varies with ethnicity and country. Active disease associated with HIV typically results from reactivation of latent infection in the setting of advanced immunosuppression with CD4$^+$ T cell counts of less than 50 cells/mm^3 (Dieterich, 1991). Other risk factors for CMV disease include plasma HIV RNA levels of more than 100,000 copies/mL and the presence of other OIs.

Before the use of ART, CMV retinitis was the most common intraocular infection in patients with AIDS, occurring in up to 40% of patients (Whitcup, 2000). Currently, the incidence of new cases of CMV end-organ disease has declined to fewer than 6 cases/100 person-years (Jabs, 2007).

Clinical Presentation and Diagnosis

CMV can infect different organs of the body. Retinitis accounts for 85% of CMV manifestations and is the leading cause of vision loss among people with AIDS. Other CMV clinical syndromes include esophagitis, colitis, polyradiculopathy, ventriculoencephalitis, pneumonitis, adrenalitis, and pancreatitis.

Chorioretinitis
CMV chorioretinitis presents with painless progressive loss of vision, floaters, and/or visual field cut defects. Symptoms are unilateral at first, but without treatment they can become bilateral. The diagnosis is exclusively made by recognition of typical retinal changes during a funduscopic examination: creamy or yellow-white granular areas with perivascular exudates and hemorrhage. These lesions initially are found in the periphery of the fundus but can later involve the macula and the optic disc, resulting in blindness.

Colitis
CMV colitis is the second most common manifestation of CMV infection in people with AIDS. Patients present with severe diarrhea, abdominal pain and cramping, anorexia, weight loss, and fever. The diagnosis is made by detection of mucosal ulcerations on endoscopic examination combined with colonoscopic or rectal biopsy. Pathology will reveal intracytoplasmatic or intranuclear inclusions. A positive culture itself does not confirm the diagnosis. Mucosal hemorrhage and perforation rarely occur, but they are life-threatening.

Esophagitis
CMV esophagitis causes odynophagia, nausea, fever, and retrosternal pain. Diagnosis is made by endoscopic examination that reveals diffuse inflammation of the esophagus and/or esophageal ulcers. Biopsy specimens also reveal intranuclear inclusions. A positive culture itself does not make the diagnosis.

CMV Polyradiculopathy
CMV polyradiculopathy presents with sacrolumbar radicular pain and lower limb paresthesia that may develop into progressive flaccid paralysis of the legs with decreasing and ultimately absent tendon reflexes. Urinary retention and stool incontinence may occur. If untreated, the condition rapidly advances up the spine, causing ascending sensory loss and growing flaccidity in the upper limbs, similar to Guillain–Barré-like paralysis. The CSF may have a pleocytosis with a predominance of polymorphonuclear cells, elevated protein, and moderately low glucose. Lumbar MRI reveals gadolinium enhancement of the cauda equina in 33% of patients. Diagnosis is made by viral culture, CMV antigen assays, and detection of CMV deoxyribonucleic acid via PCR in the CSF.

Ventriculoencephalitis
CMV ventriculoencephalitis is a late manifestation of CMV disease. It presents with fever, lethargy, confusion, and an acute course consisting of cranial nerve palsies, nystagmus, and other focal neurologic deficits that rapidly leads to death. Computed tomography (CT) and MRI scans show white matter enhancement. MRI with gadolinium may reveal a characteristic periventricular ring-like enhancement. Viral culture of the CSF is not always positive, although CMV deoxyribonucleic acid can often be detected in CSF using PCR.

Dementia
CMV dementia can present with fever, lethargy, and confusion, and it may be clinically similar to dementia caused directly by HIV. CSF reveals pleocytosis that may be polymorphonuclear, low to normal glucose, and normal to high protein. CT and MRI scans may show cerebral atrophy.

Pneumonia
CMV pneumonitis is uncommon in patients with AIDS. Symptoms include shortness of breath, dyspnea, dry nonproductive cough, and hypoxia. Imaging studies show diffuse interstitial infiltrates. A definitive diagnosis is made when multiple CMV inclusion bodies are seen in lung tissue. CMV may be isolated in bronchial washings and lavage fluid from approximately 50% of PLWH undergoing bronchoscopy secondary to viral shedding.

CMV viremia is common in asymptomatic persons with low CD4$^+$ T cell counts (<100 cells/mm^3). Viremia is typically present in active disease but may also be present in the absence of end-organ disease, so the tests are of limited value. The absence of CMV antibody may be helpful in excluding CMV disease; however, rarely, active disease can present during primary CMV infection with negative antibodies, and immunoglobin G antibody tests may revert to negative in individuals with advanced immunosuppression.

Treatment

Table 33.4 shows the current treatment recommendations from the Guidelines for the Prevention and Treatment of Opportunistic Infections (USDHHS, 2018).

For CMV chorioretinitis, treatment consists of an induction phase of high-dose drug given for at least 2 weeks. Once retinitis is stable, patients are placed on chronic maintenance therapy until there is evidence of immune recovery (sustained CD4+ T cell counts >100 cells/mm³ for ≥6 months). In the absence of antiretroviral-mediated immune reconstitution, most patients will have a reactivation of CMV infection despite suppressive therapy and will require reinduction therapy. Intraocular therapy may be useful in salvage therapy for patients who cannot tolerate systemic therapy. Any local therapy should be accompanied by systemic anti-CMV therapy. Systemic therapy has been shown to decrease CMV involvement of the contralateral eye, to reduce the risk of CMV disease in other organs, and to increase survival rates. Intraocular therapy alone has been associated with progression of CMV to the contralateral eye, as well as with systemic disease (Martin, 1994).

Ganciclovir and valganciclovir, foscarnet, and cidofovir carry significant risk for toxicity. Ganciclovir and valganciclovir can cause neutropenia, thrombocytopenia, nausea, diarrhea, renal dysfunction, and central venous catheter infection. Foscarnet more commonly causes nephrotoxicity, electrolyte abnormalities seizures, genital ulcers, and central venous catheter infection. Cidofovir, when used, is associated with nephrotoxicity and intraocular hypotony.

Prevention/Prophylaxis

In patients with CD4+ T cell count of less than 100 cells/mm³, early recognition of the manifestations of end-organ CMV disease is the primary method of prevention. Primary prophylaxis against CMV is not recommended. Patients with CD4+ T cell counts of less than 100 cells/mm³ should have annual ophthalmology exam. Secondary prophylaxis is done with valganciclovir until CD4+ T cell count has been greater than 100 cells/mm³ for 3–6 months and the lesions are not life-threatening. If CD4+ T cell count decreases to less than 100 cells/mm³, secondary prophylaxis should be reinstituted.

HUMAN HERPESVIRUS-8

The prevalence of human herpesvirus-8 (HHV-8) ranges between 1% and 5% in the general population, but it is between 20% and 77% in MSM (Pauk, 2000). HHV-8 is associated with all forms of Kaposi's sarcoma, primary

Table 33.4 CYTOMEGALOVIRUS TREATMENT RECOMMENDATIONS

CONDITION	FIRST CHOICE TREATMENT	ALTERNATIVE TREATMENT
CMV retinitis	*Sight-threatening lesions* Intravitreal injections Ganciclovir or foscarnet plus Valganciclovir 900 mg PO b.i.d. for 14–21 days, then once daily *For small peripheral lesions* Valganciclovir 900 mg PO bid for 14–21 days, then 900 mg once daily Or any of the alternative treatments	Intravitreal injections Ganciclovir or foscarnet plus Ganciclovir 5 mg/kg IV every 12 hours for 14–21 days, then 5 mg/kg IV daily or Ganciclovir 5 mg/kg IV every 12 hours for 14–21 days, then valganciclovir 900 mg PO daily Foscarnet 60 mg/kg IV every 8 hours or Foscarnet 90 mg/kg IV every 12 hours for 14–21 days, then 90–120 mg/kg IV every 24 hours or Cidofovir 5 mg/kg/week IV for 2 weeks, then 5 mg/kg every other week with saline hydration and probenecid 2 g PO 3 hours before the dose followed by 1 g 2 hours and 8 hours after the dose (total of 4 g)
Secondary prophylaxis (previously called maintenance therapy) for CMV retinitis	Valganciclovir 900 mg PO daily or Ganciclovir implant (replaced every 6–8 months if CD4+ count remains <100 cells/mm³) plus Valganciclovir 900 mg PO daily until immune recovery	Ganciclovir 5 mg/kg IV 5–7 times weekly or Foscarnet 90–120 mg/kg body weight IV once daily or Cidofovir 5 mg/kg body weight IV every other week as above
CMV colitis or esophagitis	Ganciclovir IV or Foscarnet IV for 21–28 days	
CMV neurological disease	Ganciclovir IV plus Foscarnet IV Until symptomatic improvement	

CMV, cytomegalovirus; IV, intravenous; PO, orally.

effusion lymphoma, and lymphoproliferative disorders such as multicentric Castleman's disease (see Chapter 34).

JOHN CUNNINGHAM (JC) VIRUS

JC virus causes PML, a disease characterized by focal demyelination. Approximately 85% of adults are seropositive for JC virus worldwide. The incidence of PML has decreased significantly since the widespread use of ART. However, PML has also been reported in PLWH with CD4$^+$ T cell counts of greater than 300 cells/mm^3 and as a complication of IRIS (Berger, 1998; Cinque, 2003).

Clinical Presentation

The clinical presentation of PML depends on the localization of brain lesions, and the specific deficits vary from patient to patient. Patients present with symptoms of diffuse encephalopathy to focal deficits such as ataxia, hemiparesis, or speech difficulties. Symptoms tend to progress rapidly over several weeks to months. Fever and headache may be present; seizures are seen in 20% of cases.

Diagnosis

Brain biopsy will reveal the typical findings of focal myelin loss with peculiar astrocytes and lipid-laden macrophages, and it is used to make a definitive diagnosis. MRI of the brain demonstrates distinct white matter lesions in areas of the brain corresponding to the clinical deficits. The lesions are usually white on T2 images, and they are also characteristically dark on T1 images. PCR detection of the JC virus in CSF has a diagnostic sensitivity of 70–80% and specificity of 100%.

Treatment

Initiation of effective ART is the treatment of choice. It prolongs survival and improves neurologic deficits when immune reconstitution is achieved. The early use of a five-drug antiretroviral regimen after PML diagnosis appears to improve survival (Gasnault, 2011). Other treatments have been attempted with no improvement in survival.

REFERENCES

American Thoracic Society. Targeted tuberculin testing and treatment of latent tuberculosis infection. June 2000. Available at http://www.cdc.gov/mmwr/preview/rr4906a1.htm.

Benson CA, Andersen JW, Macatangay BJC, et al. Safety and immunogenicity of Zoster [JWOY1] vaccine live in HIV-positive adults with CD4+ cell counts above 200 cells/mL virologically suppressed on antiretroviral therapy. *Clin Infect Dis*. 2018;67(11):1712–1719.

Berger JR, Levy RM, Flomenhoft D. Predictive factors for prolonged survival in acquired immunodeficiency syndrome-associated progressive multifocal leukoencephalopathy. *Ann Neurol*. 1998;44:341–349.

Berkowitz EM, Moyle G, Stellbrink HJ, et al. Safety and Immunogenicity of an Adjuvanted Herpes Zoster Subunit candidate vaccine in HIV-positive adults: a phase 1/2a randomized, placebo-controlled study. *J Infect Dis*. 2015;211(8):1279–1287.

Blanc FX, Sok T, Laureillard, D, et al. Earlier versus later start of antiretroviral therapy in HIV-positive adults with tuberculosis. *N Engl J Med*. 2011;365(16):1471–1481.

Boulware DR, Meya DB, Muzoora C, et al. Timing of antiretroviral therapy after diagnosis of cryptococcal meningitis. *N Engl J Med*. 2014;370(26):2487–2498.

Buchbinder SP, Katz MH, Hessol NA, et al. Herpes zoster and human immunodeficiency virus infection. *J Infect Dis*. 1992;166:1153–1156.

Cattamanchi A, Smith R, Steingart KR, et al. Interferon-gamma release assays for the diagnosis of latent tuberculosis infection in HIV-positive individuals: a systematic review and meta-analysis. *J AIDS*. 2011;56:230–238.

Centers for Disease Control and Prevention (CDC). Targeted tuberculin testing and treatment of latent tuberculosis infection. *MMWR*. 2000;49(RR-6).

Centers for Disease Control and Prevention (CDC). Treatment of tuberculosis. *MMWR*. 2003;52(RR-11).

Centers for Disease Control and Prevention (CDC). Guidelines for prevention and treatment of opportunistic infections in HIV-infected adults and adolescents. *MMWR*. 2009;58(RR-4).

Centers for Disease Control and Prevention (CDC). Updated guidelines for using interferon gamma release assays to detect *Mycobacterium tuberculosis* infection—United States, 2010. Available at http://www.cdc.gov/mmwr/preview/mmwrhtml/rr5905a1.htm?s_cid=rr5905a1_e.

Centers for Disease Control and Prevention (CDC). *Reported tuberculosis in the United States, 2014*. Atlanta, GA: US Department of Health and Human Services; 2011.

Centers for Disease Control and Prevention (CDC). Guidelines for prevention and treatment of opportunistic infections in HIV-positive adults and adolescents. 2015. Available at https://aidsinfo.nih.gov/guidelines/html/4/adult-and-adolescent-oi-prevention-and-treatment-guidelines/0.

Centers for Disease Control and Prevention (CDC). Tuberculosis. Available at https://www.cdc.gov/tb/statistics/default.htm. Accessed October 31, 2018.

Cinque P, Bossolasco S, Brambilla AM, et al. The effect of highly active antiretroviral therapy-induced immune reconstitution on development and outcome of progressive multifocal leukoencephalopathy: study of 43 cases with review of the literature. *J Neurovirol*. 2003;9:73–80.

Corey L, Wald A, Celum CL, et al. The effects of herpes simplex virus-2 on HIV-1 acquisition and transmission: a review of two overlapping epidemics. *J AIDS*. 2004;35:435–445.

Dieterich DT, Rahmin M. Cytomegalovirus colitis in AIDS: presentation in 44 patients and a review of the literature. *J AIDS*. 1991;4:s29–s35.

Engstrom RE Jr, Holland GN, Margolis TP, et al. The progressive outer retinal necrosis syndrome: a variant of necrotizing herpetic retinopathy in patients with AIDS. *Ophthalmology*. 1994;101:1488–1502.

Fenner L, Gagneux S, Janssens JP, et al. Tuberculosis in HIV-negative and HIV-positive patients in a low-incidence country: clinical characteristics and treatment outcomes. *PLoS One*. 2012;7(3):e34186.

Gasnault J, Costagliola D, Hendel-Chavez H, et al. Improved survival of HIV-1-infected patients with progressive multifocal leukoencephalopathy receiving early 5-drug combination antiretroviral therapy. *PLoS One*. 2011;6:e20967.

Gebo KA, Kalyani R, Moore RD, et al. The incidence of, risk factors for, and sequelae of herpes zoster among HIV patients in the highly active antiretroviral therapy era. *J AIDS*. 2005;40:169–174.

Geng EH, Kahn JS, Chang OC, et al. The effect of AIDS Clinical Trials Group Protocol 5164 on the time from *Pneumocystis jirovecii* pneumonia diagnosis to antiretroviral initiation in routine clinical practice: a case study of diffusion, dissemination, and implementation. *Clin Infect Dis*. 2011;53(10):1008–1014.

Griffith DE. Management of disease due to *Mycobacterium kansasii*. *Clin Chest Med*. 2002;23:613–621.

Griffith DE, Aksamit T, Brown-Elliott BA, et al. An official ATS/IDSA statement: diagnosis, treatment, and prevention of nontuberculous mycobacterial diseases. *Am J Respir Crit Care Med.* 2007;175:367–416.

Harrison RA, Soong S, Weiss HL, et al. A mixed model for factors predictive of pain in AIDS patients with herpes zoster. *J Pain Symptom Manage.* 1999;17:410–417.

Jabs DA, Van Natta ML, Holbrook JT, et al. Longitudinal study of the ocular complications of AIDS: 1. Ocular diagnoses at enrollment. *Ophthalmology.* 2007;114:780–786.

Jones D, Havlir DV. Nontuberculous mycobacteria in the HIV infected patient. *Clin Chest Med.* 2002;23:665–674.

Karim SSA, Naidoo K, Grobler A, et al. Integration of antiretroviral therapy with tuberculosis treatment. *N Engl J Med.* 2011;365(16):1492–1501.

Makadzange AT, Ndhlovu CE, Takarinda K, et al. Early versus delayed initiation of antiretroviral therapy for concurrent HIV infection and cryptococcal meningitis in sub-Saharan Africa. *Clin Infect Dis.* 2010;50(11):1532–1538.

Martin DF, Parks DJ, Mellow SD, et al. Treatment of cytomegalovirus retinitis with an intraocular sustained-release ganciclovir implant: a randomized controlled clinical trial. *Arch Ophthalmol.* 1994;112:1531–1539.

Martinson NA, Hoffmann CJ, RE Chaisson. Epidemiology of tuberculosis and HIV. *Proc Am Thorac Soc.* 2011;8:288–293.

Miramontes R, et al. Tuberculosis infection in the United States: prevalence estimates from the National Health and Nutrition Examination Survey, 2011–2012. *PLoS One.* 2015;10(11):e0140881. doi:10.1371/journal.pone.0140881.

Pauk J, Huang ML, Brodie SJ, et al. Mucosal shedding of human herpesvirus 8 in men. *N Engl J Med.* 2000;343:1369–1377.

Safrin S, Elbeik T, Phan L, et al. Correlation between response to acyclovir and foscarnet therapy and in vitro susceptibility result for isolates of herpes simplex virus from human immunodeficiency virus-infected patients. *Antimicrob Agents Chemother.* 1994;38:1246–1250.

Santin M, Munoz L, Rigau D. Interferon-c release assays for the diagnosis of tuberculosis and tuberculosis infection in HIV-positive adults: a systematic review and meta-analysis. *PLoS One.* 2012;7(3):e32482.

Sax PE, Sloan CE, Schackman BR, et al. Early antiretroviral therapy for patients with acute AIDS-related opportunistic infections: a cost-effectiveness analysis of ACTG A5164. *HIV Clinical Trials.* 2010;11(5):248–259.

Sungkanuparph S, Filler SG, Chetchotisakd P, et al. Cryptococcal immune reconstitution inflammatory syndrome after antiretroviral therapy in AIDS patients with cryptococcal meningitis: a prospective multicenter study. *Clin Infect Dis.* 2009;49(6):931–934.

Török ME, Yen NT, Chau TT, et al. Timing of initiation of antiretroviral therapy in human immunodeficiency virus (HIV)—associated tuberculous meningitis. *Clin Infect Dis.* June 2011;52(11):1374–1383. Available at http://www.ncbi.nlm.nih.gov/pubmed/21596680

US Department of Health and Human Services (USDHHS), Panel on Antiretroviral Guidelines for Adults and Adolescents. Guidelines for the use of antiretroviral agents in HIV-1-infected adults and adolescents. Available at https://www.aidsinfo.nih.gov/ContentFiles/AdultandAdolescentGL.pdf. Published 2018.

US Department of Health and Human Services (USDHHS), Panel on Opportunistic Infections in HIV-positive Adults and Adolescents. Guidelines for the prevention and treatment of opportunistic infections in HIV-positive adults and adolescents: recommendations from the Centers for Disease Control and Prevention, the National Institutes of Health, and the HIV Medicine Association of the Infectious Diseases Society of America. 2018. Available at https://aidsinfo.nih.gov/contentfiles/lvguidelines/adult_oi.pdf. Accessed December 17, 2015.

Whitcup S. Cytomegalovirus retinitis in the era of highly active antiretroviral therapy. *JAMA.* 2000;283:653–657.

World Health Organization (WHO). Global tuberculosis report 2015, 20th ed. 2015a. Available at http://apps.who.int/iris/bitstream/10665/191102/1/9789241565059_eng.pdf?ua=1.

World Health Organization (WHO). TB/HIV factsheet 2015. 2015b. Available at http://www.who.int/tb/challenges/hiv/tbhiv_factsheet_2015.pdf?ua=1.

Xu F, Sternberg MR, Kottiri BJ, et al. Trends in herpes simplex virus type 1 and type 2 seroprevalence in the United States. *JAMA.* 2006;296:964–973.

Zolopa A, Andersen J, Powderly W, et al. Early antiretroviral therapy reduces AIDS progression/death in individuals with acute opportunistic infections: a multicenter randomized strategy trial. *PLoS One.* 2009;4(5):e5575.

34.

MALIGNANCIES IN HIV

Eva Clark and Elizabeth Chiao

CHAPTER GOALS

- Review the epidemiology and role of antiretroviral therapy (ART) on the impact of AIDS-defining malignancies, which remain common among individuals with HIV.

- Discuss the role of human herpes virus-8 (HHV-8) in the development of Kaposi's sarcoma (KS), which remains the most common tumor associated with HIV infection.

- Discuss the role of Epstein–Barr virus (EBV) in primary central nervous system lymphoma and other HIV-associated lymphomas.

- Review the role of human papillomavirus (HPV) vaccination in virally mediated anogenital squamous cell cancers in both men and women.

- Discuss non–AIDS-defining malignancies, including lung, prostate, oropharyngeal, liver, breast, and pancreatic cancer.

- Emphasize that ART initiation is of utmost importance for all AIDS-defining malignancies and non–AIDS-defining malignancies and summarize new National Cancer Center Network Guidelines for HIV malignancies.

INTRODUCTION

LEARNING OBJECTIVE

Discuss AIDS-associated and non–AIDS-associated malignancies.

WHAT'S NEW?

Use of integrase inhibitors, the newest class of antiretrovirals, makes concurrent chemotherapeutic options safer and more feasible for many patients.

KEY POINTS

- Malignancies in HIV-positive patients remain a major health concern.

- Antiretroviral therapy (ART) continues to influence the epidemiology of malignancies, with decreasing rates overall.

Malignancies were one of the earliest recognized manifestations that led to the eventual description of the AIDS epidemic. Kaposi's sarcoma (KS) became one of the first entities described in association with AIDS (Ziegler, 1984). Subsequently, intermediate-grade and high-grade non-Hodgkin's lymphoma (NHL), invasive cervical cancer, and primary central nervous system lymphoma (PCNSL) were defined by the US Centers for Disease Control and Prevention (CDC) as "AIDS-defining conditions" (CDC, 2008). Since the advent of combination ART, several other cancers that are not AIDS-defining have been found to have an increased incidence in patients with HIV. These include, but are not limited to, Hodgkin's disease and anal, liver, lung, oropharyngeal, colorectal, and renal cancers (Patel, 2008). They are generally referred to as "non–AIDS-defining cancers" (NADCs). The increasing longevity of persons living with HIV as well as concurrent modifiable risk factors such as tobacco use may also influence the epidemiology of these malignancies.

The introduction of combination ART in the mid-1990s has significantly impacted the clinical history and outcomes of HIV infection. In addition to changing the natural history of HIV disease in terms of survival and incidence of opportunistic diseases, it has also dramatically decreased the incidence of virally mediated HIV-associated malignancies, such as KS and PCNSL (Silverberg, 2015). Even so, cancer remains a significant concern for the HIV-positive population. A large US registry linkage study during the post-ART era included 448,258 HIV-positive individuals from 1996 to 2012 (Hernández-Ramírez, 2017). It found an elevated risk for development of cancer overall (standardized incidence ratio [SIR] 1.69, 95% confidence interval [CI] 1.67–1.72), AIDS-defining cancers (KS [498.11, 477.82–519.03], NHL [11.51, 11.14–11.89], and cervical cancer [3.24, 2.94–3.56]), most other virus-related cancers (e.g., anal [19.06, 18.13–20.03], liver [3.21, 3.02–3.41], and Hodgkin's lymphoma [7.70, 7.20–8.23]), as well as several virus–unrelated cancers (e.g., lung [1.97, 1.89–2.05]) (Hernández-Ramírez, 2017). However, their SIRs significantly decreased over the study period for KS, two subtypes of NHL, and cancers of the anus, liver, and lung, although they remained elevated above that of the general population. SIRs did not increase over time for any cancer. In addition, cancer risk appears to be higher for older HIV-positive individuals. When this same dataset was stratified by age, HIV-positive individuals older than 50 years were more likely to develop KS (SIR, 103.34), NHL (3.05), Hodgkin lymphoma (7.61), and cervical (2.02), anal (14.00), lung (1.71), liver (2.91), and oral cavity/pharyngeal (1.66) cancers, but were less likely to develop breast (0.61), prostate (0.47), and colon (0.63) cancers (Mahale, 2018). Furthermore, recent data indicate that HIV-positive individuals have an increased risk for not only these cancers initially, but also for developing a second primary cancer (Hessol, 2018).

Management of malignancies in HIV-positive patients presents the clinician with many challenges, including the risk of further compromise to the immune system of these patients receiving chemotherapy, toxicities of treatment, pharmacologic interaction between ART and chemotherapy drugs, and the risk of intercurrent opportunistic infections (Mandell, 2010; Reid, 2018). The safety profile and feasibility of ART administration with concurrent chemotherapy have also improved with the introduction and increased use of integrase inhibitors during the past several years. New guidelines for managing cancer in HIV-positive patients were recently released by the National Comprehensive Cancer Network (NCCN) (Reid, 2018). They advise that HIV-positive individuals who develop cancer should be cared for by both an oncologist and an HIV specialist and should receive cancer therapy according to standard guidelines developed for the general population. The patient's ART may need to be modified if there are potential interactions with the proposed cancer therapy, but generally ART should be continued during cancer therapy.

This chapter reviews the malignancies most commonly associated with HIV, along with other non-HIV associated cancers that HIV-positive individuals often develop.

RECOMMENDED READING

Shiels MS, Islam JY, Rosenberg PS, et al. Projected cancer incidence rates and burden of incident cancer cases in HIV-infected adults in the United States through 2030. *Ann Intern Med*. June 19, 2018;168(12):866–873. doi: 10.7326/M17-2499. Epub 2018 May 8.

Silverberg MJ, Lau B, Achenbach CJ, et al. Cumulative incidence of cancer among persons with HIV in North America. *Ann Intern Med*. 2015;163(7):507–518.

Reid E, Suneja G, Ambinder RF, et al. Cancer in people living with HIV, Version 1.2018, NCCN Clinical Practice Guidelines in Oncology. *J Natl Compr Canc Netw*. August 2018;16(8):986–1017.

KAPOSI'S SARCOMA

LEARNING OBJECTIVES

- Discuss the epidemiology of KS.

- Discuss the pathogenesis and clinical manifestations.

- Review the treatments for KS, including local and systemic therapies.

WHAT'S NEW?

The incidence of KS continues to decline with the use of ART, but it remains significantly elevated in areas with endemic disease, such as sub-Saharan Africa. There are several novel therapies that have been studied for HIV-related KS.

KEY POINTS

- The presence of human herpes virus-8 (HHV-8) and advanced immunosuppression are both associated with risk of KS development and other lymphoproliferative states, such as multicentric Castleman's disease and primary body cavity lymphoma.

- Treatment for KS includes ART, local therapy, and systemic therapy.

- The goals of treatment are suppressive and generally noncurative.

Chemotherapy and radiotherapy are palliative treatments for KS. In general, treatment decisions and referrals to oncology should be based on evidence of symptomatic or systemic disease. Radiotherapy should be avoided in the pelvis and lower extremities because of damage to the lymphatics and the potential for lymphedema and skin breakdown.

EPIDEMIOLOGY

Kaposi's sarcoma was first described in 1872 by Moritz Kaposi, a Hungarian dermatologist. Four types of KS have been described: classic, endemic, transplant-associated, and AIDS-associated or epidemic KS. Classic KS is typically seen in elderly men of Mediterranean or Eastern European descent and is characterized by cutaneous lesions of the lower extremities (Iscovich, 2000). The endemic form, found primarily in sub-Saharan Africa, often is more aggressive and morbid, with visceral involvement (Friedman-Kien, 1990). Transplant-associated KS was first described in the 1970s and is seen in immunosuppressed allograft recipients. Both cutaneous disease and visceral disease are common (Penn, 1979).

AIDS-associated KS was first described in gay men in the early 1980s, at the advent of the HIV epidemic (Friedman-Kien, 1981). This malignancy disproportionately affected gay men with AIDS, who were estimated to have a 20-fold higher risk of developing KS compared to other HIV transmission risk groups (Beral, 1990; Hoover, 1993). KS is rarely reported in intravenous drug users or other HIV risk groups (Mitsuyasu, 1984; Safai, 1987).

The incidence of KS in resource-abundant countries has declined markedly since the early 1990s with the widespread use of ART. Of 85,922 cases of KS in the United States evaluated by Shiels et al. between 1990 and 2007, the proportion of KS in persons with AIDS declined from 89% in 1990 to 1995 to 67% in 2001 to 2007 ($p < 0.001$) (Shiels, 2011). Cumulative incidence of KS by age 75 years was among the highest compared to other cancers (lung, anal, colorectal, Hodgkin's lymphoma, liver, and oropharyngeal) from 1995 to 2009 at 4.1%. However, there were significant decreases in incidence of KS by 4% per year from 2005 to 2009 compared to 1996–1999 rates ($p < 0.01$) (Silverberg, 2015). Similarly, the Swiss HIV Cohort Study showed that the KS incidence was 33.3 per 1,000 patient-years (py) in 1984–1986 and did not change significantly in the subsequent periods until 1996–1998, when it declined to 5.1 per 1,000 py (95% confidence interval [CI], 3.9–6.5) and then further decreased to 1.4 per 1,000 py in 1999–2001 and remained constant thereafter (Franceschi, 2008). A Brazilian retrospective cohort also described a decreased incidence of KS from 1998 to 2010, with an incidence rate ratio per year of 0.89 (95% CI, 0.83–0.97) (Castilho, 2015). In 2010, KS accounted for approximately 12% of cancers diagnosed in HIV-positive individuals (Robbins, 2015). Despite the overall decline in KS, there remain concerning differences in improvement in traditionally underserved racial and geographic groups in the United States. Between 2001 and 2013, Royse et al. evaluated 4,455 KS cases in US men and determined that the annual percent change (APC) for KS incidence significantly decreased for white men between 2001 and 2013 (APC −4.52, $p = 0.02$) (Royse, 2017). In contrast, the APC for African American men was not significant (APC −1.84, $p = 0.09$), and the APC among Southern African American men significantly increased (+3.0, $p = 0.03$).

In areas of southern Africa where KS is endemic, this cancer reached epidemic proportions during the initial AIDS epidemic due to lack of ART. For instance, in Zimbabwe, KS was reported to represent 40% of all cancers in men (Chokunonga, 2000). A prospective cohort from 2004 to 2010 found that the incidence in Zimbabwe, Botswana, South Africa, and Zambia reached 413 per 100,000 py (95% CI, 342–497), with higher rates among age groups older than 60 years (Rohner, 2014). Despite the increased availability of ART in these countries, estimates of KS have minimally decreased in the HIV population on ART, with the incidence of KS remaining high at 164 per 100,000 py (95% CI, 151–178) (Rohner, 2014). Individuals with KS in this geographic region have high tumor burdens and aggressive disease progression, and survival from time of diagnosis is often less than 6 months (Campbell, 2003).

PATHOGENESIS

In 1994, Chang and Moore (Chang, 1994) discovered a new herpesvirus, HHV-8 or KS herpes virus (KSHV), in more than 90% of AIDS-KS tissue samples. Although the KS types vary in epidemiology and clinical presentation, all are associated with HHV-8. In 2003, HHV-8 viremia was shown to be an early marker of KS, and the risk of developing disease was demonstrated to increase with HHV-8 antibody titers (Engels, 2003; Newton, 2003). HHV-8 also is associated with rare lymphoproliferative diseases most often seen in individuals with HIV, including multicentric Castleman's disease and a rare form of NHL called primary effusion or body cavity lymphoma. Although infection with KSHV is necessary for the development of KSHV-associated disease, it is not sufficient,

and, in fact, HHV-8 viremia is prevalent only in a subset of cases. In an analysis of 335 patients with HIV-associated KS, only 130 (39%) were viremic, and the mean HHV-8 viral load was only moderate with 6,630 DNA copies/mL (Haq, 2016). Among individuals with HIV, immunosuppression confers the greatest risk and is most predictive of development of KS (Jacobson, 2000; Renwick, 1998).

The pathogenesis of KS is complex and involves viral processes and dysregulation of cytokine pathways. The HHV-8 genome encodes many homologues of human cellular gene products that are involved in inflammation, cell cycle regulation, and angiogenesis, such as viral cyclin-D1, vascular endothelial growth factor (VEGF), basic fibroblast growth factor, and interleukin-6 (IL-6) (Cannon, 2000). Much work has been done on the tumorigenesis of KS. KSHV infection leads to upregulation of Toll-like receptor 4 (TLR4), its adaptor MyD88, and coreceptors CD14 and MD2 (Gruffaz, 2018). The TLR4 pathway seems to be activated constitutively in KSHV-transformed cells, resulting in chronic induction of IL-6, IL-1β, and IL-18. IL-6 production in turn results in activation of the STAT3 pathway, an essential event for uncontrolled cellular proliferation and transformation. Gruffaz et al. have shown that TLR4 stimulation with lipopolysaccharides or live bacteria enhanced tumorigenesis while TLR4 antagonist CLI095 inhibited it. A regulatory transactivating (tat) protein of HIV is released by infected cells and guards KS cells from apoptosis (Deregibus, 2002), stimulates growth and angiogenesis (Barillari, 2002; Ensoli, 1990), and also increases the production and release of matrix metalloproteinases (MMPs) from endothelial and inflammatory cells. MMPs contribute to the angiogenesis found in KS lesions (Impola, 2003; Lafrenie, 1996).

The mechanism of HHV-8 transmissibility remains unclear. HHV-8 has been detected in semen, prostate tissue (Monini, 1996), and breast milk (Dedicoat, 2004). The virus is often shed from the oropharynx of both immunocompetent and immunocompromised men and women in areas where KSHV is endemic (Casper, 2004, 2007). Behaviors associated with exposure to saliva are correlated with a higher risk of KSHV infection, implicating both sexual and horizontal transmission (Casper, 2006; Plancoulaine, 2000). A relatively high KSHV seroprevalence has been described among injection drug users, and an increased incidence of KSHV infection has been noted among transfusion recipients in areas where KSHV is endemic, suggesting that parenteral transmission may be possible (Cannon, 2001; Hladik, 2006). Finally, transmission of KSHV from donors of solid organs has been described (Barozzi, 2003; Luppi, 2000).

CLINICAL MANIFESTATIONS

KS is an angioproliferative disease varying from an indolent to fulminant disease with potential for significant morbidity and mortality. The disease can occur in patients with a wide range of CD4[+] cell counts but becomes increasingly common as immune function declines. The progression of disease may be rapid or slow. Patients with limited disease and controlled

HIV infection usually do reasonably well. However, in the setting of uncontrolled HIV viral replication and low CD4$^+$ counts, KS progresses rapidly.

The skin is the most common site of presentation. Visceral involvement also occurs, and, as the disease progresses, KS frequently involves the gastrointestinal (GI) tract. At autopsy, almost every organ system can show involvement. Visceral disease is rare in the absence of extensive cutaneous disease.

The cutaneous presentation of KS occurs in 95% of cases. Lesions may occur anywhere on the skin. Common sites include the face (particularly the periorbital area and tip of the nose), external ear, mouth, torso, and lower extremities. They can evolve from macules or nodular tumors to large plaque-like tumor masses that involve extensive cutaneous surfaces and eventually evolve into ulcerating tumors. Their color may vary from violaceous in light-skinned individuals to brownish-black in dark-skinned individuals. These lesions are generally nonblanching, nonpruritic, and painless. Lesions of KS may become painful in the setting of immune reconstitution inflammatory syndrome (IRIS).

Lymphedema associated with KS usually appears in patients with visible cutaneous lesions, and edema may be out of proportion to the extent of visible lesions. Lymphedema also may occur in patients with no visible skin lesions. Common sites include the face, neck, external genitals, and lower extremities. A contiguous area of skin usually is involved as well.

Oral cavity involvement is seen in approximately one-third of KS patients and is the initial site of diagnosis 15% of the time (Dezube, 2004). These lesions may be flat or nodular and are red or purplish. They usually appear on the hard palate, but they may develop on the soft palate, gingival areas, and tongue. Oral lesions, if extensive, may cause tooth loss, pain, and ulceration. Involvement of the oral cavity correlates with KS in the GI tract.

Gastrointestinal KS has been reported in 40% of cases at initial diagnosis (Dezube, 2004) with any segment of the GI tract involved. Visceral spread of KS that involves the GI tract is rarely symptomatic. However, with disease progression, patients may have symptoms of abdominal pain, nausea, vomiting, or GI bleeding (Danzig, 1991). Rare cases of obstruction, perforation, or protein-losing enteropathy have been reported (Friedman, 1988). In those with advanced immunosuppression (CD4$^+$ T cell count <100 cells/mm^3), GI KS may be more severe with complications. Some believe that screening endoscopy to detect occult disease may be warranted in these patients (Nagata, 2012).

Pulmonary KS is also common; however, in contrast to KS at other visceral sites, lung involvement is generally symptomatic. Common symptoms include cough, bronchospasm, dyspnea, and hemoptysis. This complication tends to occur in the setting of advanced AIDS, with most individuals having CD4$^+$ cell counts of less than 100 cells/mm^3 (Gill, 1989) and in patients with more extensive cutaneous disease (e.g., with >50 lesions). Of note, it can occur in patients with minimal and absent cutaneous KS. The disease is often rapidly progressive when it involves the lungs, with a median survival time of only 2–6 months in the pre-ART era (Kaplan, 1988). Respiratory failure is often the cause of death. The radiographic appearance is variable, with the characteristic reticulonodular pattern seen in approximately one-third of patients (Kaplan, 1988). Otherwise, diffuse interstitial infiltrates, pleural effusions, and hilar adenopathy may be seen (Levine, 2001).

Once KS is clinically suspected, diagnosis is made by biopsy and histologic examination or by presumptive diagnosis based on the endoscopic appearance of a visceral lesion (Aboulafia, 2001). A histologic confirmation is essential to exclude other conditions that can mimic KS. Endoscopically, the classic appearance of small submucosal vascular nodules establishes the diagnosis of GI KS. It may be difficult to establish a diagnosis of GI KS by biopsy because many of the lesions are submucosal (Hengge, 2002). In patients with suspected pulmonary KS, violaceous endobronchial lesions typically are observed on bronchoscopic examination. A presumptive diagnosis of pulmonary KS can be made based on characteristic radiographic and endobronchial findings in patients who have had KS at other sites (Kaplan, 1988). Endobronchial biopsy is discouraged because of the risk of hemorrhage. Gallium scanning may be helpful in differentiating KS from pulmonary infection because KS is not gallium-avid (Kaplan, 1988).

In the pre-ART era, the AIDS Clinical Trials Group (ACTG) developed a staging system based on tumor extent (T), severity of immunosuppression (I), and the presence of systemic illness (S) (Krown, 1997). Two different risk categories were noted based on this staging system: a good risk, defined as T0I0S0; and a poor risk, defined as T1I1S1 (Table 34.1).

Based on epidemiological, clinical, staging, and survival data of patients in two Italian prospective cohort studies (*n* = 211), Nasti et al. concluded that, in the era of ART, a refinement of the ACTG staging system is needed (Nasti, 2003). Patient CD4$^+$ T cell counts in this study did not provide prognostic information, and only the combination of T1S1 identified patients with unfavorable prognosis. The 3-year survival rate for patients with T1S1 was 53%, which was significantly lower compared to the 3-year survival rates of patients with T0S0, T1S0, and T0S1, which were 88%, 80%, and 81%, respectively. Several studies have found other prognostic markers for KS. Stebbing et al. developed a prognostic index predicting poor survival. The index included the following variables: not having KS as the AIDS-defining illness, decreasing CD4$^+$ T cell count, age 50 years or older, and having another AIDS-associated illness at the same time (Stebbing, 2006). Other variables, including CD8$^+$ cell count (Stebbing, 2007) and detectable HHV-8 DNA in plasma at the time of diagnosis (El Amari, 2008), have also been associated with poor KS prognosis.

TREATMENT

Treatment of KS is generally not considered curative and was not shown to have a significant impact on survival in the pre-ART era. An older retrospective review of 194 cases of KS (Volberding, 1989) showed no significant difference in survival time between patients treated with chemotherapy or interferon-α (IFN-α) and patients not treated. In a more recent randomized trial done in South Africa of ART alone

Table 34.1 AIDS CLINICAL TRIALS GROUP (ACTG) TUMOR STAGING SYSTEM

CHARACTERISTIC	GOOD RISK (0)	POOR RISK (1)
	All of the following:	Any of the following:
Tumor (T)	Tumor confined to skin and/or lymph nodes and/or minimal oral disease[a]	Tumor-associated edema or ulceration; extensive oral KS; GI KS; other visceral KS
Immune system (I)	CD4 count ≥150 cells/mm³	CD4+ T cell count <150 cells/mm³
Systemic illness (S)	No history of OI or thrush; no systemic symptoms; Karnofsky performance status ≥70	History of OI and/or thrush; systemic symptoms; Karnofsky performance status <70; other HIV-related illnesses

[a]Non-nodular KS confined to the palate.

GI, gastrointestinal; KS, Kaposi's sarcoma; OI, opportunistic infection.

SOURCE: Adapted from Krown (1989) and incorporating revision by Krown (1997), with permission from the American Society of Clinical Oncology.

versus ART plus chemotherapy for KS, there was a significant difference in KS response but no difference in survival between the two arms (Mosam, 2012). In the United States, the primary goals of treatment for patients with KS are palliation of symptoms and improved cosmesis. Consultation with a KS-experienced oncologist or dermatologist should be considered for most patients diagnosed with this malignancy.

Impact of Antiretroviral Therapy

ART is a key component in the treatment of KS and should be initiated or optimized to achieve complete HIV RNA suppression in all patients with AIDS-associated KS. The inhibition of HIV replication, decreased production of the tat protein, restored immunity to HHV-8, and the direct antiangiogenic activity of some protease inhibitors (PIs) are among the many benefits of ART (Noy, 2003; Dubrow, 2017). Some older data suggested that PIs have an anti–KS effect (Sgadari, 2003); however, non-PI-containing ART regimens also lead to KS regression.

Combination ART has been associated with a lengthening of time to treatment failure with either local or systemic therapy for KS. A retrospective study found a median time of 20.4 months from the initiation of ART plus chemotherapy versus 6 months with just chemotherapy to detect treatment failure among HIV-positive individuals with KS (Bower, 1999). It has also been demonstrated that HIV-positive individuals who were receiving ART at KS diagnosis had a less aggressive presentation versus individuals who were ART-naïve at the time of KS diagnosis (Nasti, 2003). Another retrospective analysis from 1990 to 1999 found an 81% reduction in the risk of death among HIV-positive individuals with KS after the initiation of ART (Tam, 2002).

KS-associated IRIS has been well described. Some patients may experience painful enlarged lesions or progression of KS lesions during the first months of ART. In a prospective study of 69 patients with HIV and KSHV coinfection, approximately 12% of patients experienced IRIS-KS after initiation of ART (Letang, 2010).

Local Treatment

Local treatment should be reserved for patients with minimal or locally symptomatic disease. These patients should concurrently receive ART. Current options for local treatment include the following:

- Radiotherapy has been the mainstay of local therapy for KS. It is best suited for patients with a single or a few locally symptomatic areas or for symptomatic disease that requires rapid tumor reduction. Electron beam radiation applied to the entire face is highly effective in relief of facial edema. Radiotherapy also can be useful for treatment of dysphagia caused by pharyngeal lesions and tumor masses of the eye or the extremities (Hill, 1987). Radiotherapy, whether given as whole-body electron beam therapy, fractionated focal radiation therapy, or single treatments, has produced complete remissions in 50–80% of patients (Cooper, 1991; Pluda, 1992). Complications such as severe mucositis, radiotherapy fibrosis, loss of skin compliance, and chronic lymphedema may occur with these treatments.

- With intralesional chemotherapy, vinblastine has been most commonly used, with a reported response rate of 70% in older studies (Boudreaux, 1993). Small cutaneous lesions can be treated with intralesional chemotherapy for cosmetic purposes. Repeated treatments may be necessary. Intralesional chemotherapy can cause significant pain and areas of hyperpigmentation after treatment.

- Alitretinoin gel (Panretin) is a topical treatment that may be used for relatively asymptomatic patients with KS lesions that do not respond to ART alone and for whom the KS is predominantly an issue of cosmesis. A response rate of 49% ($n = 184$) in a phase 3 study was reported (Walmsley, 1999). Adverse effects include dry skin and light hypersensitivity.

- Cryotherapy with liquid nitrogen and laser therapy has been used successfully for the treatment of isolated small KS lesions. Given the significant mucosal toxicity associated with radiotherapy in the treatment of oral lesions, laser surgery may be substituted for radiation.

- There are several new therapies being explored for KS. One is a phase 1 trial of intralesional nivolumab therapy, which is an immune checkpoint inhibitor (NCT03316274; Bender-Ignacio, 2018).

Systemic Treatment

As mentioned earlier, although it is strongly recommended to start ART for all HIV-positive individuals with KS, adjunct therapies for patients with mild to moderate disease have not been well studied. One recent multicenter trial evaluated the use of oral etoposide (given "as needed" vs. immediately [as 8 cycles of therapy]) and found that only about 30% of patients in both groups responded to therapy overall (Hosseinipour, 2018). Immediate treatment with oral etoposide resulted in early clinical benefits that were no longer observed 48 weeks post-therapy.

Systemic intravenous chemotherapy is used for more severe disease, including symptomatic visceral disease, extensive skin involvement, significant edema, or rapidly progressive KS. As described previously, the goal of systemic chemotherapy is mainly palliation of symptoms. Large randomized studies have established liposomal anthracyclines (doxorubicin and daunorubicin) as first-line single-agent chemotherapy agents with promising results compared to combination chemotherapy treatment (Gill, 1996; Northfelt, 1998; Stewart, 1998). These studies found that liposomal anthracyclines alone can achieve response rates equal to or better than those of combination chemotherapy with a lower incidence of toxicity such as nausea, fatigue, alopecia, and neuropathy. Neutropenia, however, occurred as frequently with the liposomal agent as with the standard combination regimen. Prognosis is good; in one study of 140 patients with T1 disease who were treated with ART and liposomal anthracycline chemotherapy, the 5-year overall survival was 85% (Bower, 2014).

Paclitaxel is a highly active agent that is often used as second-line therapy. It has significant antitumor activity in patients with previously untreated (Gill, 1995) and refractory KS (Saville, 1995). The most significant side effects are hypersensitivity, myelosuppression, peripheral neuropathy, alopecia, and drug interactions with ART. This agent is the treatment of choice for refractory KS or if there are contraindications to the use of anthracyclines. Regarding comparison of liposomal anthracyclines versus taxanes, one small randomized trial comparing liposomal doxorubicin (37 patients) and paclitaxel (36 patients) found that both therapies improved symptoms such as pain and swelling in HIV-positive patients with advanced KS (Cianfrocca, 2018). A 2014 Cochrane review indicated no observed difference between liposomal doxorubicin, liposomal daunorubicin, and paclitaxel for patients on ART (Gbabe, 2014).

Several newer therapies are currently being studied for severe KS. Inhibition of the KS-activated mammalian target of rapamycin (mTOR) signaling pathway has been examined in an AIDS Malignancy Consortium (AMC) study and has shown promising therapeutic results (Krown, 2012). Imatinib, a platelet-derived growth factor receptor/c-kit inhibitor, induced responses in 10 of 30 patients with KS when given up to 1 year in a multicenter phase 2 trial (Koon, 2014). The vascular endothelial growth factor-A inhibitor, bevacizumab, was shown in another phase 2 trial to produce complete and partial responses in 3 and 2 of 16 patients, respectively (Uldrik, 2012). Two immunomodulatory agents with antiangiogenic effects, pomalidomide (oral) and lenalidomide (intravenous) were recently evaluated in phase 1/2 trials. Pomalidomide was found to be well-tolerated and active in KS regardless of HIV status (Polizzotto, 2016; NCT02659930). Lenalidomide was well-tolerated in antiretroviral-experienced patients with progressive KS previously treated with chemotherapy, but its recent phase 2 trial was halted due to lack of responses in this study population (Pourcher, 2017). Several other targeted therapies for KS are currently being evaluated in clinical trials (Bender-Ignacio, 2018).

RECOMMENDED READING

Cianfrocca M, Lee S, Von Roenn J, et al. Randomized trial of paclitaxel vs. pegylated liposomal doxorubicin for advanced human immunodeficiency virus-associated Kaposi sarcoma: evidence of symptom palliation from chemotherapy. *Cancer*. 2010;116(16):3969–3677.

Hosseinipour MC, Kang M, Krown SE, Bukuru A, et al. As-needed vs immediate etoposide chemotherapy in combination with antiretroviral therapy for mild-to-moderate AIDS-associated Kaposi sarcoma in resource-limited settings: A5264/AMC-067 randomized clinical trial. *Clin Infect Dis*. 2018;67(2):251–260.

Reid E, Suneja G, Ambinder RF, et al. Cancer in people living with HIV, Version 1.2018, NCCN Clinical Practice Guidelines in Oncology. *J Natl Compr Canc Netw*. August 2018;16(8):986–1017.

Shiels MS, Pfeiffer RM, Hall HI, et al. Proportions of Kaposi sarcoma, selected non-Hodgkin lymphomas, and cervical cancer in the United States occurring in persons with AIDS, 1980–2007. *JAMA*. 2011;305(14):1450–1459.

HIV-RELATED PRIMARY CENTRAL NERVOUS SYSTEM LYMPHOMA

LEARNING OBJECTIVES

- Review the epidemiology of PCNSL in HIV patients.
- Review the pathophysiology and clinical presentation.
- Review chemotherapeutic strategies for treatment.
- Discuss survival among these patients.

WHAT'S NEW?

Fluorodeoxyglucose–positron emission tomography (FDG-PET) and magnetic resonance spectroscopy provide less invasive strategies to characterize invasiveness of disease and distinguish from other pathologies.

KEY POINTS

- Epstein–Barr virus (EBV)-mediated oncogenesis in the setting of advanced immunosuppression is largely responsible for PCNSL.

- Treatment with ART should be initiated and maintained for all HIV patients with PCNSL.

- Despite improved survival in the ART era, overall survivability remains poor.

Primary CNS lymphoma is a rare type of NHL, accounting for 1–2% of all NHLs and less than 5% of all primary brain tumors (Lister, 2002). PCNSL has been diagnosed in 1.6–9.0% of patients with AIDS and represents the second most common intracranial mass lesion in this population (Rosenblum, 1988; Welch, 1984). The vast majority of PCNSL has been linked to EBV-infected B cells that reach the CNS during advanced immunodeficiency (Cingolani, 2005). MacMahon and colleagues noted that EBV genes important for oncogenesis are abundant in patients with primary CNS lymphoma, suggesting a pathogenic role of EBV in this setting (MacMahon, 1991). This association suggests that the pathogenesis of PCNSL might differ from systemic NHL, which has a 40–50% association with EBV (Ballerini, 1993; Hamilton-Dutoit, 1989).

EPIDEMIOLOGY

In the era before effective ART, the relative risk of PCNSL was approximately 1,000-fold and as high as 3,600-fold in individuals with AIDS compared to the general population (Cote, 1996).

The age-adjusted incidence of PCNSL in the United States had increased substantially since the 1970s, from 0.16 per 100,000 py in 1973–1984 to 0.48 per 100,000 py in 1985–1997 (Olson, 2002). However, with the introduction of ART in the mid to late 1990s, the incidence of PCNSL in AIDS has significantly decreased (Hoffman, 2001; Wolf, 2005). In the Multicenter AIDS Cohort Study, the incidence rate in 2,734 HIV-positive men declined from 4.3 to 0.4 per 100,000 py (Sacktor, 2001). In another study, PCNSL accounted for only 1% of lymphoma diagnoses in HIV-positive patients in the period 2006–2015 (Gopal, 2013). Despite this dramatic decrease in incidence, survival rates have not significantly improved, especially compared to those of HIV-negative individuals (Bayraktar, 2011; Conti, 2000).

CLINICAL PRESENTATION

The clinical presentation of CNS lymphoma is similar irrespective of HIV status. Symptoms may include headaches, confusion, lethargy, memory loss, personality changes, and seizures. On examination, patients may present with hemiparesis, aphasia, and cranial nerve palsies. Lesions are most common in the cerebrum, basal ganglia, and brainstem. More diffuse and multifocal involvement is seen in HIV-related PCNSL (Gage, 2000). These lesions are contrast-enhancing on computed tomography (CT) and MRI. Before ART, the median CD4$^+$ cell count at presentation was less than 50 cells/mm^3 (Levine, 1991).

Polymerase chain reaction (PCR) to detect EBV DNA in the cerebrospinal fluid is useful for diagnosing AIDS-associated CNS lymphoma. Identification of EBV by PCR can detect most cases of AIDS-related PCNSL with a sensitivity of 80–100% and specificity for lymphoma of 93–100% (Bossolasco, 2002). Cerebrospinal fluid cytology alone has limited utility due to poor sensitivity and specificity (Ekstein, 2006).

Single-photon emission computed tomography has been suggested as a less invasive technique for diagnosis. However, due to conflicting results in terms of sensitivity and specificity, its role in the diagnosis of PCNSL remains limited (Licho, 2002; Ruiz, 1994). FDG-PET and magnetic resonance spectroscopy are two other imaging modalities that can aid in the diagnosis of cerebral PCNSL lesions apart from other infectious CNS pathologies such as toxoplasmosis. Magnetic resonance spectroscopy typically shows decreased N-acetylaspartate and increased choline, which reflects neoplastic cell proliferation (Westwood, 2013). FDG-PET can also help identify extracerebral systemic disease involvement (Lewitschnig, 2013). Currently, the gold standard for diagnosis of PCNSL is stereotactic brain biopsy. In patients in whom a brain biopsy is unobtainable, the combination of imaging, negative toxoplasma serology, previous toxoplasmosis prophylaxis, and positive EBV cerebrospinal fluid by PCR may be sufficient to make a presumptive diagnosis.

TREATMENT AND SURVIVAL

The relative rarity of PCNSL precludes large-scale randomized trials; therefore, the optimal treatment for PCNSL has not been determined. Norden et al. showed that HIV positivity significantly reduced median overall survival to 2 months vesus 12 months in HIV-negative patients (Norden, 2011). Despite good initial response rates to treatment, median survival times with treatment remain only 2–5.5 months (Baumgartner, 1990). The previous standard treatment of patients with AIDS-related PCNSL was palliative corticosteroids and whole-brain radiation that achieved a complete response in 20–50% of patients (Cote, 1996). Radiation alone can improve symptoms and extend median survival, but this is likely affected by a patient's baseline functional status and not the dose of radiation received (Goldstein, 1991).

Regarding chemotherapy for AIDS-related PCNSL, an uncontrolled pilot study published in 1997 used high-dose intravenous methotrexate in 15 patients, including 10 with histologically confirmed PCNSL. The median time since clinical onset was 27 days (range 7–69 days), and the mean CD4$^+$ T cell count was 30 cells/mm^3. Complete responses, defined as clinical improvement and disappearance of contrast-enhancing brain abnormalities on CT or MRI, were obtained in 7 of 15 patients (3 of 10 patients with histological diagnosis and 4 of 5 patients without histological confirmation). One patient relapsed at 6 months. Six patients failed to respond, and 2 patients died of severe sepsis. The median survival time was 290 days for the 10 patients with histological diagnosis and 347 days for the 5 patients without histological confirmation. In addition, steroids were also administered and individuals ultimately received ART including a PI (Jacomet, 1997). More recently, Gupta et al. retrospectively studied 20 HIV-positive patients treated with methotrexate-based regimens (Gupta, 2017). Some of these patients were treated with high-dose methotrexate alone, some with high-dose methotrexate and rituximab, and some with regimens that included a variety of other agents. The median survival in patients treated before ART and without high-dose methotrexate was 2 months, whereas with ART and high-dose methotrexate-based regimens, the median survival had not yet been reached with a median follow-up of 27 months. In HIV-negative individuals with PCNSL, high-dose intravenous methotrexate remains the standard of care for those who can tolerate the therapy, and available evidence supports this strategy, combined with ART, in HIV-positive patients as well. In 2016, the IELSG32 trial provided a high level of evidence supporting the use of MATRix combination (methotrexate, cytarabine, and rituximab with or without thiotepa) as the new standard chemoimmunotherapy for patients aged up to 70 years with newly diagnosed PCNSL (Ferreri, 2016). A phase 2 trial is under way evaluating induction with rituximab, high-dose methotrexate, and leucovorin every 2 weeks for 6 cycles, followed by consolidation with high-dose methotrexate alone (NCT00267865). Whole-brain radiation is traditionally reserved for those with poor performance status (National Comprehensive Cancer Network [NCCN] PSCNL version 1.2015); however, in the second randomization of the IELSG32 trial, both whole-brain radiotherapy and autologous stem-cell transplantation were found to be feasible and effective as consolidation therapies after high-dose methotrexate-based chemoimmunotherapy (Ferreri, 2017).

ROLE OF ANTIRETROVIRAL THERAPY

Combination ART should be initiated in all individuals with AIDS-related PCNSL who are undertaking treatment because it is associated with significant improvement in survival. In the pre-ART era, radiotherapy prolonged survival for 2–5.5 months compared to palliative care (Donahue, 1995). McGowan and Shah (McGowan, 1998) were the first to describe a case of remission maintained for more than 2 years after treatment with ART alone in an individual who had PCNSL. Other case reports have also reported similar PCNSL response to ART (Aboulafia, 2007; Corales, 2000; Travi, 2012). In a retrospective analysis, Hoffman and colleagues (Hoffman, 2001) showed that survival times of patients receiving ART in addition to radiotherapy differed significantly from those of patients receiving radiotherapy or palliative care alone. Four of the 6 patients receiving ART survived for more than 1.5 years. In another retrospective analysis, Skiest and Crosby (Skiest, 2003) demonstrated a prolonged median survival of 667 days in individuals who received ART. These findings strongly suggest that immune recovery contributes to longer remission in HIV patients with PCNSL.

RECOMMENDED READING

Cingolani A, Fratino L, Scoppettuolo G, et al. Changing pattern of primary cerebral lymphoma in the highly active antiretroviral therapy era. *J Neurovirol.* 2005;11(Suppl 3):38–44.

Ferreri AJM, Cwynarski K, Pulczynski E, et al. Whole-brain radiotherapy or autologous stem-cell transplantation as consolidation strategies after high-dose methotrexate-based chemoimmunotherapy in patients with primary CNS lymphoma: results of the second randomisation of the International Extranodal Lymphoma Study Group-32 phase 2 trial. *Lancet Haematol.* November 2017;4(11):e510–e523.

Gupta NK, Nolan A, Omuro A, et al. Long-term survival in AIDS-related primary central nervous system lymphoma. *Neuro Oncol.* 2017;19:99–108

Westwood TD, Hogan C, Julyan PJ, et al. Utility of FDG-PETCT and magnetic resonance spectroscopy in differentiating between cerebral lymphoma and non-malignant CNS lesions in HIV-infected patients. *Eur J Radiol.* 2013;82(8):e374–e379.

SYSTEMIC NON-HODGKIN'S LYMPHOMA

LEARNING OBJECTIVES

- Review the epidemiology of NHL.
- Review the pathophysiology and clinical manifestations of NHL.
- Review the treatment of NHL and survival outcomes.

WHAT'S NEW?

- Survival for NHL continues to improve in the ART era; however, incidence continues to be significantly higher compared to that for HIV-negative persons.
- Intensive chemotherapy and autologous hematopoietic cell transplantation (HCT) are safe in patients with HIV and are associated with improved outcomes.

KEY POINTS

- NHL development is likely a multifactorial interplay among host immune factors as well as the presence of viral mediators including EBV and HHV-8. Disease can occur in a variety of nodal and extranodal sites, and some forms of NHL are more aggressive than others, such as primary effusion lymphoma (PEL).
- Prognostic factors include host immunity, the presence of injection drug use, performance status, and the degree of tumor burden.
- Treatment with ART and intensive chemotherapy with consideration of HCT are cornerstones of NHL treatment.

The first cases of AIDS-related NHL were described in 1982 (Ziegler, 1982). In 1985, NHL was added to the list of AIDS-defining malignancies. Before the ART era, it was estimated to occur in approximately 8% of all HIV cases (Kaplan,

Table 34.2 AIDS-RELATED LYMPHOMAS: WORLD HEALTH ORGANIZATION CLASSIFICATION

Lymphomas also occurring in immunocompetent patient
Burkitt's lymphoma
Diffuse large B cell lymphoma: Centroblastic, immunoblastic, and anaplastic variants
Lymphomas occurring specifically in HIV-positive patients
Primary effusion lymphoma
Plasmablastic lymphoma
Lymphomas also occurring in other immunodeficiency states
Polymorphic or posttransplant lymphoproliferative disorder-like B cell lymphoma

SOURCE: Adapted from Raphael (2008).

1989), and it is currently the second most common neoplasm occurring among HIV-positive individuals (Knowles, 2001).

The World Health Organization (WHO) has divided AIDS-related lymphomas (ARLs) into three categories (Table 34.2):

1. Lymphomas also occurring in immunocompetent patients, such as Burkitt's lymphoma and diffuse large B cell lymphoma

2. Lymphomas occurring specifically in HIV-positive patients, such as PEL and plasmablastic lymphoma

3. Lymphomas also occurring in other immunodeficiency states, such as polymorphic or posttransplant lymphoproliferative disorder–like B cell lymphoma

Diffuse large B cell lymphoma (DLBCL) and Burkitt's lymphoma are the most common ARLs, representing approximately 90% of these malignancies (Besson, 2001). Only intermediate-grade or high-grade lymphomas are considered AIDS-defining.

EPIDEMIOLOGY

Individuals with impaired cell-mediated immunity show a marked increase in the incidence of NHL. This has been best described in immunosuppressed allograft recipients. Similar trends were seen in HIV-positive individuals in the pre-ART era. The CDC examined data of 2,824 NHL cases occurring in 97,258 HIV-positive individuals between 1981 and 1989 in the United States. The risk was 60 times greater in HIV-positive individuals (Beral, 1991). The risk also varies by histologic subtype, with up to 600-fold excess risk for immunoblastic lymphoma (IBL) (Cote, 1997). In a recent study evaluating the cumulative incidence of NHL in persons with HIV living in the United States and Canada ($n = 86,620$), the incidence of NHL from 1996 to 2009 was 4.5% by age 75 years compared to only 0.7% in HIV-negative persons ($n = 196,987$) (Silverberg, 2015). Gopal and colleagues evaluated data from the US Centers for AIDS Research network including 23,050

HIV-positive patients diagnosed between 1996 and 2011 and found that lymphomas developed in 2.1% of these patients (Gopal, 2013). Most of these were DLBCL (42.2%), followed by Hodgkin lymphoma (16.6%), Burkitt lymphoma (11.8%), PCNSL (11.3%), and other NHLs (18.1%).

PATHOGENESIS

The pathogenesis of HIV NHL is most likely multifactorial, involving HIV, immune dysfunction, cytokine dysregulation, and other viral antigens, including EBV and HHV-8 (Gates, 2003). EBV is present in approximately 40–50% of cases of AIDS-related systemic NHL (Hamilton-Dutoit, 1989). This contrasts with a report by Ballerini and colleagues, who reported 100% EBV coinfection in the immunoblastic lymphoma variant of DLBCL (Ballerini, 1993). The expression of the latent EBV transforming proteins EBNA-2 and LMP-1 is known to play a central role in the initiation and maintenance of EBV-induced B cell growth and proliferation (Liebowitz, 1989). Both EBNA-2 and LMP-1 can serve as targets for cytotoxic T cells; thus, their expression induces T cell immune surveillance and regulates lymphomagenesis in individuals who are immunocompetent. With immunodeficiency states such as late-stage HIV, EBNA-2 and LMP-1 expression may become unregulated and subsequently lead to uncontrolled proliferation of EBV-infected cells (Gaidano, 1995). Genetic alterations involving oncogenes and tumor suppressor genes may also occur, and often *MYC* and *BCL6* translocations are implicated in neoplastic development (Chadburn, 2013).

Expression of HHV-8 also is associated with PEL, which often presents as malignant effusions in both the chest and the abdomen with a paucity of nodal masses. It is aggressive and often refractory to chemotherapy. HHV-8 has been universally found in malignant cells, often in conjunction with EBV (Komanduri, 1996). Neoplastic cells have an immunoblastic to plasmablastic appearance. Most PELs have lymphocyte activation markers (CD30 and CD38) without normal B cell markers (CD19 and CD20).

CLINICAL CHARACTERISTICS

Approximately two-thirds of ARLs are classified as DLBCL (Navarro, 2006). AIDS-related systemic NHL usually presented as widespread disease involving extranodal sites in the pre-ART era (Knowles, 1988). The most common sites of extranodal disease are the gastrointestinal tract, CNS, bone marrow, and liver. Ziegler et al. reported that 95% of patients from several institutions had evidence of extranodal disease, including 42% with CNS involvement and 33% with bone marrow involvement (Ziegler, 1984). In a multicenter retrospective review of pooled data from 886 HIV patients with DLBCL, CNS involvement was found in 13% of patients and was not associated with reduced overall survival (Barta, 2016). However, CNS relapse was associated with a median overall survival of only 1.6 months. GI NHL occurs in approximately 30% of HIV-positive patients with NHL. Most of these cases involve the stomach, but virtually any site in the GI tract or hepatobiliary tree can be involved (Burkes, 1986).

Interestingly, plasmablastic lymphomas are associated with characteristic development of oral cavity lesions in the majority of cases and predominate in mucosal sites (Chadburn, 2013). In the ART era, among patients with undetectable plasma HIV RNA levels, Gerard et al. found that NHL occurred at a median $CD4^+$ T cell count of 297 cells/mm^3. In addition, they found that 65% of the cases occurred within 18 months of initiating HIV treatment with ART (Gerard, 2009). Other studies have shown that PEL and immunoblastic NHL are seen in patients with lower $CD4^+$ cell counts, of older age, and with a prior diagnosis of AIDS, whereas Burkitt NHL tends to occur in patients with more preserved immune function (Knowles, 1996). In a more recent study of 23,050 patients with HIV infection diagnosed between 1996 and 2011, Gopal and colleagues found that patients with Hodgkin lymphoma and Burkitt NHL had the highest $CD4^+$ T cell counts, while patients with PCNSL had the lowest (Gopal, 2013). In 2010, NHL accounted for approximately 21% of cancers diagnosed in HIV-positive individuals (Robbins, 2015).

PROGNOSTIC FEATURES

Historically, poor prognostic factors for patients with HIV-related NHL have included age older than 35 years, $CD4^+$ T cell count of less than 100 cells/mm^3, history of injection drug use, history of AIDS-defining condition, poor performance status, elevated lactate dehydrogenase, tumor bulk or stage of disease, and International Prognostic Index (IPI) (Straus, 1998). The IPI includes clinical features that reflect the growth and invasive potential of the tumor (tumor stage, serum lactate dehydrogenase [LDH] level, and number of extranodal disease sites), the patient's response to the tumor (performance status), and the patient's ability to tolerate intensive therapy (age and performance status). The simplified model for younger patients (the age-adjusted IPI) uses a subgroup of these clinical features (tumor stage, LDH level, and performance status).

Lim and colleagues compared the prognostic factors for survival and the use of the IPI in pre- and post-ART HIV-positive individuals with DLBCL (Lim, 2005) In groups with low-, low-intermediate-, and high-intermediate-risk IPI disease, the 3-year overall survival rates were 20%, 22%, and 5% in the pre-ART era and improved to 64%, 64%, and 50% in the post-ART era, respectively.

Of note, PEL and extra-cavity PEL are known to be aggressive malignancies with a traditionally dismal prognosis. An early study found a median survival time of 6 months and few survivors beyond 12 months. Poor performance status and lack of ART portend poorer prognosis (Boulanger, 2005). However, PEL prognosis may be improving. A 2015 single-center retrospective study of 15 patients found that complete remission was achieved in 14 (93.3%) (Cattaneo, 2015). Subsequently four patients relapsed, and two patients died. The overall survival rate at 3 years was 66.7%.

More recently, Barta and colleagues have developed an AIDS-related lymphoma IPI that combines the age-adjusted IPI with an HIV severity score including $CD4^+$ T cell count, viral load, and prior history of AIDS to risk-stratify HIV-related lymphomas (Barta, 2014). Using this scoring system, this group evaluated patients enrolled in HIV-associated lymphoma trials between 2005 and 2010 and found that individual HIV-related factors such as low $CD4^+$ T cell counts (< 50 cells/mm^3) and prior history of AIDS were no longer associated with poorer outcomes (Barta, 2015).

TREATMENT

The treatment for AIDS-related lymphoma is similar to that of HIV-negative individuals, with some exceptions (Reid, 2018). Intrathecal chemotherapy prophylaxis is necessary because patients with HIV are at an increased risk for CNS involvement. Those cases include lymphomas with aggressive pathologic features, including Burkitt's lymphoma, plasmablastic lymphoma, and presentations consistent with possible CNS involvement (Chari, 2005). The use of hematopoietic stimulants such as granulocyte colony-stimulating factor (G-CSF) may aid in reducing chemotherapy-induced cytopenic complications. *Pneumocystis jirovecii* pneumonia prophylaxis is administered with standard-dose chemotherapy, irrespective of $CD4^+$ T cell count.

Chemotherapy in the Pre-ART Era

In the pre-ART era, HIV-positive individuals with NHL had a poor prognosis, were managed on low-dose chemotherapy regimens because of concern for toxicity and had a median survival of 5–8 months (Kaplan, 1997; Sandler, 1996). In addition to persistent neoplasia contributing to death, many patients in this era died due to the infectious complications of opportunistic diseases (Lowenthal, 1988).

Chemotherapy in the ART Era

In the ART era, more recent standard chemotherapy regimens have been reported without excessive toxicity due to restored immunity. The AIDS Malignancy Consortium reported on 65 patients who were given reduced doses of cyclophosphamide and doxorubicin combined with vincristine and prednisone (modified CHOP) or full doses of CHOP combined with G-CSF with concomitant ART. Complete response rates were 30% and 48% in the reduced- and full-dose groups, respectively (Ratner, 2001). No long-term outcomes were reported in this study. Other studies of CHOP-based chemotherapy and concurrent ART have reported median survival of 2 years. In patients with Burkitt's lymphoma, a particularly aggressive form of NHL, intensive chemotherapy with cyclophosphamide, doxorubicin, high-dose methotrexate/ifosfamide, etoposide, and high-dose cytarabine (CODOX-M/IVAC) resulted in rates of event-free survival and remission similar to those of their HIV-negative counterparts (Wang, 2003).

Risk-adaptive chemotherapy has also been studied comparing the post- to pre-ART era. A total of 485 HIV-positive individuals were assigned randomly to chemotherapy after risk stratification based on an HIV score (comprised of performance status, prior AIDS, and CD4$^+$ T cell counts <100 cells/mm^3). Of these patients, there were 218 good-risk patients (HIV score 0) who received doxorubicin, cyclophosphamide, vindesine, bleomycin, and prednisone (ACVBP) or CHOP; 177 intermediate-risk patients (HIV score 1) who received CHOP or low-dose CHP; and 90 poor-risk patients (HIV score 2 or 3) who received low-dose CHOP or vincristine and steroids. Five-year overall survival in the good-risk group was 51% for ACVBP versus 47% for CHOP ($p = 0.85$), that in the intermediate-risk group was 28% for CHOP versus 24% for low-dose CHOP ($p = 0.19$), and that in the poor-risk group was 11% for low-dose CHOP versus 3% for vincristine and steroid ($p = 0.14$). The significant factors in this study for overall survival were ART (relative risk [RR], 1.6; $p = 0.0002$), HIV score (RR, 1.7; $p = 0.0001$), and IPI score (RR, 1.5; $p = 0.0012$) but not the intensity of chemotherapy (Mounier, 2006).

An infusional regimen of cyclophosphamide, doxorubicin, and etoposide with or without ART (only didanosine) resulted in a complete response rate of 45% and median overall survival of 12.8 months. At the time of the analysis, 30% in the pre-ART group were alive, compared with 47% in the ART group. Furthermore, patients in the ART group experienced less nonhematologic toxicity (22% vs. 42%), thrombocytopenia (31% vs. 52%), and anemia (9% vs. 27%) (Sparano, 2004). A similar regimen, etoposide, prednisone, vincristine, and doxorubicin (EPOCH), has been used more commonly and with perhaps even more success in the latter portion of the ART era. In two retrospective pooled analyses, Barta and colleagues concluded that EPOCH is superior to CHOP (Barta, 2012; Barta, 2013), however these studies were limited by the potential confounder that experience with CHOP occurred in earlier time periods than that with EPOCH.

Regarding treatment of PEL, a 2012 multicenter retrospective study found no survival benefit from regimens that were more intensive than CHOP (Castillo, 2012). A 2015 retrospective single-institution study of 15 patients treated with CHOP or CHOP-like regimens found that complete remission was achieved in 14 patients (93.3%); four of these subsequently relapsed (Cattaneo, 2015).

Regimens That Include Rituximab

In the early 2000s, uncertainty existed around the use of rituximab in HIV-positive patients with low CD4$^+$ T cell counts due to concern for increased infection risk (Kaplan, 2003; Avivi, 2003). However, with subsequent experience there is now a general consensus that outcomes are improved when rituximab is added to the chemotherapy regimens discussed earlier, thus rituximab should be regarded as the standard of care for both DLBCL and Burkitt lymphoma. Two recent multicenter retrospective analyses of DLBCL patients with and without HIV infection treated with rituximab plus CHOP (R-CHOP) have been completed. Coutinho et al. evaluated patients treated between 2003 and 2011 and found that HIV positivity was associated with an improved 5-year overall survival rate (78% compared with 64% in patients without HIV infection) (Coutinho, 2014). In contrast,

Baptista et al. evaluated patients treated between 2001 and 2011 and found that HIV positivity was associated with a worse 5-year survival rate (56% compared with 74% in HIV-negative patients) (Baptista, 2015). However, in the latter study the HIV-positive patients had a worse performance status and higher Ann Arbor stages than did HIV-negative patients, and, when complete response rates were compared among patients with high tumor burdens, there was no difference between the two groups. Although R-CHOP has become a commonly used regimen in the developed world, there is a paucity of data from low-resource settings. Currently, a phase 2 trial of R-CHOP in HIV-positive and negative patients with DLBCL is under way in Malawi to establish the safety of this regimen in that population (NCT02660710).

Sparano et al. examined rituximab plus infusional etoposide, vincristine, doxorubicin, cyclophosphamide, and prednisone (R-EPOCH) given either concurrently or sequentially. In the concurrent arm, 35 of 48 evaluable patients (73%; 95% CI, 58–85%) had a complete response, whereas 29 of 53 evaluable patients in the sequential arm (55%; 95% CI, 41–68%) had a complete response. Toxicity was comparable in the two arms, although patients with a baseline CD4$^+$ T cell count of less than 50 cells/mm^3 had a high infectious death rate in the concurrent arm (Sparano, 2010). There is an ongoing phase 2 trial of short-course R-EPOCH in HIV-positive patients with untreated NHL (NCT00006436). It is a dose-escalation study in which patients receive treatment every 3 weeks with R-EPOCH for 1 cycle beyond complete response of all detectable tumors for a minimum of 3 and maximum of 6 cycles. Finally, there is a phase 2 trial of ibrutinib (a small molecule drug that binds permanently to Bruton's tyrosine kinase) in combination with R-EPOCH in stage II–IV DLBCL (NCT03220022). Evidence remains unclear whether R-CHOP or R-EPOCH is best for patients with AIDS-related lymphomas. A large multicenter trial recently addressed this question in the HIV-negative population and showed no difference between R-CHOP and dose-adjusted R-EPOCH in event-free survival or overall survival (Wilson, 2016). Despite a paucity of large studies in the HIV-positive population, treatment with both R-CHOP and R-EPOCH is usually effective at achieving remission in HIV patients with DLBCL, and most patients who achieve remission remain lymphoma-free.

Regarding Burkitt's lymphoma, a 2012 study examined CODOX-M, followed by IVAC with or without rituximab (Rodrigo, 2012). Most patients were on ART and had a median CD4$^+$ T cell count of 375 cells/mm^3. Ten of the 14 patients who received ART, intensive chemotherapy, and rituximab survived to the follow-up period of nearly 12 months. Complications included late neutropenia, which responded well to G-CSF. Due to predilection of herpesvirus reactivation with rituximab, prophylaxis for herpes simplex and varicella zoster and preemptive monitoring of cytomegalovirus were given. More recently, a prospective multicenter trial showed that modified CODOX-M/IVAC with rituximab was safe and effective in HIV-positive patients receiving ART, and the 2-year overall survival rate for 34 patients with HIV-related Burkitt lymphoma was 69.0% (Noy, 2015). A 2013 study of short-course low-intensity R-EPOCH in 13 patients with Burkitt lymphoma including 11 HIV-positive patients found that the overall survival at a median follow-up of 73 months was even better, 90% (Dunleavy, 2013). No randomized data are available to determine which of the two regimens is best in HIV-positive patients with Burkitt lymphoma, however both appear to be effective although the efficacy of R-EPOCH in patients with CNS involvement has not yet been established.

Intrathecal Chemotherapy for AIDS-Related NHL

CNS involvement by systemic DLBCL has long been recognized as a problem, especially in HIV-positive patients. To date there have not been any formal studies to evaluate the role of intrathecal prophylaxis in HIV patients with DLBCL. In the absence of definitive data, clinicians routinely administer prophylaxis to patients with the following characteristics: extranodal involvement of two or more sites, elevated lactate dehydrogenase levels, or bone marrow or testicular involvement.

Alternative Therapies for AIDS-Related NHL

Newer, targeted anti-cancer therapies are currently being explored for several types of uncommon but aggressive ARLs, but currently data are sparse. One systematic review published in 2017 evaluated the use of bortezomib (a 26S proteasome inhibitor that is traditionally used for multiple myeloma) in 21 patients with plasmablastic lymphoma, of whom 11 received bortezomib as initial treatment and 10 received bortezomib for relapsed disease. Eleven patients were HIV-positive and 10 were HIV-negative. The overall response rate to bortezomib-containing regimens was 100% as initial therapy and 90% in the relapsed setting, and the 2-year survival of patients treated with bortezomib initially was 55% (Guerrero-Garcia, 2017). Daratumumab, a CD38-directed human IgG1κ monoclonal antibody that is typically used for multiple myeloma, has been shown to be effective in controlling a case of refractory PEL (Shah, 2018). Pembrolizumab is a biologic agent currently in phase 1 trials for patients with advanced NHL (NCT02595866).

Hematopoietic-Cell Transplantation for AIDS-Related NHL

Autologous HCT has long been the optimal therapy for high-risk and refractory NHL in non-HIV patients, and now a sufficient number of HIV-positive individuals have undergone autologous HCT to determine that it is a safe and feasible approach for ARL patients who meet criteria for transplantation (Navarro, 2006). Most recently, a multicenter study to evaluate the safety and efficacy of autologous HCT for HIV-positive lymphoma patients evaluated 40 patients with persistent or recurrent ARLs (DLBCL, plasmablastic lymphoma, Burkitt or Burkitt-like lymphoma, or classical Hodgkin lymphoma) (Alvarnas, 2016). Overall survival and time to progression were not different for HIV-positive patients when compared

with matched HIV-negative controls. Uninterrupted ART should be continued in these patients during the peritransplant period, when feasible, to maintain virological suppression and avoid untoward effects of acute virological rebound, including acute retroviral syndrome and opportunistic infections (Woolfrey, 2008). Administration of ART is generally considered safe, with minimal effect on the transplantation course, including adverse drug–drug interactions or other significant adverse events (Johnston, 2016).

One study showed that low $CD4^+$ T cell count, marrow involvement, and poor performance status independently affected survival with HCT (Re, 2009). Overall survival has been reported to be 50–55% at 9 months (Gabarre, 2000; Re, 2003), 71% at 21 months (Diez-Martin, 2003), and 85% at 32 months (Krishnan, 2005). All studies except a French series (Diez-Martin, 2003) have required HIV disease to be under control for HCT, either by low to undetectable HIV RNA levels or by $CD4^+$ T cell counts of more than 100 cells/mm[3]. In another study, Diez-Martin et al. showed a similar incidence of relapse, overall survival, and progression-free survival in cohorts of HIV-positive and HIV-negative lymphoma patients who received HCT (Diez-Martin, 2009). Long-term survival of autologous HCT for relapsed/refractory lymphoma was examined in a 2015 retrospective review of HIV-positive survivors (Zanet, 2015). This study found a survival of 65% at 5 years for 37 patients. Among 26 patients who achieved complete remission, overall survival at 10 years was 91% and event-free survival was 36%. Nine patients developed opportunistic infections at a median of 0.4 years post-HCT.

Regarding allogeneic HCT, one famous case reported in 2009 demonstrated that allogeneic HCT with donor cells that are resistant to HIV infection (in this case, because of a homozygous deletion polymorphism in the donor's CCR5 gene) can cure HIV infection (Hutter, 2009). Although fascinating, this outcome is the exception rather than the rule with allogeneic HCT. Importantly, caution must be observed because, in typical allogeneic HCTs, the HIV reservoir disappears along with the patient's T cells but can aggressively rebound if ART is discontinued (Henrich, 2014; Sugarman, 2016). More research is required to thoroughly explore the mechanism and frequency of this phenomenon. The first prospective multicenter trial of matched related or unrelated allogeneic HCT in HIV-positive patients was recently completed and included 17 patients with acute leukemias, myelodysplasia, Hodgkin lymphomas, and NHLs (Ambinder, 2017). There were no deaths at 100 days posttransplant, and the overall survival rate at 1 year was 57%. Deaths were due to relapsed or progressive disease in 5 patients, acute graft versus host disease, adult respiratory distress syndrome, and liver failure. The overall conclusion from this trial was that allogeneic HCT should be considered the standard of care for HIV-positive patients who meet usual transplant eligibility criteria. Other studies are currently being conducted to explore gene-modified autologous and allogeneic HCT with HIV-resistant cells (DiGiusto, 2016; Lederman, 2016; Bender-Ignacio, 2018).

Chemotherapy: ART Interactions

ART interruption during cancer treatment should generally be avoided because it increases the risk of severe consequences (including immunologic compromise, opportunistic infection, and death) (El-Sadr, 2006) and it improves tolerance and outcomes of cancer treatment. However, interactions between ART and proposed anti-cancer therapeutic options must always be checked as many medications used for chemotherapy (such as cyclophosphamide and vincristine) and immunotherapy are metabolized via the CYP3A4 isoenzyme. PIs (including ritonavir), non-nucleoside reverse transcriptase inhibitors, and pharmacokinetic boosters such as cobicistat inhibit and induce CYP3A4, with the potential for altered chemotherapeutic and cytotoxic effects. Thus, chemotherapy without antiretroviral drugs has been studied due to concerns of drug interactions with chemotherapy and noncompliance with ART resulting in increased resistance (Powles, 2000). Furthermore, PIs (in ART regimens) have been associated with increased incidence of neutropenia with concomitant chemotherapy (Bower, 2004). In one study of 39 patients receiving dose-adjusted EPOCH, antiretrovirals were not given until after the final cycle of chemotherapy. A complete remission rate of 74% was achieved (Little, 2003).

There are many types of ART regimens that are unlikely to lead to problematic drug–drug interactions with chemotherapeutic agents. Among those with the fewest potential interactions are the integrase inhibitors (raltegravir, elvitegravir, dolutegravir, and bictegravir). Raltegravir, an integrase inhibitor that is metabolized via glucuronidation, has been given simultaneously with CHOP and with other antimetabolites such as gemcitabine and methotrexate, as well as with monoclonal antibodies rituximab and trastuzumab, with good tolerability and durable viral suppression (Bañon, 2014). Raltegravir improves virologic and immunologic responses in antiretroviral treatment-naïve patients and is considered in the US Department of Health and Human Services (USDHHS) ART guidelines for HIV disease as an acceptable first-line therapy; thus, it could be a suitable alternative for preventing chemotherapeutic–ART interactions (Fulco, 2010).

Impact of ART

Most studies have shown that the incidence of HIV NHL, like that for most other AIDS-defining cancers, has declined over time. In a meta-analysis by Appleby et al. (Appleby, 2000) that included 47,936 HIV-positive individuals with NHL (including PCNSL), the incidence declined from 6.2 cases per 1,000 py in the pre-ART era to 3.6 cases per 1,000 py in the post-ART era ($p < 0.0001$).

In a population-based, record-linkage study of cancer in 472,378 individuals with AIDS from 1980 to 2006, the cumulative incidence of NHL declined from 3.8% during 1990–1995 to 2.2% during 1996–2006. Of note, NHL was the most common AIDS-defining cancer during the ART era (53%) (Simard, 2011). In addition, the Swiss Cohort study examined 429 NHL cases of 12,959 HIV-positive individuals from 1993 to 2006. NHL incidence reached 13.6 per 1,000 py in 1993–1995 and declined to 1.8 in 2002–2006. Combination ART use was associated with a decline in NHL incidence (hazard ratio [HR], 0.26; 95% CI, 0.20–0.33) (Polesel, 2008).

A retrospective study using US and Canadian data from 1996 to 2009 showed a significant decline in the annual hazard rate of NHL (–8%) in HIV-positive compared to that of HIV-negative individuals, signifying a narrowing of the gap of NHL burden between HIV-positive and -negative groups (Silverberg, 2015). This reduction also represents the benefit of immunological recovery and viral control.

RECOMMENDED READING

Alvarnas JC, Le Rademacher J, Wang Y, et al. Autologous hematopoietic cell transplantation for HIV-related lymphoma: results of the BMT CTN 0803/AMC 071 trial. *Blood*. 2016;128:1050–1058.

Bañon S, Machuca I, Araujo S, et al. Efficacy, safety, and lack of interactions with the use of raltegravir in HIV-infected patients undergoing antineoplastic chemotherapy. *J Intern AIDS Soc*. 2014;17(4 Suppl 3):19590.

Zanet E, Taborelli M, Rupolo M, et al. Postautologous stem cell transplantation long-term outcomes in 26 HIV-positive patients affected by relapsed/refractory lymphoma. *AIDS*. 2015;29(17):2303–2308.

NON–AIDS-DEFINING CANCERS

LEARNING OBJECTIVES

- Review the risk factors and epidemiology of NADCs.

- Review the impact of anogenital neoplasias and squamous cell cancer of the anus (SCCA) in men and women.

- Discuss treatment of anogenital neoplasias and SCCA, including the role of ART.

WHAT'S NEW?

- Women are more recognized as a high-risk group for SCCA, and predisposing factors include positivity for high-risk human papilloma virus (HPV) serotypes.

- HPV vaccination in HIV-positive women has demonstrated durable immunogenicity and safety.

- HPV vaccination for HIV-positive men beyond recommended ages may be beneficial and cost-effective in preventing invasive neoplasia.

KEY POINTS

- Due to the aging HIV population, NADCs are responsible for an increasing number of deaths. Immunologic control with ART, however, has decreased the incidence of some cancers, including anogenital cancers.

- Screening with either cervical Papanicolaou (Pap) smear or high-risk HPV in women is a key surveillance measure for detecting precancerous lesions. Screening with anal Pap smear in men and women with risk factors is also recommended, although uptake of this practice may be contingent on the availability of high-resolution anoscopy.

- HPV vaccination for HIV-positive men and women is safe and efficacious.

Since the advent of widely available ART in the United States, HIV-positive individuals have had significantly improved survival and decreased mortality from AIDS-related infections and ADCs. However, with longer survival, it has become evident that HIV-positive individuals are now at increased risk for NADCs. Multiple risk factors for NADCs include degree and duration of viremia, low CD4+ T cell nadir, coinfection with oncogenic viruses (e.g., HPV and HBV), and personal carcinogenic exposure, which also should be considered when implementing risk mitigation strategies (Kowalkowski, 2014; Reidel, 2015; Vallet-Prichard, 2004).

Simard et al. confirmed the benefits of immunological control in a population-based, record-linkage study examining cancers in 472,378 individuals with AIDS from 1980 to 2006 (Simard, 2011). The cumulative incidence of ADCs declined sharply across three AIDS calendar periods (from 18% in 1980–1989 to 11% in 1990–1995 and 4.2% in 1996–2006). The cumulative incidence of NADC increased from 1.1% to 1.5%, with no change thereafter (1% in 1996–2006). However, the cumulative incidence increased steadily over time for specific NADCs (anal cancer, Hodgkin's lymphoma, and liver cancer) (Simard, 2011). Another study (Simard, 2010) showed an elevated incidence for the following NADCs in patients 3–10 years after the onset of AIDS: Hodgkin's lymphoma and cancers of the oral cavity and/or pharynx, tongue, anus, liver, larynx, lung and/or bronchus, and penis. These data demonstrate that having previously diagnosed advanced immunosuppression appears to increase the risk for NADCs as well as ADCs.

The increased risk of NADCs among HIV-positive individuals has been reported by Patel et al. (Patel, 2008). The incidences of the following cancers were significantly higher: anal (standardized rate ratio [SRR], 42.9; 95% CI, 34.1–53.3), vaginal (SRR, 21.0; CI, 11.2–35.9), Hodgkin's lymphoma (SRR, 14.7; CI, 11.6–18.2), liver (SRR, 7.7; CI, 5.7–10.1), lung (SRR, 3.3; CI, 2.8–3.9), melanoma (SRR, 2.6; CI, 1.9–3.6), oropharyngeal (SRR, 2.6; CI, 1.9–3.4), leukemia (SRR, 2.5; CI, 1.6–3.8), colorectal (SRR, 2.3; CI, 1.8–2.9), and renal (SRR, 1.8; CI, 1.1–2.7). The incidence of prostate cancer was significantly lower among HIV-positive persons compared to the general population (SRR, 0.6; CI, 0.4–0.8). Only the relative incidence of anal cancer increased over time (Patel, 2008). Of particular note, none of the AIDS–cancer match studies found an increased risk of breast, colon, or prostate cancer. It is unclear if there is a definite link between the level of immunodeficiency and certain NADCs. Some studies have failed to show such a relationship (Burgi, 2005). Conversely, Reekie et al. utilized data from 4,453 patients in the prospective, multinational EuroSIDA cohort (Reekie, 2010). The incidence of NADCs in this cohort from 1994 to

2007 was 4.3 per 1,000 py of follow-up. After adjustment, a higher current CD4+ T cell count was independently associated with a decreased incidence of NADCs. In addition, an increased rate of virus-related cancers and non–virus-related epithelial cancers was found in immunodeficient patients. Hodgkin's lymphoma, anal cancer, and lung cancer were all found at a higher rate in patients with lower current CD4+ T cell counts after adjustment for other demographic and traditional risk factors (Reekie, 2010). More recently, a study of the US Veterans Aging Cohort Study also showed that increased risk of lung cancer is associated with lower CD4+ T cell counts, lower CD4:CD8 ratios, and increased viral load (Sigel, 2017).

It has also been previously hypothesized that individuals with HIV are at higher risk for malignancies at younger ages. Shiels et al. (Shiels, 2010) used the national US AIDS Cancer Registry Match to demonstrate that individuals with HIV are not at increased risk for colon, prostate, or breast cancer at younger ages, but they were younger at the time of diagnosis for lung and anal cancers. They also found that the age of diagnosis of Hodgkin's lymphoma was significantly older than that of the general population. A study using data from the HIV/AIDS Cancer Match study found that HIV-positive patients with cancer tended to be younger than age 50 years compared to their uninfected counterparts, whose cancer occurred more often after age 60 years. This study also found that those with HIV presented with more advanced-stage cancers with distant disease (32.2%) compared to uninfected patients (17.7%), and they experienced higher cancer-specific mortality (Coghill, 2015). By comparing data from both the North American AIDS Cohort Collaboration on Research and Design (NAACCRD) and the SEER program, Shiels et al. found that HIV-positive individuals were diagnosed with lung cancer, anal cancer, head and neck cancer, kidney cancer, and myeloma at earlier ages than their HIV-negative counterparts (Shiels, 2017).

NADCs are responsible for an increasingly large proportion of deaths in patients with HIV disease in the ART era, which is likely due to longer survival among individuals with HIV. A study conducted by the Data Collection on Adverse Events of Anti-HIV Drugs (D:A:D) evaluated factors associated with mortality due to NADCs and ADCs (Monforte, 2008). The study included 23,437 patients followed from 1999 to 2001. It was found that the overall mortality rate due to NADCs was higher than that due to ADCs. The death rate from NADCs was 1.8 per 1,000 py of follow-up (95% CI, 1.5–2.1) compared to 1.1 per 1,000 py of follow-up (95% CI, 0.9–1.2) for ADCs. In addition, based on multivariable analysis, it was found that most recent CD4+ T cell count and increasing age were associated with an increased risk of death from ADCs and NADCs. Other factors, such as ART utilization, increased the risk of death for NADCs only. It is unlikely that HIV treatment itself increases the risk for NADCs. Rather, this finding underscores the complex relationship between prolonged survival with HIV disease, immunosuppression, and the diagnosis of and survival from NADCs.

The Mortalité study in France captured the changing patterns of AIDS-related deaths in that country (Bonnet, 2005; Lewden, 2005). Lewden reported on cancer deaths among HIV-positive individuals in the original study and found that, in 2000, NADCs were the third leading cause of death. It was also found that as the patient population increased above age 45 years, deaths due to malignant disease eclipsed those due to infectious etiologies. The study was updated in 2005 and it found that the rate of death from non-AIDS/hepatitis-related cancers increased from 38% in 2000 to 50% in 2005. A subsequent follow-up study found that the combination of ADCs and NADCs has become the leading cause of death in France (Morlat, 2014). Similarly, a more recent Tanzanian study showed that NADCs increased by 33.8% from 2002 to 2014, while the proportion of NADCs relative to all cancers significantly decreased from 6.8% in 2002 to 5.6% in 2014 (APC = −2.74%) (Campbell, 2016). Most of these increases were due to lung and liver cancers, although the number of head and neck cancers also increased.

A US retrospective study found that cancer-related mortality among HIV-positive individuals compared to HIV-negative individuals (1996–2010) was significantly elevated for colorectal cancer (HR, 1.49; 95% CI, 1.2–1.8), pancreatic cancer (HR, 1.7; CI, 1.35–2.18), lung cancer (HR, 1.28; CI, 1.17–1.3), melanoma (HR, 1.72; CI, 1.09–2.7), breast cancer (HR, 2.61; CI, 2.06–3.3), and prostate cancer (HR, 1.57; CI, 1.02–2.41) (Coghill, 2015).

Regardless of etiology, as the HIV-positive population ages, the risk of NADCs will also undoubtedly increase. Some evidence suggests that treatment of these individuals may be more difficult than that of the general population, that HIV-positive patients may present with more advanced disease, and that HIV-positive patients may not tolerate cancer therapies as well as HIV-negative patients (Bower, 2003). Screening for early signs of malignancy may be an important method for earlier diagnosis. However, no studies of screening approaches have been performed, and no specific recommendations for alternative screening practices different from what is recommended for the general population exist for HIV-positive adults for most cancers.

Most studies of treatment outcomes for NADCs in the ART era demonstrate that HIV-positive individuals have outcomes similar to those of HIV-negative individuals. Simard and Engels evaluated cause of death in the pre-ART and ART eras and showed that death from NADCs (lung, Hodgkin's lymphoma, anal cancers, and other unspecified cancers) decreased steadily from 1980 to 2006 (Simard, 2010). For all NADCs, the number of deaths per 1,000 py from 1980 to 1989 and then from 1996 to 2006 significantly declined from 2.21 to 0.84 (Simard, 2010). Due to the benefit of ART on cancer outcomes in HIV-positive individuals, it is recommended that most patients be treated similarly to those without HIV infection and that ART should be administered concurrently with chemotherapy or radiotherapy (Chiao, 2010; Reid, 2018).

ANOGENITAL NEOPLASIA

Anogenital neoplasia refers to anal and cervical carcinomas and their precursor lesions. One of the most important risk factors associated with anogenital neoplasia is HPV infection. HPV is a DNA virus and generally infects stratified squamous epithelium. More than 100 HPV serotypes have been identified to date, and at least 30 of these have a high predilection for the anogenital tract. HPV serotypes 6 and 11 have been associated with benign disease, whereas serotypes 16, 18, and 31 are associated with high-grade cervical or anal squamous intraepithelial lesions (SILs) or cervical and anal carcinomas.

In HIV, HPV infection has a well-established relationship with the increased risk of developing anogenital neoplasia (Bjorge, 2002; Palefsky, 1991). Frisch reported an increase in both invasive and in situ forms of not only cervical and anal cancer but also vulvar/vaginal and penile cancers among HIV-positive individuals (Frisch, 2000).

PATHOGENESIS OF HPV IN HIV INFECTION

The increased prevalence of HPV disease associated with HIV infection may be mediated by impaired T cell and antigen-presenting cell function. However, local effects of HIV infection may also upregulate HPV replication and oncogenesis. The HPV viral oncogenes E6 and E7 can immortalize primary keratinocytes and transform cells in culture (Barbosa, 1989; Munger, 1989). In an animal model of estrogen-stimulated HPV-induced cervical cancer, expression of E7 alone resulted in precancers and cancer, whereas the expression of E6 and E7 together resulted in larger cancers (Riley, 2003). Although the exact mechanisms of HIV-related immunosuppression and HPV coinfection have not been determined, several in vitro studies have shown that the HIV tat protein can drive the replication of HPV-16 and HPV-18 through the overexpression of E7 and other genes in the early region (Tornesello, 1993; Vernone, 1993).

EPIDEMIOLOGY OF HIV-ASSOCIATED CERVICAL INTRAEPITHELIAL NEOPLASIA

The relationship between HIV infection and increased prevalence of cervical intraepithelial neoplasia (CIN) has been shown in many studies. Mandelblatt et al. performed a meta-analysis of 15 cross-sectional studies published between 1986 and 1998 that evaluated prevalence of cervical neoplasia, HPV infection, and HIV infection among women (Mandelblatt, 1999). They found that among women infected with HPV, HIV-positive women were significantly more likely to develop cervical neoplasia, and this effect was related to the degree of immunodeficiency. Several other studies have also shown that HIV-positive women are at higher risk for CIN, including that by Ahdieh et al., who found that 13% of HIV-positive women versus 2% of HIV-negative women had abnormal cytological findings (Ahdieh, 2000). They also found that HIV-positive women had a much lower rate of HPV clearance on follow-up exams and that, in a multivariate model, the increased rate of CIN among HIV-positive women was fully accounted for by HPV persistence (Ahdieh, 2000). A 2016 study from the Kaiser group found that HIV-positive women had two-fold higher odds of cervical intraepithelial neoplasia grade 2+ (CIN2+) and CIN3+, but this was only in women with a recent CD4+ count of less than 500 cells/mm^3 (Silverberg, 2016).

EPIDEMIOLOGY OF HIV-ASSOCIATED CERVICAL CARCINOMA

Since 1993, invasive cervical cancer has been listed by the CDC as an "AIDS-defining" condition. In the United States, where the incidence of cervical cancer in general is relatively low, the incidence in HIV-positive women is 66% higher than in women without HIV (Brickman, 2015). However, in some areas of Africa, the cervical cancer incidence is much higher, nearly 168 per 100,000 women (Lince-Deroche, 2015). Cervical cancer mortality remains higher in HIV-positive women than in HIV-negative women, especially in resource-limited settings (Ferlay, 2013). However, quantifying the contribution of HIV infection to the development of cervical cancer among HIV-positive women was challenging in the pre-ART era. A 1996 study that evaluated the relationship between HIV and cervical cancer found no conclusive evidence that HIV per se increased the risk of cervical cancer among HIV-positive women (International Agency for Research on Cancer, 1996). Subsequent studies continue to yield conflicting results. In developed countries with access to ART, several studies have shown an increased risk of cervical cancer. Using a national AIDS–cancer linked registry database of cases through 1998, Frisch et al. found a relative risk of 5.4 for invasive cervical cancer among HIV-positive women compared to the general population (Frisch, 2001). However, no increased risk in cervical cancer has been noted in case–control studies from multiple sub-Saharan African countries, where endemic rates of cervical cancer are higher and women have shorter survival (Gichangi, 2002; La Ruche, 1998; Patil, 1995).

As noted previously, with the use of ART since the mid-1990s, there have been definite declines in the incidence of AIDS-related cancers. This has been attributed to the improved immune function and control of oncogenic viruses seen with ART. This declining trend has not been consistently seen in AIDS-related cervical cancer. Shiels et al. showed an increasing proportion of cervical cancers in persons with AIDS from 0.11% in 1980–1989 (95% CI, 0.08–0.13) to 0.69% in 2001–2007 (95% CI, 0.49–0.89) (Shiels, 2011).

EFFECT OF ART ON HIV-ASSOCIATED CERVICAL DYSPLASIA

Although ART has significantly improved the survival of HIV-positive individuals through immune reconstitution and has decreased the incidence of opportunistic infections, the effects of ART on HPV infection and CIN among HIV-positive women remain unclear. Whereas three older studies did not find a significant reduction in risk of cervical dysplasia among women on ART (Lillo, 2001; Moore, 2002; Orlando, 1999), a recent prospective study did find a reduction in cervical dysplasia risk related to ART (Minkoff, 2010).

The largest retrospective analysis performed by the Women's Interagency HIV Study (WIHS) group found that, among 741 HIV-positive women, those on ART were 40% (95% CI, 4–81) more likely to exhibit a regression of cervical lesions and were also significantly less likely to have progression of CIN (odds ratio [OR], 0.68) (Minkoff, 2001). The same group subsequently prospectively evaluated 286 HIV-positive women who initiated ART (Minkoff, 2010). They were assessed semiannually for HPV infection (by PCR) and SILs. Combination ART initiation among adherent women was associated with a significant reduction in HPV prevalence, incident detection of oncogenic HPV infection, and decreased prevalence and more rapid clearance of oncogenic HPV-positive SILs. Effects were smaller among nonadherent women (Minkoff, 2010). More recently, a large systematic review evaluated HIV-positive women with high-grade cervical lesions (high-grade squamous intraepithelial lesions [HSIL]-CIN2[+]) (Kelly, 2018). HIV-positive women on ART had lower prevalence of high-risk HPV than did those not on ART. Their review included 17 studies that reported the association of ART with longitudinal cervical lesion outcomes and determined that ART was associated with a decreased risk of HSIL-CIN2[+] incidence, SIL progression, and increased likelihood of SIL or CIN regression. Furthermore, three of their studies indicated that ART was associated with a reduction in invasive cervical cancer incidence. Collectively, the data suggest that treating HIV infection with ART has a beneficial effect on progression of HPV-related cervical disease.

SCREENING, TREATMENT, AND PREVENTION OF HIV-ASSOCIATED CERVICAL DYSPLASIA

Screening

Current US Public Health Service and Infectious Diseases Society of America guidelines recommend that HIV-positive women undergo a complete history and physical that includes a pelvic exam and Pap test at the time of initial evaluation. The Pap test is the primary mode for cervical cancer screening for HIV-positive women. Screening for these women should commence within 1 year of the onset of sexual activity regardless of mode of HIV transmission (e.g., sexual activity and perinatal exposure) but no later than age 21 years. Women aged 21–29 years should have a Pap test at the time of initial diagnosis with HIV. Co-testing (Pap test and HPV test) is not recommended for women with HIV younger than 30 years. If the initial Pap test for young (or newly diagnosed) HIV-positive women is normal, the next Pap test should be performed in 12 months (although some experts still recommend a repeat Pap test at 6 months after baseline testing). If the results of the three consecutive Pap tests are normal, follow-up Pap tests can be done every 3 years. For women age 30 years or older, either Pap testing alone or co-testing with both Pap and HPV are acceptable screening strategies. For women who undergo Pap testing alone, the protocol is identical to that just described for women younger than 30. For women who undergo co-testing, Pap and HPV testing should be done at the time of HIV diagnosis (or starting at age 30 years). If the Pap is normal and the HPV screening test is negative, repeat cervical cancer screening can be done in 3 years. Women who have a normal Pap test but are positive for HPV should have repeat co-testing in one year (unless genotype testing for 16 or 16/18 is positive, in which case the patient should be referred for colposcopy). If either of the co-tests at 1 year is abnormal (i.e., abnormal cytology or positive HPV), referral to colposcopy is recommended. Any HIV-positive woman with an abnormal Pap smear that shows atypical squamous cell of undetermined significance (ASCUS) or higher grade lesions should undergo colposcopy (CDC, 2015). Cervical cancer screening in HIV-positive women should continue throughout their lifetime (and not end at age 65 years, as in the general population).

Treatment

Treatment options for CIN include cryotherapy, loop electrosurgical excision procedure (LEEP), and cold knife conization (Santesso, 2016). These options are generally safe and effective. Cryotherapy is an especially important option for women living in low-resource settings. A recent South African study evaluated 220 HIV-positive women who were randomized to cryotherapy ($n = 112$) or no treatment ($n = 108$) (Firnhaber, 2017). Ninety-four percent were receiving ART, their median $CD4^+$ T cell counts were 499 cells/mm^3, and 59% were high-risk HPV-positive. Cryotherapy reduced progression to HSIL (2 of 99 [2%] progressed in the cryotherapy group vs. 15 of 103 [15%] in the no treatment group; 86% reduction [95% CI: 41–97%; $p = 0.002$]). Participants in the cryotherapy arm experienced greater regression to normal histology and improved cytologic outcomes. Of note, endocervical extension is more frequent among HIV-positive women (Foulot, 2008). Therefore, LEEP is thought to be less effective and recurrence rates are higher in HIV-positive women than in HIV-negative women, although another recent South African study found that rates of cumulative CIN2$^+$ were lower after LEEP than cryotherapy treatment at 6 months (Smith, 2017). Importantly, in this study, both treatments appeared effective in reducing CIN2+ by more than 70% at 12 months.

Invasive cervical cancer diagnosed in HIV-positive women is treated using the same criteria and protocols as those for HIV-negative women as long as no other contraindications for treatment exist (Reid, 2018). Limited data exist on the treatment of cervical cancer in HIV-positive women (Ntekim, 2015). One prospective cohort study of 348 patients with cervical cancer in Botswana compared outcomes between HIV-positive women (66%) and HIV-negative women (Dryden-Peterson, 2016). The HIV-positive group had a median $CD4^+$ T cell count of 397 cells/mm^3 (interquartile range, 264–555). HIV infection was significantly associated with an increased risk of death among all women (HR, 1.95; 95% CI, 1.20–3.17) and among the subset of those who received guideline-concordant curative therapy (HR, 2.63; 95% CI, 1.05–6.55). These results suggest that HIV infection has an adverse effect on cervical cancer survival. That this effect was greater for women with a lower $CD4^+$ T cell count ($p = 0.036$) suggests that immune suppression plays a significant role. Of note, the study was conducted in a resource-limited environment, and survival of both HIV-positive and -negative patients with cervical cancer was lower than would be expected in the United States. Regarding newer therapies, there is an ongoing phase 3 trial evaluating standard chemoradiotherapy with or without modulated electrohyperthermia (a noninvasive intervention using 13.56 MHz radiofrequency treatment) for locally advanced cervical cancer in South Africa that includes HIV-positive women (NCT03332069).

Prevention

There are currently three US Food and Drug Administration (FDA)-approved HPV vaccines: bivalent, quadrivalent, and 9-valent. All three prevent HPV-16 and HPV-18 infections and prevent precancers (and likely cancers) caused by HPV-16 and HPV-18. In addition, the quadrivalent and 9-valent HPV vaccines prevent HPV-6 and HPV-11 infections and genital warts due to these types. The 9-valent vaccine also prevents infection and precancers due to five additional types (31, 33, 45, 52, and 58). The CDC currently recommends the HPV vaccine for HIV-positive individuals 9–26 years old. For individuals 9–14 years old, the vaccine can be given as two doses 6–12 months apart (CDC, HPV Fact Sheet). Older individuals should receive the three-dose series (0, 2, and 6 months). Although the CDC has not yet released recommendations for older individuals, the FDA recently approved the HPV vaccine for individuals up to 45 years old.

EPIDEMIOLOGY OF HIV-ASSOCIATED ANAL INTRAEPITHELIAL NEOPLASIA

Unlike cervical HPV infection, which peaks in the third decade in women, anal HPV infection is highly prevalent throughout adult life among men who have sex with men (MSM) well into the sixth decade (Chin-Hong, 2004; Schiffman, 2003). Several studies have reported the prevalence of anal intraepithelial neoplasia (AIN) among HIV-positive men and women. Palefsky found that the relative risk of developing high-grade squamous intraepithelial lesions (HSIL) was 3.7 for HIV-positive compared to HIV-negative MSM (Palefsky, 2001). Sixteen studies demonstrated that between 41% and 97% of HIV-positive men are found to have anal dysplasia on anal Pap smear screening (Kiviat, 2002; Palefsky, 2001; Piketty, 2008). In a meta-analysis of 31 studies, Machalek showed that the pooled prevalence of anal HPV detected by PCR was 89% in HIV-positive compared to 53.6% in HIV-negative men ($p = 0.047$) (Machalek, 2012). In addition, the prevalence of HPV-16 and HPV-18, associated with high-grade neoplasia and malignancy, was also significantly higher in HIV-positive compared to HIV-negative men.

EPIDEMIOLOGY OF HIV-ASSOCIATED SQUAMOUS CELL CANCER OF THE ANUS

Even before the HIV epidemic, anal cancer incidence among MSM was estimated to be as high as approximately 35 cases per 100,000 py. This rate is comparable to the incidence of cervical cancer in the United States before the advent of routine cervical cytology (Daling, 1987; Melbye, 1994). In the 1960s, the annual incidence of SCCA among men in the

United States was relatively low and stable, with approximately 0.5 cases per 100,000 persons. Since then, studies have shown a steady increase. A US population-based analysis of the Surveillance, Epidemiology and End Results (SEER) program data found that the incidence of SCCA in the United States among men increased from 1.06 per 100,000 persons from 1973 to 1979 to 2.04 per 100,000 persons from 1996 to 2004 (Johnson, 2004).

Many studies have shown that the incidence of SCCA is higher in HIV-positive persons. In a meta-analysis, Machalek examined nine studies published before November 2011 reporting anal cancer incidence in MSM (Machalek, 2012). Six were linkage studies based on data obtained from HIV/AIDS and cancer registries, and three were observational cohort studies. The incidence of anal cancer was significantly higher in HIV-positive men than in HIV-negative men ($p = 0.011$). This result has been mirrored in several studies in the United States and Europe, which show that the incidence of anal cancer among HIV-positive individuals ranges from 42 to 137 cases per 100,000 py, a rate 30–100 times higher than that of the general population (D'Souza, 2008; Patel, 2008; Piketty, 2008).

Squamous cell cancers of the anus may be overlooked in the female population; however, the rate of HPV-related anal cancers among women appears to be higher than that in men (1.8 vs. 1.2 per 100,000 persons) (CDC, April 20, 2012). Other publications have found incidence rates as high as 18–30 per 100,000 persons (Piketty, 2012; Silverberg, 2012). Incidence of anal cancer in HIV-positive women in higher income countries is also high (3.9–30 per 100,000 persons) (Stier, 2015). Women with $CD4^+$ T cell counts of less than 200 cells/mm^3 have a nearly 15-fold higher risk of developing invasive SCCA compared to the general population (SIR 14.5; 95% CI, 8.8–22.4) (Chaturvedi, 2009). Like the effects of HPV on cervical endothelium, the virus can lead to high-grade precancerous lesions and anal cancer. A recent systematic review of SCCA in women revealed higher prevalence of HPV in the anus versus cervix in most studies reviewed (16–85% vs. 17–70%, respectively) and that concordant HPV genotypes were found in 9–16% of women. Risk factors for anal HPV included cervical HPV, low $CD4^+$ cell count, smoking, and perianal warts (Stier, 2015). Furthermore, Machalek et al. found that the incidence of anal cancer was actually higher in the ART era. For example, from 1996 onward, the annual incidence of SCCA was 78 per 100,000 persons compared to 22 per 100,000 persons prior to this time. The reason for this increase is unclear. Improved survival associated with ART may allow for sufficient time for men with chronic HPV infection to develop anal cancer. Increases in screening are unlikely to explain this trend because routine screening is not yet currently recommended or routinely implemented in most clinical practice settings (Machalet, 2012). However, risk factors associated with SCCA have been shown to be associated with greater immunosuppression, including nadir $CD4^+$ T cell count and median HIV RNA levels of greater than 500,000 copies/mL (Guiguet, 2009).

SCREENING, TREATMENT, AND PREVENTION OF HIV-ASSOCIATED ANAL DYSPLASIA

As discussed previously, HIV-positive individuals are at an increased risk for SCCA and AIN; however, there is no standard screening protocol for anal cancer. SCCA shares many biologic similarities with cervical cancer, including detectable dysplastic precursor lesions and high-risk HPV infection. Consequently, many have recommended annual anal Pap screening for HIV-positive patients (Bosch, 1995). Anal Pap smears are acquired by randomly obtaining squamous cells from the anal canal using a Dacron swab. They are then fixed in liquid cytology media. Like cervical cytology protocols, abnormal anal cytologic findings are confirmed by high-resolution anoscopy-directed biopsy of visualized lesions (Figure 34.1). HPV DNA testing remains controversial due to the high prevalence of high-risk HPV infection in HIV-positive persons (Berry, 2009; Benevolo, 2016). However, presence of high-risk HPV genotype 16 is associated with concurrent high-grade anal lesions in HIV-positive women (Heard, 2015, 2016). Anal cytology is categorized according to the Bethesda system for cervical cytology: ASCUS, low-grade squamous intraepithelial lesion (LSIL), and HSIL. Anal Pap smears have a similar sensitivity and specificity as cervical Pap smears. Note that there are no definitive clinical studies showing that anal Pap smears decrease SCCA-related morbidity and mortality among HIV-positive individuals. Furthermore, anal cytology should not be performed if evaluation with high-resolution anoscopy is not available for the patient. Women with a history of cervical or vulvar neoplasias are more likely to have anal HPV infection and abnormal anal cytology (Stier, 2015). The presence of anal warts or condyloma acuminata may also be an indicator for HPV infection of the anal canal and may warrant further screening. High-risk patients should be followed every 6 months for at least 5 years, ideally with periodic photographic documentation of the perianal region. There should be a low threshold to repeat biopsies of any changing lesion.

There is a lack of consensus and rigorous evidence regarding recommendations for performing annual digital rectal exam (DRE) in patients at risk for SCCA, such as MSM. The 2015 European AIDS Clinical Society (EACS) guidelines recommend DRE with or without an anal Pap smear every 1–3 years in MSM (EACS, 2015). The 2015 Guidelines for Prevention and Treatment of Opportunistic Infections in HIV-positive Adults and Adolescents suggest that annual DRE is only a class B, grade III recommendation (USDHHS, 2015). Recently, a phase 2 clinical trial was conducted to assess the feasibility of teaching MSM to recognize palpable masses in the anal canal using self or partner exams (Nyitray, 2018). Results indicated that tumors 3 mm or larger may be detectable by self or partner exams, which is significant as there is a high cure rate for tumors 10 mm or smaller.

Treatment

The surveillance of patients with AIN II and III is predominantly aimed at the identification of early invasive carcinoma

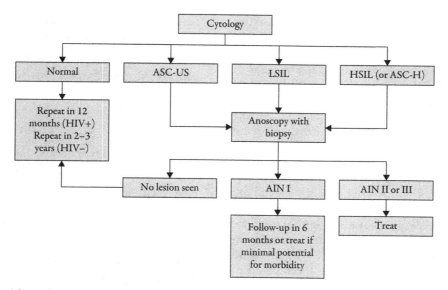

Figure 34.1 Screening protocol for anal intraepithelial neoplasia (AIN). Recommended screening protocol for anal intraepithelial neoplasia. ASC-H, atypical squamous cells, cannot rule out HSIL; ASC-US, atypical squamous cells of undetermined significance; HSIL, high-grade squamous intraepithelial lesion; LSIL, low-grade squamous intraepithelial lesion. From (Curr Infect Dis Rep. 2010 March; 12(2): 126–133).

that can be treated by local excision or localized chemotherapy and radiation. Little data exist regarding the management of AIN, but it is thought that, like CIN, if AIN can be eradicated, then malignant transformation can be prevented. Targeted biopsies using high-resolution anoscopy and 3% acetic acid to the anal canal mucosa (like colposcopy) can help identify areas of AIN.

Treatment options for anal dysplasia are similar for HIV-positive and -negative individuals. These include topical trichloroacetic acid, liquid nitrogen, imiquimod, infrared coagulation, electrocautery, carbon dioxide (CO_2) laser, and surgical excision. One randomized trial of 156 HIV-positive MSM showed that electrocautery is better than imiquimod and fluorouracil in the treatment of AIN but recognized that recurrence rates were substantial (Richel, 2013). Of note, there are several new therapies being evaluated for HIV-positive patients with anal dysplasia. These include two Australian studies: a phase 2 trial evaluating the immunomodulator pomalidomide in anal HSIL (NCT03113942) and a phase 1 study evaluating a new topical drug with direct anti-HPV activity, ABI-1968 (NCT03202992).

Currently, the recommended treatment for HIV-positive patients with anal cancer is the same as that recommended for the general population (Reid, 2018). In the general population, concurrent chemoradiotherapy with 5-fluorouracil (5-FU) infusion and mitomycin (or cisplatin) has been established as the standard-of-care regimen for nonmetastatic anal cancer. In the ART era, reports on clinical outcomes of HIV-positive patients with anal cancer have been conflicting. Some studies have shown that HIV-positive and -negative patients had comparable disease control and survival (Blazy, 2005; Chiao, 2008; Fraunholz, 2011), whereas others have suggested that HIV-positive patients may do worse in terms of treatment-related toxicity and/or an increased risk for local relapse (Oehler-Janne, 2008; Grew, 2015). Existing evidence is limited by mostly retrospective data as well as small numbers of patients studied, thus further investigation into this question would be beneficial.

Prevention

Routine vaccination with quadrivalent HPV or the 9-valent HPV vaccine is now available for all individuals aged 9–45 years to prevent genital warts and the development of precancerous and cancerous HPV-mediated lesions (FDA, 2018). Advisory Committee on Immunization Practices (ACIP) recommendations for individuals older than age 26 have not yet been updated (Advisory Committee on Immunization Practices, 2016).

EFFECT OF ART ON ANAL DYSPLASIA

Like studies evaluating the effect of ART on cervical dysplasia, studies evaluating the effect of HIV therapy on anal dysplasia have found conflicting results. This may be related to the significant design and methodological differences among these studies. There are two small case series ($n = 4$ and 26 patients, respectively) describing outcomes of HIV-associated SCCA, with 5-year survival rates of 47–60% (Jephcott, 2004; Myerson, 2001). In studies that specifically compared survival among patients with SCCA in the pre-ART versus ART eras, there was a nonsignificant trend toward improved survival, better tolerability of chemoradiotherapy, and improved local tumor control in the ART era (Bower, 2004; Cleator, 2000; Stadler, 2004).

A study linking the New York State cancer registry with the New York City HIV/AIDS registry found that in the early ART era (1990–1996), the 24-month survival was 76% for patients with AIDS compared to 78% for patients without AIDS, suggesting that, at least during this time period,

HIV-positive patients with SCCA had equivalent survival with HIV-negative patients.

Palefsky and colleagues compared the rates of progression and regression of anal dysplasia after 6 months of ART (Palefsky, 2001). They found that the likelihood of lesion progression or regression was not affected by ART initiation, but they noted that among the patients starting ART at higher CD4+ T cell counts, ART demonstrated a nonsignificant benefit on anal dysplasia lesions. In contrast, Wilkin et al. conducted a cross-sectional study evaluating anal HPV infection and anal dysplasia in 98 HIV-positive men (Wilkin, 2004). In a multivariate analysis, they found that ART and higher nadir CD4+ T cell count were significantly protective for anal dysplasia by histology but were not protective of anal HPV infection. A Canadian study retrospectively evaluated 1,691 HIV-positive MSM and found that immunosuppression with nadir CD4+ T cell count of less than 100 cells/mm³ was a risk factor for anal cancer (OR, 3.08; $p = 0.01$). They also found that men treated during the pre-ART era had a higher incidence (370 vs. 93 per 100,000 py) and shorter lead time to development of anal cancer compared to those in the post-ART era (Duncan, 2015). Therefore, it remains unclear if ART initiation influences the natural history of AIN in HIV-positive individuals. However, ART is beneficial for men undergoing treatment for HPV-related disease.

RECOMMENDED READING

Kojic EM, Kang M, Cespedes MS, et al. Immunogenicity and safety of the quadrivalent human papillomavirus vaccine in HIV-1-infected women. *Clin Infect Dis.* 2014;59(1):127–135.

Piketty C, Selinger-Leneman H, Grabar S, et al. Marked increase in the incidence of invasive anal cancer among HIV-infected patients despite treatment with combination antiretroviral therapy. *AIDS (London).* 2008;22(10):1203–1211.

Stier EA, Sebring MC, Mendez AE, et al. Prevalence of anal human papillomavirus infection and anal HPV-related disorders in women: A systematic review. *Am J Ob Gyn.* 2015;213(3):278–309.

LUNG CANCER

LEARNING OBJECTIVES

- Review the epidemiology and risks of lung cancer in those with HIV.

- Review the pathogenesis of lung cancer.

- Discuss the treatment of lung cancer.

- Discuss the treatment outcomes and mortality associated with lung cancer in HIV-positive persons.

WHAT'S NEW?

- HIV-positive patients have an increasing incidence of lung cancer during the ART era.

- Surgery, chemotherapy, and radiation are mainstays of standard treatment for patients with HIV.

- Treatment disparities between HIV and non-HIV patients may contribute to poor survivability of those with lung cancer.

KEY POINTS

- Tobacco cessation is of utmost importance in preventing lung cancers in patients with HIV.

- People with HIV have a higher incidence of lung cancer than the general population, although a predominant histology of non-small cell lung cancer is common in both groups.

- HIV-positive patients have worse survival, which may be due to frequent presentation with advanced disease.

- No specific guidelines for treating HIV patients with lung cancer exist, and more rigorous studies evaluating standards of care are needed.

Lung cancer is the leading cause of death due to cancer in the general US population, and it also represents the most common NADC (Frisch, 2001). Lung cancers in HIV are primarily non-small cell cancer (NSCLC) types, including adenocarcinoma and squamous cell carcinoma. This largely reflects the trend of histology types among the general population in Western settings (Cadranel, 2006). Mortality from lung cancer remains high in HIV-positive individuals compared to the general population, especially for patients presenting at advanced stages (Coghill, 2015; Shiels, 2010).

The incidence of lung cancer, like that of other NADCs, has increased for several reasons, including increased life expectancy in the era of ART and longer cumulative exposure to carcinogens known to be associated with lung cancer development, namely tobacco smoke. Notably, tobacco exposure in the HIV population remains a significant health problem, with disproportionate use compared to the general population (Clifford, 2012; Rahmanian, 2011; Altekruse, 2018). Due to this increased risk, smoking cessation is of utmost importance in this patient population (Shepherd, 2018). Immunosuppression may also be a contributing factor; however, this relationship is not clearly understood.

EPIDEMIOLOGY OF LUNG CANCER IN HIV

Engels et al. examined data from large HIV and cancer registries in the United States to estimate the incidence of lung cancer. They found the incidence in the HIV population to be 59 per 100,000 py during a period from 1991 to 2002 (Engels, 2008). This same study found that the incidence of lung cancer increased from 51 per 100,000 py to 126 per 100,000 py between those with HIV compared to those with an AIDS diagnosis (Engels, 2008). In another study including Canadian data, researchers found that, from 1996 to 2009, the incidence of lung cancer in HIV-positive individuals was

129 per 100,000 py compared to 45.4 per 100,000 py in HIV-negative individuals. The incidence of lung cancer was higher for persons aged 75 years than for those aged 65 years (3.4% vs. 2.2%), which supports the increased risk of cancer development as the population ages (Silverberg, 2015). Marcus et al. evaluated a Californian cohort of 24,768 HIV-positive compared to 257,600 HIV-negative individuals between 1996 and 2011 and found that the lung cancer rate was 66 per 100,000 py for HIV-positive individuals and 33 per 100,000 py for HIV-negative individuals (rate ratio 2.0, 95% CI: 1.7–2.2) (Marcus, 2017).

A Ugandan study evaluating overall cancer incidence (ADC and NADCs) in HIV-positive persons from 1988 to 2002 found the incidence over time to be increased, with a SIR of 5 (Mbulaiteye, 2006). Another study using the Swiss HIV Cohort Study and Swiss cancer registries found that cancers of the trachea, lung, and bronchus were significantly elevated compared to those of the general population, with a SIR of 3.2 (Clifford, 2005).

The impact of ART on the incidence and risk of lung cancer remains unclear. Studies attempting to evaluate the incidence of lung cancer during the pre-ART and ART eras have found mixed results, with increased incidence in both eras. The previously cited study by Silverberg et al. showed that cumulative incidence of lung cancer in North America continues to increase in the ART era (Silverberg, 2015). They found a cumulative incidence of 3.7% from 2005 to 2009 compared to 1.8% from 1996 to 2009 (Silverberg, 2015). Another study that examined data from 34 states showed similar results, with a steady increase in the number of lung cancers (35 to 283 cases) from 1991 to 2005, which largely occurred in persons older than 50 years (Shiels, 2011). This phenomenon speaks to the increasing longevity of the HIV population and accumulation of malignant comorbidities.

RISK FACTORS ASSOCIATED WITH LUNG CANCER IN HIV

Risk factors for lung cancer are multiple and include tobacco exposure, injection drug use, and possibly HIV infection itself. Other comorbid pulmonary diseases, such as chronic obstructive pulmonary disease and bacterial pneumonia, are more common in HIV-positive individuals than in HIV-negative individuals and may place HIV-positive individuals at higher risk for cancer due to persistent states of inflammation (Crothers, 2011; Shebl, 2010). Inflammatory markers circulating in the blood have been associated with theoretical risk of lung cancer; these include C-reactive protein, serum amyloid, soluble tumor necrosis factor receptor-2, lymphoid differentiation cytokine interleukin-7, and various leukocyte-derived chemokines (Shiels, 2013). However, it remains to be determined exactly how these inflammatory states that are not confounded by smoking or other traditional risks factors like pneumonia impact the risk of lung cancer.

Cigarette smoking has repeatedly been implicated as a major risk factor for lung cancer in the general population as well as in the HIV population (Altekruse, 2018; Shepherd, 2018). Prevalence of cigarette smoking among HIV-positive persons is estimated to be between 42% and 59%, and it greatly exceeds that of the general population by two- to threefold (Mdodo, 2015; Tesoriero, 2010; Altekruse, 2018). In a Swiss study, Clifford and others reported that all persons with cancer of the respiratory tract were smokers, and there was a threefold higher excess risk of these cancers (Clifford, 2005). A similar finding was demonstrated in a US study that showed patients with HIV and lung cancer were 1.3 times more likely to be current or former smokers and to have greater pack-year tobacco consumption history compared to those with HIV but without cancer (D'Jaen, 2010). Shiels et al. also examined the role of cigarette smoking in the development of lung cancer in HIV. They found that those with HIV who smoked more than 1.43 packs per day had twice the risk of lung cancer compared to those with HIV who smoked less. Compared to HIV-negative patients who smoked less than 1.43 packs per day, those with HIV and who smoked more than 1.43 packs per day had a 7.2 times higher risk of developing lung cancer (Shiels, 2010). A more recent study using the North American AIDS Cohort Collaboration on Research and Design consortium evaluated 52,441 HIV-positive individuals including 2,306 who were diagnosed with cancer between 2000 and 2015 (Altekruse, 2018). They found that HIV-positive individuals diagnosed with cancer were more likely to have been smokers (79%) compared to those without cancer (73%). Furthermore, in HIV-positive individuals smoking was associated with increased risk of cancer overall ([HR =1.33 [95% CI: 1.18–1.49]), smoking-related cancers (HR= 2.31 [1.80–2.98]), and lung cancer (HR =17.80 [5.60–56.63]). Reddy et al. recently used an HIV microsimulation model to evaluate cumulative lung cancer mortality by smoking exposure and found that HIV-positive individuals who continue to smoke have a 16.6–29.8% estimated mortality depending on sex and smoking intensity, while estimated mortality decreased to 3.7–7.9% for those who quit smoking and to 1.2–1.6% for never smokers (Reddy, 2017). Even HIV-positive individuals who were adherent to ART were 6–13 times more likely to die from lung cancer than from traditional AIDS-related causes. When the authors applied this model to the current US HIV-positive population, they found that 9.3% could die from lung cancer if their smoking habits do not change.

Other studies have not found the same association with smoking. Engels et al. studied 5,238 HIV-positive patients and found that the overall smoking-adjusted SIR for lung cancer was 2.5 times higher than that of the general population (95% CI, 1.6–3.5) (Engels, 2006). However, in an analysis that assumed that all participants smoked, the smoking-adjusted SIR was only 1.7. This suggests that smoking did not account for all excess risk of lung cancer in HIV (Engels, 2006). In the mortality analysis by Shiels et al., it was found that, after adjusting for smoking and other patient characteristics, the risk of death was 3.8 times higher for HIV-positive versus HIV-negative patients (Shiels, 2010). A large Veterans Administration study found that the incidence rate ratio (1.7) of lung cancer in HIV patients remained significantly elevated after multivariable adjustment for confounders including smoking compared to persons without HIV (Sigel, 2012). These studies suggest that, independent of smoking, HIV positivity portends a higher incidence and mortality risk for lung cancer.

Injection drug use (IDU) among HIV-positive patients has also been associated with an increased risk of lung cancer compared with that for nonusers in several studies. One study in particular demonstrated that those with IDU, with or without HIV, had an increased risk of lung cancer, with SIRs of 14.3 and 6.2, respectively (Serraino, 2000). Other studies have found little evidence to support this risk factor, however. In a study by Kirk et al. that included 2,086 participants (the AIDS Link to the Intravenous Experience Study), IDU was not associated with increased risk of lung cancer (Kirk, 2007).

HIV itself may also be associated with the development of lung cancer due to directly acting oncogenic effects. HIV-1 replication depends on tat protein expression, which can upregulate expression of protooncogenes c-myc, c-fos, and c-jun to enhance cellular proliferation, including human adenocarcinoma cell lines (El-Solh, 1997). Allelic loss and changes in microsatellites, which are short tandem repeat DNA sequences, have also been described in other malignancies, such as KS, NHL, and SCCA, and have been found in lung cancers of HIV-positive patients (Wistuba, 1998). These genetic alterations may lead to activation of oncogenes and loss of tumor suppressor genes. However, the lack of HIV viral integration into cellular DNA of somatic neoplastic cells challenges this hypothesis of oncogenesis because cancer cells can have background genetic alterations and immunosuppression can also be associated with microsatellite changes (Bedi, 1995). Poor control of HIV also could contribute to the development of lung cancer. A study of HIV-positive individuals included in the US Veterans Aging Cohort Study found that increased risk of lung cancer was associated with low $CD4^+$ T cell count, low CD4/CD8 ratio, high HIV viral load, and more cumulative episodes of bacterial pneumonia (Sigel, 2017). Another recent study similarly noted that a $CD4^+$ cell count of less than 200 cells/mm^3 was associated with a younger age at lung cancer diagnosis (Shiels, 2017). In contrast, a large Californian cohort study by Marcus et al. did not find an association between increased development of lung cancer and $CD4^+$ T cell count of less than 200 cells/mm^3 (Marcus, 2017).

Although men historically have been considered at higher risk for lung cancer, women also share a significant proportion of lung cancer diagnoses. This may be due to the increase in women tobacco smokers in the population or the increase in the number of HIV-positive women. The WIHS compared data from the National Health and Nutritional Examination (NHANES) II and SEER. Researchers found that HIV-positive women have higher lifetime cigarette consumption as well as an elevated SIR of 3 (95% CI, 1.7–5.1) compared to the general population with a SIR of 2.11 (95% CI, 0.25–7.61). Furthermore, these data did not vary by pre-ART versus ART era (Levine, 2010). A French study evaluating cancer in HIV-positive patients in the pre-ART and ART eras found that the SIR of women was three times higher than that of men in the ART era (6.28 vs. 2.12) (Herida, 2003). Several additional studies have shown greater incidence in women with SIR ranging from 1.6 to 16.7 (Calabresi, 2013; Clifford, 2005; Ramirez-Marrero, 2010).

DIAGNOSIS AND CLINICAL PRESENTATION OF LUNG CANCER IN HIV

Despite the increased risk of cancer with aging, HIV-positive persons with lung cancer tend to be younger. In several studies, age at presentation ranged from 38 to 57 years. This is far below the age of presentation among the general population, which is closer to the seventh decade of life (Winstone, 2013). Stage at presentation also tends to be advanced in HIV-positive patients, with a majority presenting with stages III or IV. This likely contributes to the poor survivability of these patients (Sigel, 2012; Winstone, 2013).

The majority of histological types mirror those of the general population, with greater than 50% consisting of NSCLC. Adenocarcinoma is the predominant non-small cell cancer (36%), followed by squamous cell carcinoma (30%) (Sigel, 2012). Many patients present with advanced disease and have symptoms of persistent cough and chest pain (Karp, 1993). Early diagnosis of lung cancer improves prognosis; however, screening with plain chest radiography at any interval has not been shown to be effective and is not recommended. Use of low-dose chest computed tomography (LDCT) may be beneficial in these patients. The recommendation of the US Preventive Services Task Force (USPTF) to screen high-risk patients for lung cancer with LDCT was based on the findings from the National Lung Screening Trial (National Lung Screening Trial Research Team, 2011). This was a large randomized trial that found a 20% reduction in lung cancer mortality after implementing annual screening by LDCT in patients aged 55–74 years and at least a 30 pack-year smoking history. Because of improved mortality benefit, current USPTF guidelines recommend lung cancer screening with LDCT for people aged 55–80 in the general population with at least a 30 pack-year smoking history and currently smoke or who have quit within 15 years, regardless of gender (Moyer, 2014). Of note, a handful of studies that have evaluated LDCT in HIV-positive patients have suggested that these patients, especially those with low $CD4^+$ counts, are more likely to have false-positive LDCT findings due to prior lung infections (Sigel, 2014; Ronit, 2017). A recent modeling study evaluating HIV-infected patients with $CD4^+$ T cell counts of at least 500 cells/mm^3 found that screening using the Centers for Medicare and Medicaid Services criteria (age 55–77, 30 pack-years of smoking, current smoker or quit within 15 years of screening) would reduce lung cancer mortality by 18.9% in this population, similar to the mortality reduction of uninfected individuals (Kong, 2018). Thus, the benefit and cost-effectiveness of LDCT in patients infected with HIV remain unknown, but following the USPTF and NCCN guidelines for the general population is reasonable after discussing risks (e.g., false positives and radiation exposure) and benefits (e.g., early detection and better prognosis) with patients (Reid, 2018). Currently, a French multicenter prospective pilot study (ANRS EP48 HIV-CHEST cohort) is evaluating the utility of LDCT in HIV-positive individuals (NCT01207986; Makinson, 2015).

Understanding the mechanisms underlying the development of lung cancer in HIV-positive individuals could lead to improved lung cancer screening methodologies. Zheng et al. recently studied the molecular mechanisms underlying the gene expression profiles of lung cancer in HIV-positive patients and identified 758 differentially expressed genes in HIV-associated lung cancer (Zheng, 2018). Specifically, they found that the expression levels of SIX1 and TFAP2A mRNA are increased in HIV-associated lung cancer and that expression levels of ADH1B, INMT, and SYNPO2 mRNA are decreased.

TREATMENT OF LUNG CANCER

There are no alternative or specific treatment guidelines for lung cancer in the HIV population. Most randomized trials for lung cancer have historically excluded HIV-positive patients due to concerns regarding immune suppression, toxicity, and drug interactions with ART (Persad, 2008). Current treatment strategies are mainly with protocols for patients without HIV and depend on tumor histology, stage of disease, and underlying host factors such as comorbidities and pulmonary function. Patients with NSCLC are staged (I–IV) based on the tumor node metastasis system, with stage I disease confined to localized tumor without invasion into the chest wall, diaphragm, mediastinum, or surrounding structures and stage IV indicating metastatic disease (Shepherd, 2007). MRI of the brain should also be pursued for stage II or higher to identify intracranial metastasis. For localized, nonmetastatic disease, surgical resection is the preferred strategy with intent to cure for those patients able to undergo surgery. Surgery (lobectomy, sublobular resection, and video-assisted thoracoscopy) may be followed by adjuvant chemotherapy or radiation for those with more advanced stages or invasion (NCCN, 2.2016). For nonsurgical candidates, ablation with radiotherapy can be considered. Studies evaluating surgery in HIV-positive patients have been described in mainly small case–control series and case reports. Patients undergoing surgery for localized disease (stage I or stage II) tolerated surgery well with minimal complications (Cadranel, 2006).

For patients with advanced NSCLC or recurrence after initial definitive therapy, goals of therapy are largely palliative. For patients with solitary metastasis or recurrence, curative intention with additional surgery or radiotherapy may be indicated and beneficial to help prolong survival. However, risks and benefits must be weighed in advanced disease to avoid undue adverse events and toxicities. Systemic therapy with combination chemotherapy using a platinum-based regimen is the mainstay agent with or without additional agents, such as the vascular endothelial growth factor inhibitor bevacizumab (NCCN, 2.2016).

Use of chemotherapy in HIV-positive patients is feasible, and it has been used in patients to treat metastatic disease and as an adjuvant therapy and in combination with radiation for locally advanced disease. One large retrospective study found similar rates of treatment modality between HIV and non-HIV patients (Sigel, 2013). Limited data from case series have provided heterogeneous results regarding use of chemotherapeutic agents, efficacy, and drug toxicities in HIV patients with lung cancer (Bower, 2003; Powles, 2003; Spano,

2004). Additional studies to evaluate efficacy, tolerability, and safety of chemotherapy in HIV patients are needed.

Additional molecular and genetic mutation analysis for potential genetic-directed therapy targets has been explored. These should be performed when possible in patients with advanced stage NSCLC, namely for the presence of epidermal growth factor receptor (EGFR) and anaplasmic lymphoma kinase (NCCN, 2.2016). Other targets include RAS family oncogenes, the mTOR signaling pathway, and the MEK signaling pathway. Treatment with EGFR tyrosine kinase inhibitors such as erlotinib may also be considered for patients with this specific EGFR mutation in the tumor. However, long-term survival has yet to be established with use of these agents (Okuma, 2014). Several novel treatment regimens are being studied in HIV-positive patients with advanced lung cancer. Immunotherapies such as nivolumab, ipilimumab, and durvalumab are being evaluated in patients with advanced solid tumors, including NSCLC (NCT03304093, NCT02408861) and (NCT03094286; Bender-Ignacio, 2018).

SURVIVAL OF LUNG CANCER IN HIV

Survival among patients with HIV and lung cancer is worse compared to that of their uninfected counterparts. Coghill et al. analyzed data from 1996 to 2010 and found that in 1,058 HIV-positive patients, all-cause mortality and cancer-specific mortality risk were respectively 85% and 28% higher for HIV patients with lung cancer compared to HIV-negative patients (Coghill, 2015). For patients with local-stage NSCLC receiving standard cancer therapy, those with HIV continued to have greater cancer-related deaths compared to HIV-uninfected patients (HR, 1.8; 95% CI, 1.21–2.7) (Coghill, 2015). Another large study utilizing SEER registry data compared 267 HIV-positive to 1,428 noninfected patients with similar cancer stage and histology of NSCLC (Sigel, 2013). Both groups with stage I to IIIA disease received surgery, chemotherapy, and radiotherapy at similar rates. Among the HIV-positive group, 82% died during follow-up compared to 66% of the uninfected group ($p < 0.001$). Median overall survival for HIV patients was only 6 months compared to 20 months for the uninfected cohort. Overall 5-year survival was also poor for HIV-positive patients at 9% compared to 23% for the noninfected group. Patients with HIV and advanced disease (stage IIIB to IV) had the worst survival, with 9–20 times greater risk of death compared to HIV patients with only localized disease. Moreover, a major proportion of those with HIV also died from non–cancer-related causes (31% vs. 9%; $p < 0.001$).

Such disparity in outcomes in the previously discussed studies may be explained by several hypotheses, including the fact that patients with HIV experience overall greater mortality than the general population. It may be that tumors behave more aggressively in patients with HIV due to tumor effect or poor immunological surveillance due to lack of fully intact cellular immunity. Recent evaluation of the North American AIDS Cohort Collaboration on Research and Design dataset found that HIV-positive individuals with a history of an AIDS-defining illness at lung cancer diagnosis had higher mortality and poorer survival after diagnosis compared to those without (Grover, 2018). Poor tolerability of surgery and chemotherapy may also contribute to worse outcomes. More studies are needed to clarify these issues.

Last, health disparities in treatment between HIV-positive and non-HIV populations may contribute to poor survivability. Data from the Texas Cancer registry from 1995 to 2009 showed that patients with HIV and NSCLC less frequently received any cancer treatments despite greater numbers presenting at younger ages and with distant-stage disease (Suneja, 2013). Patients with HIV and local-stage NSCLC were less likely to receive surgery (45.5% vs. 62.5%; $p = 0.04$) than uninfected patients. Those with regional disease and HIV were less likely to receive systemic chemotherapy. For distant disease, HIV-positive patients received less chemotherapy or radiation (31.1% vs. 45.5%; $p = 0.0009$) (Suneja, 2013).

RECOMMENDED READING

Coghill AE, Shiels MS, Suneja G, et al. Elevated cancer-specific mortality among HIV-infected patients in the United States. *J Clin Oncol.* 2015;33(21):2376–2383.

Grover S, Desir F, Jing Y, et al. Reduced cancer survival among adults with HIV and AIDS-defining illnesses despite no difference in cancer stage at diagnosis. *J AIDS.* 2018;79(4):421–429.

Sigel K, Crothers K, Dubrow R, et al. Prognosis in HIV-infected patients with non-small cell lung cancer. *Br J Cancer.* 2013;109:1974–1980.

Suneja G, Shiels MS, Melville SK. Disparities in the treatment and outcomes of lung cancer among HIV-infected Individuals. *AIDS.* 2013;27(3):459–468.

PROSTATE CANCER

LEARNING OBJECTIVES

- Review the epidemiology and risk factors for prostate cancer in men with HIV.

- Review the current screening recommendations for prostate cancer.

- Discuss the treatment options for prostate cancer in men with HIV.

WHAT'S NEW?

- Since the advent of prostate-specific antigen (PSA) testing, the incidence of prostate cancer has increased in HIV-positive men. However, the true incidence may be lower than that of HIV-negative men.

- Routine prostate cancer screening with PSA testing is not recommended.

KEY POINTS

- Prostate cancer represents a significant burden of neoplastic disease and mortality in HIV-positive men and also men in the general population.

- Prostate cancer appears to be associated with states of immunological control.

- Screening with serum PSA testing should not routinely be implemented, having a "D" recommendation by the US Preventive Services Task Force.

- Decision to treat early-stage cancer versus watchful waiting should be carefully considered because evidence of long-term mortality benefits remains unclear.

- First-line therapies include radical prostatectomy and radiation.

Prostate cancer remains the leading cancer diagnosis among men in the United States and other industrialized countries. It is the second leading cause of cancer deaths after lung cancer. Increased screening efforts in the United States led to increased incidence after the PSA test became widely available in 1992. However, screening and treatment among HIV-negative and HIV-positive patients have been controversial due to the occult and often indolent nature of untreated prostate cancer, especially in older men with limited life expectancy. The mortality benefit of diagnosis and treatment of early-stage prostate cancer remains unproved; thus, emphasis on screening and early detection has waned in recent years. Compared to other NADCs, such as lung or anal cancer, some studies have demonstrated HIV infection to be associated with a reduced risk of prostate cancer. Regardless, diagnosis of prostate cancer carries a significant clinical impact on patients' sexual, genitourinary, and overall health.

EPIDEMIOLOGY OF PROSTATE CANCER IN HIV

HIV-positive men in the United States experienced an increased incidence of prostate cancer after 1990 compared to the preceding decade, from 0.2% to 2.2% of all cancers in a retrospective study of population-based registry data (Engels, 2006). In the same study, the incidence increased during the pre-ART and post-ART eras, which may be explained by the introduction of the PSA screening test. Another study that was a large retrospective review also found that prostate cancer in HIV-positive men increased during the time from 1992 to 2003 (Patel, 2008). However, the HIV-positive group had statistically significantly lower rates of cancer compared to the general population in the pre-ART era (15 vs. 47 per 100,000 py) and the ART era (38 vs. 61 per 100,000 py) (Patel, 2008). Another study that examined the PSA testing era (1992 to 2007) found an incidence of 28 per 100,000 py in HIV-positive men. However, the incidence in HIV-positive men compared to the expected rate in the general population during this same time period was significantly reduced, with a SIR of only 0.5 (95% CI, 0.44–0.57) (Shiels, 2010). Of note, some disparity remains when prostate cancer diagnoses are compared among races. One study that evaluated men enrolled in the Multicenter AIDS Cohort Study (MACS) from 1996 to 2010 found an incidence of 169 per 100,000 py among all men 40–70 years old compared to 276 per 100,000 py among African American HIV-positive men (Dutta, 2017). In this study prostate cancer risk was similar by HIV-infection status

(IRR 1.0, 95% CI 0.55–1.82), but nearly threefold higher in African Americans compared to non-African Americans in adjusted models (IRRs 2.66 and 3.22, 95% CIs 1.36–5.18 and 1.27–8.16 for all or HIV-positive men, respectively).

RISK FACTORS FOR PROSTATE CANCER

Postulated risk factors that promote development of prostate cancer in HIV-positive men include exposure to carcinogens and use of androgen supplementation to treat hypogonadism. Coinfection with oncogenic viruses may also promote neoplasia (Montgomery, 2006). Chronic inflammatory states promoted by HIV systemically and localized to the prostate, as well as chronic prostatitis may contribute to cancer development (Leport, 1989; Smith, 2004).

Prostate cancer and risk of death have been associated with tobacco exposure in several studies. However, other studies have demonstrated conflicting data. Two large meta-analyses examined this issue and found similar results (Huncharek, 2010; Islami, 2014). Huncharek et al. found a dose-dependent relationship with incidence of prostate cancer in HIV-negative patients. The heaviest smokers had a 13% increased risk of cancer. These data were derived from 7 prospective cohort studies. Based on 19 prospective studies, Islami et al. found smoking to be associated with an increased risk of death (RR, 1.24) from prostate cancer, which was dose-dependent. The incidence of prostate cancer, however, was not statistically significant overall. In fact, baseline cigarette smoking was inversely associated with incidence of prostate cancer (Islami, 2014).

Unlike other malignancies in HIV, immunological control with increasing $CD4^+$ T cell count has been associated with increased risk of prostate cancer, with a relative risk that is threefold greater in the ART era (Shiels, 2010). In several studies, HIV-positive men with prostate cancer had robust $CD4^+$ T cell counts of greater than 300 cells/mm^3 (Hsiao, 2009; Marcus, 2014; Pantanowitz, 2008). Overall, data from numerous studies suggest that variations in prostate cancer deficits in HIV-positive men are due to differential PSA screening in this population and not to immunologic status.

PROSTATE CANCER SCREENING

The primary tools for diagnosis of prostate cancer include serum PSA measurement, DRE, and, ultimately, prostate biopsy for definitive histologic diagnosis. Both European and US guidelines have recommended against routine screening with PSA in both HIV-negative and HIV-positive men (Heidenreich, 2013; Moyer, 2012). Rather, whether to perform individual screening with PSA for early detection should be a well-informed, mutual decision between physician and patient based on possible benefits and harms of a positive PSA test. Optimal interval of PSA screening has also not been established. DRE alone has limited sensitivity (6–8%) of detecting prostate cancer (Gosselaar, 2009; Okotie, 2007). The combination of an abnormal DRE versus normal DRE with PSA level of higher than 3 ng/mL may enhance positive predictive value of cancer detection at 48% versus 22% (Gosselaar, 2008).

CLINICAL PRESENTATION

Prostate cancer diagnosis in HIV often occurs in the fifth and sixth decades of life, and patients often have a positive family history of prostate cancer (Hsiao, 2009; Ong, 2015; Shiels, 2010). Men with HIV may present more often with late-stage disease compared to the general population, although this is supported by limited data (Shiels, 2015). A large California cohort found more localized cancer compared to regional or distant disease among HIV-positive men (88% vs. 7%), which was similar to the pattern found in HIV-negative men (Marcus, 2014). Other studies have found no difference in presentation with early or advanced disease (Hsiao, 2009; Riedel, 2015). HIV-negative African Americans have a greater likelihood of presenting with advanced-stage prostate cancer in the general population (Siegel, 2012). Within the HIV population, African Americans may represent a higher risk group for prostate cancer because they comprise a large proportion of HIV prevalence and annual HIV diagnoses in the United States.

TREATMENT AND TREATMENT OUTCOMES OF PROSTATE CANCER

Treatment of prostate cancer in HIV-positive men is similar to that of HIV-negative men and is based on stage and grade of disease with use of the Gleason score (ranging from 2 to 10). For localized disease (stage I and stage II) not spread to lymph nodes or distant sites, strategies include active surveillance (PSA monitoring and/or repeat biopsy), radical prostatectomy, or radiation therapy (external beam radiation and/or brachytherapy) with or without androgen deprivation. For locally advanced disease (stage III) that has spread outside the prostate gland, surgery or radiation with androgen deprivation therapy are alternatives. A Gleason score greater than 8 represents high-risk neoplasia, even if disease is localized. The optimal choice between surgical intervention and radiation is unclear for these patients, and careful consideration of individual risks and benefits should be discussed on a case-by-case basis (Grimm, 2012).

Treatment of disseminated disease, which often involves osteoblastic lesions, typically involves androgen deprivation therapy, castration (medical or surgical), and systemic chemotherapy. Two phase 3 trials examining the use of abiraterone and enzalutamide for treatment of metastatic, castration-resistant prostate cancer have shown clinical benefit with these agents, which target the androgen-synthesis pathway (Loriot, 2015; Ryan, 2015). Chemotherapy with taxane-based regimens has also shown success in prolonging survival in men with castration-resistant prostate cancer. Docetaxel plus prednisone is currently the standard, initial cytotoxic chemotherapy used in metastatic, castration-resistant disease (Berthold, 2008).

Few studies have evaluated the safety, tolerability, and efficacy of treatments for prostate cancer in men with HIV. Most studies have been small and limited to evaluation of external beam radiation therapy (EBRT) with heterogeneity of dosing. One Veterans Administration study reported 15 patients who received an EBRT dose-escalation approach (75.6 Gy to 79.2 Gy) for localized disease. Of the 15 patients, 13 were treated with concomitant ART, and the 5-year event-free survival was 92.3% (Schreiber, 2014). Toxicities included urinary frequency and rectal bleeding. Eight patients on ART had a transient decline in CD4$^+$ cell count, which returned to near or above baseline in the follow-up period. Another study evaluating EBRT (72 Gy to 81 Gy) for localized prostate cancer in HIV-positive compared to HIV-negative men found that 26% of men with HIV had biochemical failure compared to 12% of matched HIV-negative controls. At a mean of 36 months, there were no deaths in the HIV group. Genitourinary and anal adverse events were overall mild (Kahn, 2012).

The risk of death from prostate cancer is associated with advanced disease compared to local or regional prostate cancer (Shiels, 2010). In a large retrospective study of HIV and cancer registries from 1996 to 2010, mortality of prostate cancer was significantly higher for HIV-positive patients as compared to that of HIV-negative patients (HR, 1.57; 95% CI, 1.02–2.41) even after adjusting for patient characteristics and cancer stage (Coghill, 2015). Cancer deaths were also greater in HIV-positive men after adjusting for treatment but not significantly so (HR, 1.64; 95% CI, 0.93–2.89). One study that used data from 1996 to 2002 found a 2.1-fold increased risk of death from prostate cancer in HIV-positive compared to HIV-negative men. Interestingly, in this study, HIV-positive men had more localized disease (Marcus, 2014).

RECOMMENDED READING

Coghill AE, Shiels MS, Suneja G, et al. Elevated cancer-specific mortality among HIV-infected patients in the United States. *J Clin Oncol.* 2015;33(21):2376–2383.

Marcus JL, Chao CR, Leyden WA, et al. Prostate cancer incidence and prostate-specific antigen testing among HIV-positive and HIV-negative men. *J AIDS.* 2014;66:495–502.

Moyer VA. Screening for prostate cancer: US Preventive Services Task Force recommendation statement. *Ann Intern Med.* 2012;157(2):120–135.

Shiels MS, Goedert JJ, Moore RD, et al. Risk of prostate cancer in U.S. men with AIDS. *Cancer Epidemiol Biomarkers Prev.* 2010;19(11):2910–2915.

COLORECTAL ADENOCARCINOMA

LEARNING OBJECTIVES

- Review the epidemiology of colorectal cancer in the HIV population.
- Discuss the screening methods for colorectal cancer.
- Review treatment modalities and outcomes in HIV patients with colorectal cancer.

WHAT'S NEW?

- The incidence of colon cancer has increased in the HIV population compared to the general population in the ART era, and mortality remains high compared to that of the HIV-negative population.

- Patients with HIV disproportionately receive less colorectal cancer screening than the general population.

- Standard chemoradiation and surgical approaches for treating colorectal cancer appear to be well tolerated in patients with HIV, although more research is needed in this area.

KEY POINTS

- Colorectal cancer presents a major health and mortality burden in the HIV population.

- Colorectal cancer presentation occurs often in younger patients and with more advanced disease compared to the general population.

- Significant disparities exist in screening HIV patients for colorectal cancer compared to HIV-negative patients.

- Standard treatment includes surgery and neoadjuvant and/or adjuvant chemoradiation.

- Survival is significantly worse compared to that of HIV-negative patients with colorectal cancer.

In the United States, colorectal cancer (CRC) is the third leading cause of cancer death in the general population for both men and women. It has been the focus of large-scale primary prevention screening efforts to identify patients with early disease (Siegel, 2014). Non-AIDS cancers such as colorectal adenocarcinoma in the HIV population have become increasingly recognized as a significant health problem as patients are living longer and may accrue greater risk factors for cancer development. Vigilance for neoplastic processes such as colorectal cancer must be maintained in HIV patients because they are often diagnosed at advanced stages and can be overlooked due to presentation at a younger age and lack of traditional risk factors such as family history (Chapman, 2009; Yegüez, 2003). This phenomenon was characterized by early case reports of colorectal adenocarcinoma in HIV. Patients were often males, aged 20s to 40s, and with advanced immunosuppression (Cappell, 1988; Klugman, 1994; Ravalli, 1989).

HIV patients who are considered "average" risk are offered screening less frequently than the general population (Nayudu, 2012). Furthermore, disparities in cancer treatment between HIV-positive and HIV-negative patients are also prevalent. Persons with HIV are less likely to receive treatment for colon cancer than their HIV-negative counterparts (Suneja, 2013). The lack of screening and treatment is likely to contribute to poorer outcomes and excess mortality in the HIV population.

EPIDEMIOLOGY OF COLON CANCER IN HIV

Patients with HIV have incurred a higher incidence of CRC than the general population. A large US study that examined cancer incidence in HIV patients compared to the general population from 1992 to 2003 found an increased SIR during the early time period of 1992 to 1995 (39.9 per 100,000 py) compared to the later time period of 2000 to 2003 (66.2 per 100,000 py). During both time periods, the rates were greater than those of the general population (20.4 and 21.1 per 100,000 py, respectively) (Patel, 2008). In a more recent study using US and Canadian data from 2006 to 2009, the incidence rate of CRC in HIV-positive patients was 36.4 per 100,000 py compared to 27.7 per 100,000 py in HIV-negative patients. During this study period, the cumulative incidence declined by 6% per year for HIV-negative patients but increased in those with HIV by 5% per year. This may reflect the declining death rate among persons with HIV (Silverberg, 2015).

A large Taiwanese study that used the National Health Insurance Research Database from 1998 to 2009 found that, among 1,282 persons with HIV and cancer, the incidence of CRC, excluding anal cancer, was 51 per 100,000 py with a SIR of 5.9 (95% CI, 4.15–8.37). Interestingly, colon cancer was the most common NADC in females, with an incidence of 156 per 100,000 py (Chen, 2014). In the US surveillance study using the HIV/AIDS Cancer Match Study registry data from 1991 to 2002, the incidence of CRC, excluding anal cancer, was 15 per 100,000 py (Engels, 2008).

Immunosuppression likely plays a role in the epidemiology of CRC, as demonstrated in the previously discussed case reports from the pre-ART era. A study by Silverberg et al. stratified groups by $CD4^+$ T cell count and found that those with HIV and less than 200 cells/mm^3 had an 80% higher relative risk compared to a protective effect of higher $CD4^+$ T cell counts (Silverberg, 2011). Another study that used flexible sigmoidoscopy for CRC screening in HIV patients found that patients with duration of HIV of greater than 10 years and $CD4^+$ T cell counts of less than 200 cells/mm^3 had greater odds of having distal colon neoplastic lesions compared to those with higher $CD4^+$ T cell counts (Bini, 2006). On the contrary, many other studies have not shown significant differences in rates among AIDS patients or reduction of CRC in the ART era. Several studies support increases in CRC in the ART era. The lack of reporting of CRC in advanced immunosuppression coupled with the increase in CRC in the ART era may be explained by increased longevity of the HIV population as well as an increase in screening measures allowing for more diagnoses.

An Australian study that used national HIV and cancer registry data in the pre-ART era evaluated the incidence of cancer among those with HIV. It did not find significantly increased incidence rates among HIV-positive patients before and after developing advanced immunosuppression (Gulrich, 2002). A US study examined cancer data from patients with an AIDS diagnosis from 1978 to 1996 (Frisch, 2001). It found the relative risk of colon cancer in patients with newly diagnosed AIDS to be no different in the period prior to AIDS or in the 5 years thereafter (RR, 0.9) (Frisch, 2001). A prospective study

at the University of Alabama at Birmingham followed HIV patients from 1989 to 2002. It demonstrated an incidence during that period of 60 cases of NADC, with an increase in annual incidence of 0.65 cases per 1,000 py in the pre-ART era and 2.34 cases per 1,000 py in the ART era. Although the study found an increase in the incidence of the relative risk in the ART era of 3.6 (95% CI, 0.8–16.3), this difference was not statistically significant (Bedimo, 2004). These findings can likely be attributed to improved longevity and screening methods in the ART era. However, a lack of information on screening efforts reported in many of these studies is a major limitation in accurately measuring the true incidence of colorectal cancer in the HIV population.

COLORECTAL CANCER SCREENING IN THE HIV POPULATION

Screening for CRC in HIV patients reflects that recommended for the general population with normal cancer risk. This is defined as no personal history of CRC, adenomatous polyps, or inflammatory bowel disease and no first-degree relative with a history of CRC. The US Preventive Services Task Force recommends that for adults with an average risk of CRC, screening with fecal occult blood testing, flexible sigmoidoscopy, or colonoscopy should begin at age 50 years and continue until age 75 years. The current screening interval for colonoscopy is 10 years. These recommendations have been effective for reducing the incidence and mortality of CRC. For those with increased risk, such as an immediate family member with a history of CRC, screening should begin at age 40 years or 10 years prior to the relative's age at onset of CRC, whichever occurs first (Whitlock, 2008). Interestingly, even in the general population, screening is underutilized. The CDC found that only 64.5% of screening-eligible people aged 50–75 years surveyed in the Behavioral Risk Factor Surveillance System reported having one of the recommended tests (Joseph, 2012).

Screening the HIV population based on standard guidelines has been more challenging, with significant disparity compared to the general population. A retrospective study in New York identified 565 screening-eligible HIV patients with average risk and found that only 25% underwent screening colonoscopy within 10 years of the review. The median age was 58 years, and most of these patients had well-controlled HIV compared to those who did not have colonoscopy. Among those who had colonoscopy and biopsy, 32% of biopsies were of tubular adenomas, which exceeds the detection rate of tubular adenomas in the general population for men (34%) and women (27%) (Nayudu, 2012). A prospective study performed among New York veterans from 1998 to 2003 sought to describe the prevalence of adenomas or CRC in the distal colon with flexible sigmoidoscopy (Bini, 2006). The study included 2,217 HIV-negative controls and 165 HIV-positive patients (85.5% on ART and 45.5% with undetectable HIV viral load). Among the HIV-positive group eligible for CRC screening, 91.9% underwent flexible sigmoidoscopy, which was similar to the percentage who underwent it in the HIV-negative cohort. More polyps were identified in the HIV group compared to the control group (30.9% vs. 23%; $p = 0.2$), and polyps in the HIV group were more likely to have neoplastic features compared to those of the controls (25.5% vs. 13.1%; $p < 0.001$; OR, 2.27; 95% CI, 1.57–3.29). The study found that duration of HIV more than 10 years and lower $CD4^+$ cell count was significantly associated with having distal neoplasias. Those with positive sigmoidoscopy went on to have full colonoscopy, which showed a higher prevalence of proximal colon neoplastic lesions in the HIV group compared to the HIV-negative controls (61.2% vs. 47.8%; $p = 0.07$) (Bini, 2006). Although not statistically significant, it appears that HIV-positive patients are at high risker for malignant potential compared to their HIV-negative counterparts. Another study comparing CRC screening in HIV patients and controls demonstrated similar results as those obtained in the New York veterans' study. This study compared 302 HIV-positive and 302 HIV-negative patients and found that those with HIV were significantly less likely to have any type of screening modality (55.6% vs. 77.8%; $p < 0.0001$). Undetectable HIV RNA levels, older age, and a family history were variables associated with having at least one CRC screening (Reinhold, 2005).

Appropriate use of screening for eligible persons is of utmost importance for the HIV population because polyps may have more high-risk features than those of the general population. Barriers to colonoscopy referral and screening should be identified and managed. Increased provider and patient education may also be beneficial. One pilot study that randomizing screening-eligible HIV patients to receive educational material and in-person decision-making support showed increased screening colonoscopy uptake (Ferron, 2015). Based on this evidence, efforts to increase on-time screening in eligible HIV-positive patients should be undertaken.

CLINICAL PRESENTATION

With regard to early presentations of CRC, one recent study compared the prevalence, type, and location of neoplastic lesions found on colonoscopy in 263 HIV-positive patients matched with 657 HIV-negative patients and found that HIV-positive patients were less likely to have any neoplastic lesions (21.3% vs. 27.7%, $p < 0.05$), adenoma (20.5% vs. 27.1%, $p = 0.04$), tubular adenomas greater than 10 mm (0.4% vs. 2.9%, $p = 0.02$), and serrated adenomas (0.0% vs. 2.6%, $p < 0.01$) (Fantry, 2016). They also found a nonsignificant increased prevalence of adenocarcinoma in HIV-positive individuals compared with HIV-negative individuals (1.5% vs. 0.8%, $p = 0.29$). However, at the time of diagnosis in HIV patients, CRC is often advanced and occurs in younger patients compared to the general population. Researchers from the Italian Cooperative Group AIDS and Tumors evaluated 27 HIV-positive and 54 matched, HIV-negative patients who were diagnosed with CRC between 1985 and 2003 (Berretta, 2009). The majority were diagnosed in the ART era, with a median age of 48 years in both groups. However, most patients in the HIV cohort were younger than age 45 years. Median $CD4^+$ T cell count at the time of diagnosis was 325 cells/mm³. In the HIV-positive group, the stage was predominantly

Dukes's stage D (distant metastasis) compared to those without HIV (74% vs. 35%; $p = 0.002$). Histopathology showed poorly differentiated adenocarcinoma in 66% of the HIV cohort compared to 26% in the HIV-negative matched controls (Berretta, 2009).

A case–control study from Southern California also found that CRC of HIV-positive patients occurred mainly in those younger than age 50 years (72%) and with advanced disease (stages III and IV). HIV patients had a younger to older age ratio of 3:1 compared to the population controls, whose ratio was 1.33. In most patients, biopsy findings revealed poorly differentiated adenocarcinoma (64%). Of note, the mean $CD4^+$ cell count at time of diagnosis was robust at 467 cells/mm³ (Wasserberg, 2007).

One multicenter retrospective study of 17 HIV patients with confirmed CRC from 1988 to 2003 reported that patients had a mean age of 43 years and a majority had a $CD4^+$ cell count of less than 500 cells/mm³ (not specified further) (Chapman, 2009). Most tumors arose in the right side of the colon (57%) and with advanced stage IV disease (47%) and histopathology with grade 2 or 3 adenocarcinomas (79%). Most metastatic sites were to the liver but also included lung, peritoneum, and subcutaneous sites (Chapman, 2009). Sigel et al. more recently evaluated 184 patients with CRC (38 HIV-positive and 146 HIV-negative) and found that HIV-positive patients were more likely to have smoked ($p = 0.001$), have right-sided colorectal cancer (37% vs. 14%; $p = 0.003$), and tumor-infiltrating lymphocytes (TIL) above 50/10 high-power fields (21% vs. 7%). They also evaluated Mismatch Repair Protein (MMR) expression levels between the two groups (as MMR is a marker for microsatellite instability) but found no difference between the two groups ($p = 0.6$) (Sigel, 2016). Given the presence of right-sided colonic tumors, colonoscopy in HIV patients may have a greater diagnostic yield compared to flexible sigmoidoscopy. Further prospective studies should be performed to evaluate the various screening techniques in the HIV-positive population.

TREATMENT FOR COLORECTAL CANCER IN HIV

Treatment for CRC in HIV-positive patients is the same as that for those without HIV and primarily depends on clinical staging of the malignancy, which is determined by physical exam and radiographic imaging. Computed tomography (CT) scanning is mandatory for determining regional extension, nodal involvement, or distant metastasis in the tumor, nodal, and metastatic staging system. Stages range from stage I to stage IV as the disease advances from confined disease to the colonic mucosa, regional lymph node involvement, and involvement of one or more distant organs including peritoneal seeding. For patients with stage II to IV disease, imaging with CT scan of the chest, abdomen, and pelvis is recommended (National Comprehensive Cancer Network [NCCN] Colon Cancer, 2016). Further imaging with MRI may be useful for better characterization of the liver for metastatic disease, especially in the setting of background steatosis (Shahani, 2014). Testing with the tumor marker carcinoembryonic antigen

(CEA) should be performed prior to treatment to help serve as a guide in the posttreatment follow-up. This test has not been validated for use specifically in the HIV population, nor has there been robust evidence supporting survival benefit in the general population, but CEA remains a standard pre- and posttreatment test for its prognostic utility (Locker, 2006).

Role of Surgery in Treatment of CRC

Treatment for localized disease can be curative with endoscopic resection of a carcinomatous polyp or surgical resection with simple colectomy and anastomosis. Surgery remains the cornerstone of therapy for localized disease, and margins should be free of cancer. Locally advanced disease or poorly differentiated polypoid lesions may warrant more invasive or radical surgery. If invasion involves surrounding structures, larger resection of contiguous, multivisceral structures is indicated to ensure negative margins in the affected noncolonic organs (NCCN Colon Cancer, 2.2016). This approach has yielded improved prognosis and outcomes in patients with locally advanced disease (Govindarajan, 2006; Lehnert, 2002). Tumor location is also an important aspect in consideration of surgical approach because management of CRC involving the rectum (especially the lower rectum) may compromise anal sphincter tone and genitourinary function. If the anus is involved, sphincter-sparing surgery may be considered with adjuvant or neoadjuvant chemotherapy and radiation (NCCN, 1.2016; Sauer, 2012).

Colorectal adenocarcinoma typically metastasizes to the liver, lung, lymph nodes, and peritoneum. With limited metastatic disease, curative surgery remains an option to improve survival; however, recurrence of disease is a reality for some patients (Neef, 2009; Shah, 2006).

Chemoradiotherapy in CRC

Neoadjuvant and adjuvant chemotherapies are generally considered for patients with advanced or metastatic disease when the expectation of noncurative surgery is present. Neoadjuvant chemoradiotherapy (CRT) is a standard approach to therapy in locally advanced rectal cancer (T3 or N1-2) prior to surgery or rectal cancer that is unresectable or medically inoperable. This consists of fractionated radiation therapy usually with a 5-fluorouracil (5-FU)-based regimen in combination with other agents, such as capecitabine or oxaliplatin and leucovorin (NCCN, 1.2016; Sauer, 2012). Adjuvant CRT following resection to eliminate microscopic foci of tumors and promote recurrence-free survival has been most beneficial in patients with nodal involvement (stage III), which has been shown in randomized controlled trials (Smith, 2004). Typical regimens include 5-FU/leucovorin- or capecitabine-based regimens (NCCN Colon Cancer, 2.2016). Other adjuvant therapies in metastatic disease include the vascular endothelial and epidermal growth factor inhibitor bevacizumab and cetuximab, respectively. Overall survival benefit of these agents remains controversial, and they may cause excess adverse events (da Gramont, 2012; Taieb, 2014).

TREATMENT OUTCOMES AND SURVIVAL OF PATIENTS WITH HIV AND CRC

There is a paucity of data on the efficacy, tolerability, and treatment outcomes of CRC for patients with HIV infection. Case series have provided much of the data on this population. As previously discussed, patients with HIV tend to present with more advanced disease, which may require both surgery and chemoradiation. In one case series, 10 HIV-positive patients with stage III or IV disease underwent segmental colon or rectal resection. One of these patients underwent complete pelvic exenteration (Wasserberg, 2007). All patients also received first-line adjuvant chemotherapy with 5-FU/leucovorin. Four of the patients received additional CPT-11 or irinotecan for metastatic disease. Of the patients with rectal involvement, one patient received neoadjuvant 5-FU/leucovorin-based chemoradiation, and 3 patients received adjuvant radiation. Overall, chemotherapy was tolerated well, but some patients did experience grade 3 adverse events with neutropenia and anemia (Wasserberg, 2007).

Another case series from Italy reported on 27 HIV-positive patients, the majority with metastatic CRC (Berretta, 2009). Of those with metastatic disease, 3 received neoadjuvant oxaliplatin-based chemotherapy for liver metastasis, 7 underwent palliative chemotherapy, and 2 were treated with 5-FU chemoradiation. The remaining patients with metastatic disease underwent palliation. One patient who received radiation incurred hemorrhagic proctitis, which prompted treatment cessation (Berretta, 2009). Overall, chemotherapy was tolerated well in the group, with few grade 3 neutropenic events.

Surgical resection provides the best curative treatment for localized colon cancer, and this has been demonstrated with SEER data (2005–2011) showing 5-year survival rates of 90% for localized disease. However, survival declines steeply with regional or nodal involvement (70%) and with distant metastasis (13%) (Howlader, 2015). Patients with HIV may not receive surgery when indicated, giving them a survival disadvantage. This disparity was highlighted in a follow-up study by the previously mentioned Italian group. In 2010, the group released a brief report on its experience treating HIV patients with liver metastasis (Berretta, 2010). They reported on 14 patients who had HIV and CRC-related liver metastasis. Only 3 patients initially had unresectable liver metastasis as determined by a multidisciplinary team; however, the other 11 patients underwent FOLFOX-4 treatment. Three patients in the group who were able to undergo surgery received neoadjuvant chemotherapy with FOLFOX-4 or FOLFIRI, followed by liver segmentectomy (2 patients) and liver segmentectomy plus radiofrequency ablation (1 patient). These 3 patients tolerated the treatments well, remained on ART without any grade 3 or 4 toxicities, and 2 of the 3 patients remained disease-free at 21-month follow-up. Although the number of patients was small, these researchers demonstrated that an aggressive surgical approach for metastatic CRC can be successfully performed in patients with HIV. Narrowing the treatment gap between the HIV population and the general population remains an important goal in the care of malignancies in HIV that may help improve survival outcomes for this group.

Mortality for HIV patients with CRC remains high compared to that for the general population. A large retrospective study estimated that those with HIV and CRC have a 50% higher risk of mortality compared to uninfected patients (Coghill, 2015). Smaller case–control studies have shown markedly poorer survival for HIV patients compared to negative controls, with 4-year survival of 15% and 49%, respectively (Berretta, 2009). A more recent study found that HIV-positive CRC patients had reduced overall survival ($p = 0.02$) when compared to their HIV-negative counterparts, but no difference in progression-free survival (Sigel, 2016). It has been hypothesized that HIV-positive individuals are less likely to receive therapy and therefore, on a population level, will have poorer survival. HIV positivity should not preclude delivery of the standard of care, and further studies are needed to rigorously evaluate the standard of care delivered to these patients. Disparities in screening and treatment of HIV patients with CRC are likely to perpetuate their less than optimal survival outcomes relative to those of HIV-negative patients.

RECOMMENDED READING

Berretta M, Cappellani A, Di Benedetto F, et al. Clinical presentation and outcome of colorectal cancer in HIV-positive patients: a clinical case–control study. *Onkologie.* 2009;32:319–324.

Bini EJ, Park J, Francois F. Use of flexible sigmoidoscopy to screen for colorectal cancer in HIV-infected patients 50 years of age or older. *JAMA Intern Med.* 2006;166(15):1626–1631.

IMMUNE CHECKPOINT INHIBITOR THERAPY FOR NADC

LEARNING OBJECTIVES

Review the mechanism and proposed use of immune check point inhibitor (ICPI) therapy for NADCs.

WHAT'S NEW?

ICPI therapy is currently being evaluated in HIV-positive individuals and, in patients with well-controlled HIV infection, is thought to be just as efficacious for the treatment of various NADCs as for the general population.

KEY POINTS

- ICPIs target key immune regulatory pathways and thus can untether T cell-mediated anti-tumor responses, which could help target certain cancers in HIV-positive individuals.

- ICPIs like PD-1 inhibitors may also be able to help eliminate the cells that carry HIV proviral DNA, thus contributing to elimination of the patient's HIV reservoir.

- PD-1/PD-L1 inhibitors have been approved for melanoma, NSCLC and other lung cancers, renal cell carcinoma, Hodgkin's lymphoma, head and neck squamous cell cancers, several types of breast cancers, gastric cancer, urothelial cancer, and colorectal cancer in the general population; studies evaluating their use in HIV-positive patients are ongoing.

ICPIs are a relatively new class of immunotherapy medications that inhibit suppression of effector T cell responses. In other words, they help to turn the cancer or infectious agent-suppressed cell-medicated immune on again. Most of these are monoclonal antibodies directed against immune checkpoints that block the interaction between the immune checkpoint and their respective checkpoint ligands. One type of immune checkpoint is programed cell death-1 (PD-1), which is predominantly expressed on T cells. The interaction of PD-1 with its ligands (PD-L1 and -L2) expressed on antigen-presenting cells and tumors sends a negative signal to T cells, which can lead to T cell exhaustion or dysfunction. T cell exhaustion is now recognized as a key mechanism contributing to impaired T cell responses against tumors and some pathogens.

ICPI therapies are an appealing treatment option for many cancers that express PD-1 because they have broad activity with good response rates, they frequently induce long-term disease control, and they are relatively nontoxic. So far, six monoclonal antibodies that target PD-1 or PD-L1 have been approved by the FDA. The first, a PD-1 inhibitor, pembrolizumab, was approved in September 2014 for the treatment of advanced or unresectable melanoma in patients failing other treatments and was so successful that it later became the first-line treatment (Robert, 2014). It is now approved for NSCLC (Garon, 2015), head and neck squamous cell cancers, refractory Hodgkin lymphoma, primary mediastinal large B cell lymphoma, advanced urothelial carcinoma, advanced gastric cancer, some types of colorectal cancers, and advanced cervical cancer. A second PD-1 inhibitor, nivolumab, was subsequently approved in 2015 for the treatment of melanoma and is now also approved for NSCLC, renal cell carcinoma, Hodgkin's lymphoma, head and neck squamous cell cancers, advanced urothelial carcinomas, certain colorectal cancers, and hepatocellular carcinoma. The third, fourth, and fifth approvals were for PD-L1 inhibitors (atezolizumab, durvalumab, and avelumab) for the treatment of advanced bladder cancer and NSCLC. The sixth and most recent (September 2018) approval was for cemiplimab, another PD-1 monoclonal antibody, for patients with metastatic or locally advanced cutaneous squamous cell carcinoma.

Therapies with ICPIs are an exciting prospect for HIV-positive patients because they have the potential to not only treat the patient's cancer but also to eliminate or reduce the HIV reservoirs that persist despite ART (Trautmann, 2006; Day, 2006). The concept behind this latter theoretical use is that HIV persistence is thought to stem primarily from the presence of integrated copies of the proviral genome within long-lived cells. Because active viral gene expression causes cell death due to viral cytopathic effects and the immune response, long-lived cells likely harbor transcriptionally silent, latent provirus, which is the remaining major barrier to finding a cure for HIV. Several studies offer evidence as to why PD-1 may be an important part of this process. PD-1 has been found to be upregulated on HIV-specific CD8$^+$ T cells and has been correlated with disease progression (Day, 2006). Blockade of PD-L1 was shown to enhance IFN-γ secretion by HIV-specific CD8$^+$ T cells, suggesting that PD-1 signaling might play a role in limiting T cell responses against HIV (Petrovas, 2006; Zhang, 2007). Checkpoints that are considered markers of T-cell exhaustion, such as PD-1, TIM-3, and LAG-3, have been used to predict time of viremia rebound after treatment interruption (Hurst, 2015). Another study suggested a role for the immune checkpoint TIGIT in limiting antiviral T cell responses in HIV (Chew, 2016). This study also showed that TIGIT expression was coexpressed with PD-1 and upregulated on T cells from both HIV-positive patients and simian immunodeficiency virus (SIV)-infected macaques. The AIDS Clinical Trials 5326 Study Team recently demonstrated that treatment with an anti-PD-L1 antibody enhanced HIV-specific CD8$^+$ T cell responses in two of eight HIV-infected patients on ART (Gay, 2017). Although these studies suggest that immune checkpoints may limit T cell responses during HIV infection and that immune checkpoint blockade might be beneficial in HIV-positive patients, larger studies are required to determine the therapeutic benefit of immune checkpoint blockade in HIV-positive individuals on ART.

With regard to cancer therapy, treatment with PD-1/PD-L1 inhibitors may be even more useful in HIV-positive cancer patients than in HIV-negative cancer patients because at least one study recently observed that, while PD-L1 expression is high in tumor cells from both HIV-positive and -negative patients with NSCLC, it was associated with poor prognosis only in the HIV-positive group (Okuma, 2018). However, to date, only a handful of case reports and small case series offer data about HIV-positive patients treated with these new medications (Wightman, 2015; Le Garff, 2017; Heppt, 2017; Samri, 2017; Guihot, 2018). Many of the PD-1/PDL-1 inhibitor therapies currently in use or being tested in HIV-positive individuals have been mentioned throughout the text of this chapter. In addition, there are several larger clinical trials under way that will be emphasized here (Bender-Ignacio, 2018). One of these trials will evaluate pembrolizumab in patients with HIV and advanced cancers, although it requires patients to have a CD4$^+$ T cell count of greater than 200 cells/mm^3 (NCT02595866). The Cancer Immunotherapy Trials Network (CITN) is conducting a trial of pembrolizumab in HIV-positive patients with solid tumors and Hodgkin lymphoma (NCT02595866). A French trial will evaluate therapy with nivolumab in HIV-positive patients with NSCLC; they are accepting patients with any CD4$^+$ T cell count but require a HIV viral load of less than 200 copies/mL (NCT03304093). Another French study is following HIV-positive patients who receive ICPIs as part of routine cancer care to evaluate their safety and effects on the HIV reservoir (NCT03354936). Pending the results of these trials, HIV positivity is not thought to be a contraindication to treatment with PD-1 inhibitors, although HIV-positive individuals with low CD4$^+$

T cell counts should be monitored closely both for treatment response and for IRIS.

REFERENCES

Aboulafia DM. Kaposi's sarcoma. *Clinics Derm.* 2001;19(3):269–283.

Aboulafia DM, Puswella AL. Highly active antiretroviral therapy as the sole treatment for AIDS-related primary central nervous system lymphoma: a case report with implications for treatment. *AIDS Patient Care STDS.* 2007;21(12):900–907.

Advisory Committee on Immunization Practices. Recommended adult immunization schedule: United States, 2013. *Ann Intern Med.* 2013;158:191–199.

Ahdieh L, Munoz A, Vlahov D, et al. Cervical neoplasia and repeated positivity of human papillomavirus infection in human immunodeficiency virus-seropositive and -seronegative women. *Am J Epidemiol.* 2000;151(12):1148–1157.

Altekruse SF, Shiels MS, Modur SP, et al. Cancer burden attributable to cigarette smoking among HIV-infected people in North America. *AIDS.* 2018;32(4):513–521.

Alvarnas JC, Le Rademacher J, Wang Y, et al. Autologous hematopoietic cell transplantation for HIV-related lymphoma: results of the BMT CTN 0803/AMC 071 trial. *Blood.* 2016;128:1050–1058.

Ambinder RF, Wu J, Logan B, et al. Allogeneic hematopoietic cell transplant (alloHCT) for hematologic malignancies in human immunodeficiency virus infected (HIV) patients (pts): Blood and Marrow Transplant Clinical Trials Network (BMT CTN 0903)/AIDS Malignancy Consortium (AMC-080) trial. *J Clin Oncol.* 2017;35(15 Suppl):abstr 7006.

Appleby P, Beral V, Newton R, et al. Highly active antiretroviral therapy and incidence of cancer in human immunodeficiency virus-infected adults. *Cancer Inst.* 2000;92:1823–1830.

Avivi I, Robinson S, Goldstone A. Clinical use of rituximab in hematological malignancies. *Br J Cancer.* 2003;89(8):1389–1394.

Ballerini P, Gaidano G, Gong JZ, et al. Multiple genetic lesions in acquired immunodeficiency syndrome-related non-Hodgkin's lymphoma. *Blood.* 1993;81(1):166–176.

Barillari G, Ensoli B. Angiogenic effects of extracellular human immunodeficiency virus type 1 Tat protein and its role in the pathogenesis of AIDS-associated Kaposi's sarcoma. *Clin Microbiol Rev.* 2002;15(2):310–326.

Bañon S, Machuca I, Araujo S, et al. Efficacy, safety, and lack of interactions with the use of raltegravir in HIV-infected patients undergoing antineoplastic chemotherapy. *J Intern AIDS Soc.* 2014;17(4 Suppl 3):19590.

Baptista MJ, Garcia O, Morgades M, et al. HIV-infection impact on clinical-biological features and outcome of diffuse large B-cell lymphoma treated with R-CHOP in the combination antiretroviral therapy era. *AIDS.* 2015;29:811–818.

Barbosa MS, Schlegel R. The E6 and E7 genes of HPV-18 are sufficient for inducing two-stage in vitro transformation of human keratinocytes. *Oncogene.* 1989;4(12):1529–1532.

Barozzi P, Luppi M, Facchetti F, et al. Post-transplant Kaposi sarcoma originates from the seeding of donor-derived progenitors. *Nature Med.* 2003;9(5):554–561.

Barta SK, Joshi J, Mounier N, et al. Central nervous system involvement in AIDS-related lymphomas. *Br J Haematol.* 2016;173:857–866.

Barta SK, Lee JY, Kaplan LD, et al. Pooled analysis of AIDS malignancy consortium trials evaluating rituximab plus CHOP or infusional EPOCH chemotherapy in HIV-associated non-Hodgkin lymphoma. *Cancer.* 2012;118:3977–3983.

Barta SK, Samuel MS, Xue X, et al. Changes in the influence of lymphoma- and HIV-specific factors on outcomes in AIDS-related non-Hodgkin lymphoma. *Ann Oncol.* 2015;26:958–966.

Barta SK, Xue X, Wang D, et al. Treatment factors affecting outcomes in HIV-associated non-Hodgkin lymphomas: a pooled analysis of 1546 patients. *Blood.* 2013;122:3251–3262.

Barta SK, Xue X, Wang D, et al. A new prognostic score for AIDS-related lymphomas in the rituximab-era. *Haematologica.* 2014;99:1731–1737.

Baumgartner JE, Rachlin JR, Beckstead JH, et al. Primary central nervous system lymphomas: natural history and response to radiation therapy in 55 patients with acquired immunodeficiency syndrome. *J Neurosurg.* 1990;73(2):206–211.

Bayraktar S, Bayraktar UD, Ramos JC, et al. Primary CNS lymphoma in HIV positive and negative patients: comparison of clinical characteristics, outcome and prognostic factors. *J Neurooncol.* 2011;101:257–265.

Bedi GC, Westra WH, Farzedegan H, et al. Microsatellite instability in primary neoplasms from HIV+ patients. *Nature Med.* 1995;1(1):65–68.

Bedimo R, Chen RY, Accortt NA, et al. Trends in AIDS-defining and non-AIDS defining malignancies among HIV-infected patients: 1989–2002. *Clin Infect Dis.* 2004;39(9):1380–1384.

Bender-Ignacio R, Lin LL, Rajdev L, et al. Evolving paradigms in HIV malignancies: review of ongoing clinical trials. *J Natl Compr Canc Netw.* 2018;16(8):1018–1026.

Benevolo M, Donà MG, Ravenda PS, et al. Anal human papillomavirus infection: prevalence, diagnosis and treatment of related lesions. *Expert Rev Anti Infect Ther.* 2016;14(5):465–477.

Beral V, Peterman TA, Berkelman RL, et al. Kaposi's sarcoma among persons with AIDS: a sexually transmitted infection? *Lancet.* 1990;335(8682):123–128.

Beral V, Peterman T, Berkelman R, et al. AIDS-associated non-Hodgkin lymphoma. *Lancet.* 1991;337(8745):805–809.

Berretta M, Cappellani A, Di Benedetto F, et al. Clinical presentation and outcome of colorectal cancer in HIV-positive patients: a clinical case–control study. *Onkologie.* 2009;32:319–324.

Berretta M, Zanet E, Basile F, et al. HIV positive patients with liver metastasis from colorectal cancer deserve the same therapeutic approach as the general population. *Onkkologie.* 2010;33:203–204.

Berry JM, Palefsky JM, Jay N, et al. Performance characteristics of anal cytology and human papillomavirus testing in patients with high-resolution anoscopy-guided biopsy of high-grade anal intraepithelial neoplasia. *Dis Colon Rectum.* 2009;52(2):239–247.

Berthold DR, Pond GR, Soban F, et al. Docetaxel plus prednisone or mitoxantrone plus prednisone for advanced prostate cancer: updated survival in the TAX 327 study. *J Clin Oncol.* 2008;26(2):242–245.

Besson C, Goubar A, Gabarre J, et al. Changes in AIDS-related lymphoma since the era of highly active antiretroviral therapy. *Blood.* 2001;98(8):2339–2344.

Bini EJ, Park J, Francois F. Use of flexible sigmoidoscopy to screen for colorectal cancer in HIV-infected patients 50 years of age or older. *JAMA Intern Med.* 2006;166(15):1626–1631.

Bjorge T, Engeland A, Luostarinen T, et al. Human papillomavirus infection as a risk factor for anal and perianal skin cancer in a prospective study. *Br J Cancer.* 2002;87(1):61–64.

Blazy A, Hennequin C, Gornet JM, et al. Anal carcinomas in HIV-positive patients: high-dose chemoradiotherapy is feasible in the era of highly active antiretroviral therapy. *Dis Colon Rectum.* 2005;48(6):1176–1181.

Bonnet F, Burty C, Lewden C, et al. Changes in cancer mortality among HIV-infected patients: the Mortalite 2005 Survey. *Clin Infect Dis.* 2009;48(5):633–639.

Bosch FX, Manos MM, Munoz N, et al. Prevalence of human papillomavirus in cervical cancer: a worldwide perspective. *J Natl Cancer Inst.* 1995;87(11):796–802.

Bossolasco S, Cinque P, Ponzoni M, et al. Epstein–Barr virus DNA load in cerebrospinal fluid and plasma of patients with AIDS-related lymphoma. *J Neurovirol.* 2002;8(5):432–438.

Boudreaux AA, Smith LL, Cosby CD, et al. Intralesional vinblastine for cutaneous Kaposi's sarcoma associated with acquired immunodeficiency syndrome: a clinical trial to evaluate efficacy and discomfort associated with infection. *J Am Acad Derm.* 1993;28(1):61–65.

Boulanger E, Gerard L, Gabarre J, et al. Prognostic factors and outcome of human herpesvirus 8-associated primary effusion lymphoma in patients with AIDS. *J Clin Oncol.* 2005;23(19):4372–4380.

Bower M, Dalla Pria A, Coyle C, et al. Prospective stage-stratified approach to AIDS-related Kaposi's sarcoma. *J Clin Oncol.* 2014;32:409–414.

Bower M, Fox P, Fife K, Gill J, Nelson M, Gazzard B. Highly active anti-retroviral therapy (HAART) prolongs time to treatment failure in Kaposi's sarcoma. *AIDS (London, England).* 1999;13(15):2105–2111.

Bower M, McCall-Peat N, Ryan N, et al. Protease inhibitors potentiate chemotherapy-induced neutropenia. *Blood.* 2004;104(9):2943–2946.

Bower M, Powles T, Nelson M, et al. HIV-related lung cancer in the era of highly active antiretroviral therapy. *AIDS (London).* 2003;17(3):371–375.

Bower M, Powles T, Newsom-Davis T, et al. HIV-associated anal cancer: has highly active antiretroviral therapy reduced the incidence or improved the outcome? *J AIDS.* 2004;37(5):1563–1565.

Brickman C, Palefsky JM. Review: human papillomavirus in the HIV-infected host: epidemiology and pathogenesis in the antiretroviral era. *Curr HIV/AIDS Rep.* 2015;12(1):6–15.

Burgi A, Brodine S, Wegner S, et al. Incidence and risk factors for the occurrence of non-AIDS-defining cancers among human immunodeficiency virus-infected individuals. *Cancer.* 2005;104(7):1505–1511.

Burkes RL, Meyer PR, Gill PS, et al. Rectal lymphoma in homosexual men. *Arch Intern Med.* 1986;146(5):913–915.

Cadranel J, Garfield D, Lavole A, et al. Lung cancer in HIV infected patients: facts, questions, and challenges. *Thorax.* 2006;61:1000–1008.

Calabresi A, Ferraresi A, Festa A, et al. Incidence of AIDS-defining cancers and virus-related and non-virus-related non-AIDS-defining cancers among HIV-infected patients compared with the general population in a large health district of northern Italy, 1999–2000. *HIV Med.* 2013;14(8):481–490.

Callahan MK, Postow MA, Wolchok JD. Targeting T cell co-receptors for cancer therapy. *Immunity.* 2016;44:1069–1078.

Campbell JA, Soliman AS, Kahesa C, et al. Changing patterns of lung, liver, and head and neck non-AIDS-defining cancers relative to HIV status in Tanzania between 2002–2014. *Infect Agent Cancer.* 2016;11:58.

Campbell TB, Borok M, White IE, et al. Relationship of Kaposi sarcoma (KS)-associated herpesvirus viremia and KS disease in Zimbabwe. *Clin Infect Dis.* 2003;36(9):1144–1151.

Cannon MJ. Kaposi's sarcoma-associated herpesvirus and acquired immunodeficiency syndrome-related malignancy. *Semin Oncol.* 2000;27:408–419.

Cannon MJ, Dollard SC, Smith DK, et al. Blood-borne and sexual transmission of human herpesvirus 8 in women with or at risk for human immunodeficiency virus infection. *N Engl J Med.* 2001;344(9):637–643.

Cappell MS, Yao F, Cho KC. Colonic adenocarcinoma associated with the acquired immune deficiency syndrome. *Cancer.* 1988;62:616–619.

Casper C, Carrell D, Miller KG, et al. HIV serodiscordant sex partners and the prevalence of human herpesvirus 8 infection among HIV negative men who have sex with men: baseline data from the EXPLORE Study. *Sex Transm Infect.* 2006;82(3):229–235.

Casper C, Krantz E, Selke S, et al. Frequent and asymptomatic oropharyngeal shedding of human herpesvirus 8 among immunocompetent men. *J Infect Dis.* 2007;195(1):30–36.

Casper C, Redman M, Huang ML, et al. HIV infection and human herpesvirus-8 oral shedding among men who have sex with men. *J AIDS.* 2004;35(3):233–238.

Castillo JJ, Furman M, Beltrán BE, et al. Human immunodeficiency virus–associated plasmablastic lymphoma. *Cancer.* 2012;118:5270–5277.

Castilho JL, Luz PM, Shepherd BE, et al. HIV and cancer: a comparative retrospective study of Brazilian and US clinical cohorts. *Infect Agent Cancer.* 2015;10(4):1–10.

Cattaneo C, Re A, Ungari M, et al. Plasmablastic lymphoma among human immunodeficiency virus-positive patients: results of a single center's experience. *Leuk Lymphoma.* 2015;56:267–269.

Centers for Disease Control and Prevention (CDC). AIDS-defining conditions. 2008. Available at https://www.cdc.gov/mmwr/preview/mmwrhtml/rr5710a2.htm.

Centers for Disease Control and Prevention (CDC). Human papillomavirus-associated cancers—United States, 2004–2008. *Morbid Mortal Wkly Rep*. 2012;61(15):258–261.

Centers for Disease Control and Prevention (CDC). Estimated HIV incidence in the United States, 2007–2010. *HIV Surveill Suppl Rep*. 2012;17(4).

Centers for Disease Control and Prevention (CDC). Human papilloma virus (HPV) fact sheet. Available at www.cdc.gov/std/hpv. Accessed May 11, 2016.

Chadburn A, Abdul-Nabi AM, Teruya BS, et al. Lymphoid proliferations associated with human immunodeficiency virus infection. *Arch Path Lab Med*. 2013;137(3):360–370.

Chang Y, Cesarman E, Pessin MS, et al. Identification of herpesvirus-like DNA sequences in AIDS-associated Kaposi's sarcoma. *Science*. 1994;266(5192):1865–1869.

Chapman C, Aboulafia DM, Dezube BJ, et al. Human immunodeficiency virus-associated adenocarcinoma of the colon: clinicopathologic findings and outcome. *Clin Colorectal Cancer*. 2009;8(4):215–219.

Chari A, Kaplan L, Volberding PA, et al. Diagnosis and management of non-Hodgkin's lymphoma and Hodgkin's lymphoma. 2005.

Chaturvedi AK, Madeleine MM, Biggar RJ, et al. Risk of human papillomavirus-associated cancers among persons with AIDS. *J Natl Cancer Inst*. 2009;101(16):1120–1130.

Chen YH, Lin MW, Bhatia K, et al. Cancer incidence in a nationwide HIV/AIDS patient cohort in Taiwan in 1998–2000. *J AIDS*. 2014;65(4):463–472.

Chew GM, Fujita T, Webb GM, et al. TIGIT marks exhausted T cells, correlates with disease progression, and serves as a target for immune restoration in HIV and SIV infection. *PLoS Pathog*. 2016;12:e1005349.

Chiao EY, Dezube BJ, Krown SE, et al. Time for oncologists to opt in for routine opt-out HIV testing? *JAMA*. 2010;304(3):334–339.

Chiao EY, Giordano TP, Richardson P, et al. Human immunodeficiency virus-associated squamous cell cancer of the anus: epidemiology and outcomes in the highly active antiretroviral therapy era. *J Clin Oncol*. 2008;26(3):474–479.

Chin-Hong PV, Vittinghoff E, Cranston RD, et al. Age-specific prevalence of anal human papillomavirus infection in HIV-negative sexually active men who have sex with men: the EXPLORE study. *J Infect Dis*. 2004;190(12):2070–2076.

Chokunonga E, Levy LM, Bassett MT, et al. Cancer incidence in the African population of Harare, Zimbabwe: second results from the cancer registry 1993–1995. *Int J Cancer*. 2000;85(1):54–59.

Cianfrocca M, Lee S, Von Roenn J, et al. Randomized trial of paclitaxel vs. pegylated liposomal doxorubicin for advanced human immunodeficiency virus-associated Kaposi sarcoma: evidence of symptom palliation from chemotherapy. *Cancer*. 2010;116(16):3969–3977.

Cingolani A, Fratino L, Scoppettuolo G, et al. Changing pattern of primary cerebral lymphoma in the highly active antiretroviral therapy era. *J Neurovirol*. 2005; 11(Suppl 3):38–44.

Cleator S, Fife K, Nelson M, et al. Treatment of HIV-associated invasive anal cancer with combined chemoradiation. *Eur J Cancer (Oxford: 1990)*. 2000;36(6):754–758.

Clifford GM, Lise M, Franceschi S, et al. Lung cancer in the Swiss HIV Cohort Study: role of smoking, immunodeficiency, and pulmonary infection. *Br J Cancer*. 2012;106:448–452.

Clifford GM, Polesel J, Richenbach M, et al. Cancer risk in the Swiss HIV Cohort Study: associations with immunodeficiency, smoking, and highly active antiretroviral therapy. *J Natl Cancer Inst*. 2005;97(6):425–432.

Coghill AE, Shiels MS, Suneja G, et al. Elevated cancer-specific mortality among HIV-infected patients in the United States. *J Clin Oncol*. 2015;33(21):2376–2383.

Conti S, Masocco M, Pezzotti P, et al. Differential impact of combined antiretroviral therapy on the survival of Italian patients with specific AIDS-defining illnesses. *J AIDS (1999)*. 2000;25(5):451–458.

Cooper JS, Steinfeld AD, Lerch I. Intentions and outcomes in the radiotherapeutic management of epidemic Kaposi's sarcoma. *Int J Radiat Oncol Biol Phys*. 1991;20(3):419–422.

Corales R, Taege A, Rehm S, et al. Regression of AIDS-related CNS lymphoma with HAART [Abstract MoPpB1086]. Proceedings of the XIII International AIDS Conference, Durban, South Africa, 2000.

Cote TR, Biggar RJ, Rosenberg PS, et al. Non-Hodgkin's lymphoma among people with AIDS: incidence, presentation and public health burden. *Int J Cancer*. 1997;73(5):645–650.

Cote TR, Manns A, Hardy CR, et al.; AIDS/Cancer Study Group. Epidemiology of brain lymphoma among people with or without acquired immunodeficiency syndrome. *J Natl Cancer Inst*. 1996;88(10):675–679.

Coutinho R, Pria AD, Gandhi S, et al. HIV status does not impair the outcome of patients diagnosed with diffuse large B-cell lymphoma treated with R-CHOP in the cART era. *AIDS*. 2014;28:689–697.

Cranston R, Yang M, Paczuski P, et al. Baseline data of a phase 3 trial of the quadrivalent HPV vaccine in HIV+ males and females: ACTG 5298. Paper presented at the 21st Conference on Retroviruses and Opportunistic Infections;, Boston, MA, March 3–6, 2014.

Crothers K, Huang, L, Goulet JL, et al. HIV infection and risk for incident pulmonary diseases in the combination antiretroviral therapy era. *Am J Respir Crit Care Med*. 2011;183(3):388–395.

Da Gramont A, Van Cutsem E, Schmoll HJ, et al. Bevacizumab plus oxaliplatin-based chemotherapy as adjuvant treatment for colon cancer (AVANT): a phase 3 randomised controlled trial. *Lancet Oncol*. 2012;13(12):1225–1233.

Daling JR, Weiss NS, Hislop TG, et al. Sexual practices, sexually transmitted diseases, and the incidence of anal cancer. *N Engl J Med*. 1987;317(16):973–977.

Danzig JB, Brandt LJ, Reinus JF, et al. Gastrointestinal malignancy in patients with AIDS. *Am J Gastroenterol*. 1991;86(6):715–718.

Day CL, Kaufmann DE, Kiepiela P, et al. PD-1 expression on HIV-specific T cells is associated with T-cell exhaustion and disease progression. *Nature*. 2006;443:350–354.

Dedicoat M, Newton R, Alkharsah KR, et al. Mother-to-child transmission of human herpesvirus-8 in South Africa. *J Infect Dis*. 2004;190(6):1068–1075.

Denny L, Hendricks B, Gordon C, et al. Safety and immunogenicity of the HPV-16/18 AS04-adjuvanted vaccine in HIV-positive women in South Africa: a partially-blind randomised placebo-controlled study. *Vaccine*. 2013;31(48):5743–5753.

Deregibus M, Cantalupp IV, Doublier S, et al. HIV-1-Tat protein activates phosphatidylinositol 3-kinase/AKT-dependent survival pathways in Kaposi's sarcoma cells. *J Biol Chem*. 2002;277(28):25195–25202.

Deshmukh AA, Chhatwal J, Chiao EY, et al. Long-term outcomes of adding HPV vaccine to the anal intraepithelial neoplasia treatment regimen in HIV-positive men who have sex with men. *Clin Infect Dis*. 2015;61(10):1527–1535.

Dezube BJ, Pantanowitz L, Aboulafia DM. Management of AIDS-related Kaposi sarcoma: advances in target discovery and treatment. *AIDS Reader*. 2004;14(5):236–238, 243.

Diez-Martin J, Balsalobre P, Carrion R. et al. Long term survival after autologous stem cell transplant (ASCT) in AIDS related lymphoma patients [Abstract 868]. *Blood*. 2003;247a:102.

Diez-Martin JL, Balsalobre P, Re A, et al. Comparable survival between HIV+ and HIV– non-Hodgkin and Hodgkin lymphoma patients undergoing autologous peripheral blood stem cell transplantation. *Blood*. 2009;113(23):6011–6014.

DiGiusto DL, Cannon PM, Holmes MC, et al. Preclinical development and qualification of ZFN-mediated CCR5 disruption in human hematopoietic stem/progenitor cells. *Mol Ther Methods Clin Dev*. 2016;3:16067.

D'Jaen GA, Pantanowitz L, Bower M, et al. Human immunodeficiency virus-associated primary lung cancer in the era of highly active antiretroviral therapy: a multi-institutional collaboration. *Clin Lung Cancer*. 2010;11(6):396–404.

Donahue BR, Sullivan JW, Cooper JS. Additional experience with empiric radiotherapy for presumed human immunodeficiency virus-associated primary central nervous system lymphoma. *Cancer*. 1995;76(2):328–332.

Dryden-Peterson S, Bvochora-Nsingo M, Suneja G, et al. HIV infection and survival among women with cervical cancer. *J Clin Oncol*. 2016;34:3749–3757.

D'Souza G, Wiley D, Li X, et al. Incidence and epidemiology of anal cancer in the multicenter AIDS cohort study. *J AIDS*. 2008;48:491–499.

Dubrow R, Qin L, Lin H, et al. Association of CD4+ T-cell count, HIV-1 RNA viral load, and antiretroviral therapy with Kaposi sarcoma risk among HIV-infected persons in the United States and Canada. *J AIDS*. 2017;75(4):382–390.

Duncan KC, Chan KJ, Chiu CG, et al. HAART slows progression to anal cancer in HIV-infected MSM. *AIDS*. 2015;29:305–311.

Dunleavy K, Pittaluga S, Shovlin M, et al. Low-intensity therapy in adults with Burkitt's lymphoma. *N Engl J Med*. 2013;369:1915–1925.

Dutta A, Uno H, Holman A, et al. Racial differences in prostate cancer risk in young HIV-positive and HIV-negative men: a prospective cohort study. *Cancer Causes Control*. 2017;28(7):767–777.

Ekstein D, Ben-Yehuda D, Slyusarevsky E, et al. CSF analysis of IgH gene rearrangement in CNS lymphoma: relationship to the disease course. *J Neurol Sci*. 2006;247:39–46.

El Amari EB, Toutous-Trellu L, Gayet-Ageron A, et al. Predicting the evolution of Kaposi sarcoma in the highly active antiretroviral therapy era. *AIDS*. 2008;22(9):1019–1028.

El-Sadr WM, Lundgren J, Neaton JD, et al. CD4+ count-guided interruption of antiretroviral treatment. *N Engl J Med*. 2006;355:2283–2296.

El-Solh A, Kumar NM, Nair MP, et al. An RDG-containing peptide from HIV-1 TAT-(65–80) modulates protooncogene expression in human bronchoalveolar carcinoma cell line, A549. *Immunol Invest*. 1997;26(3):351–370.

Engels EA, Biggar RJ, Hall I, et al. Cancer risk in people infected with human immunodeficiency virus in the United States. *Intern J Cancer*. 2008;123:187–194.

Engels EA, Biggar RJ, Marshall VA, et al. Detection and quantification of Kaposi's sarcoma-associated herpesvirus to predict AIDS-associated Kaposi's sarcoma. *AIDS (London)*. 2003;17(12):1847–1851.

Ensoli B, Barillari G, Salahuddin S, et al. Tat protein of HIV-1 stimulates growth of cells derived from Kaposi's sarcoma lesions of AIDS patients. *Nature*. 1990;345(6270):84–86.

European AIDS Clinical Society (EACS). Guidelines version 8.0. October 2015. Available at http://www.eacsociety.org/files/2015_eacsguidelines_8.0-english_revised-20151104.pdf. Accessed May 13, 2016.

Fantry LE, Nowak RG, Fisher LH, et al. Colonoscopy findings in HIV-infected men and women from an urban US cohort compared with non-HIV-infected men and women. *AIDS Res Hum Retroviruses*. 2016;32(9):860–867

Ferlay J, Soerjomataram I, Ervik M, et al. GLOBOCAN 2012 v1.0, Cancer incidence and mortality worldwide: IARC CancerBase No. 11. Lyon, France: International Agency for Research on Cancer. 2013. Available from: http://globocan.iarc.fr.

Ferreri AJM, Cwynarski K, Pulczynski E, et al. Chemoimmunotherapy with methotrexate, cytarabine, thiotepa, and rituximab (MATRix regimen) in patients with primary CNS lymphoma: results of the first randomisation of the International Extranodal Lymphoma Study Group-32 (IELSG32) phase 2 trial. *Lancet Haematol*. May 2016;3(5):e217–e227.

Ferreri AJM, Cwynarski K, Pulczynski E, et al. Whole-brain radiotherapy or autologous stem-cell transplantation as consolidation strategies after high-dose methotrexate-based chemoimmunotherapy in patients with primary CNS lymphoma: results of the second randomisation of the International Extranodal Lymphoma Study Group-32 phase 2 trial. *Lancet Haematol*. November 2017;4(11):e510–e523.

Ferron P, Asfour SS, Metsch LR, et al. Impact of a multifaceted intervention on promoting adherence to screening colonoscopy among persons in HIV primary care: a pilot study. *Clin Transl Sci*. 2015;8(4):290–297.

Firnhaber C, Swarts A, Goeieman B, et al. Cryotherapy reduces progression of cervical intraepithelial neoplasia grade 1 in South African HIV-infected women: a randomized, controlled trial. *J AIDS*. 2017;76(5):532–538.

Foulot H, Heard I, Potard V, et al. Surgical management of cervical intraepithelial neoplasia in HIV-infected women. *Eur J Obstet Gynecol Reprod Biol*. 2008;141:153–157.

Franceschi S, Dal Maso L, Rickenbach M, et al. Kaposi sarcoma incidence in the Swiss HIV Cohort Study before and after highly active antiretroviral therapy. *Br J Cancer*. 2008;99(5):800–804.

Fraunholz I, Rabeneck D, Gerstein J, et al. Concurrent chemoradiotherapy with 5-fluorouracil and mitomycin C for anal carcinoma: are there differences between HIV-positive and HIV-negative patients in the era of highly active antiretroviral therapy? *Radiother Oncol*. 2011;98(1):99–104.

Friedman SL. Gastrointestinal and hepatobiliary neoplasms in AIDS. *Gastroenterol Clin North Am*. 1988;17(3):465–486.

Friedman-Kien AE. Disseminated Kaposi's sarcoma syndrome in young homosexual men. *J Am Acad Dermatol*. 1981;5(4):468–471.

Friedman-Kien AE, Saltzman BR. Clinical manifestations of classical, endemic African, and epidemic AIDS-associated Kaposi's sarcoma. *J Am Acad Dermatol*. 1990; 22(6 Pt 2):1237–1250.

Frisch M, Biggar RJ, Engels EA, et al.; AIDS–Cancer Match Registry Study Group. Association of cancer with AIDS-related immunosuppression in adults. *JAMA*. 2001;285(13):1736–1745.

Frisch M, Biggar RJ, Goedert JJ. Human papillomavirus-associated cancers in patients with human immunodeficiency virus infection and acquired immunodeficiency syndrome. *J Nat Cancer Institute*. 2000;92(18):1500–1510.

Frisch M, Goodman MT. Human papillomavirus-associated carcinomas in Hawaii and the mainland U.S. *Cancer*. 2000;88(6):1464–1469.

Fulco PP, Hynicka L, Rackley D. Raltegravir-based HAART regimen in a patient with large B-cell lymphoma. *Ann Pharmacother*. 2010;44(2):377–382.

Gabarre J, Azar N, Autran B, et al. High-dose therapy and autologous haematopoietic stem-cell transplantation for HIV-1-associated lymphoma. *Lancet*. 2000;355(9209):1071–1072.

Gabarre J, Marcelin AG, Azar N, et al. High-dose therapy plus autologous hematopoietic stem cell transplantation for human immunodeficiency virus (HIV)-related lymphoma: results and impact on HIV disease. *Haematologica*. 2004;89(9):1100–1108.

Gage JT, Vance EA, Hildenbrand PG, et al. Brain lesion and AIDS. *Proc Baylor Univ Medical Center*. 2000;13(4):424–429.

Gaidano G, Dalla-Favera R. Molecular pathogenesis of AIDS-related lymphomas. *Adv Cancer Res*. 1995;67:113–153.

Garon EB, Rizvi NA, Hui R, et al. Pembrolizumab for the treatment of non-small-cell lung cancer. *N Engl J Med*. 2015;372:2018–2028.

Gates AE, Kaplan LD. Biology and management of AIDS-associated non-Hodgkin's lymphoma. *Hematol Oncol Clin North Am*. 2003;17(3):821–841.

Gay CL, Bosch RJ, Ritz J, et al. Clinical trial of the anti-PD-L1 antibody BMS-936559 in HIV-1 infected participants on suppressive antiretroviral therapy. *J Infect Dis*. June 1, 2017;215(11):1725–1733.

Gbabe OF, Okwundu CI, Dedicoat M, et al. Treatment of severe or progressive Kaposi's sarcoma in HIV-infected adults. *Cochrane Database Syst Rev*. 2014;(9):CD003256.

Gerard L, Meignin V, Galicier L, et al. Characteristics of non-Hodgkin lymphoma arising in HIV-infected patients with suppressed HIV replication. *AIDS*. 2009;23(17):2301–2308.

Gichangi P, De Vuyst H, Estambale B, et al. HIV and cervical cancer in Kenya. *Intern J Gynaecol Obst*. 2002;76(1):55–63.

Gill ON, Weinberg JR, Fisher IS, et al. Meta-surveillance—safer cyber-surveillance. *Lancet*. 1995;346(8977):776.

Gill PS, Akil B, Colletti P, et al. Pulmonary Kaposi's sarcoma: clinical findings and results of therapy. *Am J Med*. 1989;87(1):57–61.

Gill PS, Wernz J, Scadden DT, et al. Randomized phase III trial of liposomal daunorubicin vs. doxorubicin, bleomycin, and vincristine in AIDS-related Kaposi's sarcoma. *J Clin Oncol*. 1996;14(8):2353–2364.

Goldstein JD, Dickson DW, Moser FG, et al. Primary central nervous system lymphoma in acquired immune deficiency syndrome: a clinical and pathologic study with results of treatment with radiation. *Cancer.* 1991;67(11):2756–2765.

Gopal S, Patel MR, Yanik EL, et al. Temporal trends in presentation and survival for HIV-associated lymphoma in the antiretroviral therapy era. *J Natl Cancer Inst.* 2013;105:1221–1229.

Gosselaar C, Roobol MJ, Roemeling S, et al. The role of the digital rectal examination in subsequent screening visits in the European Randomized Study of Screening for Prostate Cancer (ERSPC), Rotterdam. *Eur Urol.* 2008;54:581–588.

Gosselaar C, Roobol MJ, van den Bergh RC, et al. Digital rectal examination and the diagnosis of prostate cancer—a study based on 8 years and three screenings within the European Randomized Study of Screening for Prostate Cancer (ERSPC), Rotterdam. *Eur Urol.* 2009;55(1):139–146.

Govindarajan A, Coburn NH, Kiss A, et al. Population-based assessment of the surgical management of locally advanced colorectal cancer. *J Natl Cancer Inst.* 2006; 98(20):1474–1481.

Grew D, Bitterman D, Leichman CG, et al. HIV infection is associated with poor outcomes for patients with anal cancer in the highly active antiretroviral therapy era. *Dis Colon Rectum.* 2015;58(12):1130–1136.

Grimm P, Billiet I, Bostwick D, et al. Comparative analysis of prostate specific antigen free survival outcomes for patients with low, intermediate, and high risk prostate cancer treatment by radical therapy: results from the Prostate Cancer Results Study Group. *Br J Urol Int.* 2012;109(Suppl 1):22–29.

Grover S, Desir F, Jing Y, et al. Reduced cancer survival among adults with HIV and AIDS-defining illnesses despite no difference in cancer stage at diagnosis. *J AIDS.* 2018;79(4):421–429.

Gruffaz M, Vasan K, Tan B, et al. TLR4-mediated inflammation promotes KSHV-induced cellular transformation and tumorigenesis by activating the STAT3 pathway. *Cancer Res.* December 15, 2017;77(24):7094–7108.

Guerrero-Garcia TA, Mogollon RJ, and Castillo JJ. Bortezomib in plasmablastic lymphoma: a glimpse of hope for a hard-to-treat disease. *Leuk Res.* November 2017;62:12–16.

Guiguet M, Boue F, Cadranel J, et al. Effect of immunodeficiency, HIV viral load, and antiretroviral therapy on the risk of individual malignancies (FHDH-ANRS CO4): a prospective cohort study. *Lancet Oncol.* 2009;10(12):1152–1159.

Guihot A, Marcelin, AG, Massiani MA, et al. Drastic decrease of the HIV reservoir in a patient treated with nivolumab for lung cancer. *Ann Oncol.* 2018;29(2):517–518.

Gulrich AE, Yueming L, McDonald A, et al. Rates of non-AIDS defining cancers in people with HIV infection before and after AIDS diagnoses. *AIDS.* 2002;16:1155–1161.

Gupta NK, Nolan A, Omuro A, et al. Long-term survival in AIDS-related primary central nervous system lymphoma. *Neuro Oncol.* 2017;19:99–108.

Hamilton-Dutoit SJ, Pallesen G, Karkov J, et al. Identification of EBV-DNA in tumour cells of AIDS-related lymphomas by in-situ hybridisation. *Lancet.* 1989;1(8637):554–552.

Haq IU, Dalla Pria A, Papanastasopoulos P, et al. The clinical application of plasma Kaposi sarcoma herpesvirus viral load as a tumour biomarker: results from 704 patients. *HIV Med.* 2016;17:56–61.

Hassett JM, Zaroulis CG, Greenberg ML, et al. Bone marrow transplantation in AIDS. *N Engl J Med.* 1983;309(11):665.

Heard I, Etienney I, Potard V, et al. High prevalence of anal human papillomavirus-associated cancer precursors in a contemporary cohort of asymptomatic HIV-infected women. *Clin Infect Dis.* 2015;60(10):1559–1568.

Heard I, Pizot-Martin I, Potard V, et al. Prevalence of and risk factors for anal oncogenic human papillomavirus infection among HIV-infected women in France in the combination antiretroviral therapy era. *J Infect Dis.* 2016;213(9):1455–1461.

Heidenreich A, Bastian PJ, Bellmunt J, et al. European Association of Urology (EAU) guidelines on prostate cancer: part 1. Screening, diagnosis, and local treatment with curative intent—update 2013. *Eur Urol.* 2014;65(1):124–137.

Hengge UR, Ruzicka T, Tyring SK, et al. Update on Kaposi's sarcoma and other HHV8 associated diseases: part 1. Epidemiology, environmental predispositions, clinical manifestations, and therapy. *Lancet Infect Dis.* 2002;2(5):281–292.

Henrich TJ, Hanhauser E, Marty FM, et al. Antiretroviral-free HIV-1 remission and viral rebound after allogeneic stem cell transplantation: report of 2 cases. *Ann Intern Med.* 2014;161:319–327.

Heppt MV, Schlaak M, Eigenlter TK et al. Checkpoint blockade for metastatic melanoma and Merkel cell carcinoma in HIV-positive patients. *Ann Oncol.* 2017;28(12):3104–3106.

Herida M, Mary-Krause M, Kaphan R, et al. Incidence of non-AIDS defining cancers before and during the highly active antiretroviral therapy era in a cohort of human immunodeficiency virus-infected patients. *J Clin Oncol* 2003;21;3447–3453.

Hernández-Ramírez RU, Shiels MS, Dubrow R, et al. Cancer risk in HIV-infected people in the USA from 1996 to 2012: a population-based, registry-linkage study. *Lancet HIV.* November 2017;4(11):e495–e504.

Hessol NA, Whittemore H, Vittinghoff E, et al. Incidence of first and second primary cancers diagnosed among people with HIV, 1985–2013: a population-based, registry linkage study. *Lancet HIV.* 2018;5(11):e647–e655.

Hill DR. The role of radiotherapy for epidemic Kaposi's sarcoma. *Semin Oncol.* 1987;14:1207.

Hladik W, Dollard SC, Mermin J, et al. Transmission of human herpesvirus 8 by blood transfusion. *N Engl J Med.* 2006;355(13):1331–1338.

Hoffmann C, Tabrizian S, Wolf E, et al. Survival of AIDS patients with primary central nervous system lymphoma is dramatically improved by HAART-induced immune recovery. *AIDS (London).* 2001;15(16):2119–2127.

Holland HK, Saral R, Rossi JJ, et al. Allogeneic bone marrow transplantation, zidovudine, and human immunodeficiency virus type 1 (HIV-1) infection: studies in a patient with non-Hodgkin lymphoma. *Ann Intern Med.* 1989;111(12):973–981.

Hoover DR, Black C, Jacobson LP, et al. Epidemiologic analysis of Kaposi's sarcoma as an early and later AIDS outcome in homosexual men. *Am J Epidemiol.* 1993;138(4):266–278.

Hosseinipour MC, Kang M, Krown SE, Bukuru A, et al. As-needed vs immediate etoposide chemotherapy in combination with antiretroviral therapy for mild-to-moderate AIDS-associated Kaposi sarcoma in resource-limited settings: A5264/AMC-067 Randomized clinical trial. *Clin Infect Dis.* 2018;67(2):251–260.

Howlader N, Noone AM, Krapcho M, et al. *SEER statistics review, 1975–2012.* Bethesda, MD: National Cancer Institute. 2015. Available at http://seer.cancer.gov/archive/csr/1975_2012. Accessed May 13, 2016.

Hsiao W, Anastasia K, Hall J, et al. Association between HIV status and positive prostate biopsy in a study of US veterans. *Scientific World J.* 2009;9:102–108.

Huncharek M, Haddock KS, Reid R, et al. Smoking as a risk factor for prostate cancer: a meta-analysis of 24 prospective cohort studies. *Am J Pub Health.* 2010;100(4):693–701.

Hurst J, Hoffmann M, Pace M, et al. Immunological biomarkers predict HIV-1 viral rebound after treatment interruption. *Nat Commun.* 2015;6:8495.

Hutter G, Nowak D, Mossner M, et al. Long-term control of HIV by CCR5 Delta32/Delta32 stem-cell transplantation. *N Engl J Med.* 2009;360:692–698.

Impola U, Cuccuru MA, Masala MV, et al. Preliminary communication: matrix metalloproteinases in Kaposi's sarcoma. *Br J Dermatol.* 2003;149(4):905–907.

International Agency for Research on Cancer. *Human immunodeficiency viruses and human T-cell lymphotropic viruses.* Geneva: World Health Organization; 1996.

International Collaboration on HIV and Cancer. Highly active antiretroviral therapy and incidence of cancer in human immunodeficiency virus-infected adults. *J Natl Cancer Institute.* 2000;92(22):1823–1830.

Ireland-Gill A, Espina BM, Akil B, et al. Treatment of acquired immunodeficiency syndrome-related Kaposi's sarcoma using bleomycin-containing combination chemotherapy regimens. *Semin Oncol.* 1992;19(2 Suppl 5):32–36.

Iscovich J, Boffetta P, Franceschi S, et al. Classic Kaposi sarcoma: epidemiology and risk factors. *Cancer.* 2000;88(3):500–517.

Islami F, Moreira DM, Boffetta P, et al. A systematic review and meta-analysis of tobacco use and prostate cancer mortality and incidence in prospective cohort-studies. *Eur Urol.* 2014;66(6):1054–1064.

Jacobson LP, Jenkins FJ, Springer G, et al. Interaction of human immunodeficiency virus type 1 and human herpesvirus type 8 infections on the incidence of Kaposi's sarcoma. *J Infect Dis.* 2000;181(6):1940–1949.

Jacomet C, Girard PM, Lebrette MG, et al. Intravenous methotrexate for primary central nervous system non-Hodgkin's lymphoma in AIDS. *AIDS (London).* 1997;11(14):1725–1730.

Jephcott CR, Paltiel C, Hay J. Quality of life after non-surgical treatment of anal carcinoma: a case–control study of long-term survivors. *Clin Oncol.* 2004;16(8):530–535.

Johnson LG, Madeleine MM, Newcomer LM, et al. Anal cancer incidence and survival: the surveillance, epidemiology, and end results experience, 1973–2000. *Cancer.* 2004;101(2):281–288.

Johnston C, Harrington R, Jain R, et al. Safety and efficacy of combination antiretroviral therapy in human immunodeficiency virus-infected adults undergoing autologous or allogeneic hematopoietic cell transplantation for hematologic malignancies. *Biol Blood Marrow Transplant.* 2016;22:149–156.

Joseph DA, King JB, Miller JW, et al. Prevalence of colorectal cancer screening among adults—behavioral risk factor surveillance system, United States, 2010. *MMWR.* 2012;61(2):51–56.

Kahn S, Jani A, Edelman S, et al. Matched cohort analysis of outcomes of definitive radiotherapy for prostate cancer in human immunodeficiency virus-positive patients. *Int Radiat Oncol Biol Physics.* 2012;83(1):16–21.

Kaplan LD, Abrams DI, Feigal E, et al. AIDS-associated non-Hodgkin's lymphoma in San Francisco. *JAMA.* 1989;261(5):719–724.

Kaplan LD, Hopewell PC, Jaffe H, et al. Kaposi's sarcoma involving the lung in patients with the acquired immunodeficiency syndrome. *J AIDS.* 1988;1(1):23–30.

Kaplan LD, Straus DJ, Testa MA, et al. Low-dose compared with standard-dose m-BACOD chemotherapy for non-Hodgkin's lymphoma associated with human immunodeficiency virus infection. National Institute of Allergy and Infectious Diseases AIDS Clinical Trials Group. *N Engl J Med.* 1997;336(23):1641–1648.

Karp J, Profeta G, Marantz PR, et al. Lung cancer in patients with immunodeficiency syndrome. *Chest.* 1993;103(2):410–413.

Kirk GD, Merlo C, O'Driscoll P, et al. HIV infection is associated with an increased risk for lung cancer, independent of smoking. *Clin Infect Dis.* 2007;45(1):103–110.

Kiviat NB, Hawes S, Lampinen T, et al. The effect of HAART on detection of anal HPV and squamous intraepithelial lesions among HIV infected homosexual men. Paper presented at the 6th International Conference on Malignancies in AIDS and Other Immunodeficiencies, Bethesda, MD, 2002.

Klugman AD, Schaffner J. Colon adenocarcinoma in HIV infection: a case report and review. *Am J Gastroenterol.* 1994;89(2):254–256.

Knowles DM. Etiology and pathogenesis of AIDS-related non-Hodgkin's lymphoma. *Hematol Oncol Clin North Am.* 1996;10(5):1081–1109.

Knowles DM. *Neoplastic hematopathology.* Philadelphia: Lippincott Williams & Wilkins; 2001.

Knowles DM, Chamulak GA, Subar M, et al. Lymphoid neoplasia associated with the acquired immunodeficiency syndrome (AIDS): the New York University Medical Center experience with 105 patients (1981–1986). *Ann Intern Med.* 1988; 108(5):744–753.

Komanduri KV, Luce JA, McGrath MS, et al. The natural history and molecular heterogeneity of HIV-associated primary malignant lymphomatous effusions. *J AIDS.* 1996;13(3):215–226.

Kong CY, Sigel K, Criss SD, et al. Benefits and harms of lung cancer screening in HIV-infected individuals with CD4+ cell count at least 500 cells/μl. *AIDS.* 2018;32(10):1333–1342.

Koon HB, Krown SE, Lee JY, et al. Phase II trial of imatinib in AIDS-associated Kaposi's sarcoma: AIDS Malignancy Consortium Protocol 042. *J Clin Oncol.* 2014;32(5):402–408.

Kowalkowski MA, Day RS, Chan W, et al. Cumulative HIV viremia and non-AIDs-defining malignancies among a sample of HIV-infected male veterans. *J AIDS.* 2014;62(2):204–211.

Krishnan A, Molina A, Zaia J, et al. Durable remissions with autologous stem cell transplantation for high-risk HIV-associated lymphomas. *Blood.* 2005;105(2):874–878.

Krown SE, Metroka C, Wernz JC. Kaposi's sarcoma in the acquired immune deficiency syndrome: a proposal for uniform evaluation, response, and staging criteria. AIDS Clinical Trials Group Oncology Committee. *J Clin Oncol.* September 1989;7(9):1201–1207.

Krown SE, Roy D, Lee JY, et al. Rapamycin with antiretroviral therapy in AIDS-associated Kaposi sarcoma: an AIDS Malignancy Consortium Study. *J AIDS.* 2012;59(5):447–454.

Krown SE, Testa MA, Huang J. AIDS-related Kaposi's sarcoma: prospective validation of the AIDS Clinical Trials Group staging classification. AIDS Clinical Trials Group Oncology Committee. *J Clin Oncol.* 1997;15(9):3085–3092.

La Ruche G, You B, Mensah-Ado I, et al. Human papillomavirus and human immunodeficiency virus infections: relation with cervical dysplasia–neoplasia in African women. *Int J Cancer.* 1998;76(4):480–486.

Lafrenie RM, Wahl LM, Epstein JS, et al. HIV-1-Tat modulates the function of monocytes and alters their interactions with microvessel endothelial cells: a mechanism of HIV pathogenesis. *J Immunol (Baltimore, 1950).* 1996;156(4):1638–1645.

Lederman MM, Cannon PM, Currier JS, et al. A cure for HIV infection: "not in my lifetime" or "just around the corner"? *Pathog Immun.* 2016;1:154–164.

Le Garff G, Samri A, Lambert-Niclot S, et al. Transient HIV-specific T cells increase inflammation in an HIV-infected patient treated with nivolumab. *AIDS.* 2017;31(7):1048–1051.

Lehnert T, Methner M, Pollok A, et al. Multivisceral resection for locally advanced primary colon and rectal cancer: an analysis of prognostic factors in 201 patients. *Ann Surg.* 2002;235(2):217–225.

Leport C, Rousseau F, Perronne C, et al. Bacterial prostatitis in patients infected with the human immunodeficiency virus. *J Urol.* 1989;141(2):334–336.

Letang E, Almeida J, Miró J, et al. Predictors of immune reconstitution inflammatory syndrome-associated with Kaposi sarcoma in Mozambique: a prospective study. *J AIDS.* 2010;53(5):589–597.

Levine AM, Seaberg EC, Hessol NA, et al. HIV as a risk factor for lung cancer in women: data from the Women's Interagency HIV Study. *J Clin Oncol.* 2010;28(9):1514–1519.

Levine AM, Sullivan-Halley J, Pike MC, et al. Human immunodeficiency virus-related lymphoma: prognostic factors predictive of survival. *Cancer.* 1991;68(11):2466–2472.

Levine AM, Tulpule A. Clinical aspects and management of AIDS-related Kaposi's sarcoma. *Eur J Cancer (Oxford: 1990).* 2001;37(10):1288–1295.

Lewden C, Salmon D, Morlat P, et al. Causes of death among human immunodeficiency virus (HIV)-infected adults in the era of potent antiretroviral therapy: emerging role of hepatitis and cancers, persistent role of AIDS. *Int J Epidemiol.* 2005;34(1):121–130.

Lewitschnig S, Gedela K, Toby M, et al. 18F-FDG PET/CT in HIV-related central nervous system pathology. *Eur J Nucl Mol Imaging.* 2013;40(9):1420–1427.

Licho R, Litofsky NS, Senitko M, et al. Inaccuracy of Tl-201 brain SPECT in distinguishing cerebral infections from lymphoma in patients with AIDS. *Clin Nuclear Med.* 2002;27(2):81–86.

Liebowitz D, Kieff E. Epstein–Barr virus latent membrane protein: induction of B-cell activation antigens and membrane patch formation does not require vimentin. *J Virol.* 1989;63(9):4051–4054.

Lillo FB, Ferrari D, Veglia F, et al. Human papillomavirus infection and associated cervical disease in human immunodeficiency virus-infected women: effect of highly active antiretroviral therapy. *J Infect Dis.* 2001;184(5):547–551.

Lim S-T, Karim R, Tulpule A, et al. Prognostic factors in HIV-related diffuse large-cell lymphoma: before versus after highly active antiretroviral therapy. *J Clin Oncol.* 2005;23(33):8477–8482.

Lince-Deroche N, Phiri J, Michelow P, et al. Costs and cost effectiveness of three approaches for cervical cancer screening among HIV-positive women in Johannesburg, South Africa. *PloS One.* 2015;10(11):e0141969.

Lister A, Abrey LE, Sandlund JT. Central nervous system lymphoma. *Am Soc Hematol. Educ Prog.* 2002;283–296.

Little RF, Pittaluga S, Grant N, et al. Highly effective treatment of acquired immunodeficiency syndrome-related lymphoma with dose-adjusted EPOCH: impact of antiretroviral therapy suspension and tumor biology. *Blood.* 2003;101(12):4653–4659.

Locker GY, Hamilton S, Harris J, et al. ASCO 2006 update of recommendations for the use of tumor markers in gastrointestinal cancer. *J Clin Oncol.* 2006;24(33):5313.

Loriot Y, Miler K, Sternberg CN, et al. Effect of enzalutamide on health-related quality of life, pain, and skeletal-related events in asymptomatic and minimally symptomatic, chemotherapy-naïve patients with metastatic castration-resistant prostate cancer (PREVAIL): results from a randomised, phase 3 trial. *Lancet Oncol.* 2015;16(5):509–521.

Lowenthal DA, Straus DJ, Wise Campbell S, et al. AIDS-related lymphoid neoplasia: the Memorial Hospital experience. *Cancer.* 1988;61(11):2325–2337.

Luppi M, Barozzi P, Santagostino G, et al. Molecular evidence of organ-related transmission of Kaposi sarcoma-associated herpesvirus or human herpesvirus-8 in transplant patients. *Blood.* 2000;96(9):3279–3281.

Machalek DA, Poynten M, Jin F, et al. Anal human papillomavirus infection and associated neoplastic lesions in men who have sex with men: a systematic review and meta-analysis. *Lancet Oncol.* 2012;13(5):487–500.

MacMahon EM, et al. Epstein–Barr virus in AIDS-related primary central nervous system lymphoma. *Lancet.* 1991;338(8773):969–973.

Mahale P, Engels EA, Coghill AE, et al. Cancer risk in older persons living with human immunodeficiency virus infection in the United States. *Clin Infect Dis.* 2018;67(1):50–57.

Makinson A, Cheret A, Abgrall S, et al. *Early lung cancer diagnosis in HIV infected population with an important smoking history with low-dose Ct: a pilot study (EP48 HIV CHEST).* Bethesda, MD: National Library of Medicine; 2015. Available at https://www.clinicaltrials.gov/ct2/show/NCT01207986?term=NCT01207986&rank=1. NLM Identifier: NCT 01207986.

Mandelblatt JS, Kanetsky P, Eggert L, et al. Is HIV infection a cofactor for cervical squamous cell neoplasia? *Cancer Epidemiol.* 1999;8(1):97–106.

Mandell SP, Mack CD, Bulger EM. Motor vehicle mismatch: a national perspective. *Injury Prev.* 2010;16(5):309–314.

Marcus JL, Chao CR, Leyden WA, et al. Prostate cancer incidence and prostate-specific antigen testing among HIV-positive and HIV-negative men. *J AIDS.* 2014;66:495–502.

Marcus JL, Leyden WA, Chao CR, et al. Immunodeficiency, AIDS-related pneumonia, and risk of lung cancer among HIV-infected individuals. *AIDS.* April 24, 2017;31(7):989–993.

Mbulaiteye SM, Katabira ET, Wabinga H, et al. Spectrum of cancers among HIV-infected persons in Africa: the Uganda AIDS-Center Registry Match Study. *Int J Cancer.* 2006;118(4):985–990.

McGowan JP, Shah S. Long-term remission of AIDS-related primary central nervous system lymphoma associated with highly active antiretroviral therapy. *AIDS (London).* 1998;12(8):952–954.

Mdodo R, Frazier EL, Dube SR, et al. Cigarette smoking prevalence among adults with HIV compared with the general adult population in the United States: cross-sectional surveys. *Ann Intern Med.* 2015;162(5):335–344.

Melbye M, Rabkin C, Frisch M, et al. Changing patterns of anal cancer incidence in the United States, 1940–1989. *Am J Epidemiol.* 1994;139(8):772–780.

Minkoff H, Ahdieh L, Massad, LS et al. The effect of highly active antiretroviral therapy on cervical cytologic changes associated with oncogenic HPV among HIV-infected women. *J AIDS.* 2001;15(16):2157–2164.

Minkoff H, Zhong Y, Burk RD, et al. Influence of adherent and effective antiretroviral therapy use on human papillomavirus infection and squamous intraepithelial lesions in human immunodeficiency virus-positive women. *J Infect Dis.* 2010;201(5):681–690.

Mitsuyasu RT, Groopman JE. Biology and therapy of Kaposi's sarcoma. *Semin Oncol.* 1984;11(1):53–59.

Monforte A, Abrams D, Pradier C, et al. HIV-induced immunodeficiency and mortality from AIDS-defining and non-AIDS-defining malignancies. *AIDS (London).* 2008;22(16):2143–2153.

Monini P, de Lellis L, Fabris M, et al. Kaposi's sarcoma-associated herpesvirus DNA sequences in prostate tissue and human semen. *N Engl J Med.* 1996;334(18):1168–1172.

Moore AL, Sabin CA, Madge S, et al. Highly active antiretroviral therapy and cervical intraepithelial neoplasia. *AIDS (London).* 2002;16(6):927–929.

Morlat P, Roussillon C, Henard S, et al. Causes of death among HIV-infected patients in France in 2010 (national survey): trends since 2000. *AIDS.* 2014;28(8):1181–1191.

Mosam A, Shaik F, Uldrick TS, et al. A randomized controlled trial of HAART versus HAART and chemotherapy in therapy-naive patients with HIV-associated Kaposi sarcoma in South Africa. *J AIDS.* 2012;60(2):150.

Mounier N, Spina M, Gabarre J, et al. AIDS-related non-Hodgkin lymphoma: final analysis of 485 patients treated with risk-adapted intensive chemotherapy. *Blood.* 2006;107(10):3832–3840.

Moyer VA. Screening for prostate cancer: US Preventive Services Task Force recommendation statement. *Ann Intern Med.* 2012;157(2):120–135.

Moyer VA. Screening for lung cancer. US Preventative Services Task Force recommendation statement. *Ann Intern Med.* 2014;160(5):330–338.

Munger K, Phelps WC, Bubb V, et al. The E6 and E7 genes of the human papillomavirus type 16 together are necessary and sufficient for transformation of primary human keratinocytes. *J Virol.* 1989;63(10):4417–4421.

Myerson RJ, Kong F, Birnbaum EH, et al. Radiation therapy for epidermoid carcinoma of the anal canal: clinical and treatment factors associated with outcome. *Radiother Oncol.* 2001;61(1):15–22.

Nagata N, Shimbo T, Yazaki H, et al. Predictive clinical factors in the diagnosis of gastrointestinal Kaposi's sarcoma and its endoscopic severity. *PLoS One.* 2012;7(11):1–7.

Nasti G, Martellotta F, Berretta M, et al. Impact of highly active antiretroviral therapy on the presenting features and outcome of patients with acquired immunodeficiency syndrome-related Kaposi sarcoma. *Cancer.* 2003;98(11):2440–2446.

Nasti G, Talamini R, Antinori A, et al. AIDS-related Kaposi's sarcoma: evaluation of potential new prognostic factors and assessment of the AIDS Clinical Trial Group Staging System in the HAART Era—the Italian Cooperative Group on AIDS and Tumors and the Italian Cohort of Patients Naive from Antiretrovirals. *J Clin Oncol.* 2003;21(15):2876–2882.

National Comprehensive Cancer Network. NCCN clinical practice guidelines in oncology. Primary CNS lymphoma version 1.2015. May 1, 2015. Available at https://www.nccn.org/professionals/physician_gls/pdf/cns.pdf. Accessed December 13, 2015.

National Comprehensive Cancer Network. NCCN clinical practice guidelines in oncology. Rectal cancer version 1.2016. November 4, 2015. Available at https://www.nccn.org/professionals/physician_gls/pdf/rectal.pdf. Accessed May 13, 2016.

National Comprehensive Cancer Network. NCCN clinical practice guidelines in oncology. Non-small cell lung cancer version 2.2016. November 23, 2015. Available at https://www.nccn.org/professionals/physician_gls/pdf/nscl.pdf. Accessed December 8, 2015.

National Comprehensive Cancer Network. NCCN clinical practice guidelines in oncology. Colon cancer version 2.2016. November 23,

2015. Available at https://www.nccn.org/professionals/physician_gls/pdf/colon.pdf. Accessed May 13, 2016.

National Lung Screening Trial Research Team. Reduced lung-cancer mortality with low-dose computed tomographic screening. *N Engl J Med.* 2011;365(5):395–409.

Navarro WH, Kaplan LD. AIDS-related lymphoproliferative disease. *Blood.* 2006;107(1):13–20.

Naydu SK, Balar B. Colorectal cancer screening in human immunodeficiency virus populations: are they at average risk? *World J Gastrointestinal Oncol.* 2012;4(12):259–264.

Neef H, Horth W, Makowiec F, et al. Outcome after resection of hepatic and pulmonary metastasis of colorectal cancer. *J Gastrointest Surg.* 2009;13(10):1813–1820.

Newton R, Ziegler J, Bourboulia D, et al. Infection with Kaposi's sarcoma-associated herpesvirus (KSHV) and human immunodeficiency virus (HIV) in relation to the risk and clinical presentation of Kaposi's sarcoma in Uganda. *Br J Cancer.* 2003;89(3):502–504.

Norden AD, Drappatz J, Wen PY, et al. Survival among patients with primary central nervous system lymphoma, 1973–2004. *J Neuro-Oncol.* 2011;101(3):487–493.

Northfelt DW, Dezube BJ, Thommes JA, et al. Pegylated-liposomal doxorubicin versus doxorubicin, bleomycin, and vincristine in the treatment of AIDS-related Kaposi's sarcoma: results of a randomized phase III clinical trial. *J Clin Oncol.* 1998;16(7):2445–2451.

Noy A. Update in Kaposi sarcoma. *Curr Opin Oncol.* 2003;15(5):379–381.

Noy A, Lee JY, Cesarman E, et al. AMC 048: modified CODOX-M/IVAC-rituximab is safe and effective for HIV-associated Burkitt lymphoma. *Blood.* 2015;126:160–166.

Ntekim A, Campbell O, Rothenbacher D. Optimal management of cervical cancer in HIV-positive patients: a systematic review. *Cancer Med.* 2015;4:1381–1393.

Nyitray AG, Hicks JT, Hwang LY, et al. A phase II clinical study to assess the feasibility of self and partner anal examinations to detect anal canal abnormalities including anal cancer. *Sex Transm Infect.* March 2018;94(2):124–130.

Oehler-Janne C, Huguet F, Provencher S, et al. HIV-specific differences in outcome of squamous cell carcinoma of the anal canal: a multicentric cohort study of HIV-positive patients receiving highly active antiretroviral therapy. *J Clin Oncol.* 2008;26(15):2550–2557.

Okotie OT, Roehl KA, Han M, et al. Characteristics of prostate cancer detected by digital rectal examination only. *Urology.* 2007;70(6):1117–1120.

Okuma Y, Hishima T, Kashima J, et al. High PD-L1 expression indicates poor prognosis of HIV-infected patients with non-small cell lung cancer. *Cancer Immunol Immunother.* March 2018;67(3):495–505.

Okuma Y, Hosomi Y, Imamura A. Lung cancer patients harboring epidermal growth factor receptor mutation among those infected by human immunodeficiency virus. *Onco Targets Ther.* 2014;31:111–115.

Olson JE, Janney CA, Rao RD, et al. The continuing increase in the incidence of primary central nervous system non-Hodgkin lymphoma: a surveillance, epidemiology, and end results analysis. *Cancer.* 2002;95(7):1504–1510.

Ong WL, Manohar P, Millar J, et al. Clinicopathological characteristics and management of prostate cancer in the human immunodeficiency virus (HIV)-positive population: experience in an Australian major HIV center. *Br J Urol Int.* 2015; 116(Suppl 3):5–10.

Orlando G, Fasolo MM, Schiavini M, et al. Role of highly active antiretroviral therapy in human papillomavirus-induced genital dysplasia in HIV-1-infected patients. *AIDS (London).* 1999;13(3):424–425.

Palefsky JM, Holly EA, Gonzales J, et al. Detection of human papillomavirus DNA in anal intraepithelial neoplasia and anal cancer. *Cancer Res.* 1991;51(3):1014–1019.

Palefsky JM, Holly EA, Ralston ML, et al. Effect of highly active antiretroviral therapy on the natural history of anal squamous intraepithelial lesions and anal human papillomavirus infection. *J AIDS (1999).* 2001;28(5):422–428.

Pantanowitz L, Bohac G, Cooley T, et al. Human immunodeficiency virus-associated prostate cancer: clinicopathological findings and outcome in a multi-institutional study. *Br J Urol Int.* 2008;101:1519–1523.

Park IU, Palefsky JM. Evaluation and management of anal intraepithelial neoplasia in HIV-negative and HIV-positive men who have sex with men. *Curr Infect Dis Rep.* 2010;12(2):126–133.

Patel P, Hanson DL, Sullivan PS, et al. Incidence of types of cancer among HIV-infected persons compared with the general population in the United States, 1992–2003. *Ann Intern Med.* 2008;148(10):728–736.

Patil P, Elem B, Zumla A. Pattern of adult malignancies in Zambia (1980–1989) in light of the human immunodeficiency virus type 1 epidemic. *J Tropical Med Hygiene.* 1995;98(4):281–284.

Penn I. Kaposi's sarcoma in organ transplant recipients: report of 20 cases. *Transplantation.* 1979;27(1):8–11.

Persad GC, Little RF, Grady C. Including persons with HIV infection in cancer clinical trials. *J Clin Oncol.* 2008;26(7):1027–1032.

Petrovas C, Casazza JP, Brenchley JM, et al. PD-1 is a regulator of virus-specific CD8+ T cell survival in HIV infection. *J Exp Med.* 2006;203:2281–2292.

Piketty C, Seliger-Leneman H, Bouvier AM. Incidence of HIV-related anal cancer remains increased despite long-term combined antiretroviral treatment: results from the French Hospital Database on HIV. *J Clin Oncol.* 2012;30(35):4360–4366.

Piketty C, Selinger-Leneman H, Grabar S, et al. Marked increase in the incidence of invasive anal cancer among HIV-infected patients despite treatment with combination antiretroviral therapy. *AIDS (London).* 2008;22(10):1203–1211.

Plancoulaine S, Abel L, van Beveren M, et al. Human herpesvirus 8 transmission from mother to child and between siblings in an endemic population. *Lancet.* 2000;356(9235):1062–1065.

Pluda J, Broder S, Yarchoan R. Therapy of AIDS and AIDS-associated neoplasms. *Cancer Chemother Biol Response Modif.* 1992;13:404–439.

Polesel J, Clifford GM, Rickenbach M, et al. Non-Hodgkin lymphoma incidence in the Swiss HIV Cohort Study before and after highly active antiretroviral therapy. *AIDS (London).* 2008;22(2):301–306.

Polizzotto MN, Uldrick TS, Wyvill KM, et al. Pomalidomide for symptomatic Kaposi's sarcoma in people with and without HIV infection: a phase I/II study. *J Clin Oncol.* December 2016;34(34):4125–4131.

Pourcher V, Desnoyer A, Assoumou L et al. Phase II trial of lenalidomide in HIV-infected patients with previously treated Kaposi's sarcoma: results of the ANRS 154 Lenakap Trial. *AIDS Res Hum Retroviruses.* January 2017;33(1):1–10.

Powles T, Matthews G, Bower M. AIDS related systemic non-Hodgkin's lymphoma. *Sex Transm Infect.* 2000;76(5):335–341.

Powles T, Thirwell C, Newsom-Davis T, et al. Does HIV adversely influence the outcome in advanced non-small-cell lung cancer in the era of HAART? *Br J Cancer.* 2003;89:457–459.

Rahmanian S, Wewers ME, Koletar S, et al. Cigarette smoking in the HIV-infected population. *Proc Am Thorac Soc.* 2011;8(3):313–319.

Ramirez-Marrero FA, Smit E, de la Torre-Feliciano T, et al. Risk of cancer among Hispanics with AIDS compared with the general population in Puerto Rico: 1987–2003. *Puerto Rico Health Sci J.* 2010;29(3):256–264.

Raphael M, Said J, Dorisch B, et al. Lymphomas associated with HIV infection. In: Swerdlow SH, Campo E, Harris NL, et al., eds. *World Health Organization classification of tumours of haematopoietic and lymphoid tissue.* 4th ed. Lyon, France: IARC Press; 2008:340–342.

Ratner L, Lee J, Tang S, et al. Chemotherapy for human immunodeficiency virus-associated non-Hodgkin's lymphoma in combination with highly active antiretroviral therapy. *J Clin Oncol.* 2001;19(8):2171–2178.

Ravalli S, Chabon A, Khan A. Gastrointestinal neoplasia in young HIV antibody-positive patients. *Am J Clin Pathol.* 1989;91:458–461.

Re A, Cattaneo C, Michieli M, et al. High-dose therapy and autologous peripheral-blood stem-cell transplantation as salvage treatment for HIV-associated lymphoma in patients receiving highly active antiretroviral therapy. *J Clin Oncol.* 2003;21(23):4423–4427.

Re A, Michieli M, Casari S, et al. High-dose therapy and autologous peripheral blood stem cell transplantation as salvage treatment for AIDS-related lymphoma: long-term results of the Italian Cooperative Group on AIDS and Tumors (GICAT) study with analysis of prognostic factors. *Blood.* 2009;114(7):1306–1313.

Reddy KP, Kong CY, Hyle EP, et al. Lung cancer mortality associated with smoking and smoking cessation among people living with HIV in the United States. *JAMA Intern Med*. November 1, 2017;177(11):1613–1621.

Reekie J, Kosa C, Engsig F, et al. Relationship between current level of immunodeficiency and non-acquired immunodeficiency syndrome-defining malignancies. *Cancer*. November 15, 2010;116(22):5306–5315.

Reid E, Suneja G, Ambinder RF, et al. Cancer in people living with HIV, Version 1.2018, NCCN clinical practice guidelines in oncology. *J Natl Compr Canc Netw*. 2018;16(8):986–1017.

Reinhold JP, Moon M, Tenner CT, et al. Colorectal cancer screening in HIV-infected patients 50 years of age and older: missed opportunities for prevention. *Am J Gastroenterol*. 2005;100:1805–1812.

Renwick N, Halaby T, Weverling GJ, et al. Seroconversion for human herpesvirus 8 during HIV infection is highly predictive of Kaposi's sarcoma. *AIDS (London)*. 1998;12(18):2481–2488.

Richel O, de Vries HJ, van Noesel CJ, et al. Comparison of imiquimod, topical fluorouracil, and electrocautery for the treatment of anal intraepithelial neoplasia in HIV-positive men who have sex with men: an open-label, randomised controlled trial. *Lancet Oncol*. 2013;14:346–353.

Riedel DJ, Cox ER, Stafford KA, et al. Clinical presentation and outcomes of prostate cancer in an urban cohort of predominantly African American, human immunodeficiency virus-infected patients. *Urology*. 2015;85(2):415–421.

Riedel DJ, Rositch AF, Redfield RR. Patterns of HIV viremia and viral suppression before diagnosis of non-AIDS-defining cancers in HIV-infected individuals. *Infect Agent Cancer*. 2015;38(10):1–7.

Riley RR, Duensing S, Brake T, et al. Dissection of human papillomavirus E6 and E7 function in transgenic mouse models of cervical carcinogenesis. *Cancer Res*. 2003;63(16):4862–4871.

Robbins HA, Pfeiffer RM, Shiels MS, et al. Excess cancers among HIV-infected people in the United States. *J Natl Cancer Inst*. 2015;107:pii: dju503.

Robert C, Ribas A, Wolchok JD, et al. Anti-programmed-death-receptor-1 treatment with pembrolizumab in ipilimumab-refractory advanced melanoma: a randomised dose-comparison cohort of a phase 1 trial. *Lancet*. 2014;384:1109–1117.

Rodrigo JA, Hicks LK, Cheung MC, et al. HIV-associated Burkitt lymphoma: good efficacy and tolerance of intensive chemotherapy including CODOX-M/IVAC with or without rituximab in the HAART era. *Adv Hematol*. 2012;2012:1–9.

Rohner E, Valeri F, Maskew M, et al. Incidence rate of Kaposi sarcoma in HIV-infected patients on antiretroviral therapy in southern Africa: a prospective multicohort study. *J AIDS*. 2014;67(5):547–554.

Ronit A, Kristensen T, Klitbo DM, et al. Incidental lung cancers and positive computed tomography images in people living with HIV. *AIDS*. 2017;31:1973–1977

Rosenblum ML, Levy RM, Bredesen DE, et al. Primary central nervous system lymphomas in patients with AIDS. *Ann Neurol*. 1988;23(Suppl):S13–S16.

Royse K, El Chaer F, Amirian ES, et al. Disparities in Kaposi sarcoma incidence and survival in the United States: 2000–2013. *PLoS One*. 2017;12(8):e0182750.

Ruiz A, Ganz WI, Post MJ, et al. Use of thallium-201 brain SPECT to differentiate cerebral lymphoma from toxoplasma encephalitis in AIDS patients. *Am J Neuroradiol*. 1994;15(10):1885–1894.

Ryan CJ, Smith MR, Fizazi K, et al. Abiraterone acetate plus prednisone versus placebo plus prednisone in chemotherapy-naïve men with metastatic castration-resistant prostate cancer (COU-AA-302): final overall survival analysis of a randomised, double-blind, placebo-controlled phase 3 study. *Lancet Oncol*. 2015;16(2):152–160.

Sacktor N, Lyles RH, Skolasky R, et al. HIV-associated neurologic disease incidence changes: multicenter AIDS cohort study, 1990–1998. *Neurology*. 2001;56(2):257–260.

Safai B. Pathophysiology and epidemiology of epidemic Kaposi's sarcoma. *Semin Oncol*. 1987;2:7–12.

Sandler AS, Kaplan LD. Diagnosis and management of systemic non-Hodgkin's lymphoma in HIV disease. *Hematol Oncol Clin North Am*. 1996;10(5):1111–1124.

Santesso N, Mustafa RA, Schunemann HJ, et al. World Health Organization guidelines for treatment of cervical intraepithelial neoplasia 2-3 and screen-and-treat strategies to prevent cervical cancer. *Int J Gynaecol Obstet*. 2016;132:252–258

Sauer R, Liersch T, Merkel S, et al. Preoperative versus postoperative chemoradiotherapy for locally advanced rectal cancer: results of the German CAO/ARO/AIO-94 randomized phase III trial after a median follow-up of 11 years. *J Clin Oncol*. 2012;20(16):1926–1933.

Saville M, Lietzau J, Pluda J, et al. Activity of placlitaxel (Taxol) as therapy for HIV-associated Kaposi's sarcoma. *Lancet*. 1995;346:26–28.

Schiffman M, Kjaer SK. Natural history of anogenital human papillomavirus infection and neoplasia. *JNCI Monographs*. 2003;2003(31):14–19.

Schreiber D, Chhabra A, Rineer J, et al. Outcomes and tolerance of human immunodeficiency virus-positive veterans undergoing dose-escalated external beam radiotherapy for localized prostate cancer. *Clin Genitourinary Cancer*. 2014;12(2):94–99.

Serraino D, Boschini A, Carrieri P, et al. Cancer risk among men with, or at risk of, HIV infection in southern Europe. *AIDS*. 2000;14(5):553–559.

Sgadari C, Monini P, Barillari G, et al. Use of HIV protease inhibitors to block Kaposi's sarcoma and tumour growth. *Lancet Oncol*. 2003;4(9):537–547.

Shah NN, Singavi AK, Harrington A. Daratumumab in primary effusion lymphoma. *N Engl J Med*. August 16, 2018;379(7):689–690.

Shah R, Al-Sukhni W, Kim RD, et al. Resection of hepatic and pulmonary metastasis from colorectal carcinoma. *JACS*. 2006;202(3):468–475.

Shebl FM, Engels EA, Goedert JJ, et al. Pulmonary infections and risk of lung cancer among persons with AIDS. *J AIDS*. 2010;55:375–379.

Shepherd FA, Crowley J, van Houtte P, et al.; the IASLC Lung Cancer Staging Project. Clinical staging of small cell lung cancer in the forthcoming (seventh) edition of the Tumor, Node, Metastasis Classification for Lung Cancer. *J Thoracic Oncol*. 2007;2(12):1067–1077.

Shepherd L, Ryom L, Law M, et al. Cessation of cigarette smoking and the impact on cancer incidence in HIV-positive persons: the D:A:D study. *Clin Infect Dis*. 2018;68(4):650–657. doi: 10.1093/cid/ciy508

Shiels MS, Althoff KN, Pfeiffer RM, et al. HIV infection, immunosuppression, and age at diagnosis of non-AIDS-defining cancers. *Clin Infect Dis*. 2017;64(4):468–475.

Shiels, MS, Cole SR, Mehta SH, et al. Lung cancer incidence and mortality among HIV-infected and HIV-uninfected injection drug users. *J AIDS*. 2010;55(4):510–515.

Shiels MS, Copeland G, Goodman M, et al. Cancer stage at diagnosis in patients infected with the human immunodeficiency virus and transplant recipients. *Cancer*. 2015;121(12):1063–2071.

Shiels MS, Goedert JJ, Moore RD, et al. Reduced risk of prostate cancer in US men with AIDS. *Cancer Epidemiol Biomarkers Prev*. 2010;19(11):2910–2915.

Shiels MS, Pfeiffer RM, Engels EA. Age at cancer diagnosis among persons with AIDS in the United States. *Ann Intern Med*. 2010;153(7):452–460.

Shiels MS, Pfeiffer RM, Gail MH, et al. Cancer burden in the HIV-infected population in the United States. *J Nat Cancer Institute*. 2011;103:753–762.

Shiels MS, Pfeiffer RM, Hall HI, et al. Proportions of Kaposi sarcoma, selected non-Hodgkin lymphomas, and cervical cancer in the United States occurring in persons with AIDS, 1980–2007. *JAMA*. 2011;305(14):1450–1459.

Shiels MS, Pfeiffer RM, Hildesheim A, et al. Circulating inflammation markers and prospective risk for lung cancer. *J Nat Cancer Inst*. 2013;105(24):1871–1880.

Siegel R, DeSantis C, Jemal A. Colorectal cancer statistics, 2014. *CA Cancer J Clinicians*. 2014;64(2):104–117.

Siegel R, Naishadham D, Jemal A. Cancer statistics, 2012. *CA Cancer J Clinicians*. 2012;62(1):10–29.

Sigel C, Cavalcanti MS, Daniel T, et al. Clinicopathologic features of colorectal carcinoma in HIV-positive patients. *Cancer Epidemiol Biomarkers Prev.* 2016;25:1098–1104.

Sigel K, Crothers K, Dubrow R, et al. Prognosis in HIV-infected patients with non-small cell lung cancer. *Br J Cancer.* 2013;109:1974–1980.

Sigel K, Wisnivesky J, Crothers K, et al. Immunological and infectious risk factors for lung cancer in US veterans with HIV: a longitudinal cohort study. *Lancet HIV.* 2017;4(2):e67–e73.

Sigel K, Wisnevesky J, Gordon K, et al. HIV as an independent risk factor for incident lung cancer. *AIDS.* 2012;26;1017–1025.

Sigel K, Wisnivesky J, Shahrir S, et al. Findings in asymptomatic HIV-infected patients undergoing chest computed tomography testing: implications for lung cancer screening. *AIDS.* 2014;28(7):1007–1014.

Silverberg MJ, Chao C, Leyden WA, et al. HIV infection, immunology, viral replication, and the risk of colon cancer. *Cancer Epidemiol Biomarkers Prev.* 2011;20(12):2551–2559.

Silverberg MJ, Lau B, Achenbach CJ, et al. Cumulative incidence of cancer among persons with HIV in North America. *Ann Intern Med.* 2015;163(7):507–518.

Silverberg MJ, Lau B, Justic AC, et al. Risk of anal cancer in HIV-infected and HIV-uninfected individuals in North America. *Clin Infect Dis.* 2012;54(17):1026–1034.

Silverberg MJ, Leyden W, Steven Gregorich S, et al. Is intensive cervical cancer screening justified in immunosuppressed women? [Abstract 162] Paper presented at the Conference on Retroviruses and Opportunistic Infections (CROI), Boston, February 22–25, 2016.

Simard EP, Engels EA. Cancer as a cause of death among people with AIDS in the United States. *Clin Infect Dis.* 2010;51(8):957–962.

Simard EP, Pfeiffer RM, Engels EA. Spectrum of cancer risk late after AIDS onset in the United States. *Arch Intern Med.* 2010;170(15):1337–1345.

Simard EP, Pfeiffer RM, Engels EA. Cumulative incidence of cancer among individuals with acquired immunodeficiency syndrome in the United States. *Cancer.* 2011;117(5):1089–1096.

Skiest DJ, Crosby C. Survival is prolonged by highly active antiretroviral therapy in AIDS patients with primary central nervous system lymphoma. *AIDS.* 2003;17(12):1787–1793.

Smith DM, Kingery JD, Wong JK, et al. The prostate as a reservoir for HIV-1. *AIDS.* 2004;18(11):1600–1602.

Smith JS, Sanusi B, Swarts A, et al. A randomized clinical trial comparing cervical dysplasia treatment with cryotherapy vs loop electrosurgical excision procedure in HIV-seropositive women from Johannesburg, South Africa. *Am J Obstet Gynecol.* 2017;217(2):183.e1–183.e11.

Smith RE, Colangelo L, Wieand HS, et al. Randomized trial of adjuvant therapy in colon carcinoma: 10-Year results of NSABP Protocol C-01. *J Natl Cancer Inst.* 2004;96(15):1128–1132.

Spano JP, Massiani MA, Bentata M, et al. Lung cancer in patients with HIV infection and review of the literature. *Med Oncol.* 2004;21:109–115.

Sparano JA, Lee S, Chen MG, et al. Phase II trial of infusional cyclophosphamide, doxorubicin, and etoposide in patients with HIV-associated non-Hodgkin's lymphoma: an Eastern Cooperative Oncology Group Trial (E1494). *J Clin Oncol.* 2004;22(8):1491–1500.

Sparano JA, Lee JY, Kaplan LD, et al. Rituximab plus concurrent infusional EPOCH chemotherapy is highly effective in HIV-associated B-cell non-Hodgkin lymphoma. *Blood.* 2010;115(15):3008–3016.

Stadler RF, Gregorcyk SG, Euhus DM, et al. Outcome of HIV-infected patients with invasive squamous-cell carcinoma of the anal canal in the era of highly active antiretroviral therapy. *Dis Colon Rectum.* 2004;47(8):1305–1309.

Stebbing J, Sanitt A, Nelson M, et al. A prognostic index for AIDS-associated Kaposi's sarcoma in the era of highly active antiretroviral therapy. *Lancet.* 2006;367(9521):1495–1502.

Stebbing J, Sanitt A, Teague A, et al. Prognostic significance of immune subset measurement in individuals with AIDS-associated Kaposi's sarcoma. *J Clin Oncol.* 2007;25(16):2230–2235.

Stewart S, Jablonowski H, Goebel FD, et al. Randomized comparative trial of pegylated liposomal doxorubicin versus bleomycin and vincristine in the treatment of AIDS-related Kaposi's sarcoma: International Pegylated Liposomal Doxorubicin Study Group. *J Clin Oncol.* 1998;16(2):683–691.

Stier EA, Sebring MC, Mendez AE, et al. Prevalence of anal human papillomavirus infection and anal HPV-related disorders in women: a systematic review. *Am J Ob Gyn.* 2015;213(3):278–309.

Straus DJ, Huang J, Testa MA, et al. Prognostic factors in the treatment of human immunodeficiency virus-associated non-Hodgkin's lymphoma: analysis of AIDS Clinical Trials Group protocol 142—Low-dose versus standard-dose m-BACOD plus granulocyte-macrophage colony-stimulating factor; National Institute of Allergy and Infectious Diseases. *J Clin Oncol.* 1998;16(11):3601–3606.

Sugarman J, Lewin SR, Henrich TJ, et al. Ethics of ART interruption after stem-cell transplantation. *Lancet HIV.* 2016;3:e8–e10.

Suneja G, Shiels MS, Melville SK. Disparities in the treatment and outcomes of lung cancer among HIV-infected individuals. *AIDS.* 2013;27(3):459–468.

Swedish KA, Goldstone SE. Prevention of anal condyloma with quadrivalent human papillomavirus vaccination of older men who have sex with men. *PLoS One.* 2014;9(4):e93393.

Taieb J, Tabernero J, Mini E, et al. Oxaliplatin, fluorouracil, and leucovorin with or without cetuximab in patients with resected stage III colon cancer (PETACC-8): an open-label, randomised phase III trial. *Lancet Oncol.* 2014;15(8):862–873.

Tam HK, Zhang Z-F, Jacobson LP, et al. Effect of highly active antiretroviral therapy on survival among HIV-infected men with Kaposi sarcoma or non-Hodgkin lymphoma. *Int J Cancer.* 2002;98(6):916–922.

Tesoiero JM, Gieryic SM, Carrascal A, et al. Smoking among HIV-positive New Yorkers: prevalence, frequency, and opportunities for cessation. *AIDS Behav.* 2010;14(4):824–835.

Tornesello ML, Buonaguro FM, Beth-Giraldo E, et al. Human immunodeficiency virus type 1 tat gene enhances human papillomavirus early gene expression. *Intervirology.* 1993;36(2):57–64.

Trautmann L, Janbazian L, Chomont N, et al. Upregulation of PD-1 expression on HIV-specific CD8+ T cells leads to reversible immune dysfunction. *Nat Med.* 2006;12:1198–1202.

Travi G, Ferreri A, Cinque P, et al. Long term remission of HIV-associated primary CNS lymphoma achieved with highly active antiretroviral therapy alone. *J Clin Oncol.* 2012;30(10):e119–e121.

Uldrick TS, Wyvill KM, Kumar P, et al. Phase II trial of bevacizumab in patients with HIV-associated Kaposi's sarcoma receiving antiretroviral therapy. *J Clin Oncol.* 2012;30(13):1476–1483.

US Department of Health and Human Services (USDHHS), Panel on Opportunistic Infections in HIV-Infected Adults and Adolescents. Guidelines for the prevention and treatment of opportunistic infections in HIV-infected adults and adolescents: recommendations from the Centers for Disease Control and Prevention, the National Institutes of Health, and the HIV Medicine Association of the Infectious Diseases Society of America. Updated September 24, 2015. Available at https://aidsinfo.nih.gov/contentfiles/lvguidelines/Adult_OI.pdf. Accessed May 13, 2016.

Vallet-Pichard A, Pol S. Hepatitis viruses and human immunodeficiency virus co-infection: pathogenesis and treatment. *J Hepatol.* 2004;41(1):156–166.

Vernon SD, Hart CE, Reeves WC, et al. The HIV-1 tat protein enhances E2-dependent human papillomavirus 16 transcription. *Virus Res.* 1993;27(2):133–145.

Volberding P, Kusick P, Feigal D. Effects of chemotherapy for HIV-associated Kaposi's sarcoma on long-term survival. *Proc Am Soc Clin Oncol.* 1989;3(9):abstract 11.

Walmsley S, Northfelt DW, Melosky B, et al. Treatment of AIDS-related cutaneous Kaposi's sarcoma with topical alitretinoin (9-cis-retinoic acid) gel: Panretin Gel North American Study Group. *J AIDS.* 1999;22(3):235–246.

Wang ES, Straus DJ, Teruya-Felstein J, et al. Intensive chemotherapy with cyclophosphamide, doxorubicine, high-dose methotrexate/ifosfamide, etoposide, and high-dose cytarabine (CODOX-M/IVAC) for human immunodeficiency virus-associated Burkett lymphoma. *Cancer.* 2003;98(3):1196–1205.

Wasserberg N, Nunoo-Mensah JW, Gonzalez Ruiz C, et al. Colorectal cancer in HIV-infected patients: a case control study. *Colorectal Dis.* 2007;22(10):1217–1221.

Welch K, Finkbeiner W, Alpers CE, et al. Autopsy findings in the acquired immune deficiency syndrome. *JAMA.* 1984;252(9):1152–1159.

Westwood TD, Hogan C, Julyan PJ, et al. Utility of FDG-PETCT and magnetic resonance spectroscopy in differentiating between cerebral lymphoma and non-malignant CNS lesions in HIV-infected patients. *Eur J Radiol.* 2013;82(8):e374–e379.

Whitlock EP, Lin JS, Liles E, et al. Screening for colorectal cancer: a targeted, updated systematic review for the US Preventive Services Task Force. *Ann Intern Med.* 2008:149(9):638–658.

Wightman F, Solomon A, Kumar SS et al. Effect of ipilimumab on the HIV reservoir in an HIV-infected individual with metastatic melanoma. *AIDS.* 2015;29(4):504–506.

Wilkin TJ, Palmer S, Brudney KF, et al. Anal intraepithelial neoplasia in heterosexual and homosexual HIV-positive men with access to antiretroviral therapy. *J Infect Dis.* 2004;190(9):1685–1691.

Wilson WH, Sin-Ho J, Pitcher BN, et al. Phase III randomized study of R-CHOP versus DA-EPOCH-R and molecular analysis of untreated diffuse large B-cell lymphoma: CALGB/Alliance 50303. *Blood.* 2016;128:469.

Winstone, TA, Man SF, Hull M, et al. Epidemic of lung cancer in patients with HIV infection. *Chest.* 2013;143(2):305–314.

Wistuba IL, Behrens C, Milchgrub S, et al. Comparison of molecular changes in lung cancers in HIV-positive and HIV-indeterminate subjects. *JAMA.* 1998;279(19):1554–1559.

Wolf T, Brodt H-R, Fichtlscherer S, et al. Changing incidence and prognostic factors of survival in AIDS-related non-Hodgkin's lymphoma in the era of highly active antiretroviral therapy (HAART). *Leuk Lymphoma.* 2005;46(2):207–215.

Wolf T, Kiderlen T, Atta J, et al. Successful treatment of AIDS-associated, primary CNS lymphoma with rituximab- and methotrexate-based chemotherapy and autologous stem cell transplantation. *Infection.* 2014;42:445–447.

Woolfrey AE, Malhotra U, Harrington RD, et al. Generation of HIV-1-specific CD8+ cell responses following allogeneic hematopoietic cell transplantation. *Blood.* 2008;112(8):3484–3487.

Yegüez JF, Martinez SA, Sands DR, et al. Colorectal malignancies in HIV-positive patients. *Am Surg.* 2003;69(11):981–987.

Zanet E, Taborelli M, Rupolo M, et al. Postautologous stem cell transplantation long-term outcomes in 26 HIV-positive patients affected by relapsed/refractory lymphoma. *AIDS.* 2015;29(17):2303–2308.

Zhang JY, Zhang Z, Wang X, et al. PD-1 up-regulation is correlated with HIV-specific memory CD8+ T-cell exhaustion in typical progressors but not in long-term nonprogressors. *Blood.* 2007;109:4671–4678.

Ziegler JL, Drew WL, Miner RC, et al. Outbreak of Burkitt's-like lymphoma in homosexual men. *Lancet.* 1982;2(8299):631–633.

Ziegler JL, Templeton AC, Vogel CL. Kaposi's sarcoma: a comparison of classical, endemic, and epidemic forms. *Semin Oncol.* 1984;11(1):47–52.

35.

DERMATOLOGIC COMPLICATIONS

Kudakwashe Mutyambizi

<table>
<tr><td>

CHAPTER GOAL

Upon completion of this chapter, the reader should be able to

• Review the dermatologic complications of HIV infection and treatment.
</td></tr>
</table>

OVERVIEW OF CUTANEOUS FINDINGS IN HIV INFECTION

LEARNING OBJECTIVE

Review the approach to skin findings in the context of HIV.

WHAT'S NEW?

Multiple biopsies increase diagnostic yield for identification of cutaneous complications of HIV.

KEY POINTS

• Dermatoses that are rare in the general population but common in HIV populations should prompt testing for HIV when there is no preexisting diagnosis.

• Correct diagnosis and management of skin complaints can improve the quality of life of HIV-infected patients who have increased longevity with antiretroviral therapy (ART).

• The appearance of AIDS-defining cutaneous illnesses in previously immune reconstituted patients on ART should prompt a reassessment of CD4+ T cell count and HIV RNA levels.

• In patients who have been on ART for less than 24 weeks, the appearance or worsening of dermatoses may be due to the immune reconstitution inflammatory syndrome (IRIS).

The hallmark of HIV infection is immune dysregulation and immunosuppression. As the immune system deteriorates, inflammatory dermatoses, metabolic dysregulation, adverse drug reactions, opportunistic infections, and cutaneous malignancies become more common, atypical in presentation, and recalcitrant to therapy. Both acute and chronic skin complaints contribute significantly to reduced quality of life for HIV patients (Mirmirani, 2002).

The US Centers for Disease Control and Prevention (CDC) recommends that individuals between ages 13 and 64 years be tested for HIV at least once in their lifetime, with increased screening of high-risk individuals and testing based on symptoms. The presence of dermatoses uncommon in the general population but concentrated in the HIV population, or dermatoses strikingly recalcitrant to therapy, should warrant suspicion and testing for HIV. In patients with known HIV/AIDS, there is a correlation between CD4+ T cell count and the occurrence of characteristic dermatoses (Goldstein, 1997; Rigopoulos, 2004). Direct CD4+ T cell testing is the gold standard assessment of immune function; however, the World Health Organization's (WHO) clinical staging provides guidelines regarding skin findings that should raise suspicion for immune deterioration, thus prompting CD4+ T cell testing, and have significance in international settings in which CD4+ T cell testing is of limited availability (Baveewo, 2011; Weinberg, 2010). The occurrence of AIDS-defining illnesses such as Kaposi's sarcoma or acute systemic illnesses and infections in patients previously immunocompetent by CD4+ T cell count or previously well controlled on ART should prompt an assessment of CD4+ T cell count and HIV RNA levels to evaluate for immune deterioration. In patients who have been on ART for less than 24 weeks, acute systemic illnesses may be due to IRIS or treatment toxicity and, during this period, do not closely parallel the WHO clinical staging guidelines (Ratnam, 2006). With these caveats, the dermatoses discussed in this chapter are presented along with the corresponding CD4+ T cell count at which they typically occur (Zancanaro, 2006).

HIV practitioners can competently diagnose many of the dermatological conditions discussed in this chapter as well as perform diagnostic biopsies and minor cosmetic procedures. Busy HIV practices sometimes maintain a supply of liquid nitrogen to treat warts and an electrocautery machine known as a hyfrecator to electrodessicate lesions such as molluscum contagiosum. Referral to a dermatologist is recommended when presented with diagnostic

Table 35.1 INDICATIONS FOR REFERRAL TO A
DERMATOLOGIST

Diagnostic uncertainty
Management uncertainty
Life-threatening differential diagnoses
Rapid progression
Persistence or recurrence despite therapy
Requires specialized medications
Requires specialized procedures
Suspected skin cancer
Indications for skin cancer screening
Pigmented lesions
Improve compliance
Patient request

or management uncertainty, particularly in the acutely ill patient, with common or chronic dermatoses recalcitrant to therapies familiar to the HIV practitioner, and for optimal tissue procurement when the clinician is uncertain of appropriate biopsy site or method.

It is important for HIV practitioners to be aware that a number of serious disseminated opportunistic infections, some of which may be fatal, may first manifest as an acute cutaneous eruption. Therefore, it is important for a skin biopsy to be performed in an acutely febrile HIV/AIDS patient with a newly developed skin eruption. The biopsy should be accompanied with a request for urgent processing with special stains for bacteria, atypical mycobacteria, fungi, and viruses as appropriate. Tissue is placed in 10% formalin for routine processing, but a portion should be placed in normal saline so that cultures for microorganisms can be performed for definitive diagnosis.

In general, when sampling a lesion, especially one that is papular or pustular, an early, new lesion that is not excoriated is most likely to yield tissue with changes that afford the dermatopathologist the best opportunity to make an accurate diagnosis (Altman, 2015). A pertinent exception in this population is biopsy of suspected Kaposi's sarcoma because early lesions can present a confusing picture histologically. An older, more mature lesion, if present, will have greater diagnostic yield (Maurer, 2005). When in doubt, one should consider taking multiple biopsies from the lesion in different stages of evolution and from different cutaneous sites. If the practitioner is not comfortable performing a good skin biopsy, dermatological referral for evaluation and biopsy determination should be made. Table 35.1 provides guidelines for referral.

RECOMMENDED READING

Altman K, Vanness E, Westergaard RP. Cutaneous manifestations of human immunodeficiency virus: A clinical update. *Curr Infect Dis Rep.* 2015;17(3):464.

Mirmirani P, Maurer TA, Berger TG, et al. Skin-related quality of life in HIV-infected patients on highly active antiretroviral therapy. *J Cutan Med Surg.* 2002;6(1):10–15.

INFLAMMATORY DERMATOSES AND HIV

LEARNING OBJECTIVE

Discuss the incidence, presentation, and management of inflammatory dermatoses in HIV.

WHAT'S NEW?

Traditional immunosuppressants and biologic therapies have been used safely in controlled settings and for short courses in HIV patients with refractory psoriasis and debilitating psoriatic arthritis who are on concurrent ART.

KEY POINTS

- Initiation of ART, ultraviolet B (UVB), and oral retinoids are good initial therapies for patients with psoriatic arthritis.

- Topical tacrolimus inhibitors and UV light have both been used safely in HIV patients.

- Patients receiving systemic biologics for debilitating psoriatic arthritis should be carefully selected and closely monitored.

- Papular pruritic eruption of AIDS and HIV-associated eosinophilic pustular folliculitis are HIV/AIDS-associated dermatologic illnesses and should prompt testing for HIV in a previously undiagnosed patient.

SEBORRHEIC DERMATITIS

Seborrheic dermatitis is a common skin disorder, with a prevalence of approximately 5% in the general population. It was noted to be the most common dermatosis in HIV-infected individuals, with a prevalence of greater than 83% in HIV/AIDS populations in the pre-ART era (Sadick, 1990). Seborrheic dermatitis is seen at all clinical stages of disease. *Malassezia* species are the causative organisms. The typical presentation is of episodic variably pruritic, thin, erythematous plaques with branny or greasy yellow-white scale involving the scalp and central face, particularly the eyebrows and nasolabial folds. Scalp involvement ranges from light "dandruff" to crusted plaques. Involvement of the anterior chest and groin areas is common. HIV should be considered in rapid and exaggerated presentations with thick, extensive plaques and also in cases recalcitrant to advanced treatment regimens. The clinical differential for facial seborrheic dermatitis includes rosacea; an overlapping presentation with psoriasis called *sebopsoriasis* that is often more difficult to treat than standard seborrheic dermatitis; contact dermatitis; tinea faciei; and connective tissue disease. In tinea faciei, a potassium hydroxide (KOH) preparation can identify dermatophytes exhibiting characteristic hyphae. In contrast, seborrheic dermatitis is thought to be an inflammatory response to the commensal yeast *Malassezia* species (thus, KOH evaluation has no role), with the increased presentation in HIV/AIDS patients thought to be due to a more vigorous inflammatory response as the yeast proliferate in the setting of $CD4^+$ T cell lymphopenia (Oble, 2005; Pedrosa, 2014). Seborrheic dermatitis is a clinical diagnosis; thus, biopsy is infrequently performed. Histology reveals psoriasiform hyperplasia, neutrophilic spongiosis, perifollicular mound parakeratosis with necrotic keratinocytes, and plasma cells occasionally present in HIV-associated seborrheic dermatitis (Soeprono, 1986). First-line therapy is with topical antifungals and low-potency topical steroids. ART therapy improves seborrheic dermatitis occurring in the setting of HIV/AIDS; however, patients typically continue to experience episodic flares.

PSORIASIS

Psoriasis also presents at all clinical stages of HIV, more frequently at $CD4^+$ T cell counts of less than 350 cells/ mm^3 (Bartlett, 2007). Psoriasis has a prevalence of approximately 2% or 3% in the general population, with various series suggesting a similar or higher incidence in HIV populations (Mallon, 2000; Obuch, 1992). The prevalence of psoriatic arthritis in the general population has previously been underestimated and is now thought to be approximately 11% in the US psoriasis population, and it is concentrated in the HIV-positive psoriasis population (Dover, 1991; Gelfand, 2005). Psoriasis characteristically presents as variably pruritic, episodic, well-demarcated plaques with silvery white scale anywhere on the body but with a predilection for the scalp, elbows, lower back, gluteal folds, external genitalia, and acral sites. Preexisting psoriasis can worsen with HIV infection and immune deterioration, and psoriasis can develop de novo with HIV infection. De novo psoriasis in HIV often involves palmar plantar locations with pustules, nail dystrophy, and psoriatic arthritis that can be debilitating. Inverse psoriasis (involving intertriginous areas), generalized pustular psoriasis, and erythrodermic psoriasis also occur more frequently in HIV (Obuch, 1992). Erythrodermic psoriasis can be difficult to distinguish from other causes of erythroderma, including atopic dermatitis, drug-induced erythroderma, pityriasis rubra pilaris, Sézary syndrome, and a paraneoplastic presentation or HIV presentation; thus, it typically warrants a biopsy. Histology reveals parakeratosis, collections of neutrophils in the stratum corneum and epidermis, and a diminished granular layer. Whereas increased defensins and canthelicidins in the skin of psoriatics in the general population have been associated with their relatively low frequency of bacterial superinfection compared to other chronic dermatoses that also result in a compromised skin barrier, such as atopic dermatitis, there is an increased frequency of bacterial superinfection in HIV psoriatics (Mallon, 2000; Zheng, 2007). Theories regarding the increased incidence and severity of psoriasis in HIV include the fact that overexpression of tumor necrosis factor (TNF) occurs in both psoriasis and HIV. Furthermore, $CD4^+$ T cell depletion in HIV skews the T cell population to CD8 cells, the effector cells in psoriasis, whereas the HIV tat gene directly induces epidermal proliferation (Duvic, 1990; Kim, 1992).

In treating psoriasis, exacerbating medications should be discontinued. Of note, systemic steroids exacerbate psoriasis. Topical treatments including topical steroids, vitamin D analogues, and topical calcineurin inhibitors such as tacrolimus are first-line therapies for mild to moderate plaque psoriasis. A black box warning on tacrolimus and malignancy risk has not identified a causal relationship, and studies have shown that topical calcineurin inhibitors can be safely used in the immunosuppressed HIV population (de Moraes, 2007; Toutous-Trellu, 2005). Randomized controlled studies have not been conducted to evaluate the efficacy and safety of systemic treatments for psoriasis in the HIV setting; thus, much of the following data are derived from case reports and case series. Systemic therapies can be used in combination with each other and with topical treatments to optimized efficacy. ART can effectively treat both moderate to severe psoriasis and psoriatic arthritis, and it is a first-line treatment, as is UV light, for this severity category (Duvic, 1994; Menon, 2010; Meola, 1993). UVB is preferentially used over psoralens plus UVA (PUVA) given its more favorable side-effect profile. Although in vitro studies have shown that UVB light can activate latent HIV in chronically infected monocytes, it has not been associated with short-term changes in immune function in vivo or changes in HIV RNA levels in patients receiving concomitant suppressive ART therapy (Breuer-McHam, 1999; Meola, 1993; Stanley, 1989). Oral retinoids, particularly acitretin, are an attractive second-line therapy because they are nonimmunosuppressants with efficacy for moderate to severe psoriasis and also psoriatic arthritis. Acitretin use is limited by hypertriglyceridemia; liver function test (LFT) elevation, particularly in combination with some antiretroviral medications; and an extended 3-year teratogenicity period in women of childbearing age due to reesterification to etretinate (Dogra, 2014). Patients with refractory psoriasis or debilitating psoriatic arthritis are candidates for immunosuppressant therapies that have shown efficacy in this patient population, including low-dose methotrexate and brief courses of cyclosporine and TNF-α inhibitors. In a case report, dramatic improvement of HIV-associated psoriatic arthritis was achieved, but frequent polymicrobial infections were experienced on etanercept (Aboulafia, 2000). In summary, concomitant ART therapy, strict prophylaxis against opportunistic infections, $CD4^+$ T cell counts, monitoring of HIV RNA levels, and close clinical monitoring of rigorously selected patients are advised when treating HIV-associated psoriasis with immunosuppressant therapy.

ATOPIC DERMATITIS AND XEROSIS

The prevalence of eczema in the US adult population is estimated at 10.7%, with approximately 17% of the population experiencing at least one of four eczematous symptoms (Hanifin, 2007). An atopic dermatitis-like condition occurs frequently in HIV populations, often despite never having had a history of atopic dermatitis in childhood. One series reported that 29% of HIV/AIDS patients who attended an urban HIV clinic in the pre-ART era had this condition (Lin, 1995). This atopic dermatitis-like condition is characterized by pruritus and a spectrum of generalized scaling from xerosis to ichthyosis, with variable plaques and lichenification involving extremities and flexural areas (Singh, 2003). Often, this xerotic condition initially presents when the CD4$^+$ T cell count is still higher than 400 cells/mm^3 and is thus an early clinical sign of HIV/AIDS, typically preceding the other papulosquamous disorders. The generalized ichthyotic form typically occurs with CD4$^+$ T cell counts of less than 50 cells/mm^3 (Sadick, 1990). Decreased cellular immunity and a switch to the TH2-like cytokine profile resulting in polyclonal activation of B cells with increased IgE production are thought to contribute to the increase in atopic conditions in HIV (Nissen, 1999). In addition, nutritional deficits and autonomic nervous dysfunction causing alterations in sweating, sebaceous gland secretion, and reduction in natural moisturizing factor secretion are thought to contribute to xerosis and ichthyosis (Cockerell, 2013). Biopsy, which is not regularly performed for this diagnosis, shows variable hyperkeratosis and parakeratosis, spongiosis, and superficial perivascular lymphocytic infiltrate. The clinical differential diagnosis includes scabies, psoriasis, and contact dermatitis. For erythematous plaques, topical steroid preparations, preferably ointments, and topical calcineurin inhibitors are appropriate first-line therapies. Topical keratolytics such as urea and lactic acid formulations are useful for areas of lichenification. Widespread flares may require short courses of systemic steroids, bridging to phototherapy for sustained flares. Oral antihistamines and a dry skin care regimen of short lukewarm showers, frequent use of nonallergic emollients, and avoidance of allergens should be used in conjunction. Bacterial superinfection is common and should be managed with antibiotics.

PAPULAR PRURITIC ERUPTION OF AIDS

Papular pruritic eruption (PPE) is a markedly pruritic papulosquamous eruption characterized by symmetric crops of nonfollicular, often urticarial erythematous papules involving the extensor extremities. Excoriations and prurigo nodularis are frequently associated secondary changes due to marked pruritus in this condition. PPE is uncommon in the general adult population but has a prevalence in the HIV population of 11–46%, thus the designation *PPE of AIDS* (Eisman, 2006). It has a greater prevalence in HIV/AIDS cohorts in sub-Saharan Africa than in the United States. Among other theories, PPE is hypothesized to be due to an exaggerated response to arthropod antigens that occurs in the setting of immune dysregulation (Resneck, 2004). PPE can develop well before other symptoms and serologic diagnosis of HIV is made; however, its occurrence also correlates with lower CD4$^+$ T cell counts, and it is common in patients with CD4$^+$ T cell counts of less than 100 cells/mm^3 (Boonchai, 1999; Cockerell, 2013). The clinical differential includes eosinophilic folliculitis, which, in contrast, affects the face and upper trunk, and differentiation of active lesions of PPE from

lesions of prurigo nodularis that may also be pruritic. The diagnosis is typically made clinically based on the distribution of lesions. Early lesions without secondary changes carry the highest histologic diagnostic yield, and they may show a dense perivascular and interstitial infiltrate of lymphocytes and some eosinophils and neutrophils, which may extend deeply around adnexa and vessels, although nonspecific findings occur (Calonje, 2012). The disease has a chronic waxing and waning course and is associated with decreased quality of life due to pruritus (Hevia, 1991; Liu, 2013). Given its association with low CD4$^+$ T cell counts, initiation of ART may improve the disease, although it can also flare with immune reconstitution. UVB has been shown to decrease both papules and pruritus, and it may have greater efficacy in regimens combining other modalities including oral antihistamines, pentoxifylline, topical steroids, topical tacrolimus, and topical anti-itch preparations (Bellavista, 2013). Reducing exposure to bites by wearing clothing that covers skin and application of insect repellant is also recommended.

HIV-ASSOCIATED EOSINOPHILIC PUSTULAR FOLLICULITIS

Eosinophilic pustular folliculitis (Ofugi's disease) is rare in the general adult population but common in the HIV/AIDS population, particularly once the CD4$^+$ T cell count declines below 250 cells/mm^3. HIV-associated eosinophilic folliculitis is characterized by persistent, markedly pruritic erythematous, mostly follicular papules and occasional pustules on the face, trunk, and upper extremities. Urticarial plaques and nonfollicular erythematous papules are also described. Peripheral eosinophilia can also be common along with elevated IgE levels (Rosenthal, 1991). It is thought to be an exaggerated cutaneous reaction to *Malassezia* yeast or other microorganisms colonizing the follicular infundibulum and reflects TH1/2 immune dysregulation. Recently, CD163$^+$ macrophages have been implicated in the pathogenesis (Okada, 2013). Additional theories include autoimmune activation against antigens in sebocytes in HIV-positive individuals (Fearfield, 1999). The clinical differential includes PPE as well as acne, molluscum, and drug reactions. Biopsy may be useful, with erythematous nonexcoriated follicular lesions carrying the highest diagnostic yield. Spongiosis involving the follicular epithelium and intra- and perifollicular mixed infiltrate is typically seen, with eosinophilic abscess formation in long-standing lesions. Treatment is often difficult, with pruritus contributing to reduced quality of life. Phototherapy (UVB or UVA), oral antihistamines, itraconazole, isotretinoin, and metronidazole are all reported treatments; however, no controlled clinical trials have been performed. First-line therapy with UVB phototherapy, topical steroids, and oral antihistamines is suggested.

RECOMMENDED READING

Cockerell CC, Calame A. *Cutaneous manifestations of HIV disease.* London, UK: Manson; 2013.

Toutous-Trellu L, Abraham S, Pechere M, et al. Topical tacrolimus for effective treatment of eosinophilic folliculitis associated with human immunodeficiency virus infection. *Arch Dermatol.* 2005;141(10):1203–1208.

HIV DRUG REACTIONS AND INTERACTIONS

LEARNING OBJECTIVE

Describe common or important cutaneous adverse drug reactions, and pertinent factors in their management, in the HIV population.

WHAT'S NEW?

In recent years, several adverse drug reactions to ART medications have been identified that were not observed or were underrepresented in preapproval trials.

KEY POINTS

- Non-nucleoside reverse transcriptase inhibitors (NNRTIs) are the most common antiretroviral drugs that cause morbilliform skin eruptions.

- Abacavir hypersensitivity reaction can be fatal, and predisposed patients can be identified by testing for the HLA-B5701 allele prior to commencing abacavir therapy.

- The injectable fillers poly-l-lactic acid and calcium hydroxyapatite are approved for facial fat loss treatment in HIV.

- Ritonavir, a CYP34A inhibitor often used to boost other antiretroviral drugs, increases the levels of corticosteroids, which can result in hypothalamic–pituitary–adrenal (HPA) axis dysfunction and Cushing's syndrome.

The incidence of medication-related skin rashes in the HIV-positive population is approximately 50% (Davis, 2008). Drug hypersensitivity reactions are classified into two categories: those secondary to ART regimens and those secondary to other medications taken by HIV-positive patients. Since its inception, ART has revolutionized the management of HIV/AIDS, with new drug classes and single-tablet combination formulations designed to decrease pill burden now available. However, antiretroviral drugs have been complicated by adverse drug reactions, including reactions that may not have been recognized or underrepresented in preapproval clinical trials (Introcaso, 2010). Thus, recognition of known and identification of previously unreported drug reactions are extremely important in the management of antiretroviral-related drug hypersensitivity reactions. It can be a particular challenge to differentiate between drug hypersensitivity reactions, IRIS, and worsening HIV infection when patients are commencing ART. Some of the adverse drug reactions are mediated through genetic and immunologic factors via the major histocompatibility complex (Chaponda, 2011). IgE levels increase with progression of HIV, and altered cytokine profiles are also believed to play a role (Davis, 2008). Immune dysregulation in HIV is also thought to make HIV patients more susceptible to non-ART medications. In addition, antiretroviral drugs can result in alterations in metabolism of other medications, particularly through the cytochrome P450 pathway, thus increasing their toxicity.

NON-NUCLEASE REVERSE TRANSCRIPTASE INHIBITORS

NNRTIs are the most common antiretroviral agents to cause morbilliform skin eruptions, which are usually distributed over the face, trunk, and extremities. In particular, nevirapine is well known for its ability to cause rash, particularly within the first 6 weeks of use. According to the manufacturer, 13% of patients taking nevirapine develop some degree of morbilliform eruption during early treatment; this has been reported to be as high as 28% in some populations in practice (Introcaso, 2010). Many patients with mild or moderate rash can continue therapy with close monitoring, and the rash will spontaneously resolve. Severe rash is seen in at least 8% of patients, and development of concomitant hepatitis in the drug hypersensitivity syndrome is an indication for immediate discontinuation of nevirapine given the potential for fatal hepatitis. Risk factors for the development of morbilliform eruption with the use of nevirapine include higher $CD4^+$ T cell count (>250 cells/mm^3 in women and >400 cells/mm^3 in men), lower HIV-1 RNA levels, Chinese ethnicity, and female gender (Davis, 2008). In addition, nevirapine can cause the mucocutaneous Stevens–Johnson syndrome at a rate of 0.5–1%, although patients with $CD4^+$ T cell counts of less than 200 cells/mm^3 (i.e., with AIDS) have a 1,000-fold higher risk (Warren, 1998). The incidence may be higher in sub-Saharan Africa, where nevirapine is more commonly used in antiretroviral regimens. Stevens–Johnson syndrome is characterized by flat, atypical targets or pruritic papules that are widespread or distributed on the trunk first and then spread to the neck, face, and proximal upper extremities. The palms and soles may be an early site of involvement. Bullae developing on the conjunctivae and mucous membranes of the nares, mouth, anorectal junction, vulvovaginal region, and urethral meatus are characteristic, with toxic epidermal necrolysis diagnosed when there is more than 30% body surface area skin detachment (Bolognia, 2012). In several studies, the use of prednisone and/or a 2-week lead-in dose of nevirapine 200 mg once daily failed to decrease the occurrence of the nevirapine-associated rash (Knobel, 2001). A dose escalation protocol is now recommended starting with nevirapine 200 mg/d for 2 weeks, followed by an increase to the standard 400 mg/d dose only if there is no rash or no worsening rash after the trial 2-week period (Anton, 1999).

NUCLEOSIDE REVERSE TRANSCRIPTASE INHIBITOR

Abacavir, a nucleoside reverse transcriptase inhibitor, can cause a well-documented, multiorgan, potentially life-threatening hypersensitivity reaction. This abacavir hypersensitivity reaction (AHR) is seen in 5–8% of HIV-positive patients on treatment. Symptoms consist of fever, rash, malaise, fatigue, tachypnea, pharyngitis, cough, wheezing, nausea, vomiting, and diarrhea that commence 9–11 days after initiating therapy. Symptoms that become worse with each subsequent dose are a classic characteristic of AHR. Symptoms of AHR recur within 24 hours of rechallenge and can be fatal. Therefore, the use of abacavir in any person suspected to have AHR is contraindicated. Pre-ART genetic testing has shown that the absence of the HLA-B5701 allele dramatically decreases (by 99.9%) the likelihood of developing abacavir hypersensitivity (Mallal, 2008). For this reason, the ART guidelines of both the US Department of Health and Human Services and the International Antiviral Society–USA recommend obtaining this test prior to initiation of any abacavir-containing regimen.

PROTEASE INHIBITORS

The protease inhibitors (PIs) are generally associated with lipodystrophy, abnormal fat distribution, and central adiposity, which can be an indication for discontinuation. The injectable fillers poly-l-lactic acid and calcium hydroxyapatite are approved for facial fat loss treatment in HIV (Jagdeo, 2015). Indinavir has the greatest variety of cutaneous side effects among PIs, including acute porphyria, Stevens–Johnson syndrome, hypersensitivity syndrome, morbilliform drug eruptions, gynecomastia, alopecia, pyogenic granuloma-like lesions, and paronychia (Ward, 2002). Ritonavir is a CYP34A inhibitor, and, through this mechanism, it decreases clearance of corticosteroids, thus increasing their levels and the risk of HPA axis dysfunction and Cushing's syndrome (Hyle, 2013). This should be considered when prescribing topical steroids for application to a large body surface area and systemic steroids for longer courses.

OTHER ANTIRETROVIRAL THERAPIES

Few other antiretroviral drugs have a strong association with severe adverse drug reactions. Approximately 6% of persons taking atazanavir, a PI, have reported typically mild rash not requiring treatment cessation. A hypersensitivity to the fusion inhibitor enfuvirtide has been seen in fewer than 1% of persons taking it. However, 98% of users experience injection site reactions, which are frequently symptomatic (Ball, 2003). The enfuvirtide injection site reaction is characterized by tender erythema, induration, and nodule or cyst formation. On histology, a palisaded granulomatous response may be seen, with multinucleated cells aggregated around altered collagen, and surrounding eosinophils, histiocytes, lymphocytes, plasma cells, and variable fibrosis. Recently, the package insert for raltegravir, an integrase inhibitor, was updated to include dermatological side effects including Stevens–Johnson syndrome and toxic epidermal necrolysis.

ANTIBIOTICS

Antibiotic drug reactions appear at a higher rate in HIV-positive patients than in the general population.

Trimethoprim–sulfamethoxazole is a commonly used antibiotic in HIV, especially for the prophylaxis of *Pneumocystis jirovecii* pneumonia (PCP). Given its importance in the prevention of PCP pneumonia, a desensitization schedule has been developed for those patients who have had reactions in the past and would benefit from its use. Desensitization has been successful using the following dosing schedule: an initial dose of trimethoprim 0.4 mg and sulfamethoxazole 2 mg, followed by doubling the dose daily over days 2–9 and at 10 days administering the full-strength dose (trimethoprim 160 mg/sulfamethoxazole 800 mg) (Gompels, 1999).

RECOMMENDED READING

Hyle EP, Wood BR, Backman ES, et al. High frequency of hypothalamic–pituitary–adrenal axis dysfunction after local corticosteroid injection in HIV-infected patients on protease inhibitor therapy. *J AIDS*. 2013;63(5):602–608.

Introcaso CE, Hines JM, Kovarik CL. (2010). Cutaneous toxicities of antiretroviral therapy for HIV: part II. Nonnucleoside reverse transcriptase inhibitors, entry and fusion inhibitors, integrase inhibitors, and immune reconstitution syndrome. *J Am Acad Dermatol*. 2010;63(4):563–569; quiz 569–570.

CUTANEOUS OPPORTUNISTIC INFECTIONS

LEARNING OBJECTIVE

Discuss the diagnosis and management of viral, fungal, bacterial, and parasitic opportunistic infections occurring in HIV patients.

WHAT'S NEW?

In 2014, the US Food and Drug Administration (FDA) approved the topical agents efinaconazole and tavorabole, which show some efficacy for the treatment of onychomycosis.

KEY POINTS

- Cutaneous *Cryptococcus* may manifest before systemic symptoms; therefore, prompt diagnosis and management can prevent fatal outcomes.

- Molluscum, histoplasmosis, and *Cryptococcus* may all present with umbilicated papulonodules; however, there is a central white core to the molluscum lesion, and patients are well as opposed to systemically ill with cryptococcal infection.

- Postherpetic neuralgia is very common in HIV patients who develop herpes zoster, and initiation of Neurontin along with antiviral therapy at diagnosis may mitigate neuralgia.

- The prozone effect may result in a false-negative syphilis test in HIV patients, and dilution of the assay should be requested when syphilis is suspected.

- The CDC now recommends an intensive regimen for the management of crusted scabies as follows: ivermectin dosed at 200 μg/kg taken on days 1, 2, 8, 9, and 15, and, for severe disease, also days 22 and 29, in combination with topical permethrin daily for 7 days and then twice a week until cure.

ONYCHOMYCOSIS

Onychomycosis is reported to affect approximately 2–13% of the general population (Rosen, 2015) and is very common in the HIV-positive population. Dermatophytes *Trichophyton mentagrophytes* and *T. rubrum* are responsible for most infections. Proximal subungual onychomycosis is a pattern seen commonly in HIV-positive patients, especially those with a $CD4^+$ T cell count of less than 450 cells/mm^3, and although it is not considered an AIDS-defining condition, it should prompt testing for HIV infection if not already determined. *T. rubrum* is usually the causative dermatophyte for this pattern, although it can also be caused by *T. megninii*. Superficial white onychomycosis, for example, is typically caused by *T. mentagrophytes* in the general population, whereas it is typically caused by *T. rubrum* in the HIV population. The clinical differential includes psoriasis, lichen planus, trauma, and periungual squamous cell carcinoma. Most topical antifungals do not penetrate the thick nail keratin and thus are ineffective. Efinaconazole is a topical triazole solution recently released on the market for the treatment of onychomycosis; it is applied daily for 48 weeks to affected nails. Localized dermatitis is a potential side effect. In preapproval trials, 15.2–17.8% of patients achieved complete cure of onychomycosis. Tavorabole, a boron-based agent that was FDA approved for onychomycosis in 2014, had even lower efficacy, with 6.5–9.1% of patients achieving clearance (Zeichner, 2015). Terbinafine is considered first-line systemic therapy, dosed at 250 mg/d for 3 or 4 months for toenails and 6 weeks for fingernails (~50% cure rate). Itraconazole may also be effective at 200 mg/d for 3 months for toenails and 6 weeks for fingernails or at 200 mg twice daily for 1 week per month for 3 months for toenails and 2 months for fingernails. The efficacy of fluconazole is lower than that of terbinafine and itraconazole. Patients with active liver disease should not receive terbinafine, and testing of LFTs at baseline and every 4–6 weeks is recommended given the risk of hepatotoxicity. Congestive heart disease is a contraindication to itraconazole use. In addition, itraconazole interacts with more medications compared to terbinafine (de Berker, 2009). Finally, the causative agent may differ between the general population and HIV-infected populations, which is relevant when selecting therapy. For example, nondermatophyte molds, such as *Scytalidium*, *Aspergillus*, and *Fusarium*, and yeast such as *Candida* are implicated in onychomycosis in HIV patients more often than in the general public. Much higher cure rates are achieved with itraconazole than with terbinafine for these organisms, whereas the reverse is true for dermatophytes (Cambuim, 2011; Warshaw, 2005). For these reasons, and given the potential side effects of systemic therapies, culture of nail clippings involved with onychomycosis is recommended before initiation of therapy by some dermatologists.

CANDIDIASIS

Angular cheilitis is typically caused by *Candida albicans* and presents as fissured white plaques at the angles of the lips. It occurs with some frequency in the elderly, but it may suggest HIV infection in young adults and may warrant testing if there is no other known reason for immunosuppression. Topical antifungal creams are effective and avoid systemic circulation for this focal disease. Associated burning and dysphagia suggest oral candidiasis, with atrophic or removable yellow white pseudomembranous or hyperplastic plaques typically seen on the tongue or dorsal palate. Oral candidiasis is often a harbinger of immunologic failure in patients on ART, although it can also be caused by steroids and antibiotics (Cockerell, 2013). Nystatin or clotrimazole troches, and oral antifungals such as fluconazole or ketoconazole when there is associated odynophagia, are effective. Ketoconazole should be taken with food and should be avoided in the setting of malabsorption given the risk of treatment failure.

Candida intertrigo is common in HIV-infected populations, and it can appear as eroded glistening erythematous plaques or as pustules with scale over a macerated erythematous surface within and extending from skin folds. Treatment with oral fluconazole or ketoconazole for larger or extensive plaques is suggested over topical antifungals.

CUTANEOUS CRYPTOCOCCOSIS

Cryptococcus neoformans causes a systemic infection in which there is skin involvement in 10% of cases. It is an AIDS-defining illness, with skin involvement preceding the more common central nervous system and pulmonary involvement in 10% of cases. The patient is typically febrile and very ill. Skin lesions can present as papules that may be umbilicated, nodules, pustules, ulcers, and plaques. A skin biopsy is necessary for diagnosis, revealing round yeast with narrow-based budding and a slimy capsule in a granulomatous or gelatinous background, highlighted by fungal stains. Culture is definitively diagnostic, and treatment is with amphotericin B or fluconazole; adjunctive flucytosine can also be used (Cockerell, 2013). ART has decreased the incidence of cryptococcal infection; however, institution of ART in patients with cryptococcal infection can result in fatal IRIS (Lortholary, 2005). Relapses are not uncommon, and secondary prophylaxis with fluconazole 200–400 mg/d for patients with $CD4^+$ T cell counts of less than 200 cells/mm^3 is recommended.

CUTANEOUS HISTOPLASMOSIS

Histoplasmosis manifests with cutaneous lesion secondary to pulmonary or disseminated disease; primary manifestation is rare. The rash is nonspecific, characterized by diffuse erythematous macules, papules that may be umbilicated, pustules, crusted ulcers, or psoriasisform papules. The face is most often involved, followed by truncal and extremity involvement (Cockerell, 2013). The clinical differential diagnosis includes molluscum contagiosum and cryptococcosis. HIV patients with cutaneous histoplasmosis may be well appearing on initial presentation; however, prompt diagnosis is important because they can rapidly and fatally decompensate with systemic involvement (Wheat, 1990). Diagnosis of cutaneous histoplasmosis requires tissue biopsy, which reveals spores with a pseudo-capsule (the fungal wall) parasitizing macrophages. Culture confirms the diagnosis. Mild infection in the general public is self-limiting and may not require treatment; however, treatment is indicated in HIV patients. Treating systemic disease also treats skin involvement and is typically done with itraconazole; amphotericin is reserved for meningitis or other disseminated infection (Hage, 2015). Similar to cryptococcosis, relapses can occur, and secondary prophylaxis with itraconazole in AIDS patients is advised.

MOLLUSCUM CONTAGIOSUM

Molluscum is a common viral infection in children and their caregivers, but it warrants testing for HIV in adults with limited exposure to children. Skin-colored discrete umbilicated papules are typical, although giant facial molluscum and extensive beard involvement occur with advanced immunosuppression. Giant molluscum can persist even after immune reconstitution; it is extremely difficult to treat and is stigmatizing. Molluscum is differentiated from cryptococcosis and histoplasmosis, which can also have umbilicated papules by the presence of a central core in molluscum lesions. Also, patients appear well with molluscum infection, whereas they are systemically ill with cryptococcal infection. Treatment options include cryotherapy for smaller lesions and curettage and excision for larger lesions. Topical imiquimod, cidofovir, and photodynamic therapy with 5-aminolevulinic acid have all shown efficacy in case reports (Drain, 2014; Foissac, 2014).

CONDYLOMA ACUMINATUM

Condyloma acuminatum (anogenital warts), which is caused by the human papillomavirus (HPV), is the most common sexually transmitted infection in the United States. Warts appear as flesh-colored to gray, rounded to pointy papules, frequently on a short peduncle. Podophyllin, trichloroacetic acid, and cryotherapy are three of the most commonly used treatments for genital warts. Cryotherapy and trichloroacetic acid yield a treatment success rate of 75%, whereas that of podophyllin is reported to be 20–50% (Murray, 2015). Therapies for recalcitrant anogenital warts include topical 5-fluoracil, cidofovir, intralesional interferon-α, and surgical excision (Nambudiri, 2013). Approximately 5% of men who have sex with men (MSM) and 15% of HIV-positive MSM have a history of perianal warts. Anogenital warts are more common in women, and HIV-infected women are five times more likely than their noninfected counterparts to have these warts (Hagensee, 2004). In addition, squamous epithelial lesions occur in 79% of HIV-positive women with anal HPV infection compared to 43% of HIV-negative women. The frequency of intraepithelial neoplasia within anogenital warts is higher than previously realized, warranting aggressive surveillance and treatment (McCloskey, 2007).

HERPES SIMPLEX

Herpes simplex virus (HSV) infection is caused by either HSV-1 or HSV-2 and is a common viral infection in the general population. It presents as grouped vesicles on an erythematous base. In HIV-positive patients, the infections occur more frequently and are less likely to self-resolve. When CD4+ T cells decrease below 100 cells/mm^3, the incidence of HSV outbreaks reaches 27% (Severson, 1999). Recommended treatment for an HIV-positive patient with recurrent herpes infection is valacyclovir 1 g twice daily for 5–10 days or acyclovir 200 mg five times a day for the same period. Acyclovir-resistant HSV has become a problem in patients with AIDS. Reported acyclovir resistance in HIV-positive patients is 10-fold higher than that in immunocompetent counterparts—0.6% and 6%, respectively (Lolis, 2008). Resistance to acyclovir also implies resistance to valacyclovir, and, in many cases, famciclovir is also not an effective treatment. Treatment of choice for acyclovir-resistant HSV is intravenous foscarnet or cidofovir. Topical cidofovir and foscarnet have been used as successful treatments as well (Strick, 2006).

HERPES ZOSTER

Herpes zoster, also known as shingles, is caused by the reactivation of varicella zoster virus (VZV), which also causes chickenpox. Ten to twenty percent of adults are affected by shingles. As T cell immunity wanes, with age or immunosuppression, the incidence of infection increases. Therefore, herpes zoster is very common with HIV infection, and it may be the presenting manifestation. In immunocompetent patients, the infection is usually limited to one dermatome. Pain, constitutional symptoms of fever, malaise, and headache may precede the eruptive phase, which consists of clusters of vesicles on an erythematous base within a dermatome. Involvement of multiple dermatomes is common in HIV-positive individuals, and disseminated infection is frequent. Treatment is with acyclovir 800 mg/d for 7–10 days, valacyclovir 1 g three times a day, or acyclovir 10 mg/kg when intravenous treatment is warranted. Foscarnet 40 mg/kg three times a day is used for treatment of acyclovir-resistant VZV (Cockerell, 2013). Continual pain, referred to as postherpetic neuralgia (PHN), can occur and can last months to years. Immunocompromised patients are at a higher risk of developing PHN, and initiation of gabapentin at presentation along with antivirals should be considered. Varicella vaccine is recommended in adults without varicella immunity and CD4+ T cell counts of more than 200 cells/mm^3. Zoster vaccine should be avoided in HIV-infected patients with AIDS or manifestations of HIV and CD4+ T cell counts of less than 200 cells/mm^3 or CD4+ T cell T lymphocytes 15% or less (CDC, Advisory Committee on Immunization Practices).

METHICILLIN-RESISTANT
STAPHYLOCOCCUS AUREUS

Staphylococcus aureus has acquired the mecA gene, which makes it less sensitive to many of the antibiotics typically used to treat skin and soft tissue infections. Methicillin-resistant *S. aureus* (MRSA) has grown to epidemic proportions during approximately the past decade. There is a higher rate of MRSA infection in the HIV-positive population. One study reported that the prevalence was 18 times higher in the HIV population compared to the general population (Crum-Cianflone, 2007).

Incision and drainage is the most important component of treatment for localized skin infections. Many cutaneous MRSA infections are generally sensitive to the antibiotics trimethoprim–sulfamethoxazole, doxycycline, clindamycin, and linezolid. These antibiotics are generally effective against MRSA, and culture and sensitivity data are helpful in guiding treatment.

Both skin and nasal colonization are potential reservoirs for reinfection. Studies have indicated that mupirocin can be used to eradicate nasal colonization, whereas chlorhexidine can be used for the skin (Kuehnert, 2006).

BACILLARY ANGIOMATOSIS

This infectious disease occurs rarely in HIV-infected patients, but awareness of bacillary angiomatosis (BA) is important because it is a clinical mimicker of Kaposi's sarcoma (KS) that can be treated effectively with erythromycin 500 mg four times a day; it is potentially systemic and fatal if untreated. Clinically, purple "grape-like" papules to nodules are seen in a focal or widespread distribution. In contrast to KS, they only rarely manifest as patches or plaques. BA can be distinguished from KS on histology, with a lobular capillary proliferation with an edematous stroma and clusters of neutrophils seen throughout the lesion (Cockerell, 2013). There is often an amorphous material that represents colonies of bacteria, and culture for *Bartonella* speciation has relevance given that *Bartonella quintana* is more frequently associated with neurologic sequelae compared to *B. henselae* (Gasquet, 1998).

SYPHILIS

Primary syphilis typically presents with an asymptomatic orogenital ulcer, whereas secondary syphilis is typically papulosquamous to psoriasiform but can mimic many other dermatoses. The color is characteristic, resembling a "clean-cut ham" or having a coppery tint. Palms and soles may present with classic coppery-colored scaly plaques. Temporal, irregular, "moth-eaten" alopecia of the beard, scalp, and eyebrows may occur. Of concern, syphilis has an accelerated rate of progression in HIV, with potential development of neurosyphilis, and can have atypical presentations including multiple chancres and syphilitic vasculitis. Diagnosis can be complicated by the prozone effect, in which a false-negative rapid plasma reagin or Venereal Disease Research Laboratory test is achieved due to overwhelming antibody titers interfering with formation of antigen antibody lattice network in the test.

Dilution of the assay overcomes this false-negative result, and this should be requested when syphilis is suspected and there is a negative result (Smith, 2004). Treatment is with penicillin formulations, and better response with decreased progression to neurosyphilis has been noted in HIV patients on ART (Ghanem, 2007).

SCABIES

Scabies is caused by an infestation of the skin by the *Sarcoptes scabiei* mite. The first symptom of scabies is usually pruritus, especially at night. Scabies is a very common infection, with an approximate prevalence of 300 million annual cases (CDC, 2006). Scabies mites cannot jump or fly and therefore require skin-to-skin contact for infection to occur. Scabies mites have not demonstrated the ability to transmit HIV. Diagnosis is made through clinical examination. Burrow scrapings can be examined under a microscope for scabies mites, eggs, and feces; however, the absence of these on microscopic evaluated does not eliminate the possibility of infection. Recently, dermoscopy has been shown to be a valuable tool in the diagnosis of scabies, with a characteristic "delta wing jet" appearance of burrows identified on dermoscopy (Suh, 2014).

"Norwegian" or "crusted" scabies is a more florid infection leading to crusted burrows. These crusted lesions typically occur in the web spaces of the hands and feet, over the elbows, and on the ears or temples. This typically occurs in immunocompromised patients, including HIV-infected patients with low CD4+ T cell counts. Norwegian scabies are much more infectious and can be easily spread to healthcare workers by skin-to-skin contact.

Per CDC guidelines, first-line treatment of scabies is either topical permethrin cream or oral ivermectin (Workowski, 2015). Permethrin cream is applied below the neck (and above the neck if lesions are evident) and washed off after 8–14 hours on days 1 and 14, or ivermectin 200 µg/kg is given on days 1 and 14. The updated CDC recommendation for treatment of crusted scabies to avoid treatment failure is an intensive regimen of ivermectin dosed at 200 µg/kg taken on days 1, 2, 8, 9, and 15, and, for severe disease, also days 22 and 29, in combination with topical permethrin daily for 7 days and then twice a week until cure (Ortega-Loayza, 2013). Compliance may be a challenge.

AMOEBA

Naegleria fowleri, Balamuthia mandrillaris, and *Acanthamoeba* are free-living protozoa that cause a rapidly progressive fatal infection in the immunocompromised. *Acanthamoeba* is a recognized pathogen in immunocompromised patients and has been cultured from the cornea, nasal and sinus cavities, ears, throat, lungs, and skin. *Acanthamoeba* can infect the skin directly or can spread to the skin by hematogenous dissemination from primary foci in the lungs or sinuses (Chandrasekar, 1997). More frequent sites of cutaneous involvement include the face, trunk, and extremities. The lesions typically present as nonspecific necrotic ulcers or nodules that may be quite tender or asymptomatic. Evaluations should include biopsy with histology showing trophozoites and culture for speciation. The survival rate is poor. Optimal treatment has not been determined; thus, combination therapy is recommended with miltefosine, fluconazole, and pentamidine. Trimethoprim–sulfamethoxazole, metronidazole, and a macrolide can be added to this regime in patients failing therapy (Mayer, 2011).

RECOMMENDED READING

Drain PK, Mosam A, Gounder L, et al. Recurrent giant molluscum contagiosum immune reconstitution inflammatory syndrome (IRIS) after initiation of antiretroviral therapy in an HIV-infected man. *Int J STD AIDS*. 2014;25(3):235–238.

McCloskey JC, Metcalf C, French MA, et al. The frequency of high-grade intraepithelial neoplasia in anal/perianal warts is higher than previously recognized. *Int J STD AIDS*. 2007;18(8):538–542.

Smith G, Holman RP. The prozone phenomenon with syphilis and HIV-1 co-infection. *South Med J*. 2004;97(4):379–382.

CUTANEOUS MALIGNANCIES IN HIV

LEARNING OBJECTIVE

Review the status of cutaneous malignancies in HIV patients.

WHAT'S NEW?

As life expectancy of HIV-positive patients has increased, cancers have become a more prevalent cause of morbidity and mortality.

KEY POINTS

- In the United States, first-line treatment for HIV-associated KS remains antiretroviral therapy, with chemotherapy indicated for progressive cutaneous disease or visceral involvement and radiation therapy for bulky obstructive tumors.

- There is an increased risk of metastatic disease in HIV patients with invasive melanoma, with worse outcomes associated with lower CD4+ T cell counts.

- There is a three- to fivefold increased risk of developing nonmelanoma skin cancer in HIV, and basal and squamous cell cancers are more aggressive in HIV patients.

KAPOSI'S SARCOMA

Prior to the HIV epidemic, KS was rare in the United States. It was seen mostly in elderly men from the Mediterranean or recipients of solid organ transplants. The increasing prevalence of KS in the early HIV years led to the discovery of human herpesvirus-8 (HHV-8), the causative agent of KS. Mucocutaneous violaceous patches, plaques, or nodules may be seen, with biopsy revealing a vascular proliferation on histology with confirmatory HHV-8 immunostaining. First-line treatment for HIV-associated KS is ART. IRIS can result in KS progression during the initiation of ART, and patients on ART can still develop KS (Krown, 2008). Chemotherapy is indicated for rapidly progressive cutaneous KS and when there is visceral involvement; radiation may be helpful when bulky plaques cause pain or lymphatic blockage (Murphy, 1997). There have been reports of HHV-8 reactivation and development of KS in patients exposed to topical and systemic steroids (Boudhir, 2013).

MELANOMA AND NONMELANOMA SKIN CANCERS

The non–AIDS-defining skin cancers in HIV include basal cell cancers, squamous cell cancers, and melanomas. Case reports suggest an increased incidence of melanoma in HIV patients (Wilkins, 2006). In addition, HIV patients are more likely to develop metastases with invasive melanoma, and lower CD4+ T cell count is predictive of worse prognosis (Rodrigues, 2002). Screening guidelines are the same as those for the general population. In addition, there is a three- to fivefold increased risk of developing nonmelanoma skin cancer in HIV. Basal cell carcinomas are more common than squamous cell carcinomas (SCCs), as is the case in the general population but in contrast to immunocompromised transplant patients, in whom SCCs are more common. Both basal cell carcinomas and SCCs are more aggressive in the HIV population (Wilkins, 2006).

ACKNOWLEDGMENTS

The author acknowledges John M. Curtain, PA-C, MPH, the author of this chapter in the previous edition.

RECOMMENDED READING

Wilkins K, Turner R, Dolev JC, et al. Cutaneous malignancy and human immunodeficiency virus disease. *J Am Acad Dermatol*. 2006;54(2):189–206; quiz 207–110.

REFERENCES

Aboulafia D M, Bundow D, Wilske K, Ochs UI. Etanercept for the treatment of human immunodeficiency virus-associated psoriatic arthritis. *Mayo Clin Proc*. 2000;75(10):1093–1098.

Altman K, Vanness E, Westergaard RP. Cutaneous manifestations of human immunodeficiency virus: a clinical update. *Curr Infect Dis Rep*. 2015;17(3):464.

Anton P, Soriano V, Jimenez-Nacher I, et al. Incidence of rash and discontinuation of nevirapine using two different escalating initial doses. *AIDS*. 1999;13(4):524–525.

Ball RA, Kinchelow T, ISR Substudy Group. Injection site reactions with the HIV-1 fusion inhibitor enfuvirtide. *J Am Acad Dermatol*. 2003;49(5):826–831.

Bartlett BL, Khambaty M, Mendoza N, et al. Dermatological management of human immunodeficiency virus (HIV). *Skin Therapy Lett*. 2007;12(8):1–3.

Baveewo S, Ssali F, Karamagi C, et al. Validation of World Health Organisation HIV/AIDS clinical staging in predicting initiation of antiretroviral therapy and clinical predictors of low CD4+ T cell count in Uganda. *PLoS One.* 2011;6(5):e19089.

Bellavista S, D'Antuono A, Infusino SD, Trimarco R, Patrizi A. Pruritic papular eruption in HIV: a case successfully treated with NB-UVB. *Dermatol Ther.* 2013;26(2):173–175.

Bolognia JL, Jorizzo JL, Schaffer J. *Dermatology.* 3rd ed. New York: Elsevier; 2012.

Boonchai W, Laohasrisakul R, Manonukul J, Kulthanan K. Pruritic papular eruption in HIV seropositive patients: a cutaneous marker for immunosuppression. *Int J Dermatol.* 1999;38(5):348–350.

Boudhir H, Mael-Ainin M, Senouci K, et al. [Kaposi's disease: an unusual side-effect of topical corticosteroids]. *Ann Dermatol Venereol.* 2013;140(6–7):459–461.

Breuer-McHam J, Marshall G, Adu-Oppong A, et al. Alterations in HIV expression in AIDS patients with psoriasis or pruritus treated with phototherapy. *J Am Acad Dermatol.* 1999;40(1):48–60.

Calonje E, Brenn T, Lazar A, Mckee P. *McKee's pathology of the skin* (4th ed.). St. Louis, MO: Saunders; 2012:901.

Cambuim II, Macedo DP, Delgado M, et al. Clinical and mycological evaluation of onychomycosis among Brazilian HIV/AIDS patients [in Portuguese]. *Rev Soc Bras Med Trop.* 2011;44(1):40–42.

Chandrasekar PH, Nandi PS, Fairfax MR, Crane LR. Cutaneous infections due to *Acanthamoeba* in patients with acquired immunodeficiency syndrome. *Arch Intern Med.* 1997;157(5):569–572.

Chaponda M, Pirmohamed M. Hypersensitivity reactions to HIV therapy. *Br J Clin Pharmacol.* 2011;71(5):659–671.

Cockerell C, Calame A. *Cutaneous manifestations of HIV disease.* London: Manson; 2013.

Crum-Cianflone NF, Burgi AA, Hale BR. Increasing rates of community-acquired methicillin-resistant *Staphylococcus aureus* infections among HIV-infected persons. *Int J STD AIDS.* 2007;18(8):521–526.

Davis CM, Shearer WT. Diagnosis and management of HIV drug hypersensitivity. *J Allergy Clin Immunol.* 2008;121(4):826–832, e825.

de Berker D. Clinical practice: fungal nail disease. *N Engl J Med.* 2009;360(20):2108–2116.

de Moraes AP, de Arruda EA, Vitoriano MA, et al. An open-label efficacy pilot study with pimecrolimus cream 1% in adults with facial seborrhoeic dermatitis infected with HIV. *J Eur Acad Dermatol Venereol.* 2007;21(5):596–601.

Dogra S, Yadav S. Acitretin in psoriasis: an evolving scenario. *Int J Dermatol.* 2014; 53(5):525–538.

Dover JS, Johnson RA. Cutaneous manifestations of human immunodeficiency virus infection: part II. *Arch Dermatol.* 1991;127(10):1549–1558.

Drain PK, Mosam A, Gounder L, et al. Recurrent giant molluscum contagiosum immune reconstitution inflammatory syndrome (IRIS) after initiation of antiretroviral therapy in an HIV-infected man. *Int J STD AIDS.* 2014;25(3):235–238.

Duvic M. Immunology of AIDS related to psoriasis. *J Invest Dermatol.* 1990; 95(5):38S–40S.

Duvic M, Crane MM, Conant M, et al. Zidovudine improves psoriasis in human immunodeficiency virus-positive males. *Arch Dermatol.* 1994;130(4):447–451.

Eisman S. Pruritic papular eruption in HIV. *Dermatol Clin.* 2006;24(4):449–457, vi.

Fearfield LA, Rowe A, Francis N, Bunker CB, Staughton RC. Itchy folliculitis and human immunodeficiency virus infection: clinicopathological and immunological features, pathogenesis and treatment. *Br J Dermatol.* 1999;141(1):3–11.

Foissac M, Goehringer F, Ranaivo IM, et al. Efficacy and safety of intravenous cidofovir in the treatment of giant molluscum contagiosum in an immunosuppressed patient [in French]. *Ann Dermatol Venereol.* 2014;141(10):620–622.

Gasquet S, Maurin M, Brouqui P, Lepidi H, Raoult D. Bacillary angiomatosis in immunocompromised patients. *AIDS.* 1998;12(14):1793–1803.

Gelfand JM, Gladman DD, Mease PJ, et al. Epidemiology of psoriatic arthritis in the population of the United States. *J Am Acad Dermatol.* 2005;53(4):573.

Ghanem KG, Erbelding EJ, Wiener ZS, Rompalo AM. Serological response to syphilis treatment in HIV-positive and HIV-negative patients attending sexually transmitted diseases clinics. *Sex Transm Infect.* 2007;83(2):97–101.

Goldstein B, Berman B, Sukenik E, Frankel SJ. Correlation of skin disorders with CD4+ T cell lymphocyte counts in patients with HIV/AIDS. *J Am Acad Dermatol.* 1997; 36(2 Pt 1):262–264.

Gompels MM, Simpson N, Snow M, et al. Desensitization to cotrimoxazole (trimethoprim-sulphamethoxazole) in HIV-infected patients: is patch testing a useful predictor of reaction? *J Infect.* 1999;38:111–115.

Hage CA, Azar MM, Bahr N, Loyd J, Wheat LJ. Histoplasmosis: up-to-date evidence-based approach to diagnosis and management. *Semin Respir Crit Care Med.* 2015;36(5):729–745.

Hagensee ME, Cameron JE, Leigh JE, Clark RA. Human papillomavirus infection and disease in HIV-infected individuals. *Am J Med Sci.* 2004;328(1):57–63.

Hanifin JM, Reed ML, Eczema P, et al.; Impact Working Group. A population-based survey of eczema prevalence in the United States. *Dermatitis.* 2007;18(2):82–91.

Hevia O, Jimenez-Acosta F, Ceballos PI, et al. Pruritic papular eruption of the acquired immunodeficiency syndrome: a clinicopathologic study. *J Am Acad Dermatol.* 1991;24(2 Pt 1):231–235.

Hyle EP, Wood BR, Backman ES, et al. High frequency of hypothalamic–pituitary–adrenal axis dysfunction after local corticosteroid injection in HIV-infected patients on protease inhibitor therapy. *J AIDS.* 2013;63(5):602–608.

Introcaso CE, Hines JM, Kovarik CL. Cutaneous toxicities of antiretroviral therapy for HIV: part II. Nonnucleoside reverse transcriptase inhibitors, entry and fusion inhibitors, integrase inhibitors, and immune reconstitution syndrome. *J Am Acad Dermatol.* 2010;63(4):563–569; quiz 569–570.

Jagdeo J, Ho D, Lo A, Carruthers A. A systematic review of filler agents for aesthetic treatment of HIV facial lipoatrophy (FLA). *J Am Acad Dermatol.* 2015; 73(6):1040–1054, e1014.

Kim CM, Vogel J, Jay G, Rhim JS. The HIV tat gene transforms human keratinocytes. *Oncogene.* 1992;7(8):1525–1529.

Knobel H, Miro JM, Domingo P, et al. Failure of a short-term prednisone regimen to prevent nevirapine-associated rash: a double-blind placebo-controlled trial: the GESIDA 09/99 study. *J AIDS.* 2001;28(1):14–18.

Krown SE, Lee JY, Dittmer DP; AIDS Malignancy Consortium. More on HIV-associated Kaposi's sarcoma. *N Engl J Med.* 2008;358(5):535–536; author reply 536.

Kuehnert MJ, Kruszon-Moran D, Hill HA, et al. Prevalence of *Staphylococcus aureus* nasal colonization in the United States, 2001–2002. *J Infect Dis.* 2006; 193(2):172–179.

Lin RY, Lazarus TS. Asthma and related atopic disorders in outpatients attending an urban HIV clinic. *Ann Allergy Asthma Immunol.* 1995;74(6):510–515.

Liu Z, Xie Z, Zhang L, et al. Reliability and validity of dermatology life quality index: assessment of quality of life in human immunodeficiency virus/acquired immunodeficiency syndrome patients with pruritic papular eruption. *J Tradit Chin Med.* 2013;33(5):580–583.

Lolis MS, Gonzalez L, Cohen PJ, Schwartz RA. Drug-resistant herpes simplex virus in HIV infected patients. *Acta Dermatovenerol Croat.* 2008;16(4):204–208.

Lortholary O, Fontanet A, Memain N, et al.; Cryptococcosis Study Group. Incidence and risk factors of immune reconstitution inflammatory syndrome complicating HIV-associated cryptococcosis in France. *AIDS.* 2005;19(10):1043–1049.

Mallal S, Phillips E, Carosi G, et al. HLA-B*5701 screening for hypersensitivity to abacavir. *N Engl J Med.* 2008;358(6):568–579.

Mallon E, Bunker CB. HIV-associated psoriasis. *AIDS Patient Care STDS.* 2000; 14(5):239–246.

Maurer TA. Dermatologic manifestations of HIV infection. *Top HIV Med.* 2005; 13(5):149–154.

Mayer PL, Larkin JA, Hennessy JM. Amebic encephalitis. *Surg Neurol Int.* 2011;2:50.

McCloskey JC, Metcalf C, French MA, et al. The frequency of high-grade intraepithelial neoplasia in anal/perianal warts is higher than previously recognized. *Int J STD AIDS.* 2007;18(8):538–542.

Menon K, Van Voorhees AS, Bebo BF, et al. Psoriasis in patients with HIV infection: from the medical board of the National Psoriasis Foundation. *J Am Acad Dermatol.* 2010;62(2):291–299.

Meola T, Soter NA, Ostreicher R, Sanchez M, Moy JA. The safety of UVB phototherapy in patients with HIV infection. *J Am Acad Dermatol.* 1993;29(2 Pt 1):216–220.

Mirmirani P, Maurer TA, Berger TG, et al. Skin-related quality of life in HIV-infected patients on highly active antiretroviral therapy. *J Cutan Med Surg.* 2002;6(1):10–15.

Murphy M, Armstrong D, Sepkowitz KA, et al. Regression of AIDS-related Kaposi's sarcoma following treatment with an HIV-1 protease inhibitor. *AIDS.* 1997; 11(2):261–262.

Murray H, Barber CJ, Foreman RM, et al.; GBD 2013 DALYs and HALE Collaborators. Global, regional, and national disability-adjusted life years (DALYs) for 306 diseases and injuries and healthy life expectancy (HALE) for 188 countries, 1990–2013: quantifying the epidemiological transition. *Lancet.* 2015;386:2145–2191.

Nambudiri VE, Mutyambizi K, Walls AC, et al. Successful treatment of perianal giant condyloma acuminatum in an immunocompromised host with systemic interleukin 2 and topical cidofovir. *JAMA Dermatol.* 2013;149(9):1068–1070.

Nissen D, Nolte H, Permin H, et al. Evaluation of IgE-sensitization to fungi in HIV-positive patients with eczematous skin reactions. *Ann Allergy Asthma Immunol.* 1999;83(2):153–159.

Oble DA, Collett E, Hsieh M, et al. A novel T cell receptor transgenic animal model of seborrheic dermatitis-like skin disease. *J Invest Dermatol.* 2005;124(1):151–159.

Obuch ML, Maurer TA, Becker B, Berger TG. Psoriasis and human immunodeficiency virus infection. *J Am Acad Dermatol.* 1992;27(5 Pt 1):667–673.

Okada S, Fujimura T, Furudate S, et al. Immunosuppression-associated eosinophilic pustular folliculitis (IS-EPF) developing after highly active anti-retroviral therapy (HAART): the possible mechanisms through CD163+ M2 macrophages. *Eur J Dermatol.*2013;23(5):713–714.

Ortega-Loayza AG, McCall CO, Nunley JR. Crusted scabies and multiple dosages of ivermectin. *J Drugs Dermatol.* 2013;12(5):584–585.

Pedrosa AF, Lisboa C, Goncalves Rodrigues A. Malassezia infections: a medical conundrum. *J Am Acad Dermatol.* 2014;71(1):170–176.

Ratnam I, Chiu C, Kandala NB, Easterbrook PJ. Incidence and risk factors for immune reconstitution inflammatory syndrome in an ethnically diverse HIV type 1-infected cohort. *Clin Infect Dis.* 2006;42(3):418–427.

Resneck JS Jr, Van Beek M, Furmanski L, et al. Etiology of pruritic papular eruption with HIV infection in Uganda. *JAMA.* 2004;292(21):2614–2621.

Rigopoulos D, Paparizos V, Katsambas A. Cutaneous markers of HIV infection. *Clin Dermatol.* 2004;22(6):487–498.

Rodrigues LK, Klencke BJ, Vin-Christian K, et al. Altered clinical course of malignant melanoma in HIV-positive patients. *Arch Dermatol.* 2002;138(6):765–770.

Rosen T, Friedlander SF, Kircik L. Onychomycosis: epidemiology, diagnosis, and treatment in a changing landscape. *J Drugs Dermatol.* 2015;14(3):223–233.

Rosenthal D, LeBoit PE, Klumpp L, Berger TG. Human immunodeficiency virus-associated eosinophilic folliculitis. A unique dermatosis associated with advanced human immunodeficiency virus infection. *Arch Dermatol.* 1991;127(2):206–209.

Sadick NS, McNutt NS, Kaplan MH. Papulosquamous dermatoses of AIDS. *J Am Acad Dermatol.* 1990;22(6 Pt 2):1270–1277.

Severson JL, Tyring SK. Relation between herpes simplex viruses and human immunodeficiency virus infections. *Arch Dermatol.* 1999;135(11):1393–1397.

Singh F, Rudikoff D. HIV-associated pruritus: etiology and management. *Am J Clin Dermatol.* 2003;4(3):177–188.

Smith G, Holman RP. The prozone phenomenon with syphilis and HIV-1 co-infection. *South Med J.* 2004;97(4):379–382.

Soeprono FF, Schinella RA, Cockerell CJ, Comite SL. Seborrheic-like dermatitis of acquired immunodeficiency syndrome: a clinicopathologic study. *J Am Acad Dermatol.* 1986;14(2 Pt 1):242–248.

Stanley SK, Folks TM, Fauci AS. Induction of expression of human immunodeficiency virus in a chronically infected promonocytic cell line by ultraviolet irradiation. *AIDS Res Hum Retroviruses.* 1989;5(4):375–384.

Strick LB, Wald A, Celum C. Management of herpes simplex virus type 2 infection in HIV type 1-infected persons. *Clin Infect Dis.* 2006;43(3):347–356.

Suh KS, Han SH, Lee KH, et al. Mites and burrows are frequently found in nodular scabies by dermoscopy and histopathology. *J Am Acad Dermatol.* 2014; 71(5):1022–1023.

Toutous-Trellu L, Abraham S, Pechere M, et al. Topical tacrolimus for effective treatment of eosinophilic folliculitis associated with human immunodeficiency virus infection. *Arch Dermatol.* 2005;141(10):1203–1208.

Ward HA, Russo GG, Shrum J. Cutaneous manifestations of antiretroviral therapy. *J Am Acad Dermatol.* 2002;46(2):284–293.

Warren KJ, Boxwell DE, Kim NY, Drolet BA. Nevirapine-associated Stevens–Johnson syndrome. *Lancet.* 1998;351(9102):567.

Warshaw EM, Nelson D, Carver SM, et al. A pilot evaluation of pulse itraconazole vs. terbinafine for treatment of *Candida* toenail onychomycosis. *Int J Dermatol.* 2005;44(9):785–788.

Weinberg JL, Kovarik CL. The WHO clinical staging system for HIV/AIDS. *Virtual Mentor.* 2010;12(3):202–206.

Wheat LJ, Connolly-Stringfield PA, Baker RL, et al. Disseminated histoplasmosis in the acquired immune deficiency syndrome: clinical findings, diagnosis and treatment, and review of the literature. *Medicine (Baltimore).* 1990;69(6):361–374.

Wilkins K, Turner R, Dolev JC, et al. Cutaneous malignancy and human immunodeficiency virus disease. *J Am Acad Dermatol.* 2006;54(2):189–206; quiz 209–110.

Workowski KA, Bolan GA. Sexually transmitted diseases treatment guidelines, 2015. *MMWR Recomm Rep.* 2015;64(RR-03):1–137.

Zancanaro PC, McGirt LY, Mamelak AJ, et al. Cutaneous manifestations of HIV in the era of highly active antiretroviral therapy: an institutional urban clinic experience. *J Am Acad Dermatol.* 2006;54(4):581–588.

Zeichner JA. New topical therapeutic options in the management of superficial fungal infections. *J Drugs Dermatol.* 2015;14(10):s35–s41.

Zheng Y, Niyonsaba F, Ushio H, et al. Cathelicidin LL-37 induces the generation of reactive oxygen species and release of human alpha-defensins from neutrophils. *Br J Dermatol.* 2007;157(6):1124–1131.

36.

ENDOCRINE AND METABOLIC DISORDERS

Rajagopal V. Sekhar

CHAPTER GOAL

Upon completion of this chapter, the reader should be able to

- Understand the endocrine and metabolic complications affetecting HIV infected patients, and clinical management of these complications.

- After reading this chapter, the reader should understand the mechanism and clinical management of endocrine and metabolic diseases in HIV-positive patients.

INTRODUCTION

With the advent of effective antiretroviral (ARV) therapeutic regimens, HIV infection is now recognized as a chronic disease, and people living with HIV (PLWH) have a longer life expectancy. We are now able to see the emergence of disorders in such patients who live longer, and these include an increasing prevalence of endocrine and metabolic abnormalities. The underlying etiology of these disorders can be attributed to multiple factors, including the effects of HIV itself, antiretroviral therapies (ART), inflammation, endothelial and immune dysfunction, and coinfections. Since endocrine disorders are often insidious in their development, clinical suspicion and appropriate dynamic testing are necessary for accurate diagnosis and management and should include the participation of an endocrinologist where possible. Since PLWH are now living longer, we are witnessing the evolution of HIV as a chronic disease, with new emerging phenotypes which range from an increase in the incidence and prevalence of metabolic diseases such as central obesity, metabolic syndrome, and fatty liver disease. There are also reports of "accelerated aging" afflicting PLWH, in which relatively younger PLWH develop geriatric complications typically seen in HIV uninfected people who are 20–30 years older. These include physical decline with development of impaired mitochondrial fuel oxidation, muscle weakness, inflammation, insulin resistance, and cognitive decline, but underlying mechanisms are not well understood, and interventions are lacking. This chapter will focus on endocrine and metabolic disorders in HIV infection and discuss mechanisms, specific endocrine disorders, and emerging knowledge on metabolic disease and mitochondrial impairment in PLWH.

WHAT'S NEW?

- An increasing prevalence of diabetes mellitus (DM) is seen in HIV-positive patients worldwide.

- An increased prevalence of metabolic disorders, including fatty-liver disease, abdominal obesity, and the metabolic syndrome is seen in HIV-positive patients.

- There is a high prevalence of vitamin D deficiency.

- There is a potential for reversing impaired mitochondrial fuel oxidation in HIV-positive patients, with a novel role for glutathione.

KEY POINTS

- Abnormalities in glucose and lipids are common in HIV.

- HIV patients have a higher prevalence of metabolic disorders.

- HIV infection, ARVs, and other factors play a role in the development of endocrine disease.

- For endocrine disorders in HIV, early referral to an endocrinologist is suggested.

MECHANISMS OF ENDOCRINE AND METABOLIC DISEASE IN HIV

The mechanisms through which HIV infection initiates and sustains endocrine and metabolic disorders are complex and involve abnormalities in hormonal secretion, transport, metabolism, and resistance. However, the underlying mechanisms for many of these disorders are still not completely understood, as in the case of HIV-associated lipodystrophy or accelerated aging in HIV.

An important contributing factor is inflammation and immune dysfunction in the context of HIV, with abnormalities in cytokine, chemokine, and other immune phenomena that affect endocrine function (Merrill, 1989; Salim, 1988; Tracey, 1990). For example, interleukin-1 (IL-1) has been shown to increase adrenocorticotropic hormone (ACTH) in cultured pituitary cells (Meyer, 1987; Szebeni, 1991). Other pituitary hormones may also be affected; effects include prolactin elevations (Parra, 2004) and deficient growth hormone secretion (Koutkia, 2004). HIV-positive mononuclear cells can increase interferon-α (Grunfeld, 1992) and impair glucocorticoid receptor activity (Norbiato, 1996), and abnormalities in IL-1 and tumor necrosis factor (TNF) can affect gonadal function by inhibiting gonadal steroidogenesis (Calkins, 1988; Hales, 1992; Xiong, 1993). Interestingly, results from a small pilot study showed that correcting deficiency of the endogenous antioxidant protein glutathione was associated with a striking decline in inflammation with significant decreases in hsCRP and TNF-α blood levels within 2 weeks (Sekhar, 2015), and further studies are needed to confirm and extend these findings.

Another contributor to HIV-related endocrine disease is opportunistic infections. For example, cytomegalovirus (CMV) infection predisposes to an increased risk of developing adrenalitis (Glasgow, 1985). Infections caused by mycobacterial pathogens may also affect adrenal function, whereas CMV, cryptococcal, and toxoplasma infections can affect central nervous system (CNS) function and cause retinitis, meningitis, and pituitary disease (Giampalmo, 1990). CMV infection has been reported in one instance to cause hypernatremia, likely through a reset osmostat (Keuneke, 1999). Thyroid function can be affected by opportunistic pathogens in HIV, including *Pneumocystis*, which is a rare cause of thyroiditis (Drucker, 1990).

HIV-positive patients are also experiencing an increase in the incidence and prevalence of metabolic disorders, including centripetal fat accumulation as in the metabolic syndrome, fatty liver disease, and mitochondrial dysfunction. The underlying mechanisms are not well understood, and effective interventions are lacking. There is an urgent need for exploratory studies to guide relevant clinical trials to facilitate identification of mechanisms and develop therapeutic strategies.

The development and clinical use of ART have led to significant benefits for HIV patients, including decreased early mortality, decreased opportunistic infection, and improved nutritional status. However, these benefits are associated with increases in the incidence and prevalence of endocrine and metabolic complications, most notably dyslipidemia, and changes in body morphology ranging from lipodystrophy (Carr, 1998) to central obesity in the context of metabolic syndrome. The role of ARV drugs are discussed next.

PROTEASE INHIBITORS

The initial use of protease inhibitor (PI) drugs in PLWH led to observations of abnormalities in total body fat distribution, most notably an increase in abdominal fat that was initially described by colorful names such as the "protease paunch" (Mishriki, 1998) or "Crixivan belly" (Huff, 1997–1998). Since then, the PI class of drugs has been linked to the development of abdominal obesity and biochemical abnormalities comprising severe hypertriglyceridemia, dyslipidemia, insulin resistance, and diabetes. Many PI drugs, including lopinavir/ritonavir, nelfinavir, amprenavir, and saquinavir, are metabolized by the hepatic cytochrome 450 CYP3A4 isoenzyme pathway. PI

drugs have been shown to directly impact insulin resistance. For example, indinavir can inhibit GLUT4 activity and thus impair insulin-stimulated glucose uptake and predispose to hyperglycemia (Caron, 2001; Murata, 2000). In addition to their permissive role in metabolic and glycemic abnormalities, PI drugs have also been implicated in the development of prolactin abnormalities (Hutchinson, 2000) and in osteomalacia (Cozzolino, 2003).

NUCLEOSIDE REVERSE TRANSCRIPTASE INHIBITORS

Nucleoside reverse transcriptase inhibitors (NRTIs) have also been described to induce changes in body morphology. For example, stavudine has been linked to the development of lipoatrophy in HIV (Saint-Marc, 1999). These drugs have also been linked to the development of mitochondrial dysfunction (Mallon, 2005), which could result in abnormalities of glucose and lipid metabolism (Sekhar, 2002; Shikuma, 2001).

NON-NUCLEOSIDE REVERSE TRANSCRIPTASE INHIBITORS

Non-nucleoside reverse transcriptase inhibitors (NNRTIs) have been linked to dyslipidemia (Padmapriyadarsini, 2011) and fat depletion in 3T3-L1 cells (Minami, 2011).

ENDOCRINE DISORDERS IN HIV

Any endocrine or metabolic disorder can affect PLWH, and include diabetes; metabolic syndrome; disorders of adrenal, thyroid, pituitary, and gonadal function; and bone and dyslipidemia. Bone disorders and dyslipidemia are discussed elsewhere in other chapters.

DIABETES MELLITUS

The prevalence of diabetes mellitus (DM) is increasing in PLWH worldwide (Tzur, 2015). Early reports indicate that the prevalence of DM ranges from 1.5% to 2.6% in ART-treatment naïve patients (El-Sadr, 2005; Tien, 2007) to 5.9% when coinfected with hepatitis C (Visnegarwala, 2005). However, a more recent publication estimates this to be as high as 15.1% with a relative risk of 2.4 compared to the general population (Duncan, 2018). Another study followed PLWH for 10 years in Malawi, Africa, and found the prevalence of DM to be higher in every age group (from 30 to 60+) compared to controls (Mathabire, 2018). As reported in the Multicenter AIDS Cohort Study, exposure to ART results in a 14% incidence of DM in HIV-positive men, which is fourfold higher than that for HIV-seronegative controls (Brown, 2005). However, there are reports suggesting that glycosylated hemoglobin (HbA1c) may underestimate glycemia in PLWH (Slama, 2014; Kim, 2009). One study examined HbA1c in 1,500 HIV-negative and 1,357 HIV-positive men in the MACS cohort over 13 years and found that HbA1c underestimates glycemia in HIV-positive men (Slama, 2014). Another study compared 100 HIV-positive adults with type 2 diabetes to 200 HIV-negative type 2 diabetic participants, found similar results, and linked it to use of abacavir and increased mean corpuscular volume (MCV) (Kim, 2009). The reasons for this meteoric rise in the incidence of DM are likely to be multifactorial, but a recent meta-analysis implicated ART as potentially the single most consistent determinant of DM in PLWH worldwide (Nduka, 2017). Collectively, these reports indicate a surging increase in the incidence and prevalence of DM among HIV-positive adults and suggest that relying solely on HbA1c could lead to underdiagnosing and undertreating diabetes. The implications are that it is important to carefully screen for hyperglycemia and diabetes in PLWH and to correlate HbA1c with other measures of HIV-positive glycemic control, including fasting and prandial home glucose monitoring, for a reliable assessment of glycemic status and control. The overall management of DM in PLWH is similar to that in HIV-uninfected patients and requires the combined approach of a team comprising a diabetes educator, dietitian, physician, and diabetes nursing staff and careful attention to the triumvirate of exercise, diet, and pharmacotherapy. The long-term complications of DM include retinopathy, nephropathy, neuropathy, and coronary artery disease. Interestingly, PLWH are at risk of retinitis due to opportunistic infections, to HIV-associated nephropathy (HIVAN), and to neuropathy, and also have an increased risk of cardiovascular disease. The concurrence of these end organ complications from both HIV infection and DM theoretically suggests that PLWH could be at higher risk from the twin burden of two chronic diseases, HIV and DM.

ADRENAL DISORDERS

HIV infection can involve adrenal dysfunction. The incidence of hypoadrenalism is reported to be 20% in HIV-positive PLWH (González-González, 2001), and postmortem studies have shown that up to two-thirds of people with AIDS may have adrenal involvement (Bricaire, 1988). Presentation of adrenal dysfunction may be subtle and escape clinical scrutiny, and it is relatively common in hospitalized PLWH (Membreno, 1987). The etiology of adrenal hypofunction can range from primary hypoadrenalism involving the adrenal gland, with elevations in adrenocorticotropic hormone (ACTH) levels (Villette, 1990) to secondary hypoadrenalism due to pituitary suppression due to inherent pituitary pathology or possibly suppression of the hypothalamo-pituitary-adrenal axis by exogenous steroid use (Danaher, 2009; Kaviani, 2011). PLWH have also been described to develop hyperadrenalism with iatrogenic Cushing's syndrome when administered steroids via oral, inhaled, and parenteral routes (Gray, 2010; Johnson, 2006; Samaras, 2005; Yombi, 2008).

PLWH may also have abnormalities in the mineralocorticoid axis (Stricker, 1999). HIV-positive women with the wasting syndrome may have significant shunting of adrenal steroid metabolism away from androgenic pathways and toward cortisol production (Grinspoon, 2001).

THYROID ABNORMALITIES

The clinical presentation of thyroid abnormalities in HIV infection ranges from asymptomatic hypo- or hyperthyroidism to clinically overt disease. The prevalence of thyroid dysfunction appears to be higher in PLWH. Although earlier reports suggested that thyroid dysfunction in PLWH is generally similar to that seen in HIV-negative populations (Hoffman, 2007), recent reports indicate that the prevalence of thyroid dysfunction may be much higher. A recent study evaluated thyroid function in 178 PLWH and found that 33% of patients had evidence of thyroid dysfunction (Ji, 2016). Most of these abnormalities involve hypothyroidism, ranging from an increased prevalence of subclinical hypothyroidism (Madeddu, 2006; Silva, 2015) to clinical hypothyroidism (Beltran, 2003). Factors contributing to thyroid disorders in HIV infection include, but are not limited to, ARVs, infection, and immune factors.

ARVs could play a role in the development of thyroid abnormalities in PLWH. For example, HIV-related non-autoimmune primary hypothyroidism and subclinical hypothyroidism have been linked to stavudine, decreased CD4[+] T cell counts, and male gender (Calza, 2002; Madeddu, 2006; Quirino, 2004; Silva, 2015).

HIV-related immune and other factors are also linked to the development of abnormal thyroid function tests. For example, CD4[+] T cell counts have been inversely correlated with thyroid binding globulin (Bourdoux, 1991), and diminished levels of triiodothyronine (T3) and reverse T3 with increased thyroid binding globulin may be associated with HIV progression. Hyperthyroidism can also occur in PLWH. Autoimmune Graves's disease is an anti–thyroid-stimulating hormone receptor antibody after the initiation of ART and after an increase in CD4[+] T cell count (Jubault, 2000).

Infection as an etiological factor for thyroid disease was much more prevalent in the pre-ART era and was caused by a wide variety of infectious microorganisms. However, these can still be seen in patients not on ART, those with ART drug resistance, or those who are nonadherent to medications.

Although the clinical presentation of thyroid abnormalities ranges from asymptomatic hypo- or hyperthyroidism to clinically overt disease, the diagnostic workup is similar to that in HIV-negative patients and should begin with evaluations of thyroxine and thyrotropin, with additional testing for thyroiditis antibodies where appropriate.

PARATHYROID DISORDERS

Hyperparathyroidism is a condition marked by elevated secretion of parathyroid hormone. Hyperparathyroidism can be primary due to abnormalities within the parathyroid gland itself, most often due to adenoma, and rarely due to cancer. Secondary causes of hyperparathyroidism are due to conditions such as renal impairment and vitamin D deficiency. The etiology of primary hyperparathyroidism in the HIV-positive population is similar to the general population and typically presents as hypercalcemia; this should be appropriately investigated with the final treatment being surgical removal of the parathyroid adenoma. However, vitamin D deficiency is reported to impact a third of HIV patients (Van den Bout, 2008) and is a common cause for secondary hyperparathyroidism (Dao, 2011; Mueller, 2010) with referrals to endocrinologists. Antiretroviral drugs such as efavirenz have been implicated in the increased prevalence of vitamin D deficiency in the HIV-positive population (Nylén, 2016), but other factors such as CD4$^+$ T cell counts and advanced disease may also play a role (Theodorou, 2014). Other ARV drugs such as tenofovir disoproxil fumarate have also been linked to secondary hyperparathyroidism in PLWH (Noe, 2018).

GONADAL DYSFUNCTION

Gonadal dysfunction is common in PLWH (Crum, 2005; Rietschel, 2000). In male patients, decreased levels of testosterone may be associated with fatigue, muscle wasting and sarcopenia, decreased bone density, low libido, weight loss, decreased strength (Grinspoon, 1996; Wanke, 2000), and impotence (Mylonakis, 2001). In a study of 300 PLWH, 17% were found to be hypogonadal, and all patients with low testosterone had secondary hypogonadism. Interestingly, there was no correlation between hypogonadism and erectile dysfunction, but increasing age and a higher body mass index were positively correlated with hypogonadism, whereas smoking was negatively correlated (Crum-Cianflone, 2007). Although underlying causes are not fully understood, elevated levels of prolactin have been implicated in the development of male hypogonadism (Collazos, 2009). Treatment of patients with AIDS wasting syndrome with testosterone or placebo was associated with a sustained increase in lean mass only with testosterone after a 6-month period (Grinspoon, 1999). Testosterone therapy, especially in older patients, should involve careful monitoring of prostate-specific antigen levels, liver profiles, and hematocrit levels.

HIV-positive women have increased rates of oligomenorrhea and amenorrhea. HIV has been shown to infect the cervix, uterus, and fallopian tubes (Howell, 1997). In one study, 8% of women living with HIV had evidence of early menopause and 48% had anovulatory cycles, whereas women who ovulated had higher CD4$^+$ T cell counts (Chirgwin, 1996). In a recent study from Nigeria reporting abnormalities in premenopausal women living with HIV, mean serum levels of the FSH, LH, progesterone, and estradiol did not differ between the follicular and luteal phase of the menstrual cycle, suggesting loss of hormonal regulation, and the researchers linked these abnormalities to hypothyroidism, which could be corrected with treatment (Ukibe, 2017).

Gynecomastia

Males living with HIV have a 2.9% incidence of developing gynecomastia, which is not linked to progression of HIV disease (Biglia, 2004) but is linked to hypogonadism, lipoatrophy, hepatitis C (Manfredi, 2001), and also to lipodystrophy (Biglia, 2004). The role of ARVs in the development of gynecomastia is controversial, with no correlation found in some studies (Manfredi, 2001), whereas other studies have linked gynecomastia with PI-based ARV regimens (Manfredi, 2004; Peyriere, 1999; Toma, 1998). When associated with PI therapy, gynecomastia does not resolve after cessation of ART, and underlying mechanisms are not clear. Treatment of gynecomastia includes removal of any identifiable cause and, in extreme cases, surgical removal.

Pituitary Disease

The pituitary gland is located in the sella turcica and comprises the anterior pituitary (adenohypophysis) and posterior pituitary (neurohypophysis). The adenohypophyseal hormones are intimately involved in controlling thyroid, adrenal, and gonadal function; growth; and milk secretion. The neurohypophysis primarily controls water balance, acting via antidiuretic hormone. Many pituitary hormones are regulated by prohormones secreted by the hypothalamus which are delivered to the pituitary via a portal system through the pituitary stalk (e.g., corticotropin releasing hormone [CRH]; growth hormone releasing hormone [GHRH]; thyrotropin releasing hormone [TRH]; gonadotropin releasing hormone [GnRH]; and vasopressin), with the sole exception being prolactin which is under inhibitory control by dopamine. Therefore, pituitary disease can be caused by pathology at the level of the hypothalamus, pituitary stalk compression, or disease in the pituitary gland itself.

Growth Hormone Disorders

Disorders of growth hormone (GH) are reported in HIV infection. Adult patients with HIV-associated lipodystrophy are described to have GH deficiency with reduced pulse and amplitude of GH secretion, which may be related to an increased somatostatin tone, decreased ghrelin, and increased circulatory free fatty acid concentrations (Koutkia, 2004). HIV-positive children and adults with AIDS wasting syndrome have low levels of insulin-like growth factor-1 (IGF-1) and IGF binding protein 3 and increased concentrations of GH, suggesting resistance to GH (Frost, 1996; Pinto, 2000; Ratner Kaufman, 1997; Rondanelli, 2002).

Pituitary Adrenal Disorders

Iatrogenic Cushing's syndrome, together with secondary hypoadrenalism, is a frequent observation in PLWH who receive steroid therapy (Danaher, 2009; Gray, 2010; Johnson, 2006; Kaviani, 2011; Samaras, 2005; Yombi, 2008). This is likely caused by the effect of several ARV drugs (almost entirely ritonavir or cobicistat boosting) on the hepatic cytochrome P450 system, which prolongs the half-life of steroids. This results in elevated levels of exogenously administered steroids and suppression of ACTH and thereby of endogenous cortisol production, resulting in iatrogenic Cushing's syndrome together with endogenous adrenal insufficiency. Because sudden withdrawal of exogenous steroids in this situation could precipitate a catastrophic adrenal crisis, caution must be exercised while discontinuing steroids, and a gentle taper is recommended.

Prolactin Disorders

PLWH have been reported to have disturbances in basal and rhythmic prolactin secretions associated with CD4⁺ T lymphocytes (Parra, 2004). Elevation in serum prolactin is described in PLWH (Collazos, 2002), and hyperprolactinemia in HIV-positive men has been linked to hypogonadism and gynecomastia (Collazos, 2009). Although the etiology of the hyperprolactinemia is unclear, use of PIs has been linked to elevations in prolactin (Ram, 2004).

Posterior Pituitary Disorders

Posterior pituitary disorders are caused by excess secretion of antidiuretic hormone (ADH), resulting in hyponatremia, or a paucity of ADH, resulting in diabetes insipidus. In one report, 33% of people living with AIDS were found to have hyponatremia primarily due to the syndrome of inappropriate ADH secretion (Agarwal, 1989). PLWH may also develop hypernatremia caused by diabetes insipidus due to intracranial pathology—a recently published case report highlights the role of CNS lymphoma in a person living with HIV who presented with diabetes insipidus (Tavares-Bello 2017).

METABOLIC DISORDERS IN HIV

METABOLIC SYNDROME

With increased longevity in PLWH, there is also an increasing risk of developing metabolic syndrome, with central obesity, insulin resistance, hypertriglyceridemia, and hypertension, which could predispose to an increase risk of cardiovascular disease (Hadigan, 2001). Whereas the prevalence of metabolic syndrome in non-HIV-positive individuals is 3%, HIV-positive people taking ART have a prevalence of 16–18% (Samaras, 2007). HIV-positive women appear to have an even higher burden of metabolic syndrome, with a 33% prevalence compared to 22% for HIV-seronegative women (Sobieszczyk, 2008).

Clinically, the previously discussed data translate into HIV-positive patients having an increased incidence and prevalence of abdominal obesity, insulin resistance, dyslipidemia, and hypertension, all of which contribute to elevated cardiometabolic risk in PLWH. Treatment of these disorders involves a combination of patient education; adherence to dietary control; encouragement of physical activity and exercise, where possible; and appropriate pharmacotherapy targeting glycemic control, blood pressure, and lipids.

NONALCOHOLIC FATTY LIVER DISEASE

Liver disease is an important contributor to morbidity and mortality among PLWH. Despite the success with therapeutic interventions to cure hepatitis C viral coinfection, there is an increase in the prevalence of nonalcoholic fatty liver disease (NAFLD), defined as liver fat accumulation (causing fatty liver) in the absence of other causes of liver disease such as excess alcohol consumption, viral hepatitis, or any other specific hepatic pathology. NAFLD ranges from simple hepatic steatosis at one end of the spectrum, to nonalcoholic steatohepatitis (NASH) and hepatic fibrosis, which progresses to cirrhosis and hepatocellular carcinoma on the other end. NASH is now the third most common indication for liver transplantation in the United States. The prevalence of NAFLD and NASH is increasing in PLWH. A study examining HIV-positive patients with altered transaminases found the prevalence of NASH reported up to 55% (Morse, 2015). NAFLD in HIV may have a more aggressive progression to NASH: a recently published study examined the clinical and histological differences between HIV-associated NAFLD and primary NAFLD, and reported that HIV-associated NAFLD was associated with increased severity of liver disease and higher prevalence of NASH (Vodkin, 2015). Furthermore, the presence of NAFLD is linked to the development of systemic inflammation, insulin resistance, diabetes, and cardiovascular disease. Conversely, NAFLD is a well-recognized complication of type 2 diabetes, with reported prevalence as high as 80–85%, and, given the rising incidence and prevalence of type 2 diabetes in PLWH, NAFLD and NASH could soon become the most significant metabolic complication of HIV infection. Thus, the combination of high prevalence of NAFLD/NASH in PLWH with increased severity of NASH makes it an extremely urgent public health concern, especially since mechanisms are not well understood and effective interventions are lacking.

HIV AND MITOCHONDRIAL IMPAIRMENT

PLWH are well described to have an impairment in mitochondrial fat oxidation. Mitochondrial impairment is also well described in other HIV-uninfected conditions which include type 2 diabetes, obesity, and aging, but underlying mechanisms are unclear and currently there are no viable or effective interventions to reverse mitochondrial dysfunction in any human condition. It is from this perspective that the results of a small pilot study that investigated mechanisms and reported reversibility of mitochondrial impairment are relevant (Nguyen, 2014). Based on their discoveries in rodents and older humans (Nguyen, 2013) that adequate availability of the endogenous antioxidant protein glutathione is critically necessary for optimal mitochondrial fatty acid oxidation, the investigators evaluated and found that HIV-positive patients with impaired mitochondrial fat oxidation and oxidative stress had severe deficiency of glutathione, which, in turn, was caused by deficient synthesis due to decreased availability of two of its precursor amino acids, cysteine and glycine. When these amino acids were supplemented in the diet for 2 weeks, it corrected their deficiency, restored glutathione synthesis rates, increased glutathione concentrations, and lowered oxidative stress. This was associated with a significant improvement of mitochondrial fuel oxidation in the fasted and fed states, together with a 31% decrease in insulin resistance, decrease in total body fat and waist circumference (Nguyen, 2014), and in inflammation (Sekhar, 2015). Further large trials are needed to confirm and extend these results. If true, this discovery could have profound implications for improving the metabolic health of PLWH by using nutritional supplementation of oral cysteine and glycine to correct glutathione deficiency.

CONCLUSION

PLWH can be affected by endocrine and metabolic abnormalities. Although the more common disorders are dyslipidemia, diabetes, metabolic syndrome, and insulin resistance, other disorders affecting bone, adrenal glands, pituitary, and thyroid function may also be present. For rapid diagnosis and treatment of endocrine disorders in HIV-positive patients, both early referral to and working together with an endocrinologist are recommended.

REFERENCES

Agarwal A, Soni A, Ciechanowsky M, et al. Hyponatremia in patients with the acquired immunodeficiency syndrome. *Nephron.* 1989;53:317–321.

Beltran S, Lescure FX, Desailloud R, et al. Increased prevalence of hypothyroidism among human immunodeficiency virus-infected patients: a need for screening. *Clin Infect Dis.* 2003;37:579–583.

Biglia A, Blanco JL, Martínez E, et al. Gynecomastia among HIV-positive patients is associated with hypogonadism: a case–control study. *Clin Infect Dis.* 2004; 39(10):1514–1519.

Bourdoux PP, De Wit SA, Servais GM, et al. Biochemical thyroid profile in patients infected with human immunodeficiency virus. *Thyroid.* 1991;1:147–149.

Bricaire F, Marche C, Zoubi D, et al. Adrenocortical lesions and AIDS. *Lancet.* 1988;1:881.

Brown TT, Cole SR, Li X, et al. Antiretroviral therapy and the prevalence and incidence of diabetes mellitus in the multicenter AIDS cohort study. *Arch Intern Med.* 2005;165:1179–1184.

Calkins JH, Siegel MM, Nankin HR, et al. Interleukin-1 inhibits Leydig cell steroidogenesis in primary cell culture. *J Clin Endocrinol Metab.* 1988;123:1605–1610.

Calza L, Manfredi R, Chiodo F. Subclinical hypothyroidism in HIV-positive patients receiving highly active antiretroviral therapy. *J AIDS.* 2002;31:361–363.

Caron M, Auclair M, Vigouroux C, et al. The HIV protease inhibitor indinavir impairs sterol regulatory element-binding protein-1 intranuclear localization, inhibits preadipocyte differentiation, and induces insulin resistance. *Diabetes.* 2001;50:1378–1388.

Carr A, Samaras K, Burton S, et al. A syndrome of peripheral lipodystrophy, hyperlipidaemia and insulin resistance in patients receiving HIV protease inhibitors. *AIDS.* 1998;12(7):F51–F58.

Chirgwin KD, Feldman J, Muneyyirci-Delale O, et al. Menstrual function in human immunodeficiency virus-infected women without acquired immunodeficiency syndrome. *J AIDS Hum Retrovirol.* 1996. 12:489–494.

Collazos J, Esteban M. Has prolactin a role in the hypogonadal status of HIV-positive patients? *J Int Assoc Physicians AIDS Care (Chic).* 2009;8(1):43–46.

Collazos J, Ibarra S, Martinez E, et al. Serum prolactin concentrations in patients infected with HIV. *HIV Clin Trials.* 2002;3:133–138.

Cozzolino M, Vidal M, Arcidiacono MV, et al. HIV-protease inhibitors impair vitamin D bioactivation to 1,25-dihydroxyvitamin D. *AIDS.* 2003;17:513–520.

Crum NF, Furtek KJ, Olson PE, et al. A review of hypogonadism and erectile dysfunction among HIV-infected men during the pre- and post-HAART eras: diagnosis, pathogenesis, and management. *AIDS Patient Care STDS.* 2005;19(10):655–671.

Crum-Cianflone NF, Bavaro M, Hale B, et al. Erectile dysfunction and hypogonadism among men with HIV. *AIDS Patient Care STDS.* 2007;21:9–19.

Danaher PJ, Salsbury TL, Delmar JA. Metabolic derangement after injection of triamcinolone into the hip of an HIV-infected patient receiving ritonavir. *Orthopedics.* 2009;32(6):450.

Dao CN, Patel P, Overton ET, et al. Low vitamin D among HIV-infected adults: prevalence of and risk factors for low vitamin D Levels in a cohort of HIV-infected adults and comparison to prevalence among adults in the US general population. *Clin Infect Dis.* 2011;52:396.

Drucker DJ, Bailey D, Rotstein L. Thyroiditis as the presenting manifestation of disseminated extrapulmonary Pneumocystis carinii infection. *J Clin Endocrinol Metab.* 1990;71:1663–1665.

Duncan AD, Goff LM, Peters BS. Type 2 diabetes prevalence and its risk factors in HIV: a cross-sectional study, *PLOS One.* 2018;13(3):e0194199.

El-Sadr WM. Effects of HIV disease on lipid, glucose and insulin levels: results from a large antiretroviral-naive cohort. *HIV Med.* 2005;6:114–121.

Frost RA, Fuhrer J, Steigbigel R. Wasting in the acquired immune deficiency syndrome is associated with multiple defects in the serum insulin-like growth factor system. *Clin Endocrinol (Oxf).* 1996: 44:501.

Giampalmo A, Buffa D, Quaglia AC. AIDS pathology: Various critical considerations (especially regarding the brain, the heart, the lungs, the hypophysis and the adrenal glands). *Pathologica.* 1990;82(1982):663–677.

Glasgow BJ, Steinsapir KD, Anders K, et al. Adrenal pathology in the acquired immune deficiency syndrome. *Am J Clin Pathol.* 1985;84:594–597.

González-González JG, de la Garza-Hernández NE, Garza-Morán RA, et al. Prevalence of abnormal adrenocortical function in human immunodeficiency virus infection by low-dose cosyntropin test. *Int J STD AIDS.* 2001;12(12):804–810.

Gray D, Roux P, Carrihill M, et al. Adrenal suppression and Cushing's syndrome secondary to ritonavir and budesonide. *S Afr Med J.* 2010;100(5):296–297.

Grinspoon S, Corcoran C, Anderson E, et al. Sustained anabolic effects of long-term androgen administration in men with AIDS and wasting. *Clin Infect Dis.* 1999;28:634–636.

Grinspoon S, Corcoran C, Lee K, et al. Loss of lean body and muscle mass correlates with androgen levels in hypogonadal men with acquired immunodeficiency syndrome and wasting. *J Clin Endocrinol Metab.* 1996;81:4051–4058.

Grinspoon S, Corcoran C, Stanley T, et al. Mechanisms of androgen deficiency in human immunodeficiency virus-infected women with the wasting syndrome. *J Clin Endocrinol Metab.* 2001;86:4120–4126.

Grunfeld C, Pang M, Doerrler W, et al. Lipids, lipoproteins, triglyceride clearance, and cytokines in human immunodeficiency virus infection and the acquired immunodeficiency syndrome. *J Clin Endocrinol Metab.* 1992;74:1045–1052.

Hales DB. Interleukin1 inhibits Leydig cell steroidogenesis primarily by decreasing 17α-hydroxylase/C17–20 lyase cytochrome P450 expression. *Endocrinology.* 1992;131:2165–2172.

Hoffman CJ, Brown TT. Thyroid function abnormalities in HIV infected patients. *Clin Infect Dis.* 2007;45:488–494.

Howell AL, Edkins RD, Rier SE, et al. Human immunodeficiency virus type 1 infection of cells and tissues from the upper and lower human female reproductive tract. *J Virol.* 1997;71:3498–3506.

Huff A. Protease inhibitor side effects take people by surprise. *GMHC Treat Issues.* 1997–1998 Winter;12(1):25–27.

Hutchinson J, Murphy M, Harries R, et al. Galactorrhoea and hyper-prolactinoma associated with protease inhibitors. *Lancet.* 2000;356:1003–1004.

Ji S, Jin C, Hoxtermann S, et al. Prevalence and Influencing factors of thyroid dysfunction in HIV-positive patients. *Biomed Res Int.* 2016;3874257.

Johnson SR, Marion AA, Vrchoticky T, et al. Cushing syndrome with secondary adrenal insufficiency from concomitant therapy with ritonavir and fluticasone. *J Pediatr.* 2006;148(3):386–388.

Jubault V, Penformin F, Schillo F, et al. Sequential occurrence of thyroid autoantibodies and Grave's disease after immune restoration in severely immunocompromised human immuno-deficiency virus-1 infected patients. *J Clin Endocrinol Metab.* 2000;85:4254–4257.

Kaviani N, Bukberg P, Manessis A, et al. Iatrogenic osteoporosis, bilateral HIP osteonecrosis, and secondary adrenal suppression in an HIV-positive man receiving inhaled corticosteroids and ritonavir-boosted highly active antiretroviral therapy. *Endocr Pract.* 2011;17(1):74–78.

Keuneke C, Anders HJ, Schlöndorff D. Adipsic hypernatremia in two patients with AIDS and cytomegalovirus encephalitis. *Am J Kidney Dis.* 1999;33(2):379–382.

Kim PS, Woods C, Georgoff P, et al. A1c underestimates glycemia in HIV infection. *Diabetes Care.* 2009;32(9):1591–1593.

Koutkia P, Meininger G, Canavan B, et al. Metabolic regulation of growth hormone by free fatty acids, somatostatin, and ghrelin in HIV-lipodystrophy. *Am J Physiol Endocrinol Metab.* 2004;286(2):E296–E303.

Madeddu G, Spanu A, Chessa F, et al. Thyroid function in human immunodeficiency virus patients treated with highly active antiretroviral therapy (HAART): a longitudinal study. *Clinical Endocrinology Oxf).* 2006;64(4):375–383.

Mallon PW, Unemori P, Sedwell R, et al. In vivo, nucleoside reverse-transcriptase inhibitors alter expression of both mitochondrial and lipid metabolism genes in the absence of depletion of mitochondrial DNA. *J Infect Dis.* 2005;191(10):1686–1696.

Manfredi R, Calza L, Chiodo F. Gynecomastia associated with highly active antiretroviral therapy. *Ann Pharmacother.* 2001;35(4):438–439.

Manfredi R, Calza L, Chiodo F. Another emerging event occurring during HIV infection treated with any antiretroviral therapy: Frequency and role of gynecomastia. *Infez Med.* 2004;12(1):51–59.

Mathabire Rücker SC, Tayea A, Bitilinyu-Bangoh J, et al. High rates of hypertension, diabetes, elevated low-density lipoprotein cholesterol, and cardiovascular disease risk factors in HIV-positive patients in Malawi. *AIDS.* 2018;32(2):253–260.

Membreno L, Irony I, Dere W, et al. Adrenocortical function in acquired immunodeficiency syndrome. *J Clin Endocrinol Metab.* 1987;65:482–487.

Merrill JE, Koyanagi Y, Chen ISY. Interleukin-1 and tumor necrosis factor α can be induced from mononuclear phagocytes by human immunodeficiency virus type 1 binding to the CD4 receptor. *J Virol.* 1989;63:4404–4408.

Meyer WJ, Smith EM, Richards GE, et al. In vivo immunoreactive adrenocorticotropin (ACTH) production by human mononuclear leukocytes from normal and ACTH-deficient individuals. *J Clin Endocrinol Metab.* 1987;64:98–105.

Minami R, Yamamoto M, Takahama S, et al. Comparison of the influence of four classes of HIV antiretrovirals on adipogenic differentiation: the minimal effect of raltegravir and atazanavir. *J Infect Chemother.* 2011;17(2):183–188.

Mishriki YY. A baffling case of bulging belly: protease paunch. *Postgrad Med.* 1998;104(3):45–46.

Morse CG, McLaughlin M, Matthews L, et al. Nonalcoholic steatohepatitis and hepatic fibrosis in HIV-1-monoinfected adults with elevated aminotransferase levels on antiretroviral therapy. *Clin Infect Dis.* 2015;60(10):1569–1578.

Mueller NJ, Fux CA, Ledergerber B, et al. High prevalence of severe vitamin D deficiency in combined antiretroviral therapy-naive and successfully treated Swiss HIV patients. *AIDS.* 2010;24:1127.

Murata H, Hruz PW, Mueckler M. The mechanism of insulin resistance caused by HIV protease inhibitor therapy. *J Biol Chem.* 2000;275:20251–20254.

Mylonakis E, Koutkia P, Grinspoon S. Diagnosis and treatment of androgen deficiency in human immunodeficiency virus-infected men and women. *Clin Infect Dis.* 2001;33:857–864.

Nduka CU, Stranges S, Kimani PK, et al. Is there sufficient evidence for a causal association between antiretroviral therapy and diabetes in HIV patients? A meta-analysis. *Diabetes Metab Res Rev.* 2017;33(6):e2902.

Nguyen D, Hsu JW, Jahoor F, et al. Effect of increasing glutathione with cysteine and glycine supplementation on mitochondrial fuel oxidation, insulin sensitivity, and body composition in older HIV-infected patients. *J Clin Endocrinol Metab.* 2014;99(1):169–177.

Nguyen D, Samson SL, Reddy VT, et al. Impaired mitochondrial fatty acid oxidation and insulin resistance in aging: a novel protective role of glutathione. *Aging Cell.* 2013;12(3):415–425.

Noe S, Oldenbuettel C, Heldwein S, et al. Secondary hyperparathyroidism in patients in Central Europe. *Horm Metab Res.* 2018;50(4):317–324.

Norbiato G, Bevilacqua M, Vago T, et al. Glucocorticoids and interferon-alpha in the acquired immunodeficiency syndrome. *J Clin Endocrinol Metab.* 1996;81:2601–2606.

Nylén H, Habtewold A, Makonnen E, et al. Prevalence and risk factors for efavirenz-based antiretroviral treatment-associated severe vitamin D deficiency: a prospective cohort study. *Medicine (Baltimore).* 2016;95(34):e4631.

Padmapriyadarsini C, Ramesh Kumar S, et al. Dyslipidemia among HIV-infected patients with tuberculosis taking once-daily nonnucleoside reverse-transcriptase inhibitor-based antiretroviral therapy in India. *Clin Infect Dis.* 2011;52(4):540–546.

Parra A, Reyes-Terán G, Ramírez-Peredo J, et al. Differences in nocturnal basal and rhythmic prolactin secretion in untreated compared to treated HIV-infected men are associated with CD4+ T-lymphocytes. *Immunol Cell Biol.* 2004;82(1):24–31.

Peyriere H, Mauboussin JM, Rouanet I, et al. Report of gynecomastia in five male patients during antiretroviral therapy for HIV infection. *AIDS.* 1999;13:2167–2169.

Pinto G, Blanche S, Thiriet I, et al. Growth hormone treatment of children with human immunodeficiency virus-associated growth failure. *Eur J Pediatr.* 2000;159:937–938.

Quirino T, Bongiovanni M, Ricci E, et al. Hypothyroidism in HIV-infected patients who have or have not received HAART. *Clin Infect Dis.* 2004;38:596–597.

Ram S, Acharya S, Fernando JJ, et al. Serum prolactin in HIV infection. *Clin Lab.* 2004;50:617–620.

Ratner Kaufman F, Gertner JM, Sleeper LA, et al. Growth hormone secretion in HIV-positive versus HIV-negative hemophilic males with abnormal growth and pubertal development. The Hemophilia Growth and Development Study. *J AIDS Hum Retrovirol.* 1997;15:137–144.

Rietschel P, Corcoran C, Stanley T, et al. Prevalence of hypogonadism among men with weight loss related to human immunodeficiency virus infection who were receiving highly active antiretroviral therapy. *Clin Infect Dis.* 2000;31:1240–1244.

Rondanelli M, Caselli D, Arico M, et al. Insulin-like growth factor 1 (IGF-1) and IGF-binding protein 3 response to growth hormone is impaired in HIV-infected children. *AIDS Res Hum Retroviruses.* 2002;18:331–339.

Saint-Marc T, Partisani M, Poizot-Martin I, et al. A syndrome of peripheral fat wasting (lipodystrophy) in patients receiving long-term nucleoside analogue therapy. *AIDS.* 1999;13(13):1659–1667.

Salim YS, Faber V, Wiik A, et al. Anticorticosteroid antibodies in AIDS patients. *APMIS.* 1988;96:889–894.

Samaras K, Pett S, Gowers A, et al. Iatrogenic Cushing's syndrome with osteoporosis and secondary adrenal failure in human immunodeficiency virus-infected patients receiving inhaled corticosteroids and ritonavir-boosted protease inhibitors: six cases. *J Clin Endocrinol Metab.* 2005;90(7):4394–4398.

Samaras K, Wand H, Law M, et al. Prevalence of metabolic syndrome in HIV infected using International Diabetes Foundation and Adult Treatment Panel III criteria: associations with insulin resistance, disturbed body fat compartmentalization, elevated C-reactive protein, and hypoadiponectinemia. *Diabetes Care*. 2007;30:113–119.

Sekhar RV, Jahoor F, White AC, et al. Metabolic basis of HIV-lipodystrophy syndrome. *Am J Physiol Endocrinol Metab*. 2002;283(2):E332–E337.

Sekhar RV, Liu CW, Rice S. Increasing glutathione concentrations with cysteine and glycine supplementation lowers inflammation in HIV patients. *AIDS*. 2015;29(14):1899–1900.

Shikuma CM, Hu N, Milne C, et al. Mitochondrial DNA decrease in subcutaneous adipose tissue of HIV-infected individuals with peripheral lipoatrophy. *AIDS*. 2001;15:1801–1809.

Silva GA, Andrade MC, Sugui Dde A, et al. Association between antiretrovirals and thyroid diseases: a cross-sectional study. *Arch Endocrinol Metab*. 2015;59(2):116–122.

Slama L, Palella FJ, Abraham AG, et al. Inaccuracy of haemoglobin A1c among HIV-infected men: effects of CD4 cell count, antiretroviral therapies and haematological parameters. *J Antimicrob Chemother* 2014;69(12):2260–2267.

Sobieszczyk ME, Hoover DR, Anastos K, et al. Prevalence and predictors of metabolic syndrome among HIV-infected and HIV-uninfected women in the Women's Interagency HIV Study. *J AIDS*. 2008;48:272–280.

Stricker RB, Goldberg DA, Hu C, et al. A syndrome resembling primary aldosteronism (Conn syndrome) in untreated HIV disease. *AIDS*. 1999;13:1791–1792.

Szebeni J, Dieffenbach C, Wahl SM, et al. Induction of alpha interferon by human immunodeficiency virus type 1 in human monocyte–macrophage cultures. *J Virol*. 1991;65:6362–6364.

Tavares-Bello C, Sousa Santos F, Sequiera Duarte J, et al. Diabetes insipidus and hypopituitarism in HIV: an unexpected cause. *Endocrinol Diabetes Metab Case Rep*. 2017;17–24.

Theodorou M, Serste T, Van Gossum M, et al. Factors associated with vitamin D deficiency in a population of 2044 HIV-infected patients. *Clin Nutr*. 2014;33(2):274–279.

Tien PC, et al. Antiretroviral therapy exposure and incidence of diabetes mellitus in the Women's Interagency HIV study. *AIDS*. 2007;21:1739–1745.

Toma E, Therrien R. Gynecomastia during indinavir antiretroviral therapy in HIV infection. *AIDS*. 1998;12:681–682.

Tracey KJ, Cerami A. Metabolic responses to cachectin/TNF: A brief review. *Ann N Y Acad Sci*. 1990;587:325–331.

Tzur F, Chowers M, Agmon-Levin N, et al. Increased prevalence of diabetes mellitus in a non-obese adult population: HIV-infected Ethiopians. *Isr Med Assoc J*. 2015;17(10):620–623.

Ukibe NR, Ukibe SN, Emelumadu OF, et al. Impact of thyroid function abnormalities on reproductive hormones during menstrual cycle in premenopausal HIV infected females at NAUTH, Nnewi, Nigeria. *PLoS One*. 2017;12(7):e0176361.

Van den Bout-Van Den Beukel, C, Fievez L, Michels M, et al. Vitamin D deficiency among HIV type 1-infected individuals in the Netherlands: effects of antiretroviral therapy. *AIDS Res Hum Retrovir*. 2008;24:1375–1382.

Villette JM, Bourin P, Doinel C, et al. Circadian variations in plasma levels of hypophyseal, adrenocortical and testicular hormones in men infected with human immunodeficiency virus. *J Clin Endocrinol Metab*. 1990;70:572–577.

Visnegarwala F, Chen L, Raghavan S, et al. Prevalence of diabetes mellitus and dyslipidemia among antiretroviral naïve patients co-infected with hepatitis C virus (HCV) and HIV-1 compared to patients without co-infection. *J Infect*. 2005;50:331–337.

Vodkin I, Valasek MA, Bettencourt R, et al. Clinical, biochemical and histological differences between HIV-associated NAFLD and primary NAFLD: a case-control study. *Aliment Pharmacol Ther*. 2015;41(4):368–378.

Wanke CA, Silva M, Knox TA, et al. Weight loss and wasting remain common complications in individuals infected with human immunodeficiency virus in the era of highly active antiretroviral therapy. *Clin Infect Dis*. 2000;31:803.

Xiong Y, Hales DB. The role of the tumor necrosis factor-alpha in the regulation of mouse Leydig cell steroidogenesis. *Endocrinology*. 1993;132:2438–2444.

Yombi JC, Maiter D, Belkhir L, et al. Cushing's syndrome and secondary adrenal insufficiency after a single intra-articular administration of triamcinolone acetonide in HIV-infected patients treated with ritonavir. *Clin Rheumatol*. 2008; 27(Suppl 2):S79–S82.

37.

NONOPPORTUNISTIC INFECTIONS

RESPIRATORY COMPLICATIONS

Karen J. Vigil

CHAPTER GOAL

Upon completion of this chapter, the reader should be able to

- Demonstrate knowledge regarding the diagnosis and treatment of respiratory complications in patients living with HIV infection.

LEARNING OBJECTIVE

Review and characterize the respiratory complications related to HIV infection to provide early and accurate diagnosis and treatment.

KEY POINTS

Nonspecific Interstitial Pneumonitis

- Nonspecific interstitial pneumonitis (NSIP) encompasses several lymphocytic pulmonary syndromes including follicular bronchiolitis, lymphocytic bronchiolitis, lymphocytic interstitial pneumonitis (LIP), and diffuse infiltrative CD8+ lymphocytosis syndrome (DILS). Patients may be asymptomatic or present with dyspnea, nonproductive cough, and fever in a patient with CD4+ T cell counts greater than 200 cells/mm³. X-ray findings are nonspecific but characteristically show bilateral reticulonodular "interstitial" infiltrates.

- The diagnosis of NSIP requires histologic confirmation by biopsy. The optimum treatment remains unclear.

Lymphocytic Interstitial Pneumonitis

- LIP is a common respiratory complication of HIV infection in children but a rare complication in HIV-infected adults.

- It presents with slowly progressive dyspnea and nonproductive cough. X-ray findings are nonspecific but characteristically show bilateral reticulonodular "interstitial" infiltrates with a basal lung predominance.

- The diagnosis requires histologic confirmation by biopsy. Antiretroviral therapy (ART) has been used with success for treatment.

Pulmonary Arterial Hypertension

- The prevalence of pulmonary arterial hypertension (PAH) is higher in HIV-infected patients compared to the general population.

- The clinical presentation is similar to that in the general population, with progressive dyspnea, nonproductive cough, chest pain, and sometimes syncope or near syncope. These symptoms should prompt evaluation for early diagnosis.

- The diagnosis is first suggested by chest radiograph revealing prominent pulmonary arteries or by electrocardiogram. Right heart catheterization is the standard of diagnosis.

- Potential therapies for HIV-associated PAH include ART, oxygen, diuretics, and directed therapy. Prostanoids (epoprostenol, treprostinil, and iloprost), endothelin receptor antagonists (bosentan), and phosphodiesterase-5 inhibitors (sildenafil) are used in patients with HIV-associated PAH and have improved mortality.

NONSPECIFIC INTERSTITIAL PNEUMONITIS

The prevalence of NSIP is unknown. It was found in 48% of asymptomatic patients with AIDS in the 1980s (Ognibene, 1988) and in 38% of patients with AIDS and pulmonary symptoms or abnormal imaging studies (Suffredini, 1987). Different from LIP, it has been characterized only in adults and not in children.

The etiology of NSIP is unknown. It encompasses several lymphocytic pulmonary syndromes in patients living with HIV: follicular bronchiolitis, lymphocytic bronchiolitis, LIP, and DILS. Histologically, it is characterized by the presence of perivascular and peribronchial interstitial lymphocytes, plasma cells, and macrophages; however, these are also found along the pleura and interlobar fibrous septate (Travis, 1992).

Clinical symptoms are minimal or nonexistent; dyspnea, nonproductive cough, and fever have been reported (Suffredini, 1987). Physical exam may reveal crackles. Imaging studies may be normal or may show diffuse interstitial infiltrates (reticular, reticulonodular, or alveolar). Pleural effusions may also be seen. High-resolution computed tomography (CT) is also unspecific. Ground-glass pattern, consolidations, and honeycombing have been described. Similar to LIP, spirometry typically shows decreased diffusing capacity. Definitive diagnosis is made by histologic confirmation. The treatment is unclear. It can remain stable for many years or regress on its own. Theoretically, ART may improve its symptoms, but there is no pathological evidence to support this theory.

HIV LYMPHOCYTIC INTERSTITIAL PNEUMONITIS

LIP is a rare histopathologic disease that accounts for 40% of lung diseases in children with AIDS but only 1% or 2% of lung diseases in HIV-infected adults (Anderson, 1988; Stover, 1985).

Histologically, LIP is characterized by diffuse infiltration with polyclonal lymphocytes and occasionally plasma cells and histiocytes into the alveolar septae and along lymphatic vessels (Halprin, 1972). Type II pneumocyte hyperplasia and germinal center within lymphoid follicles are commonly found. Biopsies show CD8[+] and CD20[+] cells predominance. Fibrosis may develop in advanced cases.

Although the etiology of LIP is not clear, it has been suggested that Epstein–Barr virus (EBV) may play a role. EBV DNA samples have been found in fragments of lung tissues taken from children with LIP (Reddy, 1988). Contrarily, other studies have not shown any difference in the frequency of EBV in lung biopsies when comparing adult HIV-infected patients with LIP and control groups (van Zyl-Smit, 2015). HIV itself may play a role in the pathology of LIP, as has been demonstrated in a transgenic mouse model in which HIV induced a lymphoid interstitial pneumonitis syndrome (Hanna, 1998). HIV RNA copies have been obtained in lung biopsy samples of patients with LIP, and HIV-specific IgG is frequently present in the bronchoalveolar lavage fluid (Resnick, 1987). Human T-lymphotropic virus type I (HTLV-I) has been linked to LIP in Japan (Setoguchi, 1991).

The clinical presentation of LIP is similar in adults and children. Cough is the predominant symptom associated with slowly progressive dyspnea. Symptoms are usually present for several months. Fever, chest pain, weight loss, and arthralgias have also been reported. Physical exam may be completely normal or may reveal crackles. Children may have clubbing, salivary gland enlargement, lymphadenopathy, and hepatosplenomegaly.

Chest X-rays are normal or show bilateral reticular or nodular opacities. Focal areas of confluent pulmonary opacifications have been described as well as pulmonary cysts and patchy consolidations, the latter being less common. Chest CT shows diffuse ground-glass opacities with small nodules (2–3 mm) in a peribronchovascular distribution (Pitcher, 2010). Similar to other diffuse interstitial lung diseases, spirometry typically shows decreased total lung capacity and decreased diffusing capacity.

There is no consensus regarding the optimal treatment for LIP in HIV-infected patients. Corticosteroids at a dosage of 1 mg/kg/d are recommended. However, in several case reports, ART has been demonstrated to be effective by itself (Garcia Lujan, 2004; Innes, 2004; Ripamonti, 2003).

DIFFUSE INFILTRATIVE CD[+]8 LYMPHOCYTE SYNDROME

DILS is a rare multisystemic syndrome characterized by CD8[+] T cell lymphocytosis associated with a CD8[+] T cell infiltration of multiple organs. It is primarily characterized by parotid gland enlargement, xerophthalmia, xerostomia, and LIP. Respiratory clinical manifestations include nonproductive cough and dyspnea. Diffuse lymphadenopathy, hepatosplenomegaly, lymphocytic gastritis, and seventh cranial nerve palsy have also been described.

Histologic examination demonstrates visceral lymphocytic infiltration that could be a direct consequence of the large amount of CD8[+] cells. Lymphoid follicles with CD8[+] germinal centers are seen in salivary and parotid glands biopsies. HIV has been detected in macrophages within germinal center of lymphoid tissues; therefore, ART plays a major role on treatment. Immunosuppression with steroids is also recommended,

PULMONARY ARTERIAL HYPERTENSION

PAH has a higher prevalence among HIV-infected patients compared to the general population. It was reported to be 0.5% in 1991 (Speich, 1991) and remains the same in the ART era (Opravil, 2008; Sitbon, 2008; Zuber, 2004).

The occurrence of PAH in HIV-infected patients is not related to the CD4[+] T cell count. No risk factors have been found. However, a small study reported that chronic hepatitis C, drug addiction, and female sex increased by threefold the risk of developing PAH (Quezada, 2012). In a series that compared PAH in HIV-infected patients and PAH in non–HIV-infected participants, the HIV-infected patients were significantly younger and had milder disease (50% vs. 75% had New York Heart Association functional class III or IV, respectively) (Petipretz, 1994).

The clinical presentation of patients with HIV and PAH is similar to that of uninfected patients. Patients experience symptoms related to right heart dysfunction, such as progressive shortness of breath, pedal edema, nonproductive cough, fatigue, syncope, and chest pain. Physical exam may reveal increased intensity of the pulmonary second heart sound, third and fourth sound gallop, tricuspid and pulmonary regurgitation murmurs, elevated jugular venous pressure, and peripheral edema.

The diagnosis is usually made 6 months after the development of symptoms. Chest X-rays may show cardiomegaly and enlarged pulmonary artery, but clear lung fields. Transthoracic Doppler echocardiogram shows systolic flattening of the interventricular septum, enlargement of the right atrium and the right ventricle, and a reduction in both left ventricular systolic and left ventricular diastolic dimensions. It is important to note that a thorough evaluation should be done to exclude other causes of pulmonary hypertension.

Right heart catheterization is still the standard for diagnosing HIV PAH and for assessing its severity and response to treatment. PAH is defined by an mPAP of 25 mm Hg or higher, a mean pulmonary capillary wedge pressure of 15 mm Hg or less, and a normal or reduced cardiac output (Galie, 2009).

Treatment of HIV-associated PAH is similar to that of PAH in non–HIV-infected patients. Supportive therapy includes exercise, oxygen administration, diuretics, and digoxin. Oxygen is recommended if arterial blood oxygen pressure is 60 mm Hg or less. Diuretics reduce the right ventricular preload and are recommended in patients with right ventricular failure. The role of digoxin is controversial; however, it has been shown to improve cardiac output in patients with acutely right ventricular dysfunction attributable to PAH. Patients should be counseled against smoking and pregnancy. Anticoagulation is not routinely recommended in HIV-infected patients as there are no direct data of its benefit. Similarly, calcium channel blockers are of limited efficacy as vasoreactivity has been shown in only a small number of patients. Although there is no conclusive evidence of the effect of antiretrovirals on the progression of HIV-associated PAH, it is recommended to start ART in all patients with PAH regardless of the CD4[+] cell count, as supported by current guidelines. ART has been demonstrated to cause improvements in pressure gradient over time and to significantly reduce the risk of death in patients with HIV-associated PAH.

Specific therapy for PAH has also been evaluated in patients with HIV-associated PAH. Although there are no controlled clinical trials, prostanoids (epoprostenol, treprostinil, and iloprost), endothelin receptor antagonists (bosentan), and phosphodiesterase-5 inhibitors (sildenafil) have been used in patients with HIV-associated PAH and have been shown to improve symptoms and hemodynamic parameters. Caution should be taken with the use of these medications due to possible severe drug interactions, particularly with protease inhibitors and cobicistat.

PAH is an independent risk factor for death among HIV-infected patients (Opravil, 2008). However, with the advent of ART and the new treatment modalities, the overall survival rate at 1 year is 88% and 72% at 3 years (Degano, 2010).

REFERENCES

Anderson V, Lee H. Lymphocytic interstitial pneumonitis in pediatric AIDS. *Pediatr Pathol.* 1988;8:417–421.

Degano B, Guillaume M, Savale L, Montani D, et al. HIV-associated pulmonary arterial hypertension: survival and prognostic factors in the modern therapeutic era. *AIDS.* 2010;24:67–75

Galie N, Hoeper M, Humbert M. Guidelines for the diagnosis and treatment of pulmonary hypertension. *Eur Heart J.* 2009;30:2493–2537.

Garcia Lujan R, Echave-Sustaeta J, Garcia Quero C, et al. Lymphoid interstitial pneumonia resolved through antiretroviral therapy in an adult infected by human immunodeficiency virus. *Arch Bronconeumol.* 2004;40:537–539.

Halprin G, Ramirez J, Pratt O. Lymphoid interstitial pneumonia. *Chest.* 1972;62:418–423.

Hanna Z, Kay DG, Cool M et al. Transgenic mice expressing human immunodeficiency virus Type 1 in immune cells develop a severe AIDS-like disease. *J Virol.* 1998;72:121–132.

Innes A, Huang L, Nishimura S. Resolution of lymphocytic interstitial pneumonitis in an HIV infected adult after treatment with HAART. *Sex Transm Infect.* 2004;80:417–418.

Ognibene F, Masur H, Rogers P, et al. Nonspecific interstitial pneumonitis without evidence of *Pneumocysitis carinii* in asymptomatic patients infected with human immunodeficiency virus (HIV). *Ann Intern Med.* 1988;109:874–879.

Opravil M, Sereni D. Natural history of HIV-associated pulmonary arterial hypertension: trends in the HAART era. *AIDS.* 2008;22:35–40.

Petipretz P, Brenot F, Azarian R. Pulmonary hypertension in patients with human immunodeficiency virus infection: comparison with primary pulmonary hypertension. *Circulation.* 1994;89:2722–2727.

Pitcher R, Beningfield S, Zar H. Chest radiographic features of lymphocytic pneumonitis in HIV-infected children. *Clin Radiol.* 2010;65:150–154.

Quezada M, Martin-Carbonero L, Soriano V, et al. Prevalence and risk factors associated with pulmonary hypertension in HIV-infected patients on regular follow-up. *AIDS.* 2012;26:1387–1392.

Reddy A, Lyall E, Crawford D. Epstein–Barr virus and lymphoid interstitial pneumonitis: an association revisited. *Pediatr Infect Dis J.* 1998;17:82–83.

Resnick L, Pitchenik A, Fisher E, et al. Detection of HTLVIII/LAV specific IgG and antigen in bronchoalveolar lavage fluid from two patients with lymphocytic interstitial pneumonitis associated with AIDS related complex. *Am J Med.* 1987;82:553–556.

Ripamonti D, Rizzi M, Maggiolo F, et al. Resolution of lymphocytic interstitial pneumonia in a human immunodeficiency virus infected adult following the start of highly antiretroviral therapy. *Scand J Infect Dis.* 2003;35:348–351.

Setoguchi Y, Takahashi S, Nukiwa T, et al. Detection of human T-cell lymphotropic virus type I-related antibodies in patients with lymphocytic interstitial pneumonia. *Am Rev Respir Dis.* 1991;144:1361–1365.

Sitbon O, Lascoux-Combe C, Delfraissy JF, et al. Prevalence of HIV-related pulmonary arterial hypertension in the current antiretroviral therapy era. *Am J Respir Crit Care Med.* 2008;177:108–113.

Speich R, Jenni R, Opravil M, et al. Primary pulmonary hypertension in HIV infection. *Chest.* 1991;100:1268–1271.

Stover D, White D, Romano P, et al. Spectrum of pulmonary diseases associated with the acquired immune deficiency syndrome. *Am J Med.* 1985;78:429–437.

Suffredini A, Ognibene F, Lack E, et al. Nonspecific interstitial pneumonitis: a common cause of pulmonary disease in the acquired immunodeficiency syndrome. *Ann Intern Med.* 1987;107:7–13.

Travis W, Fox C, Devaney K. Lymphoid pneumonitis in 50 adult patients infected with the human immunodeficiency virus: lymphocytic interstitial pneumonitis versus nonspecific interstitial pneumonitis. *Hum Pathol.* 1992;23:529–541.

van Zyl-Smit RN, Naidoo J, Wainwright H, et al. HIV associated Lymphocytic Interstitial Pneumonia: a clinical, histological and radiographic study from an HIV endemic resource-poor setting. *BMC Pulm Med.* 2015;15:38–44.

Zuber J, Calmy A, Evison J. Pulmonary arterial hypertension related to HIV infection improved hemodynamics and survival associated with antiretroviral therapy. *Clin Infect Dis.* 2004;38:1178–1185.

38.

PSYCHIATRIC ILLNESS AND TREATMENT IN HIV POPULATIONS

Elizabeth David and Rakel Beall Wilkins

CHAPTER GOAL

Upon completion of this chapter, the reader should be able to

- Discuss the psychiatric concomitants of HIV illness and the role of psychiatric care in the overall treatment of HIV populations.

INTRODUCTION

From the earliest recognized AIDS deaths in 1981 to the commencement of highly active antiretroviral therapy (HAART) in the mid-1990s and the simpler combination ART regimens now available, HIV has remained a disease and an epidemic in constant evolution. For many years a near-certain death sentence, it has become a treatable chronic condition, with issues of HIV-associated dementia and rapid death by opportunistic infection generally replaced by treatment of "premature" aging and slow neurological decline and questions of maximizing adherence to treatment. Issues that have not changed include the tremendous psychosocial burden to the individual and family and the economic cost to the patient and society, as well as factors of stigmatization and marginalization of HIV populations. Many HIV-positive individuals were already stigmatized before contracting this illness. The prevalence of HIV infection is much higher in gay/bi/transsexual populations, in people of color, in substance abusers, in prison populations, in the homeless, in individuals with histories of physical and emotional trauma, and in people with mental illness (Whetten, 2008). HIV infection then adds to the burden through the psychological manifestations it causes (demoralization, depression, mania, anxiety, insomnia, and neurocognitive deficits), through disturbances in appearance (wasting, lipodystrophy, and Kaposi's sarcoma) and function (kidney disease, diabetes, and chronic pain), and through tremendous losses (people, independence, health, employment, and sense of control). From the earliest days of the epidemic, it has been recognized that mental illness and HIV infection are closely related (Hoffman, 1984), with some estimates of comorbidity as high as 50–70% (Blashill, 2011; Gaynes, 2008). Psychiatric illnesses are in and of themselves potentially lethal conditions, with increased rates of suicide and increased rates of illness and death from other conditions, including cancer, diabetes, and cardiovascular and cerebrovascular disease. They are associated with tremendous costs in terms of quality of life, lost productivity, and treatment. In combination with HIV-related illness, these issues are magnified.

Addressing these complex mental health issues is central to prevention, diagnosis, and treatment of HIV-related illness. Psychiatric illness is both a risk factor for disease and a barrier to adequate treatment. Substance abuse and "triple diagnosis" patients (HIV, substance abuse, and mental illness) have been particularly problematic (see Chapter 31). The chronically mentally ill are both overrepresented in this population and more difficult to reach and treat due to homelessness, distrust, and the unstructured nature of their lives. Survivors of physical and emotional trauma are a group increasingly recognized as both vulnerable to HIV infection and difficult to treat. They are prone to risk behaviors but slow to establish trusting relationships with treaters. In addition to these issues of primary mental illness is the factor of secondary mental health problems—those caused by the virus and/or its treatment.

LEARNING OBJECTIVES

- Discuss the bidirectional causes of the close association between HIV infection and psychiatric illness/symptoms.

- Recognize symptoms suggesting the presence of a psychiatric component to the clinical picture.

- Describe general principles of treatment and when specific intervention by mental health professionals is advised.

WHAT'S NEW?

This chapter has been updated to reflect terminology from the fifth edition of the *Diagnostic and Statistical Manual of Mental Disorders* (DSM-5; American Psychiatric Association, 2013), and additional recommendations regarding in- and outpatient psychiatric consultation have been added.

MENTAL ILLNESS AND HIV INFECTION

The interaction between HIV and mental illness is complex. For many individuals, the psychiatric condition is a preexisting one, predisposing to HIV infection through behavioral factors and risk environment (Rhodes, 2002). The risk factors for HIV are well-established and involve blood/bodily fluid contact with infected individuals through unprotected sexual behaviors, needle sharing, multiple sexual partners, and fetal/natal exposure. Individuals with preexisting psychiatric illness often engage in risky behaviors with little thought or fear of consequences. This relates to increased emotional immaturity and impulsivity (bipolar disorder, personality disorders, anxiety conditions, and posttraumatic stress disorder [PTSD]), poor contact with reality (schizophrenia and other psychotic conditions), denial and disinhibition (substance use disorders), cognitive dysfunction (major neurocognitive disorders and dementia), active thoughts of self-harm (depression), and victimization or impaired judgment (Kent, 2011; Owe-Larssom, 2009). Barriers to treatment, such as distrust of authority (including fear of legal consequences), poor communication skills, limited access (financial and transportation), lack of motivation, and unstructured lifestyle, all result in poor overall health care and delayed diagnosis of all health issues. Diagnosis of mental health issues is frequently challenging, and adherence to treatment is frequently impacted by these same factors.

Even for patients without psychiatric illness, the diagnosis of serious medical illness is a significant emotional blow. Freud stated that emotional health involves the ability to integrate and balance aspects of love, work, and play (Freud, 1910). What could more thoroughly disrupt this balance and integration than an illness such as HIV, with so many devastating consequences, such a complex regimen of treatment, and so many far-reaching biological, psychological, and social consequences? Every day, every pill, every medical visit, and every secret kept from family, friends, and coworkers is a reminder that one is compromised, vulnerable, damaged, not normal. In her landmark work, Kubler-Ross discussed this trauma and the individual's response to it through repetitive processes of denial, anger, bargaining, and depression before (ideally) reaching a degree of acceptance (Kubler-Ross, 1969). Treaters see the negative aspect of this emotional upheaval in its behavioral correlates: unrealistic anger at medical staff, equally unrealistic expectations of outcomes, guilt, fear, increased substance use, demoralization/hopelessness/amotivation, poor adherence to treatment, suicidal thoughts/suicide, and helplessness/neediness. We can help through building a positive and supportive treatment alliance that facilitates communication, acknowledges the huge cost to the patient, tolerates some of the stress behaviors, and does not take these behaviors personally but also sets limits of appropriateness. Timely referral to a psychiatrist or a psychotherapist is essential when stress becomes distress and behavior goes beyond those limits of appropriateness or when the patient becomes dangerous to him- or herself or others.

HIV enters the central nervous system (CNS) very early in the course of systemic infection, and the brain becomes an important site of damage in patients with HIV/AIDS (Ho, 1985). This causes many of those infected to develop neurological and psychological symptoms with etiology posited to relate to the presence of viral particles, neuroimmunological and neuroinflammatory responses, disruption of dopamine pathways and dopamine depletion (Kumar, 2011), and cytokine activation (Brafanca, 2011). Accelerated aging from HIV infection and HIV treatments, damage caused by opportunistic infections or comorbid medical conditions (e.g., hepatitis C virus), and concomitant use of drugs of abuse (Gannon, 2011) also play important roles. AIDS mania and a continuum of neurocognitive deficits from very subtle to frank and debilitating dementia are well-defined psychiatric syndromes directly related to the presence of virus, but depression, insomnia, and anxiety are also among the mental health symptoms that result from the infection itself. This part of disease progression seems to be less amenable to treatment with HAART compared to the more peripheral manifestations (Heaton, 2010), although antiretrovirals with higher levels of CNS penetration may promote improvement in some functions (Cysique, 2004). Unfortunately, those agents capable of crossing the blood–brain barrier are also the medications most likely to have psychiatric symptomatology as a side effect of use—a Pyrrhic victory in many ways.

Regardless of etiology, the presence of psychiatric symptoms and substance abuse is associated with poorer outcomes in HIV illness—lower levels of treatment adherence, slower virologic suppression, less subjective quality of life, increased morbidity and mortality, and increased utilization of medical services (Blashill, 2011; Carrico, 2011; Leserman, 2008; Nel, 2011; Pence, 2007). Adequate treatment of the psychiatric illness, however, improves outcome across all categories (Cook, 2006; Horberg, 2008; Mellins, 2009; Walkup, 2008). Although most of the literature cited in this chapter relates to HIV-positive adults, the diagnostic descriptions and treatments can, for the most part, be applied to adolescents and children (Benton, 2010; Rao, 2007).

PSYCHIATRIC DISORDERS AND TREATMENT

Careful diagnosis is essential given the complex interaction between psychiatric illness, HIV infection, substance abuse, comorbid medical conditions, and side effects of medications. Psychiatric illness cannot be diagnosed if these others medical factors play the primary role in causing symptoms (i.e., delirium), and psychiatric medications will seldom be of benefit in those cases. The following brief descriptions are based on the criteria from DSM-5 (American Psychiatric Association, 2013). The context of HIV infection results in no appreciable changes from the usual clinical manifestations of psychiatric disorders, with the possible exception of AIDS mania. Equally, pharmacological and nonpharmacological approaches to the treatment of psychiatric illness in the context of HIV illness are not radically different from those in HIV-negative populations. HIV-positive patients do seem to have some increased sensitivity to the side effects of the older "first-generation" antipsychotic drugs, even absent antiretroviral treatment (Kent, 2011). Because many psychopharmacologic agents are metabolized by the same elements of the cytochrome P450 isoenzyme system that metabolize protease inhibitors (PIs) and non-nucleoside/nucleotide reverse transcriptase inhibitors (NNRTIs), there were many fears early on that they could not be used concomitantly. In fact, however, there are surprisingly few clinically significant interactions except as specifically noted in the following sections. As in all clinical situations, however, a "start low and go slow" philosophy is warranted, and the relative risks and benefits of treatment must be carefully weighed.

Stress and Adjustment Disorders

There are multiple stressors associated with living with a serious and debilitating illness. Some kinds of emotional and behavioral reactions to this stress are normal, short-lived, and do not require treatment beyond support, reassurance, education, and therapeutic optimism. Assistance with access to resources and support networks or with informing family or significant others of the diagnosis can be "curative." Such reactions typically occur immediately after diagnosis and at periods of acute change in the illness (opportunistic infections, deteriorating CD4/viral load indices, initiation of ART, and onset of other comorbid medical complications) or in social circumstances (loss and financial problems). Typically, patients with these acute stress reactions are able to attribute the onset and nature of their symptoms to specific life events. They can also be distracted from their emotions and symptoms and are capable of feeling pleasure and interest in other things. *Adjustment reactions* (normal responses to stressful circumstances) are typically treated with supportive counseling and psychotherapy. It is only when stress reactions—anger, worry, guilt, sadness, and insomnia—are sustained for months, reach a point that they interfere with normal life functioning, or actually threaten survival (substance abuse, high-risk activities, and self-destructive thoughts/behaviors) that they require intervention. *Adjustment disorders* may also respond to support and psychotherapy, but they may necessitate psychiatric medications and/or hospital admission. The specific medication used depends on the symptoms being manifested. A complex of sadness, guilt, and insomnia frequently responds to use of antidepressants, particularly the more sedating ones (sertraline and mirtazapine). Symptoms on the anxiety continuum may benefit from use of almost any medication with a sedating side effect. Low-dose trazodone or antihistamine (hydroxyzine or diphenhydramine are commonly used) can be helpful, although caution must be used because these agents tend to cause drying of mucous membranes, which can exacerbate oral thrush. The use of benzodiazepines is rarely indicated (see later discussion). Because of the known relationship between stress and compromised immune function, early appropriate intervention is important (Leserman, 2008).

Anxiety Disorders and PTSD

This group of illnesses includes generalized anxiety disorder (persistent feelings of anxiety), the phobias (irrational fear of a particular thing or behavior), panic disorder (spontaneous attacks of intense anxiety), and obsessive–compulsive disorder (intrusive anxiety-provoking thoughts that compel ritualized behaviors thought to alleviate that anxiety). PTSD (anxiety-related thoughts and behaviors connected to memories of past traumatic life experiences) was formerly included in this group, but it has been separated into its own category in DMS-5. All involve activation of the sympathetic nervous system (psychological and physiological fight–flight–freeze responses) in situationally inappropriate circumstances because there is no current emergency. Careful diagnosis requires that endocrine disorders (especially thyroid-related), substance use (including caffeine, steroids, and psychostimulants), agitated depression, dementia, and delirium be eliminated as primary etiological factors. HIV-positive individuals have rates of anxiety disorders greater than those of the general population (Gaynes, 2008; Klinkenberg, 2004; Martinez, 2002), as well as an increased incidence of past traumatic experiences (Pence, 2009). Treatment ideally consists of a combination of psychotherapy (supportive, interpersonal, mindfulness, cognitive–behavioral, biofeedback, exposure and response prevention, flooding, etc.) and psychopharmacotherapy with antidepressants and/or anti-anxiety agents. Because therapeutic benefit with antidepressant is delayed in onset, it may be useful to supplement early treatment with low-dose benzodiazepine—lorazepam or other short-acting agent for panic disorder or phobias (used as needed at onset of panic attack or exposure to phobic object, but no more than three or four times a day) and clonazepam or other long-acting medication for generalized anxiety. Benzodiazepines are rarely the regimen of choice for more than the first 2–4 weeks, however, and should be discontinued at the earliest time practical. Some alternative treatments have also been shown to be effective, including relaxation/meditation, breath training, acupuncture, and guided imagery. All of the antidepressants except bupropion have efficacy in anxiety disorders, and selection of a specific medication should be based on safety (the serotonin and serotonin/norepinephrine reuptake inhibitors [SNRIs] are overall much safer than tricyclics or monoamine oxidase inhibitors), side-effect profile (relative sedation vs. excitation, potential for gastric symptoms, appetite stimulation vs. suppression, anticholinergic effects, concerns for liver function, assistance with pain control, etc.), and past response to medications in the patient or a family member. The selective serotonin reuptake inhibitors (SSRIs) can increase dream and flashback symptoms in patients with past traumatic experiences, although small doses of prazosin can mitigate this effect. As noted previously, antianxiety agents include benzodiazepines, antihistamines, buspirone, and small doses of antidepressants (e.g., trazodone) or atypical antipsychotics (e.g., Seroquel—an off-label use). All except buspirone work by sedating the patient, and they can be taken at the onset of anxiety symptoms. (Buspirone, like the antidepressants, must be taken on a regular basis to be effective.) The benzodiazepines also disinhibit behaviors, cause various degrees of cognitive impairment including amnesia and motor slowing/incoordination (a serious issue in a population already at risk for neurocognitive impairment), increase the risk of falls, and can trigger relapse or increased substance use in patients with substance abuse problems. They are meant for temporary use only and can usually be discontinued when the antidepressants have become effective (2–4 weeks). A consensus survey of psychiatrists treating HIV revealed clonazepam to be the most frequently used benzodiazepine, followed by lorazepam (Freudenreich, 2010). Alprazolam, midazolam, and triazolam should be avoided due to their high potential for addiction and their adverse interactions with antiretrovirals (ARVs). Again, the byword for concomitant use of any psychopharmacologic agent with an ARV is "Start low. Go slow."

Affective Disorders

Disorders of mood, particularly depression, are the most common psychiatric manifestations of HIV disease, with rates much higher in HIV-positive individuals than in the general population (Berger-Greenstein, 2007; Gaynes, 2011; Treisman, 2007) and increasing frequency with advancing disease (Atkinson, 2008). Depression hinders treatment of HIV-positive individuals, thus increasing risk of disease progression and spread (Benton, 2008; Villes, 2007), and it may have direct effects on immune responses (Alciati, 2007). Risk of suicidal ideation and attempts is significantly increased (Fermamdez, 2006), as is successful suicide (Carrico, 2010). Adequate treatment, however, reverses all these trends for both depression (Horberg, 2008; Mellins, 2009; Walkup, 2008) and bipolar disorder (Walkup, 2011).

Major depression consists of a constellation of symptoms related to persistent low mood (crying spells, guilt, low self-esteem, negative ruminations, social isolation, and loss of pleasure and interest), mental slowing (poor attention, concentration, memory, and energy; loss of libido; and motor retardation), and changes in behavior (increased or decreased sleep or appetite). Those with severe illness may also have psychotic symptoms—hallucinations and delusions—usually with depressive content. Careful diagnosis is essential because many of these symptoms might also be caused by serious medical illness, major neurocognitive impairment (dementia and delirium), side effects of medications, substance abuse, or grief and loss. Unlike adjustment disorders, patients with major depression generally cannot cite a precipitating event nor be distracted from their negative emotions. It is the relentless nature of the symptoms that results in a sense of hopelessness and despair, with a progressive narrowing of emotional focus until it may seem that death (suicide) is the only way out. Treatment ideally consists of combined psychotherapy and psychopharmacology with antidepressant medications, sometimes adding augmenting agents (a second antidepressant from another class, lithium, testosterone, thyroid medications, psychostimulants, and mood stabilizers). Low doses of antipsychotics are indicated on a temporary basis if psychotic features are present. Ketamine in very low doses is being used in some centers, but it must be used with extreme caution in patients on ARV treatment. Alternative treatments including exercise, meditation/relaxation, acupuncture, and herbal medications have been found to be helpful. Patients on St. John's wort should be cautioned, however, because this popular herbal antidepressant has significant adverse clinical interactions with multiple ARVs, anticancer drugs, anti-inflammatory agents, antibiotics, psychopharmacologic agents, cardiovascular drugs, anti-hypoglycemics, oral contraceptives, proton pump inhibitors, statins, and anti-asthmatic medications (Di, 2008). All of the normal antidepressant drugs show efficacy in the HIV-positive population, and choice of a particular medication should be based on safety (Watkins, 2011), side-effect profile, and past response to medications in the patient or a family member. A consensus study revealed that the SSRIs are the most common first-line drugs, with citalopram the number one choice (Freudenreich, 2010), although this may be changing with newer US Food and Drug Administration warnings about QT prolongation caused by this medication in higher doses. The SSRIs do have an anticoagulant effect, and, used long term, they can result in significant decreases in bone density. They can also cause bruxism and extrapyramidal side effects as well as sexual dysfunction. Switching drugs within a pharmacologic class is of benefit if patients find specific side effects intolerable. If a medication in any given class of antidepressants fails to show therapeutic benefit (8- to 12-week trial of adequate doses), a switch to another class of drugs is advised because agents within any given class have similar efficacy (Warden, 2007), so a switch to an SNRI (venlafaxine and duloxetine) and then to bupropion is a useful algorithm when there is treatment failure (Freudenreich, 2010). Particular caution is suggested in using bupropion (either as an antidepressant or in smoking cessation) in combination with the PIs (especially saquinavir or indinavir) or NNRTIs (especially efavirenz) because metabolism of bupropion can be inhibited, thus increasing the risk of seizures. Lopinavir/ritonavir, on the other hand, increases metabolism of bupropion, so bupropion doses must be increased when used with this antiretroviral combination (Hogeland, 2007). Currently, mirtazapine is considered to be a second-line choice, although it can be particularly useful for patients with chronic pain, weight loss, nausea, and vomiting (especially from chemotherapy regimens). Monoamine oxidase inhibitors (MAOIs) are not generally used in this population, and they are contraindicated for concomitant use with other antidepressants and most antipsychotics. (Remember that the antibiotic linezolid is also an MAOI.) All antidepressant regimens take several weeks to have therapeutic benefit, and the symptoms may not all resolve simultaneously. For this reason, particular caution and close observation are warranted in the early weeks of treatment: if energy, motivation, and a sense of agency return before suicidal thoughts and impulses disappear, a person who has had suicidal thoughts but insufficient energy to act on them may suddenly find the energy to act. The use of antidepressants in children and younger adolescents is particularly fraught with danger of suicide, and most antidepressant medications now carry a black box warning for this population. Inpatient psychiatric treatment is necessary if there are questions of safety, and this is obviously a situation in which it is best to err on the side of caution. Duration of treatment is a significant question. In the general population, an individual with a single episode of depression is generally treated for 4–6 months, whereas individuals with more than two episodes receive protracted therapy with antidepressants. Because of concurrent medical illnesses, stress, and the propensity for HIV virus to cause/exacerbate affective symptoms, long-term use of antidepressants is frequently necessary.

Bipolar disorder is defined by intermittent episodes of low (depressive) and high (hypomanic or manic) moods, each lasting days, weeks, or months and in a continuum of severity from mild to disabling. These mood swings are not a reaction to life events. The lows are identical to the depressive episodes described previously. The high episodes consist of persistent elevated mood tone (euphoric or irritable), increased energy (racing thoughts that bounce from topic to topic, little need for sleep, rapid speech, and increased libido), and an inflated sense of self-worth, and they often lead to engaging in risky behaviors. In mania, there is frank psychosis, with delusions (usually grandiose), disorganized thinking, and hallucinations leading to severe impairment in functioning and judgment. Psychopharmacologic treatment consists of mood stabilizer medications (lithium, valproic acid, carbamazepine, lamotrigine, and "second-generation" antipsychotic medications), with antidepressants and antipsychotics added if these symptoms are prominent. Some clinicians believe that long-acting benzodiazepine can be helpful in the first days of treatment for active mania, but these agents can further disinhibit and should be used only on a short-term basis. All of these medications are effective and reasonably safe in HIV populations. Lithium has a very narrow window of safety, and it is eliminated by the kidney. Particular caution is necessary in patients with kidney dysfunction, diarrhea, electrolyte disturbances, or cognitive impairment, but there are no specific interactions with ARVs. Lithium can cause or exacerbate thyroid dysfunction, tremor, acne, and psoriasis. Valproic acid appears to have few clinically significant drug interactions with the ARVs. However, it is metabolized by the liver, and it can increase liver enzymes and cause ammonemia. In addition, there is risk of severe hepatitis, weight gain, thrombocytopenia, nystagmus, and tremor. The use of carbamazepine is more complicated: it is metabolized by the cytochrome P450 system, and it induces its own metabolism. There have been reports of clinically significant carbamazepine toxicity when used in combination with ritonavir and other potent CYP3A4 inhibitors and also of virologic failure caused by enzyme induction. In addition, carbamazepine causes a significant risk for bone marrow suppression. Lamotrigine is effective particularly for depressive symptoms and appears to be safe when used in combination with ART. Initiation and discontinuation of this agent must be managed very carefully due to the risk of life-threatening rashes (Stevens–Johnson syndrome). It should be remembered that use of antidepressants without a mood stabilizer in a bipolar patient can trigger a manic episode.

AIDS mania is a specific manifestation of late-stage HIV infection. The mood is more likely to be irritable, sullen, and withdrawn than euphoric and hypertalkative, and there is frequently no prior personal or family history of psychiatric illness. Otherwise, the symptoms are typical of mania. Episodes, however, tend to be protracted, frequently with a prodrome of progressive cognitive decline. Symptoms do not usually respond to the usual psychopharmacological approaches, nor is there spontaneous remission if the condition is left untreated. The treatment of choice is initiation of aggressive ART.

Psychotic Disorders

The psychotic disorders are defined by loss of contact with reality (hallucinations and delusions) as well as by varying degrees of disorganized thinking and behavior. Insight and judgment are compromised, and it is frequently difficult to communicate clearly with these individuals because they can seem lost in their own, sometimes quite bizarre, world. Symptoms can be present on a temporary/episodic basis (brief psychotic episode and schizophreniform disorder) or may be more chronic (schizophrenia). Although disruption of thinking and behavior are most typical, any psychotic illnesses may involve some affective symptoms, even if only because patients recognize that they are somehow damaged and different. When symptoms of an emotional nature (depression or excitation) are a prominent and invariate part of the psychosis, schizoaffective disorder must be considered. Differential diagnosis includes affective disorder with psychotic features, medical illness (psychosis secondary to a medical condition such as HIV), side effects of medications, delirium/dementia, and substance abuse. Initial medical workup of anyone with a new-onset psychosis should probably include a urine drug screen (although many of the newer synthetic substances do not appear on standard tests), serology, endocrine screen, liver function tests, and computed tomography and/or magnetic resonance imaging of the brain. Visual hallucinations are rare in primary psychiatric illness, and they should also prompt a more complete medical evaluation. The chronically mentally ill are at increased risk of exposure to HIV due to factors such as homelessness, poor insight/judgment, lack of knowledge, victimization, and increased rates of substance abuse and other high-risk behaviors. Without adequate psychiatric treatment, their psychosis is a serious barrier to medical treatment due to poor adherence, difficulties communicating with providers, and unstable lifestyle (Carrico, 2011). Treatment consists of control of symptoms with medications along with psychosocial support. All of the antipsychotic medications work in HIV-positive patients. As previously noted, HIV-positive individuals, even without ARV treatment, seem to be somewhat more sensitive to the dopamine-mediated extrapyramidal side effects of these drugs. These side effects are most common with the high-potency first-generation antispychotics (i.e., haloperidol and fluphenazine). Both the first-generation and newer antipsychotics have significant risk for metabolic, cardiac (prolonged QT intervals), and endocrine side effects, and all are metabolized by the liver. They do not seem to have clinically significant interactions with ARV treatments, with the possible exception of lurasidone, but the issue of QT prolongation should be closely monitored because some of the ARVs also have this side effect. In the consensus survey, quetiapine was the most commonly used agent for psychosis, perhaps because it is also useful in mood stabilization and sedation (Freudenreich, 2010). A recent meta-analysis also revealed that quetiapine is the safest of the antipsychotic drugs to use for psychosis and behavioral control in demented patients (Kales, 2012). Clozapine and the low-potency first-generation medications (chlorpromazine and thioridazine) are seldom used (Freudenreich, 2010), although certainly not contraindicated. Use of depo injections tends to result in fewer side effects than seen with daily oral formulations and can be particularly useful in individuals for whom compliance with antipsychotic medication is problematic. It is safest, however, to initiate treatment with oral medication and then switch to the long-acting forms later.

Personality Disorders and the Difficult-to-Treat Patient

Personality can be thought of as enduring patterns of behavior, and this is partly what we refer to when we say we "know" a person—he or she has somewhat predictable responses to given circumstances, a familiar emotional tone, consistent belief systems, and a well-formed sense of identity and agency. When these patterns are stable and healthy, one's responses to adversity (coping techniques) help to mitigate stress, and one can modulate emotional responses to fit the circumstances, thus maintaining a stable sense of self and other and control over one's world. In personality disorders, an individual is stuck in repetitive patterns that do not work: coping techniques that actually escalate stressful situations, relationship paradigms that result in little perceived support and an increasing sense of frustration by and with others, spiraling loss of emotional control, and, ultimately, the fearful recognition that one is out of control of both internal and external worlds. Borderline and antisocial personality disorders are common in HIV-positive populations because these individuals tend to engage in high-risk behaviors that expose them to contracting the virus. The presence of these character pathologies also complicates treatment adherence (Hansen, 2009). They tend to be easily frustrated, to expect immediate gratification, to want sure-fire/magical interventions, and to demand "special" treatment from everybody. They also challenge authority and have limited ability to adequately and consistently structure their own lives. As difficult and challenging as it can be to work with these individuals, it is important to remember that their behavior is not intentional—it is their best effort to adjust to and control their chaotic world (Groves, 1978). Frequently, the emotions they engender in others are only reflections of the emotional turmoil within themselves. These are patients for whom referral to psychotherapy and the presence of a strong, consistent treatment team with a clearly delineated treatment contract are essential to preserve coherent participation in medical care. Because their psychological symptoms tend to be so reactive to events in the environment, switching rapidly and wildly, caution should be used in initiating medications. Although consistent use of an SSRI or a mood stabilizer may be useful, chasing symptoms with medications is contraindicated. It is generally much more useful to help these patients understand that their problems are related to their own patterns of response and poor behavioral choices than to teach them that some medication is going to provide them with internal peace or a sense of purpose, meaning, security, and attachment.

Substance Use Disorders

For a full discussion of this topic, see Chapter 31. Suffice it to say here that concurrent substance abuse complicates diagnosis and treatment of all other psychiatric conditions as well as HIV-related illnesses. These complications, as well as problems with adherence to treatment and overall morbidity and mortality, are additive in nature. It is essential to good treatment of HIV illness that clinicians screen for substance abuse and address it consistently and aggressively.

Major Neurocognitive Disorders (Delirium and Dementia)

HIV infection is associated with a number of CNS complications that may be temporary (delirium) or permanent (the continuum of neurocognitive deficits from asymptomatic to frank dementia). Dementia is a common manifestation of HIV illness, and it is discussed in Chapter 45. Delirium is a potentially life-threatening medical condition, generally of sudden and rapid onset and pursuing a waxing and waning course. Neurologists call this *encephalopathy*, and it is the most common neuropsychiatric diagnosis in hospitalized or critically ill HIV patients, with an estimated frequency of 40–65% (Gallago, 2011). It can manifest with any psychiatric symptom (anxiety, depression, mania, and psychosis) but most frequently includes disturbances in orientation, awareness/alertness, reality testing (hallucinations, including visual—which are very unusual in primary psychiatric conditions), communication (mumbled, incoherent speech), and motor behavior (lethargy, agitation, and picking at skin/clothing/intravenous lines). Several screening tools are used to diagnose delirium, of which the Cognitive Assessment Measurement Scale (CAMS and CAMS-ICU) is probably the most thoroughly researched. Definitive treatment involves correction of the underlying medical condition (infection, electrolyte disturbance, medication side effect, endocrine imbalance, intoxication, etc.). *Temporary* use of low-dose antipsychotic medications can be helpful, but they should be tapered and discontinued as the delirium resolves. Avoid the use of any anticholinergic agents and of antipsychotics with high anticholinergic side effects (Thorazine and thioridazine). Olanzapine, a sedating antipsychotic, may help with agitation but has been reported to cause, exacerbate, and/or prolong delirium in some cases. Use of benzodiazepines is also generally counterproductive, with the obvious exception of delirium caused by alcohol or benzodiazepine withdrawal. Measures that improve the patient's connection with reality can be very helpful. These include constant soft lighting (patients tend to misperceive shadows), quiet and soothing background noise, a visible clock and/or calendar in the room, a written list of names of nursing staff and others, and repeated self-introduction of caregivers and visitors.

Sexual Dysfunction

Sexual dysfunctions are very common in HIV illness. Disorders of desire (hypoactive sexual desire disorder) may be almost universal in HIV-positive men and women, and erectile dysfunction is very common in men with AIDS (Shindel, 2011). Although certainly related to stress, depression, and uncertainties about spreading the disease to sexual partners, it also seems likely that the virus itself, the myriad comorbid conditions (including hypogonadism, diabetes, and peripheral neuropathy), and the multiple medications used to treat all these conditions play a role. Treatment, therefore, is obviously complex. To the degree that these disorders are due to secondary issues, efforts can be made to change those conditions. Depression, stress, and comorbid conditions can be treated, and sometimes medications can be changed or doses modified to minimize sexual side effects. Sexual counseling and therapy are helpful in teaching the patient that sexual behavior and loving are not always about intercourse. Medications for erectile dysfunction (sildenafil, vardenafil, and tadalafil) can be used in this population, but doses must be reduced when given in the context of ART because metabolism is delayed. This obviously increases the probability of adverse side effects from the erectile dysfunction drugs, including visual changes, priapism, hypotension, and myocardial infarct. As with all medications, risks and benefits must be carefully weighed by the patient and the clinician.

SLEEP DISTURBANCE

Insomnia is defined as difficulty initiating and/or maintaining sleep or overall non-restful sleep. It tends to impair daytime function, and it is even more common in HIV-positive individuals than in the general population. This condition has been linked to poor quality of life and nonadherence to treatment (Saberi, 2011). Stress and depression play a role in etiology, and some ARVs disrupt sleep continuity. Efavirenz, a medication from the NNRTI class, is most consistently associated with sleep disturbances, including delayed sleep initiation, impaired sleep maintenance, and vivid nightmares. However, it appears that insomnia may be a primary symptom of viral presence, with changes in sleep architecture and decreased sleep efficiency noted even prior to onset of any symptoms of HIV/AIDS (Norman, 1992). Pharmacological treatment of insomnia includes the use of benzodiazepines, nonbenzodiazepine hypnotics, antihistamines, antidepressants, and antipsychotics. Of the benzodiazepines, clonazepam, lorazepam, oxazepam, and temazepam are relatively safe, although, as previously noted, their use in patients with current or past substance abuse is problematic. Use of alprazolam, flurazepam, quazepam, and triazolam is contraindicated with ARVs and ketoconazole and also in patients with kidney or hepatic disease. Sustained use of benzodiazepine medications is rarely, if ever, indicated. All of the nonbenzodiazepine hypnotics (eszopiclone, zaleplon, and zolpidem) are relatively safe in HIV populations, although dosages of zolpidem should be reduced if it used with PIs, even in boosting dosages. Dosages of all nonbenzodiazepine hypnotics should also be reduced in patients with hepatic disease. Antihistamines (especially diphenhydramine and hydroxyzine) are effective in many patients, and they are safe in HIV populations. However, it should be remembered that some patients have paradoxical excitatory responses to these medications. Sleep induction is an off-label use

for any antidepressant or antipsychotic. Nonetheless, low-dose tricyclics (especially doxepin and amitriptyline) and mirtazapine can be very useful in this regard. They can also help with control of neuropathic pain, which can improve sleep quality. In higher doses, all are associated with weight gain, which can be beneficial in some cases. Trazodone is frequently used to induce and maintain sleep in normal populations, but its use in HIV-positive patients on ART is problematic because final metabolism of the trazodone is slowed and untoward side effects (sleep disruption, vivid dreams, increased sedation, anxiety, and hypotension) occur. Of the antipsychotics, quetiapine and olanzapine are frequently used, although again, this is an off-label usage. As previously noted, HIV-positive individuals are much more sensitive to the extrapyramidal side effects of these medications. They also cause endocrine disturbances (prolactinemia) and metabolic side effects that may be cumulative with those of ART, such as lipodystrophy, hyperlipidemia, and insulin resistance (Omonuwa, 2009).

PSYCHIATRIC EFFECTS OF ANTIRETROVIRAL THERAPY

Many of the ARV agents have prominent psychiatric side effects that have been discussed previously. The most prominent of these psychiatric symptoms is vivid dreams and nightmares. Unfortunately, these issues seem to be more common, problematic, and sustained in individuals who are already vulnerable or experiencing psychiatric symptoms—that is, those with chronic mental illness. The vivid dreams and nightmares can be especially troubling for individuals with PTSD or past traumatic experiences. Although psychiatric diagnoses should not be a contraindication for use of these agents when indicated, special caution and close follow-up are certainly warranted. As with PTSD, low-dose prazosin can sometimes ameliorate the sleep disturbance experienced.

USE OF PSYCHIATRIC CONSULTATION

Mental health issues in HIV-positive individuals are very common. In an ideal world, mental health professionals would be integrated into every HIV treatment setting, and patients suspected of having significant illness or distress could be seen rapidly and frequently after referral. In reality, this is rarely the case, and even when psychiatrists and other mental health providers are on-site, visits are commonly delayed due to sheer numbers of patients. So when is referral most warranted and useful? First and foremost, the patient must be aware of and agree to mental health evaluation. Exceptions to this relate to those individuals who are incapable of understanding the need for assessment and treatment, who are imminently dangerous to self or other, or who are systematically destroying themselves and their treatment/treatment team by their behavior. Beyond that, the first part of a decision for referral rests on the primary problem and referring to the correct person. Certain individuals will benefit most from referral to support groups of like-minded people with similar problems, and many actually prefer this form of treatment. Although there are certainly exceptions, most psychiatrists are not the primary resource for either substance abuse counseling or for individual/marital/group psychotherapy. The first task is handled, in general, by specific substance abuse counselors and by self-help groups (Alcoholics Anonymous, Narcotics Anonymous, etc.). Psychotherapy is also more frequently done by behavioral specialists other than psychiatrists—psychologists, social workers, licensed counselors, etc. Pain management and medical management of substance detox and sobriety are also frequently handled by other caregivers. In most settings, it is possible to refer directly to these providers, who can then screen for cases requiring specific psychiatric intervention. Psychologists are specifically trained in diagnostic processes (including psychological and neuropsychological testing and screening) and in psychotherapeutic interventions. Psychiatrists, although trained in behavioral interventions and therapy techniques, are medical doctors, and they are the first-line resource for evaluation of individuals with complex psychiatric/medical issues, those who will probably require psychotropic medications, and those who have not responded to conventional psychotropic medications. Although psychiatrists can be helpful in diagnosing delirium and can assist in behavioral management of symptoms, the presence of these major neurocognitive disorders (including acute intoxication) generally makes it impossible to ascertain if there is true psychiatric illness underlying the current medical process. The final caveat is this: When in doubt, consult. I know I would much rather be included when I am not needed than absent when I could be of help, and I think most psychiatrists feel the same.

CULTURAL CONSIDERATIONS IN TREATING COMORBID HIV AND PSYCHIATRIC ILLNESS

The stigma associated with living with HIV is very well known, as is the stigma associated with psychiatric illness, but when the two are combined the consequences can be multiplicative and mutually reinforcing. Often it is fear of marginalization and/or discrimination that causes individuals to avoid HIV and mental health screenings and to be poorly adherent to treatment once diagnoses are made. These obstacles are further magnified when the individuals impacted by comorbid HIV and psychiatric illness belong to historically marginalized demographic groups. Whether it is because of their gender, ethnicity, or sexual orientation, individuals may encounter challenges in both navigating the healthcare system and receiving care that is uniquely suited to their needs. For instance, African and Caribbean black women have been found to experience higher rates of HIV related stigma and are more likely to report being marginalized or discriminated against based on racist and sexist stereotypes (Loutfy, 2012). This finding is of particular concern and importance in the United States, as African American women continue to be disproportionately represented among new HIV cases (CDC, 2014). Despite these statistics and the best efforts of public health clinicians, many HIV/mental

health interventions lack sufficient cultural sensitivity and are therefore less likely to be effective across different demographic groups. A 2016 cohort study of 31,000 HIV-infected individuals found that while 47% of respondents had an indication for antidepressant treatment, black non-Hispanics, Hispanics and other non-white ethnicities were significantly less likely to initiate antidepressant treatment than their white non-Hispanic peers (Bengtson, 2016). These findings suggest a strong cultural component to acceptance of mental health treatment, one that may be mediated by historical mistrust of the healthcare system and/or a reliance on alternative methods of emotional support. In 2016, respondents in a qualitative study of primary care providers who treat African American adults with HIV reported that their patients were more likely to seek emotional support from family or their spiritual community rather than seeking formal mental health treatment (Le, 2016). Accordingly, interventions aimed at identifying and preventing adverse HIV and mental health outcomes in these vulnerable groups should be tailored to address these pervasive cultural stigmas and norms. Neither HIV treatment nor mental health treatment are a one-size-fits-all endeavor, and clinicians should continue to enlist the input of patients, families, and spiritual and community leaders to develop programs that suit the diversity and cultural sensitivities of the people they seek to help and heal.

CONCLUSION

From the earliest days of the AIDS epidemic, it has been apparent that large numbers of HIV-positive people also have psychiatric illness. This, of course, raises the question of the direction of relatedness: Is psychiatric illness a risk factor for HIV infection, or does the HIV virus cause or predispose to psychiatric symptoms? The answer seems to be "yes"—the association goes both ways. Individuals with psychiatric illness (depression, bipolar disorders, anxiety disorders, PTSD, schizophrenia, dementia, and substance use disorders) tend to engage in behaviors that place them at increased risk for exposure to the HIV virus. Contracting HIV infection results in numerous psychosocial stressors that trigger or exacerbate expression of psychological symptoms in vulnerable individuals. The virus itself precipitates changes in the CNS that cause psychiatric manifestations. Finally, treatment with certain of the current ARV agents can result in psychiatric/behavioral symptoms. In turn, the presence of these psychiatric symptoms creates additional problems with diagnosis and treatment of HIV-related illnesses. All HIV-positive individuals should be screened for the presence of psychiatric illness. Fortunately, HIV-positive individuals respond well to traditional psychopharmacological and psychotherapeutic approaches to mental distress and illness, and, with adequate psychiatric treatment, they have good adherence and response to HIV treatment. Psychiatric illness alone is no longer considered to be a contraindication to full treatment of HIV or AIDS.

REFERENCES

Alciati A, Gallo L, Monforte AD, et al. Major depression-related immunological changes and combination antiretroviral therapy in HIV-seropositive patients. *Hum Psychopharmacol.* 2007;22(1):33–40.

American Psychiatric Association. *Diagnostic and statistical manual of mental disorders.* 5th ed. Arlington, VA: American Psychiatric Publishing; 2013.

Atkinson JH, Heaeton RK, Patterson TL, et al. Two-year prospective study of major depressive disorder in HIV-positive men. *J Affect Disord.* 2008;108:225–233.

Bengtson AM, Pence BW, Crane HM, et al. Disparities in depressive symptoms and antidepressant treatment by gender and race/ethnicity among people living with HIV in the United States. *PLoS One.* 2016;11(8):e0160738.

Benton TD. Depression and HIV/AIDS. *Curr Psychiatry Rep.* 2008;10(3):280–285.

Benton TD. Psychiatric considerations in children and adolescents with HIV/AIDS. *Child Adolesc Psychiatr Clin North Am.* 2010;19(2):387–400.

Berger-Greenstein JA, Cuevas CA, Brady SM, et al. Major depression in patients with HIV/AIDS and substance abuse. *AIDS Patient Care STDS.* 2007;21:942–949.

Blashill AJ, Perry N, Safren SA. Mental health: a focus on stress, coping, and mental illness as it relates to treatment retention, adherence, and other health outcomes. *Curr HIV/AIDS Rep.* 2011;8(4):215–222.

Brafanca M, Palha A. HIV associated neurocognitive disorders. *Actas Esp Psiquiatr.* 2011;39(6):374–383.

Carrico A. Elevated suicide rate among HIV-positive persons despite benefits of antiretroviral therapy: implications for a stress and coping model of suicide. *Am J Psychiatry.* 2010;167:117–119.

Carrico AW, Bangsberg DR, Weisner SD, et al. Psychiatric correlates of HAART utilization and viral load among HIV-positive impoverished persons. *AIDS.* 2011; 25(8):1113–1118.

Centers for Disease Control (CDC). HIV Among African Americans Online 2014. Available at http://www.cdc.gov/hiv/group/racialethnic/africanamericans/index.html.

Cook JA, Burke-Miller J, Anastos K, et al. Effects of treated and untreated depressive symptoms on highly active antiretroviral therapy use in a US multi-site cohort of HIV-positive women. *AIDS Care.* 2006;18(2):3–100.

Cysique LA, Maruff P, Brew BJ. Prevalence and pattern of neuropsychological impairment in human immunodeficiency virus-infected/acquired immunodeficiency syndrome (HIV/AIDS) patients across pre- and post-highly active antiretroviral therapy eras: a combined study of two cohorts. *J Neurovirol.* 2004;10(6):350–357.

Di YM, Li CG, Xue CC, et al. Clinical drugs that interact with St. John's wort and implication in drug development. *Curr Pharm Des.* 2008;14(17):1723–1742.

Fernandez F, Ruiz P. *Psychiatric aspects of HIV/AIDS.* Philadelphia: Lippincott Wilkins & Williams; 2006.

Freud S. Five lectures on psycho-analysis. *Am J Psychol.* 1910;21.

Freudenreich O, Goforth HW, Cozza KL, et al. Psychiatric treatment of persons with HIV/AIDS: an HIV psychiatry consensus survey of current practices. *Psychosomatics.* 2010;51:480–488.

Gallego L, Barreiro P, Lopez-Ibor JJ. Diagnosis and clinical features of major neuropsychiatric disorders in HIV infection. *AIDS Rev.* 2011;13:171–179.

Gannon P, Khan MZ, Kolson DL. Current understanding of HIV-associated neurocognitive disorders pathogenesis. *Curr Opin Neurol.* 2011;24(3):275–283.

Gaynes BN, Farley JF, Dusetzina SB, et al. Does the presence of accompanying symptom clusters differentiate the comparative effectiveness of second-line medication strategies for treating depression? *Depress Anxiety.* 2011;28(11):989–998.

Gaynes BN, Pence BW, Eron JJ Jr, et al. Prevalence and comorbidity of psychiatric diagnoses based on reference standard in an HIV+ population. *Psychosom Med.* 2008;70:505–511.

Groves, JE. Taking care of the hateful patient. *N Engl J Med.* 1978;298:883–887.

Hansen N, Vaughan E, Cavanaugh C, et al. Health-related quality of life in bereaved HIV-positive adults: relationships between HIV symptoms, grief, social support, and axis II indication. *Health Psychol.* 2009;28:249–257.

Heaton RK, Clifford DB, Franklin DR, et al. HIV-associated neurocognitive disorders persist in the era of potent antiretroviral therapy: CHARTER study. *Neurology.* 2010;75(23):2087–2096.

Ho D, Tota TR, Schooley RT, et al. Isolation of HTV-III from cerebrospinal fluid and neural tissues of patients with neurologic syndromes relate to the acquired immunodeficiency syndrome. *N Engl J Med.* 1985;313(24):1493–1497.

Hoffman, RS. Neuropsychiatric complications of AIDS. *Psychosomatics.* 1984;25:393–395.

Hogeland GW, Swindells S, McNabb JC, et al. Lopinavir/ritonavir reduces bupropion plasma concentrations in healthy subjects. *Clin Pharmacol Ther.* 2007;81(1):69–75.

Horberg MA, Silverberg MJ, Hurley LB, et al. Effects of depression and selective serotonin reuptake inhibitor use on adherence to highly active antiretroviral therapy and on clinical outcomes in HIV-positive patients. *J Acquir Immune Defic Syndr.* 2008;7(3):384–390.

Kales HC, Kim HM, Zivin K, et al. Risk of mortality among individual antipsychotics in patients with dementia. 2012;169:71–79.

Kent LK, Blumenfield M. Psychodynamic psychiatry in the general medical setting. *J Am Acad Psychoanal Dyn Psychiatry.* 2011;9(1):41–62.

Klinkenberg WD, Dacks SL;HIV/AIDS Treatment Adherence, Health Outcomes and Cost Study Group. Mental disorders and drug abuse in persons living with HIV/AIDS. *AIDS Care.* 2004;16(Suppl 1):S22–S42.

Kubler-Ross E. *On death and dying.* New York: Macmillan; 1969.

Kumar AM, Ownby RL, Waldrop-Valverde D, et al. Human immunodeficiency virus infection in the CNS and decreased dopamine availability: relationship with neuropsychological performance. *J Neurovirol.* 2011;17:26–40.

Le H-N, Hipolito MMS, Lambert S, et al. Culturally sensitive approaches to identification and treatment of depression among HIV infected African American adults: a qualitative study of primary care providers' perspectives. *J Depress Anxiety.* 2016;5(2):223.

Leserman J. Role of depression, stress and trauma in HIV disease progression in HIV. *Psychosom Med.* 2008;70:539–545.

Loutfy MR, Logie CH, Zhang Y, et al. Gender and ethnicity differences in HIV-related stigma experienced by people living with HIV in Ontario, Canada. *PLoS One.* 2012;7(12): e48168.

Martinez A, Israelski BS, Walker C, et al. Posttraumatic stress disorder in women attending human immunodeficiency virus outpatient clinics. *AIDS Patient Care STDs.* 2002;98:9–17.

Mellins CA, Havens JF, McDonnell C et al. Adherence to antiretroviral medications and medical care in HIV-positive adults diagnosed with mental and substance abuse disorders. *AIDS Care.* 2009;21(2):168–177.

Nel A, Kagee A. Common mental health problems and antiretroviral therapy adherence. *AIDS Care.* 2011;23(11):1360–1365.

Norman SE, Cheick AD, Freeman C, et al. Sleep disturbances in men with asymptomatic human immunodeficiency (HIV) infection. *Sleep.* 1992;15:150–155.

Omonuwa TS, Goforth HW, Preud'homme X, et al. The pharmacologic management of insomnia in patients with HIV. *J Clin Sleep Med.* 2009;5(3):251–262.

Owe-Larssom B, Sall, L, Allgulander C. HIV infection and psychiatric illness. *Afr J Psychiatry.* 2009;115–128.

Pence BW. The impact of mental health and traumatic life experiences on antiretroviral treatment outcomes for people living with HIV/AIDS. *J Antimicrob Chemother.* 2009;63(4):636–640.

Pence BW, Miller WC, Gaynes BN, et al. Psychiatric illness and virologic response in patients initiating highly active antiretroviral therapy. *J Acquir Immune Defic Syndr.* 2007;44(2):159–165.

Rao R, Sagar R, Kabra SK, et al. Psychiatric morbidity in HIV-positive children. *AIDS Care.* 2007;19(6):828–833.

Rhodes T. The "risk environment": a framework for understanding and reducing drug-related harm. *Int J Drug Policy*. 2002;13:85–94.

Saberi P, Neilands TB, Johnson MO. Quality of sleep: associations with antiretroviral nonadherence. *AIDS Patient Care STDS*. 2011;26(9):517–524.

Shindel A, Horberg M Smith J, et al. Sexual dysfunction, HIV, and AIDS in men who have sex with men. *AIDS Patient Care STD*. 2011;25:41–49.

Treisman G, Angelinno A. Interrelation between psychiatric disorders and the prevention and treatment of HIV infection. *Clin Infect Dis*. 2007;45(Suppl 4):S313–S317.

Villes V, Spire B, Lewden C, et al. The effect of depressive symptoms at ART initiation on HIV clinical progression and mortality: implications in clinical practice. *Antivir Ther*. 2007;12:1067–1071.

Walkup J, Wei W, Sambamoorthi U, et al. Antidepressant treatment and adherence to combination antiretroviral therapy among patients with AIDS and diagnosed depression. *Psychiatr Q*. 2008;79(1):43.

Walkup JT, Akincigil A, Chakravarty S, et al. Bipolar medication use and adherence to antiretroviral therapy among patients with HIV-AIDS and bipolar disorder. *Psychiatr Serv*. 2011;62(3):313–316.

Warden D, Rush AJ. The STAR*D project results: a comprehensive review of findings. *Curr Psychiatry Rep*. 2007;9(6):449–459.

Watkins CC, Pieper AA, Treisman GJ. Safety considerations in drug treatment of depression in HIV-positive patients: an updated review. *Drug Saf*. 2011;34(8):623–639.

Whetten K, Reif S, Whetten R, et al. Trauma, mental health, distrust and stigma among HIV-positive persons: implications for effective care. *Psychosom Med*. 2008;70(5):531–538.

39.

NEUROLOGICAL EFFECTS OF HIV INFECTION

Rodrigo Hasbun, Richard Dunham, Rituparna Das, Karen Nunez-Wallace,
Lydia J. Sharp, Doris Kung, and Joseph S. Kass

LEARNING OBJECTIVE

Discuss the clinical features, differential diagnosis, and management of HIV-associated neurocognitive disorders.

WHAT'S NEW?

- CD8[+] T cell encephalitis has been described as a severe form of HIV-associated neurocognitive disorder (HAND).

- The central nervous system (CNS) penetration effectiveness score has been correlated with cerebrospinal fluid (CSF) viral escape.

- CSF viral escape occurred in 7.2% of 1,063 patients, with the most important predictor being a regimen composed of protease inhibitors (PIs) (especially atazanavir) and nucleoside reverse transcriptase inhibitors (NRTIs). Neurocognitive impairment has been associated with lack of retention in care in older adults, with virologic failure, and, when coupled with frailty, it is associated with greater risk for falls, disability, and death.

- The impact of the CNS-targeted combination antiretroviral therapy (ART) on HAND is currently being explored.

KEY POINTS

- There is a high prevalence of HAND in ART-naïve patients and in patients treated with ART with virological suppression.

- Rapid screening tools such as the Montreal Cognitive Assessment test and the Frontal Assessment Battery test have been evaluated for their use in diagnosing HAND in the clinic.

- HAND is associated with significant cognitive, behavioral, and motor abnormalities that can impact ART compliance, retention in care in older individuals, virological success, and quality of life.

- CNS-targeted ART can be considered in patients with HAND, and corticosteroids can be considered in patients with CD8[+] T cell encephalitis.

Despite the use of combination ART, up to 39% of patients currently experience HAND (Robertson, 2007), and up to 42% of patients have at least 1 copy/mL of HIV-1 RNA in the CSF (Anderson, 2017). It is unclear if inadequate CSF penetration by the majority of the ARVs accounts for the high prevalence and whether CNS-active ART improves cognitive impairment. However, higher CSF penetration scores have been correlated with a lower probability of detectable CSF HIV RNA levels (Hammond, 2014; Anderson, 2017). A recent study documented that CSF viral escaped occurred in 7.2% of 1,063 patients with the most important predictor being a regimen composed of PIs (especially atazanavir) and NRTIs (Mukerji, 2018).

HIV causes a chronic form of encephalitis (HIVE) that is clinically characterized by either dementia or mild neurocognitive impairment. Since the introduction of ART in 1996, the incidence of HIV dementia has decreased by 50% (McArthur, 2005), but the prevalence of mild neurocognitive disorder (MND) has increased up to 39% (Robertson, 2007). HIVE is the result of direct microglial infection, interruption of trophic factors, or caused by inflammatory cytokines (Boisse, 2008). HIV enters the brain primarily by the "Trojan horse mechanism": it is carried by monocytes and lymphocytes that cross the blood–brain barrier. HIV has a predilection for the basal ganglia, deep white matter, and hippocampus, resulting in a subcortical dementia. Brain computed tomography (CT) scanning or magnetic resonance imaging (MRI) typically show cerebral atrophy and symmetrical white matter lesions. HIV dementia is a diagnosis of exclusion; other coinfections (e.g., JC virus-associated progressive multifocal leukoencephalopathy, hepatitis C, neurosyphilis, and cryptococcal meningitis), cerebrovascular disease, malnutrition, and drug abuse should be ruled out before making the diagnosis. In patients receiving ART with immunological response, a novel condition called *CD8[+] T cell encephalitis* was recently described (Lescure, 2013). Patients can present with HAND, headache, focal neurological deficits, and seizures, with MRI

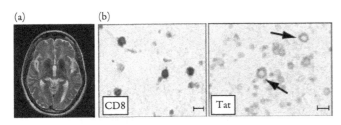

Figure 39.1 (A) Magnetic resonance imaging of an HIV-positive patient with virological suppression for 4 years with biopsy-proven CD8+ T cell encephalitis. (B) The presence of CD8+ T cells and HIV Tat antigens on brain biopsy. From Johnson TP (2013).

of the brain showing bilateral white matter lesions. CSF usually shows a lymphocytic pleocytosis with CD8+ T cells greater than 65%. A brain biopsy, if performed, shows pronounced CD8+ T cell infiltration with the presence of scant HIV antigens (Figure 39.1) (Johnson, 2013). Patients improve dramatically with corticosteroids and with improved CNS penetration of their ART regimen. The optimal dose and duration of corticosteroids are currently unknown.

Neuropsychological impairment is a surrogate marker for the presence of HIVE on autopsy (Cherner, 2002). Cognitive impairment has also been associated with ART nonadherence (Maggiolog, 2007), lack of retention in care in older adults (Jacks, 2015), and a negative impact on quality of life. In the pre-ART era, it was shown to be an independent predictor of death (Ellis, 1997). Furthermore, CSF HIV RNA levels are increased in HIV-1–infected individuals with neurocognitive impairment, as are several CSF biomarker levels, such as tumor necrosis-α, neurofilament light, neopterin, β_2 microglobulin, and monocyte chemotactic protein-1 (Boisse, 2008). A recent clinical model identified the following variables as associated with detectable CSF viral load: detectable serum HIV RNA on polymerase chain reaction (PCR), a CNS penetration score lower than 9, non-Caucasian race, less than 95% ART adherence, depression, and less than 36 months of ART duration (Hammond, 2014).

CLINICAL MANIFESTATIONS OF HAND

The clinical features of HAND are related to the involvement of HIV in the subcortical structures. The following can occur: slowing of processing speed; motor and psychomotor abnormalities; and executive, planning, or multitasking dysfunction (Valcour, 2011a). HAND affects the following three areas:

- *Cognitive*: Memory, concentration, mental processing speed, and comprehension

- *Behavioral*: Apathy, depression, agitation, and sometimes mania

- *Motor function*: Unsteady gait, poor coordination, abnormal tone, and tremors

In addition, patients with CD8+ T cell encephalitis can also manifest with new-onset seizures, status epilepticus, and altered mental status. Furthermore, HAND is associated with virological failure (Shahani, 2018), and, when combined with frailty, it is associated with greater risk for falls, disability, and death (Erlandson, 2018).

RISK FACTORS

Several studies have documented host genetic factors (polymorphisms in apolipoprotein E4, chemokine receptor CCR2, and monocyte chemoattractant protein-1), HIV-specific disease factors (history of AIDS-defining illness or low CD4+ T cell nadir, particular HIV variants, HIV RNA levels in CSF, duration of HIV infection, and older age at conversion), and comorbidities (>50 years of age, anemia, vascular disease, metabolic abnormalities, and hepatitis C coinfection) associated with HAND (Alfahad, 2013).

SCREENING TOOLS FOR COGNITIVE IMPAIRMENT

Despite the high prevalence of HAND in HIV clinics, it has not become routine to screen patients for cognitive impairment or to consider more CNS-active ART for those affected, even though there are now recommendations from an international consortium to do so (Mind Exchange Working Group, 2013). Screening tools that have been evaluated in HAND include several versions of the HIV dementia scale, the Mini Mental Status Exam (MMSE), standardized questionnaires that assess symptoms such as the Medical Outcomes survey, and the Montreal Cognitive Assessment (MoCA) and Frontal Assessment Battery test. The dementia scales are reliable but only in severe cases of HAND, the MMSE is not sensitive enough to detect HAND, and the subjective reporting of cognitive symptoms will miss patients due to poor insight or due to mood disturbances (Valcour, 2011a, 2011b). The MMSE is now proprietary. Recent studies have shown that the MoCA is a rapid, reliable, and sensitive test to detect cognitive impairment in HIV-1–infected individuals (Hasbun, 2012). A recent large study comparing different screening tools for HAND showed the Frontal Assessment Battery test had the highest correct classification rate (Triunfo, 2018).

DEFINITIONS OF NEUROCOGNITIVE DISORDERS

In 2007, the diagnostic criteria for HIV-associated neurocognitive disorders were revised (Antinori, 2007). Three HANDs were defined in these new criteria: asymptomatic neurocognitive impairment (ANI), MND, and HIV-associated dementia (HAD). ANI was defined as having a combination of the following: (1) an acquired mild to moderate impairment in cognitive function documented by a score of at least 1 standard deviation (SD) below demographically corrected norms on tests on at least two different cognitive domains, (2) the functional impairment has been seen for more than 1 month, (3) the impairment does not meet criteria for delirium or dementia, and (4) the cognitive impairment is not fully explained by comorbid conditions.

The definition of MND is identical to that of ANI, but it also includes interference with activities of daily living. The diagnosis of HAD includes a marked impairment of cognitive impairment.

CEREBROSPINAL FLUID ACTIVITY OF ANTIRETROVIRALS

There are currently more than 30 US Food and Drug Administration (FDA)-approved ARVs or combinations in six mechanistic classes for treatment of HIV infection, but only some have adequate CSF penetration (US Department of Health and Human Services [USDHHS], 2016). The CNS penetration-effectiveness score has been designed to classify the different ARVs with regard to their capability of lowering CSF RNA levels (Letendre, 2011). ARVs were assigned a score of from 1 to 4 based on their chemical properties, CSF penetration, and/or effectiveness in CNS studies (Table 39.1). A higher CNS penetration score was associated with higher virological suppression in the CSF (Letendre, 2010). Furthermore, a study showed that 10% of patients with virological suppression in the serum had viral escape (detectable CSF viral loads) (Edén, 2010). In addition, a higher CSF penetration score is associated with a lower rate of neurocognitive impairment (Carvalhal, 2016).

Very few randomized studies have evaluated the impact of CNS active ARVs in HIV neurocognitive disorders. In the pre-ART era, zidovudine (AZT) demonstrated efficacy in the treatment of HIV-associated dementia in a randomized clinical trial. AIDS Clinical Trial Group Study 005 randomized HIV patients with dementia to 2,000 mg/d of AZT, 1,000 mg/d AZT, or placebo (Sidtis, 1993). The greatest neuropsychological improvement was seen in those patients treated with high-dose AZT. In the ART era, a trial involving 49 patients found no neurocognitive benefit of CNS-targeted ART (Ellis, 2014). Future HIV treatment guidelines are anticipated to change and recommend cognitive screening and CNS ART as part of patients' evaluations.

RECOMMENDED READING

Calcagno A, Di Perri G, Bonora S. Pharmacokinetics and pharmacodynamics of antiretrovirals in the central nervous system. *Clin Pharmacokinet.* 2014;53(10):891–906. Available at https://www.ncbi.nlm.nih.gov/pubmed/25200312.
Letendre SL, Mills AM, Tashima KT, et al. ING116070: a study of the pharmacokinetics and antiviral activity of dolutegravir in cerebrospinal fluid in HIV-1-infected, antiretroviral therapy-naïve subjects. *Clin Infect Dis.* 2014;59(7):1032–1037. Available at https://www.ncbi.nlm.nih.gov/pubmed/24944232.

MYELOPATHY

LEARNING OBJECTIVE

Discuss the clinical presentation, differential diagnosis, and management of HIV-associated vacuolar myelopathy in HIV-positive patients.

WHAT'S NEW?

The incidence of HIV-associated vacuolar myelopathy (VM) has been reduced significantly. It remains a cause of disability in end-stage HIV and has a poor prognosis.

KEY POINTS

- VM is an uncommon complication of HIV infection and tends to occur in the late stages of HIV infection.

Table 39.1 CENTRAL NERVOUS SYSTEM PENETRATION-EFFECTIVENESS SCORE OF DIFFERENT ANTIRETROVIRALS (CPE SCORE)

DRUG CLASS	CPE SCORE			
	4	3	2	1
NRTIs	Zidovudine	Abacavir Emtricitabine	Didanosine Lamivudine Stavudine	Tenofovir Zalcitabine
NNRTIs	Nevirapine	Delavirdine Efavirenz	Etravirine	
Protease inhibitors	Indinavir	Darunavir/r Fosamprenavir/r Indinavir Lopinavir/r	Atazanavir Atazanavir/r Fosamprenavir	Nelfinavir Ritonavir Saquinavir Saquinavir/r Tipranavir/r
Entry/fusion inhibitors		Maraviroc		Enfuvirtide
Integrase inhibitors		Raltegravir Dolutegravir		

NRTI, nucleoside reverse transcriptase inhibitor; NNRTI, non-nucleoside reverse transcriptase inhibitor.
Adapted from Letendre (2011)

- Acute transverse myelitis and inflammatory CSF are unlikely to be VM.

- Human T cell lymphotropic virus type 1 (HTLV-1) infection is another infectious cause of myelopathy, and it should be considered in endemic geographic areas and in cases of co-infection with HIV.

- HIV and HTLV-1 can both cause a chronic myelopathy involving dorsal and lateral columns.

- The workup for a myelopathic patient includes MRI of the spine with and without contrast and may include CSF analysis and investigations for nutritional deficiencies and toxic agents.

HIV-ASSOCIATED VACUOLAR MYELOPATHY

Spinal cord injury, nonspecifically referred to as either *myelopathy* or *myelitis*, is a neurologic complication of HIV infection. Myelopathies in HIV-positive individuals can be due to either the direct effect of HIV invasion of the spinal cord, referred to as *HIV-associated VM*, or a secondary process such as an opportunistic infection or neoplasm that either invades or compresses the spinal cord.

VM is a chronic myelopathy seen in the late stages of HIV infection and affects 10–15% of untreated AIDS patients. Patients typically experience a slow, painless progression of neurologic symptoms over several months, most commonly lower extremity weakness and spasticity (Di Rocco, 1999). Patients also complain of progressive weakness or clumsiness in the lower extremities, as well as leg cramps and difficulty walking. Urinary symptoms such as frequency and urgency are also common, as is difficulty in achieving and maintaining an erection. Sensation in the legs, particularly proprioception and vibratory sense, is usually impaired, but a clear sensory level on the trunk is unusual. Arms are typically spared until advanced-stage disease. Localized back pain is not a common feature. Patients are also typically hyperreflexic in the lower extremities (hyperreflexia may spread to the upper extremities if the cervical cord is involved) and exhibit extensor plantar responses. VM patients present very similarly to patients with subacute combined degeneration due to vitamin B_{12} deficiency. Acute transverse myelitis, a prominent sensory level, or high numbers of inflammatory cells in the CSF should suggest another diagnosis. Although new HIV infections have been associated with acute myelopathy, this acute inflammatory process is a different entity from VM. Acute transverse myelitis associated with HIV seroconversion may respond well to steroids, intravenous immunoglobulin (IVIG), and ART (Hamada, 2011).

VM is the result of a chronic inflammatory degeneration with vacuolization and myelin pallor of the lateral and posterior tracts, typically affecting the thoracic cord most severely. On histologic examination, the lateral and dorsal columns demonstrate axonal injury and macrophage infiltration with lipid-laden macrophages and microglia infected with HIV (Dal Pan, 1997; Petito, 1994; Tyor, 1993). As many as 20–50% of AIDS patients may have pathological evidence of VM

at autopsy (Dal Pan, 1994; Di Rocco, 1998; McArthur, 2005). However, it is relatively uncommon clinically, affecting only 6.5–10% of HIV-positive patients (Cho, 2012).

There is no effective treatment for VM. Patients with VM often have coexisting HIV-associated dementia and peripheral neuropathies. Rehabilitation is helpful to maximize physical capacity. ART does not appear to alter the natural history of the disease (Banks, 2002). Antispasmodic agents such as baclofen, tizanidine, and botulinum toxin can be used for symptomatic relief.

The differential diagnosis for myelopathy in an HIV patient is broad and includes the following categories: (1) infections, including HTLV-1-associated myelopathy/tropical spastic paraparesis (HAM/TSP; discussed later), tuberculosis (TB) spondylitis or meningomyelitis, cytomegalovirus (CMV) radiculomyelitis, varicella zoster myelitis, toxoplasma myelopathy, neurosyphilis with tabes dorsalis, and bacterial epidural abscess (particularly among intravenous drug users); (2) neoplastic diseases, especially lymphoma and spinal metastases from systemic neoplasms; (3) nutritional deficiencies such as B_{12}, folate, copper, thiamine (presenting as beriberi), and vitamin E; and (4) toxic etiologies such as lathyrism (Di Rocco, 1998). Thus, an MRI of the spinal cord with and without contrast, lumbar puncture with CSF analysis, and serum analysis for vitamin and mineral deficiencies will be needed to evaluate for these etiologies (Chong, 1999).

Clinicians should consider common infectious causes initially. One study from Cape Town, Africa—an area known for a high prevalence of TB and HIV—reviewed 216 cases of myelopathy and cauda equina syndrome in HIV-positive patients (median $CD4^+$ count 185 cell/mm^3). Investigators found that 68% of myelopathy cases were due to TB (Candy, 2014). This large number of TB-related myelopathy cases in HIV patients has also been seen in other small studies in Africa (Bhigjee, 2001; Modi, 2011). TB spondylitis could be diagnosed radiographically with a high degree of certainty using MRI, and the diagnosis was confirmed with either CSF analysis or open biopsy.

HTLV-1–ASSOCIATED MYELOPATHY/TROPICAL SPASTIC PARAPARESIS

HTLV-1 is a retrovirus that is T cell-tropic and causes a proliferation of T cells (Manns, 1999). Although its full disease spectrum remains unknown, this virus is associated with adult T cell leukemia/lymphoma, uveitis, and HAM, which is also referred to as TSP. The prevalence of HTLV-1 infection increases with age, and it is more common in women than in men. It is also geographically clustered, with high rates in southern Japan, the Caribbean, areas of Africa, the Middle East, South America, the Pacific Melanesian Islands, and Papua New Guinea. Among low-risk groups in the United States and Europe, seroprevalence is approximately 1%. The majority of these patients remain asymptomatic during their lifetime. Approximately 1% of these HTLV-positive patients develop a myelopathy (Pillat, 2011). Given the overlapping risk factors for both HIV infection and HTLV-1 infection, it is important to consider HIV and HTLV-1 coinfection in HIV patients presenting with a slowly progressive myelopathy.

HAM patients present with progressive muscle weakness in the legs, hyperreflexia, clonus, extensor plantar responses, sensory disturbances, urinary incontinence, impotence, and lower back pain. HTLV-1 antibodies are present in both plasma and the CSF, as well as in brain and spinal cord tissue.

The diagnostic approach to HAM/TSP is similar to that outlined previously for VM, including MRI of the spine with and without contrast, lumbar puncture, and an investigation for nutritional deficiencies and toxic exposures. Definitive diagnosis requires an assay to detect HTLV-1 antibodies in plasma and CSF, including an assay capable of distinguishing between HTLV-1 and HTLV-2.

There is evidence that immune-modulating therapy, such as corticosteroids and IVIG, may be beneficial in the treatment of HTLV-1 myelopathy. Research is under way to develop new therapies in addition to preventive and therapeutic vaccines for HTLV-1 (Martin, 2011), but currently prevention education, particularly regarding breastfeeding and sexual behavior, is the only known method of reducing incidence.

MRI IN HIV-ASSOCIATED VACUOLAR MYELOPATHY

MRI of the spinal cord in VM is nonspecific and thus lacks pathognomonic features to differentiate it from non–HIV-related spinal cord disease. The spinal cord may appear normal, but the most affected spinal cords appear atrophic with or without hyperintensities on T_2-weighted images (Chong, 1999; Yousem, 2010).

RECOMMENDED READING

Di Rocco A. Diseases of the spinal cord in human immunodeficiency virus infection. *Semin Neurol*. 1999;19:151–155.
Manns A, Hisada M, La Grenade L. Human T-lymphotropic virus type I infection. *Lancet*. 1999;353:1951–1958.

INTRACRANIAL LESIONS

LEARNING OBJECTIVE

Discuss the clinical presentation, differential diagnosis, and treatment of intracranial lesions in HIV-positive patients.

WHAT'S NEW?

Due to concern for drug–drug interactions, particularly in patients receiving ART, most clinicians favor levetiracetam as the first line for managing seizures. In the setting of status epilepticus, phenytoin remains the recommended therapeutic intervention for cessation of clinical and subclinical seizures. Of note, it may be important to avoid enzyme-inducing antiepileptic drugs in people on ARV regimens that include protease inhibitors or non-nucleoside reverse transcriptase inhibitors (NNRTIs).

KEY POINTS

- Intracranial focal lesions in HIV specifically occur in patients with CD4$^+$ T cell counts less than 200 cell/mm³.

- The most common focal mass lesion is toxoplasmosis. The use of prophylactic agents such as trimethoprim–sulfamethoxazole can decrease the incidence of toxoplasmosis.

- Primary central nervous system lymphoma (PCNSL) is the most common brain neoplasm seen in HIV patients. On imaging studies, it is usually a solitary intracranial mass lesion in the setting of a negative toxoplasmosis serology.

- Progressive multifocal leukoencephalopathy (PML) on neuroimaging is a nonenhancing lesion of the white matter involving the subcortical U-fibers without edema or mass effect.

Intracranial mass lesions are common neurologic findings and account for as much as half of the neurologic disorders seen in HIV patients. Although intracranial mass lesions typically occur in patients with known HIV infections with advanced immunosuppression (CD4$^+$ counts <200 cells/mm³), an intracranial lesion can occasionally be the initial presenting symptom of AIDS. Intracranial lesions in HIV-positive patients can be broadly categorized into three groups: opportunistic infections, neoplasms, and cerebrovascular disease (American Academy of Neurology [AAN], 1998).

The clinical presentation of intracranial lesions varies depending on the underlying etiology. Typical presenting clinical symptoms include alteration in level of awareness and consciousness as well as focal neurologic deficits. In developed countries such as the United States, the most common etiologies include toxoplasmosis, PCNSL, bacterial and fungal abscesses, and PML. Additional differential diagnosis includes primary brain tumor, brain metastasis from systemic cancer, tuberculoma, and lesions of fungal origin. Differentiating among this large differential diagnosis of intracranial lesions can be challenging, especially with regard to use of biopsy for establishing the diagnosis. However, in patients with large lesions with mass effect and impending herniation, open biopsy with decompression is recommended. Nevertheless, making the correct diagnosis is paramount to effectively managing the causal pathogen in a timely manner. Achieving this goal requires a knowledge-based diagnostic algorithm that accounts for the relative frequency of various etiologies of intracranial lesions. Figure 39.2 provides a useful process of differential considerations based on level of immunosuppression, typical clinical and radiographic presentation, management options, and prognosis with or without empirical treatment (AAN, 1998).

Cerebral toxoplasmosis is the most common cause of space-occupying intracranial focal mass lesions in HIV/AIDS and typically results from reactivation of latent infection of

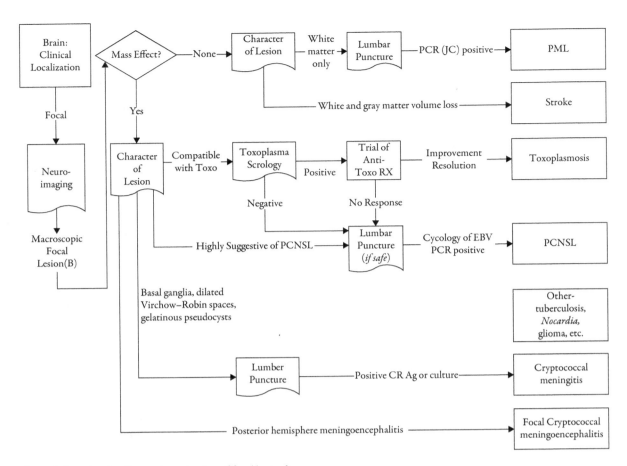

Figure 39.2 General algorithm for diagnostic evaluation of focal brain diseases.

Toxoplasma gondii, an obligate intracellular parasite (AAN, 2000a). In the United States, there has been a decline in the incidence of cerebral toxoplasmosis due to widespread use of prophylaxis agents such as trimethoprim–sulfamethoxazole and ART in HIV-positive patients (AAN, 1998).

Toxoplasmosis often presents with subacute changes in level of consciousness, fever, headaches, seizures, and focal neurologic deficit. It should be suspected in any HIV patient with an intracranial mass lesion, especially if the patient has a CD4^{+n} T cell count of less than 100 cells/mm^3, is not receiving toxoplasmosis prophylaxis, and has immunoglobulin G antibodies to *T. gondii* (AAN, 2000a). Investigative studies such as CSF analysis, toxoplasma serology, or imaging studies do not always provide a definitive diagnosis. In this patient population, obtaining lumbar puncture is often contraindicated due to the presence of lesions with mass effect and increased risk of herniation. In cases in which CSF is obtained, analysis frequently shows nonspecific mild mononuclear pleocytosis with elevated protein. PCR can increase utility of CSF analysis. PCR can detect *T. gondii* with high specificity (100%) but variable sensitivity (30–50%) (AAN, 2002). Consequently, whereas a positive PCR result is highly suggestive of the diagnosis, a negative result does not exclude it.

Imaging studies can also provide supportive information. MRI with or without contrast has greater sensitivity than contrast-enhanced CT, especially for detecting multiple lesions, subcortical lesions, and posterior fossa involvement. However, neither imaging modality alone is sufficient enough to make a diagnosis because there is no pathognomonic radiographically distinguishing feature of toxoplasmosis compared to PCNSL. Toxoplasmosis typically presents as multiple, homogeneous, ring-enhancing lesions with cerebral edema and mass effect. It has a predilection for the basal ganglia and corticomedullary junction, with involvement of both white and gray matter (AAN, 2000a). Although a solitary mass lesion with edema is often observed in PCNSL, it can also be seen in toxoplasmosis (AAN, 2000a). Thallium single-photon emission computed tomography (SPECT) and positron emission tomography (PET) can be useful in distinguishing toxoplasmosis from lymphoma. Lymphoma has increased thallium uptake on SPECT and hypermetabolism of glucose and methionine on PET. Toxoplasma is hypometabolic on PET and does not show uptake of thallium (AAN, 2000a). As a result of the limitation of the investigative modalities mentioned previously, diagnosis of toxoplasmosis is often presumptive and based on clinical and radiographic findings, as well as clinical and radiographic response to empirical treatment within the first 2 weeks. Open or stereotactic brain biopsy can yield a definitive diagnosis; however, there is morbidity and even mortality associated with the procedure due to subsequent intracranial hemorrhage. Biopsy is often pursued as a last resort in patients who do not improve with empirical management, have large mass effect with impending herniation, and require a rapid definitive diagnosis.

Empirical anti-toxoplasma therapy is usually started once toxoplasmosis is suspected. First-line treatment includes the use of sulfadiazine, pyrimethamine, and folinic acid (leucovorin) (AAN, 2000a). Folinic acid must be given to counteract myelosuppression from use of pyrimethamine. Treatment duration is at least 6 weeks before resuming secondary prophylaxis. Recrudescence occurs in up to 30% of patients, usually due to poor adherence to secondary prophylaxis; however, it can occur despite good adherence to the treatment plan (AAN, 2000a). In patients with sulfa allergy or intolerance, clindamycin is an alternative to sulfadiazine; however, use of clindamycin is associated with a slightly increased incidence of recrudescence. If the patient is intolerant to both sulfadiazine and clindamycin, alternatives include high-dosed trimethoprim–sulfamethoxazole, azithromycin, and atovaquone. Atovaquone is less tolerated due to gastrointestinal side effects. There is usually clinical improvement within the first 10–14 days of treatment. Clinical improvement occurs prior to radiographic evidence of improvement, which may be noted within 2 or 3 weeks. Lack of improvement within the first 2 weeks should raise suspicion for an alternative diagnosis.

The use of adjunctive corticosteroids, such as dexamethasone, should be brief, and they should be implemented only in very particular circumstances, such as when there is clinical evidence of midline shift or impending herniation, signs of critically elevated intracranial pressure, or clinical deterioration within the first 48 hours of therapy. Under these circumstances, the benefits of steroids outweigh the many risks of steroid administration. The use of steroids can be a diagnostic confounder because it can improve the clinical presentation, making it difficult to distinguish between effects of steroid use and the therapeutic effectiveness of empiric treatment. In addition, steroid anti-inflammatory actions affect the radiographic presentation by decreasing the intensity of contrast enhancement and surrounding edema, thus interfering with reliable comparative interpretation of subsequent radiographic images. Steroids can also complicate the pathological diagnosis of PCNSL if a biopsy is needed, rendering the biopsy falsely negative for the presence of lymphoma. Aside from more acute steroid complications such as avascular necrosis, hyperglycemia, and psychiatric symptoms, the prolonged use of steroids can also make the patient susceptible to other opportunistic infections.

An important differential diagnosis is PCNSL. It is one of the four AIDS-defining neoplasms, which include systemic non-Hodgkin's lymphoma, Kaposi's sarcoma, and invasive cervical carcinoma. PCNSL is commonly seen in HIV patients with $CD4^+$ T cell counts of less than 50 cells/mm^3 and is rarely the initial presenting symptom of AIDS. The pathogenesis is also strongly related to reactivation of latent Epstein–Barr virus (EBV) infection. The clinical presentation is very similar to that of toxoplasmosis, with alteration of the level of consciousness, impaired cognitive function, seizures, and focal neurologic deficits such as aphasia and hemiparesis. Investigative studies such as CSF analysis and imaging are often utilized. Lumbar puncture should only be obtained

if there are no contraindications, such as risk of herniation. CSF analysis, particularly cytology, can be helpful, but it has a very low sensitivity. PCR assay of CSF for EBV DNA can be diagnostic. PCR for EBV has a sensitivity greater than 80% and a specificity greater than 95%. As with toxoplasmosis, MRI often provides higher diagnostic yield than CT scan, but CT with contrast remains useful particularly in patients who have contraindication for getting an MRI. PCNSL can present with single or multiple well-defined, ring or patchy enhancing lesions with edema and mass effect. It often involves supratentorial regions such as the corpus callosum and periventricular or periependymal areas (PCNSL in AIDS) (AAN, 2000b). As previously mentioned, SPECT and PET can be useful in differentiating lymphoma from other etiologies, including toxoplasmosis. Although PET and SPECT have limited sensitivity, they have high specificity. A diagnosis is often made using a combination of CSF cytology, toxoplasmosis serologic testing, failure of trial of empirical antibiotics usually for treatment of toxoplasmosis, and positive CSF PCR for EBV; if necessary, a brain biopsy is obtained (AAN, 2000b). Open or stereotactic brain biopsy is typically required prior to whole-brain irradiation, which is the current mainstay treatment for PCNSL. Whole-brain radiation appears to be able to prevent further neurologic progression or produce reversal of deficits. However, the treatment plan is based on the patient's overall health status. There can be spread of lymphoma with involvement of the eyes; therefore, a complete ophthalmologic examination including a slit-lamp examination should be performed (AAN, 2000b).

Other etiologies of intracranial mass lesions include other neoplasms, cerebrovascular disease, and opportunistic infections. Kaposi's sarcoma may rarely manifest as an intracranial lesion. Furthermore, patients with HIV may also develop brain lesions unrelated to immunocompromised status, such as glioma or metastatic disease.

In addition to toxoplasmosis, patients with HIV may develop parasitic, fungal, or bacterial infections that present as a mass lesion. Most of these opportunistic infections present with meningitis and focal neurological signs and symptoms related to the presence of a mass lesion. Although neurocysticercosis (NCC) is not more common in patients with HIV, the incidence of HIV infection is growing in countries where NCC is endemic. Coinfection has been rarely reported, but reports of concomitant infection with HIV, NCC, and an additional pathogen have been reported. Furthermore, in the setting of immunocompromise, interpretation of imaging findings may be particularly difficult. On imaging studies, the appearance of neurocysticercosis varies depending on the stage of infection. MRI is favored over CT scan, especially for evaluation of intraventricular and cisternal/subarachnoidal cysts as well as cystic degeneration and pericystic inflammatory reaction (Serpa, 2007).

Common bacterial mass lesions include abscess from *Mycobacterium tuberculosis, Nocardia, Listeria monocytogenes*, and *Treponema pallidum*. In developing countries, particularly in highly endemic areas such as Southeast Asia and Africa, tuberculous meningitis is common. Due to its proclivity for the basal meninges, tuberculous meningitis often presents clinically with multiple cranial neuropathies and hydrocephalus (AAN, 2000a). Neuroimaging may show masses, which are often tuberculomas. Intracranial tuberculomas can be seen on MRI as hypointense or isointense due to varying amounts of caseous necrosis. This variable appearance of intracranial tuberculoma is attributed to the changing nature of the granulomatous lesion (Park, 2008). The diagnosis of tuberculous meningitis can be challenging and requires a combination of CSF analysis including culture for TB, acid-fast bacilli stain, and TB PCR along with a clinical evaluation for systemic TB.

Common etiologies of fungal abscesses include *Cryptococcus neoformans, Candida albicans*, aspergillosis, mucormycosis histoplasmosis, and coccidioidomycosis. Of these fungi, cryptococcosis is the most common opportunistic fungal infection in HIV-positive patients and arises from an acquired infection from *C. neoformans*, an encapsulated yeast. The widespread use of fluconazole as prophylaxis has resulted in a decrease in incidence. Neuroimaging, usually a contrast-enhanced brain MRI, may show cryptococcomas—multiple enhancing lesions of various sizes most often seen within perivascular spaces. These lesions usually resolve with treatment. A definitive diagnosis is made by a positive CSF culture for *C. neoformans*, a positive CSF India ink stain, or a reactive CSF cryptococcal antigen test. For additional information, see Chapter 33.

PML is characterized by multifocal areas of demyelinating often in subcortical and periventricular areas. The pathogenesis is reactivation of JC virus infecting oligodendroglia in the setting of advanced immunosuppression. On imaging studies, the lesions are usually nonenhancing with contrast and do not produce any edema or mass effect. The subcortical U fibers are involved. However, in the setting of immune reconstitution inflammatory syndrome (IRIS), on MRI with contrast, PML can present with contrast enhancement, focal edema, and mass effect (Tan, 2009).

HIV-positive patients with intracranial lesions are at heightened risk for developing seizures. Antiepileptic drugs (AEDs) should not be given for routine prophylaxis to patients with a CNS mass lesion because not all patients with CNS lesions will develop seizures. However, once the patient experiences a seizure, chronic AED administration is appropriate. In 2012, the American Academy of Neurology (AAN) issued an evidence-based guideline for clinicians about AED selection for people with HIV/AIDS (Birbeck, 2012). The guideline describes the strength of evidence for each of its recommendations based on the quality of evidence available from clinical investigations. The vast majority of the recommendations in this guideline were rated as having weak evidence.

The AAN guideline states that it may be important to avoid enzyme-inducing AEDS (EI-AEDs) in people on ARV regimens that include protease inhibitor (PI) or non-nucleotide reverse transcriptase inhibitors (NNRTIs) because pharmacokinetic interactions may result in virologic failure (Birbeck, 2012). Examples of EI-AEDs include phenobarbital, phenytoin, and carbamazepine. The guideline identifies circumstances in which specific dose adjustments to the ARV regimen of the AED are advised to maintain adequate serum levels of the mediations. For example, patients concurrently on phenytoin and lopinavir/ritonavir may need a 50% dosage increase in lopinavir/ritonavir to maintain adequate serum levels of the PI and virologic control. Patients coadministered atazanavir/ritonavir and lamotrigine may require a 50% increase in lamotrigine dose to maintain adequate serum levels of the AED and seizure control. Patients taking both zidovudine and the P450 inhibitor valproic acid may require a zidovudine dose reduction to maintain unchanged zidovudine levels (Birbeck, 2012). Although not specifically recommended in the guideline, renally excreted medications such as levetiracetam are often favored for patients on ARVs given their lack of drug–drug interactions. However, in the setting of status epilepticus, the use of intravenous phenytoin or fosphenytoin remains the recommended therapeutic intervention for cessation of clinical and subclinical seizures.

Using the approach discussed in this chapter, common etiologies of intracranial mass lesion can be systemically evaluated in order to make a diagnosis and institute therapy. In settings with limited resources such as sophisticated neuroimaging, CSF PCR, and biopsy, clinical findings on history and physical combined with the prevalence of infectious etiologies should guide the diagnosis and subsequent empiric therapeutic intervention.

MENINGITIS

LEARNING OBJECTIVE

Review the differential diagnosis and clinical management of meningitis in HIV-positive patients.

WHAT'S NEW?

- Timing of ART should be deferred in cryptococcal meningitis.

- Meningococcal A vaccine has decreased the burden of meningitis in Africa.

KEY POINTS

- The differential diagnosis is broad.

- Meningitis in HIV-positive patients is usually treatable, and a cause should be investigated.

- A meta-analysis of studies of meningitis in HIV-positive patients in Africa documented that the three most common causes were *C. neoformans, M. tuberculosis*, and bacterial meningitis.

- The differential diagnosis of meningitis in HIV-positive individuals is broad (viral, bacterial, fungal, mycobacterial, lymphomatous, etc.) (Table 39.2).

Table 39.2 CAUSES OF MENINGITIS IN HIV-POSITIVE PATIENTS

Viral	Acute HIV seroconversion, CD8$^+$ T cell encephalitis, enterovirus, herpes simplex virus, arboviruses (West Nile virus, St. Louis encephalitis), cytomegalovirus, varicella zoster virus, influenza virus, Epstein–Barr virus, lymphocytic choriomeningitis virus, mumps
Bacterial	Bacterial meningitis, endocarditis, parameningeal focus (e.g., epidural abscess and mastoiditis), syphilis, Lyme disease, *Mycoplasma pneumoniae*, *Bartonella henselae*, *Brucella* species, *Ehrlichia*, *Rickettsia*, leptospirosis, *Mycobacterium tuberculosis*
Fungal	*Cryptococcus neoformans*, *Coccidioides immitis*, *Histoplasma capsulatum*, *Aspergillus* species, zygomycosis
Parasitic	*Naegleria/Acanthamoeba*, *Taenia solium*, *Angiostrongylus cantonensis*, *Toxoplasma gondii*
Noninfectious	Medications (e.g., antibiotics and nonsteroidal anti-inflammatory drugs), meningeal carcinomatosis (lymphoma and leukemia), vasculitis, chemical meningitis (intrathecal injections and spinal anesthesia), seizures

NEUROLOGIC EVENTS IN EARLY STAGE HIV INFECTION

Acute HIV infection may manifest as an "aseptic meningitis" presentation, but this is most likely an underdiagnosed as only 30% of adults with meningitis are tested for HIV and only few have an HIV-1 RNA level done (Shukla, 2017). Patients with recent HIV exposure present with severe headache, stiff neck, diffuse macular rash, photophobia, and a lymphocytic pleocytosis in the CSF. Patients typically have positive HIV RNA levels and/or a positive HIV p24 antigen.

Approximately one-third of patients with HIV who present with meningitis do so during the early stages of the HIV disease (i.e., CD4+ T cells >200 cells/mm³) (Vigil, 2018). The most common causes of meningitis in these patients are *herpes simplex* type 2, *varicella zoster virus* (VZV) and arboviruses (West Nile, St. Louis encephalitis). *Herpes simplex* type 2 can present with the initial genital outbreak of herpes or in patients with recurrent episodes of aseptic meningitis (Mollaret's meningitis). Arboviruses should be suspected in the summer and fall in patients with fever and recent mosquito bites. Unfortunately, viral PCR and arboviral serologies are obtained in the minority of patients with meningitis (Nesher, 2016). Other less common causes of meningitis in the HIV-positive patient include VZV, syphilis, and bacterial meningitis. VZV can present with a dermatomal vesicular rash and an aseptic meningitis presentation, and it should prompt screening for HIV. In more advance stages of HIV infection, it can present as disseminated VZV. It can also present without a rash (*zoster sine herpete*); with the Ramsay–Hunt syndrome; or with stroke, myelopathy, retinitis, or encephalitis.

The diagnosis is made using CSF VZV PCR, CSF anti-VZV antibody, or by culturing the virus from a vesicular lesion, if present. CSF VZV PCR has a specificity of greater than 95% but a sensitivity of only 30%. A positive VZV PCR confirms the diagnosis but a negative test does not rule out the diagnosis. CSF anti-VZV antibody is the more sensitive test, with a 98% sensitivity (Osiro, 2017; Nagel, 2007; DeBiasi, 2004; Aberle, 2005). Treatment is with high-dose intravenous acyclovir.

Syphilis can also present as an aseptic meningitis syndrome in patients with a diffuse rash that involves the palms and soles. A serum rapid plasma reagin (RPR) of greater than 1:32 and a CD4$^+$ T cell count of less than 350 cells/mm³ are associated with neurosyphilis and should prompt the performance of a lumbar puncture (Marra, 2004). Bacterial meningitis represents a diagnostic consideration in all stages of HIV, but its incidence has decreased with the advent of the conjugate vaccines (Lopez, 2014). If bacterial meningitis is suspected, intravenous dexamethasone and antibiotic therapy with vancomycin, ceftriaxone, and ampicillin should be started to cover for *Streptococcus pneumoniae*, *Neisseria meningitides*, and *Listeria monocytogenes* until CSF cultures are negative (Tunkel, 2004). Recently, delayed cerebral injury has been documented in 4% of patients with bacterial meningitis with an association with the use of steroids (Gallegos, 2018). Despite this, dexamethasone should continue to be used in pneumococcal meningitis where it is associated with a decrease in mortality (Hasbun, 2017).

NEUROLOGIC EVENTS IN LATE STAGE HIV INFECTION (CD4$^+$ T CELL COUNT <200 CELLS/MM³)

The most common cause of meningitis in patients with advance immunosuppression is *Cryptococcus neoformans, TB, CMV*, and *toxoplasmosis*. In cryptococcal meningitis, the CSF examination typically shows a lymphocytic pleocytosis but inflammation may be absent. CSF India ink examination is positive in up to 50% of cases, and the CSF cryptococcal antigen test is positive in approximately 90% of cases. An opening pressure should be documented because its elevation is associated with higher CSF fungal burden and also higher neurological morbidity and mortality (Gambarin, 2002). The preferred therapy for cryptococcal meningitis is a combination of intravenous amphotericin B deoxycholate at 0.7–1 mg/kg/d plus flucytosine 100 mg/kg/d divided in four doses for 2 weeks followed by fluconazole 400 mg/d PO to decrease the intracranial hypertension (i.e., >25 cm of H$_2$O) by either repeat lumbar punctures or temporary percutaneous lumbar drains or ventriculostomy if persistent elevations occur (Perfect, 2012). If flucytosine is not available or the patient experiences drug toxicity, the patient can be treated with a combination of amphotericin B with fluconazole either 400 mg or 800 mg once daily for 14 days. A repeat lumbar puncture should be done at the end of the 2-week period to document a negative CSF fungal culture. Intravenous amphotericin B should be continued if the patient has persistently positive CSF cultures, is clinically deteriorating or comatose, or has persistent elevated and symptomatic intracranial pressures (Perfect, 2012). A therapeutic lumbar puncture to decrease intracranial pressure was associated with a reduced risk of death in a study performed in Africa (Rolfes, 2014). The same study also documented that ART should be delayed until 5 weeks after initial presentation to avoid an increase in mortality (Boulware, 2014).

CMV can cause meningitis, ventriculitis, polyradiculitis, polyradiculomyelopathy, retinitis, esophagitis, and colitis in patients with advanced HIV disease (CD4$^+$ T cell count <50 cells/mm^3). It is treated initially with intravenous ganciclovir 5 mg/kg every 12 hours, and then the patient is switched to oral valganciclovir when stable (US Department of Health and Human Services [USDHHS], 2016). MRI of the brain typically shows periventricular enhancement, and CSF can demonstrate either a lymphocytic (encephalitis) or neutrophilic (polyradiculitis) pleocytosis, hypoglycorrhachia, and mild elevations of the protein. A positive CMV PCR in the CSF makes the diagnosis.

Mycobacterial TB can occur at any stage of the HIV illness, but extrapulmonary disease (e.g., meningitis, lymphadenitis, pleuritis, and pericarditis) occurs more frequently in patients with CD4$^+$ T cell counts of less than 200 cells/mm^3. The incidence of TB has declined in the United States, and there are fewer than 1,000 cases of coinfection reported annually (USDHHS, 2016). TB and HIV must be treated together rather than sequentially, particularly in patients with low CD4$^+$ T cell counts. Tuberculous meningitis usually has a subacute to chronic presentation, lymphocytic pleocytosis, a low CSF glucose, and basilar involvement with cranial nerve palsies and altered mental status. A Thwaites's diagnostic score less than 4 (5 parameters—age, duration of illness, white blood cell count, total CSF white blood cell count, and percentage of CSF neutrophils) or a Lancet consensus score of greater than 6 (20 parameters divided in four categories: clinical, CSF, CNS imaging, and evidence of TB elsewhere) indicate possible TB meningitis, and patients with these scores should be considered for empiric therapy. The CSF acid-fast bacilli smear is insensitive, and CSF cultures are positive in only 38–88% of cases (Thwaites, 2012). Caution should be used in areas with neurobrucellosis as patients may also have suggestion scores for TB meningitis (Erdem, 2015). A CSF *M. tuberculosis* PCR and an adenosine deaminase level can also aid in the diagnosis. Duration of treatment is 1 year. The mortality is higher for HIV-positive patients than HIV-negative patients with TB meningitis (51.3% vs. 23% (Thao, 2013). Prognostic factors for death in HIV coinfected patients include severity of illness, lower CSF pleocytosis, lower weight, lower CD4+ T cell counts, and abnormal sodium levels (Thao, 2018).

Finally, toxoplasmosis may also present with a meningitis/encephalitis presentation in patients with advanced AIDS (Opintan, 2017). Toxoplasmosis classically presents with fever, focal neurological signs, seizures, and headaches, with MRI of the brain showing multiple ring-enhancing lesions with restriction of diffusion on diffusion-weighted imaging (DWI). Toxoplasmosis is a very unlikely cause of disease if the serum toxoplasma IGG is negative (Rosenow, 2003). If the serology is negative or the neuroimaging is not suggestive of toxoplasmosis, an early brain biopsy is advocated (Rosenow, 2007).

MENINGITIS IN HIV-POSITIVE VERSUS HIV-NEGATIVE PATIENTS

A recent study of 549 adults with community-acquired meningitis who were tested for HIV revealed that 25% were infected (Vigil, 2018). HIV-positive patients presented with less meningeal symptoms (headache, neck stiffness, and Kernig's sign), but with higher rates of hypoglycorrhachia, elevated CSF protein, and an abnormal cranial imaging. HIV-positive patients also were more likely to have cryptococcal meningitis, neurosyphilis, and VZV than those without HIV. Patients with HIV coinfection were also more likely to have a pathogen identified (57%) than those without HIV (31%). An adverse clinical outcome was seen in approximately 25% of patients with abnormal neurological exam and hypoglycorrhachia being identified as predictors. HIV coinfection was not associated with an adverse outcome.

IMMUNE RECONSTITUTION SYNDROME IN HIV

IRIS occurs after the initiation of combination ART and either "unmasks" a previous subclinical infection or worsens a known infection despite appropriate therapy (paradoxical reaction). In the CNS, IRIS can develop with many opportunistic processes, most commonly cryptococcal meningitis, TB meningitis, and progressive multifocal leukoencephalopathy (Huis in't Veld, 2012). The two most common and serious CNS IRIS events are cryptococcal and tuberculous meningitis. TB IRIS usually presents between a few weeks to 3 months after the initiation of ART, and it can present with meningitis or tuberculomas or both. Risk factors include low CD4$^+$ cell counts, disseminated TB, and extrapulmonary TB. Treatment should consist of adjunctive steroids. CSF acid-fast bacilli cultures are typically negative. Cryptococcal IRIS can develop between 1 and 10 months after initiating ART and can present as culture-negative meningitis, cryptococcomas, pneumonitis, and/or lymphadenopathy. Adjunctive steroids should be considered. Additionally, CD8$^+$ T cell encephalitis syndrome has been described in patients receiving ART with low or undetectable serum HIV viral loads (Lescure, 2013). These patients usually have a low CD4$^+$ T cell nadir and a history of opportunistic infections, and they usually present with high CD4$^+$ T cell counts. They can present with memory disturbances, headaches, diplopia, ataxia, and, sometimes, seizures. MRI of the brain shows bilateral white matter lesions, and CSF shows lymphocytic pleocytosis with detectable CSF HIV viral loads. The treatment is corticosteroids and optimizing the CNS penetration of ART.

MENINGITIS IN RESOURCE-LIMITED COUNTRIES

A review of 1,303 episodes of meningitis with confirmed etiologies in HIV-positive patients in sub-Saharan Africa showed that 52% had cryptococcal meningitis, 19.6% had TB, 14.2% had bacterial meningitis, and 14.2% had other etiologies (Veltman, 2014). Mortality rates were high, ranging from 25% to 68% in the different studies.

DISTAL SYMMETRICAL POLYNEUROPATHY

WHAT'S NEW?

High-concentration capsaicin dermal patch has shown efficacy in patients with painful HIV distal symmetric polyneuropathy (SDP) and in one study produced a sustained reduction in pain over 12 weeks.

KEY POINTS

- DSP is the most common neurologic complication of HIV infection, occurring in 30–60% of patients.

- ARV toxic neuropathy is associated with use of older NRTI therapy, especially for didanosine and stavudine.

- Treatment includes removal of neurotoxins and management of pain/discomfort.

DSP occurs in 30–60% of all HIV-positive patients (Ellis, 2010; Evans, 2011), making it the most common neurologic complication in HIV disease. Its incidence increases to as high as 62% in advanced HIV/AIDS (Schifitto, 2002; Simpson, 2006). DSP may develop at any time after the onset of HIV infection, with a mean time of developing neuropathy at 9.5 years after HIV diagnosis (Robinson-Papp, 2009). However, a smaller study suggested that signs of neuropathy may be detected in as many as 35% of patients with a median of only 3.5 months after HIV transmission (Wang, 2014). Although the etiology of DSP is still under investigation, it is most likely an indirect result of HIV infection, probably through immune-mediated mechanisms (Pardo, 2001). Risk factors for DSP in HIV-positive individuals include increased age, Caucasian race, lower hemoglobin levels, hypertriglyceridemia, lower CD4$^+$ cell count nadir, current combination ART use, and past use of the dideoxynucleoside drugs (didanosine, stavudine, and zalcitabine) (Banerjee, 2011; Ellis, 2010; Simpson, 2006; Tagliati, 1999).

Neuropathy associated with NRTIs, especially didanosine, stavudine, and zalcitabine, is the only neurologic complication that has increased since the introduction of ART (Keswani, 2002). The risk of ARV toxic neuropathy (ATN) appears to be substantially higher when didanosine and stavudine are used together, especially when combined with hydroxyurea (Moore, 2000). There are no discrete distinguishing features between DSP and ATN (Pardo, 2001; Price, 1999), and a current hypothesis is that mitochondrial dysfunction mediates NRTI toxicity (Kallianpur, 2009).

Symmetrical spontaneous and evoked pains predominantly in the feet and progressing to the upper extremities are typical symptoms, along with tingling, numbness, stabbing sensations, and burning (Figure 39.3) (Cornblath, 1988; DeVivo, 2000; Price, 1999; Wulff, 1999a). Deep

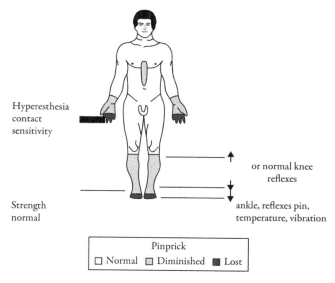

Figure 39.3 Typical signs and symptoms of distal sensory polyneuropathy (DSP).

tendon reflexes at the ankles are typically diminished or absent, and appreciation of temperature may be decreased (Wulff, 1999a).

The pathology of DSP includes damage to and loss of both large- and small-caliber sensory nerve fibers, with macrophage infiltration in the dorsal root ganglia and along the nerve trunks (Keswani, 2002). Sural nerve biopsies obtained from patients with ATN have shown severe axonal destruction, prominent in unmyelinated fibers (Dalakas, 1996). Different possible pathogenetic mechanisms of DSP in HIV have been studied. Activation of macrophages and production of proinflammatory cytokines appear to play a significant role (Pardo, 2001). Secreted viral proteins such as the envelope glycoprotein gp120 may also contribute to HIV neurotoxicity (Keswani, 2003). DNA damage in the mitochondria of distal axons may also add to the distal degeneration of sensory nerve fibers (Lehmann, 2011). Prominent mitochondrial abnormalities have more significantly been noted in association with NRTIs, supporting the suggestion that neuronal mitochondrial damage underlies ATN (Chen, 1991). Further support for this concept is derived from in vitro observations of graded inhibition of γ-DNA polymerase by different NRTIs (Martin, 1994). Dideoxynucleosides (didanosine, zalcitabine, and stavudine) are the most potent inhibitors of this enzyme in vitro (Martin, 1994), and zidovudine, lamivudine, abacavir, emtricitabine, and tenofovir have only minimal effects. Mitochondrial DNA content in lymphocytes, however, does not correlate with the presence of ATN (Simpson, 2006).

The differential diagnosis of DSP/ATN includes other toxic neuropathies, including those caused by other medications commonly used in HIV/AIDS patients such as metronidazole, dapsone, vincristine, isoniazid (DeVivo, 2000), and fluoroquinolones (Cohen, 2001), as well as diabetes mellitus, vitamin B$_{12}$ deficiency, diffuse infiltrative lymphocytosis syndrome, alcohol abuse, hepatitis C, and uremia (DeVivo, 2000; Williams, 2002).

DSP or ATN is usually diagnosed on clinical grounds. Marra et al. reported that a brief screening examination, performed at a single center by trained nonphysicians, correlated well with the diagnosis of DSP as made by an experienced AIDS neurologist (Marra, 1998). In a multicenter study, however, nonphysician neurological findings were less reliable (Simpson, 2006). Nerve conduction studies can be useful, typically showing axonal neuropathy with absent or reduced sensory nerve action potentials, although they might be normal in either mild cases or when the neuropathy is restricted to small fibers (DeVivo, 2000). Punch skin biopsies have been used to identify reduced densities of unmyelinated nerve fibers in HIV-associated sensory neuropathies. Skin biopsy analysis is now available in some settings, and it is particularly helpful either when symptoms of burning pain are more prominent than actual neurologic signs or when a nonorganic cause of sensory symptoms is suspected (Polydefkis, 2002). Quantitative sudomotor axon reflex test may also be performed to document small-fiber neuropathy. In a study of 102 patients with HIV, autonomic dysfunction was present in 62% of participants (Robinson-Papp, 2013). Sural nerve biopsy is rarely indicated except when mononeuritis multiplex is present.

Diagnosis of neurotoxic neuropathy can be confirmed by withdrawal of the suspected neurotoxin and monitoring for attenuation of symptoms. Symptoms typically improve or resolve over 2–10 weeks in approximately two-thirds of patients (Blum, 1996). When ARV alternatives are not available, one can "treat through"—maintain the ARV regimen and add adjuvant pain-modifying agents. If the ARV regimen must be switched to remove the offending agent, this is usually feasible except in heavily treated patients. Symptoms may not always subside upon stopping the offending agent—or if they do, recovery may be only partial (Price, 1999; Wulff, 1999a).

Treatment of HIV sensory neuropathies focuses on removing neurotoxins and managing pain and discomfort. One study showed that 40% of HIV-positive patients have severe pain, with a numeric pain rating scale of 5 or greater out of 10, and 90% experience some pain (Smyth, 2007). Although there is no FDA-approved treatment for the pain often associated with DSP caused by HIV, various pain-modifying agents have been used for HIV sensory neuropathies, as they have for diabetic polyneuropathy, including antidepressants, anticonvulsants, and narcotics. In mild neuropathies, over-the-counter treatments such as acetaminophen can be helpful (DeVivo, 2000; Wulff, 1999a). One randomized control study demonstrated evidence of efficacy for topical capsaicin 8% (Simpson, 2008). Night splints may also be useful in the management of neuropathic pain with improvement of sleep (Sandoval, 2010). Although pain-modifying anticonvulsants and antidepressants have been useful clinically (DeVivo, 2000; Wulff, 1999a) and can improve quality of life and function for many patients with HIV sensory neuropathies (Simpson, 2003), placebo-controlled trials on neuropathic pain have shown no significant benefit from amitriptyline, low-dose topical capsaicin, pregabalin, gabapentin, subcutaneous recombinant human nerve growth factor, subcutaneous prosapeptide, intranasal peptide T, or lamotrigine (Phillips,

2010). Lamotrigine did show some superiority to placebo in the neurotoxic ARV-exposed stratum as a secondary outcome measure of the study. Although placebo-controlled trials have been negative, tricyclic antidepressants (e.g., desipramine and amitriptyline) occasionally can be useful. Sedation is common with some, particularly amitriptyline, so these are more useful for control of nighttime neuropathic pain. Daytime sedation can generally be avoided by using small doses and escalating slowly. Pain-modifying anticonvulsants have also been useful clinically (DeVivo, 2000; Wulff, 1999a) and can improve quality of life and function for many patients with HIV sensory neuropathies (Simpson, 2003). Use of opiate medication must be approached with caution due to the prevalence of risk factors for aberrant prescription opiate use that is often found in this population (Chou, 2009). Alternative treatments include acupuncture and hypnosis (Dorfman, 2013). Further management details are provided by Verma et al. (Verma, 2004).

CONSIDERATIONS FOR RESOURCE-LIMITED SETTINGS

Cherry et al. have shown that a brief peripheral neuropathy screen, which can be easily performed in resource-limited settings, can reliably diagnose peripheral neuropathy (Cherry, 2005). ART regimens containing neurotoxic dideoxynucleosides are rapidly declining overall. One of the worst offenders, stavudine, is no longer a common component of such therapy in less-developed areas in the world where ATN might be expected to remain a common problem.

INFLAMMATORY DEMYELINATING POLYNEUROPATHY

LEARNING OBJECTIVE

Discuss the clinical features, differential diagnosis, and management of acute and chronic inflammatory demyelinating polyneuropathy in HIV-positive patients.

WHAT'S NEW?

The differential diagnosis of acute inflammatory demyelinating polyneuropathy (AIDP) includes disorders of the spinal cord, such as transverse myelitis, acute spinal cord compression, and acute infarction of the spinal cord; disorders affecting anterior horn cells, including poliomyelitis and West Nile virus; acute peripheral neuropathies such as tick paralysis, porphyria, Lyme disease, and lead or arsenic poisoning; and neuromuscular junction disorders such as botulism, myasthenia gravis, or Lambert–Eaton myasthenic syndrome.

KEY POINTS

- Acute and chronic inflammatory demyelinating polyneuropathies (AIDP/CIDP) are not common

HIV-associated peripheral neuropathies. Their cause is autoimmune-induced inflammation and breakdown of peripheral nerve myelin.

- AIDP has rapid onset and progression and often develops during HIV seroconversion or before immunosuppression has evolved.

- AIDP/CIDP in HIV-positive patients is not associated with CSF albuminocytological dissociation. These patients often have a CSF lymphocytic pleocytosis.

- AIDP is usually treated with plasmapheresis or intravenous immunoglobulin and with ganciclovir/foscarnet/cidofovir if CMV is detected as a causative agent.

- CIDP is treated with corticosteroids or intermittent courses of either plasmapheresis or intravenous immunoglobulin that may be continued long term until therapeutic response.

Peripheral neuropathy is the most common neurologic manifestation in patients with HIV/AIDS and can manifest in a number of ways: distal symmetric polyneuropathy, inflammatory polyneuropathy (AIDP/CIDP), mononeuritis multiplex, autonomic neuropathy, and progressive polyradiculopathy (Wulff, 1999b, 2000). Whereas distal symmetric polyneuropathy is the most common presentation and can occur secondary to direct HIV infection or as a side effect of NRTIs (Parry, 1997; Wulff, 2000), inflammatory demyelinating neuropathies in patients with HIV are much less common (Leger, 1989).

Inflammatory demyelinating polyradiculopathies are classified as either acute or chronic based on the duration of symptom progression. AIDP, also known as Guillain–Barré syndrome (GBS), is defined as progressive, usually ascending weakness and sensory symptoms with symptom nadir by 4 weeks. In contrast, CIDP is classified by progressive proximal and distal weakness and sensory loss with symptom progression for longer than 8 weeks.

The association between inflammatory polyneuropathies and HIV was first reported in 1985 by Lipkin et al. (Lipkin, 1985). AIDP typically occurs in the early stages of HIV infection during the seroconversion stage or during early HIV infection before seroconversion has evolved (Markarian, 1998; Mishra, 1985; Wulff 1999b). In patients with relatively intact immune function, AIDP may be the first clinical manifestation of HIV infection (Parry, 1997). Miller–Fischer/GBS overlap syndrome has been reported in advanced AIDS, with elevated anti-GQ1b antibody titer despite severe immunosuppression (Hiraga, 2007). GBS has also been reported as an immune reconstitution syndrome in patients treated with combination ART and a dramatic increase in CD4[+] T cell counts (Piliero, 2003; Rauschkaa, 2003). CIDP generally occurs later during the advanced stage of HIV infection (Verma, 2000, 2001).

PATHOGENESIS

Both AIDP and CIDP are thought to be due to an underlying autoimmune inflammatory response against peripheral nerve myelin-associated antigens, resulting in breakdown of peripheral nerve myelin (Radziwill, 2002). Rarely, HIV infection has been reported in association with an acute axonal motor neuropathy, where the pathology is thought to be associated with an immune response against the peripheral nerve axon (Dardis, 2015; Goldstein, 2013; Jadhav, 2014; Wagner, 2007).

CLINICAL FEATURES

AIDP is frequently associated with a preceding illness, such as upper respiratory infection or acute enterocolitis. AIDP commonly presents with paresthesias, followed by back pain, ascending symmetric numbness and weakness, and absent reflexes. Patients may also experience facial weakness, ophthalmoplegia, and autonomic dysfunction (commonly labile blood pressures and tachycardia).

CIDP can present with progressive or relapsing proximal and distal weakness, sensory loss, and absent reflexes. Pain is a less common presentation (Dimachkie, 2014).

CEREBROSPINAL FLUID ANALYSIS

CSF is characteristically acellular in AIDP without HIV infection. Protein levels may be normal during the first week of the illness, but there will be an increase in protein 2 or 3 weeks after symptom onset. Elevated CSF protein has been associated mainly with increased permeability of the blood–CSF barrier (Winer, 2001). On the other hand, AIDP seen with HIV infection may be associated with lymphocytic pleocytosis. In a study of 10 patients with HIV-associated AIDP, CSF white blood cell count ranged from 2 to 17 cells/mm[3] (Brannagan, 2003). The presence of increased protein in the CSF is useful for the diagnosis, and a lymphocytic CSF pleocytosis (10–50 cells/mm[3]) distinguishes HIV-associated inflammatory demyelinating neuropathies from those without HIV infection (Wulff, 1999b). However, the absence of CSF pleocytosis does not rule out HIV infection and hence warrants testing HIV in all patients with AIDP (Brannagan, 2003). In addition, either elevated CSF protein or cell counts may be found in asymptomatic patients with HIV infection (Marshall, 1988). Generally, CSF pleocytosis is suggestive of either inflammatory/infectious etiology or underlying malignancy. Markedly elevated cell counts or the presence of CSF polymorphonuclear granulocytes in a patient with AIDP/CIDP should alert the physician to seriously consider alternative diagnoses (Hughes, 1991). Enterovirus myelitis, West Nile myelitis, European tick-borne encephalitis virus, and herpes virus infection (CMV, VZV, EBV, and HSV-1 and -2) may show an initial polymorphonuclear pleocytosis. Lyme disease and HIV infection need to be considered with a lymphocytic pleocytosis (Rauschkaa, 2003).

The mean CD4[+] T cell count was 367 cells/mm[3] (range, 55–800 cells/mm[3]) in a series of 10 HIV-positive patients with GBS as reported by Brannagan and Zhou. An acute polyradiculapathy in patients with CD4[+] cell counts of less than 50 cells/mm[3] may be secondary to CMV infection, and empiric ganciclovir is indicated (Brannagan, 2003).

Diagnosis is aided by nerve conduction studies showing features of demyelination—that is, slowing of nerve conduction velocities, prolonged distal latencies, temporal dispersion, conduction block, and prolonged F-wave latencies.

BIOPSY

Nerve biopsies are rarely done to diagnose either AIDP or CIDP, but biopsy may be considered if the clinical or physiologic picture is atypical. Pathology includes macrophage-mediated segmental demyelination and an inflammatory infiltrate (Cornblath, 1987).

DIFFERENTIAL DIAGNOSIS

The differential diagnosis of AIDP includes disorders of the spinal cord such as transverse myelitis, acute spinal cord compression, and acute infarction of the spinal cord (which in the initial phases may present with flaccid areflexia below the level of the lesion due to spinal shock); disorders affecting anterior horn cells, including poliomyelitis and West Nile virus; acute peripheral neuropathies such as tick paralysis, porphyria, Lyme disease, and lead or arsenic poisoning; and neuromuscular junction disorders such as botulism, myasthenia gravis, or Lambert–Eaton myasthenic syndrome (Wakerly, 2015). In patients with subacute/chronic neuropathy and HIV infection with CD4+ T cell counts of less than 50 cells/mm³, mononeuritis multiplex, distal symmetric polyneuropathy, and CMV-related polyradiculomyelitis or polyradiculitis need to be considered in the differential diagnosis.

TREATMENT

AIDP is treated with either high-dose IVIG therapy or plasmapheresis. These treatments enhance recovery and arrest clinical progression (Cornblath, 1987; Hadden, 1998; Plasma Exchange/Sandoglobulin Guillain–Barré Syndrome Trial Group, 1997). IVIG and plasma exchange have been shown to be equally effective in treating HIV-negative AIDP (Plasma Exchange/Sandoglobulin Guillain–Barré Trial Group, 1997; van der Meche, 1992). In 2015, Rosca et al. reported improvement in CD4+ and CD8+ counts and HIV RNA levels in their patient treated with IVIG for HIV-associated GBS (Rosca, 2015). Due to the possibility of CMV polyradiculomyelitis or polyradiculitis, patients with severe immunosuppression (CD4+ T cell counts <50 cells/mm³) should be treated with intravenous ganciclovir, foscarnet, or cidofovir or a combination of these, in addition to the standard treatment. CIDP is treated with oral prednisone, pulse intravenous high-dose methylprednisolone or dexamethasone, or intermittent courses of plasmapheresis or IVIG. A randomized controlled study confirmed the benefit of prednisone in HIV-related CIDP, although this treatment approach may worsen immunosuppression (Lindenbaum, 2001). Acute relapses in CIDP are treated with either IVIG or plasmapheresis.

Initial clinical course and response to pharmacological treatment in AIDP is similar in HIV-seropositive and -seronegative patients (Verma, 2001). Schreiber (2011) reported on a patient with GBS as the initial presentation of HIV infection, who recovered fully using IVIG and rehabilitation without initiation of ART, suggesting that patients with GBS early in the course of HIV infection may behave like those with GBS without HIV infection. Compared to HIV-negative patients, HIV-associated GBS patients may experience relapses and may be more likely to develop CIDP (Brannagan, 2003). With CIDP, although treatment can halt the progression of the disease and remyelination of the peripheral nerves can occur, there is evidence that unrecoverable secondary axonal damage can occur in some cases (Hughes, 1991).

NEUROLOGICAL COMPLICATIONS OF HIV PATIENTS WITH CYTOMEGALOVIRUS INFECTION

LEARNING OBJECTIVE

Discuss the clinical syndromes, differential diagnosis, and management of neurological complications of CMV infection in HIV-positive patients.

KEY POINTS

- CMV CNS disease occurs late in the course of HIV and it may involve different parts of the central nervous system.

- Diagnosis is based on the clinical findings, results of imaging and virological markers.

- The treatment should be started empirically while awaiting the CSF PCR results.

CMV, a member of the herpesvirus family, is a frequent opportunistic viral infection in HIV-positive patients and occurs when the CD4+ T cell count is less than 100 cells/mm³ due to reactivation of latent infection. CMV infection of the nervous system accounts for fewer than 1% of CMV infections in HIV patients (McCutchan, 1995) and often develops concurrently with other, more common CMV extraneural disease such as retinitis or gastrointestinal involvement. Clinical syndromes of CMV infection in the nervous system include encephalitis, polyradiculomyelitis, polyradiculitis, and multifocal neuropathy (Anders, 1999). Although these syndromes are uncommon, recognition, treatment with antivirals, and restoring immune response are paramount to reduce the risk of death.

CMV encephalitis is the most common manifestation of CNS infection due to CMV. Clinically, infection can present as diffuse encephalitis, ventriculoencephalitis, or focal encephalitis. Diffuse encephalitis develops over several weeks and thus presents subacutely with memory loss, attention and concentration difficulties, and delirium. Focal neurological deficits may also be seen. Pathologically, microglial nodules may be found in the cortex, brainstem, cerebellum, and basal ganglia, occurring most commonly in gray matter (Morgello, 1987). On neuroimaging, MRI may show a variety of patterns. The brain may appear normal, or it may show hyperintense T2 lesions in the areas described previously and nodular lesions with or without enhancement on T1 post-contrast images (Maschke, 2002).

Ventriculoencephalitis presents with lethargy, confusion, cranial nerve deficits, ataxia, and focal neurological deficits, and it sometimes occurs concomitantly with CMV polyradiculitis. Ventriculoencephalitis may be more insidious in onset and have a poorer prognosis (Maschke, 2002). CMV encephalitis has been reported to occur even while patients are on treatment with ganciclovir for extra-CNS disease (Bermann, 1994). Pathologically, necrotizing lesions are seen in the ventricular system, and imaging shows periventricular enhancement with or without ventriculomegaly. The third and less common type of CMV encephalitis, focal encephalitis, presents with focal neurological deficits corresponding to a cerebral mass lesion. MRI will show ring-enhancing lesions with surrounding edema.

CSF PCR for CMV DNA confirms the diagnosis of CMV encephalitis. The CSF may also show pleocytosis with either a polymorphonuclear or a mononuclear predominance, along with elevated protein and decreased glucose levels. Viral culture is rarely positive. The detection of other viruses often confounds the diagnosis; thus, the index of suspicion must be based on the presentation and imaging findings in the context of profound immunosuppression. The differential diagnosis for CMV encephalitis must include HIV encephalitis, PML, and neurosyphilis. When CMV encephalitis presents as a ring-enhancing lesion, the differential diagnosis expands to other etiologies known to present similarly, such as toxoplasmosis, primary CNS lymphoma, and tuberculous meningitis with tuberculomas (Offiah, 2006).

CMV polyradiculitis (or polyradiculomyelitis if the infection involves not only the nerve roots but also the spinal cord) typically presents as an ascending weakness beginning in the lower extremities with areflexia, sensory loss, and weakness. Patients typically experience urinary retention and decreased anal sphincter tone. MRI of the spine with contrast demonstrates enhancement of the nerve roots, typically involving the cauda equina. Nerve conduction studies will show low compound muscle action potentials and mildly slowed conduction velocity corresponding to axonal involvement. Electromyography will show acute denervation with spontaneous activity and decreased recruitment. CSF studies in CMV polyradiculitis usually reveal a polymorphonuclear-predominant pleocytosis, elevated protein, and decreased glucose levels. CSF PCR for CMV DNA can confirm the diagnosis.

The differential diagnosis of CMV polyradiculitis includes GBS, which may be clinically indistinguishable and only differentiated on nerve conduction studies showing a more demyelinating pattern (Corral, 1997). Other opportunistic infections, including TB, toxoplasmosis, and HSV-2, can

present in a similar manner. Syphilis and lymphoma can also cause polyradiculitis.

Treatment for both CMV encephalitis and CMV polyradiculitis/polyradiculomyelitis is similar. Induction treatment with either intravenous ganciclovir or foscarnet is the usual first-line treatment option. Sometimes in severe encephalitis cases, combination treatment with both ganciclovir and foscarnet has been used (Portegies, 2004; Silva, 2010). Cidofovir can be used as an alternate treatment option. Empiric treatment of CMV infection is often advised because CSF results may be delayed. Maintenance treatment with ganciclovir has been recommended, but the duration of treatment has not been well studied. Of note, patients with CMV polyradiculitis/polyradiculomyelitis have been shown to be more responsive to treatment compared to CMV encephalitis patients (Cinque, 1998).

The best described CMV infection of the peripheral nervous system is an asymmetric multifocal neuropathy, observed in HIV patients with low CD4+ counts. Infection affects individual peripheral nerves, with the radial, ulnar, peroneal, and lateral cutaneous nerves of the thigh being most commonly involved (Anders, 1999). Rapid progression has been reported and can become confluent (Robinson-Papp, 2009). Electrodiagnostic studies of the nerves show multifocal sensory and motor nerve dysfunction in an axonal pattern with acute denervation. CSF studies may or may not be positive for CMV PCR, and nerve biopsy may also fail to reveal CMV. Empiric treatment is warranted when clinical suspicion is high, especially in the setting of concomitant CMV infection affecting other organs. Treatment is also with either ganciclovir or foscarnet as the first-line option. The differential diagnosis should include mononeuropathy multiplex in HIV patients with high CD4+ counts, hepatitis C with cryoglobulinemia, mononeuropathy multiplex due to vasculitis in association with B cell lymphoma, and distal sensory polyneuropathy associated with either HIV or ARV treatment with dideoxynucleoside reverse transcriptase inhibitors.

RECOMMENDED READING

Aberle SW, Aberle JH, Steininger C, et al. Quantitative real time PCR detection of varicella-zoster virus DNA in cerebrospinal fluid in patients with neurological disease. *Med Microbiol Immunol.* 2005;194:7–12.

Alfahad T, Nath A. Update on HIV-associated neurocognitive disorders. *Curr Neurol Neurosci Rep.* 2013;13:387.

American Academy of Neurology (AAN). Evaluation and management of intracranial mass lesions in AIDS: report of the Quality Standards Subcommittee of the American Academy of Neurology. *Neurology.* 1998;50:21–26.

American Academy of Neurology (AAN). Opportunistic infections: toxoplasmosis. The Neurologic complications of AIDS. *Neurol Continuum.* 2000a;6(5):128–149.

American Academy of Neurology (AAN). Primary central nervous system lymphoma in AIDS: the neurologic complications of AIDS. *Neurol Continuum.* 2000b;6(5):177–185.

American Academy of Neurology (AAN). Opportunistic and fungal infections of the central nervous system. *Neurol Continuum.* 2002;8(3):125.

Anders HJ, Goebel FD. Neurological manifestations of cytomegalovirus infection in the acquired immunodeficiency syndrome. *Int J STD AIDS*. 1999;10:151–161.

Anderson AM, Muñoz-Moreno JA, McClernon DR, et al. Prevalence and correlates of persistent HIV-1 RNA in cerebrospinal fluid during antiretroviral therapy, *J Infect Dis* 2017;215(1):105–113.

Antinori A, Arendt G, Becker JT, et al. Updated research nosology for HIV-associated neurocognitive disorders. *Neurology*. 2007;69(18):1789–1799.

Banerjee S, McCutchan JA, Ances BM, et al. Hypertriglyceridemia in combination antiretroviral-treated HIV-positive individuals: potential impact on HIV sensory polyneuropathy. *AIDS*. 2011;25(2):F1–F6.

Banks LT, Geraci A, Liu M, et al. A natural history of HIV myelopathy in the HAART era. *Neurology*. 2002;58:A441.

Bermann SM, Kim RC. The development of cytomegalovirus encephalitis in AIDS patients receiving ganciclovir. *Am J Med*. 1994;96:415–419.

Bhigjee AI, Madurai S, Bill PL, et al. Spectrum of myelopathies in HIV seropositive South African patients. *Neurology*. 2001;57:348–351.

Birbeck G, French J, Perucca E, et al. Evidence-based guideline: antiepileptic drug selection for people with HIV/AIDS: report of the Quality Standards Subcommittee of the American Academy of Neurology and the Ad Hoc Task Force of the Commission on Therapeutic Strategies of the International League Against Epilepsy. *Neurology*. 2012;78(2):139–145.

Blum AS, Dal Pan GJ, Feinberg J, et al. Low-dose zalcitabine-related toxic neuropathy: frequency, natural history, and risk factors. *Neurology*. 1996;46(4):999–1003.

Boisse L, Gill MJ, Power C. HIV infection of the central nervous system: clinical features and neuropathogenesis. *Neurol Clin*. 2008;26:799–819.

Boulware DR, Meya DB, Muzoora C, et al. Timing of antiretroviral therapy after diagnosis of cryptococcal meningitis. *N Engl J Med*. 2014;370:2487–2498.

Brannagan TH 3rd, Zhou Y. HIV associated Guillain–Barré syndrome. *J Neurol Sci*. 2003;208(1–2):39–42.

Candy S, Chang G, Andronikous S. Acute myelopathy or cauda equine syndrome in HIV positive adults in a tuberculosis endemic setting: MRI, clinical, and pathologic findings. *AJNR*. 2014;35(8):1634–1641.

Carvalhal A, Gill MJ, Letendre SL, et al. Central nervous system penetration effectiveness of antiretroviral drugs and neuropsychological impairment in the Ontario HIV Treatment Network Cohort Study. *J Neuroviral*. 2016;22(3):349–357.

Chen CH, Vazquez-Padua M, Cheng YC. Effect of anti-human immunodeficiency virus nucleoside analogs on mitochondrial DNA and its implication for delayed toxicity. *Mol Pharmacol*. 1991;39(5):625–628.

Cherner M, Masliah E, Ellis RJ, et al. Neurocognitive dysfunction predicts postmortem findings of HIV encephalitis. *Neurology*. 2002;59(10):1563–1567.

Cherry CL, Wesselingh SL, Lal L, et al. Evaluation of a clinical screening tool for HIV-associated sensory neuropathies. *Neurology*. 2005;65(11):1778–1781.

Cho T, Vaitkevicius H. Infectious myelopathies. *Continuum*. 2012;18(6):1351–1373.

Chong J, Di Rocco A, Tagliati M, et al. MR findings in AIDS-associated myelopathy. *Am J Neuroradiol*. 1999;20(8):1412–1416.

Chou R, Fanciullo GJ, Fine PG, et al. Opioids for chronic noncancer pain: prediction and identification of aberrant drug-related behaviors: a review of the evidence for an American Pain Society and American Academy of Pain Medicine clinical practice guideline. *J Pain*. 2009;10(2):131–146.

Cinque P, Cleator GM, Weber T, et al. Clinical review diagnosis and clinical management of neurological disorders caused by cytomegalovirus in AIDS patients. *J Neuro Virol*. 1998;4:120–132.

Cohen JS. Peripheral neuropathy associated with fluoroquinolones. *Ann Pharmocother*. 2001;35(12):1540–1547.

Cornblath DR, McArthur JC. Predominantly sensory neuropathy in patients with AIDS and AIDS-related complex. *Neurology*. 1988;38(5):794–796.

Cornblath DR, McArthur JC, Kennedy PGE, et al. Inflammatory demyelinating peripheral neuropathies associated with human T-cell lymphotropic virus type III infection. *Ann Neurol*. 1987;21:32040.

Corral I, Quereda C, Casado JL, et al. Acute polyradiculopathies in HIV-positive patients. *J Neurol*. 1997;244:499–504.

Dalakas MC, Cupler EJ. Neuropathies in HIV infection. *Baillieres Clin Neurol*. 1996;5(1):199–218.

Dal Pan GJ, Berger JR. Spinal cord disease in human immunodeficiency virus infection. In Berger JR, Levy RM, eds. *AIDS and the nervous system*. 2nd ed. Philadelphia: Lippincott-Raven; 1997:173–187.

Dal Pan GJ, Glass JD, McArthur JC. Clinicopathologic correlations of HIV-1-associated vacuolar myelopathy: an autopsy-based case–control study. *Neurology*. 1994;44(11):2159–2164.

Dardis C. Acute motor axonal neuropathy in a patient with prolonged CD4 depletion due to HIV: a local variant of macrophage activation syndrome? *Oxford Med Case Rep*. 2015;2:200–2002.

DeBiasi RL, Tyler KL. Molecular methods diagnosis of viral encephalitis. *Clin Microbiol Rev*. 2004;17(4):903–925.

DeVivo DC, Percy AK, Chiriboga CA, et al. Neuromuscular disorders in HIV-1 infection. *Continuum*. 2000;6:73–76.

Dimachkie MM, Barohn RJ. Distal myopathies. *Neurol Clin*. 2014;32(3):817–842.

Di Rocco A. Diseases of the spinal cord in human immunodeficiency virus infection. *Semin Neurol*. 1999;19:151–155.

Di Rocco A, Simpson, DM. AIDS-associated vacuolar myelopathy. *AIDS Patient Care STDs*. 1998;12(6):457–461.

Dorfman D, George MC, Schnur J, et al. Hypnosis for treatment of HIV neuropathic pain: a preliminary report. *Pain Med*. 2013;14:1048–1056.

Echerarria JM, Casas I, Tenorio A, et al. Detection of varicella zoster virus-specific DNA sequences in cerebrospinal fluid from patients with asceptic meningitis and no cutaneous lesions. *J Med Virol*. 1994;43:331–335.

Edén A, Fuchs D, Hagberg L, et al. HIV-1 viral escape in cerebrospinal fluid of subjects on suppressive treatment. *J Infect Dis*. 2010;202(12):1819–1825.

Ellis R, Deutsch R, Heaton RK, et al. Neurocognitive impairment is an independent risk factor for death in HIV infection: San Diego HIV Neurobehavioral Research Center Group. *Arch Neurol*. 1997;54(4):416–424.

Ellis RJ, Letendre SL, Vaida F, et al. Randomized trial of central nervous system targeted antiretrovirals for HIV-associated neurocognitive disorder. *Clin Infect Dis*. 2014;58(7):1015–1022.

Ellis RJ, Rosario D, Clifford DB, et al. Continued high prevalence and adverse clinical impact of human immunodeficiency virus-associated sensory neuropathy in the era of combination antiretroviral therapy: the CHARTER Study. *Arch Neurol*. 2010;67(5):552–558.

Erdem H, Senbayrak S, Gencer S, et al. Tuberculosis and brucellosis meningitis differential diagnosis. *Travel Med Infect Dis*. 2015;13(2):185–191.

Erlandson KM, Perez J, Abdo M, et al. Frailty, neurocognitive impairment, or both in predicting poor health outcomes among adults living with human immunodeficiency virus. *Clin Infect Dis*. 2018.

Evans SR, Ellis RJ, Chen H, et al. Peripheral neuropathy in HIV: prevalence and risk factors. *AIDS*. 2011;25(7):919–928.

Gallegos, C, Tobolowsky F, Nigo M, Hasbun R. Delayed cerebral thrombosis in adults with bacterial meningitis: a novel complication of adjunctive steroids? *Crit Care Med*. 2018;46(8):e 811–e814.

Gambarin KH, Hamill RJ. Management of increased intracranial pressure in cryptococcal meningitis. *Curr Infect Dis Rep*. 2002;4(4):332–338.

Goldstein JM, Azizi SA, Booss J, et al. Human immunodeficiency virus-associated motor axonal polyradiculoneuropathy. *Arch Neurol*. 1993;50:1316–1319.

Hadden RD, Cornblath DR, Hughes RA, et al.; Plasma Exchange/Sandoglobulin Guillain–Barré Syndrome Trial Group. Electrophysiological classification of Guillain–Barré syndrome: clinical associations and outcome. *Ann Neurol*. 1998;44(5): 780–788.

Hamada Y, Watanabe K, Aoki T, et al. Primary HIV infection with acute transverse myelitis. *Intern Med*. 2011;50:1615–1617.

Hammond ER, Crum RM, Treisman GJ, et al. The cerebrospinal fluid HIV risk score for assessing central nervous system activity in persons with HIV. *Am J Epidemiol*. 2014;180(3):297–307.

Hasbun R. The acute aseptic meningitis syndrome. *Curr Infect Dis Rep*. 2000;2(4):345–351.

Hasbun R, Eraso J, Ramireddy S, et al. Screening for neurocognitive impairment in HIV individuals: the utility of the Montreal Cognitive Assessment Test. *J AIDS Clinic Res*. 2012;3:10.

Hasbun R, Rosenthal N, Balada-Llasat JM, et al. Epidemiology of meningitis and encephalitis in the United States, 2011–2014. *Clin Infect Dis*. 2017;65(3):359–363.

;Hiraga A, Kuwabara S, Nakamura A, et al. Fisher/Guillain–Barré overlap syndrome in advanced AIDS. *J Neurol Sci*. 2007;258(1–2):148–150.

Hughes RA. Inflammatory neuropathy: sixth meeting of the Peripheral Neuropathy Association. St. Catherine's College, Oxford, England, August 14–18, 1990. *Neurology*. 1991;41(5):758–759.

Huis in't Veld D, Sun HY, Hung CC, Colebunders R. The immune reconstitution inflammatory syndrome related to HIV co-infections: a review. *Eur J Clin Microbiol Infect Dis*. 2012;31(6):919–927.

Ismail Z, Rajji TK, Shulman KL. Brief cognitive screening instruments: an update. *Int J Geriatr Psychiatry*. 2010;25(2):111–120.

Jacks A, Wainwright D, Salazar L, et al. Neurocognitive deficits increase lack of retention in care among older with newly diagnosed HIV infection. *AIDS*. 2015;29(13):1711–1714.

Jadhav S, Agrawal M, Rathi S. Acute motor axonal neuropathy in HIV infection. *Indian J Pediatr*. 2014;81:193.

Johnson TP, Patel K, Johnson KR, et al. Induction of IL-17 and nonclassical T-cell activation by HIV-Tat protein. *Proc Natl Acad Sci USA*. 2013;110:13588–13593.

Kallianpur AR, Hulgan T. Pharmacogenetics of nucleoside reverse-transcriptase inhibitor-associated peripheral neuropathy. *Pharmacogenomics*. 2009;10(4):623–637.

Keswani SC, Pardo CA, Cherry CL, et al. HIV-associated sensory neuropathies. *AIDS*. 2002;16(16):2105–2117.

Keswani SC, Polley M, Pardo CA, et al. Schwann cell chemokine receptors mediate HIV-1 gp120 toxicity to sensory neurons. *Arch Neurol*. 2003;54(3):287–296.

Leger JM, Bouche P, Bolgert F, et al. The spectrum of polyneuropathies in patients infected with HIV. *J Neurol Neurosurg Psychiatry*. 1989;52(12):1369–1374.

Lehmann HC, Chen W, Borzan J, et al. Mitochondrial dysfunction in distal axons contributes to human immunodeficiency virus sensory neuropathy. *Arch Neurol*. 2011;69(1):100–110.

Lescure FX, Moulignier A, Savatovsky J, et al. CD8 encephalitis in HIV-positive patients receiving cART: a treatable entity. *Clin Infect Dis*. 2013;57(1):101–108.

Letendre S. Central nervous system complications in HIV disease: HIV-associated neurocognitive disorder. *Top Antivir Med*. 2011;19(4):137–142.

Letendre S, Fitzsimons C, Ellis R, et al. Correlates of CSF viral loads in 1221 volunteers of the CHARTER Cohort [Abstract 172]. Paper presented at the 17th Conference on Retrovirus and Opportunistic Infections, San Francisco, February 16–19, 2010.

Lindenbaum Y, Kissel JT, Mendell JR. Treatment approaches for Guillain–Barré syndrome and chronic inflammatory demyelinating polyradiculopathy. *Neurol Clin*. 2001;19(1):187–204.

Lipkin WI, Parry G, Kiprov D, et al. Inflammatory neuropathy in homosexual men with lymphadenopathy. *Neurology*. 1985;35(10):1479–1483.

Lopez Castelblanco R, Lee M, Hasbun R. Epidemiology of bacterial meningitis in the US: a population-based study. *Lancet Infect Dis*. 2014;14:813–819.

Maggiolo F, Airoldi M, Kleinloog HD, et al. Effect of adherence to HAART on virologic outcome and on the selection of resistance-conferring mutations in NNRTI- or PI-treated patients. *HIV Clin Trials*. 2007;8(5):282–292.

Manns A, Hisada M, La Grenade L. Human T-lymphotropic virus type I infection. *Lancet*. 1999;353(9168):1951–1958.

Markarian Y, Wulff EA, Simpson DM. Peripheral neuropathy in HIV disease. *AIDS Clin Care*. 1998;10(12):89–91, 93, 98.

Marra C, Maxwell CL, Smith SL, et al. Cerebrospinal fluid abnormalities in patients with syphilis: association with clinical and laboratory features. *J Infect Dis*. 2004;189(3):369–376.

Marra CM, Boutin P, Collier AC. Screening for distal sensory peripheral neuropathy in HIV-positive persons in research and clinical settings. *Neurology*. 1998;51(6):1678–1681.

Marshall DW, Brey RL, Cahill WT, et al. Spectrum of cerebrospinal fluid findings in various stages of human immunodeficiency virus infection. *Arch Neurol*. 1988;45:954–958.

Martin F, Taylor GP. Prospects for the management of human T-cell lymphotropic virus type 1-associated myelopathy. *AIDS Rev*. 2011;13(3):161–170.

Martin JL, Brown CE, Matthews-Davis N, et al. Effects of antiviral nucleoside analogs on human DNA polymerases and mitochondrial DNA synthesis. *Antimicrob Agents Chemother*. 1994;38(12):2743–2749.

Maschke M, Kastrup O, Diener HC. CNS manifestations of cytomegalovirus infections diagnosis and treatment. *CNS Drugs*. 2002;16(5):303–315.

McArthur JC, Brew BJ, Nath A. Neurological complications of HIV infection. *Lancet Neurol*. 2005;4(9):543–555.

McCutchan JA. Cytomegalovirus infections of the nervous system in patients with AIDS. *Clin Infect Dis*. 1995;20(4):747–754.

Mind Exchange Working Group. Assessment, diagnosis, and treatment of HIV-associated neurocognitive disorder: a consensus report of the Mind Exchange Program. *Clin Infect Dis*. 2013;56(7):1004–1017.

Mishra BB, Sommers W, Koski CL, et al. Acute inflammatory demyelinating polyneuropathy in the acquired immune deficiency syndrome. *Ann Neurol*. 1985;18:131–132.

Modi G, Ranchhod J, Hari K, et al. Non-traumatic myelopathy at the Chris Hani Baragwanath Hospital, South Africa—the influence of HIV. *QJM*. 2011: 104:697–703.

Moore RD, Wong WM, Keruly JC, et al. Incidence of neuropathy in HIV-positive patients on monotherapy versus those on combination therapy with didanosine, stavudine and hydroxyurea. *AIDS*. 2000;14(3):273–278.

Morgello S, Cho ES, Nielsen S, et al. Cytomegalovirus encephalitis in patients with acquired immunodeficiency syndrome: an autopsy study of 30 cases and a review of the literature. *Hum Pathol*. 1987;18:289–297.

Mukerji SS, Misra V, Lorenz D, et al. Impact of antiretroviral regimens on cerebrospinal fluid viral escape in a prospective multicohort study of antiretroviral therapy-experience Human immunodeficiency virus-1-infected adults in the United States. *Clin Infect Dis*. 2018.

Nesher L, Hadi CM, Salazar L, et al. Epidemiology of meningitis with a negative CSF Gram-stain: underutilization of available diagnostic tests. *Epidemiol Infect*. 2016; 144(1):189–197.

Offiah CE, Turnbull IW. The imaging appearances of intracranial CNS infections in adult HIV and AIDS patients. *Clin Radiol*. 2006;61:393–401.

Opintan JA, Awadzi BK, Biney IJK, et al. High rates of cerebral toxoplasmosis in HIV patients presenting with meningitis in Accra, Ghana. *Trans R Soc Trop Med Hyg*. 2017;111(10):;464–471.

Osiro S, Salomon N. Varicella-zoster (VZV) multifocal vasculopathy in a patient with systemic lupus erythematosus—a diagnostic and treatment dilemma. *IDCases*. 2007;81–83.

Pardo CA, McArthur JC, Griffin JW. HIV neuropathy: insights in the pathology of HIV peripheral nerve disease. *J Peripheral Nerv Syst*. 2001;6(1):21–27.

Park H, Song Y. Multiple tuberculoma involving the brain and spinal cord in a patient with miliary pulmonary tuberculosis. *J Korean Neurosurg Soc*. 2008;44(1):36–39.

Parry O, Mielke J, Latif AS, et al. Peripheral neuropathy in individuals with HIV infection in Zimbabwe. *Acta Neurol Scand*. 1997;96(4):218–222.

Perfect JR, Dismukes WE, Dromer F, et al. Clinical practice guidelines for the treatment of cryptococcal disease: 2010 update from the Infectious Diseases Society of America. *Clin Infect Dis*. 2012;50:291–322.

Petito CK, Vecchio D, Chen YT. HIV antigen and DNA in AIDS spinal cords correlate with macrophage infiltration but not with vacuolar myelopathy. *J Neuropathol Exp Neurol*. 1994;53(1):86–94.

Phillips TJ, Cherry CL, Cox S, et al. Pharmacological treatment of painful HIV-associated sensory neuropathy: a systematic review and meta-analysis of randomised controlled trials. *PLoS One*. 2010;5(12):e14433.

Piliero PJ, Fish DG, Preston S, et al. Guillain–Barré syndrome associated with immune reconstitution. *Clin Infect Dis*. 2003;36(9):e111–e114.

Pillat MM, Bauer ME, de Oliveira AC, et al. HTLV-1-associated myelopathy/tropical spastic paraparesis (HAM/TSP): still an obscure disease. *Cent Nerv Syst Agents Med Chem*. 2011;11(4):239–245.

Plasma Exchange/Sandoglobulin Guillain–Barré Syndrome Trial Group. Randomised trial of plasma exchange, intravenous immunoglobulin, and combined treatments in Guillain–Barré syndrome. *Lancet*. 1997;349:225–230.

Polydefkis M, Yiannoutsos CT, Cohen BA, et al. Reduced intraepidermal nerve fiber density in HIV-associated sensory neuropathy. *Neurology*. 2002;58(1):115–119.

Portegies P, Solod L, Cinque P, et al. EFNS Task Force guidelines for the diagnosis and management of neurological complications of HIV infection. *Eur J Neurol*. 2004;11:297–304.

Price RW, Yiannoutsos CT, Clifford DB, et al. Neurological outcomes in late HIV infection: adverse impact of neurological impairment on survival and protective effect of antiviral therapy. AIDS Clinical Trial Group and Neurological AIDS Research Consortium Study Team. *AIDS*. 1999;13(13):1677–1685.

Radziwill AJ, Kuntzer T, Steck AJ. Immunopathology and treatments of Guillain–Barré syndrome and of chronic inflammatory demyelinating polyneuropathy. *Rev Neurol (Paris)*. 2002;158(3):301–310.

Rauschkaa H, Jellingerb K, Lassmannc H, et al. Guillain–Barré syndrome with marked pleocytosis or a significant proportion of polymorphonuclear granulocytes in the cerebrospinal fluid: neuropathological investigation of five cases and review of differential diagnoses. *Eur J Neurol*. 2003;10:479–486.

Robertson KR, Smurzynski M, Parsons TD, et al. The prevalence and incidence of neurocognitive impairment in the HAART era. *AIDS*. 2007;21:1915–1921.

Robinson-Papp J, Gonzalez-Duarte A, Simpson DM, et al. The roles of ethnicity and antiretrovirals in HIV-associated polyneuropathy: a pilot study. *J Acquir Immune Defic Syndr*. 2009;51(5):569–573.

Robinson-Papp J, Sharma S, Simpson DM, et al. Autonomic dysfunction is common in HIV and associated with distal symmetric polyneuropathy. *J Neurovirol*. 2013;19:172–180.

Robinson-Papp J, Simpson DM. Neuromuscular diseases associated with HIV-1 infection. *Muscle Nerve*. 2009;40(6):1043–1053.

Rolfes MA, Hullsiek KH, Rhein J, et al. The effect of therapeutic lumbar punctures on acute mortality from cryptococcal meningitis. *Clin Infect Dis*. 2014;59(11):1607–1614.

Rosca EC, Rosca O, Simu M. Intravenous immunoglobulin treatment in a HIV-1 positive patient with Guillain–Barré syndrome. *Int Immunopharmacol*. 2015;29(2):964–965.

Rosenow JM, Hirschfeld A. Utility of brain biopsy in patient with acquired immunodeficiency syndrome before and after introduction of highly active antiretroviral therapy, *Neurosurgery*. 2007;61(1):130–141.

Sandoval R, Runft B, Roddey T. Pilot study: does lower extremity night splinting assist in the management of painful peripheral neuropathy in the HIV/AIDS population? *J Int Assoc Phys AIDS Care (Chic)*. 2010;9(6):368–381.

Schifitto G, McDermott MP, McArthur JC, et al.; Dana Consortium on the Therapy of HIV Dementia and Related Cognitive Disorders. Incidence of and risk factors for HIV-associated distal sensory polyneuropathy. *Neurology*. 2002;58(12):1764–1768.

Schreiber AL, Norbury JW, DeSousa EA. Functional recovery of untreated human immunodeficiency virus-associated Guillain–Barré syndrome: a case report. *Ann Phys Rehabil Med*. 2011;54:519–524.

Serpa JA, Moran A, Goodman JC, Giordano TP, and White AC. Neurocysticercosis in the HIV era: a case report and review of the literature. *Am J Trop Med Hyg*. 2007;77(1):113–117.

Shahani L, Salazar L, Woods SP, Hasbun R. Baseline neurocognitive functioning predicts viral load suppression at 1-year follow-up among newly diagnosed HIV infected patients. *AIDS Behav*. 2018.

Shukla B, Aguilera EA, Salazar L, Wootton SH, Kaewpoowat Q, Hasbun R. Aseptic meningitis in adults and children: diagnostic and management challenges. *J Clin Virol*. 2017;94:110–114.

Sidtis JJ, Gatsonis C, Price RW, et al.;AIDS Clinical Trials Group. Zidovudine treatment of the AIDS dementia complex: results of a placebo-controlled trial. *Ann Neurol*. 1993;33:343–349.

Silva CA, Penalva de Oliveira AC, Vilas-Boas L, et al. Neurologic cytomegalovirus complications in patients with AIDS: retrospective review of 13 cases and review of the literature. *Rev Inst Med Trop Sao Paulo*. 2010;52(6):305–310.

Simpson DM, Brown S, Tobias J;NGX-4010 C107 Study Group. Controlled trial of high-concentration capsaicin patch for treatment of painful HIV neuropathy. *Neurology*. 2008;70:2305–2313.

Simpson DM, Kitch D, Evans SR, et al.; ACTG A5117 Study Group. HIV neuropathy natural history cohort study: assessment measures and risk factors. *Neurology*. 2006;66(11):1679–1687.

Simpson JK 3rd. Chronic neuropathic pain. *N Engl J Med*. 2003;348(26):2688–2689;author reply 2688–2689.

Smyth K, Affandi JS, McArthur JC, et al. Prevalence of and risk factors for HIV-associated neuropathy in Melbourne, Australia 1993–2006. *HIV Med*. 2007;8:367–373.

Tagliati M, Grinnell J, Godbold J, et al. Peripheral nerve function in HIV infection: clinical, electrophysiologic, and laboratory findings. *Arch Neurol*. 1999;56(1):84–89.

Tan K, Roda R, et al. PML-IRIS in patients with HIV infection: clinical manifestations and treatment with steroids. *Neurology*. 2009;72(17):1458–1464.

Thao LTP, Heemskerk AD, Geskus RB, et al. Prognostic models for 9-month mortality in tuberculous meningitis. *Clin Infect Dis*. 2018;66(4):523–532.

Thwaites GE. The management of suspected encephalitis. *BMJ*. 2012;344.

Triunfo M, Vai D, Montrucchio C, et al. Diagnostic accuracy of new and old cognitive screening tools for HIV-associated neurocognitive disorders. *HIV Med*. 2018;19:455–464.

Tunkel AR, Glaser CA, Bloch KC, et al. The management of encephalitis: clinical practice guidelines by the Infectious Diseases Society of America. *Clin Infect Dis*. 2004;47(3):303–327.

Tyor WR, Glass JD, Baumrind N, et al. Cytokine expression of macrophages in HIV-1-associated vacuolar myelopathy. *Neurology*. 1993;43(5):1002–1009.

US Department of Health and Human Services (USDHHS), Panel on Antiretroviral Guidelines for Adults and Adolescents. Guidelines for the use of antiretroviral agents in HIV-1-infected adults and adolescents. October 25, 2018. Available at https://aidsinfo.nih.gov/guidelines/html/1/adult-and-adolescent-treatment-guidelines/0.

US Department of Health and Human Services (USDHHS), Panel on Opportunistic Infections in HIV-positive Adults and Adolescents. Guidelines for the prevention and treatment of opportunistic infections in HIV-positive adults and adolescents: recommendations from the Centers for Disease Control and Prevention, the National Institutes of Health, and the HIV Medicine Association of the Infectious Diseases Society of America. Available at https://aidsinfo.nih.gov/contentfiles/lvguidelines/adult_oi.pdf. Accessed September 20, 2018.

Valcour V, Paul R, Chiao S, et al. Screening for cognitive impairment in human immunodeficiency virus. *Clin Infect Dis*. 2011a;53(8):836–842.

Valcour V, Sithinamsuwan P, Letendre S, et al. Pathogenesis of HIV in the central nervous system. *Curr HIV/AIDS Rep*. 2011;8(1):54–61.

Valcour VG. Evaluating cognitive impairment in the clinical setting: practical screening and assessment tools. *Top Antivir Med*. 2011b;19(5):175–180.

Van der Meche FG, Schitz PI; Dutch Guillain–Barré Study Group. A randomized trial comparing intravenous immune globulin and plasma exchange in Guillain–Barré syndrome. *N Engl J Med*. 1992;326(17):1123–1129.

Vanheule S, Desmet M, Groenvynck H, et al. The factor of the Beck Depression Inventory-II: an evaluation. *Assessment*. 2008;15(2):177–187.

Veltman JA, Bristow CC, Klausner JD. Meningitis in HIV-positive patients in sub-Saharan Africa: a review. *J Int AIDS Soc*. 2014;17:19184.

Verma A. Epidemiology and clinical features HIV-1 associated neuropathies. *J Peripheral Nerv Syst*. 2001;6(1):8–13.

Verma A, Bradley WG. HIV-1 associated neuropathies. *CNS Spectrums*. 2000;5(5):66–67.

Verma S, Estanislao L, Mintz L, et al. Controlling neuropathic pain in HIV. *Curr HIV/AIDS Rep*. 2004;1(3):136–141.

Vigil KJ, Salazar L, Hasbun R. Community-Acquired Meningitis in HIV-infected Patients in the United States. *AIDS Patient Care STDS*. 2018;32(2):42–47.

Wagner JC, Bromber MB. HIV infection presenting with motor axonal variant of Guillain–Barré syndrome. *J Clin Neuromusc Disord*. 2007;9:303–305.

Wakerly BR, Yuki N. Mimics and chameleons in Guillain–Barré and Miller–Fisher syndromes. *Practical Neurol*. 2015;15:90–99.

Wang SX, Ho EL, Grill M, et al. Peripheral neuropathy in primary HIV infection associates with systemic and CNS immune activation. *J Acquir Immune Defic Syndr*. 2014;66(3):303–310.

Weekly Epidemiological Record. Meningococcal disease control in countries of the African meningitis belt, 2014. *Wkly Epidemiol Rec*. 2015;90(13):123–131.

Winer JB. Guillain–Barré syndrome. *J Clin Pathol*. 2001;54:381–385.

Wulff EA, Simpson DM. Neuromuscular complications of the human immunodeficiency virus type 1 infection. *Semin Neurol*. 1999a;19(2):157–164.

Wulff EA, Simpson DM. Neuromuscular complications of HIV-1 infection. *Curr Infect Dis Rep*. 1999b;1(2):192–197.

Wulff EA, Wang AK, Simpson DM. HIV-associated peripheral neuropathy: epidemiology, pathophysiology and treatment. *Drugs*. 2000;59(6):1251–1260.

Yousem DM, Grossman RI. *The requisites: neuroradiology*. 3rd ed. Philadelphia: Mosby; 2010:209.

40.

HIV AND HEPATITIS COINFECTION

Ana Monczor, Margaret Hoffman-Terry, and Karen J. Vigil

CHAPTER GOALS

Upon completion of this chapter, the reader should be able to

- Discuss the clinical presentation, diagnosis, treatment, and treatment complications of hepatitis B and hepatitis C in HIV-infected patients.

INTRODUCTION

Hepatitis B (HBV) infection is common in people living with HIV, and all patients with HIV should be screened for HBV infection. The most common route of transmission worldwide is through perinatal or early childhood exposure, but adult transmission of HBV is often by routes similar to those for HIV, including sexual contact and injection drug use. Although it varies by exposure route, approximately 10% of people living with HIV also have chronic HBV infection, and up to 90% have serologic evidence of past exposure to HBV (Alter, 2006). Long-term complications of HBV infection can include cirrhosis, end-stage liver disease, and hepatocellular carcinoma (HCC).

LEARNING OBJECTIVE

Discuss the clinical presentation, diagnosis, treatment, and treatment complications of HBV in HIV-positive patients.

WHAT'S NEW?

- All patients with HIV/HBV coinfection should receive treatment for both viruses, regardless of $CD4^+$ T cell count or independent need for HBV treatment.

- Tenofovir alafenamide (TAF) demonstrated similar efficacy in HBeAg-positive and HBeAg-negative patients and less bone density and renal function decline than tenofovir disoproxil fumarate (TDF) in two large phase 3 clinical trials among HIV-negative patient with chronic HBV infection.

KEY POINTS

- All HIV-positive patients should have a complete evaluation for HBV infection.

- Patients without evidence of prior immunity or current HBV infection should be vaccinated against HBV.

- HBV treatment in coinfected patients should include two active agents against HBV, in the context of fully suppressive antiretroviral therapy (ART) against HIV.

DIAGNOSIS AND EVALUATION

Initial testing for HBV should include serologic testing for surface antigen (HBsAg), core antibody (anti-HBc total), and surface antibody (anti-HBs). HBsAg can usually be detected approximately 4 weeks after exposure. Resolution of acute HBV is characterized by negative HBsAg and the presence of anti-HBs and anti-HBc, but reactivation may recur with severe immunosuppression. Chronic HBV is defined as the presence of HBsAg for at least 6 months. For patients with chronic HBV, tests for HBV DNA, HBeAg, and anti-HBeAb are recommended.

Patients with HBeAg usually have high HBV DNA and elevated alanine aminotransferase (ALT) levels and are at high risk of future liver complications. A conversion from HBeAg to anti-HBe can imply a transition from active disease to an inactive carrier state, but this occurs less commonly in people coinfected with HIV. This inactive carrier state is also characterized by HBV DNA of less than 2000 IU/mL and normal ALT. These patients do remain at risk for reactivation of HBV and liver disease progression but at a lower rate than that of patients with active disease. Finally, there also exists a state of HBeAg-negative active hepatitis, which is a result of mutations in the pre-core and core promoter regions. These patients are at significant risk of progressive liver disease, and HBV DNA levels should be monitored regularly, with treatment instituted as recommended (Hadziyannis, 2006).

A sometimes confusing situation, especially common in HIV/HBV coinfected people, is the presence of anti-HBc alone, with negative results for HBsAg and anti-HBs. This may represent the "window phase" of acute HBV infection between loss of HBsAg and emergence of anti-HBs, prior infection with subsequent loss of anti-HBs, a false-positive anti-HBc, or "occult HBV infection," with a positive HBV DNA. The clinical significance of this situation is unclear, but it may be prudent to test these patients for HBV DNA and treat if positive and vaccinate if negative. Patients with occult HBV are at increased risk of HBV reactivation, and it is also associated with increased risk of HCC (Shire, 2004).

Elevations of hepatic transaminases are suggestive of inflammation, and hepatic synthetic function is measured by serum albumin and coagulation factors. An assessment of the degree of liver fibrosis is important, and options for this include liver biopsy or noninvasive testing such as transient elastography or an increasing array of serum biomarker tests. Patients with cirrhosis should have HCC screening by ultrasound every 6–12 months, and all patients with cirrhosis should be comanaged with a hepatologist (Lok, 2009).

Authoritative guidelines have been published regarding treatment of HBV (Terrault, 2018), but it should be emphasized that current HIV guidelines recommend treatment of all HIV-positive patients, regardless of CD4$^+$ T cell status, and that coinfected patients with HBV should be a priority group for HIV treatment. Thus, it follows that all HIV/HBV coinfected patients should be treated for both HIV and HBV with combination ART that includes two drugs with activity against HBV, such as tenofovir alafenamide (TAF) or tenofovir disoproxil fumarate (TDF) plus emtricitabine or lamivudine, regardless of the exact stage of HBV or degree of liver fibrosis.

Symptoms and Signs

Acute hepatitis typically occurs 2–5 months after exposure and can be asymptomatic or manifest as symptoms of fatigue, fever, right upper quadrant pain, and nausea with or without jaundice. Initial studies are positive for HBsAg and immunoglobulin M (IgM) antibody to HBV core antigen (IgM anti-HBc), although IgM anti-HBc may also be seen in some patients with reactivation of chronic HBV. HBV DNA and HBeAg levels rise, and elevated levels of serum liver transaminases (ALT and aspartate aminotransferase [AST]) develop. With successful clearance of acute infection, HBV DNA, HBsAg, and HBeAg will resolve, and the antibodies anti-HBs, anti-HBe, and anti-HBc IgG will develop.

Fewer than 10% of immunocompetent adults and approximately 20% of HIV patients will fail to clear an acute HBV infection, do not produce antibody to HBsAg, and thus develop chronic infection. These patients may develop chronic fatigue or extrahepatic manifestations of hepatitis, such as glomerulonephritis or arthritis, or they may be asymptomatic until the development of cirrhosis years or decades later.

Coinfection Considerations

In general terms, the presence of HIV coinfection worsens outcomes related to HBV. HIV-positive patients are less likely to resolve acute HBV exposure and have higher levels of HBV DNA compared to patients without HIV (Colin, 1999). HIV coinfection is associated with more rapid progression of HBV-related cirrhosis, HCC, and fatal hepatic failure (Thio, 2002). Indeed, HBV infection was associated with a relative risk of 3.73 for liver-related deaths in HIV coinfected participants in the Data Collection on Adverse Events of Anti-HIV Drugs (D:A:D) study (Weber, 2006).

Because the immune response plays a key role in both HBV clearance and the immune damage associated with chronic HBV infection, HIV coinfection impacts the course of HBV infection. HIV-induced immunosuppression increases the risk of reactivation of quiescent HBV, and initiation of ART may result in exacerbation of HBV liver disease (hepatitis flares) or fulminant hepatitis (Sulkowski, 2001).

Stopping antiretroviral agents with activity against HBV (lamivudine, emtricitabine, and TDF or TAF) may lead to frequent HBV rebound, sometimes accompanied by a severe flare of HBV and hepatocellular damage (Dore, 2010). Thus, when coinfected patients change ART regimens, it is crucial to maintain agents with anti-HBV activity. If anti-HBV treatment is discontinued, serum transaminase levels should be monitored regularly; if a hepatic flare occurs, then HBV therapy should be restarted immediately because this could be life-saving (US Department of Health and Human Services [USDHHS], Panel on Opportunistic Infections, 2018) .

HBV Prevention

HIV-positive patients should be counseled about transmission risks for HBV, including sexual transmission, sharing of needles and syringes, and tattooing or body piercing. Patients at risk for HBV should be advised to avoid these behaviors associated with transmission (USDHHS, Panel on Opportunistic Infections, 2018).

HBV vaccination is the most effective way to prevent HBV infection. If there is no evidence of chronic infection or previous vaccination (anti-HBs <10 IU/mL), then a hepatitis B vaccination series should be administered (USDHHS, 2018). Patients who are positive for anti-HBs and anti-HBc have a resolved infection and do not require vaccination. Patients with "isolated anti-HBc" (see previous description) who have an undetectable HBV DNA should receive a complete HBV vaccine series.

Unfortunately, the preventive HBV vaccination is less effective in people living with HIV, with efficacy rates in this population of approximately 65%, and those with a CD4$^+$ T cell count less than 350 cells/mm^3 have even lower response rates. HBV vaccination of all nonimmune HIV-positive individuals is currently recommended regardless of CD4$^+$ T cell count, and vaccination should not be deferred in patients with CD4$^+$ T cell counts of less than 350 cells/mm^3 (USDHHS, Panel on Opportunistic Infections, 2018). Various revaccination strategies are available for patients who do not respond to an initial series, and research attempting to determine the optimal vaccine series for initial vaccination to improve response rates is ongoing (Launay, 2011). A repeat three-dose vaccination series or a double dose of vaccine is recommended in HIV-positive nonresponders (Terrault, 2018).

The use of HBV active antiretroviral agents to prevent acquisition of HBV in HIV-infected patients who have not responded to a vaccine series is an emerging idea. In one study, tenofovir use was particularly protective against acquisition of primary HBV infection in HIV-positive patients (Heuft, 2014).

HIV/HBV-coinfected patients should also be vaccinated against hepatitis A if susceptible, and they should avoid alcohol consumption.

Goals of Treatment

The goals of treatment for HBV infection are to achieve sustained suppression of viral replication to below detectable levels and to improve or stabilize the degree of liver disease in order to prevent cirrhosis, hepatic failure, and HCC. Measurements of response to therapy include the decline in HBV DNA levels to undetectable levels, loss of HBeAg or gain of anti-HBe antibody (termed seroconversion), normalization of serum ALT, and improvement in liver histology. Functional cure is represented by an undetectable HBsAg, which may reduce progression to cirrhosis and liver cancer (Sherman, 2015).

HIV Treatment Recommendations in the Setting of HBV Coinfection

Because coinfection with HIV is associated with more rapid progression of HBV-related liver disease and there is evidence that earlier treatment of HIV may slow the development of liver disease by improving immune function and reducing HIV-related inflammation and immune activation, current HIV treatment guidelines recommend that all coinfected patients start ART and that the ART regimen include drugs with activity against both viruses (USDHHS, Panel on Antiretroviral Guidelines for Adults and Adolescents, 2018).

The Panel on Opportunistic Infections makes the following recommendations for HIV/HBV-coinfected patients (USDHHS, Panel on Opportunistic Infections, 2018, and American Association for the Study of Liver Disease [AASLD] 2018 Hepatitis B Guidance, Terrault, 2018):

- Regardless of CD4+ T cell count or the need for HBV treatment, ART that includes agents active against both HIV and HBV is recommended for all coinfected patients.

- ART must include two drugs active against HBV, preferably TDF or TAF and emtricitabine or lamivudine, regardless of the level of HBV DNA.

- If the patient refuses HIV treatment, then there are few options available to treat HBV because entecavir given without suppressive ART may result in HIV resistance, and telbivudine and adefovir are not recommended. A 48-week course of pegylated interferon-α-2a can be considered in such circumstances (Terrault, 2018).

- In circumstances in which tenofovir use is not acceptable as part of the ART regimen, the alternate recommendation is to use entecavir in addition to a fully suppressive ART.

- Chronic use of lamivudine or emtricitabine as the single active agent against HBV should be avoided because of the high rate of subsequent HBV resistance.

Patients being treated for HBV should have HBV DNA measured every 12–24 weeks. If the HBV DNA is greater than 1,000 IU/mL after 1 year, then adherence to medication should be assessed and HBV resistance testing considered. Viral failure and resistance are more common in HIV-coinfected patients with HBV, especially when lamivudine is used alone for treatment. The risk of resistance has declined with the use of more potent drugs such as tenofovir and entecavir (Luetkemeyer, 2011). Unfortunately, even with long-term suppression of HBV DNA, the loss of HBsAg (functional cure) of HBV is not common in patients with HIV coinfection (Sherman, 2015), and indefinite treatment is usually recommended.

SPECIAL CONSIDERATIONS

Immune Reconstitution Inflammatory Syndrome

Immune reconstitution during the course of HIV treatment can lead to a severe flare of chronic HBV infection, with significant increases in hepatic transaminases, perhaps due to enhanced host immune responses against HBV. HBV-associated immune reconstitution inflammatory syndrome (IRIS) is most likely to occur during the first few weeks after starting ART and can present as acute hepatitis. Careful monitoring of hepatic transaminases after the initiation of ART is helpful (Audsley, 2011). Development of signs of hepatic synthetic dysfunction, such as elevated prothrombin time or low albumin, should prompt evaluation by a hepatologist. Distinguishing between HBV-related IRIS and drug-induced liver toxicity can be challenging and may require examination of liver histology and consultation with a hepatologist. Very little information is available regarding the best treatment for HBV-related IRIS, and the decision regarding whether to continue, modify, or interrupt therapy should be individualized based on the severity of hepatic injury.

Treatment Interruptions

Due to the overlap in anti-HIV and HBV activity of emtricitabine, lamivudine, and tenofovir, interruption of treatment should be avoided in HIV/HBV coinfection to avoid potentially severe flares of HBV with hepatic inflammation and necrosis. In particular, when there is a need to discontinue one of the HBV-active drugs in the HIV treatment regimen, careful follow-up of liver function tests (LFTs) is required, and addition of a second agent with anti-HBV activity should be considered. If there is a need to change ART due to HIV resistance and HBV suppression is maintained despite HIV treatment failure, the antiretrovirals with activity against HBV should be continued for HBV treatment in addition to other appropriate antiretroviral agents.

TREATMENT OPTIONS FOR HEPATITIS B INFECTION

The US Food and Drug Administration (FDA)-approved and AASLD-preferred drugs for the treatment of HBV infection include interferon-α (IFN-α; standard and pegylated), entecavir, TDF, and TAF, while the nonpreferred drugs include lamivudine, adefovir, and telbivudine. The fixed-dose combination of tenofovir–emtricitabine or emtricitabine alone are not FDA-approved for use to treat HBV, but they have demonstrated activity (USDHHS, Panel on Opportunistic Infections, 2018).

Interferons

Pegylated IFN-α (Peg-IFN) is an alternative therapy for the treatment of chronic HBV for patients who refuse ART. There are limited data on the treatment of HIV/HBV coinfected patients, with lower rates of success and more toxicities compared to those of HBV monoinfected populations. Toxicities include psychiatric reactions, fatigue, headache, and cytopenias.

Nucleoside/Nucleotide Analogs

Lamivudine
Lamivudine is effective in treating HBV infection in mono-infected patients, but the development of HBV resistance to lamivudine through YMDD mutations is more common in the setting of HIV/HBV coinfection. By the fourth year of lamivudine monotherapy, greater than 90% of coinfected patients develop HBV resistance. Thus, it is recommended that lamivudine always be used in combination with another anti-HBV drug.

Emtricitabine
Emtricitabine has an overlapping resistance profile with lamivudine and a longer half-life. It is used generally in combination with tenofovir, in a fixed-dose tablet.

Tenofovir Disoproxil Fumarate
Tenofovir disoproxil fumarate (TDF) is a nucleotide analog with potent anti-HIV and anti-HBV activity. In coinfected patients, it has shown success in suppressing HBV replication even in the presence of lamivudine resistance. It has greater activity than adefovir in both monoinfected and coinfected populations (Peters, 2006). TDF in combination with emtricitabine or lamivudine is the initial recommended treatment option as part of a fully suppressive HIV treatment regimen for coinfected patients whose creatinine clearance (CrCl) is 60 mL/min or greater (USDHHS, Panel on Opportunistic Infections, 2018).

Tenofovir Alafenamide
Tenofovir alafenamide (TAF) is also a prodrug of tenofovir that is preferentially concentrated in lymphoid tissue, and, combined with emtricitabine, it is the preferred treatment for patients whose CrCl is 30 mL/min or greater, for treatment of HIV/HBV-coinfection. Two large international trials evaluated the safety and efficacy of TAF compared to TDF in HIV-, HCV-, and HVD-negative patients with chronic HBV infection. One study enrolled 873 HBeAg-positive patient and the second one enrolled 426 HBeAg-negative patients randomized to TAF 25 mg/d or TDF 300 mg/d in a 2:1 ratio. The 96-week analysis show similar rates of viral suppression in HBeAg-positive patients treated with TAF or TDF (73% vs. 3.9%, respectively, $p = 0.47$) and in HBeAg-negative patients treated with TAF or TDF (90% vs. 91%, respectively, $p = 0.84$). Patients treated with TAF have less bone density and renal function decline than TDF (Agarwal, 2018). TAF is FDA approved at an oral dose of 25 mg/d for the treatment of chronic HBV infection in HIV-negative adults with compensated liver disease and CrCl above 15 mL/min. Switching from a TDF- to a TAF-containing regimen maintained HBV suppression in coinfected patients (Gallant, 2016).

Adefovir Dipivoxil
Adefovir dipivoxil is a nucleotide analog with modest anti-HIV activity only at higher doses (120–300 mg/d) and anti-HBV activity at a lower dose of 10 mg/d. It is less potent than other treatment choices, and since resistance can develop with monotherapy (Lok, 2009), it can be combined with lamivudine or emtricitabine. This regimen is associated with high incidence of renal toxicity: therefore, it is not recommended for HBV/HIV-coinfected patients.

Entecavir
Entecavir is a nucleoside analog with high anti-HBV activity. Resistance to entecavir develops at a more rapid rate in lamivudine-resistant strains of HBV. Due to rare but confirmed reports of the development of the M184V mutation in the HIV reverse transcriptase gene and evidence of anti-HIV activity in vivo, entecavir in patients with HIV/HBV coinfection must be given with a fully suppressive HIV treatment regimen.

Telbivudine
Telbivudine is a thymidine analog with little HIV activity and potent anti-HBV activity. There is a significant risk of development of resistance and cross-resistance with lamivudine with monotherapy. Few data are available regarding its use in HIV/HBV-coinfected patients. It has been associated with elevations of creatine kinase and myopathy.

SUMMARY

Hepatitis B infection is a common and potentially severe comorbidity for people with HIV infection. Screening for HBV infection, vaccination, and careful assessment of chronic HBV infection are important components of HIV care. Consideration of chronic HBV status when selecting HIV treatment regimens is essential in optimizing management of both infections. Monitoring for response to treatment for HBV and screening for complications such as cirrhosis or HCC are part of the ongoing care of the HIV/HBV-coinfected patient.

HIV AND HEPATITIS C COINFECTION

Margaret Hoffman-Terry and Karen J. Vigil

LEARNING OBJECTIVE

Discuss the clinical presentation, diagnosis, and treatment of hepatitis C virus (HCV) in patients coinfected with HIV.

WHAT'S NEW?

- The treatment of HCV has changed dramatically during the past few years. The emergence of new interferon-free, oral, direct-acting antivirals (DAAs) achieves a cure of greater than 90% of persons with chronic HCV infections. Injectable Peg-IFN has been fully replaced by safer, more efficacious, and much better tolerated all-oral DAA combinations.

- Because ART may slow the progression of HCV-related liver disease, it should be considered for all HIV/HCV-coinfected patients, regardless of CD4+ T cell count. If treatment with the new DAAs is planned, the ART regimen may need to be modified to reduce the potential for drug–drug interactions and/or drug toxicities that may develop during the period of concurrent HIV and HCV treatment.

KEY POINTS

- Programs serving HIV/HCV-coinfected patients can expect to experience an almost 70% higher rate of utilization in this group.

- The coinfection epidemic is evolving. The Swiss HIV Cohort Study (SHCS) group has observed an 18-fold increase in HIV/HCV coinfection in men who have sex with men (MSM) from 1998 to 2011, in association with a history of unsafe sex, a past syphilis history, and chronic HBV.

- Multiple DAAs have been approved by the FDA.

- Although HCV treatment regimens are now much simpler and all oral, factors such as renal disease, drug–drug interactions, disease severity, and especially cost considerations remain.

With many of the 1.2 million HIV-positive Americans already in care for their HIV, HIV providers are in a unique position to treat and likely cure HCV in those who are also coinfected with this virus. Rapid progress in HCV therapeutics has benefited greatly from the framework that previous HIV research laid down during the past 30 years, rocketing along at breakneck speed and condensing into years what previously would have taken decades. HIV providers, with their intimate knowledge of virology, resistance, drug–drug interactions, and the psychosocial needs of this population, stand in unique stead to treat HCV.

EPIDEMIOLOGY

As ART continues to extend the life span of HIV-positive persons by decades, HCV coinfection has become an increasingly important cause of both morbidity and mortality. Liver disease has emerged as the leading cause of non–AIDS-related deaths in HIV-positive persons coinfected with HCV or HBV (Centers for Disease Control and Prevention [CDC], 2014). HCV coinfection places a growing burden on the HIV healthcare delivery system, as evidenced by an analysis conducted by the AIDS Clinical Trials Group (ACTG) Longitudinal Linked Randomized Trials (ALLRT) cohort. When controlling for age, race, sex, history of AIDS-defining events, and current CD4+ T cell count and HIV RNA levels, the relative risk of hospitalization, emergency department visits, and disability days for HIV/HCV coinfected versus HIV mono-infected participants was 1.8 (95% confidence interval [CI], 1.3–2.5), 1.7 (95% CI, 1.4–2.1), and 1.6 (95% CI, 1.3–1.9), respectively. Based on the ACTG's study findings, programs serving coinfected patients can expect to experience an almost 70% higher rate of utilization for this group (Linas, 2011). A study from the New York City Department of Health and Mental Hygiene using death certificate data showed HIV/HCV-coinfected persons to be at exceptionally high risk for premature death (median age, 52.0 years) compared to those living with HCV alone (median age, 60.0 years) or those with neither virus (median age, 78.0 years). Decedents had an odds ratio of 2.2 for death from liver cancer and 3.1 for drug-related causes, with 53.6% of deaths attributed to HIV/AIDS and 94% occurring prematurely (defined as younger than age 65 years) (Pinchoff, 2014).

HCV is a single-stranded RNA virus transmitted primarily through blood exposure and, less commonly, through sexual or vertical transmission. Because HIV and HCV share similar routes of transmission, approximately one-fourth of all HIV-positive persons in the United States are also infected with HCV. This percentage increases to 80% for people who inject drugs (PWID) (CDC, 2014). Heterosexual transmission risk is low and generally quoted as less than 1% per year, although high-risk sex practices such as aggressive anal intercourse and multiple sex partners increase transmission risk. Vertical transmission is possible, with pregnant women coinfected with HIV/HCV having a 15–20% chance of passing HCV to their infants compared to the 5–15% rate seen in infants born to HCV mono-infected mothers (Bevilacqua, 2009; Mast, 2005). Most studies to date do not support elective cesarean delivery for HCV-positive women. Breastfeeding is not known to transmit HCV, but because breastfeeding may transmit HIV, it is contraindicated for coinfected mothers in the United States.

In recent years, coinfection has been a changing epidemic, as evidenced by data from the Swiss Cohort Study. What was once a disease of PWID and hemophiliacs has become a sexually transmitted disease of MSM. The 4.1 cases per 100 person-years seen in MSM in 2011 in the Swiss Cohort Study represented an 18-fold increase from 1998, with HCV seen in association with a history of unsafe anal sex, a past syphilis history, and chronic HBV (Wandeler, 2012). In 2011, a report was published that included 5-year data from 74 HIV-positive MSM who had no history of injectable drug use (IDU) and had newly elevated ALT levels with a positive HCV antibody test (Fierer, 2012). This matched case–control study was conducted beginning in July 2007 and examined men who were within 12 months of the clinical onset of HIV infection and who had no IDU history. HIV-positive MSM newly infected with HCV were significantly more likely to have had receptive anal intercourse (mOR, 24.87) or insertive anal intercourse (matched odds ratio [mOR], 2.62) with no condom use and with ejaculation, engaged in group sex (mOR, 19.2), engaged in sex while high on drugs (mOR, 11.37), previously had syphilis (mOR, 8.8), and had sex while using crystal methamphetamine (mOR, 26.8). HIV coinfection results in increased HCV RNA levels, which are thought to increase the infectiousness of HCV acquired through sexual contact. HIV-positive patients should be counseled that unprotected sex can transmit other infections, including HCV.

The connection between prescription narcotic abuse, HIV, and HCV was highlighted by a community outbreak of HIV linked to IDU of oxymorphone in a rural county of Indiana. Prior to this investigation, only 5 HIV cases per year were reported. As of April 21, 2015, 135 persons had confirmed or probable HIV infection in a community of 4,200 persons. Mean age was 35 years, with 54.8% being males, 80% reporting IDU, and 17% who had not yet been interviewed. All reported their drug of choice was injectable crushed oxymorphone, sometimes with other illicit drugs. Of these, 7.4% were female commercial sex workers. Strikingly, coinfection with HCV was found in 84.4% of patients (Conrad, 2015). Those interviewed reported an average of 9 syringe-sharing or sex partners and social contacts who may be at risk. Of the 230 contacts tested, 109 (47.4%) were positive for HIV. Injectable drug use in this community is multigenerational, with the crushed oxymorphone (40 mg tablets are not designed to resist crushing) dissolved in nonsterile water and injected via insulin syringes with the syringes often shared. This outbreak highlights the vulnerability of many resource-poor rural communities that traditionally have low rates of HIV and HCV and the need for community interventions at multiple levels. This is a reminder of how often concomitant transmission of the two viruses continues to occur, particularly in vulnerable PWID and MSM.

CLINICAL COURSE

The most striking feature of HCV when acquired by a person infected with HIV is its ability to cause chronic hepatitis in as much as 90% of patients within 6 months. This occurs due to the lack of CD4$^+$ T cell responses and significantly reduced IFN-γ ELISpot responses against HCV (Elliott, 2006). Between 60% and 70% of chronically infected persons will have fluctuating serum ALT levels because this is the enzyme most associated with liver cell injury in HCV. Less than 20% have nonspecific symptoms, including fatigue and generalized weakness. There are significant similarities and differences between HIV and HCV. Both are RNA viruses with rapid replication rates (10 trillion HCV virions vs. 10 billion HIV virions produced daily). Both are prone to frequent mutations and exist as heterogeneous quasispecies to avoid the immune system. Both viruses incite abundant but ineffective antibody responses. Although both have many reservoirs in the human body, HCV exists primarily in the cytoplasm of hepatocytes and can be eradicated from the body. HIV is integrated into the nuclei of CD4$^+$ T lymphocytes and long-lived memory cell reservoirs and therefore cannot be eradicated with current ART. HCV RNA levels are only broadly predictive of long-term prognosis, whereas HIV RNA is very predictive of clinical events in untreated patients.

There are six different HCV genotypes (1–6) at various prevalence rates throughout the world. In the United States, genotype (GT) 1 accounts for two-thirds of cases, with GTs 2–4 occurring less commonly.

DIAGNOSIS

HCV may be diagnosed earlier in asymptomatic HIV patients with elevated ALT/AST levels due to greater frequency of lab monitoring (Mohsen, 2003). Coinfection with HIV greatly impacts the natural history of HCV infection. Coinfected patients are less likely to spontaneously clear HCV, have increased HCV RNA, and progress more rapidly to cirrhosis and end-stage liver disease (ESLD) (Asselah, 2006). Predictors of severe liver fibrosis include age older than 40 years at time of infection, alcohol consumption of more than 50 g/d, daily marijuana use, high body mass index, male gender, postmenopausal status, and longer duration of infection (Poynard, 1997). Although ART may slow this rate, it continues to exceed that seen in persons with HCV mono-infection. Low CD4$^+$ T cell counts also appear to magnify the progression. A meta-analysis of eight studies that examined the role of HIV with HCV found that coinfected patients had approximately two times the risk of cirrhosis on liver biopsy and six times the risk of decompensated liver disease with ascites, varices, or encephalopathy compared to HCV mono-infected patients (Poynard, 1997). A Veterans Health Administration study examined 4,820 coinfected and 6,079 HCV mono-infected patients in care from 1997 to 2010. All had detectable HCV RNA levels and were HCV treatment-naïve. Hepatic decompensation was significantly greater at 10 years in the coinfected group (7.4% vs. 4.8%; $p < 0.001$) (Lo, 2014). Coinfected patients had a higher rate of hepatic decompensation (hazard ratio [HR] 1.56 when accounting for competing risks), even when HIV RNA levels were maintained under 1,000 copies/mL (HR, 1.44). Approximately one-third of patients with chronic HCV will progress to cirrhosis at a median time of less than 20 years (Thomas, 2000). Once cirrhosis has developed, 50% will decompensate within the first 5 years, with ascites being the usual first sign. Approximately 1–4% of cirrhotic patients per year will develop HCC. Median survival time is 35 months versus 65 months for those without HIV (Beretta, 2011).

Although the average time from infection to fibrosis is shortened from 35 to 25 years in HIV-coinfected patients, Fierer's group at Mt. Sinai School of Medicine (New York City) found that HIV-positive MSM who developed HCV had a much more rapid onset of fibrosis. In a 2008 analysis, 9 of 11 (82%) men had stage 2 (moderate) fibrosis at a median of only 4 months after diagnosis (Fierer, 2012). In 2013, Fierer et al. reported on 4 patients who developed decompensated cirrhosis and death within 2–8 years post-HCV infection (Fierer, 2013). The authors noted that the order in which the infections are acquired is important. When HCV is acquired after HIV, there is accelerated progression to fibrosis that may be proportional to the degree of immunosuppression. However, not all studies have seen such rapid progression. The European NEAT cohort evaluated fibrosis rates in 41 HIV-positive patients who subsequently developed HCV. Most were MSM on ART with a mean CD4+ T cell count of 500 cells/mm³. FibroScan transient elastometry (used to assess liver stiffness) over a maximum follow-up of 8 years found no significant hepatic changes (Boesecke, 2014).

Deferring HCV treatment in the age of DAAs may lead to increased rates of HCC and death. Data from the SHCS and published HCV data were used for mathematical modeling to predict the decrease in progression to cirrhosis, HCC, and death in the HIV/HCV-coinfected population. If therapy was initiated during stages F0 or F1, the percentage of liver-related-deaths was 2%. However, if treatment was deferred until F3 or F4 stage, mortality increased to 7% and 22%, respectively. If patients are not treated immediately, they remain infectious. Important from a public health perspective, those treated between 1 month and 1 year after diagnosis remained infectious from a HCV standpoint for approximately 5 years, compared to 12 years for stage 2, 15 years for stage 3, and nearly 20 years for stage 4 (Zahnd, 2016).

DECISION TO TREAT

According to the Infectious Disease Society of America's "Primary Care Guidelines for HIV," all HIV-positive persons should be screened for HCV with antibody testing upon entry into care and annually thereafter for those at risk and whenever HCV infection is suspected (Aberg, 2013). HCV RNA levels should be tested in all those with a positive antibody test to assess for active disease because antibodies persist for a lifetime even in patients who have cleared the virus. Infants born to coinfected mothers should also have antibody testing performed. Seronegative at-risk individuals, along with those with evidence of past HCV infection, should undergo annual screening. HCV transmission may be facilitated by the presence of genital erosions related to sexually transmitted diseases. Reinfection with HCV can occur, necessitating that patients be aware that high-risk behaviors put them at risk for reinfection (Danta, 2008). Patients with HCV/HIV coinfection should be advised to avoid alcohol consumption and to avoid sharing razors, toothbrushes, syringes, and so on to prevent spread of infection to others. Those who are susceptible to hepatitis A or hepatitis B should be vaccinated against these viruses because dual or triple infections are typically more severe (Low, 2008).

Although the increased likelihood of ART-associated liver toxicity with underlying HCV infection may complicate HIV treatment, this must be balanced against the increased risk of fibrosis with lower CD4+ T cell counts (Sulkowski, 2000). It should not discourage HIV providers from following USDHHS treatment guidelines, given the improved survival of coinfected patients on ART and the fact that newer ART agents are much less likely to cause hepatotoxicity. The benefit of HIV treatment on HCV was noted in 10,900 ART-naïve HIV/HCV coinfected patients in the Veterans Aging Cohort Study's Virtual Cohort (Anderson, 2014). This study examined incident or new cases of liver decompensation occurring from 1996 to 2010. The cohort was 60% black, median age was 47 years, and one-third had baseline CD4+ T cell counts of less than 200 cells/mm³. During a median 3.1 years of follow-up, 69% initiated ART and 36% started IFN-based HCV treatment. During the 46,444 person-years of follow-up, 645 liver decompensation events occurred in 6% of participants. Those starting ART by prescription refill history had a significantly lower rate of liver decompensation (HR, 0.72, or 28% risk reduction). When examining those with HIV RNA of more than 400 copies/mL at baseline (making the assumption that those with lower HIV RNA were on unreported ART), the risk reduction was even more dramatic (HR, 0.59, or 41% risk reduction). The study authors concluded that all HIV/HCV-coinfected persons should receive ART to lower the risk of ESLD. This is in keeping with current USDHHS treatment guidelines for ART in HIV infection.

The provider and patient must weigh many variables when deciding to treat HCV, including disease severity, extrahepatic manifestations, risk of side effects, comorbid conditions such as renal disease, and likelihood of cure with the availability of more effective and well tolerated DAA HCV regimens. Treatment goals should include viral eradication, prevention of disease progression, improved quality of life, increased rates of survival, decreased risk of cirrhosis and HCC, and normalization of liver enzymes to simplify chronic ART. For most HIV/HCV-coinfected patients, even those with cirrhosis, the potential for preservation of immune function, reduction of immune activation and inflammation, and slowing progression of liver disease outweighs the risk of drug-induced liver injury, so ART should always be considered regardless of the CD4+ T cell count. If CD4+ T cell count is less than 200 cells/mm³, HIV treatment to improve the immune status must take precedence. Initial ART regimens for HIV/HCV-coinfected people are similar to people living with HIV without HCV infection. However, drug–drug interactions between antiretroviral drugs and DDA should be considered when choosing the initial therapy or when switching a suppressive antiretroviral regimen in order to start treatment for HCV.

Testing for HCV RNA by polymerase chain reaction is the only reliable way to diagnose acute HCV infection because approximately 30% of patients do not have detectable antibodies at the onset of symptoms. A positive HCV antibody test with history of a prior negative HCV antibody test is also indicative of recent seroconversion. More than 90% will have antibodies by 3 months postexposure, with less than 5% of coinfected patients (usually those with advanced immunosuppression) failing to produce detectable HCV antibodies. Acute HCV is asymptomatic in 70–80% of cases, but cure rates are significantly higher with acute disease. It is therefore important to routinely screen at-risk individuals and promptly investigate elevated hepatic transaminase levels. Acutely infected HCV patients who are symptomatic have a higher likelihood of spontaneous viral clearance, so they should be monitored for 12 weeks before initiating HCV therapy. Asymptomatic patients have a lower rate of spontaneous clearance, so they may benefit from early therapy. If HCV RNA remains elevated at 12 weeks post-seroconversion, treatment should be strongly considered. If RNA is still present at 6 months, spontaneous clearance is unlikely, and the infection is considered chronic. Due to high efficacy and safety, the same DAA regimens used to treat chronic HCV may now be used to treat acute HCV. Acute HCV infection may present with flu-like symptoms, nausea, abdominal pain, and jaundice. Infrequently, severe hepatic dysfunction with transaminases up to 10 times normal is seen, but fulminant hepatitis is rare (USDHHS, Panel on Antiretroviral Guidelines for Adults and Adolescents, 2018).

Prior to initiating HCV treatment in the coinfected patient, specific baseline lab tests should be conducted. These include a complete blood count (CBC) with platelets, hepatic function panel including ALT, AST, alkaline phosphatase, albumin, and total bilirubin, prothrombin time/international normalized ratio (PT/INR), calculated glomerular filtration rate (eGFR), HIV and HCV RNA, CD4[+] T cell count, and HCV genotype and subtype. A pregnancy test is recommended for all females of childbearing potential if RBV use is planned because RBV is a known teratogen. Counseling against alcohol consumption is key because this can rapidly worsen fibrosis. HBV and hepatitis A virus vaccination should be offered to all patients without evidence of exposure to these infections.

A screening ultrasound is recommended to rule out cirrhosis and HCC in those with laboratory or clinical evidence of significant fibrosis or cirrhosis. Conventional computed tomography, magnetic resonance imaging, or single-photon emission computed tomography (SPECT) may be used but are generally reserved for evaluation of liver masses or screening patients with more advanced fibrosis/cirrhosis. Although liver biopsy has been considered the gold standard in assessing disease stage, it is invasive, uncomfortable, and has bleeding risk (1/10,000 experience severe bleeding or fatality). Biopsies are generally scored 0–4 based on degree of inflammation (grade) and degree of fibrosis (stage). Metavir scoring is one of the most common systems for interpreting a liver biopsy and is shown in Figure 40.1.

Because of the risks associated with biopsy, alternatives such as FibroScan and FibroSURE have rapidly risen in popularity and acceptance in clinical practice. FibroScan utilizes

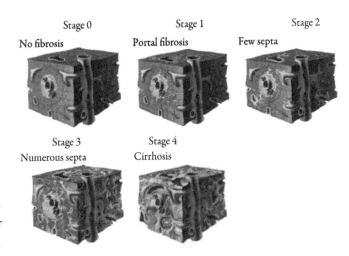

Figure 40.1 Metavir histologic staging.

a mild-amplitude, low-frequency vibration transmitted through the liver to measure tissue "stiffness." This noninvasive and less expensive monitoring tool has been used in Europe for more than a decade and has been approved in the United States since 2013 for clinical use. FibroSURE uses six blood serum tests (α_2-macroglobulin, haptoglobin, apolipoprotein A1, γ-glutamyl transferase, ALT, and total bilirubin) along with age and gender to generate a score that correlates with degree of liver disease. Other noninvasive biomarker formulas, such as APRI, which incorporates platelet counts with tests of coagulation and transaminases, and fibrosis-4 (FIB-4) may also be used to evaluate degree of fibrosis. APRI and FibroSURE have been validated in coinfection and predict no disease versus cirrhosis accurately but are not as accurate in the mid-range of the disease spectrum (Rallon, 2011; Schneider, 2014).

Several formulas are used to assess the degree of cirrhosis. The Child–Turcotte–Pugh score uses encephalopathy, ascites, bilirubin, albumin, and PT or INR to classify severity of cirrhosis (class A, 5–6 points; class B, 7–9 points; and class C, 10–15 points). The Model for End-stage Liver Disease (MELD) score uses serum creatinine, bilirubin, and INR and two or more dialysis sessions within the previous week to predict probability of survival for patients with ESLD. This is the formula currently used for liver allocation by the United Network of Organ Sharing and predicts the 3-month mortality rate. A MELD calculator is provided on the Mayo Clinic website (http://www.mayoclinic.org/medical-professionals/model-end-stage-liver-disease/meld-model). The HALT-C formula for predicting cirrhosis uses platelet count, INR, AST, and ALT to predict the probability of a biopsy demonstrating cirrhosis (Lok, 2009).

THERAPEUTIC MODALITIES

Multiple, all-oral combinations of DAAs are now available as the recommended regimens for treatment (Table 40.1). Injectable Peg-IFN has been fully replaced by safer, more efficacious, and much better tolerated all-oral combinations, with guidelines no longer recommending its use except in alternative regimens to shorten treatment. Coinfected patients cured

Table 40.1 CURRENT DIRECT ANTIRETROVIRAL AGENTS FOR HEPATITIS C

DIRECT ANTIVIRAL AGENT	GENOTYPES TREATED	CLASS	GFR	COMMENTS
Elbasvir/grazoprevir Zepatier®	1 and 4	NS5A inhibitor + NS3/4A protease inhibitor	No dose adjustment in patients with renal impairment including those on hemodialysis	NS5A testing is required in patients with GT 1a
Ledipasvir/ sofosbuvir Harvoni®	1 to 6	NS5A inhibitor + nucleotide polymerase inhibitor (NS5B)	No dosage recommendation for patients with glomerular filtration rate less than 30 mL/min/1.73 m2)	First fixed oral combination
Sofosbuvir/ velpatasvir Epclusa®	1 to 6	Nucleotide polymerase inhibitor (NS5B) + NS5A inhibitor	No dosage recommendation for patients with glomerular filtration rate less than 30 mL/min/1.73 m2)	
Sofosbuvir/ velpatasvir/ voxilapresvir Vosevi®	1 to 6	Nucleotide polymerase inhibitor (NS5B)+ NS5A inhibitor+ NS3/4A protease inhibitor	No dosage recommendation for patients with glomerular filtration rate less than 30 mL/min/1.73 m2)	For patients who have failed therapy with a NS5A inhibitor–containing regimen
Glecaprevir/ pibrentasvir Mavyret®	1 to 6	HCV NS3/4A protease inhibitor + HCV NS5A inhibitor	No dose adjustment in patients with renal impairment including those on hemodialysis.	
Daclatasvir (Daklinza)® + Sofosbuvir (Sovaldi®) (alternative regimen)	1 and 3	NS5A inhibitor + nucleotide polymerase inhibitor (NS5B)	No dosage adjustment is required for patients with any degree of renal impairment	Several drug interactions with antiretroviral treatments

of their HCV with Peg-IFN and RBV had lower rates of liver-related morbidity and mortality, and we expect to see the same results with the DAAs.

Monitoring of treatment should include a week 4 HCV RNA. Most HCV treatment-naïve patients will be undetectable by this point unless they are cirrhotic. If detectable at 4 weeks, a follow-up at week 6 HCV RNA should be done. If it is rising by 1 $\log_{10}$ or more, treatment should be stopped. The HCV RNA at 12 weeks posttreatment is crucial because this determines cure (SVR12).

Excellent cure rates result in a dramatic decrease in the rate of complications from HCV such as fibrosis and HCC, extrahepatic manifestations such as cryoglobulinemia, and debilitating symptoms such as fatigue. Evidence supports treating all patients with HCV unless their life expectancy is less than 12 months because of a non–liver-related condition. As such, current guidelines recommend treatment for all HCV-infected persons. The guidelines also note that "immediate treatment" is assigned the highest priority in patients with advanced fibrosis/compensated cirrhosis, organ transplant, type 2/3 mixed cryoglobulinemia with end organ manifestations, and renal complications such as nephrotic syndrome. HIV places patients in the "high priority" for treatment category given the increased risk of fibrosis and HCC. Of great importance is the knowledge that treatment response is similar in coinfected and mono-infected patients. As such, HIV/HCV-coinfected persons should be treated and retreated in the same manner as those who are not coinfected with HIV, but with constant attention to potential drug–drug interactions.

Drug–drug interactions increase the complexity of treating HCV in the HIV-positive patient on ART, as does the issue of renal function. Based on current evidence, the preferred treatment for patients with CKD stage 4 or 5 (eGFR <30 mL/min or end stage renal disease) cis either elbasvir (50 mg)/grazoprevir (100 mg) or glecaprevir (300 mg)/pibrentasvir (120 mg). ART switches may need to occur prior to treatment

for HCV. Patients may return to their prior regimen after treatment is completed. Although choosing a regimen to avoid drug interactions may seem daunting, interrupting ART while on HCV treatment is not recommended. Treatment interruption is associated with increased cardiovascular events as well as fibrosis progression and liver-related events. Because this area is in constant flux, see "Guidelines for the Use of Antiretroviral Agents in HIV-1-Infected Adults and Adolescents" (USDHHS, Panel on Antiretroviral Guidelines for Adults and Adolescents, 2018) under the HIV/HCV coinfection section and "AASLD/IDSA HCV Guidance: Recommendations for Testing, Managing and Treating Hepatitis C" under the Management of Unique Populations section, for current advice on ART for HIV when treating HCV.

The standard of care for chronic HCV infection in HIV-positive patients was Peg-IFN-α-2a or -2b and RBV with a cure rate around 50%. Coinfected cure rates with Peg/RBV were never as good as those in mono-infected patients. Peg-IFN plus RBV worked by nonspecifically stimulating the body's immune response. Side effects were severe and will usually preclude treatment completion. IFN commonly caused flu-like symptoms, depression, anxiety, neutropenia, thrombocytopenia, reversible mild hair loss, and altered thyroid or glucose metabolism. RBV typically caused a drop in hemoglobin (~2 g in the first month of treatment), teratogenicity, cough/dyspnea, rash/pruritus, insomnia, and anorexia. Fortunately, these drugs represent the past rather than the future of hepatitis C treatment. RBV is used only in limited cases.

The oral DDAs are the current drugs for HCV treatment. DAAs were engineered to work at multiple HCV-specific sites, such as the protease and polymerase enzymes (Figure 40.2). The first generation, boceprevir and telaprevir, were NS3/4A PIs. Although briefly state-of-the-art between their licensure in 2010 and 2012, they are no longer recommended in the United States because more efficacious and less toxic drugs have been developed. The second wave of HCV therapies

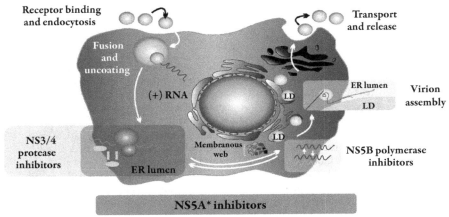

Figure 40.2 Hepatitis C virus (HCV) life cycle and antiviral therapy for patients with HCV.

have simple rules for use, shorter duration of therapy, fewer drug–drug interactions and side effects, and are highly effective in both HCV–mono-infected patients and HIV/HCV-coinfected patients. The results in HIV/HCV-coinfected patients have been so impressive and so similar to those seen in mono-infection that many researchers are calling for a halt to separate trials in HIV-positive patients.

DIRECT ACTING AGENTS

The HCV genome encodes 10 polyproteins, seven nonstructural proteins, and three structural proteins (NS3/4A, NS5A, NS5B) that play an important role in HCV replication and are the target of current DAA (Figure 40.3).

Sofosbuvir (SOF) and simeprevir (SIM) were the initial second-generation DAA approved in the United States. SIM was discontinued in May 2018 due to decreased utilization. However, SOF has become the cornerstone of most of the current combination treatments for hepatitis C.

NS5B Polymerase Inhibitor(s)

NS5B polymerase is required for viral replication, acting as a chain terminator. SOF is a nucleotide analog inhibitor of this enzyme. The NS5B site is highly conserved among all genotypes; SOF is pangenotypic. It is given as 400 mg once daily. It is not metabolized by the CYP450 enzyme complex and thus is an ideal candidate for use in HIV/HCV coinfection.

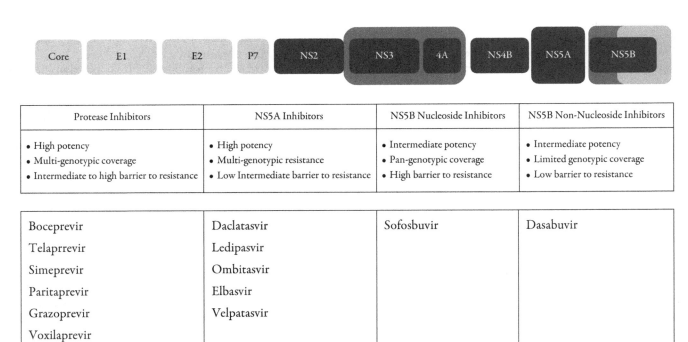

Protease Inhibitors	NS5A Inhibitors	NS5B Nucleoside Inhibitors	NS5B Non-Nucleoside Inhibitors
• High potency • Multi-genotypic coverage • Intermediate to high barrier to resistance	• High potency • Multi-genotypic resistance • Low Intermediate barrier to resistance	• Intermediate potency • Pan-genotypic coverage • High barrier to resistance	• Intermediate potency • Limited genotypic coverage • Low barrier to resistance
Boceprevir Telaprrevir Simeprevir Paritaprevir Grazoprevir Voxilaprevir Glecaprevir	Daclatasvir Ledipasvir Ombitasvir Elbasvir Velpatasvir	Sofosbuvir	Dasabuvir

Figure 40.3 Hepatitis C polyprotein structure and therapeutic targets for direct-acting antiviral drug development. From Poordad (2012).

The non-nucleoside polymerase inhibitors, as a class, are less potent and have a lower genetic barrier to resistance. The only currently approved drug is dasavuvir. It is coformulated with ombitasvir, paritaprevir, and ritonavir as a fixed-dose combination.

NS3/4A Protease Inhibitors

Glecaprevir, grazoprevir, paritaprevir, and voxileprevir are the current DAAs available in this class. They are noncovalent inhibitors of the NS3/4A serine protease of HCV.

NS5A Inhibitors

The exact mechanism of action of the NS5A inhibitors is not completely understood. However, some studies showed that they bind to the N-terminal domain of NS5A, causing structural distortion and inhibiting both viral RNA replication and virion assembly at an early stage. Daclatasvir, elbasvir, ledipasvir, ombitasvir, pibrentasvir, and velpastavir are antivirals in this class. With the exception of daclatasvir, all others are coformulated in fixed-dose combinations.

Daclatasvir is an NS5A inhibitor that was evaluated in the ALLY-2 study, an open-label trial of 151 HCV treatment-naïve and 52 treatment-experienced HIV-positive patients. HCV treatment-naïve patients were randomized in a 2:1 ratio to 12 or 8 weeks at a standard dose of 60 mg/d with dose adjustment for concomitant ART as needed. All patients received SOF 400 mg once daily. All treatment-experienced patients received 12 weeks of therapy at the same doses. The primary end point was SVR12 posttreatment in the HCV GT 1 treatment-naïve patients. HCV GT 1–4 were enrolled with 83% having GT 1; 14% were compensated cirrhotics, and 98% were on ART.

The most commonly reported adverse events in the ALLY-2 study were fatigue (17%), nausea (13%), and headache (11%), with no study drug discontinuations due to adverse events. Declines in HCV VL were rapid, with 92–98% of patients at less than 25 IU/mL by week 4 of treatment. No effect on HIV suppression or $CD4^+$ T cell count was noted. On treatment, HCV responses were similar in the 8- and 12-week groups, but relapse was more common after 8 weeks of treatment. Nine of the 12 patients with HCV relapses (7 of 10 in the 8-week group) received concurrent darunavir (DRV)/ritonavir (RTV) with daclatasvir at a reduced 30 mg dose. Current data suggest that the 60 mg dose is the ideal when given with DRV or LPV. The researchers also suggest that HIV-1 may adversely affect outcomes with the truncated course of therapy.

Drug–drug interactions affect dosing of this compound. Daclatasvir is a substrate of both CYP3A4 and P-gp. Strong or moderate inducers of CYP3A4 and P-gp may decrease plasma levels and the therapeutic effect of daclatasvir, so coadministration with strong inducers is contraindicated, whereas administration with moderate inducers requires dose adjustment. Strong inhibitors of CYP3A4 may increase plasma daclatasvir levels, so dose adjustment of daclatasvir is needed. Coadministration with inhibitors of P-gp is likely to have a limited effect on daclatasvir exposure. Daclatasvir should be decreased to 30 mg/d when given with RTV-boosted atazanavir or cobicistat, and it should be increased to 90 mg/d when given with efavirenz. Daclatasvir should not be given with the rifamycins or the older seizure drugs.

FIXED-DOSE COMBINATIONS

Ledipasvir/Sofosbuvir

Ledipasvir/sofosbuvir (LDV/SOF, trade name Harvoni), LDV 90 mg/SOF 400 mg, was the first interferon- and ribavirin-free once-daily, single-tablet regimen for HCV approved by the FDA (on October 14, 2014).

The ION-4 study was a phase 3, multicenter, open-label trial of 335 HIV/HCV-coinfected patients. Enrolled participants had GT 1 and 4 (75% GT 1a, 23% GT 1b, and 2% GT 4), 20% had compensated cirrhosis, and 55% were treatment-experienced. Based on drug–drug interaction data available at the beginning of the trial, ARTs allowed in study patients were emtricitabine (FTC)/TDF with efavirenz (EFV), RPV, or raltegravir (RAL). The primary end point was SVR12 posttreatment, with SVR24 as the secondary end point.

No difference in response rates at week 12 of treatment was seen with GT 1a versus GT 1b based on sex, treatment history, concomitant ART, or cirrhosis status. Thirteen patients (4%) did not achieve SVR. One person died at week 4 of treatment, 2 had breakthrough on treatment that was believed to likely be related to poor adherence by treating physicians, and 10 relapsed after treatment. All 10 relapsers were black, with 7 having the TT allele in the gene encoding IL28B (which confers an increased risk of failure with IFN-containing regimens). Black race and the presence of the TT allele were found as a significant association in the univariate analysis. Black race alone in the multivariate analysis was significantly associated with relapse. The association of lower SVR with black race, which comprised 34% of the study population, was not seen in the studies of LDV/SOB in HCV–mono-infected persons and was not related to the CYP2B6 polymorphism, which is more common in blacks and results in increased EFV levels (Naggie, 2015).

LDV/SOF increases exposure to TDF by approximately 40%. Patients on RTV-containing regimens may experience a relative increase of 30–60% in TDF exposure and so were excluded from the trial along with those on cobicistat-containing combinations. Although 77% of patients had an adverse event, these were usually mild to moderate and resulted in no premature study discontinuations. Headache (25%), fatigue (21%), and diarrhea (11%) were the most common adverse events. Eight patients experienced 15 serious adverse events, with HCC in 2 patients and portal vein thrombosis in 2 patients—all being reported in cirrhotics. Three patients experienced serious infections. Grade 3 laboratory abnormalities occurred in 9% and grade 4 laboratory abnormalities in 2% of patients, with elevations in lipase, creatinine phosphokinase, and serum glucose being most common.

Ombitasvir/Paritaprevir/Ritonavir/Dasabuvir (Viekira Pak)

Approved on December 19, 2014, ombitasvir is an NS5A inhibitor, paritaprevir an NS3/4A protease inhibitor, and RTV is a CYP3A inhibitor that increases plasma concentrations of paritaprevir. Dasabuvir is a non-nucleoside NS5B polymerase inhibitor. Several CYP enzymes (3A4 and 2C8) and several drug transporters are involved in the metabolism of this drug combination; therefore, complex drug–drug interactions are likely to occur. It is currently considered an alternative regimen in the AASLD/IDSA Hepatitis C Guidance. The product will be discontinued January 2019.

Elbasvir/Grazoprevir

Elbasvir/grazoprevir (ELB/GRZ, trade name Zepatier)I is a fixed-dose combination of 50 mg of elbasvir, an NS5A inhibitor, and 100 mg of grazoprevir, an NS3/4A protease inhibitor, taken once a day with or without food for the treatment of chronic HCV GT 1 or 4 infection in adults. Treatment is typically 12 weeks. RBV is added and treatment extended to 16 weeks if baseline NS5A polymorphisms are found in a GT 1a patient. RBV may be added in GT 1a or 1b patients who are Peg/RBV/PI-experienced. GT 4 patients who are Peg/IFN/RBV-experienced also receive 16 weeks of treatment. RBV is given as two daily doses depending on baseline NS5A polymorphisms and treatment experience. No dosage adjustment for ELB/GRZ is needed for renal impairment, including those on hemodialysis, although the RBV may need adjustment per guidelines. It is contraindicated in those with Child–Pugh B or C disease. ELB/GRZ is contraindicated with OATP1B1/3 inhibitors and strong CYP3A inducers such as EFV. Other contraindicated drugs include phenytoin and carbamazepine, rifampin, and St. John's wort. Coadministration with nafcillin, ketoconazole, bosentan, modafinil, entecavir (ETV), and cobicistat-containing compounds is not recommended. The risk of ALT elevations may be elevated with zidovudine (ATZ), DRV, lopinavir (LPV), and cyclosporine. Statins also interact with ELB/GRZ. Thus, atorvastatin should not exceed 20 mg; rosuvastatin should not exceed 10 mg; and the lowest possible dose of fluvastatin, lovastatin, and simvastatin should be used. Tacrolimus levels may be increased by ELB/GRZ.

ELB/GRZ was approved for the treatment of GT 1 and 4 only based on results from the C-EDGE study. A total of 299 patients were enrolled with GT 1, 4, and 6. The SVR 12 was only 92% in patients with GT 1 a, but 99% in patients with GT 1 b and 100% in GT 4. Further analysis demonstrated lower SVR 12 rates in patients with baseline NS5A resistance associated variants (at positions 28, 30, 31, and 93) associated with more than fivefold loss in elbasvir susceptibility. Therefore, a baselines resistance test is recommended in patients with GT 1a. If baselines resistance mutations are found, treatment should be extended for 16 weeks and RBV should be added.

In the C-EDGE Coinfection trial—a phase 3, open-label trial involving 218 HCV treatment-naïve HCV/HIV patients who received ELB/GRZ one tablet daily for 12 weeks—95.0% of patients achieved a cure, with six relapses and one reinfection. The drug worked equally well in GT 1a or 1b and GT 4. Seven percent reported fatigue, 7% headache, 5% nausea, 5% insomnia, and 5% diarrhea. No serious adverse events occurred (Rockstroh, 2015).

It should be noted that the FDA has issued a black box warning that ELB/GRZ could cause LFT elevations of more than 5 times the upper limit of normal. Therefore, it is recommended to monitor LFTs while on treatment.

Sofosbuvir/Velpatasvir

Sofobuvir/velpatasvir (SOF/VEL, trade name Epclusa) is a pangenotypic regimen approved on June 28, 2016, to be given as a once-daily fixed-dose combination tablet for 12 weeks in patients without cirrhosis or with compensated cirrhosis. In patients with decompensated cirrhosis it must be used with ribavirin. Velpatasvir is a HCV NS5A inhibitor required for viral replication.

The ASTRAL-1 study was a randomized, double-blinded, placebo-controlled study that evaluated 12 weeks of treatment with SOF/VEL compared to placebo in treatment naïve and Peg-IFN treatment-experienced patients without cirrhosis or with compensated cirrhosis. Patients with all genotypes were included. Of 328 patients with GT 1, 98% achieved SVR12. Rates were similar in patients with compensated cirrhosis. Even in previously treatment-experienced patients with IFN-based regimens and first-generation protease inhibitors, this combination achieved more than 96% efficacy (Pianko, 2015). In the ASTRAL-5 study, velpatasvir/sofosbuvir was given to 106 people with HIV/HCV coinfection, virally suppressed on ART containing raltegravir, rilpivirine, or ritonavir boosted protease inhibitors either with tenofovir or abacavir. Genotypes 1 to 4 were included; 18% of participants had compensated cirrhosis. Patient SVR 12 was achieved in 95% of the patients and was well tolerated. The most commonly reported side effects were fatigue, headaches, nausea, and insomnia.

Glecaprevir/Pibrentasvir

Glecaprevir (GLE) 200 mg and pibrentasvir (PIB) 120 mg comes as three tablets to be taken once a day (GLE/PIB, trade name Mavyret). This combination has several advantages compared to others. Not only is it pangenotypic, but it could also be used in patients with chronic kidney disease and is approved for 8 weeks in treatment-naïve patients with no cirrhosis based on data from ENDURANCE-1 and ENDURANCE-3 studies.

In ENDURANCE-1 and ENDURANCE-3, out of 1,208 patients with GT 1 and 3 treated for 8 weeks, 99.1% (95% CI, 98–100) of patients with GT 1 and 95% (95% CI, 91–98; 149 of 157 patients) of patients with GT achieved SVR 12 (Zeuzem, 2018). It is also approved for use in treatment-experienced patients for a total of 8–16 weeks based on cirrhosis stage and previously used DAA. Of note, this combination is contraindicated in patients with advanced cirrhosis (Child-Pugh B or C). The EXPEDITION-2 study evaluated the 8 weeks of GLE/PIB in HIV/HCV-coinfected patients. Overall SVR 12 rate was 98%.

Sofosbuvir/Velpatasvir/Voxilaprevir

Sofosbuvir/velpatasvir, voxileprevir (SOF/VEL/VOX, trade name Vosevi) is a 12-week pangenotypic, single, fixed-dose DAA indicated in patients with HCV GT 1a who have failed therapy with a NS5A inhibitor–containing regimen.

Voxileprevir is a reversible potent inhibitor of the NS3/4A protease required for the cleavage of the HCV encoded polyprotein. The single-tablet regimen consists of 400 mg of sofosbuvir, 100 mg velpatasvir, and 100 mg voxileprevir. It is administered once daily with food. Patients with advanced liver disease (Child Pugh B and C) should not take this regimen.

POLARIS-1 and POLARIS-4 assessed the efficacy and safety of SOF/VEL/VOX for 12 weeks in patients with HCV infection and who had previously received unsuccessful treatment with DAA-based regimens. All HCV genotypes were included; 46% of patients had cirrhosis. The most common NS5A inhibitors used in previous unsuccessful treatment were ledipasvir (55% of patients), daclatasvir (23%), and ombitasvir (13%) in POLARIS-1 while in POLARIS-4, it was sofosbuvir (85%). SVR rates were 96% and 100% for genotypes 1a ($n = 101$) and 1b ($n = 45$), respectively. In POLARIS-1 and POLARIS-4, 83% and 49% of participants had baseline viral substitutions associated with resistance to NS3 inhibitors or NS5A inhibitors. SVR 12 was achieved in 97% (199 of 205) of participants in POLARIS-1 and 100% (83 of 83) in POLARIS-4.

In a phase 2, open-label study, 49 patients with HCV genotype 1 infection who previously failed to achieve sustained virologic response on a DAA-based regimen were randomized to receive SOF/VEL/VOX with or without RBV for 12 weeks. The primary efficacy endpoint was the proportion of patients who achieved SVR 12. SVR12 was achieved by 24 of 24 patients (100%; 95% CI, 86–100) receiving sofosbuvir-velpatasvir-voxilaprevir alone and 24 of 25 (96%; 95% CI, 80–100) receiving the same treatment with RBV. Virological response was achieved by 13 of 13 (100%) patients without baseline RASs and by 34 of 35 (97%) with baseline RASs. No large randomized control studies in HIV/HCV-coinfected patients have been done.

TREATMENT FAILURES

For those who fail HCV treatment, assessment for disease progression should be done every 6–12 months with a hepatic function panel, CBC, and INR. If they have F3 or F4 disease, HCC surveillance every 6 months with ultrasound is advised. If cirrhotic, they should have endoscopic evaluation for varices. As new treatments become available, they should be considered for these patients.

Liver transplantation is a possibility in patients in whom HCV therapy is contraindicated due to decompensated cirrhosis. As long as the $CD4^+$ T cell count is greater than 100 cells/mm^3 and HIV RNA levels are less than 400 copies/mL and without other contraindications (e.g., metastatic disease, ongoing alcohol or drug abuse, and active opportunistic infection), patients may be appropriate for referral to a transplant center for evaluation. Studies have shown higher rates of waitlist mortality and posttransplant mortality, as well as more severe recurrent HCV disease (Terrault, 2012). Data from a prospective multicenter trial showed lower 3-year survival (60% vs. 79%; $p < 0.001$) in HIV/HCV-coinfected versus HCV–monoinfected patients, as well as lower graft survival (53% vs. 74%; $p < 0.001$). Graft rejection was more common in coinfection (35% vs. 18%), likely related to the difficulties of managing immunosuppressive drugs in this population (Zahnd, 2015).

New DAA drug therapy in HCV mono-infected and HIV/HCV coinfected individuals has shown pretransplant and posttransplant virologic responses of 70–93% in some trials.

RESISTANCE

Resistance-associated variants (RAVs) may exist at the start of treatment in a small number of patients. Routine monitoring is recommended in (1) patients who have failed treatment with a prior NS5A inhibitor–containing regimen, (2) GT 1a patients planning to receive elbasvir/grazoprevir, and (3) GT 3 cirrhotic patients planning to receive sofosbuvir/velpatasvir. This area is currently in great flux, so change in these guidelines is expected. HCV resistance testing is recommended to search for RAVs that may confer decreased susceptibility to NS3/4A protease inhibitors and NS5A complex inhibitors.

SUMMARY

The world of HIV/HCV coinfection is in rapid flux, with many new and exciting agents being released. Similar to HIV treatment, a combination of oral agents that disrupt the HCV virus at various sites of the life cycle has the best chance for decreasing viral replication long-term and curing infection. Questions regarding optimal combination as well as drug access and costs will need to be addressed in the next several years if the majority of HIV/HCV-coinfected patients are to be effectively treated.

ACKNOWLEDGMENTS

The authors acknowledge Aimee Wilkin, MD, MPH, the author of the first section of this chapter in the previous edition.

REFERENCES

Aberg JA, Gallant JE, Ghanem KG, et al. Primary care guidelines for the management of persons infected with HIV: 2013 update by the HIV Medicine Association of the Infectious Diseases Society of America. *Clin Infect Dis*. 2014;58(1):e1–e34.

Agarwal K, Brunetto M, Seto WK, et al. 96 weeks treatment of tenofovir alafenamide vs. tenofovir disoproxil fumarate for hepatitis B virus infection [published online ahead of print January 17, 2018]. *J Hepatol*. 2018;68(4):672–681. doi:10.1016/j.jhep.2017.11.039.

Alter MJ. Epidemiology of viral hepatitis and HIV Coinfection. *J Hepatol*. 2006;44(1 Suppl):S6–S9.

Alvarez D, Dieterich DT, Brau N, et al. Zidovudine use but not weight-based ribavirin dosing impacts anemia during HCV treatment in HIV-positive persons. *J Virol Hepatol*. 2006;13:683–689.

AASLD-IDSA. Recommendations for testing, managing, and treating hepatitis C. Available at: http://www.hcvguidelines.org. Accessed October 2018.

Anderson JP, Tchetgen EJ, Lo R, et al. Antiretroviral therapy reduces the rate of hepatic decompensation among HIV and hepatitis C virus-coinfected veterans. *Clin Infect Dis*. 2014;58(5):719–727.

Asselah T, Rubbia-Brandt L, Marcellin P, et al. Steatosis in chronic hepatitis C: why does it really matter? *Gut*. 2006;55(1):123–130.

Audsley J, Seaberg E, Sasadeusz J, et al. Factors associated with elevated ALT in an international HIV/HBV coinfected cohort on long-term HAART. *PLoS One*. 2011;6(11):e26482.

Beretta M, Garlassi E, Cacopardo B, et al. Hepatocellular carcinoma in HIV-infected patients: check early, treat hard. *Oncologist.* 2011;16(9):1258–1269.

Bevilacqua E, Fabris A, Floreano P, et al. Genetic factors in mother-to-child transmission of HCV infection. *Virology.* 2009;390(1):64–70.

Boesecke C, Ingiliz P, Mandoerfer M, et al.; the NEAT Study Group. Is there long-term evidence of advanced liver fibrosis after acute hepatitis C in HIV coinfection? [Abstract 644]. Paper presented at the 21st Conference on Retroviruses and Opportunistic Infections, Boston, March 3–6, 2014.

Centers for Disease Control and Prevention (CDC). HIV/AIDS and viral hepatitis fact sheet. Available at http://www.cdc.gov/hepatitis/populations/hiv.htm. Accessed January 15, 2016.

Colin J, Cazals-Hatem D, Loriot M, et al. Influence of human immunodeficiency virus infection on chronic hepatitis B in homosexual men. *Hepatology.* 1999;29(4):1306–1310.

Conrad C, Bradley H, Broz D, et al. Community outbreak of HIV infection linked to injection drug use of oxymorphone—Indiana, 2015. *MMWR.* 2015;64(16):443–444.

Danta M, Dusheiko GM. Acute HCV in HIV-positive individuals—a review. *Curr Pharm Des.* 2008;14(17):1690–1697.

Dore G, Soriano V, Rockstroh J, et al. Frequent hepatitis B virus rebound among HIV-hepatitis B virus coinfected patients following antiretroviral therapy interruption. *AIDS.* 2010;24(6):857–865.

Elliott LN, Lloyd A, Ziegler JB, et al. Protective immunity against hepatitis C virus infection. *Immunol Cell Biol.* 2006;84:239–249.

Fierer DS, Dieterich DT, Fiel MI, et al. Rapid progression to decompensated cirrhosis, liver transplant, and death in HIV-infected men after primary hepatitis C virus infection. *Clin Infect Dis.* 2013;56(7):1038–1043.

Fierer DS, Mullen MP, Dieterich DT, et al. Early-onset liver fibrosis due to primary hepatitis C virus infection is higher over time in HIV-infected men. *Clin Infect Dis.* 2012;55(6):887–888;author reply, 888–889.

Gallant J, Brunetta J, Crofoot G, et al. Brief Report: Efficacy and Safety of Switching to a Single-Tablet Regimen of Elvitegravir/Cobicistat/Emtricitabine/Tenofovir Alafenamide in HIV-1/Hepatitis B–Coinfected Adults. *J Acquir Immune Defic Syndr.* 2016;73(3):294–298.

Hadziyannis S, Papatheodoridis G. Hepatitis B e antigen-negative chronic hepatitis B: natural history and treatment. *Semin Liver Dis.* 2006;26:130–141.

Heuft M, Houba S, van den Berk G, et al. Protective effect of hepatitis B virus-active antiretroviral therapy against primary hepatitis B virus infection. *AIDS.* 2014;28(7):999–1005.

Launay O, Van der Vliet D, Rosenberg A, et al. Safety and immunogenicity of 4 intramuscular double doses and 4 intradermal low doses vs. standard hepatitis B vaccine regimen in adults with HIV-1: a randomized controlled trial. *JAMA.* 2011;305(14):1432–1440.

Lawitz E, Ghalib R, Rodriguez-Torres M, et al. COSMOS Study: SVR4 results of a once-daily regimen of simeprevir (TMC435) plus sofosbuvir (GS-7977) with or without ribavirin in HCV genotype 1 null responders [Abstract 155LB]. Presented at the 20th Conference on Retroviruses and Opportunistic Infections, Atlanta, GA, March 3–6, 2013.

Lawitz E, Sulkowski M, Ghalib R, et al. Simeprevir plus sofosbuvir, with or without ribavirin, to treat chronic infection with hepatitis C virus genotype 1 in non-responders to pegylated interferon and ribavirin and treatment-naive patients: the COSMOS randomised study. *Lancet.* 2014;384(9956):1756–1765.

Linas BP, Wang B, Smurzynski M, et al. The impact of HIV/HCV coinfection on health care utilization and disability: results of the ACTG Longitudinal Linked Randomized Trials (ALLRT) Cohort. *J Viral Hepat.* 2011;18(7):506–512.

Lo Re III V, Kallan M, Tate J, et al. Hepatic decompensation in antiretroviral-treated patients coinfected with HIV and hepatitis C virus compared with hepatitis C virus-monoinfected patients: a cohort study. *Ann Intern Med.* 2014;160(6):369–379.

Lok AS, McMahon BJ. Chronic hepatitis B: update 2009. *Hepatology.* 2009;50(3):661–662.

Low E, Vogel M, Rockstroh J, et al. Acute hepatitis C in HIV-positive individuals. *AIDS Rev.* 2008;10(4):245–253.

Luetkemeyer A, Charlebois E, Hare C, et al. Resistance patterns and response to entecavir intensification among HIV–HBV-coinfected adults with persistent HBV viremia. *J AIDS.* 2011;58(3):e96–e99.

Mast EE, Hwang LY, Seto DS, et al. Risk factors for perinatal transmission of hepatitis C virus (HCV) and the natural history of HCV infection acquired in infancy. *J Infect Dis.* 2005;192(11):1880–1889.

Mohsen AH, Easterbrook P. Hepatitis C testing in HIV infected patients. *Sex Transm Infect.* 2003;79(1):76.

Naggie S, Cooper C, Saag M, et al. Ledipasvir and sofosbuvir for HCV in patients coinfected with HIV-1. *N Engl J Med.* 2015;373(8):705–713.

Peters M, Andersen J, Lynch P, et al. Randomized controlled study of tenofovir and adefovir in chronic hepatitis B virus and HIV infection: ACTG 5127. *Hepatology.* 2006;44(5):1110–1116.

Pianko S, Flamm SL, Shiffman ML, et al. Sofosbuvir plus velpatasvir combination therapy for treatment-experienced patients with genotype 1 or 3 hepatitis C virus infection: a randomized trial. *Ann Intern Med.* 2015;163(11):809–817.

Pinchoff J, Drobnik A, Bornschlegel K, et al. Deaths among people with hepatitis C in New York City, 2000–2011. *Clin Infect Dis.* 2014;58(8):1047–1054.

Poynard T, Bedossa P, Opolon P. Natural history of liver fibrosis progression in patients with chronic hepatitis C. The OBSVIRC, METAVIR, CLINIVIR, and DOSVIRC groups. *Lancet.* 1997;349(9055):825–832.

Rallon NI, Soriano V, Naggie S, et al. IL28B gene polymorphism and viral kinetics in HIV. HCV coinfected patients treated with pegylated interferon and ribavirin. *AIDS.* 2011;25(8):1025–1033.

Rockstroh JK, Nelson M, Katlama C, et al. Efficacy and safety of grazoprevir (MK-5172) and elbasvir (MK-8742) in patients with hepatitis C virus and HIV coinfection (C-EDGE COINFECTION): a non-randomised, open-label trial. *Lancet HIV.* 2015;2(8):e319–e327.

Schneider MD, Sarrazin C. Commentary: antiviral therapy of hepatitis C in 2014: do we need resistance testing? *Antivir Res.* 2014;105:64–71.

Sherman K. Management of the hepatitis B virus/HIV-coinfected patient. *Top Antivir Med.* 2015;23(3):111–114.

Shire N, Rouster S, Rajicic N, et al. Occult hepatitis B in HIV-infected patients. *J AIDS.* 2004;36(3):869–875.

Sulkowski M, Thomas D, Chaisson R, et al. Reactivation of hepatitis B virus replication accompanied by acute hepatitis in patients receiving highly active antiretroviral therapy. *Clin Infect Dis.* 2001;32(1):144–148.

Sulkowski MS, Mast EE, Seeff LB, et al. Hepatitis C virus infection as an opportunistic disease in persons infected with human immunodeficiency virus [review]. *Clin Infect Dis.* 2000;30(Suppl 1):S77–S84.

Sulkowski MS, Naggie S, Lalezari J, et al. Sofosbuvir and ribavirin for hepatitis C in patients with HIV coinfection. *JAMA.* 2014;312(4):353–361. Erratum in: *JAMA.* November 12, 2014;312(18):1932.

Sulkowski MS, Thomas DL, Chaisson RE, et al. Hepatotoxicity associated with antiretrovirals in adults infected with HIV and the role of hepatitis C or B infection. *JAMA.* 2000;283:74–80.

Terrault N, Lok A, McMahon B, et al. Update on Prevention, Diagnosis, and Treatment of Chronic Hepatitis B: AASLD 2018 Hepatitis B Guidance. *Hepatology.* 2018;67:1560–1599.

Thio C, Seaberg E, Skolasky R Jr, et al. HIV-1, hepatitis B virus, and risk of liver-related mortality in the Multicenter Cohort Study (MACS). *Lancet.* 2002;360(9349):1921–1926.

Thomas DL, Strathdee SA, Vlahov D. Long-term prognosis of hepatitis C virus infection. *JAMA.* 2000;284(20):2592.

Wandeler G, Gsponer T, Bregenzer A, et al. Hepatitis C virus infections in the Swiss HIV Cohort Study: a rapidly evolving epidemic. *Clin Infect Dis.* November 15, 2012;55(10):1408–1416.

Weber R, Sabin CA, Friis-Moller N, et al. Liver-related deaths in persons infected with the human immunodeficiency virus: the D:A:D study. *Arch Intern Med.* 2006;166(15):1632–1641.

Zahnd C, Salazar-Vizcaya L, Dufour JF, et al. Modelling the impact of deferring HCV treatment on liver-related complications in HIV coinfected men who have sex with men. *J Hepatol.* 2016;65(1):26–32.

Zeuzem S, Foster GR, Wwang S, et al. Glecaprevir–pibrentasvir for 8 or 12 weeks in HCV genotype 1 or 3 infection. *N Engl J Med.* 2018;378(4):354.

41.

OCULAR COMPLICATIONS

James P. Dunn

CYTOMEGALOVIRUS

LEARNING OBJECTIVE

Describe the incidence, screening, diagnosis, management, and referral indication for HIV-infected patients with cytomegalovirus (CMV) retinitis in the era of antiretroviral therapy (ART).

WHAT'S NEW?

As therapy for HIV has improved, CMV retinitis has become a less common opportunistic infection. However, patients with advanced HIV disease may still present with CMV retinitis. There is no evidence that routine screening can prevent disease in these patients.

KEY POINTS

- Symptoms of CMV retinitis are nonspecific and include floaters, light flashes, peripheral visual field loss, and blurred central vision. Pain, redness, and photophobia are not features, and central vision is often good.

- Immune recovery uveitis occurs in 10–15% of eyes with CMV retinitis in patients who respond to ART, with blurred vision as the most common symptom.

- Anti-CMV therapy is associated with increased survival in patients who remain immunosuppressed.

- Screening for CMV disease does not improve the diagnosis or survival of patients.

INCIDENCE AND SCREENING

Before the era of ART, CMV retinitis was the most common ocular opportunistic infection in patients with AIDS, occurring in up to 30% of patients (Jabs, 1995). The incidence of CMV retinitis, its natural history, and the indications for and response to therapy depend in part on whether at-risk patients are taking ART (Jabs, 2002). Patients taking ART, especially those with immune recovery, are at lower risk of CMV retinitis than are patients who remain profoundly immunosuppressed, and so they do not need to be screened as often.

The recent demographic shifts in the AIDS epidemic (resulting in HIV infection in more women and minorities) have been reflected by a similar demographic shift in cases of CMV retinitis (Jabs, 2002); its incidence has decreased by up to 90% in the ART era but has reached a plateau of approximately 0.2/person-year of follow-up (Sugar, 2012; Yust, 2004). A $CD4^+$ T cell count of less than 50 cells/mm^3 at the clinical visit prior to CMV retinitis evaluation is the most important risk factor for developing retinitis (Sugar, 2012). In a large European study of patients with CMV disease, 64% had CMV retinitis, 27% had extraocular CMV disease (primarily gastrointestinal and neurologic), and 8% had both (Yust, 2004).

Primary prophylaxis for CMV retinitis is not generally recommended because of its uncertain efficacy, cost, and potential toxicity (Kaplan, 2002). Therefore, patients who have $CD4^+$ counts of less than 100 cells/mm^3 must be educated about signs and symptoms of CMV retinitis and encouraged to seek timely evaluation if they occur (Whitley, 1998). Prompt and regular ophthalmologic screening for retinitis is appropriate for any patient with a $CD4^+$ count of less than 50 cells/mm^3 because of the high incidence of ocular disease and the fact that most affected patients are asymptomatic (Kaplan, 2002; Nishijima, 2015; Whitley, 1998; Wohl, 2000). Routine dilated funduscopic examinations in patients at high risk may allow early diagnosis in asymptomatic patients. No study has shown, however, that regular screening improves final visual outcomes in patients with CMV retinitis compared to those who are not seen until they are symptomatic.

It is particularly important to examine CMV-seropositive children who have advanced HIV infection for possible eye disease every 4–6 months (Kaplan, 2002). Although the incidence of eye disease is low in this group (Hammond, 1997),

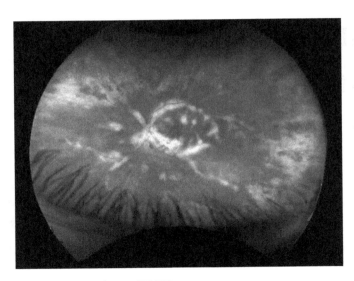

Figure 41.1 Cytomegalovirus (CMV) retinitis. From the New York State Department of Health AIDS Institute Clinical Guidelines Development Program (2000–2004).

children are less likely than adults to express symptoms of infection.

DIAGNOSIS

The majority of patients have no visual symptoms at diagnosis (Wohl, 2000), such as light flashes, loss of central or peripheral visual fields, and blurred or distorted vision (Whitley, 1998). There is typically no pain, redness, or photophobia (Jabs, 2002; Whitley, 1998). Approximately 70–80% of patients had visual acuity of 20/40 or better at the time of diagnosis in one mostly pre-ART study (Whitley, 1998). The diagnosis is based on characteristic features seen on indirect or slit-lamp funduscopy, including yellow-white areas of retinal necrosis, a dry-appearing granular border, and edema with vascular distribution, often with a hemorrhagic component (Jabs, 2002; Whitely, 1998; see Figure 41.1).

Several diagnostic screening tests have been evaluated, including quantitative plasma CMV DNA polymerase chain reaction (PCR) (Mizushima, 2015), and CMV viral load in plasma and leukocytes (Jabs, 1999), but their cost-effectiveness remains unproved, and none is in widespread clinical use. CMV viral load has limited clinical utility because of its low positive predictive value (Jabs, 2005).

MANAGEMENT

Management of CMV retinitis depends on patient factors (e.g., underlying medical conditions, concomitant medications, living conditions, and lifestyle preferences), characteristics of the ophthalmic disease (e.g., location and extent of lesions), and characteristics of available therapies (e.g., their relative efficacies, risks of toxic effects and adverse outcomes, and quality-of-life issues) (Whitley, 1998). Successful management requires close collaboration between treating physicians and ophthalmologists.

The most effective treatment for CMV retinitis is an ART regimen containing a protease inhibitor, which is associated with markedly prolonged times to relapse and improved survival (Kempen, 2003). Oral valganciclovir, the prodrug of

ganciclovir, has largely replaced intravenous therapy (ganciclovir, foscarnet, or cidofovir) (Martin, 2002) because of its excellent bioavailability and convenient dosing regimen. Adverse effects of valganciclovir include neutropenia, anemia, thrombocytopenia, nausea, and diarrhea. Regular monitoring of blood chemistry and hematology values is important during both induction and maintenance therapy. Foscarnet and cidofovir may still be indicated in patients with ganciclovir-resistant CMV retinitis, which is associated with worse visual outcomes (Jabs, 2003) and increased mortality (Jabs, 2010). Both drugs are nephrotoxic, and the dosage must be adjusted for renal status. Cidofovir can cause uveitis and must be given with probenecid, which itself may cause severe malaise and weakness (Whitley, 1998).

Regional anti-CMV therapy is an option in patients who cannot tolerate systemic therapy. Intravitreal ganciclovir 2 mg/0.1 mL or foscarnet 2.4 mg/0.1 mL injections are also effective and avoid the risk of systemic toxicity, but they must be repeated at least weekly (Teoh, 2012). It is important to understand, however, that systemic anti-CMV therapy, compared to only intraocular therapy, is associated with significantly lower mortality, less visceral CMV disease, and reduced risk of second-eye involvement (Jabs, 2013; Sittivarakul, 2016).

The ganciclovir ocular implant was another appropriate choice for initial therapy, and many experts chose this for patients who had immediately sight-threatening disease (Whitley, 1998). However, the implant was voluntarily taken off the market in 2013 due to poor sales.

In patients not taking ART, the combination of systemic therapy and the ganciclovir implant reduces the risk of new CMV disease and delays the progression of retinitis beyond that achieved with systemic therapy alone (Martin,1999), although either systemic or implant therapy appears comparably effective in patients with immune recovery (Kempen, 2003). The use of ART is associated with a 60% reduction in retinal detachment, with the greatest benefit among patients who have an immunologic response to highly active antiretroviral therapy (HAART) (Kempen, 2001) and a 50% reduction in retinitis progression (Jabs, 2003). In a large retrospective series (Kempen, 2003), ART was associated with 81% lower mortality, reflecting a 98% reduction in patients with immune recovery and a 49% reduction in those without. The use of systemic anti-CMV treatment was independently associated with a 28% lower mortality rate than use of ART alone.

The most common causes of visual loss in patients with CMV retinitis are retinitis near the optic disc or fovea (zone 1 involvement), retinal detachment, cataract, and macular edema (Thorne, 2006).

Approximately 10–15% of patients who have controlled CMV retinitis have decreased vision and/or floaters after initiating ART because of immune recovery uveitis (Jabs, 2002; Kempen, 2006). Eyes with immune recovery uveitis have a significantly higher risk of cystoid macular edema and epiretinal membrane than do eyes of patients without immune recovery uveitis. Risk factors for immune recovery uveitis include large CMV lesions (25% or more of the total retinal area) and the use of intravitreous cidofovir. Reports conflict as to whether the continued use of anti-CMV therapy reduces the risk of immune recovery uveitis (Kempen, 2006; Kosobucki, 2004).

The use of ART has created distinct groups of patients based on their potential for immunologic improvement (Martin, 1999). In patients already taking ART, physicians must reevaluate this therapy if CMV retinitis develops because this can indicate progressing immune dysfunction (Martin, 1999). The previously discussed treatment options for CMV retinitis apply whether or not patients with CMV are receiving ART (Martin, 1999), but the length of therapy is affected by the response to ART. In one retrospective analysis of patients whose maintenance therapy was stopped after showing immune recovery (Curi, 2001), reactivation and progression did not occur after 20.4 months of follow-up. Maintenance anti-CMV therapy can often be discontinued in patients taking ART for at least 6 months with CD4[+] counts of greater than 100–150 cells/mm[3] for at least 3 months. Close follow-up is recommended, however, especially in patients with sight-threatening lesions (Wohl, 2005).

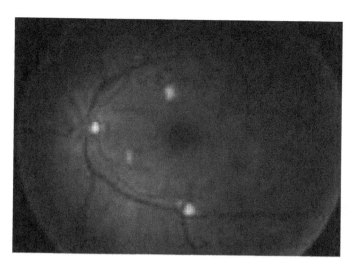

Figure 41.2 HIV microangiopathy. From the New York State Department of Health AIDS Institute Clinical Guidelines Development Program (2000–2004).

HIV RETINOPATHY

LEARNING OBJECTIVE

Discuss the diagnosis and significance of HIV retinopathy.

WHAT'S NEW?

The presence of HIV-related retinal microangiopathy is associated with the development of systemic CMV disease.

KEY POINT

- HIV retinopathy is asymptomatic, usually easily diagnosed, and serves as a marker of immunosuppression and the development of CMV retinitis.

INTRODUCTION TO HIV RETINOPATHY

Noninfectious retinal microvasculopathy, also called *AIDS retinopathy* or *background HIV retinopathy*, is the most common ocular manifestation of HIV infection, and it was present in 50% of patients in one retrospective series (Jabs, 1995). It typically occurs without CMV retinitis, and immunosuppression alone cannot account for it (Glasgow, 1994). However, given that it usually occurs only in patients who have CD4[+] counts of less than 200 cells/mm[3] (Jabs, 1995), it serves as a clinical marker of advanced immunosuppression. The presence of HIV-related retinal microangiopathy is associated with the development of systemic CMV disease (Iwasaki, 2013).

Clinical features are usually limited to the posterior pole and thus are often visible on direct ophthalmoscopy. The most common findings are cotton-wool spots (Jabs, 1995). They are usually asymptomatic and often resolve spontaneously, typically within 2 months (Kuppermann, 1993). The cause is unknown. Less often noted are intraretinal hemorrhages—which can appear as flame-shaped hemorrhages posteriorly, dot-blot hemorrhages, or punctate intraretinal hemorrhages peripherally—as well as microaneurysms, telangiectasias, and Roth spots (white-centered hemorrhages). In one study, fluorescein angiography revealed microvasculopathy in 100% of patients with AIDS (Newsome, 1984; see Figure 41.2).

Noninfectious retinal vascular occlusion (retinal vein and, less often, retinal artery occlusion) was found in 1.3% of patients with AIDS in one study (Dunn, 2005). A significant association with microvasculopathy was found. The visual prognosis is often poor.

One study described uveitis with chronic multifocal (mostly peripheral) retinal infiltrates as a distinct clinical entity of unknown cause in HIV-infected patients (Levinson, 1998). Cases of similar infiltrates with diffuse interstitial lymphocytosis syndrome have been seen in which parotid gland swelling improved markedly with ART, but the retinal infiltrates did not. The visual prognosis is good. A similar pattern is often seen in African children with AIDS (Kestelyn, 2000).

HIV RETINOPATHY COMPARED WITH CMV RETINITIS

CMV retinitis is not thought to occur unless there is microvasculopathy that disrupts the barrier between the blood supply and the retina, allowing CMV into the retina. There, CMV typically takes hold in parts of the retina damaged previously by HIV microvasculopathy (Glasgow, 1994). The diagnosis of CMV retinitis is clinical and based on the appearance of a focal necrotizing retinitis (Whitley, 1998). A small area of retinitis may resemble cotton-wool spots, a nerve-fiber layer infarct that will resolve in time. Therefore, retinal changes are more profound in HIV-infected patients who have CMV retinitis compared to those who have HIV retinopathy (including capillary destruction), and peripheral retinitis is more frequent than macular infection (Glasgow, 1994).

OTHER OCULAR INFECTIONS

LEARNING OBJECTIVE

Discuss the ocular manifestations of varicella zoster virus (VZV), including progressive outer retinal necrosis.

Non-CMV ocular infections such as herpetic retinitis, toxoplasmosis retinitis, and choroiditis are less common than CMV retinitis and can occur over a wide range of CD4 counts.

KEY POINTS

- In HIV-infected patients, VZV infection is a significant cause of ocular morbidity. Herpes zoster ophthalmicus and progressive outer retinal necrosis are the most important clinical manifestations.

- In people at risk for HIV, herpes zoster ophthalmicus may be a marker of infection; aggressive treatment with acyclovir or valacyclovir is recommended.

- Progressive outer retinal necrosis (PORN) is a rapidly progressive, necrotizing retinitis that occurs in severely immunocompromised patients; intravenous combination therapies have been successful in some cases.

Non-CMV ocular infections such as herpetic retinitis, toxoplasmosis retinitis, and choroiditis are approximately one-tenth as common as CMV retinitis, and the range of CD4+ counts among affected patients is also much wider than that for patients with CMV retinitis (Gangaputra, 2013). VZV can cause eye infections in both anterior and posterior segments of the eye in HIV-infected patients, and it is a significant cause of ocular morbidity. Herpes zoster ophthalmicus and necrotizing herpetic retinopathy are the most important clinical manifestations.

Because herpes zoster ophthalmicus can also occur in patients who are immunocompetent, it is not an AIDS-defining condition. It is more common, however, in HIV-infected patients (Hodge, 1998), and it can serve as an important early clinical marker for HIV infection when it occurs in young patients from high-risk groups (Hodge, 1998). One study found that of 112 patients with herpes zoster ophthalmicus, 29 patients (26%) were infected with HIV; all were younger than age 50 years (Sellitti, 1993). Small case series have suggested that peripheral ulcerative keratitis and neuro-ophthalmologic complications (e.g., encephalitis and cranial nerve palsies) might be more common in patients with AIDS who have herpes zoster ophthalmicus (Neves, 1996). Bilateral herpes zoster ophthalmicus has also been reported (Neves, 1996).

A study of HIV-associated herpes zoster ophthalmicus described 48 patients (Margolis, 1998). The median CD4+ count at diagnosis was 48 cells/mm³ (range, 2–490 cells/mm³). Fifteen patients (31%) had mild or no ocular involvement, whereas 17 patients (35%) had mostly mild stromal keratitis. Serious complications occurred in 20% of patients, including postherpetic neuralgia in 2 patients (4%), chronic infectious pseudodendritic keratitis in 2 patients (4%), elevated intraocular pressure in 3 patients (6%), and central nervous system disease in 2 patients (4%). Aggressive treatment with intravenous acyclovir, high-dose oral acyclovir, or valganciclovir is recommended for all patients.

There are two forms of necrotizing herpetic retinitis—acute retinal necrosis and PORN—with substantial clinical overlap (Engstrom, 1994; Holland, 1994). Acute retinal necrosis presents as a peripheral retinitis, spreads rapidly in a centrifugal manner, and can occur at any CD4+ T cell count and in patients without immune compromise (Holland, 1994). It may be caused by either herpes simplex virus or VZV. PORN often presents with posterior pole involvement, spreads even more rapidly, occurs largely among patients with severe immune compromise (CD4+ T cells <50 cells/mm³), and has a worse prognosis (Engstrom, 1994; Gangaputra, 2013; Margolis, 1998). VZV is almost always the causative agent (Engstrom, 1994). It is a rapidly progressive, necrotizing retinitis characterized by deep retinal lesions but minimal or no retinal vasculitis, vitreitis, or iritis (Engstrom, 1994). A "cracked-mud" perivascular pattern may be seen (Figure 41.3). This pattern is caused by early removal of necrotic debris or edema from retinal tissue adjacent to blood vessels (Engstrom, 1994). Bilateral involvement is common. It has been emphasized that PORN is a variant of the necrotizing herpetic retinopathy that occurs in severely immunocompromised patients, whereas acute retinal necrosis tends to occur in the eyes of patients who have less severe immunosuppression (Guex-Crosier, 1997). Patients with PORN usually have a low CD4+ count, with a median of 25 cells/mm³ (Engstrom, 1994). The diagnosis of both acute retinal necrosis and PORN is usually made clinically, but it can be facilitated by PCR testing from the anterior chamber or vitreous (Knox, 1998).

One study found that 67% of patients with PORN had a history of cutaneous zoster (Engstrom, 1994). Another study found that 2 of 48 patients (4%) with herpes zoster ophthalmicus developed PORN (Margolis, 1998). Retrobulbar optic neuritis can occur before the onset of visible retinal lesions (Shayegani, 1996). In contrast to CMV retinitis, PORN progresses more rapidly and often has a dismal visual prognosis; two-thirds of affected eyes develop legal blindness within 4 weeks of diagnosis because of retrobulbar optic neuritis, retinal detachment, or central retinal necrosis (Engstrom, 1994). Some reports have linked PORN with

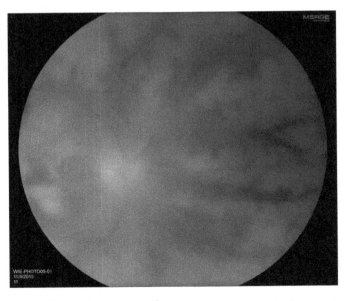

Figure 41.3 Progressive outer retinal necrosis. From the New York State Department of Health AIDS Institute Clinical Guidelines Development Program (2000–2004).

VZV encephalitis (Neves, 1996; van den Horn, 1996). The mortality of patients with herpetic retinitis approaches that of patients with CMV retinitis (Gangaputra, 2013).

Intravenous acyclovir alone is usually ineffective in treating PORN (Engstrom, 1994). Case reports have described successful outcomes with combined intravenous ganciclovir and foscarnet (Moorthy, 1997), intravitreal ganciclovir plus intravenous acyclovir (Meffert, 1997), ganciclovir implants (no longer available) plus intravenous acyclovir and intravitreal foscarnet injections (Roig-Melo, 2001), and intravenous cidofovir as salvage therapy (Schliefer, 1999). Most investigators recommend some type of combined therapy (Kim, 2007).

Chronic suppressive antiviral therapy is needed to prevent disease recurrence, which manifests as increased border opacification of formerly inactive lesions or the appearance of new lesions. Repair of PORN-associated retinal detachment with pars plana vitrectomy, endolaser photocoagulation, and silicone oil tamponade (along with antiviral therapy) may yield ambulatory vision in some cases (Weinberg, 1997).

Ocular complications of syphilis infection are discussed in Chapter 44.

RECOMMENDED READING

Ciulla TA, Danis RP. Repair of retinal detachments due to herpes varicella-zoster virus retinitis. *Ophthalmology*. 1998;105:390–391.

Dunn JP. Viral retinitis. *Ophthalmol Clin North Am*. 1999;12:109–121.

Goldberg DE, Smithen LM, Angelilli A, et al. HIV-associated retinopathy in the ART era. *Retina*. 2005;25:633–649.

Kappel PJ, Charonis AC, Holland GN, et al. Outcomes associated with ganciclovir implants in patients with AIDS-related cytomegalovirus retinitis. *Ophthalmology*. 2006;113:673–668.

REFERENCES

Curi AL, Muralha A, Muralha L, et al. Suspension of anticytomegalovirus maintenance therapy following immune recovery due to highly active antiretroviral therapy. *Br J Ophthalmol*. 2001;85:471–473.

Dunn JP, Yamashita A, Kempen JH, et al. Retinal vascular occlusion in patients infected with human immunodeficiency virus. *Retina*. 2005;25:759–766.

Engstrom RE Jr, Holland GN, Margolis TP, et al. The progressive outer retinal necrosis syndrome: a variant of necrotizing herpetic retinopathy in patients with AIDS. *Ophthalmology*. 1994;101:1488–1502.

Gangaputra S, Drye L, Vaidya V, et al.; Studies of the Ocular Complications of AIDS (SOCA) Research Group. Non-cytomegalovirus ocular opportunistic infections in patients with acquired immunodeficiency syndrome. *Am J Ophthalmol*. 2013;155:206–212.

Glasgow BJ, Weisberger AK. A quantitative and cartographic study of retinal microvasculopathy in acquired immunodeficiency syndrome. *Am J Ophthalmol*. 1994;118(1):46–56.

Guex-Crosier Y, Rochat C, Herbort CP. Necrotizing herpetic retinopathies: a spectrum of herpes virus-induced diseases determined by the immune state of the host. *Ocul Immunol Inflamm*. 1997;5:259–265.

Hammond CJ, Evans JA, Shah SM, et al. The spectrum of eye disease in children with AIDS due to vertically transmitted HIV disease: clinical findings, virology, and recommendations for surveillance. *Graefes Arch Clin Exp Opthalmol*. 1997;235:125–129.

Hodge WG, Seiff SR, Margolis TP. Ocular opportunistic infection incidences among patients who are HIV positive compared to patients who are HIV negative. *Ophthalmology*. 1998;105:895–900.

Holland GN. Standard diagnostic criteria for the acute retinal necrosis syndrome: Executive Committee of the American Uveitis Society. *Am J Ophthalmol*. 1994;117:663–667.

Iwasaki Y, Yamamoto N, Kawaguchi T, et al. Human immunodeficiency virus-related retinal microangiopathy and systemic cytomegalovirus disease association. *Jpn J Ophthalmol*. 2013;57:372–378.

Jabs DA. Ocular manifestations of HIV infection. *Trans Am Ophthalmol Soc*. 1995;93:623–683.

Jabs DA, Ahuja A, Van Natta M, et al.; Studies of the Ocular Complications of AIDS Research Group. Comparison of treatment regimens for cytomegalovirus retinitis in patients with AIDS in the era of highly active antiretroviral therapy. *Ophthalmology*. 2013;120:1262–1270.

Jabs DA, Forman M, Enger C, et al.; Cytomegalovirus Retinitis and Viral Resistance Study Group. Comparison of cytomegalovirus loads in plasma and leukocytes of patients with cytomegalovirus retinitis. *J Clin Microbiol*. 1999;37:1431–1435.

Jabs DA, Martin BK, Forman MS; Cytomegalovirus Retinitis and Viral Resistance Research Group. Mortality associated with resistant cytomegalovirus among patients with cytomegalovirus retinitis and AIDS. *Ophthalmology*. 2010;117:128–132.

Jabs DA, Martin BK, Forman MS, et al.; Cytomegalovirus Retinitis and Viral Resistance Study Group. Cytomegalovirus resistance to ganciclovir and clinical outcomes of patients with cytomegalovirus retinitis. *Am J Ophthalmol*. 2003;135:26–34.

Jabs DA, Martin BK, Forman MS, Ricks MO. Cytomegalovirus (CMV) blood DNA load, CMV retinitis progression, and occurrence of resistant CMV in patients with CMV retinitis [published correction appears in *J Infect Dis*. 2004:192:1310]. *J Infect Dis*. 2005;192:640–649.

Jabs DA, Van Natta ML, Kempen JH, et al. Characteristics of patients with cytomegalovirus retinitis in the era of highly active antiretroviral therapy. *Am J Ophthalmol*. 2002;133:48–61.

Kaplan JE, Masur H, Holmes KK; USPHS; Infectious Disease Society of America. Guidelines for preventing opportunistic infections among HIV-infected persons—2002. Recommendations of the US Public Health Service and the Infectious Diseases Society of America. *MMWR Recomm Rep*. 2002;51(RR-8):1–52.

Kempen JH, Jabs DA, Dunn JP, et al. Retinal detachment risk in cytomegalovirus retinitis related to acquired immunodeficiency syndrome. *Arch Ophthalmol*. 2001;119:33–40.

Kempen JH, Jabs DA, Wilson LA, et al. Mortality risk for patients with cytomegalovirus retinitis and the acquired immunodeficiency syndrome. *Clin Infect Dis*. 2003;37:1365–1373.

Kempen JH, Min Y-I, Freeman WR, et al. Risk of immune recovery uveitis in patients with AIDS and cytomegalovirus retinitis. *Ophthalmology*. 2006;113:684–694.

Kestelyn P, Lepage P, Karita E, et al. Ocular manifestations of infection with the human immunodeficiency virus in an African pediatric population. *Ocul Immunol Inflamm*. 2000;8:263–273.

Kim SJ, Equi R, Belair ML, et al. Long-term preservation of vision in progressive outer retinal necrosis treated with combination antiviral drugs and highly active antiretroviral therapy. *Ocul Immunol Inflamm*. 2007;15:425–427.

Knox CM, Chandler D, Short GA, et al. Polymerase chain reaction-based assays of vitreous samples for the diagnosis of viral retinitis: use in diagnostic dilemmas. *Ophthalmology*. 1998;105:37–45.

Kosobucki BR, Goldberg DE, Bessho K, et al. Valganciclovir therapy for immune recovery uveitis complicated by macular edema. *Am J Ophthalmol*. 2004;137:636–638.

Kuppermann BD, Petty JG, Richman DD, et al. Correlation between CD4+ counts and prevalence of cytomegalovirus retinitis and human immunodeficiency virus-related noninfectious retinal vasculopathy in patients with acquired immunodeficiency syndrome. *Am J Ophthalmol.* 1993;115:575–582.

Levinson RD, Vann R, Davis JL, et al. Chronic multifocal retinal infiltrates in patients infected with human immunodeficiency virus. *Am J Ophthalmol.* 1998;125:312–324.

Margolis TP, Milner MS, Shama A, et al. Herpes zoster ophthalmicus in patients with human immunodeficiency virus infection. *Am J Ophthalmol.* 1998;125:285–291.

Martin DF, Dunn JP, Davis JL, et al. Use of the ganciclovir implant for the treatment of cytomegalovirus retinitis in the era of potent antiretroviral therapy: recommendations of the International AIDS Society–USA panel. *Am J Ophthalmol.* 1999;127:329–339.

Martin DF, Sierra-Madero J, Walmsley S, et al.; Valganciclovir Study Group. A controlled trial of valganciclovir as induction therapy for cytomegalovirus retinitis. *N Engl J Med.* 2002;346:1119–1126.

Meffert SA, Kertes PJ, Lim PL, et al. Successful treatment of progressive outer retinal necrosis using high-dose intravitreal ganciclovir. *Retina.* 1997;17:560–562.

Mizushima D, Nishijima T, Yashiro S, et al. Diagnostic utility of quantitative plasma cytomegalovirus DNA PCR for cytomegalovirus end-organ diseases in patients with HIV-1 infection. *J AIDS.* 2015;68:140–146.

Moorthy RS, Weinberg DV, Teich SA, et al. Management of varicella-zoster virus retinitis in AIDS. *Br J Ophthalmol.* 1997;81:189–194.

Neves RA1, Rodriguez A, Power WJ, et al. Herpes zoster peripheral ulcerative keratitis in patients with the acquired immunodeficiency syndrome. *Cornea.* 1996;15:446–450.

Newsome DA, Green WR, Miller ED, et al. Microvascular aspects of acquired immune deficiency syndrome retinopathy. *Am J Ophthalmol.* 1984;98:590–601.

Nishijima T, Yashiro S, Teruya K, et al. Routine eye screening by an ophthalmologist is clinically useful for HIV-1-infected patients with CD4 count less than 200/μl. *PLoS One.* 2015;10:e0136747.

Roig-Melo EA, Macky TA, Heredia-Elizondo ML, et al. Progressive outer retinal necrosis syndrome: successful treatment with a new combination of antiviral drugs. *Eur J Ophthalmol.* 2001;11:200–202.

Schliefer K, Gümbel HO, Rockstroh JK, et al. Management of progressive outer retinal necrosis with cidofovir in a human immunodeficiency virus-infected patient. *Clin Infect Dis.* 1999;29:684–685.

Sellitti TP1, Huang AJ, Schiffman J, et al. Association of herpes zoster ophthalmicus with acquired immunodeficiency syndrome and acute retinal necrosis. *Am J Ophthalmol.* 1993;116:297–301.

Shayegani A, Odel JG, Kazim M, et al. Varicella-zoster virus retrobulbar optic neuritis in a patient with human immunodeficiency virus. *Am J Ophthalmol.* 1996;122:586–588.

Sittivarakul W, Benjhawaleemas T, Aui-Aree N, et al. Incidence rate and risk factors for contralateral eye involvement among patients with AIDS and cytomegalovirus retinitis treated with local therapy. *Ocul Immunol Inflamm.* 2016;24:530–536.

Sugar EA, Jabs DA, Ahuja A, et al.; Studies of the Ocular Complications of AIDS Research Group. Incidence of cytomegalovirus retinitis in the era of highly active antiretroviral therapy. *Am J Ophthalmol.* 2012;153:1016–1024.

Teoh SC, Ou X, Lim TH. Intravitreal ganciclovir maintenance injection for cytomegalovirus retinitis: efficacy of a low-volume, intermediate-dose regimen. *Ophthalmology.* 2012;119(3):588–595.

Thorne JE, Jabs DA, Kempen JH, et al.; Studies of Ocular Complications of AIDS Research Group. Causes of visual acuity loss among patients with AIDS and cytomegalovirus retinitis in the era of highly active antiretroviral therapy. *Ophthalmology.* 2006;113:1441–1445.

van den Horn GJ, Meenken C, Troost D. Association of progressive outer retinal necrosis and varicella zoster encephalitis in a patient with AIDS. *Br J Ophthalmol.* 1996;80:982–985.

Weinberg DV, Lyon AT. Repair of retinal detachments due to herpes varicella-zoster virus retinitis in patients with acquired immune deficiency syndrome. *Ophthalmology.* 1997;104:279–282.

Whitley RJ, Jacobson MA, Friedberg DN, et al. Guidelines for the treatment of cytomegalovirus diseases in patients with AIDS in the era of potent antiretroviral therapy: recommendations of an international panel. International AIDS Society–USA. *Arch Intern Med.* 1998;158:957–969.

Wohl DA, Kendall MA, Owens S, et al. The safety of discontinuation of maintenance therapy for cytomegalovirus (CMV) retinitis and incidence of memory recovery uveitis following potent antiretroviral therapy. *HIV Clin Trials.* 2005;6:136–146.

Wohl DA, Pedersen S, van der Horst CM. Routine ophthalmologic screening for cytomegalovirus retinitis in patients with AIDS. *J AIDS.* 2000;23:438–439.

Yust I, Fox Z, Burke M, et al.; EuroSIDA. Retinal and extraocular cytomegalovirus end-organ disease in HIV-infected patients in Europe: a EuroSIDA study, 1994–2001. *Eur J Clin Microbiol Infect Dis.* 2004;23:550–559.

42.

CARDIOVASCULAR DISEASE

David A. Wohl and Jeffrey T. Kirchner

CHAPTER GOALS

Upon completion of this chapter, the reader should be able to

- To gain a greater understanding of the pathophysiology of CVD and myocardial infarction in persons living with HIV infection.

- To understand the link of chronic HIV infection as it relates to increased risk of CVD and myocardial infarction.

- To understand the potential association between specific antiretroviral drugs, CVD risk and myocardial infarction.

- To assess CVD risk in persons with HIV infection by application of the AHA/ACC ASCVD 10-year risk calculator.

- To become familiar with medical therapies including statins and non-statins to lower the risk of CVD and myocardial infarction in patients living with HIV infection.

- To become familiar with lifestyle interventions including diet, exercise and smoking cessation to lower the risk of CVD and myocardial infarction in patients living with HIV infection.

INTRODUCTION

There is considerable evidence that PLWH are at increased risk for CVD, including MI and stroke. Epidemiological studies have repeatedly demonstrated higher rates of CVD, especially MI and stroke, among HIV-infected compared to HIV-uninfected patients (Triant, 2009; Freiberg, 2013). Premature atherosclerosis in HIV-infected patients was noted more than 15 years ago in autopsy studies of HIV-infected adults (Morgello, 2002). More recent studies have found a greater frequency of coronary artery disease in PLWH, including those treated with ART and having suppressed viremia relative to uninfected controls (Post, 2014; Metkus, 2015).

Most of these studies acknowledge a higher prevalence of known traditional risk factors for CVD among PLWH and typically adjust for confounding variables. Cigarette smoking, in particular, is several-fold greater in HIV-infected individuals versus the general population. After accounting for such traditional risks, significant differences between PLWH and those without HIV infection generally persist—although the more factors added to these models, the greater the attenuation between HIV infection and CVD (Post, 2014).

Other factors, including poor diet, sedentary lifestyle, substance abuse, and even stress and mental illness, can increase the risk of CVD and could account for some of the excess CVD burden among PLWH. However, data on these confounders are not typically collected (Khambaty, 2016; White, 2015; Freiberg, 2010).

Biologically plausible explanations for higher CVD risk accompanying HIV do exist. Findings of relatively higher levels of markers of immune activation and inflammation among infected patients with suppressed viremia compared to uninfected controls and a correlation between such markers and adverse events suggest infection-related pathogenic mechanisms for CVD in HIV (Deeks, 2013; Hunt, 2012). Moreover, although ART has been found to consistently reduce surrogate markers for inflammation, endothelial dysfunction, and immune activation, there remains a concern that certain drugs can also contribute to CVD. In the large Data Collection on Adverse Events of Anti-HIV Drugs (D:A:D) cohort study of PLWH, lopinavir, darunavir, and abacavir have been associated with CVD (Worm, 2010; Monforte, 2013; Ryom, 2018). It remains unclear if such associations are affected by co-confounding variables and, if truly contributing, what are the mechanisms by which they act to cause CVD. The heightened risk for CVD in people living with HIV infection, regardless of etiology, requires healthcare providers to be diligent in assessing for this risk and intervening, when appropriate, using evidence-based guidelines developed for the general population.

LEARNING OBJECTIVE

Review the prevalence, prognosis, and management of cardiovascular disease in HIV-infected patients and understand its relationship to HIV infection and antiretroviral therapy (ART).

WHAT'S NEW?

- In all persons with HIV, regardless of age, clinicians should emphasize a heart-healthy lifestyle to reduce atherosclerotic cardiovascular disease (ASCVD0—the assessment of cardiovascular risk serves to facilitate the clinician–patient discussion regarding medical and nonmedical interventions.

- In patients with clinical ASCVD who are 75 years of age or younger, high-intensity statin therapy should be initiated or continued with the aim of achieving a 50% or greater reduction in LDL-C levels.

- In adults 40–75 years of age without diabetes and a 10-year risk of 7.5–19.9%, risk-enhancing factors including family history of premature ASCVD, LDL-C of greater than 160 mg/dL, metabolic syndrome, and chronic HIV favors initiation of statin therapy.

- The presence of risk-enhancing factors for ASCVD may favor statin therapy at a 10-year risk of 5–7.5%.

- Half of myocardial infarctions (MI) occurring in people living with HIV (PLWH) may be type 2 (vasospasm, endothelial dysfunction), caused by illicit substance use (e.g., cocaine) or sepsis. Type 1 MIs (thromboembolic) account for the majority of remaining acute CVD events among PLWH.

- In addition to MI, heart failure is being seen more commonly in PLWH.

KEY POINTS

- PLWH are at increased risk for CVD, including MI, stroke, and heart failure.

- Reasons for an increased CVD risk are multiple and include a combination of traditional risk factors, along with substance use, chronic inflammation, immune activation, and effects of ART.

- Patients with HIV infection should undergo screening for established CVD risk factors, including hypertension, diabetes mellitus, dyslipidemia, and cigarette smoking and family history.

- Proven interventions to lower the risk of CVD and MI include diet, exercise, smoking cessation, and the use of lipid-lowering agents and anti-hypertensive medications to treat modifiable risk factors.

- Patients with HIV infection should be assessed for their 10-year cardiovascular risk by using the American College of Cardiology/American Heart Association (ACC/AHA) risk calculator. Depending on risk score and the presence of ASCVD risk-enhancing factors, many may be eligible for medical therapy with a high- or moderated-intensity statin with a goal of lowering LDL-C by 30–50%.

- Non-statin therapies (e.g. fibrates, niacin, omega-3 fatty acids, and ezetimibe) are not routinely recommended by clinical guidelines as first-line therapy due to a lack of conclusive data for improving cardiovascular outcomes.

- Changing ART to improve lipid profiles in patients with hyperlipidemia should be a consideration for select patients but should not compromise virologic or immunologic control.

EVIDENCE OF EXCESS RISK FOR CARDIOVASCULAR DISEASE IN HIV

One of the largest epidemiological studies examining differential rates of CVD among HIV-infected and HIV-uninfected persons was conducted within a registry of patients receiving care in Boston that included 3,851 HIV-infected and 1,044,589 HIV-uninfected patients (Triant, 2009). The difference in acute MI rates between HIV and non-HIV patients was significant, with a relative risk (RR) of 1.75 (95% confidence interval [CI], 1.51–2.02; $p < 0.0001$), adjusting for age, gender, race, hypertension, diabetes, and dyslipidemia. Importantly, complete smoking data, however, were not available, thus limiting the analysis given the several-fold higher rates of smoking in HIV-infected persons compared to age-matched uninfected controls (Triant, 2009).

Similar studies of the incidence of MI and stroke were conducted by the Kaiser Permanente system in California (Klein, 2014, 2015). Rates of both conditions were historically higher for HIV-infected compared to HIV-uninfected members. However, a convergence over time in the rates of MI and stroke experienced by infected and uninfected patients has been observed. Improved detection and the management of CVD risk factors and more aggressive treatment of HIV infection are hypothesized to account for the decline in CVD rates in this cohort of patients. Similar declines in the rates of CVD over the past decade have been reported from cohorts in Europe and British Columbia (Cheung, 2016; Hatleberg, 2016).

A paper from the Veterans Aging Cohort Study (VACS) that reported on 81,000 participants (33% HIV-positive) found that HIV-infected veterans had twice the risk of acute MI compared to those who were HIV-negative (Paisible, 2015). However, it also found a low prevalence of optimization of cardiac health in this high-risk Veterans Administration population, including blood pressure control, treatment of hyperlipidemia, and smoking cessation. This alone may account for the increased risk of MI, and not HIV infection.

Most recently, a 2018 paper by Shah included data from 80 studies of 793,000 persons with HIV and a follow-up of 3.5 million person-years. The authors of this study reported a 2.16 relative risk of CVD in persons with HIV-infected compared to uninfected individuals (Shah, 2018). This is comparable to a relative risk of 2.48 with hypertension and 2.95 with smoking found in the multinational INTERHART study (Yusuf, 2004).

In contrast, a retrospective cohort study from Spain examined data on 3,760 HIV-infected patients who were in care from 1983 to 2011 (Echeverria, 2014). The prevalence of coronary events in this "Mediterranean cohort" was only 2.15%, which is actually lower compared to that in other similar studies of HIV-infected adults. The authors noted that the majority of patients with cardiac disease in this cohort had other CVD risk factors that were not being optimally treated, including hyperlipidemia.

Beyond cohort studies, pathophysiological evidence of excess CVD accompanying HIV infection has been pursued. Relatively high levels of inflammation within the aorta, possibly mediated by monocyte activation, were demonstrated by fluorodeoxyglucose positron emission tomography (FDG-PET) scanning in a small study of ART-receiving HIV-infected patients without known CVD compared to uninfected controls with similar CVD risks. These data were later correlated with vulnerable coronary plaques (Subramanian, 2012; Tawakol, 2014). Similarly, a larger cross-sectional study from the Multicenter AIDS Cohort Study (MACS) examined coronary calcium scores and coronary plaque morphology in HIV-infected and -uninfected men who have sex with men and found that plaque was highly prevalent in both groups (Post, 2014). After adjustment for major confounders, there remained a higher prevalence of plaque in the HIV-infected men (prevalence ratio [PR], 1.13; 95% CI, 1.04–1.23), who were also more likely to have noncalcified plaques (the most vulnerable to rupture) (PR, 1.25; 95% CI, 1.10–1.43). Older age was associated with noncalcified plaque in HIV-infected but not HIV-uninfected men. This factor seemed to drive the overall differences between these groups. Adjustment for additional confounders reduced the association between HIV infection and noncalcified plaques.

The concept of HIV causing "accelerated" aging with CVD and other conditions accompanying growing older occurring earlier in those infected with HIV has been countered by data from the US Veterans Administration Aging Cohort and a study using large registries of HIV-infected and HIV-uninfected persons in Denmark (Althoff, 2015; Rasmussen 2015). In both groups, excess risk of CVD with HIV infection was observed. However, this was detected at similar ages in HIV-positive and HIV-negative persons, and, over time, there was no observed increase in overall risk for those with HIV. Other research has highlighted the substantial contribution of more traditional risks for CVD to excess disease among PLWH. Data from large European observational studies including the D:A:D cohort and MAGNIFICENT Consortium indicate that the main drivers of CVD in PLWH are not related to HIV infection or its therapy (Friis-Moller, 2010; Rotger, 2013). Age, male gender, family history, smoking, lipid profile, diabetes mellitus, and hypertension were significantly more associated with CVD events than ART composition. In the North American NA-ACCORD cohort, the attributable risk of type 1 MI was much greater with smoking, hypertension, and total cholesterol than CD4+ cell count, plasma HIV RNA level, or a diagnosis of AIDS (Althoff, 2017). Consequently, modeling studies have found that interventions that target the management of blood pressure, glucose, and lipid levels, as well as smoking cessation, can be expected to have a much greater clinical impact than earlier initiation of HIV therapy or avoidance of ART that has been associated with risk of CVD (Smit, 2018).

Recent data also suggest that MI that occur in PLWH may, in as much as half of the cases, be type 2 MI, which are related to vasospasm and endothelial dysfunction (Crane, 2017). In one study, this type of MI was more often observed in younger PLWH, and in those with lower CD4+ cell counts, lipid levels, and Framingham Risk Scores than those with type 1 MI (Crane, 2017). Illicit substance use, especially with cocaine, and sepsis, which increases the demand for coronary blood supply, were found to be risks for type 2 MI in this study.

In recent years it is also becoming apparent that heart failure may also be more common in PLWH. In the HIV-Heart Study being conducted within the Kaiser Permanente healthcare system, the rate of incident heart failure was compared between 39,000 PLWH and more than 387,000 matched control (1:10)

patients without HIV infection. Incident heart failure was significantly higher among PLWH (4% vs. 3%) with a hazard ratio indicating a 66% greater risk in the fully adjusted model that accounted for coronary syndrome events, suggesting an independent mechanism independent of atherosclerosis (Go, 2018).

PROPOSED MECHANISMS

While traditional and non-HIV-related factors appear to be driving much of the CVD events that PLWH experience, factors related to HIV infection and treatment may play a role. Numerous mechanistic studies have examined the association between CVD (i.e., plaque, coronary calcium, arterial inflammation, and endothelial dysfunction) and markers of inflammation, immune activation, and microbial translocation across the gut (Deeks, 2013; Hunt, 2012). In the FDG-PET study, aortic wall inflammation was significantly correlated with markers of monocyte and macrophage activation, suggesting that these cell lines play a role in the observed changes. The monocyte activation marker soluble CD163 was also correlated with a noncalcified coronary plaque in HIV-infected men and women with well-controlled HIV. In the MACS coronary imaging study, as in most other cohorts, smoking rates were higher among those who were HIV-positive. That smoking interacts with HIV and aging to accelerate CVD was observed by an examination of carotid intima-media thickness, suggesting HIV infection modifies the effect of smoking and age on cardiovascular health (Fitch, 2013). In a related report, smoking and obesity were each significantly associated with levels of inflammatory markers including interleukin-6 (IL-6), sCD14, and sTNFR-I and -II (Krishnan, 2014). Similar findings linking smoking and inflammation were seen in the SUN cohort of HIV-infected patients (Cioe, 2014). In that study, heavy alcohol intake was also associated with elevations of the coagulation marker D-dimer.

Data from Hsue and colleagues regarding T cell activation and inflammation suggest that this is yet another pathogenic means of developing vascular disease (Hsue, 2010). Residual immune activation secondary to incomplete control of HIV infection (despite undetectable viremia), coinfections (e.g., cytomegalovirus and hepatitis C virus), and irreversible translocation of microbial products across an altered gut lumen has been demonstrated in HIV-infected patients. They may collectively or individually promote a pro-inflammatory milieu that is pro-atherogenic (Deeks, 2013). Consistent findings of a relationship between nadir CD4+ T cell count and risk for CVD (as well as other end-organ diseases) add support for a role of long-term systemic inflammation in cardiovascular health of persons with HIV infection.

A number of studies have also shown that the risk of CVD among persons with HIV infection may also be influenced by immunodeficiency—specifically, low CD4+ T cell counts (Drozd, 2015). In the NA-ACCORD observational cohort, lower current CD4+ T cells, as well as a history of AIDS and detectable plasma HIV RNA levels, were predictors of primary MI in a time-updated model. This analysis also was consistent with other studies in finding a strong link between impaired renal function and CVD (Palella, 2015; Ryom, 2015).

The pathogenesis of heart failure in the setting of HIV infection remains unclear. One hypothesis is that HIV acts directly on the myocardium, as well as indirectly via inflammation and autoimmunity (Remick, 2014). Some antiretroviral drugs, including nucleoside reverse transcriptase inhibitors (NRTIs) in this theoretical model could be contributing to the pathogenesis.

THE EFFECT OF ANTIRETROVIRAL THERAPY ON CARDIOVASCULAR DISEASE

Multiple retrospective and prospective studies have evaluated the impact of ART on CVD. As in the epidemiological studies, these are often challenged by factors that confound analyses and/or lack an appropriate control group. The Strategies for Management of Antiretroviral Therapy (SMART) study, a randomized trial comparing continuous versus intermittent ART (based on $CD4^+$ T cell count), found continuous ART to be significantly associated with a decreased risk of mortality. Intermittent therapy ("treatment interruption") heightened the risk for developing CVD, renal disease, and hepatic events—which led to an understanding of the adverse effects of viremia on organ function (SMART, 2006). Other work demonstrating reductions in markers of inflammation, endothelial dysfunction, and immune activation following initiation of ART has further cemented the concept that treatment of HIV, on the whole, reduces the risk of CVD (McComsey, 2012; Torriani, 2008).

Despite its benefits vis-à-vis countering the impact of ongoing viral replication on health, ART may carry an inherent risk for CVD, as suggested by the effects of some agents on lipids (e.g., increased low-density lipoprotein [LDL] cholesterol and triglyceride levels). To date, the most influential data on this issue is from the D:A:D cohort. This is a large, ongoing, prospective, single-arm, observational cohort study of tens of thousands of HIV-infected patients, mostly in Europe.

In 2003, D:A:D investigators first reported the incidence of MI to be increased significantly with prolonged exposure to combination antiretroviral therapy (cART) (Friis Moller, 2003). The adjusted risk rate per year of exposure to cART ranged from 0.32 for no medication use to 2.93 for at least 6 years of use. However, although there was a significant relative risk of MI with cART, the absolute risk of MI was low (over a period of 36,199 person-years, 126 patients had an MI). The initial association between ART and MI was mainly driven by protease inhibitor (PI) therapy (D:A:D Study Group, 2007; Sabin, 2104). While some of the earliest analyses conducted by the D:A:D group found PI therapy to be associated with CVD; recent work has differentiated this risk by more modern agents of the PI class. (Ryom, 2018). Similar to lopinavir and older PIs, in 2018, newer data from D:A:D found that ritonavir-boosted darunavir was associated with a 51% relative increased risk of MI and 49% increased risk of stroke over a 5-year period (Ryom, 2018). Conversely, another PI-boosted atazanavir was not associated with an increased MI risk. This may be due to the indirect hyperbilirubinemia

that occurs with atazanavir. Other studies actually found a cardio-protective effect of higher bilirubin levels in the blood. A retrospective analysis conducted within the VACS found that patients with and without HIV infection with elevated bilirubin levels had lower rates of CVD and heart failure after adjustment for traditional risk factors (Marconi, 2018).

An earlier link between treatment with the NRTI abacavir and MI ushered in a series of subsequent investigations that have reached mixed conclusion. Possible biomolecular mechanisms for this association have been sought and include increased platelet reactivity and/or endothelial cell and leukocyte interactions (that may be induced by abacavir), but these remain to be proved (Baum, 2011; De Pablo, 2012). In a recent study of patients switching from abacavir to tenofovir alafenamide fumarate, changes in assessments of platelet reactivity and collagen interaction suggest abacavir causes platelet dysfunction. The investigators believe this could explain the findings of an association between abacavir and CVD (Mallon, 2018). Per the latest US Department of Health and Human Services (USDHHS) and International Antiretroviral Association (IAS)-USA HIV treatment guidelines, abacavir should be avoided in patients with or at high risk for cardiovascular disease (USDHHS, 2018; Saag, 2018). As HIV therapy evolves and exposure to new agents accumulate, the D:A:D investigators and other cohorts will regularly reexamine the risks associated with CVD events.

SCREENING AND ASSESSING CARDIOVASCULAR RISK

Given the higher risk of CVD among people living with HIV infection, the standard of HIV care must include baseline screening for traditional CVD risk factors and appropriate attention to management. This includes blood pressure control and maintaining a normal body mass index (BMI). Laboratory parameters should include a lipid panel (total cholesterol [TC], high-density lipoprotein [HDL], LDL, and triglycerides [TG]) and fasting blood glucose level or hemoglobin A1C. Baseline renal and hepatic function should be measured as well (Aberg, 2014). Patients started on ART should have a lipid profile repeated approximately 3 months after they are stabilized on therapy. If the baseline and subsequent values are normal, then repeating a lipid panel yearly is recommended (Aberg, 2014). Risks for CVD and dyslipidemias should generally be managed according to the most recent ACC/AHA guidelines (Goff, 2014; Grundy 2018).

As mentioned earlier, evidence suggests that the effects of smoking on CVD are magnified in those with HIV infection. Therefore, there is particular urgency for HIV care providers to incorporate evidence-based interventions to facilitate cessation of smoking into their practice (see later discussion). Data from the D:A:D cohort indicate a significant reduction in CVD incidence among HIV-infected individuals who quit smoking (Petoumenos, 2011). Similarly, other modifiable CVD risks (hyperlipidemia, hypertension, diabetes mellitus, and obesity) should be sought and acted on (see later discussion).

In the past, CVD risk for patients was usually assessed via the Framingham (MA) heart study risk calculator (available at https://www.easycalculation.com/medical/framingham.

php) Older studies have used this with HIV-infected persons and found it generally performed well in assessing the 10-year risk of CVD. However, it may underestimate risk compared to use in HIV-uninfected patients (Law, 2006). The newer 10-year CVD risk AHA/ACC risk calculator (available at http://www.cardiosource.org/science-and-quality/practice-guidelines-and-quality-standards/2013-prevention-guideline-tools.aspx) has become the standard of care in the United States (Grundy, 2018) (Box 42.1). However, similar to the Framingham risk calculator, the ACC/AHA calculator may actually underestimate the risk of CVD in HIV-infected patients (Regan, 2015; Thompson, 2015, Triant, 2018). More prospective data to validate these guidelines in patients with HIV disease are needed for the development of a CVD risk calculator that could include HIV-specific factors and may further stratify patients based on sex.

Although several inflammatory biomarkers have been studied for their potential role in identifying HIV-infected persons at increased risk for coronary disease, the clinical utility of measuring these has not been determined. These markers include the highly sensitive C-reactive protein (hsCRP), D-dimer, IL-6, amyloid, and adiponectin (Triant, 2009). In several studies, such as SMART, they correlated with the risk of MI and mortality. However, their predictive value for individual patients has not been established. Other diagnostic techniques that may be surrogate markers or provide direct evidence of coronary artery disease (CAD) in patients with HIV include carotid artery intima-media thickness and coronary artery calcification (Hsu, 2010; Baker, 2011; Grinspoon, 2017). Similar to the inflammatory biomarkers, current utilization of these tests should follow practice standards and guidelines as applied to the general population.

Box 42.1 FACTORS INCLUDED IN THE AHA/ACA RISK CALCULATOR

10-Year ASCVD Risk: Pooled Cohort Equation

DEMOGRAPHICS

- Age (40–79 Year)
- Gender
- Race

HISTORY

- HTN
- DM
- Tobacco

MEASUREMENTS

- Total cholesterol
- HDL
- systolic blood pressure

Original Content from http://www.cvriskcalculator.com/

Age (years)	40-79
Gender	⦿ Male ○ Female
Race	○ African American ⦿ Other
Total cholesterol (mg/dL)	150-320
HDL cholesterol (mg/dL)	20-100
Systolic blood pressure (mmHg)	90-200
Diastolic blood pressure (mmHg)	50-140
Treated for high blood pressure	⦿ No ○ Yes
Diabetes	⦿ No ○ Yes
Smoker	⦿ No ○ Yes
	Calculate

Adapted from http://www.cvriskcalculator.com/

INTERVENTIONS AND MANAGEMENT

There is currently no robust evidence base on which to determine if the management of CVD risks in HIV-infected persons should differ from the general population. Modifiable risk factors, including dyslipidemia, smoking, hypertension, diabetes mellitus, and obesity, remain very important in patients who have HIV infection, and possibly even more so than for the general population. As noted previously, the ACC/AHA risk calculator may actually underestimate the risk of heart disease in HIV-infected persons (Triant, 2018). Nonetheless, risk-based assessment for CVD in persons with HIV disease remains a rational starting point to guide counseling, drug therapy (including statins and aspirin), and other risk-reduction interventions (Grundy, 2018).

Aggressively treating the patient's HIV infection with full viral suppression should remain the primary objective, even in the presence of CVD risk factors or established CAD. Older data from the SMART study noted earlier, as well as the ATHENA cohort (Van Lelyveld, 2010), found that ongoing viremia and incomplete immune recovery increase the risk of cardiovascular events. In addition, a National Institutes of Health (NIH)-sponsored study of 6,517 patients, of whom 273 sustained an acute MI, found immunologic control was the most important HIV-related factor associated with acute MI (Triant, 2010).

Because of their potential effects on cholesterol (and thus CVD risk), the choice of ART should take into consideration a patient's individual CVD risk factors. Some combination ART regimens, such as ritonavir-boosted PIs, will increase lipid subsets, including LDL-C and triglycerides. This could further increase CVD risk in addition to those seen with PIs in the D:A:D cohort. The pharmacological booster cobicistat appears to increase LDL cholesterol, similar to ritonavir, but with a smaller impact on triglycerides. The NRTI abacavir increases LDL cholesterol and triglycerides, whereas tenofovir disoproxil fumarate (TDF) has been observed to lower LDL cholesterol levels (Tungsiripat, 2010). However, as noted earlier, in some studies, including D:A:D and SMART, abacavir has been associated with an increased risk of CVD and MI. (SMART, 2008; Dorjee, 2018). In clinical trials, the newer NRTI tenofovir alafenamide (TAF) produced increases in fasting lipid parameters (TC, HDL, direct LDL, and TGs) compared to TDF (Sax, 2014). The more widely used integrase strand inhibitors (INSTIs) raltegravir, dolutegravir, elvitegravir, and bictegravir have not been found to significantly affect lipid levels (Dorjee, 2018).

In patients with moderate to severe dyslipidemia and increased CVD risk, switching ART to a regimen with less effects on cholesterol and/or triglycerides should be considered. This should not be done at the expense of compromising virologic control. In the SPRIAL study, patients with stable HIV disease were switched from a ritonavir-boosted PI-based regimen to raltegravir, leading to significant improvement in patients' lipid profiles (Martinez, 2010). In the SPIRIT study, changing from a ritonavir-boosted PI plus dual nucleoside regimen to rilpivirine plus TDF/emtricitabine led to significant reductions in LDL cholesterol (Palella, 2014). In the MARCH study, patients switched from a boosted-PI to maraviroc had significant reductions in mean total cholesterol over 96 weeks (Pett, 2018). Last, in the NEAT022 study, patients over the age of 50 years or over 18 years with a 10-year CVD risk score of greater than 10% switched from a ritonavir-boosted PI to dolutegravir. At 48 weeks, patients switched to dolutegravir (DTG) had significant improvements in total cholesterol and other lipid fractions (Gatell, 2017). Viral suppression was 93% in the DTG group and 95% in the PI-ritonavir group.

Management of lipid disorders in patients with HIV infection should follow guidelines established for the general population. Attention should be also paid to the potential for drug–drug interactions between lipid-lowering and antiretroviral drugs. There are several sets of cholesterol guidelines, but most practitioners in the United States currently follow those of AHA/ACC (Figure 42.1 and Table 42.1). Pharmacologic treatment is often needed to reduce a patient's risk for CVD. The most recent US recommendations for the management of cholesterol are based on several factors, including 10-year risk of ASCVD, presence of diabetes mellitus, baseline LDL-C levels, and chronic inflammatory conditions including HIV infection (Grundy, 2018). Depending on individual risk and the presence of risk-enhancing factors, this may include "high-intensity" or "moderate-intensity" dosing with statin therapy and/or the use of additional lipid-lowering agents (see later discussion). In addition, the most recent guidelines note that if ASCVD risk is uncertain, coronary artery calcium

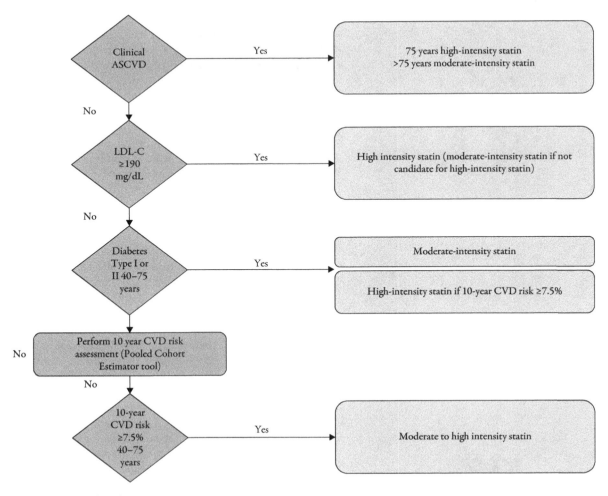

Figure 42.1 ACC/AHA statin benefit groups. SOURCE: Adapted from Stone (2014).

Table 42.1 THE 2018 KEY RECOMMENDATION FOR REDUCING THE RISK OF ATHEROSCLEROTIC CARDIOVASCULAR DISEASE (ASCVD) THROUGH CHOLESTEROL MANAGEMENT

- In all patients, regardless of age, emphasize a heart-healthy lifestyle to reduce ASCVD risk. In young adults 20–39 years of age, an assessment of lifetime risk facilitates the clinician–patient risk discussion.

- In patients with clinical ASCVD, the goal is to reduce low-density lipoprotein cholesterol (LDL-C) by >50% with high-intensity statin therapy or maximally tolerated statin therapy.

- In very-high-risk patients (history of multiple major ASCVD events or 1 event and multiple risk factors), with an LDL-C of >70 mg/dL on maximal statin therapy, consider adding ezetimibe. In patients whose LDL-C remains ≥70 mg/dL on maximally tolerated statin and ezetimibe, adding a PCSK9 inhibitor is reasonable following a clinician–patient discussion about the net benefit, safety, and cost.

- In patients with severe primary hypercholesterolemia (LDL-C level ≥190 mg/dL), begin high-intensity statin therapy without calculating 10-year ASCVD risk. If the LDL-C level remains ≥100 mg/dL, adding ezetimibe is reasonable. If the LDL-C on statin plus ezetimibe remains ≥100 mg/dL and the patient has multiple factors that increase the risk of ASCVD events, a PCSK9 inhibitor may be considered.

- In patients 40–75 years of age *with* diabetes mellitus and LDL-C ≥70 mg/dL, start moderate-intensity statin therapy without calculating 10-year ASCVD risk.

- In adults 40–75 years of age *without* diabetes mellitus with LDL-C ≥70 mg/dL and a 10-year ASCVD risk of ≥7.5%, start moderate-intensity statin if a discussion of treatment options favors statin therapy. If risk status is uncertain, consider using coronary artery calcium (CAC) to improve specificity. If CAC is zero, treatment with statin therapy may be withheld (except in cigarette smokers, diabetes mellitus, or strong family history of premature ASCVD). A CAC score of 1 to 99 favors statin therapy, especially in those ≥55 years of age. If the CAC score is ≥100 Agatston units, statin therapy is indicated unless deferred by clinician–patient risk discussion.

- In adults 40–75 years of age *without* diabetes mellitus and 10-year risk of 7.5–19.9% risk-enhancing factors (family hx, LDL-C >160mg/dL, metabolic syndrome, chronic kidney disease, premature menopause) favors statin therapy. The presence of inflammatory disorders including HIV with other risk-enhancing factors may favor statin therapy in patients at 10-year risk of only 5–7.5%.

- Assess adherence and response to lifestyle changes and cholesterol-lowering medications with repeat lipid measurement 4–12 weeks after statin initiation repeated every 3–12 months.

SOURCE: Adapted from Grundy (2018).

(CAC) may be used to determine indication for statin therapy (Grundy, 2018).

STATIN THERAPY

The initial choice for CVD risk reduction is a 3-hydroxy-3-methylglutaryl coenzyme A reductase inhibitor ("statin").

These agents are very effective in lowering TC and LDL cholesterol (LDL-C) but vary in potency. There are a multitude of clinical trials supporting their role for primary and secondary prevention of ASCVD (Grundy, 2018). Preferred statins for patients with HIV disease include pravastatin, fluvastatin, atorvastatin, rosuvastatin, and pitavastatin. Of note, simvastatin and lovastatin should not be used in patients taking PIs. They are both metabolized by cytochrome P3A4 isoenzyme, and inhibition of this enzyme system results in elevated statin levels with an increased risk of rhabdomyolysis and hepatic toxicity. Conversely, the non-nucleoside reverse transcriptase inhibitor (NNRTI) efavirenz reduces the level of simvastatin and lovastatin and thus decreases efficacy.

There are concerns regarding statin intolerance due to adverse effects of these drugs including fatigue, myalgias, and myopathy—the latter is associated with elevation in creatinine kinase (CK). Myalgias are reported by about 15% of persons taking statins but most do not have elevations in CK (Guyton, 2014). As statins remain the best drugs for CVD risk reduction, before considering a patient to be truly statin-intolerant it is prudent to rule out other causes of muscle-related symptoms such as hypothyroidism, vitamin B_{12} or vitamin D deficiency, or other inflammatory musculoskeletal disorders. Re-challenging a statin-intolerant patient with a different agent or alternative dosing strategy (once weekly dosing) can also be done (Backes, 2017).

There was a concern for hepatoxicity with statins, but in 2012 the US Food and Drug Administration (FDA) removed the recommendation for period monitoring of liver function tests in patients on statin therapy. Hepatic transaminase levels should be checked at baseline and only as clinically indicated thereafter. For HIV-infected patients who are coinfected with HBV or HCV, it may be prudent to monitor at least biannually for elevations in liver enzymes.

Rosuvastatin use was associated with a small but significant increase in the risk of diabetes mellitus in the JUPITER trial of HIV-uninfected patients (Ridker, 2012). A meta-analysis has confirmed this risk but also found it to be dose-dependent. It was also determined that treating 255 patients with statin therapy for 4 years would result in just one case of diabetes (Navarese, 2013). The FDA currently considers new-onset diabetes to be a class effect of statins, but it likely varies with individual agent and dosing.

Regarding trials of statin efficacy, there are growing data supporting the use of statins in HIV-infected persons (Eckard, 2016; Mosepele, 2018). A retrospective cohort study of 700 HIV-infected patients taking atorvastatin, pravastatin, or rosuvastatin found that after a year of therapy on one of these agents, decreases in TC and LDL-C were significantly greater with atorvastatin and rosuvastatin compared to pravastatin (Sing, 2011). The likelihood of achieving treatment goals for non–HDL-C at that time was higher with rosuvastatin (odds ratio [OR], 2.3) but not atorvastatin (OR, 1.5) or pravastatin. Toxicity rates were low and were the same for all three agents. In addition, a recent study by Aberg compared 4 mg/d of pitavastatin to 40 mg/d of pravastatin in HIV-infected adults (n = 252) who were taking ART for at least 6 months. This study found that after 12 weeks of statin therapy, LDL cholesterol decreased by 31% in the pitavastatin group compared to 21% in the pravastatin group. At 52 weeks, adverse events, discontinuations (5% vs. 4%), and virologic failures (3% vs. 4%) were similar in both groups. The authors believe these data support pitavastatin as the "preferred drug" for dyslipidemia in persons with HIV (Aberg, 2017).

In terms of studies using statins for non–lipid-lowering reasons (i.e., anti-inflammatory), the SATURN trial randomized HIV-infected patients on ART with evidence of heightened immune activation or inflammation (hsCRP ≥2 mg/L) to rosuvastatin or placebo (McComsey, 2014). Rosuvastatin was associated with a significant decline in a number of markers of inflammation and immune activation, including monocyte activation markers, as well as increased hip bone density. However, rosuvastatin was associated with significant increases in fasting glucose, fasting insulin, and insulin resistance.

The REPRIEVE trial was initiated by the NIH in 2015. This study is evaluating the use of pitavastatin versus placebo in 7,500 HIV-infected adults aged 40–75 years (https://clinicaltrials.gov/ct2/show/NCT02344290?term=REPRIEVE&rank=4 Clinical Trials.gov, 2018). Numerous primary outcomes will be measured including the time to the first event of a composite of major cardiovascular events (including atherosclerotic or other CVD death, nonfatal MI, unstable angina hospitalization, coronary arterial revascularization, nonfatal stroke, or transient ischemic attack [TIA]). Secondary outcomes (change in lipid levels, inflammatory biomarkers, and all-cause mortality) are also being evaluated. Also embedded in REPRIEVE will be a sub study of 800 patients who undergo coronary computed tomography to assess formation of coronary plaque. There may be preliminary data forthcoming, but the study is not expected to close until 2022 (https://clinicaltrials.gov/ct2/show/NCT02344290?term=REPRIEVE&rank=4 Clinical Trials.gov, 2018).

Statins are recommended as first-line therapy from primary and secondary prevention of CVD in persons with HIV. Intensity of therapy should be determined by baseline risk and comorbidities (see Table 42.2). Statins that are not metabolized by the CYP450 system (pravastatin and pitavastatin) may be the preferred agents in patients with HIV to reduce the potential for drug–drug interactions.

Table 42.2 LEVELS OF HIGH- AND MODERATE-INTENSITY STATIN THERAPY

HIGH-INTENSITY STATIN THERAPY	MODERATE-INTENSITY STATIN THERAPY
Lowers LDL-C by ~≥50%	Lowers LDL-C by ~30–49%
Atorvastatin 40–80 mg	Atorvastatin 10–20 mg
Rosuvastatin 20–40 mg	Fluvastatin 40 mg bid
	Fluvastatin XL 80 mg
	Lovastatin 40 mg [a]
	Pitavastatin 1-4 mg
	Pravastatin 40 mg (80 g)
	Rosuvastatin (5 mg) 10 mg
	Simvastatin 20–40 mg [a]

LDL-C, low-density lipoprotein cholesterol.
[a] Should not be used with protease inhibitors.
SOURCE: Adapted from Grundy (2018).

FIBRIC ACID DERIVATIVES

In HIV-infected patients with hypertriglyceridemia, fibric acid derivatives including clofibrate, gemfibrozil, or fenofibrate may be considered for treatment. They are generally recommended in patients with fasting triglyceride levels of 500 mg/dL or higher. These drugs effectively lower triglycerides but have little effect on LDL and HDL cholesterol. Data from D:A:D suggested a very minor association between elevated triglycerides and MI after adjusting for other lipid and nonlipid risk factors. However, the D:A:D: study group also concluded that use of fibrates alone to lower triglycerides is unlikely to have a major impact on the incidence of MI (D:A:D, 2011). In the past, fibrates were also used to lower triglycerides in patients with HIV due to the potential for acute pancreatitis with triglyceride levels of greater than 1,000 mg/dL.

The current ACC/AHA treatment guidelines do not recommend this class of medications for dyslipidemia (Grundy, 2018). They cite a lack of data supporting an effect on CVD outcomes and note that their role in the primary prevention of CVD is less clear as it relates to a reduction in triglyceride levels. They do note that in adults with fasting triglycerides of 500 mg/dL or higher, and especially fasting triglycerides of 1,000 mg/dL or more, it is important to identify and address causes of hypertriglyceridemia. If triglycerides are persistently elevated or increasing, they recommend of a very-low-fat diet, avoidance of refined carbohydrates and alcohol, consumption of omega-3 fatty acids, and, if necessary, to prevent acute pancreatitis, fibrate therapy (Grundy, 2018). A Cochrane review from 2016 concluded that there is "moderate-quality" evidence suggesting fibrates lower the risk of CVD and coronary events in primary prevention, but the absolute risk reduction was less than 1% (Jacob, 2016). Other guidelines, including those from Europe and the American Association of Clinical Endocrinologists (AACE), note that fibrates "may be considered" in select patients with TGs of greater than 200 mg/dL or if they sustain recurrent ASCVD events despite statin therapy (Baer, 2017). The ACC/AHA guidelines state that the combination of gemfibrozil with a statin should be avoided due to an increased risk for myopathy (Grundy, 2018).

EZETIMIBE

Ezetimibe is a drug that selectively inhibits gastrointestinal cholesterol absorption within the small intestine. Overall, this drug is safe, usually well-tolerated, and effective in reducing LDL-cholesterol by an additional 12–19% when taken with a statin therapy. Studies with ezetimibe have been performed in persons with HIV disease. They have examined ezetimibe as both monotherapy and adjunctive therapy for lipid management but did not specifically assess CVD outcomes (Grandi, 2014; Leyes, 2014; Saeedi, 2015, Wohl, 2008).

A recent study from Thailand of HIV patients on a PI plus a statin for at least 6 months found the addition of 10 mg/d of ezetimibe produced a significant decline in mean serum total cholesterol, LDL, and TGs (Boonthos, 2018). Moreover, there were no adverse events or abnormal lab parameters noted in study participants. The IMPROVE-IT trial demonstrated that ezetimibe significantly reduces the risk of major cardiovascular events in a group of high-risk patients with known CVD and already low LDL-C levels. In this trial, there was an absolute risk reduction of 2% in the cardiovascular event rate (32.7% vs. 34.7%) with the addition of ezetimibe in patients on simvastatin compared to those on simvastatin monotherapy (Cannon 2015; Hammersley, 2017).

The ACC/AHA guidelines as well as the National Institute for Care Excellence (NICE) guidelines from the UK only recommend ezetimibe monotherapy for primary hyperlipidemia in patients for whom a statin is contraindicated or if they cannot tolerate statin therapy (NICE, 2016; Grundy, 2018). This is based on the lack of CVD outcome trials of ezetimibe monotherapy. A 2017 US update on non-statin therapies suggests the addition of 10 mg/d of ezetimibe for patients whom additional lowering of LDL-C is desired (Lloyd-Jones, 2017). The newest US guidelines note that it is "reasonable" to add ezetimibe in very high-risk patients with an LDL-C of greater than 70 mg/dL despite maximal statin therapy (Grundy, 2018). In a similar manner, the NICE guidelines from the UK and the European Society of Cardiology support ezetimibe as add-on therapy in "high or very high-risk patients" who fail to meet specific LDL targets.

OMEGA-3 FATTY ACIDS

Three to five grams per day of omega-3 fatty acids ("fish oil") generally can produce a 30–50% reduction in triglyceride levels. Their low cost, good tolerability, and lack of drug–drug interactions have made these agents potentially attractive for use in the general population, including persons with HIV infection. There are data, including a recent study, to support the use of omega-3 fatty acids to lower triglycerides in patients with HIV disease who were taking ART (Vieira, 2017; De Truchis, 2007; Gerber, 2008; Wohl, 2005). The study by Vieira was a systematic review with a meta-analysis of randomized clinical trials of patients with baseline TG levels of great than 200 mg/dL. The average combined reduction in TGs in patients taking omega-3 fatty acids was −114 mg/dL. Other studies have looked at the use of fish oil supplements in HIV patients to assess their effect on inflammatory biomarkers and oxidative stress—both with potential relationships to CAD and found either no change or clinical benefit (Swanson, 2018; Amador-Licona, 2016, Oliveira 2015).

The relationship between circulating TG levels and atherosclerosis is still unclear. Current US cholesterol guidelines cite a lack of any randomized controlled trials (RCTs) evaluating this class of drugs and with no proof of beneficial CVD outcomes. They may prevent pancreatitis in patients with severe triglyceride elevations (>1,000 mg/dL) but have been associated with adverse events, including gastrointestinal upset, skin conditions (rash and pruritus), and bleeding. Recent data from the British ASCEND trial found that 1 g of omega-3 fatty acid daily did not reduce non-fatal MI or stroke, TIA, or CVD death compared to an olive-oil placebo (8.9% vs. 9.2%) (Bowman, 2018). Therefore, the collective evidence suggests little or no role for omega-3 fatty acid supplementation for primary or secondary prevention of CVD, with no apparent effect on major cardiac events, sudden cardiac death, or all-cause mortality (Rogers, 2018).

NIACIN

The most recent ACC/AHA guidelines do not recommend any formulations of oral niacin therapy for lipid-lowering or CVD prevention (Grundy, 2018). The past cholesterol guidelines note that if niacin is to be used as adjunctive therapy with a statin, any CVD risk reduction benefit should be weighed against the risks for niacin-associated adverse events, including flushing, hyperglycemia, elevated liver enzymes, peptic ulcer disease, and acute gout. A study by Dube found that despite improvements in lipids, niacin treatment for 24 weeks did not improve endothelial function or inflammatory markers in persons with well-controlled HIV infection and low HDL-C (Dube, 2015). A systematic review of niacin therapy concluded that it does not decrease mortality in patients with low HDL or CAD and should not be prescribed alone or in combination with a statin (Garg, 2017). An evidence-based review of several studies with niacin concluded that it does not reduce CVD morbidity or mortality in patients with established heart disease (Lazzopina, 2018).

PCSK9 INHIBITORS

In 2015, the FDA approved two drugs in this class for use in select patient populations. The agents alirocumab (Praluent) and evolocumab (Repatha) are indicated for the treatment of high LDL cholesterol. These medications are humanized monoclonal antibodies that inactivate proprotein convertase subtilisin-kexin type 9 (PCSK9) (Shahreyar, 2018). This inactivation results in decreased LDL-receptor degradation, increased recirculation of the receptor to the surface of hepatocytes, and consequent lowering of LDL cholesterol levels in the bloodstream (Everett, 2015). These drugs can lower LDL cholesterol by approximately 60%, and are generally safe and generally well tolerated. They are administered as a subcutaneous injection either every 2 weeks or once a month.

There are now several studies providing evidence that PCKS9 inhibitors reduce CVD events when added to statin therapy (Sabatine, 2017; Giugliano, 2017). However, these agents are very expensive, currently costing approximately $14,000 per patient/year. In patients with ASCVD, this class of drugs exceeds the generally accepted cost threshold of $100,000–150,000 per quality-adjusted life year (Kazi, 2016). Until the cost can be justified with more data and clinical outcomes from longer term studies, the PCSK9 inhibitors should be limited to very high-risk ASCVD patients—those with familial hypercholesterolemia or with known ASCVD who need further lowering of LDL despite maximal statin and ezetimibe therapy (Lloyd Jones, 2017; Grundy, 2018). Of note, PSCK9 levels are elevated in HIV-positive persons, and, in ART-naïve patients, are positively associated with immunodeficiency and severity of HIV disease but the role of treatment remains unknown (Boccara, 2017).

ASPIRIN

Aspirin (acetylsalicylic acid or ASA) is often recommended by healthcare providers for the prevention of CVD and associated clinical events, including MI and stroke. Worth noting, aspirin is not FDA approved for the prevention of CAD or MI (Truong, 2015). However, recent surveillance data from the CDC found that 27% of US adults were taking aspirin for primary prevention and 74.9% for secondary CVD prevention (Wall, MMWR, 2018). While the benefit of aspirin has been clearly demonstrated for people with established CVD, this risk-benefit equation is more complex in primary prevention of CVD and related clinical outcomes such as MI. Aspirin irreversibly inhibits cyclooxygenase-1 (COX-1) and blocks the formation and release of thromboxane A2, a strong platelet activator. The COX-1 enzyme is also responsible for producing prostaglandins that protect gastric mucosa, thus patients who take aspirin may be susceptible to gastrointestinal bleeding. Risk factors for GI bleeding with aspirin include higher dose and longer duration of use, history of gastrointestinal ulcers, bleeding disorders, renal failure, advanced liver disease, and thrombocytopenia. Other factors that increase the risk for bleeding with low-dose aspirin use include concurrent anticoagulation or the use of nonsteroidal anti-inflammatory drugs (NSAIDs).

The evidence for aspirin in the primary prevention of CVD, MI, or stroke remains limited, and there are very little data in PLWH (O'Brien, 2013; Suchindran, 2014). At the time of its last update in 2016, the US Preventive Services Task Force (USPSTF) noted that, for primary prevention, "aspirin modestly reduces nonfatal MI/coronary events and major CVD events, but increases major GI bleeding risk (Whitlock, 2016). More precise real-world estimates for bleeding events (GI, CNS) are necessary to calculate the net benefit." The USPSTF notes that at some absolute risk for 10-year CVD events, benefits could outweigh bleeding risks, but models and further studies to identify these populations are needed (Guirguis-Blake, 2016; Bibbins-Domingo, 2016). The USPSTF currently recommends the use of aspirin in person ages 50–59 years who have a 10% or greater 10-year CVD risk (http://tools.acc.org/ASCVD-Risk-Estimator), who are not at risk of bleeding, have a life expectancy of at least 10 years, and are willing to take low-dose aspirin for at least 10 years. The recommendation for aspirin as primary prevention of CVD in persons less than 50 years or greater than 70 years of age is given an "I" grade, meaning there is insufficient evidence to support this practice (see Table 42.3).

There are several ongoing primary prevention trials with aspirin that should provide guidance in the future regarding the use of aspirin. The Aspirin in Reducing Events in the Elderly (ASPREE) trial includes patients older than 70 years and is being conducted in Australia and the United States. The ACCEPT-D trial is looking at low-dose aspirin plus simvastatin in diabetics (Walker, 2018). The Aspirin to Reduce Risk of Initial Vascular Events (ARRIVE) trial from Europe randomized more than 12,500 adults with presumed moderate CVD risk to aspirin 100 mg/d or placebo. During 5 years of follow-up there was no reduction in CVD events by intent-to-treat analysis (Gaziano, 2018). There was a 19%

Table 42.3 US PREVENTIVE SERVICES TASK FOR RECOMMENDATION FOR ASPIRIN THERAPY

ADULTS AGED 50–59 YEARS WITH A ≥10% 10-YEAR CVD RISK

The USPSTF recommends initiating low-dose aspirin for primary prevention of CVD in adults aged 50–59 years who have a 10% or greater 10-year CVD risk, are not at increased risk for bleeding, have a life expectancy of at least 10 years, and are willing to take low-dose aspirin daily for at least 10 years. [level of evidence = B]

ADULTS AGED 60–69 YEARS WITH A ≥10% 10-YEAR CVD RISK

The decision to initiate low-dose aspirin use for the primary prevention of CVD in adults aged 60–69 years who have a 10% or greater 10-year CVD risk should be an individual one. Persons not at increased risk for bleeding, have a life expectancy of at least 10 years, and are willing to take low-dose aspirin daily for at least 10 years are more likely to benefit. Persons who place a higher value on the potential benefits than the potential harms may choose to initiate low-dose aspirin. [level of evidence = C]

ADULTS YOUNGER THAN 50 YEARS

Current evidence is insufficient to assess the balance of benefits and harms of aspirin use for primary prevention of CVD. [level of evidence = I]

ADULTS AGED 70 YEARS OR OLDER

Current evidence is insufficient to assess the balance of benefits and harms of aspirin use for primary prevention of CVD. [level of evidence = I]

Adapted from Guirguis-Blake, 2016

relative reduction in the composite endpoint of CVD events in patients who actually took ASA but also a doubling in the rate of GI bleeding (0.5% in absolute terms). Last, ASCEND is a study from the UK which looked at 100 mg/d of aspirin in diabetics without known CVD. The results of the ASCEND trial were recently published ($N = 15,480$), and, during a mean follow-up of 7.4 years, serious vascular events occurred in a significantly lower percentage of participants in the aspirin group than in the placebo group—8.5% vs. 9.6% ($p = 0.01$). However, major bleeding events occurred in a greater number of participants (4.1% vs. 3.2%, $P = 0.003$) in the aspirin group compared with the placebo group, with most being gastrointestinal bleeding and extracranial bleeding (Bowman, 2018).

For *secondary prevention*, numerous studies have evaluated the role of aspirin in acute treatment of cardiac events and secondary prevention of CVD. There are strong data demonstrating that low-dose daily aspirin effectively reduces the risk of recurrence of vascular events in patients with a history of a previous MI, stroke, or TIA by approximately 20%. There has been FDA-approved labeling for this indication since the 1980s (Paikin, 2012). Because of this consistently reported benefit, which has been found to outweigh the risk of major bleeding, aspirin therapy for secondary prevention is part of standard clinical practice.

The optimal dose of aspirin to prevent CVD events is not known. Primary prevention trials demonstrate some benefit with doses ranging from 75 mg/d and 100 mg/d or 325 mg every other day. A dose of 75 mg/d is as effective as higher doses, and the risk for GI bleeding increases with the dosage. A pragmatic approach consistent with the evidence is to prescribe 81 mg/d, which is the most commonly recommended dose in the United States.

BLOOD PRESSURE CONTROL

Hypertension has become more prevalent as the HIV population ages. It is one of the most important CVD risk factors and is strongly associated with CAD, stroke, and heart failure. The prevalence varies with different HIV cohorts but is estimated to range from 10% to 50% (Boccara, 2017). Data from the CDC's Medical Monitoring Project found that 42% of PLWH had hypertension ($N = 8.631$), but only 49% had their blood pressured controlled (Olaiya, 2018). The global incidence of HIV-infected adults with hypertension is estimated to be 35% compared to 30% of HIV-uninfected adults (Fahme, 2018).

Factors associated with elevated blood pressure in the HIV-infected population appear similar to those of the general population and include older age; male sex; African American, African, and Caribbean ethnicities; higher BMI; diabetes; and chronic kidney disease. Although less commonly seen than in the past, lipodystrophy and metabolic syndrome have also been associated with hypertension in HIV-infected adults (Fahme, 2018). Older studies of blood pressure changes in the D:A:D study and a US cohort found no evidence that ART increased the risk of hypertension (Thiebault, 2005; Medina-Torne, 2012). Conversely, other studies have implicated both PIs and duration of ART as being associated with hypertension (Boccara, 2017). Some researchers also believe that immune activation and chronic inflammation contribute to the pathophysiology of hypertension in persons with HIV disease (van Zoest, 2017).

It is reasonable to screen and manage hypertension in HIV-infected adults per the current national guidelines (Elton, 2018). It should be noted, however, that the newest US hypertension guidelines have been controversial and not collectively endorsed by all professional societies. The 2017 recommendation is for a diagnosis of "hypertension" rather than "prehypertension" for adults with a systolic BP of 130 mm Hg or greater. They also recommend drug treatment for "high-risk" people with hypertension. These include those with existing CVD or a calculated 10-year CVD risk of 10% or greater, or another high-risk condition such as chronic kidney disease or diabetes (Whelton, 2017). Some feel that by following the new ACC/AHA guidelines a large number of people will be subject to medical treatment with little or no benefit in terms of CVD risk reduction and mortality (Bell, 2018; Brunstrom, 2018). They believe the threshold for treating hypertension should remain at 140 mm Hg. Regardless, for those for whom medical therapy is deemed necessary, it is important to be aware of potential drug–drug interactions with ART and antihypertensive agents. There have not been any large-scale studies of specific blood pressure–lowering medications in HIV-infected adults. However, there are small studies of renin-angiotensin antagonists showing very favorable results, and many adult patients with HIV infection will likely need two or more medications to reached recommended blood pressure goals (Fahme, 2018).

SMOKING CESSATION

Smoking prevalence is very high in many HIV-infected cohorts, and smoking cessation remains a very important part of CVD risk reduction. There is also an increased risk of lung cancer in PLWH which is directly influenced by smoking as well as immunosuppressive and inflammatory aspects of HIV (Sigel, 2017). Getting patients to stop smoking has been shown to significantly reduce their AHA/ACA risk scores by 50% or greater. Counseling, including the "5 A strategy" (ask, advise, assess, assist, arrange follow-up), has proved successful. In addition, pharmacologic interventions including nicotine replacement, bupropion, and varenicline are all potentially

BP Category	Systolic BP		Diastolic BP	Treatment or Follow-up
Normal	<120 mm Hg	and	<80 mm Hg	Evaluate yearly; encourage healthy lifestyle changes to maintain normal BP
Elevated	120-129 mm Hg	and	<80 mm Hg	Recommend healthy lifestyle changes and reassess in 3-6 months

Hypertension Stage 1	130-139 mm Hg	or	80-89 mm Hg	Assess the 10-year risk for heart disease and stroke using the atherosclerotic cardiovascular disease (AVSCD risk calculator
				• If risk is <10%, start with healthy lifestyle recommendations and reassess in 3-6 months
				• If risk is >10% or the patient has known clinical CVD, diabetes mellitus, chronic kidney disease, recommend lifestyle changes and BP-lowering medication (1 medication); reassess in 1 month for effectiveness of medication therapy
				  – If goal is met after 1 month, reassess in 3-6 months
				  – If goal is not met after 1 month, consider different medication or titration and continue monthly follow-up until control is achieved

Hypertension Stage 2	≥140 mm Hg	or	≥90 mm Hg	Recommend healthy lifestyle changes and BP-lowering medication (2 medications of different classes); reassess in 1 month for effectiveness • If goal is met in 1 month; reassess in 3-6 months • If goal is not met after 1 month, consider different medications or titration and continue follow-up until control is achieved

Figure 42.2 ACC/AHA Guidelines for Diagnosis and Management of Hypertension. SOURCE: Whelton PK, 2018.

effective therapies to assist patients with smoking cessation (see Box 42.2).

A large multinational study of more than 8,000 adult smokers recently looked at the safety of varenicline, bupropion, and 21 mg nicotine patches in regards to adverse cardiovascular effects. There was a very low incidence of cardiovascular events (<0.5%) during 12 weeks of treatment and at 12 more weeks of follow-up (Benowitz, 2018). These data support these therapeutic interventions by themselves or in combination to help patients stop smoking. A study from France of HIV-infected adults found varenicline significantly more effective than placebo in helping them maintain continuous abstinence at 48 weeks (Mercie, 2018). A Cochrane review of 12 studies assessing the effectiveness of interventions (behavioral and pharmacotherapy) to motivate and assist tobacco use cessation in PLWH found moderate evidence that combined interventions were effective for long-term abstinence (Pool, 2016). The authors concluded that tobacco cessation should be offered to all PLWH as even non-sustained periods of abstinence are beneficial.

NONPHARMACOLOGICAL INTERVENTIONS

The process of atherosclerosis is thought to begin at a young age and progress over many decades before clinical CVD (e.g., acute coronary syndromes, stable or unstable angina, MI) becomes evident. As noted earlier, for many reasons, this progression may be accelerated in PLWH due to disease- and ART-related factors.

Lifestyle modifications including a healthy diet, regular physical activity, maintaining a normal BMI, limited alcohol use, and not smoking have been associated with improvements in CVD risk. Regarding physical activity, the ACC/AHA guidelines for cholesterol and high blood pressure both recommend that adults should be advised to engage in aerobic physical activity 3–4 sessions per week, lasting on average 40 minutes per session and involving moderate- to vigorous-intensity physical activity (Grundy, 2018; Whelton 2017). These behaviors can lead to improvements in TC, LDL, HDL, blood glucose, and blood pressure—and ultimately lower 10-year and lifetime rates of CVD. Several published studies have found variable results in terms of exercise in PLWH. One systematic review found that lower levels of physical activity in persons with HIV disease were consistently associated with older age, lower educational level, lower CD4 count, exposure to ART, and the presence of lipodystrophy. Other important barriers were the presence of bodily pain and depression (Vancamfort, 2018). As persons with HIV disease are living much longer, it is important to encourage engagement in multiple aspects of a healthy lifestyle, including a regular physical activity.

RECOMMENDED READING

Martins Pinto DA, Lopez Vaz da Silva MJ. Cardiovascular disease in the setting of human immunodeficiency virus infection. *Curr Cardiol Rev.* 2018; 14:25–41.

REFERENCES

Aberg JA, Gallant JE, Ghanem KG, et al. Primary care guidelines for the management of persons infected with HIV: 2013 update by the HIV Medicine Association of the Infectious Diseases Society of America. *Clin Infect Dis.* 2014 Jan; 58(1):1–34.

Aberg JA, Sponseller CA, Ward DJ et al. Pitavastatin versus pravastatin in adults with HIV-1 infection and dyslipidemia (INTREPID): 12 week and 52-week results of a phase 4, multicenter, randomized double-blind, superiority trial. *Lancet HIV* 2017; 4(7); e284–e294.

Althoff KN, McGinnis KA, Wyatt CM, et al. Comparison of risk and age at diagnosis of myocardial infarction, end-stage renal disease, and non-AIDS defining cancer in HIV-infected versus uninfected adults. *Clin Infect Dis.* 2015; 60:627–638.

Althoff KN, Palella FJ, Gebo K, et al. Impact of smoking, hypertension and cholesterol on myocardial infarction in HIV+ adults. CROI 2017. Boston, Abstract# 130.

Amador-Licona N, Díaz-Murillo TA, Gabriel-Ortiz G et al., Omega 3 Fatty Acids Supplementation and Oxidative Stress in HIV-Seropositive Patients. A Clinical Trial. *PLoS One.* 2016 Mar 25; 11(3): e0151637.

Backes JM, Russinger JF, Gibson CA, Moriarity PM. Statin-associated muscle symptoms—managing the highly intolerant. *J Clin Lipidol.* 2017; 11(1):24–33.

Baer, J. AACE and EAS Lipid Guidelines. *Am J Cardiol* 2017/08/11/08. https://www.acc.org/latest-in-cardiology/articles/2017/08/11/08/35/aace-and-eas-lipid-guidelines.

Baker JV, Henry WK, Patel P, et al.; Study to Understand the Natural History of HIV/AIDS in the Era of Effective Therapy Investigators. Progression of carotid intima-media thickness in a contemporary human immunodeficiency virus cohort. *Clin Infect Dis.* 2011 Oct; 53(8):826–835.

Baum PD, Sullam PM, Stoddart CA, et al. Abacavir increases platelet reactivity via competitive inhibition of soluble guanylyl cyclase. *AIDS.* 2011; 25(18):2243–2248.

Bell, KJ. Incremental Benefits and Harms of the 2017 American College of Cardiology American Heart Association High Blood Pressure Guideline. *JAMA Intern Med.* 2018; 178(6):755–757.

Benowitz NL, Pipe A, West R et al. Cardiovascular safety of varenicline, bupropion, and nicotine patches in smokers. A randomized controlled trial. *JAMA Intern Med* 2018; 178(5):622–631.

Bibbins-Domingo K; U.S. Preventive Services Task Force. Aspirin Use for the Primary Prevention of Cardiovascular Disease and Colorectal Cancer: U.S. Preventive Services Task Force Recommendation Statement. *Ann Intern Med.*2016 Jun 21; 164(12):836–845.

Boccara F. Cardiovascular health in an aging HIV population. AIDS 2017; 31(suppl 2): S157–S163.

Boccara F, Ghislain M, Meyer L et al. Impact of protease inhibitors on circulating PCSK9 levels in HIV-infected antiretroviral-naïve patients from an ongoing prospective cohort. ANRS-COPANA Study Group. *AIDS* 2017; 31(17):2367–2376.

Boonthos K, Puttilerpong C, PenssuparpT. Short-term efficacy and safety of adding ezetimibe to current regimen of lipid-lowering drugs in HIV-infected Thai patients treated with protease inhibitors. *Japan J Infect Dis* 2018; 71:220–224.

Bowman L, Marion Mafham M, Wallendszus K et al. Effects of Aspirin for Primary Prevention in Persons with Diabetes Mellitus the ASCEND Study Collaborative Group*. August 26, 2018, at *NEJM. org.* DOI: 10.1056/NEJMoa1804988

Brunstrom M. Carlberg B. Association of blood pressure lowering with mortality and cardiovascular disease across blood pressure levels: a systematic review and meta-analysis. *JAMA Intern Med.* 2018; 178(1):28–36.

Cannon C, Blazing M, Giugliano R et al. Ezetimibe added to statin therapy after acute coronary syndromes. *N Engl J Med* 2015; 372:2387–2397.

Cheung CC, Ding E, Sereda P, et al. Reductions in all-cause and cause-specific mortality among HIV-infected individuals receiving antiretroviral therapy in British Columbia, Canada: 2001-2012. *HIV Med.* 2016 Oct; 17(9):694–701.

Cioe PA, et al. Soluble CD14 and D-dimer are associated with smoking and heavy alcohol use in HIV-infected adults. CROI 2014, Boston, MA, Abstract # 732.

Clinical Trials.gov. https://clinicaltrials.gov/ct2/show/NCT02344290?term=REPRIEVE&rank=4.

Crane HM, Paramsothy P, Drozd DR, et al. Types of Myocardial Infarction Among Human Immunodeficiency Virus-Infected Individuals in the United States. *JAMA Cardiol.* 2017;2(3):260–267.

D:A:D Study Group. Class of antiretroviral drugs and the risk of myocardial infarction. *N Engl J Med.* 2007; 356:1723–1735.

Data Collection on Adverse Events of Anti-HIV Drugs (D:A:D) Study Group. The impact of fasting on the interpretation of triglyceride levels for predicting myocardial infarction risk in HIV-positive individuals: The D:A:D study. *J Infect Dis.* 2011; 204(4):521–525.

De Pablo C, Orden S, Calatayud S, et al. Differential effects of tenofovir/emtricitabine and abacavir/lamivudine on human leukocyte recruitment. *Antivir Ther.* 2012; 17(8):1615–1619.

De Truchis P, Kirstetter M, Perier A, et al. Reduction in triglyceride level with N-3 polyunsaturated fatty acids in HIV-infected patients taking potent antiretroviral therapy: A randomized prospective study. *J Acquir Immun Defic Syndr.* 2007; 44(3):278–285.

Deeks S, Lewin SR, Havlir DA. The end of AIDS: HIV infection as a chronic disease. *Lancet.* 2013; 283(9903):1525–1533.

Dorjee K, Choden T, Baxi SM, et al. Risk of Cardiovascular Disease Associated with Exposure to Abacavir Among Individuals With HIV: A Systematic Review and Meta-analyses Of Results from Seventeen Epidemiologic Studies. Int J Antimicrob Agents. 2018 Jul 21. Pii: S0924-8579(18)30201-2.

Drozd DR, Kitahata MM, Althoff KN, et al. Incidence and risk of myocardial infarction (MI) by type in the NA-ACCORD. CROI 2015, Seattle, WA, Abstract # 748.

Dubé MP, Komarow L, Fichtenbaum CJ et al. Extended-Release niacin versus Fenofibrate in HIV-Infected participants With Low HDL Cholesterol: Effects on Endothelial Function, Lipoproteins, and Inflammation. *Clin Infect Dis.* 2015 Sep 1; 61(5):840–849.

Echeverria P, Domingo P, Llibre JM, et al. Prevalence of ischemic heart disease and management of coronary risk in daily clinical practice: Results from a Mediterranean cohort of HIV-infected patients. *Biomed Research Int.* 2014; 823058:1–8.

Eckard AR, Meissner EG, Singh I et al. Cardiovascular disease, statins, and HIV. J Infect Dis 2016; 214(suppl 2): S83–S92.

Elton PK, Carey RM, Aronow WS et al. ACC/AHA/AAAP/ABC/ACPM/AGS/ASH/ASPC/NMA/PCNA. Guideline for the Prevention, Detection, and Management of High Blood Pressure in Adults. *Hypertension.* 2018; 71: e13–e115.

Everett BM, Smith RJ, Hiatt WR. Reducing LDL with PCSK9 Inhibitors—The clinical benefit of lipid drugs. *N Engl J Med.* 2015; 373:1588–1591.

Fahme SA, Bloomfield GS, Peck R. Hypertension and HIV-Infected Adults. Novel Pathophysiologic mechanisms. *Hypertension 2018; 72:44–55.*

Fitch KV, Looby SE, Rope A, et al. Effects of aging and smoking on carotid intima-media thickness in HIV-infection. *AIDS.* 2013; 27(1):49–57.

Freiberg MS, McGinnis KA, Kraemer K, et al. The association between alcohol consumption and prevalent cardiovascular diseases among HIV-infected and HIV-uninfected men. *J Acquir Immune Defic Syndr.* 2010 Feb;53(2):247–253.

Freiberg MS, Chang CC, Kuller LH, et al. HIV infection and the risk of acute myocardial infarction. *JAMA Intern Med.* 2013 Apr 22;173(8):614–622.

Friis-Moller, Sabin, Weber, et al.; the Data Collection on Adverse Events of Anti-HIV Drugs (D: A:D) study group. *N Engl J Med.* 2003; 349:1993–2003.

Friis-Møller N, Thiébaut R, Reiss P, et al. Predicting the risk of cardiovascular disease in HIV-infected patients: the data collection on adverse effects of anti-HIV drugs study. Eur J Cardiovasc Prev Rehabil. 2010 Oct;17(5):491–501

Garg A, Sharma A, Krishnamoorthy P, et al. Role of niacin in current clinical practice: a systematic review. *Am J Med 2017; 130(2):173–187.*

Gatell JM, Assoumou L, Moyle G et al. Switching from a ritonavir-boosted protease inhibitor to a dolutegravir-based regimen for maintenance of viral suppression in patients with high cardiovascular risk. *AIDS* 2017; 31:2503–2514.

Gaziano JM, Brotons C, Coppolecchia R. Use of aspirin to reduce the risk of initial vascular events in patients at moderate risk of cardiovascular disease. (ARRIVE): a randomized double-blind placebo-controlled trial. *Lancet.* 2018 Aug 24. pii: S0140-6736(18)31924-X. doi: 10.1016/S0140-6736(18)31924-X. [Epub ahead of print].

Gerber JG, Kitch DW, Fichtenbaum CJ, et al. Fish oil and fenofibrate for the treatment of hypertriglyceridemia in HIV-infected subjects on antiretroviral therapy: Results of ACTG A5186. J *Acquir Immun Defic Syndr.* 2008; 47(4):459–466.

Giugliano RP, Keech A, Murphy SA. Clinical efficacy and safety of evolocumab in High-Risk patients receiving a statin: Secondary analysis of patients with Low LDL cholesterol levels and in those already receiving a maximal-potency statin in a randomized clinical Trial. *JAMA* 2017 Dec 1;2(12):1385–1391.

Go AS, Horberg M, Reynolds K, et al. HIV infection independently increases the risk of developing heart failure: The HIV HEART study. AIDS 2018: 22nd International AIDS Conference, Amsterdam, Netherlands, July 23–27, 2018. Abstract THAB0103.

Goff DC Jr, Lloyd-Jones DM, Bennett G, et al. 2013 ACC/AHA guideline on the assessment of cardiovascular risk: A report of the American College of Cardiology/American Heart Association Task Force on Practice Guidelines. *J Am Coll Cardiol.* 2014; 63:2935–2959.

Grandi AM, Nicolini E, Rizzi L, et al. Dyslipidemia in HIV-positive patients: A randomized, controlled, prospective study on ezetimibe + fenofibrate versus pravastatin monotherapy. *J Int AIDS Soc.* 2014; 17:19004.

Grinspoon S, Hoffman U. Cardiovascular disease imaging in HIV. Novel phenotypes and new targets for risk reduction. *Circ Cardiovasc Imaging* 2017;10: e006710.

Grundy SM, Stone NJ, Bailey AL et al. 2008 AHA/ACC guideline on the management of blood cholesterol: a report of the American College of Cardiology/ American Heart Association Task Force on Clinical Practice Guidelines. *Circulation* 2018; DOI:10.1161

Guirguis-Blake JM, Evans CV, Senger CA, et al. Aspirin for the primary prevention of cardiovascular events: A systematic evidence review for the U.S. Preventive Services Task Force. *Ann Intern Med* 2016. 164(12):804–813.

Guyton JR, Bays HE, Grundy SM et al. An assessment of the Statin Intolerance Panel: 2014 update. *J Clin Lipidol* 2014; 8(3 suppl): S72–S81.

Hatleberg CI, Ryom L, El-Sadr W, et al. Improvements over time in short-term mortality following myocardial infarction in HIV-positive individuals. AIDS. 2016 Jun 19;30(10):1583–1596

Hammersley D, Signy M. Ezetimibe: an update on its clinical usefulness in specific patient groups. *Ther Adv Chronic Dis.* 2017 Jan; 8(1): 4–11.

Hsue P, Hunt P, Schnell A., et al. Inflammation is associated with endothelial dysfunction among individuals with treated and suppressed HIV infection. CROI 2010, San Francisco, CA, 2010, Abstract #708.

Hunt PW. HIV and inflammation: Mechanisms and consequences. *Curr HIV/AIDS Rep.* 2012; 9(2):139–147.

Jakob T, Nordmann AJ, Schandelmaier S, et al. Fibrates for primary prevention of cardiovascular events. *Cochrane Database Syst Rev.* 2016; 16;11:CD009753.

Kazi DS, Moran AE, Coxson PG et al. Cost-effectiveness of PCSK9 Inhibitor Therapy in patients with heterozygous familial hypercholesterolemia or Atherosclerotic Cardiovascular Disease. *JAMA.* 2016; 16; 316(7):743–753.

Khambaty T, Stewart JC, Gupta SK, et al. Association Between Depressive Disorders and Incident Acute Myocardial Infarction in Human Immunodeficiency Virus-Infected Adults: Veterans Aging Cohort Study. *JAMA Cardiol.* 2016 Nov 1;1(8):929–937.

Klein DB, Leyden WA, Chao CR. No difference in the incidence of myocardial infarction for HIV+ and HIV− individuals in recent years. *Clin Infect Dis.* 2015; 60(8):1278–1285.

Klein DB, Marcus JL, Leyden WA, et al. Infection and immunodeficiency as risk factors for ischemic stroke. CROI 2014, Boston, MA, 2014. Abstract #741.

Krishnan S, Bosch RJ, Rodriguez B, et al. Correlates of inflammatory biomarkers one year after suppressive ART. CROI 2014, Boston, MA, March 3–6, 2014. Abstract 757.

Law M, Friis-Moller N, El-Sadr WA, et al. The use of the Framingham equation to predict myocardial infarctions in HIV-infected patients: Comparison with observed events in the D: A:D study. *HIV Med.* 2006; 7:218–230.

Lazzopina P, Mounsey A, Handler R. Does niacin decrease cardiovascular morbidity and mortality in CVD patients? *J Fam Pract* 2018; 67(5):314–319.

Leyes P, Martinez E, Larrousse M, et al. Effects of ezetimibe on cholesterol metabolism in HIV-infected patients with protease inhibitor-associated dyslipidemia: A single-arm intervention trial. *BMC Infect Dis.* 2014; 11:14:497.

Lloyd-Jones DM et al.2017 Focused update of the 2016 ACC Expert Consensus Decision pathway on the role of non-statin therapies for LDL-Cholesterol lowering in the management of atherosclerotic cardiovascular disease. *J Amer Coll Cardiol* 2017; 70(14):1785–1822.

Mallon P et al. Platelet function upon switching to TAF vs continuing ABC: a randomized sub study. 25th CROI Boston, abstract # 80, 2018.

Marconi VC, Duncan MS, So-Armah K. et al. Bilirubin Is Inversely Associated with Cardiovascular Disease among HIV-Positive and HIV-Negative Individuals in VACS (Veterans Aging Cohort Study). *J Am Heart Assoc.* 2018 May 2; 7(10). e007792.

Martinez E, Larrousse M, Llibre JM, et al. Substitution of raltegravir for ritonavir-boosted protease inhibitors in HIV-infected patients: The SPIRAL study. *AIDS.* 2010; 24(11):1697–1707.

McComsey GA, Kitch D, Daar ES, et al. Inflammation markers after randomization to abacavir/lamivudine or tenofovir/emtricitabine with efavirenz or atazanavir/ritonavir. *AIDS.* 2012 Jul 17; 26(11):1371–8573.

McComsey GA, Jiang Y, Erlandson KM, et al. Rosuvastatin improves hip bone mineral density but worsens insulin resistance. CROI 2014, Boston, MA, March 3–6, 2014. Abstract 134.

Medical Letter on Drugs and Therapeutics. Drugs for Tobacco Dependence. *JAMA* 2018; 320(9):926–927.

Medina-Torne S, Ganesan A, Barahona I, et al. Hypertension is common among HIV-infected persons, but not associated with HAART. *J Int Assoc Physicians AIDS Care (Chic).* 2012 Jan–Feb; 11(1):20–25.

Mercie P, Arsandaux J, Katalama C et al. Efficacy and safety of varenicline for smoking cessation in people living with HIV I France. (ANRS 144 Inter-ACTIV): a randomized controlled phase 3 clinical trial. *Lancet HIV* 2018; 5(3):126–135.

Metkus TS, Brown T, Budoff M, et al. HIV infection is associated with an increased prevalence of coronary noncalcified plaque among participants with a coronary artery calcium score of zero: Multicenter AIDS Cohort Study (MACS). *HIV Med.* 2015 Nov;16(10):635–639.

Monforte A, Reiss P, Ryom L, et al. Atazanavir is not associated with an increased risk of cardio- or cerebrovascular disease events. *AIDS.* 2013 Jan 28; 27(3):407–415.

Morgello S, Mahboob R, Yakoushina T, et al. Autopsy findings in human immunodeficiency virus-infected populations over 2 decades. *Arch Path Lab Med.* 2002; 126:182–190.

Mosepele, M., Molefe-Baikai, O.J., Grinspoon, S.K. et al. Benefits and Risks of Statin Therapy in the HIV-Infected Population. *Curr Infect Dis Rep* (2018) 20: 20. https://doi.org/10.1007/s11908-018-0628-7

Navarese EP, Buffon A, Andreotti F, et al. Meta-analysis of the impact of different types and doses of statins on new-onset diabetes mellitus. *Am J Cardiol* 2013; 111(8):1123–1130.

NICE (2016) Ezetimibe for treating primary heterozygous familial and non-familial hypercholesterolemia. Guide TA385. http://nice.org.uk/guidance.

O'Brien S, Montenont E, Hu L, et al. Aspirin attenuates platelet activation and immune activation in HIV-1-infected subjects on antiretroviral therapy: A pilot study. *J Acquir Immune Defic Syndr.* 2013 Jul 1; 63(3):280–288.

Olaiya O, Weiser J, Zhou W et al. Hypertension among persons living with HIV in medical care in the United States—Medical Monitoring Project 2013-2014. *Open Forum Infectious Diseases*, Volume 5, Issue 3, 1 March 2018, ofy028, https://doi.org/10.1093/ofid/ofy028 Accessed August 26, 2018. https://academic.oup.com/ofid

Oliveira JM, Rondo PH, Lima LR et al. Effects of low dose fish oil on inflammatory markers of Brazilian HIV-infected adults on antiretroviral therapy: A randomized parallel. Placebo-controlled trial. *Nutrients* 2015; 7(8):6520–6528.

Paikin JS, Eikelboom JW. Cardiology patient page: Aspirin. *Circulation.* 2012 Mar 13; 125(10): e439–e442.

Paisible AL, Chang CH, So-Armah KA, et al. HIV infection, cardiovascular disease risk factor profile, and risk for acute myocardial infarction. *J AIDS.* 2015; 68:209–216.

Palella F, et al. NA-ACCORD: Recent abacavir use and risk of MI. *CROI 2015, Seattle, WA, Abstract #749 LB.*

Palella FJ Jr, Fisher M, Tebas P, et al. Simplification to rilpivirine/emtricitabine/tenofovir disoproxil fumarate from ritonavir-boosted protease inhibitor antiretroviral therapy in a randomized trial of HIV-1 RNA-suppressed participants. *AIDS.* 2014 Jan 28; 28(3):335–344

Panel on Antiretroviral Guidelines for Adults and Adolescents. Guidelines for the Use of Antiretroviral Agents in Adults and Adolescents Living with HIV. Department of Health and Human Services. Available at http://www.aidsinfo.nih.gov/ContentFiles/AdultandAdolescentGL.pdf. Accessed March 20, 2019.

Petoumenos K, Worm S, Reiss P, et al.; DAD Study Group. Rates of cardiovascular disease following smoking cessation in patients with HIV infection: Results from the D:A:D study. *HIV Med.* 2011 Aug; 12(7):412–421.

Pett SL, Amin J, Horban A et al. Week 96 results of the randomized, multicenter Maraviroc Switch (MARCH) Study. *HIV Medicine* 2018; 19:65–71.

Pool ER, Dogar O, Lindsay RP. Et al. Interventions for tobacco use cessation in people living with HIV and IADS. *Cochrane Database Syst Rev.* 2016; 13(6): CD011120.

Post WS, et al. Associations between HIV infection and subclinical coronary atherosclerosis. *Ann Intern Med.* 2014; 160:458–467.

Rasmussen LD, May MT, Kronborg G, et al. Time trends for risk of severe age-related diseases in individuals with and without HIV infection in Denmark: A nationwide population-based cohort study. *Lancet HIV.* 2015; 2(7):e288–e298.

Regan S, Meigs JB, Massaro J, et al. Evaluation of the ACC/AHA CVD risk prediction algorithm among HIV-infected patients. CROI 2015, Seattle, WA, Abstract # 751.

Remick J, et al. Heart failure in patients with human immunodeficiency virus infection: epidemiology, pathophysiology, treatment, and future research. *Circulation.* 2014 Apr 29;129(17):1781–1789.

Ridker PM, Pradhan A, MacFadyen JG, et al. Cardiovascular benefits and diabetes risks of statin therapy in primary prevention: An analysis from the JUPITER trial. *Lancet.* 2012 Aug 11; 380(9841):565–571.

Rogers TS, Seehusen DA. Omega-3 fatty acids and cardiovascular disease. *Amer Fam Phys* 2018; 97(9):562–564.

Rotger M, Glass TR, Junier T, et al. Contribution of genetic background, traditional risk factors, and HIV-related factors to coronary artery disease events in HIV-positive persons. *Clin Infect Dis.* 2013; 57:112–121.

Ryom L, Lundgren JD, Reiss P, et al. Relationship between confirmed eGFR and cardiovascular disease in HIV-positive persons. *CROI 2015, Seattle WA,* Abstract # 742.

Ryom L. Lundgren JD, El-Sadr W et al. Cardiovascular disease and use of contemporary protease inhibitors: The D:A:D international prospective multicohort study. *Lancet HIV,* 2018;6: e291–e300.

Saag MS, Benson CA, MD; Gandhi RT, et al. Antiretroviral Drugs for Treatment and Prevention of HIV Infection in Adults 2018 Recommendations of the International Antiviral Society–USA Panel. *JAMA.* 2018; 320(4):379–396.

Sabatine MS, Giugliano RP, Keech AC et al. Evolocumab and clinical outcomes in patients with cardiovascular disease. *N Engl J Med* 2017; 376:1713–1722.

Sabin C, Reiss P, Ryom L, et al. Is there continued evidence for an association between abacavir and myocardial infarction risk? CROI 2014, Boston, MA, Abstract #747.

Saeedi R, Johns K, Frohlich J, et al. Lipid-lowering efficacy and safety of ezetimibe combined with rosuvastatin compared with titrating rosuvastatin monotherapy in HIV-positive patients. *Lipids Health Dis.* 2015; 14:57.

Sax PC. Zolopa A, Eleon R. Tenofovir alafenamide vs. tenofovir disoproxil fumarate in single tablet regimens for initial HIV-1 therapy: A randomized phase 2 study. *J Acquir Immune Defic Syndr.* 2014; 67(1):52–58.

Shah ASV, Stelze D, Lee KK et al. Global burden of atherosclerotic vascular disease in people living with HIV: Systematic review and meta-analysis. *Circulation* 2018; 138:1100–1112.

Shahreyar M, Salem SA, Nayyar M. Hyperlipidemia: Management with proprotein convertase Subtilisin/Kexin Type 9 (PCSK9) Inhibitors. *J Am Board Fam Med.* 2018; 31(4):628–634.

Sigel K, Makinson A, Thaler J. Lung cancer in persons with HV. *Curr Opin HIV AIDS* 2017; 12(1):31–38.

Sing S, Willig JH, Mugavero MJ, et al. Comparative efficacy and toxicity among statins in HIV-infected patients. *Clin Infect Dis.* 2011; 52(3):387–395.

Smit M, van Zoest RA, Nichols BE, et al. Cardiovascular Disease Prevention Policy in Human Immunodeficiency Virus: Recommendations from a Modeling Study. *Clin Infect Dis.* 2018 Feb 10;66(5):743–750.

Strategies for Management of Antiretroviral Therapy (SMART) Study Group. CD4$^+$ count-guided interruption of antiretroviral therapy. *N Engl J Med.* 2006; 355:2283–2296.

Strategies for Management of Antiretroviral Therapy (SMART)/INSIGHT/D:A:D Study Groups. Use of nucleoside reverse transcriptase inhibitors and risk of myocardial infarction in HIV-infected patients. *AIDS.* 2008; 22: F17–F24.

Subramanian S, Tawakol A, Burdo TH, et al. Arterial Inflammation in patients with HIV. *JAMA. 2012; 308:379–386.*

Suchindran S, Regan S, Meigs JB, et al. Aspirin use for primary and secondary prevention in human immunodeficiency virus (HIV)-infected and HIV-uninfected patients. *Open Forum Infect Dis.* 2014 Oct 20; 1(3): ofu076.

Swanson B, Keithley J, Baum L, et al. Effects of Fish Oil on HIV-Related Inflammation and Markers of Immunosenescence: A Randomized Clinical Trial. *J Altern Complement Med.* 2018 Jul; 24(7):709–716.

Tawakol A, Lo J, Zanni MV, et al. Increased arterial inflammation relates to high-risk coronary plaque morphology in HIV-infected patients. *J Acquir Immune Defic Syndr.* 2014; 66(2):164–171.

Thiebaut R, El-Sadr W, Friis-Moller N, et al.; the D:A:D Study Group. Predictors of hypertension and changes in blood pressure in HIV-infected patients. *Antiviral Ther.* 2005; 10:811–823.

Thompson-Paul A, et al. Evaluation of the ACC/AHA CVD risk prediction algorithm among HIV-infected patients. *CROI* 2015, Seattle, WA, Abstract # 747.

Torriani FJ, Komarow L, Parker RA, et al. Endothelial function in human immunodeficiency virus-infected antiretroviral-naive subjects before and after starting potent antiretroviral therapy: The ACTG (AIDS Clinical Trials Group) Study 5152s. *J Am Coll Cardiol.* 2008; 52(7):569–576.

Triant V, Meig J, Grinspoon S. Association of C-reactive protein and HIV infection with acute myocardial infarction. *J Acquir Immune Defic Syndr.* 2009; 51(3):268–273.

Triant V, Regan S, Lee H, et al. Association of immunologic and virologic factors with myocardial infarction rates in the U.S. health care system. *J Acquir Immune Defic Syndr.* 2010; 55(5):615–619.

Triant V, Perez J, Regan S et al. Cardiovascular risk prediction functions underestimate risk in HIV infection. *Circulation* 2018; 137(21):2203–2214.

Truong C. Low-dose acetylsalicylic acid for the primary prevention of cardiovascular disease: Do not misinterpret the recommendations. *Can Fam Phys.* 2015; 61(11):971–972.

Tungsiripat M, Kitch D, Glesby MJ, et al. A pilot study to determine the impact on dyslipidemia of adding tenofovir to stable background antiretroviral therapy: ACTG 5206. *AIDS.* 2010 Jul 17; 24(11):1781–1784.

van Zoest RA, van den Born BH, Reiss P. Hypertension in people living with HIV. *Curr Opin HIV AIDS.* 2017; 12(6):513–522.

Vancampfort D, Mugisha J, Richards J, et al. Physical activity correlates in people living with HIV/AIDS: systematic review of 45 studies. *Disabil Rehabil.* 2018; 40(14):1618–1629.

Van Lelyveld SF, Gras L, Kesselring A, et al. ATHENA national observational cohort study: Long-term complications in patients with poor immunological recovery despite virological successful HAART in Dutch ATHENA cohort. *AIDS.* 2012; 26(4):465–474.

Vieira AD, Silveira GR. Effectiveness of n-3 fatty acids in the treatment of hypertriglyceridemia in HIV/AIDS patients: a meta-analysis. *Cien Saude Colet.* 2017; 22(8):2659–2669.

Walker J, Hutchinson P, Ge J et al. Aspirin: 120 Years of Innovation. A report from the 2017 Scientific Conference of the IAF. 2017, Charité, Berlin. *Ecancermedicalscience* 2018; 20:12:813.

Wall HK, Ritchey MD, Gillespie C, et al. *Vital Signs*: Prevalence of Key Cardiovascular Disease Risk Factors for Million Hearts 2022—United States, 2011–2016. *MMWR Morb Mortal Wkly Rep* 2018; 67:983–991.

Whelton PK, Carey RM, Aronow WS, et al. 2017 ACC/AHA/AAPA/ABC/ACPM/AGS/APhA/ASH/ASPC/NMA/PCNA Guideline for the Prevention, Detection, Evaluation, and Management of High Blood Pressure in Adults: Executive Summary: A Report of the American College of Cardiology/American Heart Association Task Force on Clinical Practice Guidelines. *Circulation* 2018; 138(17): e426–e483.

White JR, Chang CC, So-Armah KA et al. Depression and HIV infection are risk factors for incident heart failure among veterans: VACS. *Circulation* 2015;132(17):1630–1638.

Whitlock EP, Burda BU, Williams SB, et al. Bleeding Risks with Aspirin Use for Primary Prevention in Adults: A Systematic Review for the U.S. Preventive Services Task Force. *Ann Intern Med.* 2016; 164(12):826–835.

Wohl DA, Tien HC, Busby M, et al. Randomized study of the safety and efficacy of fish oil (omega-3 fatty acid) supplementation with dietary and exercise counseling for the treatment of antiretroviral therapy-associated hypertriglyceridemia. *Clin Infect Dis.* 2005; 41(10):1498–1504.

Wohl D, Waters D, Simpson R et al. Ezetimibe alone reduces low-density lipoprotein cholesterol in HIV-infected patients receiving combination antiretroviral therapy. *Clin Infect Dis* 2008; 47:1105–1108.

Worm S, Sabin C, Weber R, et al.; D:A:D Study Group. Risk of myocardial infarction in patients with HIV infection exposed to specific individual antiretroviral drugs from 3 major drug classes. *J Infect Dis.* 2010; 201:318–330.

Yusuf S, Hawken S, Ounpuu S et al. Effect of potentially modifiable risk factors associated with myocardial infarction in 52 countries (The INTERHEART Study): case-control study. *Lancet* 2004; 364:937–952.

Young J, Xiao Y, Moodier EE, et al. Effect of cumulating exposure to abacavir on the risk of cardiovascular disease events in patients from the Swiss HIV Cohort Study. *J AIDS.* 2015; 69(4): 413–421.

43.

RENAL COMPLICATIONS

Steven Menez, Derek M. Fine, and Sana Waheed

NEPHROPATHY

LEARNING OBJECTIVE

Discuss the epidemiology, risk factors, broad pathologic spectrum, and current therapeutic interventions for HIV-related renal disease.

WHAT'S NEW?

- The renal effect of integrase inhibitors, specifically dolutegravir and the newest integrase inhibitor bictegravir, have been further elucidated.

- Further data have been obtained regarding cystatin-C–based kidney function and HIV.

RISK FACTORS

- With improved life expectancy and antiretroviral therapy (ART)-related metabolic abnormalities, chronic kidney disease has become a significant comorbidity in HIV-positive patients.

- Risk factors for kidney disease include African American race, CD4⁺ T cell counts of less than 200 cells/mm³, HIV RNA levels of greater than 10,000 copies/mL, family history of chronic kidney disease (CKD), diabetes mellitus, hypertension, and hepatitis C coinfection.

- Compared to the general population, patients with AIDS have a 16-fold higher incidence of requiring renal replacement therapy.

PATHOLOGIC SPECTRUM OF DISEASE

Although HIV-associated nephropathy (HIVAN) used to be the predominant form of renal involvement in HIV patients, this pattern has changed and other pathologies, such as immune complex disease, diabetic glomerulosclerosis, and classic focal segmental glomerulosclerosis (vs. the collapsing form of focal segmental glomerulosclerosis [FSGS] seen in HIVAN) are being seen more frequently in persons with HIV-disease.

Acute kidney injury is nearly twice as common in HIV-positive patients compared to patients without HIV, and it is associated with a sixfold increase in mortality.

PATHOGENESIS

The *ApoL1* gene, which encodes a factor to lyse *Trypanosoma brucei*, is the key susceptibility allele in HIVAN. Two HIV genes, *nef* and *vpr*, appear to contribute to podocyte dysregulation in HIVAN.

TREATMENT

- ART and angiotensin inhibition slow progression of renal disease.

- Corticosteroids may have benefit in glomerular diseases, but prospective trials are lacking.

- Renal transplantation in HIV-positive patients appears to have good outcomes but requires intensive monitoring.

Renal disease is a major cause of mortality from non–AIDS-related conditions in HIV-positive patients, along with malignancy and cardiovascular and liver disease (Mocroft, 2010). Renal pathology in HIV patients was originally reported in 1984 and was called "acquired immune deficiency syndrome (AIDS) nephropathy." The histopathology on kidney biopsy showed a collapsing type of focal and segmental glomerulosclerosis, and the clinical presentation was that of proteinuria, usually nephrotic, and rapid progression to end-stage renal disease (ESRD) (Rao, 1984). Subsequently, HIVAN became more commonly recognized as a major cause of renal disease in HIV-positive patients. In the United States, the incidence of HIVAN peaked in the mid-1990s and dropped significantly with the introduction of highly active antiretroviral therapy (HAART) by the late 1990s (Ross, 2002). Most recent data show the annual incidence of ESRD to be about 800–900 cases per year (Cohen, 2017).

EPIDEMIOLOGY

Although the incidence of HIVAN is declining, the overall prevalence of kidney disease in HIV-1–positive individuals is increasing as a result of improved patient survival (Mocroft, 2003). Consequently, the spectrum of kidney disease is being driven by metabolic risk factors including as obesity, diabetes, hypertension, the use of medications with nephrotoxic potential, and aging of the HIV-positive population (Waheed, 2014).

Despite widespread use of ART, HIV patients remain at a higher risk of renal insufficiency, cardiovascular disease, and overall mortality than matched cohorts of HIV-negative people (Kalayjian, 2011; Post, 2009). Up to 30% of patients infected with HIV are at risk of developing proteinuria—a key marker of renal disease. Moreover, cross-sectional cohorts from Europe, Asia, and North America have demonstrated high rates of chronic kidney disease (CKD) in HIV-positive patients, with 5.5% of HIV patients having stages 3–5 CKD (Post, 2009). In a large US cohort of predominantly African American HIV-positive patients with CKD, 35% progressed to ESRD (Lucas, 2008). Based on another large sample of US veterans, the incidence rate of ESRD in African Americans with HIV is even higher than that of patients with diabetes (incidence rates per 1,000 person-years [py]: 71.1 for HIV, 59.9 for diabetes mellitus, and 27.9 for patients with neither HIV nor diabetes) (Choi, 2007). Compared to the general population, patients with AIDS have a 16-fold higher risk of requiring renal replacement therapy (Lucas, 2007).

RISK FACTORS FOR NEPHROPATHY

Risk factors for the development of kidney disease in patients with HIV include African American race, diabetes mellitus, hypertension, hepatitis C coinfection, cardiovascular disease, and family history of CKD (Mocroft, 2015; Naicker, 2010).

Moreover, patients with advanced untreated HIV infection with $CD4^+$ T cell counts of less than 200 cells/mm^3 and viral load of more than 30,000 copies/mL are at high risk for developing HIVAN (Bige, 2012; Lescure, 2012).

GENETIC PREDISPOSITION

The major genetic risk factor for developing HIVAN and non-HIVAN FSGS in patients of African descent is the presence of polymorphisms in the apolipoprotein 1 (*APOL1*) gene, which is also located on chromosome 22 (Bige, 2012; Genovese, 2010; Lescure, 2012; Tzur, 2010). Two *APOL1* risk alleles, G1 and G2, are associated with the increased susceptibility for the development of HIVAN (Genovese, 2010; Papeta, 2011). The association of *APOL1* genetic variation in FSGS and HIVAN has been studied by Kopp and

colleagues (Kopp, 2011). Individuals carrying the high-risk alleles had a 29-fold greater risk of developing HIVAN and had a 17-fold higher risk of developing FSGS. In patients who carry the two *APOL1* risk alleles, this alone can explain 35% of cases of HIVAN and 18% of FSGS cases (Kopp, 2011). Indeed, *APOL1* homozygosity, present in 13% of the general African American population, was noted in more than 60% of African Americans with HIVAN and non-HIVAN FSGS (Kopp, 2011). Recently, a G3 haplotype has been identified, but further studies are needed to understand its importance in the pathogenesis of HIVAN (Ko, 2013). *ApoL1* encodes a serum factor that lyses *Trypanosoma brucei*. Thus, selective mutations in Africans to counter an endemic parasite may have contributed to the current rates of HIVAN and FSGS in African American populations.

PATHOGENESIS

In animal models, HIV gene expression within kidney cells is required for the development of HIVAN (Bruggeman, 1997). Even in HIVAN patients with undetectable plasma HIV-RNA levels, proviral DNA is found in the renal tissue of all patients (Izzedine, 2011). This implies that the kidney acts as a separate compartment from blood, allowing HIV to replicate in the kidney even in patients who achieve viral suppression in their plasma with treatment (Medapalli, 2011). It has been shown that the expression of nonstructural gene products of HIV, negative effector (*nef*) and viral protein r (*vpr*), in a murine model results in HIVAN (Zuo, 2006). HIV induces apoptosis of cells in addition to causing cytopathic effects. These effects, in combination with cytokine release, are thought to play a role in the development of HIVAN (Kimmel, 2003).

Studies have also shown that HIV infection downregulates expression of microRNAs in human podocytes (Cheng, 2013). HIV-infected podocytes reenter the cell cycle, as evidenced by an increased expression of markers of proliferation and decreased expression of cyclin-dependent kinase inhibitors (Barisoni, 1999). These cells have increased vascular endothelial growth factor expression and persistent activation of NF-κB, which also contributes to podocyte proliferation (Korgaonkar, 2008).

MARKERS OF RENAL INJURY

Markers of renal injury include elevated serum creatinine, proteinuria, glycosuria, and an increased fractional excretion of uric acid (Kalayjian, 2011). Risk factors for proteinuria include older age, African American race, insulin resistance, hypertension, and a low $CD4^+$ T cell count (Post, 2009). The presence of albuminuria and overt proteinuria is associated with increased cardiovascular morbidity and mortality in this population (George, 2010; Wyatt, 2011). In a study of HIV patients with albuminuria, the 5-year mortality rate was 20% in patients with albuminuria and 48% in patients with a glomerular filtration rate (GFR) of less than 60 mL/min and albuminuria (Choi, 2010).

Like the general population, kidney damage in patients with HIV is assessed by using creatinine-based estimates of glomerular filtration rate (eGFR) with the Cockroft–Gault equation, Modification of Diet in Renal Disease (MDRD), and CKD Epidemiology Collaboration (CKD-EPI) equation, but none of these estimates has been systematically validated in patients with HIV.

Cystatin C is an alternative marker of eGFR that does not depend on muscle mass and is more sensitive for kidney damage than creatinine-based formulas. In a cross-sectional study comparing 250 HIV-positive patients in the Nutrition for Healthy Living cohort compared to more than 2,628 participants from the NHANES cohort, cystatin-C based measurement of eGFR compared to standard creatinine-based measures led to a higher prevalence of kidney disease diagnosis (Jones, 2008). The authors partly attribute this to the underestimation of eGFR with Cr in the HIV population due to malnutrition, and thus cystatin C may be a better marker. However, it has been suggested that cystatin C levels are higher with active HIV replication, and this can overestimate eGFR, thus limiting its usefulness in HIV patients (Mauss, 2008). In addition, it appears that cystatin C-based eGFR is affected by HIV treatment factors and markers of T cell activation (Bhasin, 2013). Recently, Dragović and colleagues have shown that cystatin C may be elevated in HIV-positive patients with metabolic syndrome (Dragović, 2018). Out of 89 HIV-positive patients, the 33 individuals with metabolic syndrome had a statistically significantly higher cystatin C level compared to those without. Notably, there were no significant differences with respect to CD4 level, time on ART, smoking status, or HBV/HCV status. Currently, cystatin C is not recommended as a screening or diagnostic tool in clinical practice.

PATHOLOGIC SPECTRUM OF DISEASE

HIV-positive patients can develop multiple forms of renal involvement, including acute kidney injury (AKI), HIVAN, immune complex disease (HIVICK), thrombotic microangiopathy (TMA), and medication-induced nephrotoxicity (see Box 43.1) (Cohen, 2009). Therefore, a renal biopsy is indicated in most HIV patients with kidney disease to determine the underlying renal pathology because treatment strategies often differ based on kidney biopsy findings (Fine, 2008).

Acute Kidney Injury

Poor nutritional state of patients, dehydration, polypharmacy, and the risk of opportunistic infections in HIV patients predisposes them to development of AKI, with incidence rates as high as 5.9 per 100 pys (Franceschini, 2005). In a retrospective study of HIV-infected hospitalized patients, patients had an increased incidence of AKI in both the pre-HAART era (odds ratio [OR], 4.6) and the post-HAART era (OR, 2.8) (Franceschini, 2005). Higher incidence of AKI is also

---

Box 43.1 PATHOLOGIC SPECTRUM OF KIDNEY DISEASE IN HIV PATIENTS

Glomerular diseases:

- HIVAN; collapsing FSGC (specifically HIV-induced)
- HIVICK (HIV-associated immune complex disease)
- IgA nephropathy
- Membranoproliferative glomerulonephritis
- Membranous nephropathy
- Lupus-like glomerulonephritis
- Thrombotic microangiopathy[a]
- Classic FSGS (primary or secondary)
- Hypertensive nephrosclerosis
- Diabetic nephropathy
- Membranous glomerulopathy
- Membranoproliferative glomerulonephritis (frequently hepatitis C-related)
- Amyloidosis
- Minimal change disease
- Fibrillary glomerulonephritis

Tubular diseases:

- Acute tubular necrosis
- Drug-related tubular dysfunction
- Nephrolithiasis (primary or drug-related)
- Tumor lysis syndrome
- Obstruction

Interstitial diseases

- Interstitial nephritis
- Pyelonephritis

---

associated with advanced age, diabetes mellitus, CKD, acute or chronic liver failure, CD4+ T cell counts of less than 200 cells/mm^3, HIV-1 RNA levels of more than 10,000 copies/mL, and hepatitis coinfection (Franceschini, 2005; Wyatt, 2006). Common causes of AKI in HIV-1-positive patients are similar to those in HIV-negative individuals, with pre-renal states and acute tubular necrosis accounting for 39% and 37% of cases, respectively (Franceschini, 2005).

Rare causes of AKI in HIV patients include obstruction from lymphadenopathy related to malignancy, tumor lysis syndrome, and polyoma virus-induced renal dysfunction. Regardless of the etiology, AKI is associated with a sixfold increase in overall mortality in HIV patients (Kalim, 2008).

HIV-Associated Nephropathy

HIVAN is the most aggressive form of kidney disease associated with HIV infection and generally presents in patients with advanced HIV infection who exhibit rapidly declining GFR and significant proteinuria (Berliner, 2008). The incidence of HIVAN declined after the widespread use of ART, but it still remains a leading cause of ESRD in young African American patients. HIVAN is pathologically characterized by a collapsing form of focal and segmental sclerosis, prominent tubular microcysts, and tubulointerstitial inflammation (D'Agati, 1989).

HIV-Associated Immune Complex Kidney Disease

Various immune complex kidney diseases have been reported in patients with HIV-1 infection, such as postinfectious glomerulonephritis, membranoproliferative glomerulonephritis, membranous nephropathy, immunoglobulin A nephropathy, and lupus-like glomerulonephritis, collectively referred to as HIVICK (Balow, 2005; Kalayjian, 2011). Patients with HIVICK tend to have a better prognosis with a lower incidence of ESRD compared to patients with HIVAN (Foy, 2013).

Thrombotic Microangiopathy

TMA is a rare complication of HIV-1 infection, with an incidence of isolated renal TMA as low as 0.3% (Becker, 2004). It manifests as thrombocytopenia, microangiopathic hemolytic anemia, with or without fever and neurological deficits. Opportunistic infections, high plasma HIV viral load, low CD4 counts, and various drugs used in advanced disease can all contribute to development of TMA (Bachmeyer, 1995).

TREATMENT

Recommendations regarding therapy are limited due to the lack of randomized prospective controlled trials. Most of the treatment options, including supportive care, ART, inhibition of renin–angiotensin–aldosterone system (ACE inhibitors), and corticosteroids, are based on retrospective studies and nonrandomized trials.

Antiretroviral Therapy

Multiple observational studies have supported the benefit of ART in slowing the progression or reversing renal disease in patients with HIVAN (Elewa, 2011). In a large Johns Hopkins Clinic cohort of 4,000 HIV-positive patients, ART was associated with a 60% risk reduction for HIVAN, with 6.8 and 26.4 episodes per 1,000 pys in AIDS patients who did or did not receive ART, respectively. In addition, no patients developed HIVAN when ART was initiated before the development of AIDS (Lucas, 2004).

Consistent evidence demonstrates preservation of renal function with ART in HIV patient populations. In the Strategies for Management of Antiretroviral Therapy (SMART) group study,

continuous therapy versus episodic use of ART was evaluated in 5,472 patients with $CD4^+$ T cell counts of more than 350 cells/μL. In the continuous use group, fewer patients developed renal disease compared to the episodic use group (0.2 vs. 0.1 events/100 pys) (Strategies for Management [SMART], 2006). In addition, in a prospective, multicenter cohort involving 1,776 HIV patients, ART intervention in patients with CKD stage 2 or greater and low $CD4^+$ T cell counts led to an average increase of 9.2 mL/min in GFR at a median follow-up of 160 weeks. These results were magnified in those with a lower baseline GFR and greater decrease in viral load (Longenecker, 2009). Similar results have been demonstrated by other large African studies (Peters, 2008; Reid, 2008).

Angiotensin II Blockade

Multiple randomized controlled trials in CKD patients have demonstrated the efficacy of ACE inhibitors and angiotensin receptor blockers in slowing the progression of kidney disease, decreasing proteinuria, and decreasing the incidence of cardiovascular disease and death (Casas, 2005; Jafar, 2003). However, data regarding their use in HIV population are scarce. An older study of 18 patients with biopsy-proven HIVAN, of whom 9 patients treated with captopril, had an enhanced renal survival compared to controls (mean renal survival, 156 ± 71 vs. 37 ± 5 days; $p < 0.002$) (Kimmel, 1996). In a study of 44 consecutive patients with biopsy-proven HIVAN, patients treated with ACE inhibition had significantly less progression to ESRD compared to those without therapy (14% vs. 100% at 5 years) (Wei, 2003). Based on these results, angiotensin II blockade is recommended for most CKD and glomerular diseases in HIV patients in the absence of contraindications.

Corticosteroids

In patients with HIVAN, tubulointerstitial inflammation improves after treatment with steroids (Briggs, 1996). However, there are no randomized clinical trials to support steroid use in this population. In a retrospective cohort study of 21 patients, of which 13 received corticosteroids, the relative risk for progressive renal failure with corticosteroid treatment at 3 months was 0.20 ($p < 0.05$) (Eustace, 2000). This association remained significant despite adjustment in separate logistical regression analyses for baseline creatinine; 24-hour proteinuria; $CD4^+$ count; and history of intravenous drug use, hepatitis B, and hepatitis C coinfection (Eustace, 2000). However, there were 18 infections in corticosteroid-treated patients compared to 8 in the non–corticosteroid-treated group. In addition, steroid use has been associated with an increased risk of avascular necrosis of the femoral head (Elewa, 2011). Larger studies are needed to further elucidate the value of steroids in patients with HIV-related kidney disease, although some experts recommend a short course of corticosteroid therapy in those with a new diagnosis of HIVAN (Atta, 2008; Fine, 2008). Risks of further immunosuppression should always be weighed against the benefits when steroids are use in persons with HIV-disease.

Novel Therapies

In animal models, all-*trans*-retinoic acid has been shown to reverse the *nef*-induced signaling pathway with improvement in proteinuria and glomerulosclerosis (Ratnam, 2011). Moreover, when phosphodiesterase inhibitors are used in combination, they increase the renal protective effect of retinoids in animal models (Zhong, 2012). However, further studies are needed before their use can be recommended. There are some data to support the use of plasma exchange or eculizumab in patients with TMA (Cohen, 2017).

Renal Replacement Therapy (Dialysis)

Overall survival of HIV patients on dialysis historically was worse compared to that of the general ESRD population, potentially due to increased risk of infections (Atta, 2007). Older age, lower serum albumin level, lower CD4$^+$ T cell count, and lack of ART have all been associated with poor survival in HIV-1–positive patients undergoing hemodialysis or peritoneal dialysis (Kimmel, 1993). It appears that the incidence of ESRD has plateaued, but the prevalence of patients with HIV undergoing dialysis in the United States has increased (Cohen, 2017). Survival among these patients receiving dialysis is now noted to be similar to persons without HIV disease (Razzak, 2015).

Renal Transplantation

Renal transplantation was previously contraindicated in HIV patients due to the concern of immunosuppressive agents in patients with a dysregulated immune system. However, there is increasing data showing that renal transplantation is both safe and effective in patients with HIV (Qiu, 2006; Roland, 2008; van Maarseveen, 2012). In a prospective study of 150 patients, overall patient survival at 1 and 3 years was 95% and 88%, respectively, with allograft survival of 90% and 74%, respectively. The rate of rejection was higher in these patients, with 1- and 3-year rejection rates of 31% and 41%, respectively, compared to a 1-year rejection rate of 12% as reported by the US Scientific Registry of Transplant Recipients for the general population (Stock, 2010).

A single-center study examined the transplant outcomes of 16 patients with HIV infection and a renal transplant. Despite higher rates of acute rejection at 1 and 3 years (18% and 27%, respectively), 1- and 3-year graft survival rates were 100% and 81%, respectively (Waheed, 2015). Initially, renal transplantation in HIV patients was performed without induction therapy. However, the use of antithymocyte globulin as induction therapy is associated with a 2.6-fold lower risk of rejection, as shown in a study of 516 HIV-positive patients (Locke, 2014). Many of the agents used in posttransplantation immunosuppression have antiretroviral properties. Mycophenolate mofetil has virostatic properties through depletion of guanosine nucleosides necessary for the viral life cycle. Calcineurin inhibitors (tacrolimus and cyclosporine) selectively inhibit infected cell growth, and sirolimus disrupts infective viral replication through suppression of antigen-presenting cell function.

Patients considered eligible for renal transplant should have a CD4$^+$ T cell count great than 200/mm^3 and an undetectable viral load while on a stable ART regimen. There is concern for drug–drug interactions between some antiretroviral drugs and immunosuppressive agents. This is especially true for ritonavir or cobicistat-boosted protease inhibitors (PI) that are metabolized through the cytochrome P450 system. Thus, although kidney transplantation appears to be effective, it requires intensive monitoring of drug levels and rejection risk. The HIV Organ Policy Equity Act that allows for the transplantation of kidneys and other organs from HIV-infected donors to HIV-positive recipients should increase the donor pool and may make transplant a viable option for a greater number of patients with ESRD (Cohen, 2017).

RECOMMENDED READING

Muller E, Barday Z, Mendelson M, Kahn D. HIV-positive-to-HIV-positive kidney transplantations: results at 3 to 5 years. *N Engl J Med.* 2015;372:613–620.

ANTIRETROVIRAL THERAPY-RELATED RENAL COMPLICATIONS

LEARNING OBJECTIVE

Discuss renal complications of antiretroviral therapy.

WHAT'S NEW?

Tenofovir alafenamide fumarate (TAF), approved by the recently US Food and Drug Administration (FDA) in 2015, is a prodrug of tenofovir disoproxil fumarate (TDF) and has shown effective anti–HIV-1 activity with fewer renal side effects in clinical trials.

KEY POINTS

- ART can contribute to renal toxicities in HIV-positive patients.

- TDF may cause AKI, CKD, and/or proximal tubular dysfunction.

- Indinavir, atazanavir, and other PIs can cause nephrolithiasis.

- Cobicistat and dolutegravir can increase serum creatinine by inhibiting its tubular secretion, but they do not change the actual GFR.

PRESENTATION

Elevation in serum creatinine. Proximal tubular renal dysfunction with decreased serum phosphorus or increased urinary phosphorus excretion. Hematuria and pain with nephrolithiasis.

DIAGNOSIS

- Evaluate cause of renal insufficiency.
- Monitor renal insufficiency closely.

MANAGEMENT

- The majority of renal toxicities are treated with supportive therapy.
- The offending medication should be changed in most patients.
- Evaluate the need for adjusting doses of antiretroviral medications in renal insufficiency.

Although the overall incidence is low, ART in HIV patients can cause renal dysfunction in 0.3–2% of patients (Kalyesubula, 2011). In a study by Franceschini and colleagues, drugs associated with tubular injury, interstitial nephritis, and crystalluria accounted for 32% of all cases of AKI (Franceschini, 2005). Moreover, indinavir, atazanavir, and tenofovir have been implicated in the development of chronic kidney disease (Atta, 2008).

NUCLEOS(T)IDE REVERSE TRANSCRIPTASE INHIBITORS

TDF is a nucleotide reverse transcriptase inhibitor (NRTI) that is commonly used in HIV patients and has often been implicated as a cause of renal disease. It is cleared by the kidneys via active proximal tubular secretion and glomerular filtration.

Due to high renal toxicity rates of its acyclic nucleotide predecessors adefovir and cidofovir, both of which cause AKI and proximal tubular toxicity, there was concern regarding the potential renal toxicity of TDF. Initial studies did not reveal significant toxicity related to TDF, but after FDA approval, case reports emerged of Fanconi syndrome, renal failure, and diabetes insipidus (Gaspar, 2004; Karras, 2003; Rollot, 2003). Fanconi syndrome is characterized by proximal tubular kidney dysfunction, with decreased tubular reabsorption and urinary wasting of phosphate, glucose, amino acids, bicarbonate, and sodium. This solute loss leads to acidosis, bone disease, and electrolyte abnormalities. The exact mechanism of nephrotoxicity is unknown, but it is hypothesized that apoptosis of tubular cells and inhibition of mitochondrial DNA replication in proximal tubular cells are involved (Gitman, 2007). Fanconi syndrome is the most common manifestation of mitochondrial diseases, which supports the hypothesis that tenofovir exposure causes mitochondrial dysfunction (Kalyesubula, 2011). Most patients do not develop the full Fanconi syndrome but instead manifest primarily with urinary phosphate wasting and, hence, hypophosphatemia in most cases (Waheed, 2015). This may occur in isolation or in conjunction with AKI. Urinary phosphate wasting is a more sensitive marker of TDF-induced nephrotoxicity because hypophosphatemia is not present in all cases.

Patients with low $CD4^+$ T cell counts, advanced age, lower body weight, and higher serum creatinine are most at risk for developing TDF-induced nephrotoxicity (Kalyesubula, 2011).

In numerous clinical trials, TDF did not demonstrated significant renal toxicity, but many of these were conducted in patients without significant comorbidities and with baseline creatinine clearance (CrCl) of greater than 50 mL/min (Gallant, 2006). However, in a retrospective study of 948 patients with HIV, tenofovir use in 294 patients was associated with a greater decrease in calculated CrCl compared to that in patients treated with a non–tenofovir-containing antiretroviral regimen (difference of 6.8 mL/min; $p = 0.02$) (Winston, 2006). In an observational cohort, use of tenofovir ($n = 344$) was associated with a greater decline in renal function (13.3 mL/min in the tenofovir group and 7.5 mL/min in the alternate group) compared to that with an alternative nucleoside analogue ($n = 314$) (Gallant, 2005). In another large study of 10,841 HIV-positive patients from the Veterans Health Administration, over a 10-year period, each year of tenofovir exposure was associated with a 33% (range, 18–51%; $p < 0.0001$) increased risk of CKD (Scherzer, 2012). The HEAT Trial, which compared abacavir/lamivudine or tenofovir/emtricitabine administered with lopinavir/ritonavir, showed no significant difference in renal function between the groups. However, 1% of the patients on tenofovir developed proximal tubular kidney dysfunction (Smith, 2009).

A recent long-term follow-up of 23,905 patients in the Data Collection on Adverse Events of Anti-HIV Drugs (D:A:D) study cohort who initiated antiretrovirals with normal eGFR (>90 mL/min/1.73 m²) showed a significant increase in the development of CKD with exposure to tenofovir, ritonavir-boosted atazanavir, and ritonavir-boosted lopinavir but not other ritonavir-boosted PIs or abacavir (Mocroft, 2015). These findings are similar to those of previous studies in the cohort and add to an expanding literature on the long-term effects of antiretroviral agents on the kidney (Fine, 2013).

Some studies have shown that TDF use in conjunction with PIs can increase the risk of renal injury (Sax, 2011). This was considered to be a result of tenofovir accumulation in renal tubular cells as a consequence of tenofovir–ritonavir interaction. Tenofovir is secreted via the multidrug resistance protein (MRP) efflux pump on the luminal side of the proximal tubular cells. It was initially believed that tenofovir secretion was through MRP2. Ritonavir is a potent inhibitor of MRP2-mediated transport, and that could have led to accumulation of tenofovir in the tubular cells (Rollot, 2003). It has since been determined that MRP4 and possibly MRP2 are responsible for tenofovir secretion, and secretion is not affected by ritonavir (Ray, 2006). Because ritonavir is often used as salvage therapy, the link of ritonavir–tenofovir nephrotoxicity may actually reflect advanced disease in these patients, who have a higher risk of adverse events (Winston, 2006).

TAF is a prodrug of TDF and has demonstrated potent anti–HIV-1 activity and higher intracellular tenofovir levels compared with TDF while maintaining lower plasma tenofovir exposure at 40 mg and good tolerability (Markowitz, 2014). Tenofovir released from TDF undergoes active renal secretion via organic anion transporters (OAT1 and OAT3), leading to higher exposure of renal proximal tubules to tenofovir and a potential for renal adverse effects. Unlike TDF, TAF does not interact with renal transporters OAT1 and OAT3 and therefore it has a better renal safety profile (Bam, 2014). In a recent randomized controlled trial of HIV-1–positive patients who had achieved virologic suppression (viral load <50 mL/min) on a TDF-based regimen with a GFR of 50 mL/min or higher, patients were randomly assigned to continue the same ART or were switched to a TAF-based regimen (in combination with elvitegravir, cobicistat, and emtricitabine). The TAF-containing regimen led to continued viral suppression with improvement in bone mineral density and renal function (Mills, 2016).

Based on current knowledge of TDF toxicities, there is still no clear consensus regarding how frequently to monitor kidney function in patients on TDF, with some authors recommending a GFR-based approach (Holt, 2014). Others advocate periodic monitoring of these markers in all patients on tenofovir regardless of GFR (Fine, 2013). In those with low serum phosphate, fractional excretion of phosphate in the urine can be used to confirm decreased tubular reabsorption of phosphate (Kinai, 2005).

Although the renal toxicity of TDF is mostly reversible with the cessation of this drug, patients often do not achieve their pre-TDF CrCl levels (Waheed, 2015; Wever, 2010). With the increased availability of single-table ART regimens that contain TAF, the use of TDF in the United States has declined. Current US Department of Health and Human Services (USDHHS) HIV guidelines note that TAF has fewer bone and kidney toxicities than TDF, whereas TDF is associated with lower lipid levels; therefore safety, costs, and access should be considered when choosing between the two drugs (USDHHS, 2018). Clinicians should be vigilant regarding monitoring patients for renal toxicity, with early change in regimen when toxicity is identified.

PROTEASE INHIBITORS

The PIs indinavir and atazanavir can commonly induce urolithiasis. This was most frequently seen with indinavir but has also been observed with other PIs (Huynh, 2011; Rockwood, 2011). Indinavir was also associated with progression of CKD; however, this drug is rarely used to treat HIV so its toxicity has become of historical importance (McLaughlin, 2018).

Several studies have suggested nephrotoxicity associated with atazanavir use. The largest included 22,603 D:A:D cohort participants with normal baseline kidney function (eGFR >90 mL/min). The decline in eGFR by more than 20 mL/min to less than 70 mL/min was associated with the use of not only tenofovir but also ritonavir-boosted atazanavir.

An earlier study of the EuroSIDA cohort (a subset of the D:A:D cohort) demonstrated similar results in a smaller population ($N = 6843$) (Mocroft, 2010). In a study of a large Veterans Health Administration population, Scherzer et al. (2012) showed an association between atazanavir use and rapid GFR decline. A plausible mechanism for this potential toxicity may be related to the predilection for atazanavir to crystallize. The formation of kidney stones with atazanavir use is well described (Chan-Tack, 2007). In a Japanese study, the use of ritonavir-boosted atazanavir was shown to be associated with a higher incidence of renal stones; however, the composition of these stones was not analyzed (Hamada, 2012). With many of studies confirming an association of nephrotoxicity with use of boosted atazanavir, close monitoring of renal function in atazanavir-treated patients is recommended. If a decline in GFR or other nephrotoxicity is noted, atazanavir should be discontinued. If a PI is needed to maintain viral suppression, switching to an alternative agent such as darunavir, which has not been associated with kidney stones or nephrotoxicity, is recommended (McLaughlin, 2018).

PHARMACOKINETIC ENHANCER

Several antiretrovirals are coformulated with cobicistat (COBI), a cytochrome P450 inhibitor. COBI increases serum levels of the active agent and allows once-daily dosing of these drugs (Johnson, 2014). Although cobicistat has no inherent nephrotoxicity, it inhibits the cationic renal transporter MATE1 (multidrug and toxin extrusion protein-efflux) at the apical membrane of the proximal tubular cells, which blocks tubular secretion of creatinine (see Figure 43.1) (Lepist, 2011). This leads to an increase in plasma creatinine concentration without any effect on the actual GFR. This was evaluated in a study of 36 patients in which COBI use was associated with an increase in serum creatinine and an approximately 10 mL/min decrease in eGFR, but the decrease in eGFR was reversible upon discontinuation of the medication, thus highlighting that this drug has no adverse effect on the actual GFR (German, 2010). The timing of the increase in creatinine and subsequent resolution after discontinuation of cobicistat was consistent with altered proximal tubular creatinine secretion.

INTEGRASE STRAND TRANSFER INHIBITORS

There have been several studies looking at the effect of raltegravir (RAL), the first FDA-approved integrase strand transfer inhibitor (INSTI) on renal function (McLaughlin, 2018). A retrospective study of 29 HIV-infected patients started on RAL there was a small but nonsignificant increase in serum creatinine. In both studies the authors concluded there was no evidence of nephrotoxicity and that the increases were likely due to inhibition of renal organic cation transporter 2 (OCT2) (Lindeman, 2016).

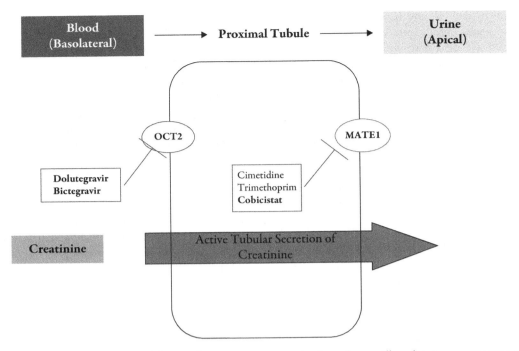

Figure 43.1 Effect of drugs on creatinine secretion. Inhibition of creatinine transporter by drugs shown will result in increase in serum creatinine without GFR effects. Model for effect of tested drugs on creatinine secretion. BCRP, breast cancer resistance protein; MATE, multidrug and toxin extrusion protein; MRP, multidrug resistance protein; OCT, organic cation transporter; OCTN, organic cation/ergothioneine transporter; Pgp, P-glycoprotein.   From Lepist (2011), poster A1-1724.

In a similar fashion, it has been found that dolutegravir (an INSTI) inhibits the tubular secretion of creatinine through the organic cation transporter 2 (OCT2) at the basolateral membrane of the proximal tubular cells. This raises serum creatinine concentration without affecting the actual GFR (Rathbun, 2014). A phase 1 study by Koteff included 34 healthy patients who received 50 mg of dolutegravir twice daily or placebo for 14 days. Participants received iohexol, which is freely filtered, and para-aminohippurate (PAH) on days 1, 7, and 14 to see if dolutegravir impacted GFR or renal blood flow. Additional tubular function biomarkers including albumin, cystatin C, and total protein were measured. The authors determined that dolutegravir increased serum creatinine levels by 10–14% but did not impact renal blood flow or glomerular filtration (Koteff, 2013).

In both the SPRING-1 and SPRING-2 trials, a noticeable rise in serum creatinine was noted with dolutegravir, although without any significant clinical adverse effects in antiretroviral-naïve HIV-positive patients (Stellbrink, 2013; Raffi, 2013). The rise in creatinine was typically seen in the first week and then stabilized thereafter. In the VIKING Trial, a similar pattern was noted for HIV-positive patients resistant to RAL and switched to dolutegravir (Eron, 2013).

Elvitegravir is primarily metabolized by the liver into two metabolites. A very small amount is excreted unchanged in the urine (McLaughlin, 2018). It is therefore not felt to prevent any risks of nephrotoxicity. However, it is coadministered with COBI, so an increase in serum creatinine in patients taking this drug would not be unexpected.

Bictegravir is a second-generation integrase inhibitor that has been evaluated in several large phase 3 clinical trials, with in vitro studies showing relatively higher barrier to resistance compared to other ART regimens. Coformulated bictegravir, emtricitabine, and tenofovir alafenamide was compared to dolutegravir-based combination ART in two noninferiority trials (Gallant, 2017; Sax, 2017). In these studies, the estimated GFR declined by −7.0 mL/min in the bictegravir arm and −11.3 mL/min in the dolutegravir arm at week 48, but there were no discontinuations due to kidney-related adverse events and no cases of tubulopathy.

The following year, the efficacy and safety of switching to a bictegravir-based combination regimen from either a dolutegravir-based or PI-based regimen was also assessed in two additional large phase 3 trials (Daar, 2018; Molina, 2018). In all four studies, there was no discontinuation of therapy due to renal adverse effects. Changes in serum creatinine, serum eGFR, and urinary markers such as albumin-to-creatinine ratio, were not significant.

DOSE ADJUSTMENT IN RENAL INSUFFICIENCY

Most non-nucleoside reverse transcriptase inhibitors (NNRTIs), integrase inhibitors, and PIs can be used safely and do not require dose modification in CKD or ESRD. Although TDF should generally be avoided in those with a CrCl level of less than 50 mL/min or stopped in those with declining eGFR, there may be instances in which other options are not available, and dose adjustment can be made. Any drug containing TDF will need dose adjustment at CrCl of less than 50 mL/min. In general, the availability of TAF now makes this less of a clinical issue for most patients.

Patient who are taking combination single-tablet regimens may still require separation of the component drugs for individual dosing if they have a decline in renal function (Kalyesubula, 2011). However, recent data from a small study found using single-table elvitegravir/cobicistat/emtricitabine/tenofovir alafenamide maintained virologic suppression at 24 weeks, was very well tolerated, and was more convenient in adult patients with ESRD on dialysis (Eron, 2018).

In summary, renal abnormalities can develop in patients on various ART regimens and cannot always be attributed to a single drug. Renal function should be monitored every 3–6 months in HIV patients receiving ART. Appropriate dose adjustments or changes in therapy should be made based on observed changes in serum creatinine or GFR.

RECOMMENDED READING

Atta MG, Deray G, Lucas GM. Antiretroviral nephrotoxicities. *Semin Nephrol.* 2008;28(6):563–575.

REFERENCES

Atta MG, Fine DM, Kirk GD, et al. Survival during renal replacement therapy among African Americans infected with HIV type 1 in urban Baltimore, Maryland. *Clin Infect Dis.* 2007;45(12):1625–1632.

Atta MG, Lucas GM, Fine DM. HIV-associated nephropathy: epidemiology, pathogenesis, diagnosis and management. *Expert Rev Anti Infect Ther.* 2008;6(3):365–371.

Bachmeyer C, Blanche P, Sereni D, et al. Thrombotic thrombocytopenic purpura and hemolytic uremic syndrome in HIV-infected patients. *AIDS (London).* 1995;9(5):532–533.

Balow JE. Nephropathy in the context of HIV infection. *Kidney Int.* 2005;67(4):1632–1633.

Bam RA, Birkus G, Babusis D, et al. Metabolism and antiretroviral activity of tenofovir alafenamide in CD4+ T-cells and macrophages from demographically diverse donors. *Antivir Ther.* 2014;19(7):669–677.

Barisoni L, Kriz W, Mundel P, et al. The dysregulated podocyte phenotype: a novel concept in the pathogenesis of collapsing idiopathic focal segmental glomerulosclerosis and HIV-associated nephropathy. *J Am Soc Nephrol.* 1999;10(1):51–61.

Becker S, Fusco G, Fusco J, et al. HIV-associated thrombotic microangiopathy in the era of highly active antiretroviral therapy: an observational study. *Clin Infect Dis.* 2004;39(Suppl 5):S267–S275.

Berliner AR, Fine DM, Lucas GM, et al. Observations on a cohort of HIV-infected patients undergoing native renal biopsy. *Am J Nephrol.* 2008;28(3):478–486.

Bhasin B, Lau B, Atta MG, et al. Viremia and T-cell activation differentially affect the performance of glomerular filtration rate equations based on creatinine and cystatin C. *PloS One.* 2013;8(12):e82028.

Bige N, Lanternier F Viard JP, et al. Presentation of HIV-associated nephropathy and outcome in HAART-treated patients. *Nephrol Dial Transplant.* 2012;27(3):1114–1121.

Briggs WA, Tanawattanacharoen S, Choi MJ, et al. Clinicopathologic correlates of prednisone treatment of human immunodeficiency virus-associated nephropathy. *Am J Kidney Dis.* 1996;28(4):618–621.

Bruggeman LA, Dikman S, Meng C, et al. Nephropathy in human immunodeficiency virus-1 transgenic mice is due to renal transgene expression. *J Clin Invest.* 1997;100(1):84–92.

Casas JP, Chua W, Loukogeorgakis S, et al. Effect of inhibitors of the renin–angiotensin system and other antihypertensive drugs on renal outcomes: systematic review and meta-analysis. *Lancet.* 2005;366(9502):2026–2033.

Chan-Tack KM, Truffa MM, Struble KA, et al. Atazanavir-associated nephrolithiasis: cases from the US Food and Drug Administration's Adverse Event Reporting System. *AIDS.* 2007;21(9):1215–1218.

Cheng K, Rai P, Plagov A, et al. MicroRNAs in HIV-associated nephropathy (HIVAN). *Exp Mol Pathol.* 2013;94(1):65–72.

Choi A, Scherzer R, Bacchetti P, et al. Cystatin C, albuminuria, and 5-year all-cause mortality in HIV-infected persons. *Am J Kidney Dis.* 2010;56(5):872–882.

Choi AI, Rodriguez RA, Bacchetti P, et al. The impact of HIV on chronic kidney disease outcomes. *Kidney Int.* 2007;72(11):1380–1387.

Cohen SD, Kimmel PL. Renal biopsy is necessary for the diagnosis of HIV-associated renal diseases. *Nat Clin Pract Nephrol.* 2009;5(1):22–23.

Cohen SD, Kopp JB, Kimmel PL. Kidney diseases associated with human immunodeficiency virus infection. *N Engl J Med.* 2017;377(24):2363–2375.

Daar ES, DeJesus E, Ruane P, et al. Efficacy and safety of switching to fixed-dose bictegravir, emtricitabine, and tenofovir alafenamide from boosted protease inhibitor-based regimens in virologically suppressed adults with HIV-1: 48-week results of a randomised, open-label, multicenter, phase 3, non-inferiority trial. *Lancet HIV.* 2018;5(7):347–356.

D'Agati V, Suh J, Carbone L, et al. Pathology of HIV-associated nephropathy: a detailed morphologic and comparative study. *Kidney Int.* 1989;35(6):1358–1370.

Dragović G, Srdić D, Al Musalhi K, et al. Higher levels of cystatin C in HIV/AIDS patients with metabolic syndrome. *Basic Clin Pharmacol Toxicol.* 2018;122:396–401.

Elewa U, Sandri AM, Rizza SA, et al. Treatment of HIV-associated nephropathies. *Nephron Clin Pract.* 2011;118(4):c346–c354.

Eron J. Safety and efficacy of E/C/F.TAF in HIV-infected adults on chronic hemodialysis [Abstract 732]. Presented at the Conference on Retroviruses and Opportunistic Infections, Boston, March 4–7, 2018.

Eron JJ, Clotet B, Katlama C, et al. Safety and efficacy of dolutegravir in treatment-experienced subjects with ratlegravir-resistant HIV type 1 infection: 24-week results of the VIKING Study. *J infect Dis.* 2013;207(5):740–748.

Eustace JA, Nuermberger E, Choi M, et al. Cohort study of the treatment of severe HIV-associated nephropathy with corticosteroids. *Kidney Int.* 2000;58(3):1253–1260.

Fine DM, Gallant JE. Nephrotoxicity of antiretroviral agents: is the list getting longer? *J Infect Dis.* 2013;207(9):1349–1351.

Fine DM, Perazella MA, Lucas GM, et al. Kidney biopsy in HIV: beyond HIV-associated nephropathy. *Am J Kidney Dis.* 2008;51(3):504–514.

Foy MC, Estrella MM, Lucas F, et al. Comparison of risk factors and outcomes in HIV immune complex kidney disease and HIV-associated nephropathy. *Clin J Am Soc Nephrol.* 2013;8(9):1524–1532.

Franceschini N, Napravnik S, Eron J Jr, et al. Incidence and etiology of acute renal failure among ambulatory HIV-infected patients. *Kidney Int.* 2005;67(4):1526–1531.

Gallant JE, DeJesus E, Arribas JR, et al. Tenofovir DF, emtricitabine, and efavirenz vs zidovudine, lamivudine, and efavirenz for HIV. *N Engl J Med.* 2006;354:251–260.

Gallant JE, Lazzarin A, Mills A, et al. Bictegravir, emtricitabine, and tenofovir alafenamide versus dolutegravir, abacavir, and lamivudine for initial treatment of HIV-1 infection (GS-US-380-1489): a double-blind, multicentre, phase 3, randomised controlled non-inferiority trial. *Lancet.* 2017;390(10107):2063–2072.

Gallant JE, Parish MA, Keruly JC, et al. Changes in renal function associated with tenofovir disoproxil fumarate treatment, compared with nucleoside reverse-transcriptase inhibitor treatment. *Clin Infect Dis.* 2005;40:1194–1198.

Gaspar G, Monereo A, Garcia-Reyne A, et al. Fanconi syndrome and acute renal failure in a patient treated with tenofovir: a call for caution. *AIDS*. 2004;18:351–352.

Genovese G, Friedman DJ, Ross MD, et al. Association of trypanolytic ApoL1 variants with kidney disease in African Americans. *Science*. 2010;329(5993):841–845.

George E, Lucas GM, Nadkarni GN, et al. Kidney function and the risk of cardiovascular events in HIV-1-infected patients. *AIDS (London)*. 2010;24(3):387–394.

German P, Warren D, West S, et al. Pharmacokinetics and bioavailability of an integrase and novel pharmacoenhancer-containing single-tablet fixed-dose combination regimen for the treatment of HIV. *J AIDS*. 2010;55(3):323–329.

Gitman MD, Hirschwerk D, Baskin CH, et al. Tenofovir-induced kidney injury. *Expert Opin Drug Saf*. 2007;6(2):155–164.

Hamada Y, Nishijima T, Watanabe K, et al. High incidence of renal stones among HIV-infected patients on ritonavir-boosted atazanavir than in those receiving other protease inhibitor-containing antiretroviral therapy. *Clin Infect Dis*. 2012;55(9):1262–1269.

Holt SG, Gracey DM, Levy MT, et al. A consensus statement on the renal monitoring of Australian patients receiving tenofovir based antiviral therapy for HIV/HBV infection. *AIDS Res Ther*. 2014;11:35.

Huynh J, Hever A, Tom T, et al. Indinavir-induced nephrolithiasis three and one-half years after cessation of indinavir therapy. *Int Urol Nephrol*. 2011;43(2):571–573.

Izzedine H, Acharya V, Wirden M, et al. Role of HIV-1 DNA levels as clinical marker of HIV-1-associated nephropathies. *Nephrol Dial Transplant*. 2011;26(2):580–583.

Jafar TH, Stark PC, Schmid H, et al. Progression of chronic kidney disease: the role of blood pressure control, proteinuria, and angiotensin-converting enzyme inhibition: A patient-level meta-analysis. *Ann Intern Med*. 2003;139(4):244–252.

Johnson LB, Saravolatz LD. The quad pill, a once-daily combination therapy for HIV infection. *Clin Infect Dis*. 2014;58(1):93–98.

Jones CY, Jones CA, Wilson IB, et al. Cystatin C and Creatinine in an HIV Cohort: the Nutrition for Healthy Living Study. *Am J Kidn Dis*. 2008;51(6):914–924.

Kalayjian RC. Renal issues in HIV infection. *Curr HIV AIDS Rep*. 2011;8(3):164–171.

Kalim S, Szczech LA, Wyatt CM. Acute kidney injury in HIV-infected patients. *Semin Nephrol*. 2008;28(6):556–562.

Kalyesubula R, Perazella MA. Nephrotoxicity of HAART. *AIDS Res Treat*. 2011;2011:562790.

Karras A, Lafaurie M, Furco A, et al. Tenfovir-related nephrotoxicity in human immunodeficiency virus-infected patients: three cases of renal failure, Fanconi syndrome, and nephrogenic diabetes insipidus. *Clin Infect Dis*. 2003;36:1070–1073.

Kimmel PL. HIV-associated nephropathy: virologic issues related to renal sclerosis. *Nephrol Dial Transplant*. 2003;18(Suppl 6):vi59–vi63.

Kimmel PL, Mishkin GJ, Uman WO. Captopril and renal survival in patients with human immunodeficiency virus nephropathy. *Am J Kidney Dis*. 1996;28(2):202–208.

Kimmel PL, Umana WO, Simmens S, et al. Continuous ambulatory peritoneal dialysis and survival of HIV-infected patients with end-stage renal disease. *Kidney Int*. 1993;44(2):373–378.

Kinai E, Hanabusa H. Renal tubular toxicity associated with tenofovir assessed using urine-beta 2 microglobulin, percentage of tubular reabsorption of phosphate and alkaline phosphatase levels. *AIDS*. 2005;19(17):2031–2033.

Ko WY, Pajan P, Gomez F, et al. Identifying Darwinian selection acting on different human APOL1 variants among diverse African populations. *Am J Hum Genet*. 2013;93(1):54–66.

Kopp JB, Nelson GW, Sampath K, et al. Genetic variants in focal segmental glomerulosclerosis and HIV-associated nephropathy. *J Am Soc Nephrol*. 2011;22(11):2129–2137.

Korgaonkar SN, Feng X, Ross MD. HIV-1 upregulates VEGF in podocytes. *J Am Soc Nephrol*. 2008;19(5):877–883.

Koteff J, Borland J, Chen S, et al. A phase 1 study to evaluate the effect of dolutegravir on renal function via measured iohexol and PAH clearance in healthy subjects. *Br J Clin Pharmacol*. 2013;75:990–996.

Lepist EI, Murray BP, Tong L, et al. Effect of cobicistat and ritonavir on proximal renal tubular cell uptake and efflux transporters [Abstract A1-1724]. Presented at the 51st Interscience Conference on Antimicrobial Agents and Chemotherapy (ICAAC), Chicago, September 17–20, 2011.

Lescure FX, Flateau C, Pacanowski J, et al. HIV-associated kidney glomerular diseases: changes with time and HAART. *Nephrol Dial Transplant*. 2012;27:2349–2355.

Lindeman TA, Dugan JM, Sahloff EG. Evaluation of serum creatinine changes with integrase inhibitor use in HIV-1 infected adults. *Open Forum Infect Dis*. 2016;3(2):1–3.

Locke JE, James NT, Mannon RB, et al. Immunosuppression regimen and the risk of acute rejection in HIV-infected kidney transplant recipients. *Transplantation*. 2014;97(4):446–450.

Longenecker CT, Scherzer R, Bacchetti P, et al. HIV viremia and changes in kidney function. *AIDS (London)*. 2009;23(9):1089–1096.

Lucas GM, Eustace JA, Sozio S, et al. Highly active antiretroviral therapy and the incidence of HIV-1-associated nephropathy: a 12-year cohort study. *AIDS (London)*. 2004;18(3):541–546.

Lucas GM, Lau B, Atta MG, et al. Chronic kidney disease incidence, and progression to end-stage renal disease, in HIV-infected individuals: a tale of two races. *J Infect Dis*. 2008;197(11):1548–1557.

Lucas GM, Mehta SH, Atta MG, et al. End-stage renal disease and chronic kidney disease in a cohort of African-American HIV-infected and at-risk HIV-seronegative participants followed between 1988 and 2004. *AIDS (London)*. 2007;21(18):2435–2443.

Markowitz M, Zolopa A, Squires K, et al. Phase I/II study of the pharmacokinetics, safety and antiretroviral activity of tenofovir alafenamide, a new prodrug of the HIV reverse transcriptase inhibitor tenofovir, in HIV-infected adults. *J Antimicrob Chemother*. 2014;69(5):1362–1369.

Mauss S, Berger F, Kuschak D, et al. Cystatin C as a marker of renal function is affected by HIV replication leading to an underestimation of kidney function in HIV patients. *Antiviral Ther*. 2008;13(8):1091–1095.

McLaughlin MM, Guerrero AJ, Merker A. Renal effects of non-tenofovir antiretroviral therapy in patients living with HIV. *Drugs Context*. 2018;7:1–15.

Medapalli RK, He JC, Klotman JP. HIV-associated nephropathy: pathogenesis. *Curr Opin Nephrol Hypertens*. 2011;20(3):306–311.

Mills A, Arribas JR, Andrade-Villanueva J, et al. Switching from tenofovir disoproxil fumarate to tenofovir alafenamide in antiretroviral regimens for virologically suppressed adults with HIV-1 infection: a randomised, active-controlled, multicentre, open-label, phase 3, non-inferiority study. *Lancet Infect Dis*. 2016;16(1):43–52.

Mocroft A, Kirk O, Reiss P, et al. Estimated glomerular filtration rate, chronic kidney disease and antiretroviral drug use in HIV-positive patients. *AIDS (London)*. 2010;24(11):1667–1678.

Mocroft A, Ledergerber B, Katlama C, et al.; EUROSIDA Study Group. Decline in the AIDS and death rates in the EUROSIDA study: an observational study. *Lancet*. 2003;362(9377):22–29.

Mocroft A, Lundgren JD, Ross M, et al.; D:A:D Study Group Royal Free Hospital Clinic Cohort, Insight Study Group, Smart Study Group and Espirit Study Group. Development and validation of a risk score for chronic kidney disease in HIV infection using protective cohort data from the D:A:D study. *PLoS Med*. 2015;12(3): e1001809.

Molina JM, Ward D, Brar I, et al. Switching to fixed-dose bictegravir, emtricitabine, and tenofovir alafenamide from dolutegravir plus abacavir and lamivudine in virologically suppressed adults with HIV-1: 48 week results of a randomised, double-blind, multicentre, active-controlled, phase 3, non-inferiority trial. *Lancet HIV*. 2018;5(7):357–365.

Naicker S, Fabian J. Risk factors for the development of chronic kidney disease with HIV/AIDS. *Clin Nephrol*. 2010;74(Suppl 1): S51–S56.

Papeta N, Kiryluk K, Patel A, et al. APOL1 variants increase risk for FSGS and HIVAN but not IgA nephropathy. *J Am Soc Nephrol*. 2011;22(11):1991–1996.

Peters PJ, Moore DM, Mermin J, et al. Antiretroviral therapy improves renal function among HIV-infected Ugandans. *Kidney Int*. 2008;74(7):925–929.

Post FA, Holt SG. Recent developments in HIV and the kidney. *Curr Opin Infect Dis.* 2009;22(1):43–48.

Qiu J, Terasaki PI, Waki J, et al. HIV-positive renal recipients can achieve survival rates similar to those of HIV-negative patients. *Transplantation.* 2006;81(12):1658–1661.

Raffi F., Rachlis A, Stellbrink HJ, et al. Once-daily dolutegravir versus raltegravir in antiretroviral-naïve adults with HIV-1 infection: 48-week results from the randomized, double-blind, non-inferiority SPRING-2 Study. *Lancet.* 2013;381(9868):735–743.

Rao TK, Filippone EJ, Nicastri AD, et al. Associated focal and segmental glomerulosclerosis in the acquired immunodeficiency syndrome. *N Engl J Med.* 1984;310(11):669–673.

Ratnam KK, Feng W, Chuang PY, et al. Role of the retinoic acid receptor-alpha in HIV-associated nephropathy. *Kidney Int.* 2011;79(6):624–634.

Rathbun RC, Lockhart SM, Miller MM, et al. Dolutegravir, a second-generation integrase inhibitor for the treatment of HIV-1 infection. *Ann Pharmacother.* 2014;48(3):395–403.

Ray AS, Cihlar T, Robinson KL, et al. Mechanism of active tubular secretion of tenofovir and potential for a renal drug-drug interaction with HIV protease inhibitors [Abstract 39]. Program and abstracts from the 7th Workshop on Clinical Pharmacology on HIV Therapy, Lisbon, Portugal, April 20–22, 2006.

Razzak CS, Workeneh BT, Montez-Rath ME, et al. Trends in the outcomes of end-stage renal disease secondary to HIV-associated nephropathy. *Nephrol Dial Transplant.* 2015;30:1734–1740.

Reid A, Stohr W, Walker AS, et al. Severe renal dysfunction and risk factors associated with renal impairment in HIV-infected adults in Africa initiating antiretroviral therapy. *Clin Infect Dis.* 2008;46(8):1271–1281.

Rockwood N, Mandalia S, Bower M, et al. Ritonavir-boosted atazanavir exposure is associated with an increased rate of renal stones compared with efavirenz, ritonavir-boosted lopinavir and ritonavir-boosted darunavir. *AIDS.* 2011;25(13):1671–1673.

Roland ME, Barin B, Carlson ML, et al. HIV-infected liver and kidney transplant recipients: 1- and 3-year outcomes. *Am J Transplant.* 2008;8(2):355–365.

Rollot F, Nazal EM, Chauvelot-Moachon L, et al. Tenofovir-related Fanconi syndrome with nephrogenic diabetes insipidus in a patient with acquired immunodeficiency syndrome: the role of lopinavir-ritonavir-didanosine. *Clin Infect Dis.* 2003;37:3174e–3176.

Ross MJ, Klotman PE. Recent progress in HIV-associated nephropathy. *J Am Soc Nephrol.* 2002;13(12):2997–3004.

Sax PE, Pozniak A, Montes ML, et al. Co-formulated bictegravir, emtricitabine, and tenofovir alafenamide versus dolutegravir with emtricitabine and tenofovir alafenamide, for initial treatment of HIV-1 infection (GS-US-380-1490): a randomised, double-blind, multicentre, phase 3, non-inferiority trial. *Lancet.* 2017;390(10107):2073–2082.

Sax PE, Tierney C, Collier AC, et al. Abacavir/lamivudine versus tenofovir DF/emtricitabine as part of combination regimens for initial treatment of HIV: final results. *J Infect Dis.* 2011;204(8):1191–1201.

Scherzer R, Estrella M, Li Y, et al. Association of tenofovir exposure with kidney disease risk in HIV infection. *AIDS.* 2012;26(7):867–875.

Smith KY, Patel P, Fine D, et al. Randomized, double-blind, placebo-matched, multicenter trial of abacavir/lamivudine or tenofovir/emtricitabine with lopinavir/ritonavir for initial HIV treatment. *AIDS.* 2009;23(12):1547–1556.

Stellbrink HJ, Reynes J, Lazzarin A, et al. Dolutegravir in antiretroviral-naive adults with HIV-1: 96-week results from a randomized dose-ranging study. *AIDS.* 2013;27(11):1771–1778.

Stock PG, Barin B, Murphy B, et al. Outcomes of kidney transplantation in HIV-infected recipients. *N Engl J Med.* 2010;363(21):2004–2014.

Strategies for Management of Antiretroviral Therapy (SMART) Study Group. CD4+ count-guided interruption of antiretroviral treatment. *N Engl J Med.* 2006;355(22):2283–2296.

Tzur S, Rosset S, Shemer R, et al. Missense mutations in the APOL1 gene are highly associated with end stage kidney disease risk previously attributed to the MYH9 gene. *Hum Genet.* 2010;128(3):345–350.

Van Maarseveen EM, Rogers CC, Trofe-Clark J, et al. Drug–drug interactions between antiretroviral and immunosuppressive agents in HIV-infected patients after solid organ transplantation: a review. *AIDS Patient Care STDs.* 2012;26(10):568–581.

Waheed S, Atta MG. Predictors of HIV-associated nephropathy. *Expert Rev Anti-Infect Ther.* 2014;12(5):555–563.

Waheed S, Sakr A, Chheda N, et al. Outcomes of renal transplantation in HIV-1 associated nephropathy. *PLoS One.* 2015;10(6):e0129702.

Wei A, Burns G, Williams CM, et al. Long-term renal survival in HIV-associated nephropathy with angiotensin-converting enzyme inhibition. *Kidney Int.* 2003;64(4):1462–1471.

Wever K, van Agtmael MA, Carr A. Incomplete reversibility of tenofovir-related renal toxicity in HIV-infected men. *J AIDS.* 2010;55(1):78–81.

Winston A, Amin J, Mallon PWG, et al. Minor changes in calculated creatinine clearance and anion-gap are associated with tenofovir disoproxil fumarate-containing highly active antiretroviral therapy. *HIV Med.* 2006;7:105–111.

Wyatt CM, Arons RR, Klotman PE, et al. Acute renal failure in hospitalized patients with HIV: risk factors and impact on in-hospital mortality. *AIDS (London).* 2006;20(4):561–565.

Wyatt CM, Hoover DR, Shi Q, et al. Pre-existing albuminuria predicts AIDS and non-AIDS mortality in women initiating antiretroviral therapy. *Antiviral Ther.* 2011;16(4):591–596.

Zhong Y, Wu Y, Liu R, et al. Roflumilast enhances the renal protective effects of retinoids in an HIV-1 transgenic mouse model of rapidly progressive renal failure. *Kidney Int.* 2012;81(9):856–864.

Zuo Y, Matsusaka T, Zhong J, et al. HIV-1 genes Vpr and Nef synergistically damage podocytes, leading to glomerulosclerosis. *J Am Soc Nephrol.* 2006;17(10):2832–2843.

44.

BODY COMPOSITION CHANGES, FRAILTY, AND MUSCULOSKELETAL COMPLICATIONS OF HIV

Amanda L. Willig and Edgar T. Overton

CHAPTER GOAL

Upon completion of this chapter, the reader should be able to

- Discuss changing epidemiology in HIV from wasting to obesity, the concepts of frailty and sarcopenia, as well as other musculoskeletal consequences of HIV infection.

INTRODUCTION

With the advancement of HIV therapies, HIV infection has become a mangeable chronic illness with a distinct change in the metabolic manifesations from a wasting disease to a disease of obesity and its complications. Here, we review the changing epidemiology of metabolic disease associated with HIV and potential interventions to mitigate these metabolic derangements.

LEARNING OBJECTIVES

- Discuss the changing paradigm of AIDS wasting to HIV-associated obesity

- Highlight the emergence of frailty in the setting of HIV.

- Highlight the growing literature on HIV-associated frailty syndrome and sarcopenia in HIV.

- Discuss interventions to prevent aging-related complications of HIV disease.

WHAT'S NEW?

- From 1998 to 2010, the proportion of people living with HIV (PLWH) who were obese at the time of antiretroviral therapy (ART) initiation doubled from 9% to 18% (Koethe, 2016).

- Within 3 years of ART initiation, the proportion of obese PLWH doubled from 18% to 36% (Koethe, 2016).

- Excess adiposity in PLWH is associated with a significant increase in inflammatory biomarkers (Koethe, 2018).

- Increased central adiposity in PLWH is associated with excess risk for hepatic steatosis, diabetes, and cardiovascular disease.

- Integrase inhibitors, particularly dolutegravir, have been linked to excess weight with ART initiation or ART switch in some but not all PLWH (Taramasso, 2017; Menard, 2017; Norwood, 2017).

- Excess adiposity in PLWH is associated with an increase in markers of inflammation, indicating negative consequences for ART-associated weight gain (Koethe, 2018).

KEY POINTS

- Obesity, frailty, and sarcopenia are complications of greater prevalence among the aging HIV population. These conditions have implications for both life span and health span, being associated with decreased functional status, excess inflammation, and excess mortality risk.

- Women with HIV are disproportionately affected by obesity.

- Treatments for these entities are limited but often require behavioral interventions, including alterations in diet or exercise initiatives.

WASTING AND OBESITY

OBESITY

Before suppressive ART, PLWH often developed opportunistic infections and AIDS wasting. However, with widespread use of ART, obesity has emerged as a common comorbidity in HIV clinics, similar to the general population. As many as 2 of every 3 PLWH in US and African populations are overweight or obese (Tate, 2012; Malaza, 2012; Wrottesley, 2014; Crum-Cianflone, 2010). In a rural South African population, obesity was more than sixfold more common among women with HIV when compared to men with HIV (Malaza, 2012). Similarly, in a US-based cohort of PLWH followed after ART initiation, women experienced greater weight gain than men (8.6 vs. 3.6 kg, $p = 0.04$) (Lakey, 2013). Notably, the greatest amount of weight gain was reported among persons diagnosed with advanced HIV disease. These findings are supported by similar results from another US population of PLWH and lower baseline CD4 counts (<50 cells/mm³) (Tate, 2012).

With numerous non-AIDS comorbidities associated with obesity (hepatitis steatosis, diabetes mellitus, cardiovascular disease, obstructive sleep apnea), efforts are needed to better understand and manage weight gain and obesity after virologic suppression.

Recent data highlight that the prevalence of obesity at time of ART initiation doubled from 9% to 18% from 1998 to 2010 (Koethe, 2016). Furthermore, after 3 years of ART, the prevalence of obesity increased from 18% to 36% in this same cohort. In another analysis, Koethe et al. demonstrated that this excess adiposity was strongly correlated with an increase in inflammatory biomarkers associated with non-AIDS events and excess mortality (Koethe, 2018). PLWH are developing significant increases in central adiposity, with negative consequences in terms of inflammation and associated metabolic complications.

Some degree of weight gain is common with most ART initiation but appears heightened with the newer integrase strand transfer inhibitor (INSTI)-based regimens (Taramasso, 2017). A recent report highlighted that 10% of persons starting a dolutegravir-based regimen discontinue this drug due to adverse events, with excessive weight gain being the most common reason provided (Menard, 2017). For persons on dolutegravir-based ART for more than 6 months, the average weight gain was 3 kg. with 20% of the cohort experiencing a greater than 10% weight gain from baseline. Similar data were reported by Norwood and colleagues. A cohort of 459 PLWH on stable efavirenz-based ART were included in this analysis. Of the cohort, 136 patients were switched to an INSTI-based regimen and, over 18 months, gained 2.9 kg compared to a 0.9 kg gain in persons remaining on efavirenz (Norwood, 2017).

Unintended weight gain comes at a significant cost. As noted earlier, excess adiposity has been linked to an increase in markers of inflammation with associated metabolic complications and heightened CVD risk (Perazzo, 2018; Koethe, 2018). These data will require further analysis to understand the mechanisms behind excess weight gain and what can be done to mitigate the process. Given the cardiometabolic and quality of life consequences of obesity, interventions are definitely needed to prevent the epidemic of obesity currently affecting the HIV population.

MUSCULOSKELETAL DISORDERS

WHAT'S NEW?

- Frailty among PLWH is increasingly linked to other aging-related comorbidities, including CVD (Tibuakuu, 2018) and neurocognitive impairment (NCI) (Paul, 2018; Oppenheim, 2018).

- Frailty is associated with decreased volumetric measurements of the brain, including cerebellar white matter and subcortical gray matter (Kallianpur, 2016).

- The combination of frailty and NCI markedly increases risk for negative outcomes including falls, loss of independence, and all-cause mortality (Erlandson, 2018, Brothers, 2017).

- Host genetics likely predisposes certain individuals to a greater risk for declines in physical performance (Sun, 2018).

- Frailty among PLWH is associated with an increase in inflammation, particularly activation of the innate immune system and an altered lipidemic profile (Yeoh, 2017).

- In an analysis from the MACS cohort, frailty remains more common among men with HIV compared to HIV-negative men (16% vs. 8%) and is strongly associated with both central adiposity and sarcopenia (Hawkins, 2018).

- In aging PLWH (median age 52 years), 26% had sarcopenia, which was more common with advancing age and female sex (Echeverria, 2018).

- Treatments for sarcopenia and frailty are limited, but resistance training can both improve muscle health (Vingren, 2018) and decrease inflammation (Zanetti, 2016).

- Despite advances in ART, neuromuscular diseases remain common among PLWH (Prior, 2018).

KEY POINTS

- The frailty phenotype is recognized frequently among aging PLWH with increased morbidity and mortality.

- Persistent inflammation of HIV is a driver of frailty and sarcopenia.

- Exercise, specifically weight-bearing exercise, can improve muscle function and reduce inflammation in PLWH.

- HIV myopathy is a rare proximal muscle disorder that can occur in HIV-infected patients.

- Some antiretroviral drugs, including zidovudine and raltegravir, can cause myopathy with an elevation in creatine kinase (CK).

- Vitamin D deficiency appears to increase the risk of statin-associated myalgias and myopathy.

FRAILTY AND PHYSICAL FUNCTION

Despite effective viral suppression with ART, declines in physical function and frailty are more common in HIV-infected populations than expected for a given age (Piggott, 2013). These accelerated functional declines are associated with an increased risk of falls, hospitalizations, and mortality (Desqulbet, 2011; Erlandson, 2012; Onen, 2010). Additionally, this combination of impaired physical function with HIV infection is associated with excess mortality when compared to either HIV infection or impaired function alone (Greene, 2014; Pigott, 2015). This accelerated mobility-disability is an emerging quality of life issue for the aging HIV population, and additional research to improve physical function is needed.

Frailty is a well-described phenotype in the geriatric field (Fried, 2001). It is characterized as a terminal state of loss of functional homeostasis that leaves a person unable to cope with and recover from various stressors. Frailty is associated with poor health outcomes, including excess mortality (Newman, 2001). In the geriatric literature, frailty and physical function impairments are associated with excess inflammation and markers of immune senescence. Impaired physical function and low muscle mass are associated with increased interleukin-6 (IL-6), a pro-inflammatory cytokine released systemically by T cells and macrophages, as well as tumor necrosis factor (TNF-α) (van Hall, 2008; De Pablo-Bernal, 2014). A recent publication described a genetic predisposition to frailty among PLWH (Sun, 2018). Whether there are overlapping genetic factors that contribute to both persistent inflammation and frailty remains to be elucidated. Regardless, inflammatory pathways are involved in the maintenance of muscle health, and excess inflammation detrimentally affects muscle quality and function. In the setting of chronic inflammatory states like HIV, loss of physical function is a concerning consequence of persistent inflammation.

The derangements in inflammatory biomarkers that characterize HIV infection, including persistent, low-grade inflammation and immune activation (De Pablo-Bernal, 2014), are strongly associated with a heightened risk for CVD, osteoporosis, anemia, physical function impairments, and frailty, among other non-AIDS events and mortality (McKibben et al., 2015; Burdo, 2011; Nordell, 2014; Hileman, 2014; Borges, 2014; Tenorio, 2014; Tien, 2010). This pro-inflammatory state is believed to be multifactorial, driven in part by low-level HIV replication and/or coinfection with other pathogens such as cytomegalovirus (CMV) (Erlandson, 2015). Recently, frailty among PLWH has been demonstrated to alter both inflammatory pathways and induce an altered lipidome profile (Yeoh et al., 2017). These inflammatory and metabolic pathways may be the link between frailty and other aging-related comorbidities.

Recent data from the Multicenter AIDS Cohort (MAC) confirm the association between frailty and aging-related comorbidities. Tibuakuu and colleagues explored the relationship between sarcopenia, low muscle mass, and CVD in a subset of this cohort that included 369 men with HIV and 144 men without HIV. The prevalence of low thigh muscle mass was similar by HIV serostatus (20%). However, low muscle mass was associated with a 2.5-fold higher prevalence of obstructive coronary stenosis, even after adjusting for traditional coronary artery disease (CAD) risk factors. This association also remained significant after adjustment for adiposity, inflammation, and physical activity (Tibuakuu, 2018).

Several recent publications have linked frailty and sarcopenia to neurocognitive impairment (Paul, 2018; Oppenheim, 2018). This relationship has been augmented by findings that highlight a reduction in volumetric brain measurements in PLWH with frailty, indicating that the overt presentation of frailty likely has underlying irreversible neurologic consequences (Kallianpur, 2016). These findings are particularly concerning as the combination of frailty with NCI markedly increases the risk of falls, loss of independence, and all-cause mortality (Erlandson, 2018; Brothers, 2017).

With the recognition of an increased prevalence of frailty and sarcopenia among PLWH at an earlier age than HIV uninfected adults, clinicians and patients are seeking treatments that may prevent or reverse these detrimental changes in physical function and muscle mass. Two recent pilot studies have specifically evaluated resistance training as a treatment for HIV-related sarcopenia (Vingren, 2018; Zanetti, 2016). Zanetti and colleagues randomized 30 PLWH to resistance training or standard of care for 12 weeks. At the end of the intervention, the intervention group had decreased subcutaneous body fat and waist circumference and increased muscle mass ($P < 0.05$ for all). Furthermore, markers of inflammation (IL-6, TNF-α, IL-1β) decreased from baseline in the intervention group ($P < 0.05$ for all). Vingren and colleagues randomized PLWH to 3 days of resistance training per week or standard of care for 6 weeks. Muscle mass, strength, and power all increased in the intervention group ($p < 0.05$ for all) but not the control group. There were no changes in markers of inflammation, likely related to the relatively short intervention period. Taken together, these studies indicate that frailty in PLWH may be reversible with simple interventions that are easily implemented. Larger studies to confirm these findings are needed, although, based on these data, it appears reasonable to recommend resistance exercises for older PLWH.

Muscle disorders can be debilitating in HIV-infected patients. Myopathies can have a range of presentation from myalgias to rhabdomyolysis. HIV-associated myopathy and polymyositis is rare in the modern ART era. This entity is a slowly progressive, symmetrical proximal muscle weakness with the diagnosis confirmed by an elevated CK, electromyography characteristics, and often a muscle biopsy. Histopathology of muscle tissue will show inflammatory infiltrates of CD8[+] T cells and macrophages surrounding major histocompatibility complex-1-expressing muscle fibers. Treatment is with immunomodulatory regimens, including corticosteroids and intravenous immunoglobulin.

Myalgias and elevated CK can occur from many other etiologies in HIV-infected patients. Substance use (cocaine), antibiotics (ciprofloxacin, trimethoprim–sulfamethoxazole) and vigorous exercise have all been associated with rhabdomyolysis. Statin-induced myopathy occurs at similar rates in PLWH as the general population, although the presence of vitamin D deficiency may increase the risk (Calza, 2017). With a growing number of PLWH becoming "statin eligible" based on national cholesterol guidelines, this may become more of an issue in the future.

Despite advances in ART, neuromuscular diseases remain common among PLWH (Prior, 2018). Drug-related myopathy remains a potential complication of ART. Zidovudine and stavudine may cause HIV treatment-associated myopathy although these agents are now rarely used to treat HIV. Inhibition of DNA polymerase-γ in mitochondria has been implicated as a probable mechanism. Elevated CK has been seen in HIV-infected patients on other antiretrovirals including protease inhibitors and integrase inhibitors. The INSTI raltegravir has been associated with muscle alterations ranging from asymptomatic creatine phosphokinase (CK) increases to rhabdomyolysis. Grade 2–4 CK elevations reported in the BENCHMARK 1 and 2 trials were similar for raltegravir versus placebo when combined with optimized background regimen at 9% versus 6%, respectively (Isentress [raltegravir] package insert, https://www.merck.com/

product/usa/pi_circulars/i/isentress/isentress_pi.pdf). Post-marketing evaluation in Italy among 496 patients showed that 5.2% of patients on raltegravir had muscle symptoms, and, of these, 1.4% discontinued the drug (Madeddu, 2015). The muscle symptoms and CK elevations seen with raltegravir do not appear to be prominent side effects of the second-generation integrase inhibitors, dolutegravir and bictegravir. When patients develop myopathy or rhabdomyolysis on a suspected HIV medication, consideration should be given to stopping that drug but also considering other causes for the patient's symptoms.

RECOMMENDED READING

Fukui SM, Piggott DA, Erlandson KM. Inflammation strikes again: frailty and HIV. *Curr HIV/AIDS Rep.* February 2018;15(1):20–29.

Hawkins KL, Brown TT, Margolick JB, Erlandson KM. Geriatric syndromes: new frontiers in HIV and sarcopenia. *AIDS.* June 1, 2017;31 Suppl 2:S137–S146

Robinson-Papp J, Simpson DM. Neuromuscular diseases associated with HIV-1 infection. *Muscle Nerve.* 2009;40(6):1043–1053.

Warriner AH, Burkholder GA, Overton ET. HIV-related metabolic comorbidities in the current ART era. *Infect Dis Clin North Am.* 2014 Sep;28(3):457–476.

REFERENCES

Borges ÁH, Weitz JI, Collins G, et al.; INSIGHT SILCAAT Scientific Committee. Markers of and activation of coagulation are associated with anaemia in antiretroviral-treated HIV disease. *AIDS* 2014;28:1791–1796.

Brothers TD, Kirkland S, Theou O, et al. Predictors of transitions in frailty severity and mortality among people aging with HIV. *PLoS One.* 2017;12(10): e0185352.

Burdo TH, Lo J, Abbara S, et al. Soluble CD163, a novel marker of activated macrophages, is elevated and associated with noncalcified coronary plaque in HIV-infected patients. *J Infect Dis.* 2011;204:1227–1236.

Calza L, Magistrelli E, Colangeli V, et al. Significant association between statin-associated myalgia and vitamin D deficiency among treated HIV-infected patients. *AIDS.* 2017;31(5):681–688.

Crum-Cianflone N, Roediger MP, Eberly L, et al.; Infectious Disease Clinical Research Program HIV Working Group. Increasing rates of obesity among HIV-infected persons during the HIV epidemic. *PLoS One.* 2010;5(4):e10106.

De Pablo-Bernal RS, Ruiz-Mateos E, Rosado I, et al. TNF-alpha levels in HIV-infected patients after long-term suppressive cART persist as high as in elderly, HIV-uninfected subjects. *J Antimicrob Chemother* 2014;69:3041–3046.

Desquilbet L, Jacobson LP, Fried LP, et al. A frailty-related phenotype before HAART initiation as an independent risk factor for AIDS or death after HAART among HIV-infected men. *J Gerontol Biol Sci Med Sci.* 2011;66:1030–1038.

Echeverría P, Bonjoch A, Puig J, et al. High prevalence of sarcopenia in HIV-infected individuals. *Biomed Res Int.* 2018;2018:5074923.

Erlandson KM, Allshouse AA, Jankowski CM, et al. Risk factors for falls in HIV-infected persons. *J AIDS.* 2012;61:484–489.

Erlandson KM, Allshouse AA, Rapaport E, et al. Physical function impairment of older, HIV-infected adults is associated with cytomegalovirus immunoglobulin response. *AIDS Res Hum Retroviruses.* 2015;31:905–912.

Erlandson KM, Perez J, Abdo M, et al. Frailty, neurocognitive impairment, or both in predicting poor health outcomes among adults living with HIV [published online ahead of print May 18, 2018]. *Clin Infect Dis.* doi: 10.1093/cid/ciy430. PMID: 29788039

Fried LP, Tangen CM, Walston J, et al.; Cardiovascular Health Study Collaborative Research Group. Frailty in older adults: evidence for a phenotype. *J Gerontol a Biol Sci Med Sci.* 2001;56:M146–M156.

Greene M, Covinsky K, Astemborski J, et al. The relationship of physical performance with HIV disease and mortality. *AIDS.* 2014;28:2711–2719.

Hawkins KL, Zhang L, Ng DK, et al. Abdominal obesity, sarcopenia, and osteoporosis are associated with frailty in men living with and without HIV. *AIDS.* 2018;32(10):1257–1266.

Hileman CO, Labbato DE, Storer NJ, et al. Is bone loss linked to chronic inflammation in antiretroviral-naive HIV-infected adults? A 48-week matched cohort study. *AIDS.* 2014;28:1759–1767.

Kallianpur KJ, Sakoda M, Gangcuangco LM, et al. Frailty characteristics in chronic HIV patients are markers of white matter atrophy independently of age and depressive symptoms: a pilot study. *Open Med J.* 2016;3:138–152.

Koethe JR, Jenkins CA, Furch BD, et al. Brief report: circulating markers of immunologic activity reflect adiposity in persons with HIV on antiretroviral therapy. *J AIDS.* 2018;79(1):135–140. PMID: 29794823

Koethe JR, Jenkins CA, Lau B, et al.; North American AIDS Cohort Collaboration on Research and Design (NA-ACCORD). Rising obesity prevalence and weight gain among adults starting antiretroviral therapy in the United States and Canada. *AIDS Res Hum Retroviruses.* 2016;32(1):50–58.

Lakey W, Yang LY, Yancy W, et al. Short communication: from wasting to obesity: initial antiretroviral therapy and weight gain in HIV-infected persons. *AIDS Res Hum Retroviruses.* 2013;29(3):435–440.

Madeddu G, De Socio GVL, Ricci E, et al. Muscle symptoms and creatine phosphokinase elevations in patients receiving raltegravir in clinical practice: results from the SCOLTA project long-term surveillance. *Int J Antimicrob Agents.* 2015;45(3):289–294.

Malaza A, Mossong J, Bärnighausen T, Newell ML. Hypertension and obesity in adults living in a high HIV prevalence rural area in South Africa. *PLoS One.* 2012;7(10):e47761.

McKibben RA, Margolick JB, Grinspoon S, et al. Elevated levels of monocyte activation markers are associated with subclinical atherosclerosis in men with and those without HIV infection. *J Infect Dis.* 2015;211(8):1219–1228. PMID: 25362192.

Menard A, Meddeb L, Tissot-Dupont H, et al. Dolutegravir and weight gain: an unexpected bothering side effect? *AIDS.* 2017;31(10):1499–1500.

Newman AB, Gottdiener JS, Mcburnie MA, et al.;Cardiovascular Health Study Research Group. Associations of subclinical cardiovascular disease with frailty. *J Gerontol A Biol Sci Med Sci.* 2001;56(3):M158–M166.

Nordell AD, McKenna M, Borges AH, et al. Severity of cardiovascular disease outcomes among patients with HIV is related to markers of inflammation and coagulation. *J Am Heart Assoc.* 2014;3(3):e000844.

Norwood J, Turner M, Bofill C, et al. Brief report: weight gain in persons with HIV switched from efavirenz-based to integrase strand transfer inhibitor-based regimens. *J AIDS.* 2017;76(5):527–531.

Onen NF, Overton ET, Seyfried W, et al. Aging and HIV infection: a comparison between older HIV-infected persons and the general population. *HIV Clin Trials.* 2010;11(2):100–109.

Oppenheim H, Paolillo EW, Moore RC, et al.; HIV Neurobehavioral Research Program (HNRP). Neurocognitive functioning predicts frailty index in HIV. *Neurology.* 2018;91(2): e162–e170.

Paul RH, Cooley SA, Garcia-Egan PM, Ances BM. Cognitive performance and frailty in older HIV-positive adults. *J AIDS.* 2018;79(3):375–380.

Perazzo H, Cardoso SW, Yanavich C, et al. Predictive factors associated with liver fibrosis and steatosis by transient elastography in patients with HIV mono-infection under long-term combined antiretroviral therapy. *J Int AIDS Soc.* 2018;21(11): e25201.

Piggott DA, Muzaale AD, Mehta SH, et al. Frailty, HIV infection, and mortality in an aging cohort of injection drug users. *PLoS One.* 2013;8(1): e54910. PMID: 23382997

Piggott DA, Varadhan R, Mehta SH, et al. Frailty, inflammation, and mortality among persons aging with HIV infection and injection drug use. *J Gerontol a Biol Sci Med Sci.* 2015;70:1542–1547.

Prior DE, Song N, Cohen JA. Neuromuscular diseases associated with human immunodeficiency virus infection. *J Neurol Sci.* 2018;387:27–36.

Sun J, Brown TT, Samuels DC, et al. The role of mitochondrial DNA variation in age-related decline in gait speed among older men living with human immunodeficiency virus. *Clin Infect Dis.* 2018;67(5):778–784. PMID: 29481608

Taramasso L, Ricci E, Menzaghi B, et al.; CISAI Study Group. Weight gain: a possible side effect of all antiretrovirals. *Open Forum Infect Dis.* November 3, 2017;4(4): ofx239.

Tate T, Willig AL, Willig JH, et al. HIV infection and obesity: where did all the wasting go? *Antivir Ther.* 2012;17:1281–1289.

Tenorio AR, Zheng Y, Bosch RJ, et al. Soluble markers of inflammation and coagulation but not T-cell activation predict non-AIDS-defining morbid events during suppressive antiretroviral treatment. *J Infect Dis.* 2014;210:1248–1259.

Tibuakuu M, Zhao D, Saxena A, et al. Low thigh muscle mass is associated with coronary artery stenosis among HIV-infected and HIV-uninfected men: the Multicenter AIDS Cohort Study (MACS). *J Cardiovasc Comput Tomogr.* 2018;12(2):131–138.

Tien PC, Choi AI, Zolopa AR, et al. Inflammation and mortality in HIV-infected adults: analysis of the FRAM study cohort. *J Acquir Immune Def Syndr.* 2010;55:316–322.

van Hall G, Steensberg A, Fischer C, et al. Interleukin-6 markedly decreases skeletal muscle protein turnover and increases nonmuscle amino acid utilization in healthy individuals. *J Clin Endocrinol Metab.* 2008;93:2851–2858.

Vingren JL, Curtis JH, Levitt DE, et al. Adding resistance training to the standard of care for inpatient substance abuse treatment in men with human immunodeficiency virus improves skeletal muscle health without altering cytokine concentrations. *J Strength Cond Res.* 2018;32(1):76–82.

Wrottesley SV, Micklesfield LK, Hamill MM, et al. Dietary intake and body composition in HIV-positive and -negative South African women. *Public Health Nutr.* 2014;17(7):1603–1613.

Yeoh HL, Cheng AC, Cherry CL, et al. Immunometabolic and lipidomic markers associated with the frailty index and quality of life in aging HIV+ men on antiretroviral therapy. *EBioMedicine.* 2017;22:112–121.

Zanetti HR, Cruz LG, Lourenço CL, et al. Non-linear resistance training reduces inflammatory biomarkers in persons living with HIV: a randomized controlled trial. *Eur J Sport Sci.* 2016;16(8):1232–1239. PMID: 2702789

45.

SEXUALLY TRANSMITTED DISEASES

Karen J. Vigil

LEARNING OBJECTIVE

Upon completion of this chapter, the reader should be able to demonstrate knowledge regarding the diagnosis and treatment of most prevalent sexual transmitted diseases in patients living with HIV infection, in order to decrease rate of transmission.

INTRODUCTION

Sexually transmitted diseases (STDs) are common in PLWH. Education and counseling on changes in sexual behaviors of patients with STDs and their sexual partners, identification of asymptomatically infection, and effective diagnosis and treatment form the cornerstone for prevention.

In the United States, most young, sexually active patients who have genital, anal, or perianal ulcers have either genital herpes or syphilis, with herpes being the most prevalent. Less common causes include chancroid and donovanosis.

SYPHILIS

WHAT'S NEW?

- Syphilis incidence continues to increase and is more prevalent in people living with HIV (PLWH) and men who have sex with men (MSM).

- PLWH with syphilis should have a detailed neurologic examination. Patients with abnormal signs or symptoms should undergo cerebrospinal fluid (CSF) analysis.

KEY POINTS

- Syphilis incidence continues to increase and is more prevalent in PLWH and MSM.

- Clinical manifestations are similar to HIV-negative people, but complications may be more common (condyloma lata and lues maligna).

- Special attention to neurologic site involvement is required as laboratory-defined neurosyphilis may be more common among PLWH.

- Although CSF abnormalities are more likely in PLWH with CD4$^+$ T cell counts of 350 cells/mm^3 or less and

a rapid plasma reagin (RPR) score of 1:32 or higher, lumbar puncture is only recommended if there any sign or symptom of neurologic involvement.

- Penicillin is the treatment of choice for syphilis; alternatives have not been well studied in PLWH; PLWH with syphilis require more intensive clinical and serologic follow-up.

Syphilis is a systemic disease caused by *Treponema pallidum*. The rates of primary and secondary syphilis in the United States have been significantly increasing. Between 2005 and 2013, the number of reported cases of primary and secondary syphilis nearly doubled. The annual rate increased from 2.9 to 5.3 cases per 100,000 population (Center for Disease Control and Prevention [2014]). In 2012, MSM account for 83.9% of cases. Coinfection with HIV has been reported as much as 50–70% among MSM with a high HIV seroconversion rate in patients with primary and secondary syphilis (Su, 2011).

Most recently, the US Centers for Disease Control and Prevention (CDC) reported 9.5 cases of primary and secondary syphilis per 100,000 population in 2017. This represents a 10.5% increase compared with 2016 and a 72% increase compared with 2013. There is a high rate of HIV coinfection, particularly in MSM. Data from 2017 showed that 45% of MSM with syphilis had HIV, compared with 8% of men who have sex with women and 4.5% of women

PRIMARY SYPHILIS

Primary syphilis refers to the chancre: a single, painless lesion with a clean base and indurated, raised borders. Chancres appears 1 week to 1 month after exposure. They are usually in the genital area but can occur anywhere on the body, including the oral cavity.

SECONDARY SYPHILIS

Secondary syphilis is characterized by a maculopapular erythematous rash that may involve the palms and soles. It typically occurs 3 weeks to 3 months after exposure. In PLWH, rash could present with other several forms, including papulosquamous, vesicular, and pustular forms. Condyloma lata (broad-based, fleshy, wart-like lesions that occur in moist, warm body areas) and lues maligna (pustular ulceronodular syphilide) are complications of secondary syphilis and are more frequent in PLWH.

LATENT SYPHILIS

Latent syphilis is defined by positive serological test in the absence of any clinical signs or symptoms of syphilis. Early latent syphilis is defined as the one acquired within the preceding year. All other forms are either late latent syphilis or latent syphilis of unknown duration. The importance of this classification is secondary to transmission, being possible in any stages until early latent syphilis, and duration of treatment.

NEUROSYPHILIS

Central nervous system involvement may occur at any stage of syphilis. CSF laboratory abnormalities are common in persons with early syphilis, even in the absence of neurologic signs or symptoms. No evidence exists to support variation from recommended treatment for early syphilis for patients found to have such abnormalities. If clinical evidence of neurologic involvement is observed, a CSF examination should be performed.

Neurosyphilis can take any of several other forms, including cranial neuropathies (auditory dysfunction), uveitis, retinitis, or central nervous system vasculitis. A lumbar puncture and CSF examination should be performed for all patients with syphilitic eye disease to identify those with abnormalities; patients found to have abnormal CSF test results should be provided follow-up CSF examinations to assess treatment response.

The 2015 CDC treatment guidelines (Workowski, 2015) recommend CSF examination:

- If there is evidence of neurologic symptoms
- If there are ophthalmologic or auditory signs or symptoms
- In patients with clinical presentation of tertiary syphilis (e.g., aortitis or gumma)
- In patients with treatment failure

CSF abnormalities are most likely in PLWH with syphilis of any stage when CD4$^+$ T cell count is 350 cells/mm^3 or less and a serum RPR titer is greater than 1:32 (Libois, 2007; Marra, 2004). However, CSF examination has not been associated with improved clinical outcomes in the absence of neurologic signs and symptoms.

Other presentation of tertiary syphilis includes cardiovascular syphilis and gummatous syphilis. Cases of rapid progression after initial infection have been reported with both entities (Maharajan, 2005; Weinert, 2008).

DIAGNOSIS

Primary chancre could be diagnosed by visualization of spirochetes under darkfield microscopic examination, although this test is no longer routinely available in clinical practice. This applies to genital lesions and not oral lesions because of the presence of nonpathogenic spirochetes in the mouth.

Nontreponemal antigen tests (VDRL and RPR) detect antibodies to antigens in the host after modification by T. pallidum. They become positive 4–6 weeks after infection or 1–3 weeks after the appearance of a primary lesion.

Treponemal tests (TPHA, TPPA, and FTA-ABS) detect antibodies that react with T. pallidum antigens. They are confirmatory for syphilis.

The diagnosis of neurosyphilis in HIV-infected patients is difficult since HIV itself cause CSF abnormalities. Classic CSF findings in neurosyphilis are lymphocytic pleocytosis, total protein elevation, and a positive VDRL test. CSF VDRL may be false negative in 30–70% of cases of neurosyphilis.

TREATMENT

PLWH who have early syphilis might be at increased risk for neurologic complications (CDC, 2007) and might have higher rates of serologic treatment failure with currently recommended regimens than non–HIV-infected people. No treatment regimens for syphilis have been demonstrated to be more effective in preventing neurosyphilis in PLWH than the syphilis regimens recommended for HIV-negative people (Rolfs, 1997). Careful follow-up after therapy is essential. The recommended and alternative treatment regimens for syphilis (Workowski, 2015) in PLWH are summarized in Table 45.1.

FOLLOW-UP

PLWH should be evaluated clinically and serologically for treatment failure at 3, 6, 9, 12, and 24 months after therapy. If the patient meets the criteria for treatment failure (signs or symptoms that persist or recur or persons who have a sustained fourfold increase in nontreponemal test titer), a new lumbar puncture with CSF examination should be performed and new treatment should be initiated. CSF examination and retreatment also should be strongly considered for PLWH whose nontreponemal test titers do not decrease fourfold within 6–12 months of therapy. If CSF examination is normal, treatment with benzathine penicillin G administered as 2.4 million units IM each at weekly intervals for 3 weeks is recommended.

For neurosyphilis, if CSF pleocytosis was present initially, a CSF examination should be repeated every 6 months until the cell count is normal. Research studies suggest that CSF improvement might occur much more slowly in PLWH, especially those with more advanced immunosuppression. If the CSF cell count has not decreased after 6 months or if the CSF is not normal after 2 years, retreatment should be considered.

PREVENTION

Annual serologic screening is recommended for all PLWH who are sexually active. More frequent screening should be performed in people with other associated risk behaviors

Table 45.1 RECOMMENDED AND ALTERNATIVE TREATMENT REGIMENS FOR SYPHILIS IN HIV-INFECTED PATIENTS

	RECOMMENDED REGIMEN	ALTERNATIVE REGIMEN
Primary, secondary and early latent syphilis	Benzathine penicillin G, 2.4 million units IM in a single dose.	
Late latent syphilis or syphilis of unknown duration	Benzathine penicillin G, at weekly doses of 2.4 million units for 3 weeks	
Neurosyphilis	Aqueous crystalline penicillin G 18–24 million units per day, administered as 3–4 million units IV every 4 hours or continuous infusion, for 10–14 days	Procaine penicillin 2.4 million units IM once daily PLUS Probenecid 500 mg orally four times a day, both for 10–14 days

such as multiple or anonymous sexual partners, injection drug users, or engaging in sex in exchange of money.

GONORRHEA

WHAT'S NEW?

- Dual therapy for gonorrhea with ceftriaxone and azithromycin is recommended to hinder the development of antimicrobial-resistant *N. gonorrhoeae.*

KEY POINTS

- Gonococcal infection remains an important cause of urethritis, cervicitis, pharyngitis, and proctitis in sexually active PLWH.

- Asymptomatic infection with gonorrhea and chlamydia is common at the female cervical site and male pharyngeal and rectal sites such that routine, periodic screening for this STD is required to detect such cases.

- Nucleic acid–based testing offers high sensitivity, ease of sample collection, and use of noninvasively acquired specimens (i.e., urine), although such tests are not cleared by the US Food and Drug Administration (FDA) for use with all specimen types.

- Antimicrobial resistance to fluoroquinolone and oral cephalosporins has been reported.

- Fewer antimicrobials are available to treat gonorrhea. Dual therapy for gonorrhea and chlamydia is recommended, not only because patients usually infected with *N. gonorrhoeae* are coinfected with *Chlamydia trachomatis,* but also to hinder the development of antimicrobial-resistant *N. gonorrhoeae*

Gonorrhea is caused by *Neisseria gonorrhoeae.* In 2017, 555,608 cases of gonorrhea were reported to the CDC (CDC: Gonorrhea—CDC Fact Sheet. 2018), accounting for an 18% increased rate since 2016 and 75% since 2009.

HIV-infected men are significantly more likely to have gonorrhea than HIV-uninfected men (Kent, 2005).

CLINICAL PRESENTATION

Acute urethritis is the main manifestation of gonorrhea. In men, urethral discharge—initially scant and later purulent—and dysuria are the major symptoms. The incubation period ranges from 1 to 10 days. In men, local complications include acute epididymitis, penile edema, penile lymphangitis, periurethral abscess, acute prostatitis, seminal vesiculitis, or infections of Tyson's and Cowper's glands. In women, gonorrhea presents as cervicitis and/or asymptomatic urethritis. However, physical exam may show purulent or mucopurulent cervical exudates.

N. gonorrhoeae may also cause rectal infection that could be asymptomatic or manifest as proctitis (rectal pain, discharge, bleeding, or anal itching). Up to one-third of MSM who have gonorrhea have positive rectal cultures (Handsfield, 1980). Additionally, pharyngeal infection should also be considered in a patient with sore throat, although it could be asymptomatic.

Disseminated gonococcal infection results from bacteremic dissemination of *N. gonorrhoeae.* Patients present with purulent arthritis or the triad of tenosynovitis, dermatitis, and migratory polyarthralgias that primarily involves an asymmetric distribution in the knees, elbows, and more distal joints. Pustules, often with a hemorrhagic component, could be present in approximately 75% of patients.

DIAGNOSIS

Urethra's discharge Gram stain reveals gram-negative diplococci during the first week after onset in men. In women, this is less common. Although cultures are the gold standard for diagnosis, nucleic acid amplification tests (NAAT) in cervical swab, urethral swab, or urine has excellent sensitivity and specificity.

TREATMENT

Quinolone-resistant *N. gonorrhoeae* strains are widely disseminated throughout the United States and the world.

Treatment failure to oral cephalosporins has been reported in Asia, Europe, Africa, and Canada (Unemo, 2012; Lewis, 2013). Therefore, quinolones and oral cephalosporins are no longer recommended regimens for the treatment of gonorrhea in the United States. The recommended treatment regimens for gonorrhea infection (Workowski, 2015) in PLWH are summarized in Table 45.2. There are limited data on alternative treatment for people with cephalosporin- or IgE-mediated penicillin allergy. Either gentamicin 240 mg or gemifloxacin 320 mg plus 2 g of azithromycin are possible options. However, consultation with an infectious disease specialist is recommended (Kirkaldi, 2014).

FOLLOW-UP

If failure to ceftriaxone is suspected, patients should be retreated with at least 250 mg of ceftriaxone intramuscularly or intravenously; partner treatment should be ensured and the situation reported to the CDC.

CHLAMYDIA INFECTIONS

WHAT'S NEW?

Due to the high prevalence of *C. trachomatis* infection in women and men who were treated for chlamydial infection during the preceding several months, *Chlamydia*-infected women and men should be retested approximately 3 months after treatment, regardless of whether they believe that their sex partners were treated.

KEY POINTS

- Most infections are asymptomatic. Therefore, routine periodic screening for *C. trachomatis* is recommended for all sexually active PLWH at exposed anatomic sites, at initial evaluation, and every 12 months thereafter or more frequently as indicated by risk.

- Nucleic acid–based testing offers high sensitivity, ease of sample collection, and use of noninvasively acquired specimens (i.e., urine), although such tests are not FDA-cleared for use with all specimen types.

- Rectal *C. trachomatis* infection is especially common among men who have sex with men; in this population, the *C. trachomatis* subtypes that cause lymphogranuloma venereum (LGV) should be included in the differential diagnosis of those with severe symptoms of proctitis, especially when *C. trachomatis* is found to be the cause.

Chlamydia is the most commonly reported STD in the United States in men and women. Rates continue to increase. In 2017, a total of 1,708,569 chlamydial infections were reported to CDC from 50 states and the District of Columbia (CDC: Chlamydia—CDC Fact Sheet, 2018). However, underreporting might be substantial as the disease maybe asymptomatic. Chlamydia infection is more frequent in younger age groups, racial/ethnic minorities, MSM, and incarcerated populations (Burstein, 1998; Rietmeijer, 2008; Satterwhite, 2008). Genital and ocular chlamydial infection are caused by serotypes D to K, while serotypes L1, L2, and L3 cause LGV.

Table 45.2 RECOMMENDED TREATMENT REGIMENS FOR GONORRHEA INFECTION IN HIV-INFECTED PATIENTS

	RECOMMENDED REGIMEN	ALTERNATIVE REGIMEN
Uncomplicated gonococcal infections of the cervix, urethra, and rectum	Ceftriaxone 250 mg IM in a single dose PLUS Azithromycin 1 g orally in a single dose	Cefixime 400 mg PO in a single dose PLUS Azithromycin 1 g orally in a single dose
Uncomplicated gonococcal infections of the pharynx	Ceftriaxone 250 mg IM in a single dose PLUS Azithromycin 1 g orally in a single dose	
Disseminated gonococcal infection (DGI)	Ceftriaxone 1 g IM or IV daily for at least 7–14 days depending on the site of infection, overall health of the patient and treatment response PLUS Azithromycin 1 g orally in a single dose	
Gonococcal meningitis and endocarditis	Ceftriaxone 1–2 g IV every 12 hours For 10–14 days for meningitis and for at least 4 weeks for endocarditis PLUS Azithromycin 1 g orally in a single dose	

CLINICAL PRESENTATION

Chlamydial genital infection secondary to serotypes D to K causes urethritis in men and cervicitis in women. Although most of the patients are asymptomatic, men may present with purulent urethral discharge (milder than gonorrhea), epididymitis, and prostatitis. Women may complain of vaginal discharge, intermenstrual bleeding, dyspareunia, and/or abdominal pain. Two to five percent of women could develop pelvic inflammatory disease that could lead to infertility, ectopic pregnancies, and chronic abdominal pain.

Serovars L1–L3 cause LGV. LGV is not endemic in the United States. Southeast Asia, the Caribbean, Latin America, and Africa are areas of more prevalence. It presents as one or more genital ulcers or papules followed by the development of unilateral or bilateral fluctuant inguinal lymphadenopathy called buboes. Since 2003, there have been reports of outbreaks in Western Europe and in the United States of *Chlamydia* L2 serotype proctitis, particularly in MSM. Reactive arthritis and Reiter syndrome (uveitis, arthritis, and urethritis) are seen in fewer than 1% of cases.

DIAGNOSIS

NAAT for *Chlamydia* genital infections (by polymerase chain reaction assay or transcription-mediated amplification) have great sensitivity and specificity and can be performed on first-catch urine or vaginal swab without the requirement of a urethral swab. The diagnosis of LGV is challenging. Cell culture is the only diagnostic test approved by the FDA. Serology helps in the diagnosis as titers are typically elevated at the time of presentation.

Diagnosis of LGV proctitis is even more difficult. NAAT may be used if a local laboratory has validated them. The CDC recommends that where LGV is suspected, the provider should collect a specimen and send the sample to the local state health department for referral to the CDC. If this is not possible, an antibiotic regimen effective against LGV should be included in empiric treatment for proctitis.

TREATMENT

Oral azithromycin 1 g single dose or doxycycline 100 mg twice a day for 7 days are the treatments of choice. For proctitis, a prolonged treatment with doxycycline for at least 21 days is recommended.

HUMAN PAPILLOMA VIRUS

WHAT'S NEW?

A 9-valent human papilloma virus (HPV) vaccine targets HPV types 6, 11, 16, 18, 31, 33, 45, 52, and 58.

KEY POINTS

- HPV is the most common STD in the United States. There are more than 100 HPV types; however, certain strains are associated with genital warts and others with intraepithelial lesions and high-grade neoplasia.

- Persons living with HIV have higher rates of HPV-related lesions; genital warts can be more aggressive and difficult to eradicate. A variety of patient- and provider-applied therapies are available.

There are three types of HPV vaccines: Cervarix (a bivalent vaccine that targets HPV types 16 and 18), Gardasil (a quadrivalent HPV vaccine that targets HPV types 6, 11, 16, and 18), and Gardasil-9 (a 9-valent vaccine that targets in addition HPV types 31, 33, 45, 52, and 58, which cause approximately 20% of cervical cancers that were not covered by Gardasil). Gardasil and Gardasil-9 are indicated in males and females 9 through 26 years of age. Cervarix is indicated in girls and women 9 through 25 years of age.

HPV is a double-stranded DNA virus that may infect the genital tract. There are more than 100 types of HPV; more than 40 may infect the genital area. HPV may cause two major clinical syndromes: genital warts (condyloma acuminata), associated mainly to types 6 and 11; and cervical epithelial or anal neoplasia linked to serotypes 16 and 18 (for more information on cervical and anal neoplasia, refer to Chapter 34).

HPV detection is significantly more common among HIV-seropositive women and men than among HIV-seronegative women and men (Mbulawa, 2009). Several studies have demonstrated that HPV increases the risk of HIV acquisition (Smith, 2010).

CLINICAL PRESENTATION

In most cases, HPV infection is transient, has no clinical manifestation or sequelae, and is self-limited. Genital warts typically present as single or multiple soft, fleshy, papillary or sessile painless keratinized growths in the vulvovaginal area, penis, anus, urethra, or perineum. Women living with HIV have a higher prevalence of genital warts, which may progress more rapidly in the presence of a declining immune status. Additionally, there are higher rates of Pap smear–detected abnormalities, dysplasia, and progression to cervical cancer relative to uninfected women.

DIAGNOSIS

Diagnosis of warts is made clinically; laboratory confirmation is not needed. In PLWH, MSM have an especially significantly increased risk of anal cancer due to oncogenic HPV types; therefore, routine anal Pap screening in HIV care settings is recommended. However, screening should not be done without the availability of referral for high-resolution anoscopy.

TREATMENT

The main indications for treatment of vulvovaginal warts are bothersome symptoms and/or psychologic distress. Vulvar biopsy to exclude precancerous or cancerous lesions is indicated when warts are identified in immunocompromised or

Table 45.3 RECOMMENDED TREATMENT REGIMENS FOR HPV/WARTS IN PEOPLE LIVING WITH HIV

External Genital Warts Patient-Applied	Podofilox 0.5% solution or gel OR Imiquimod 5% cream OR Sinecatechins 15% ointment
External Genital Warts. Provider-Administered	Cryotherapy with liquid nitrogen or cryoprobe. Repeat applications every 1--2 weeks. OR Trichloroacetic acid (TCA) or Bichloroacetic acid (BCA) 80%--90% OR Surgical removal either by tangential scissor excision, tangential shave excision, curettage, or electrosurgery
Vaginal Warts	Cryotherapy with liquid nitrogen. OR TCA or BCA 80%--90% applied to warts OR surgical removal
Urethral Meatus Warts	Cryotherapy with liquid nitrogen OR Surgical removal
Anal Warts	Cryotherapy with liquid nitrogen OR TCA or BCA 80%--90% applied to warts OR Surgical removal

postmenopausal women, when the lesions are visually atypical, or when warts fail to respond to standard therapy. The recommended treatment regimens for HPV in PLWH are summarized in Table 45.3.

PREVENTION OR PROPHYLAXIS

Routine vaccination in people with HIV is recommended for boys and girls aged 9–26 years. Women could receive any of the currently available HPV vaccines, while only the quadrivalent or 9-valent are recommended routinely for men. The vaccines are not licensed for use in people older than 26 years. The CDC emphasizes that immunocompromised or immunosuppressed patients, including patients with HIV, gay and bisexual men should also be vaccinated.

REFERENCES

Burstein GR, Waterfield G, Joffe A, Zenilman JM, Quinn TC, Gaydos CA. Screening for gonorrhea and chlamydia by DNA amplification in adolescents attending middle school health centers. Opportunity for early intervention. *Sex Transm Dis.* 1998;25:395.

Centers for Disease Control and Prevention (CDC). *Sexually transmitted disease surveillance 2014.* Atlanta, GA: US Department of Health and Human Services; 2015.

Centers for Disease Control and Prevention (CDC). Symptomatic early neurosyphilis among HIV-positive men who have sex with men: four cities, United States, January 2002—June 2004. *MMWR Morb Mortal Wkly Rep.* 2007;56:625–628.

Centers for Disease Control and Prevention (CDC). Primary and secondary syphilis—United States 2005–2013. *MMWR.* 2014;63(18):402–406. Available at http://www.cdc.gov/mmwr/preview/mmwrhtml/mm6318a4.htm). Accessed September 30, 2018.

Handsfield HH, Knapp JS, Diehr PK, KK. H. Correlation of auxotype and penicillin susceptibility of Neisseria gonorrhoeae with sexual preference and clinical manifestations of gonorrhea. *Sex Transm Dis.* 1980;7:1–5.

Kent CK, Chaw JK, Wong W, et al. Prevalence of rectal, urethral, and pharyngeal chlamydia and gonorrhea detected in 2 clinical settings among men who have sex with men: San Francisco, California, 2003. *Clin Infect Dis.* 2005;41:67–74.

Kirkcaldy RD, Weinstock HS, Moore PC, et al. The efficacy and safety of gentamicin plus azithromycin and gemifloxacin plus azithromycin as treatment of uncomplicated gonorrhea. *Clin Infect Dis.* 2014;59:1083–1091.

Lewis DA, Sriruttan C, Muller EE, et al. Phenotypic and genetic characterization of the first two cases of extended-spectrum cephalosporin-resistant *Neisseria gonorrhoeae* infection in South Africa and association with cefixime treatment failure. *J Antimicrob Chemother.* 2013;68:1267–70.

Libois A, De Wit S, Poll B, et al. HIV and syphilis: when to perform a lumbar puncture. *Sex Transm Dis.* 2007;34:141–144.

Maharajan M, Sampath K. Cardiovascular syphilis in HIV infection: a case-control study at the Institute of Sexually Transmitted Diseases, Chennai, India. *Sex Transm Infect.* 2005;81:361.

Marra CM, Maxwell CL, Smith SL, et al. Cerebrospinal fluid abnormalities in patients with syphilis: association with clinical and laboratory features. *J Infect Dis.* 2004;189:369–376.

Mbulawa ZZ, Coetzee D, Marais DJ, et al. Genital human papillomavirus prevalence and human papillomavirus concordance in heterosexual couples are positively associated with human immunodeficiency virus coinfection. *J Infect Dis.* 2009;199:1514.

Rietmeijer CA, Hopkins E, Geisler WM, Orr DP, CK K. Chlamydia trachomatis positivity rates among men tested in selected venues in the United States: a review of the recent literature. *Sex Transm Dis.* 2008;35:S8.

Rolfs RT, Joesoef MR, Hendershot EF, et al. A randomized trial of enhanced therapy for early syphilis in patients with and without human immunodeficiency virus infection. The Syphilis and HIV Study Group. *N Engl J Med.* 1997;337:307–314.

Satterwhite CL, Joesoef MR, Datta SD, H W. Estimates of Chlamydia trachomatis infections among men: United States. *Sex Transm Dis.* 2008;35:S3.

Smith JS, Moses S, Hudgens MG, et al. Increased risk of HIV acquisition among Kenyan men with human papillomavirus infection. *J Infect Dis.* 2010;201:1677.

Su JR, Weinstock H. Epidemiology of co-infection with HIV and syphilis in 34 states, United States—2009. In: Proceedings of the 2011 National HIV Prevention Conference, Atlanta, GA, August 13–17, 2011.

Unemo M, Golparian D, Nicholas R, et al. High-level cefixime- and ceftriaxone-resistant Neisseria gonorrhoeae in France: novel penA mosaic allele in a successful international clone causes treatment failure. *Antimicrob Agents Chemother.* 2012;56:1273–80.

Weinert LS, Scheffel RS, Zoratto G, et al. Cerebral syphilitic gumma in HIV-infected patients: case report and review. *Int J STD AIDS.* 2008;19:62.

Workowski KA, Bolan GA. Sexually transmitted diseases treatment guidelines, 2015. *MMWR Recomm Rep.* 2010;64:1–138.

46.

HIV AND BONE HEALTH

Edgar Turner Overton

CHAPTER GOAL

Upon completion of this chapter, the reader should be able to

- Familiar with the concept that metabolic bone disease is a common manifestation of HIV infection leading to an increased risk of fracture.

- The reader should also recognize key risk factors for metabolic bone disease and strategies to mitigate this risk.

INTRODUCTION

With improved long-term survival among populations of people living with HIV (PLWH), aging-related comorbidities, including osteoporosis, are becoming more prevalent (Justice, 2014; Ofotokun, 2011). There is increasing evidence that cardio-vascular, renal, and bone disease and neurocognitive deficits may be more common among long-term survivors of HIV infection. Data from cohort and prospective randomized studies suggest that PLWH are at increased risk of metabolic bone disease and related fractures (Battalora, 2016; Womack, 2011; Young, 2011).

LEARNING OBJECTIVES

- Discuss the prevalence of diseases of bone mineral density (BMD) and fractures in HIV-positive populations.

- Describe the risk factors associated with fractures.

- Discuss potential treatment strategies for low BMD in PLWH.

- Effectively communicate diagnostic and treatment strategies of bone diseases to patients.

WHAT'S NEW?

- A large meta-analysis of 29 studies confirms that HIV infection is associated with a 2.4- to 3.4-fold increase of osteopenia or osteoporosis at both the lumbar spine and hip (Goh, 2018).

- In a cohort of 97 suppressed PLWH, the rate of BMD loss slows after 96 weeks of antiretroviral therapy (ART) but remains at a rate of loss higher than a cohort of 614 HIV-negative adults (Grant, 2016).

- Women with HIV experience a twofold higher rate of bone loss than men living with HIV (Erlandson, 2018).

- Women with HIV in the Women's Interagency HIV Study (WIHS) Study have similar BMD as an HIV-negative cohort matched for socioeconomic status; however, the microarchitecture or quality of bone in women with HIV was significantly worse than in HIV-negative women (Sharma, 2018).

- Incidence rates for fracture vary among cohorts, but HIV infection consistently is associated with a twofold increased risk of fracture (Premaor, 2018).

- Asymptomatic vertebral fractures are common among PLWH over 50 years of age, occurring in 20% of an observational cohort. Spinal and lumbar X-rays should be considered for older PLWH (Llop, 2018).

- Tenofovir disoproxil fumarate (TDF) appears to alter the normal physiologic relationship between vitamin D and parathyroid hormone (PTH) that regulates bone homeostasis. In persons taking TDF, a higher vitamin D target may be required to prevent hyperparathyroidism and subsequent bone loss (Havens, 2018a).

- Women with HIV appear to be at greater risk of TDF-induced kidney injury (phosphate wasting) as a mechanism for BMD loss than men living with HIV (Kalayjian, 2018).

- HIV can infect osteoclasts and disrupt the normal balance of bone homeostasis. The HIV protein nef appears to increase osteoclast activity, leading to excess bone degradation (Raynaud-Messina, 2018).

- B cell dysfunction is another mechanism through which HIV infection increases bone turnover through excess expression of the cytokine RANK-ligand that activates osteoclasts (Titanji, 2017).

- High-dose vitamin D supplementation is associated with improvement in lumbar spine BMD in young PLWH. The effect appears to be mediated through a decline in PTH and bone turnover markers (Havens, 2018b).

- Zoledronic acid is safe and effective for PLWH on suppressive ART with low BMD, with greater benefit than a switch from TDF-based therapy (Hoy, 2018).

- Multiple cohort studies have found a higher than expected prevalence of low BMD in populations of adults living with HIV.

- Fracture prevalence is greater in PLWH compared to the general population. Incident fractures rates among PLWH in the HIV Outpatient Study (HOPS) were increased nearly threefold compared to those for the US general population.

- Asymptomatic vertebral fractures are highly prevalent among PLWH over the age of 50.

- Cohort studies suggest that, in addition to traditional factors such as age, smoking, and hepatitis C virus (HCV) coinfection, HIV disease-associated factors and ART factors are predictive indicators of fracture risk in PLWH.

- ART initiation is associated with a BMD decrease of 2–6%, with the largest decrease occurring in the first 6–12 months of treatment and then stabilizing.

- Greater BMD losses occur with initiation of zidovudine, TDF, and certain protease inhibitors.

- There are limited HIV-specific evidence-based recommendations regarding screening for bone disease, although extrapolation of screening recommendations from the general population is, at a minimum, reasonable. Several organizations recommend using dual-energy X-ray absorptiometry (DXA) and/or the Fracture Risk Assessment Tool (FRAX) for screening of HIV-infected persons at risk of fractures.

DEFINITIONS AND EPIDEMIOLOGY

BONE MINERALIZATION ABNORMALITIES

The World Health Organization (WHO) defines two categories of bone abnormalities based on comparison with the mean BMD of young healthy women (T-score): (1) osteoporosis—low bone mass and microarchitectural deterioration of bone tissue, BMD value more than 2.5 standard deviations below the mean BMD of young adult women (BMD T-score < –2.5); and (2) osteopenia—low bone mass, BMD value between 1 and 2.5 standard deviations below the mean BMD of young adult women (–2.5 < bone mineral density T-score < –1) (World Health Organization [WHO], 1994; Woolf, 2003). Osteomalacia is a third type of bone mineralization abnormality and refers to softening of bones due to impaired bone mineralization typically resulting from severe vitamin D deficiency (McComsey, 2010; WHO, 2002). Osteonecrosis or avascular necrosis is yet another bone abnormality resulting from interrupted blood supply to a bone or part of a bone, commonly occurring as a complication of trauma or fracture and typically located at the articular end of a bone (WHO, 2002).

In the general population, BMD peaks at approximately 22–35 years of age (Orwoll, 1995). BMD appears to decrease by 2–6% during the first 1–2 years of ART (Brown, 2009). Until recently, it was believed that PLWH subsequently experienced relative stability regarding BMD although a recent longitudinal study contradicts this dogma. Grant and colleagues followed 97 PLWH for a median of 7.5 years after ART initiation and compared their BMD data to that from 614 HIV-negative controls (Grant, 2016). While the rate of BMD loss after week 96 slowed in the cohort of PLWH, the decline in lumbar spine BMD remained significantly greater than that seen in the HIV-negative cohort. These data suggest ongoing metabolic bone disease despite HIV suppression with ART. The long-term metabolic consequences of HIV and ART need further evaluation. Additional data highlight significant differences between men and women living with HIV. A recent study included 839 female and 1,759 male PLWH with two or more DXA scans. The group reflected the aging HIV epidemic, with 82% older than 50 years of age and 76% with virologic suppression (<50 cp/mL). BMD loss was associated with ART exposure, hepatitis C (HCV) coinfection, lower physical activity, and vitamin D insufficiency. Among the women, BMD at the femoral neck declined twice as fast as among men after adjusting for traditional risk factors. More attention needs to be paid to aging-associated diseases among women with HIV.

Bone strength is a function of bone density and bone quality. Bone quality refers to rate of remodeling, microarchitecture, size, shape, amount of mineralization in the bone, and matrix quality (Yin, 2012a). Rate of remodeling is measured from serum levels of the bone turnover markers osteocalcin (OCN; a formation marker) and N-terminal telopeptide (NTX; a resorption marker). Microarchitecture is observed with computed tomography (CT) imaging. Mineralization quantity and matrix quality are determined by biopsy (Yin, 2012a). The importance of considering the microarchitecture or quality of bone was highlighted in a recent study from the WIHS (Sharma, 2018). In this analysis including 319 women with HIV and 118 without HIV, loss of BMD by DXA was similar between the two groups. However, the bone microarchitecture or quality of bone was significantly worse in the women with HIV. The effects of HIV on bone health are more complex than mere quantification by DXA.

PREVALENCE OF LOW BONE MINERAL DENSITY IN THE HIV POPULATION

Multiple cohort studies have found a higher than expected prevalence of low BMD in populations of adults living with HIV (Brown, 2006). Notably, these studies represent diverse populations of HIV-infected individuals, including antiretroviral treatment-naïve and -experienced people (Bedimo, 2012; Escota, 2015; Looker, 1998; McComsey, 2011; Tebas, 2000). A recent meta-analysis of 29 studies of BMD in PLWH confirmed the preceding statement (Goh, 2018). The prevalence of osteopenia and osteoporosis was 2.4–3.4 times higher in

PLWH compared to HIV-uninfected adults depending on site (lumbar spine and hip). Traditional risk factors (low BMI, history of fracture, older age, being Hispanic or Caucasian, low testosterone levels, smoking, low $CD4^+$ T cell counts, low lean and fat mass, and lipodystrophy) were associated with low BMD. Tenofovir-treated individuals were more likely to have low BMD compared to nonusers (53% vs. 43%), but the difference was not statistically significant.

Using data from the Study to Understand the Natural History of HIV and AIDS in the Era of Effective Therapy (SUN Study)—a prospective, observational cohort study funded by the Centers for Disease Control and Prevention (CDC)—Escota et al. determined that low BMD at the hip femoral neck was significantly more prevalent in PLWH than in matched controls from NHANES (47% vs. 29%; $p < 0.001$). In this cohort of 653 participants (77% male, 29% black, median age 41 years, median $CD4^+$ T cell count 464 cells/mm^3, and 89% with HIV RNA levels <400 copies/mL), 51% of participants had osteopenia and 10% had osteoporosis at baseline (Escota, 2015).

Postmenopausal HIV-infected women demonstrate a greater decline in BMD. In a longitudinal study of bone loss in postmenopausal women with HIV (Yin, 2011), higher rates of bone loss at the spine and forearm were observed in postmenopausal HIV-infected women than in HIV-negative minority women. Thus, higher rates of bone loss at the spine and forearm of postmenopausal women with HIV described in this study coupled with increased fracture prevalence among PLWH (Triant, 2008) suggest that an increased rate of fractures in postmenopausal women with HIV is a concern (Yin, 2011). Similarly, higher rates of bone loss were observed in men with HIV older than age 50 years (Orwoll, 1995). There are very few data on bone loss for women and men with HIV older than age 65 years, the period in which fractures are prevalent in the general population (Yin, 2012b).

There are limited data from resource-limited setting regarding low BMD in HIV-infected populations. In one South African cohort of 444 HIV-infected individuals (median age, 35 years; interquartile range [IQR], 30–40) years; 77% women), low BMD (Z-score <–2 standard deviations [SD]) was found in 17% of participants at the lumbar spine and 5% of participants at the total hip (Dave, 2015). Dave and colleagues reported that median total hip BMD was lower among those receiving ART than in ART-naïve participants (0.909 [SD 0.123] vs. 0.956 [SD 0.124] g/cm^2; $p = 0.0001$). Similarly, femoral neck BMD was lower among ART-receiving compared to ART-naïve participants (0.796 [SD 0.130] vs. 0.844 [SD 0.120] g/cm^2; $p = 0.0001$). In addition, vitamin D deficiency was found in 15% of cohort participants and associated with efavirenz use (adjusted odds ratio, 2.04; 95% confidence interval [CI], 101–4.13). In multivariate analysis, exposure to efavirenz- or lopinavir/ritonavir-based ART was associated with lower total hip BMD; higher weight, being male, and higher vitamin D concentration were associated with higher total hip BMD (adjusted $R^2 = 0.28$). Factors independently associated with lumbar spine BMD included age, weight, sex, and efavirenz use ($R^2 = 0.13$) (Dave, 2015).

Hoy recently reported results from the Strategic Timing of Antiretroviral Treatment (START) BMD substudy (Hoy, 2015; INSIGHT START Study Group, 2015). The primary START study enrollment consisted of 4,685 HIV-infected adult participants in 35 countries with $CD4^+$ T cell counts of greater than 500 cells/mm^3; the median age was 36 years, and 27% were female (INSIGHT START Study Group, 2015). Participants were randomized to start ART at study entry or delay therapy until $CD4^+$ T cell count fell below 350 cells/mm^3 or development of AIDS or another condition that dictated the use of ART (deferred-initiation group). In the BMD substudy of this primary START study, 193 participants were randomized to the early ART group and 204 participants to the deferred ART group (Hoy, 2015). Substudy participants underwent DXA scans of the lumbar spine, total hip, and femoral neck at baseline and annually thereafter. Mean follow-up time was 2.2 years. Hoy reported significantly greater loss of BMD at both the hip and the spine in participants randomized to early ART. There was no evidence of difference in development of osteoporosis between groups (or fractures in the main START study) (Hoy, 2015). More data are needed on the change in BMD among persons who initiate ART at a very high $CD4^+$ T cell count, as in the START trial.

HIGHER PREVALENCE AND INCIDENCE OF FRACTURES IN HIV POPULATION

Several recent studies have concluded that PLWH are at greater risk of bone fractures. Triant and colleagues presented findings that fracture prevalence is greater in HIV-infected women and men compared to the general population (Triant, 2008). Based on an analysis of more than 11 years of data from a large US single healthcare database, she determined that PLWH had a higher number of vertebral, hip, wrist, and combined fractures compared with non–HIV-infected participants. These findings were consistent across age, race, and sex categories, but no correlations were made as to specific risk factors due to lack of data. A recent review article highlighted that the heterogeneity and small sample size of studies of fractures among PLWH often make this a challenging topic to study (Premaor, 2018). However, despite a wide range of incident fractures among PLWH, ranging from 0.1/1,000 person-years (py) to 8.4 fractures/1,000 py, HIV is consistently associated with a twofold increased risk of fracture.

Subsequently, several large observational cohort studies published findings correlating fracture incidence in HIV-positive individuals compared to control groups. Differences in population, controls, and fracture definitions (i.e., fracture and fragility fracture definitions) were unique to each study.

The WIHS reported fracture incidence in 1,728 HIV-infected and 663 HIV-negative predominantly premenopausal women (Yin, 2010). Rates of fracture were not increased in women with HIV compared to HIV-negative women, and, in the women with HIV, the history of AIDS-defining illness was a more predictive indicator of fracture than ART.

Incident fractures rates among PLWH in the HOPS study were increased nearly threefold compared to rates in the US general population between 2000 and 2006 (Young, 2011). Rates of first fractures at any anatomic site were analyzed in 5,826 participants (median baseline age of 40 years, 79% male, 52% white, and 73% ART). Rates of fracture were indirectly standardized to the general population by age and sex using data from outpatients in the National Hospital Ambulatory Medical Care Survey (NHAMCS-OPD). Greater proportions of fractures were located at the hip, wrist, or spine in PLWH; fractures were associated with lower CD4+ T cell count nadir, duration of HIV diagnosis, and hepatitis C coinfection. The study suggested that younger PLWH, particularly those between ages 25 and 54 years, are at an increased risk of bone fracture compared to the general population. The authors recommended regular assessment of PLWH for fracture risk and particularly those with low nadir CD4+ T cell counts and other established fracture risk factors.

In the all-male Veterans Aging Cohort Study Virtual Cohort (VACS-VC) study, Womack and colleagues reported that men with HIV were at greater risk for fragility fracture compared to their HIV-negative counterparts (Womack, 2011). In this study of 119,318 men—of whom 33% were HIV-positive, 34% of this group were 50 years or older at baseline, and 55% were black or Hispanic—fracture risk factors included age, race, alcohol dependency, liver disease, tobacco smoking, or current use of corticosteroids or proton pump inhibitors.

Hansen and colleagues studied the incidence of fragility fractures in HIV-infected individuals not undergoing treatment with ART and PLWH undergoing treatment with ART in the Danish HIV Cohort Study (Hansen, 2012). In this comparative, sex- and age-matched study involving 5,306 HIV-positive participants and a general population cohort of 26,530 HIV-negative participants, the PLWH were observed to have an increased overall rate of fractures, increased risk of low-energy fractures but not high-energy fractures in HIV-infected participants without HCV coinfection, and moderate risk of low-energy fracture in PLWH undergoing ART when controlled for traditional osteoporosis risk factors of age, comorbidity, and smoking.

In the AIDS Clinical Trials Group (ACTG) A5224s, a substudy of ACTG A5202, McComsey and colleagues concluded that fracture rates increased in 269 PLWH during the first 2 years of ART initiated during the clinical trial compared to additional years of therapy. Although differences in BMD change were observed between patients who initiated different ART regimens, no significant differences in fracture rate were reported, although the cohort was young and follow-up was limited (McComsey, 2011; Yin, 2011).

Osteoporotic fractures were associated with cumulative exposure to TDF and ART in a large retrospective cohort study (56,600 patients) with a mean age of 45 years (Bedimo, 2012). Ninety-five percent of this cohort was male, limiting the ability to generalize the conclusion to females.

Another recent publication highlighted an underappreciated fracture: asymptomatic vertebral fractures (Llop, 2018). In this cohort of 93 male and 35 female PLWH with a mean age of 57 years, with more than 70% having low BMD at both hip and spine by DXA, 20% of the cohort was identified with an asymptomatic vertebral fracture. Factors associated with these fractures included older age, longer time since HIV diagnosis, and kidney insufficiency. Spine and lumbar X-rays should be considered in the aging HIV population.

Shiau and coworkers performed a meta-analysis of all studies on bone health and HIV published through September 2012 and concluded that HIV infection is associated with a modest increase in incident fracture, and they confirmed the consistent relationship of HCV coinfection as a risk factor (Shiau, 2013).

Findings from recent cohort studies have contributed to the developing field of fracture incidence in the HIV-infected population. Among 1,006 participants from two CDC-funded cohorts (median age, 43 years [IQR, 36–49]; 83% male; 67% non-Hispanic white; median CD4+ T cell count 461 cells/mm³ [IQR, 311–658]), osteopenia was determined in 36% ($n = 358$) of participants and osteoporosis in 4% ($n = 37$) of participants. A prior fracture was documented in 67 participants. During 4,068 py of observation after DXA scanning, 85 incident fractures occurred, predominantly rib/sternum ($n = 18$), hand ($n = 14$), foot ($n = 13$), and wrist ($n = 11$). Low BMD (osteopenia and/or osteoporosis) was determined in nearly 40% of the participants. Factors associated with osteopenia or osteoporosis included older age, lower nadir CD4+ T cell count, male–male sex HIV transmission risk, and history of fracture. Fourfold higher fracture rates were observed in HIV-positive participants with osteoporosis compared to HIV-positive participants with normal BMD. In multivariable analyses, osteoporosis (adjusted hazard ratio [aHR], 4.02; 95% CI, 2.02–8.01) and current/prior tobacco use (aHR, 1.59; 95% CI, 1.02–2.50) were associated with incident fracture (Battalora, 2016).

Results of new fracture risk and FRAX 10-year probability of fracture among the same CDC-combined cohort of 1,006 participants described previously were presented in poster format at CROI 2014. Battalora reported that increasing baseline FRAX 10-year probability was consistently associated with increased rates of incident fractures in this HIV-infected cohort. Participants with FRAX 10-year probability of 3% or more compared with less than 3% had higher rates of major and incident fracture (Battalora, 2014a).

In addition to traditional risk factors such as older age, smoking, and HCV coinfection, HIV-associated factors (CD4+ T cell count nadir) and ART factors are important predictive indicators of fracture risk in HIV-infected individuals (Yin, 2012). In the 2014 *Clinician's Guide to Prevention and Treatment of Osteoporosis*, the National Osteoporosis Foundation (NOF) included AIDS/HIV as disease risk factors for osteoporosis and fragility fractures (Battalora, 2014b; NOF 2014).

SPECIFIC TREATMENTS FOR BONE LOSS

Overton reported on results from the 48-week prospective, randomized, double-blind, placebo-controlled ACTG A5280 study evaluating the effect of high-dose vitamin D₃

(4,000 IU/d) plus calcium supplementation (1,000 mg/d calcium carbonate) on BMD in 142 HIV-infected participants (90% male; 37% non-Hispanic white, 33% non-Hispanic black, 25% Hispanic; median age, 33 years; body mass index, 24.4 kg/m^2; CD4$^+$ cell count, 341 cells/mm^3; HIV-1 RNA level, 4.5 log$_{10}$ copies/mL; and 25(OH) vitamin D, 23 ng/mL) with DXA scan data at baseline and week 48 initiating ART with efavirenz/emtricitabine/tenofovir. Vitamin D/calcium supplementation mitigated the loss of BMD seen with ART initiation of efavirenz/emtricitabine/tenofovir, particularly at the total hip (Overton, 2014).

The effect of vitamin D supplementation has been corroborated. Most notably, Havens and colleagues reported on a randomized control trial of high-dose vitamin D (Havens, 2018). In this randomized clinical trial (RCT) of 214 young PLWH (median age 22 years), high-dose vitamin D supplementation (50,000 units D3 monthly) was associated with a significant increase in lumbar spine BMD (1.2% increase vs. no change in the placebo arm). No effect was seen on the hip BMD. The group receiving vitamin D experienced a significant decline in PTH and bone turnover markers and an increase in serum vitamin D levels.

Several studies have demonstrated that oral alendronate is safe and effective for the treatment of low BMD in the setting of HIV (Mondy, 2005; McComsey, 2007). A recent publication evaluated the potential for intravenous zoledronic acid to mitigate the bone loss associated with ART (Hoy, 2018). This RCT identified PLWH on TDF with low BMD and randomized them to a switch from TDF or administration of a single dose of zoledronic acid. Zoledronic acid was safe and well-tolerated and was associated with a greater increase in BMD at the hip and lumbar spine (4.6% vs. 2.6% and 7.4% vs. 2.9%, respectively). Bisphosphonates can be safely administered to PLWH with excellent short-term results. Long-term data remain unavailable.

PATHOPHYSIOLOGY AND RISK FACTORS

Bone loss in PLWH is likely multifactorial, involving three common elements: the host, the virus, and ART. Lower bone density in PLWH is often attributable to host risks, including smoking, alcohol consumption, exposure to glucocorticoids, decreased activity, lipodystrophy, HCV coinfection, vitamin D deficiency, weight loss, hypogonadism, and chronic kidney disease. HLA supertype, particularly HLA-DQ3, has been associated with bone density status in one cohort study of HIV-positive adults (Haskelberg, 2014). HIV may directly affect bone cells by viral protein induction of osteoclastogenesis or by causing osteoblast apoptosis (Raynaud-Messina, 2018). Moreover, T cell and B cell activation during HIV infection results in increased circulating cytokines, including tumor necrosis factor-α, interleukin-6 (IL-6), and RANKL, which appear to induce osteoclast bone resorption (Titanji, 2017). In a recent study, elevated levels of IL-6 were associated with risk of progression to osteoporosis among PLWH (Hileman, 2014). Similar increases in cytokine levels have been reported in other chronic inflammatory diseases (e.g., rheumatoid arthritis).

ART initiation is associated with a BMD decrease of 2–6%, with the largest decrease occurring in the first 6–12 months of treatment and then stabilizing (Brown, 2009). Greater BMD losses occur with initiation of zidovudine (van Vonderen, 2009), TDF (McComsey 2011; Yin, 2011), and certain protease inhibitors (Duvivier, 2009; McComsey, 2011). Younger HIV-positive men and women on established ART had stable BMD (Yin, 2012). Among postmenopausal women, higher rates of loss of BMD were observed among the recipients of TDF-containing ART (Yin, 2011). Fracture rates, both fragility and nonfragility, are higher in PLWH and associated with HCV coinfection and possibly ART use (Bedimo, 2012; Maalouf, 2013; Yin, 2012; Young, 2011). Currently, the fracture incidence is estimated to be approximately 3–5 per 1,000 py, but this will likely increase as the population of HIV-infected individuals chronologically ages.

CLINICAL MANAGEMENT

SCREENING FOR BONE DISEASE

There are limited HIV-specific evidence-based recommendations regarding screening for bone disease, although extrapolation of screening recommendations from the general population is, at a minimum, reasonable.

The NOF published recommendations to clinicians for postmenopausal women and men aged 50 years or older (NOF, 2014). The reader is advised to consult the complete list of recommendations in the NOF *Clinician's Guide to Prevention and Treatment of Osteoporosis*. A brief listing of major recommendations is provided here:

- Counsel patient on risk of osteoporosis and related fractures.

- Check for secondary causes of osteoporosis.

- Advise patient on adequate amounts of calcium (at least 1,200 mg/d) and vitamin D (800–1,000 IU/d), including supplements if necessary, for individuals aged 50 years or older.

- Recommend regular weight-bearing and muscle-strengthening exercise to reduce risk of falls and fractures.

- Advise against tobacco smoking and excessive alcohol consumption.

- Recommend BMD testing in women aged 65 years or older and men aged 70 years or older.

- In postmenopausal women and men aged 50–69 years, recommend BMD testing based on risk factor profile.

- In postmenopausal women and men older than age 50 years who have had an adult-age fracture, diagnose and determine degree of osteoporosis.

- Initiate treatment in patients with hip or vertebral (clinical or morphometric) fractures.

- Initiate therapy in patients with BMD T-scores of −2.5 or less at the femoral neck or spine by DXA, after appropriate evaluation.

- Initiate treatment in postmenopausal women and men aged 50 years or older with low bone mass (T-score between −1.0 and −2.5, osteopenia) at the femoral neck or spine and a 10-year hip fracture probability 3% or greater or a 10-year major osteoporosis-related fracture probability of 20% or greater based on the US-adapted WHO absolute fracture risk model FRAX.

- Current US Food and Drug Administration (FDA)-approved pharmacologic options for osteoporosis are bisphosphonates (alendronate, alendronate, ibandronate, risedronate, and zoledronic acid), calcitonin, estrogen agonist/antagonist (raloxifene), estrogens and/or hormone therapy, tissue-selective estrogen complex (conjugated estrogens/bazedoxifene; PTH [1–34], teriparatide), and the RANKL inhibitor denosumab.

- BMD testing performed in DXA centers using accepted quality assurance measures is appropriate for monitoring bone loss.

- Patients taking FDA-approved medications should have laboratory and bone density reevaluation after 2 years or more frequently when medically appropriate (NOF, 2014).

Brown et al. recently published recommendations for evaluation and management of bone disease in HIV infection based on contributions from 34 HIV specialists from 16 countries (Brown, 2015). Noting global variation in practice and thus difficulty in determining one set of recommendations for evaluation and management of bone disease, use of FRAX without BMD is recommended for assessment of fracture risk in resource-limited settings (Brown, 2015). The reader is referred to the publication for a complete listing of recommendations and rationale.

SCREENING FOR VITAMIN D INSUFFICIENCY

Vitamin D testing and supplementation remains an area of intense debate among specialists. Three institutions have provided guidance for vitamin D deficiency. The Institute of Medicine (IOM) published dietary reference intakes for calcium and vitamin D but did not provide screening recommendations or specific reference intakes for PLWH (IOM, 2011). The Endocrine Society (EOS) and the European AIDS Clinical Society (EACS) recommended screening at-risk patients and those on ART and having risk factors for low vitamin D or fracture risks (European AIDS Clinical Society [EACS], 2015; Endocrine Society [EOS], 2011). There are limited data on vitamin D supplementation in HIV-positive patients although several studies have demonstrated benefit for BMD and reduction in PTH and bone turnover markers (Overton, 2015; Havens, 2018).

SCREENING FOR FALL RISK

Fall Risk Assessment Tools

Fall risk assessment tools are used to determine the probability of future falls. Typical categories of the assessment tools include fall risk factors (e.g., recent falls, medications, psychological, cognitive status, vision, mobility, transfer, behaviors, activities of daily living, environment, nutrition, continence, and other risk factors).

SCREENING FOR FRACTURE RISK

FRAX

FRAX was developed by the WHO Metabolic Bone Disease Group to assess fractures with more optimal predictors of fracture risk compared to T-scores (van den Bergh, 2010; WHO Metabolic Bone Disease Group, 2008). This assessment tool is not HIV-specific. FRAX provides the 10-year probability of hip fracture and the 10-year probability of a major osteoporotic fracture (hip, spine, shoulder, or forearm). Probability is estimated based on clinical risk factors (CRFs) and BMD values from the femoral neck (WHO Metabolic Bone Disease Group, 2008). Models have been developed based on location (i.e., Asia, Europe, Middle East and Africa, North America, Latin America, and Oceania) and ethnicity. CRFs included in the calculation tool are age, sex, weight (kilograms), height (centimeters), previous fracture, parent fractured hip, current tobacco smoking, exposure to glucocorticoids, rheumatoid arthritis, secondary osteoporosis, alcohol intake of three or more units per day, and BMD (g/cm^2) or, alternatively, T-score based on the NHANES III female reference data (Kanis, 2007).

The International Osteoporosis Foundation, the NOF, the American Society for Bone and Mineral Research, and the International Society for Clinical Densitometry endorse the use of FRAX (van den Bergh, 2010). NOF recommends using FRAX for postmenopausal women and men aged 50 years or older who are not on treatment, who have not had spine or hip fractures, and who have T-scores between −1.0 and −2.5 SD (NOF, 2014; van den Bergh, 2010). If the FRAX 10-year probability exceeds 20% for major osteoporotic fractures or 3% risk for hip fracture, NOF guidelines recommend drug treatment (NOF, 2014).

Increasing baseline FRAX 10-year probability was consistently associated with increased rates of incident fractures in a large cohort of HIV-infected adults (Battalora, 2014). Although FRAX may underestimate fracture risk in HIV-infected persons, EACS recommends FRAX screening in all persons older than age 40 years (EACS, 2015).

DUAL-ENERGY X-RAY ABSORPTIOMETRY

BMD measurements are widely obtained using DXA scan. Relevant measurement locations include the hip, spine, and forearm. DXA is a two-dimensional system in which the size of the specimen is directly proportional to the estimate of area density. Overestimation of BMD values obtained from larger patients is a concern (Amorosa, 2006a). Of greater concern is that DXA has not been validated for fractures among PLWH. Furthermore, fewer data exist on younger adults. Additional concerns are the application of WHO definitions for osteoporosis and osteopenia to populations and skeletal sites other than those serving as the basis for the DXA correlations on which these bone abnormality definitions are described (Amorosa, 2006b).

DXA is noninvasive and convenient, but it does not assess bone condition, bone structure, or bone quality, a factor directly linked to load-bearing strength (Ofotokun, 2011). It is suggested that DXA may underestimate fracture risk in HIV-positive persons (Ofotokun, 2011). In 2007, Nguyen and colleagues demonstrated that approximately 50% of postmenopausal women experiencing a fracture do not meet the clinical definition of osteoporosis based on DXA values (Ofotokun, 2011).

Other BMD measurement tools exist and assist in the prediction of fragility fracture risk but have inherent limitations. Quantitative CT scanning (QCT) detects volumetric density and in some clinical studies has been shown to detect a higher occurrence of osteoporosis and osteopenia (Pitukcheewanont, 2005). However, QCT costs more than DXA, requires a higher radiation dose, and is mainly used in research settings (Amorosa, 2006a). Other tools, including quantitative ultrasound and analysis of biochemical and hormonal markers, may prove increasingly useful in the future (Amorosa, 2006a).

NOF recommends DXA screening for osteoporosis in the general population of women aged 65 years or older and men aged 70 years or older, regardless of clinical risk factors (NOF, 2014). Postmenopausal women older than age 65 years, women in menopausal transition, and men aged 50–69 years with CRFs for fracture should also be screened. Men and women aged 50 years or older who have had a fracture after age 50 years and for whom other risk factors, including rheumatoid arthritis or glucocorticoid use, are observed should be screened (NOF, 2014). NOF does not provide HIV-specific guidelines for DXA screening.

The Infectious Diseases Society of America (IDSA) and HIV Medicine Association (HIVMA) recommend baseline DXA screening in HIV-positive postmenopausal women and men aged 50 years or older. Periodic monitoring of risk factors for premature bone loss is recommended thereafter (Aberg, 2014). Risk factors include white race, small body habitus, sedentary lifestyle, cigarette smoking, alcoholism, phenytoin therapy, corticosteroid therapy, hyperparathyroidism, vitamin D deficiency, thyroid disease, and hypogonadism (Aberg, 2014).

McComsey and colleagues recommend DXA screening in HIV-positive men and women aged 50 years or older because the majority of PLWH have an additional risk factor, and fracture data suggest that HIV and ART are linked to increased fracture risk (McComsey, 2010).

EACS recommends DXA screening for any patient with one or more of the following conditions, preferably prior to initiation of ART (EACS, 2015):

- Postmenopausal women
- Men aged 50 years or older
- History of low-impact fracture or high risk for falls
- Clinical hypogonadism
- Oral glucocorticoid use

TREATMENT

Treatment of low BMD depends on multiple factors, including the patient profile, risk factor reduction, and drug regimen adherence.

BEHAVIORAL AND LIFESTYLE ADVICE

Several lifestyle factors are associated with low BMD and/or fractures in the general population. Modification of diet to optimize calcium and vitamin D intake, increasing weight-bearing exercise, and smoking cessation are prudent in general but especially among persons at increased risk of low BMD or fractures. In addition, because excess alcohol consumption (>3 units/d) and substance dependency are associated with fracture risk, strategies to reduce consumption are reasonable.

IDENTIFY AND TREAT SECONDARY CAUSES OF LOW BONE MINERAL DENSITY

For persons with fragility fractures or *T*-scores of 1 or less, clinicians should evaluate and address secondary causes of osteoporosis, particularly in cases in which vitamin D deficiency or phosphate wasting are observed. These conditions can cause osteomalacia or bone mineralization deficiency, and they are difficult to differentiate from osteoporosis based on DXA scans (Yin, 2012).

VITAMIN D AND CALCIUM REPLACEMENT

Vitamin D deficiency is common among PLWH and may contribute to low BMD and/or fractures. Although there are no standardized guidelines for vitamin D and calcium replacement, the IOM published a report brief in November 2010 (revised in March 2011) providing suggested Dietary Reference Intakes for calcium and vitamin D (IOM, 2011). It suggests 1,000 mg/d of calcium for most adults aged 19–50 years and for men up to age 71 years. No more than 1,200 mg/d of calcium is suggested for women older than age 50 years and for both men and women aged 71 years or older (IOM, 2011).

Assuming minimal sun exposure in geographic regions consisting of the United States and Canada, the IOM suggests

600 IU/d of vitamin D for most persons aged 1–70 years and 800 IUs for persons aged 71 years or older (IOM, 2011).

These recommendations are not specific to HIV-infected persons. However, it appears reasonable to monitor 25-hydroxyvitamin D levels in HIV-infected individuals and provide supplementation in situations of ART initiation and continued therapy (Overton, 2014; Yin, 2012).

TESTOSTERONE REPLACEMENT

Testosterone deficiency is common among men living with HIV and is associated with increased risk of low BMD in the general population. A recent publication identified the BMD benefits of testosterone supplementation in a cohort of men living with and without HIV (Grant, 2018). Testosterone use was more frequently reported in HIV-positive men compared to HIV-negative men (4% vs. 2%, $P < 0.001$). In the overall study population, testosterone use was associated with significantly higher BMD at both the lumbar spine and hip when compared to men not receiving testosterone. Clinicians should assess the risks and benefits of testosterone replacement in persons with low BMD and low testosterone levels.

PHARMACOLOGIC INTERVENTIONS

Currently, there are no specific guidelines for the treatment of BMD disorders among PLWH. Rather, the management of bone disease among the HIV population follows guidance from the general population. The NOF recommends pharmacologic treatment of postmenopausal women and men aged 50 or older with hip or vertebral fractures or a T-score of –2.5 or less at the femoral neck or spine after evaluation to exclude secondary causes (NOF, 2014). In addition, patients with a T-score between –1.0 and –2.5 at the femoral neck or spine and 10-year probability fracture by FRAX of 3% or greater at the hip and of 20% or greater for any osteoporosis-related fracture should be considered for treatment (NOF, 2014).

Bisphosphonates are indicated for prevention and treatment of osteoporosis and other bone diseases, including Paget's disease (US Food and Drug Administration [FDA], 2013). Bisphosphonates inhibit osteoclast resorption and have been shown to reduce vertebral and nonvertebral fractures by 25–50% in HIV-negative individuals.

The effectiveness of antiresorptive therapy in HIV-infected patients has been evaluated in numerous placebo-controlled RCTs. Five studies evaluated patients with T-scores not within the osteoporotic range (Bolland, 2007; Guaraldi, 2004; Huang, 2009; McComsey, 2007; Mondy, 2005), and one trial studied patients with T-scores of less than –2.5 (Rozenberg, 2012). Resulting data showed significant increases in BMD at the lumbar spine in all six studies and a large increase at the hip in three (Bolland, 2007; Huang, 2009; McComsey, 2007). The 2-year treatment trials (Bolland, 2007; Rozenberg, 2012) demonstrated the greatest change in BMD. Notably, an increase in BMD was detected in the placebo groups that were also given calcium and vitamin D.

Adverse effects of bisphosphonates include osteonecrosis of the jaw (<1 case per 100,000 py of exposure) and subtrochanteric fractures or atypical femoral shaft fractures (uncommon in patients with <5 years of treatment) (Yin, 2012). Thus, only patients with a strong indication for treatment should be administered bisphosphonates, and the FDA expert panel recommends treatment up to 5 years (Yin, 2012).

Other treatments for osteoporosis include teriparatide, which is a recombinant form of PTH that stimulates osteoblasts and is used in patients who do not respond to bisphosphonates. However, no data exist on teriparatide's efficacy in PLWH (Yin, 2012). Denosumab, a monoclonal RANKL antibody, blocks the RANKL/RANKL interaction but may increase the likelihood of infection (Yin, 2012). For this reason, more data are needed to determine the safety of denosumab in PLWH (NOF, 2014; Yin, 2012). Hormone replacement including estrogen and raloxifene for women may be appropriate in some cases; however, there exists a risk of cardiovascular side effects (Yin, 2012).

ROLE OF ANTIRETROVIRAL THERAPY SELECTION AND SWITCH

Because TDF is associated with greater initial loss of BMD compared to other antiretrovirals, the US Department of Health and Human Services (USDHHS) HIV guidelines recommend the avoidance of TDF in patients with osteoporosis (USDHHS, 2018). Tenofovir alafenamide (TAF), a prodrug of tenofovir, is associated with less BMD loss compared to TDF in both initial and ART switch settings, and it may mitigate the BMD effect of TDF (Mills, 2016; Sax, 2014).

There are limited data on the efficacy of ART switch strategies. HIV clinicians may consider avoidance of TDF or ritonavir-boosted protease inhibitors in high-risk patients. Short-term studies showed that switching virologically suppressed patients to abacavir or raltegravir resulted in improvement in BMD compared to TDF (Haskelberg, 2012; Martin, 2009; Yin, 2012).

The field of metabolic bone disease remains a critical area of focus as the populations living with HIV are successfully aging into the seventh and eighth decades of life and beyond. Additional data are needed to identify the ideal preventive and treatment strategies for osteoporosis and fragility fractures for PLWH.

ACKNOWLEDGMENTS

The author would like to acknowledge Linda A. Battalora and Benjamin Young, who contributed to the prior version of this chapter.

REFERENCES

Aberg JA, Gallant JE, Ghanem KG, et al. Primary care guidelines for the management of persons infected with HIV: 2013 update by the HIV Medicine Association of the Infectious Diseases Society of America. *Clin Infect Dis.* January 2014;58(1):e1–e34.

Amorosa V, Tebas P. Bone disease and HIV infection. *Clin Infect Dis.* 2006a;42(1):108–114.

Amorosa V, Tebas P. Reply to Rojo and Ramos and to Vignolo et al. *Clin Infect Dis.* 2006b;43(1):113–114.

Battalora L, Buchacz K, Armon C, et al. Low bone mineral density is associated with increased risk of incident fracture in HIV-infected adults. *Antivir Ther.* 2016;21(1):45–54.

Battalora L, Buchacz K, Armon C, et al. New fracture risk and FRAX 10-year probability of fracture in HIV-infected adults. Presented at Poster Session P-Q5, Conference on Retroviruses and Opportunistic Infections (CROI), March 6, 2014a, Boston, MA. Abstract 778.

Battalora LA, Young B, Overton ET. Bones, fractures, antiretroviral therapy and HIV. *Curr Infect Dis Rep.* February 2014b;16(2):393.

Bedimo R, Maalouf NM, Zhang S, et al. Osteoporotic fracture risk associated with cumulative exposure to tenofovir and other antiretroviral agents. *AIDS.* April 24, 2012;26(7):825–831.

Bolland MJ, Grey AB, Horne AM, et al. Annual zoledronate increases bone density in highly active antiretroviral therapy-treated human immunodeficiency virus-infected men: a randomized controlled trial. *J Clin Endocrinol Metab.* April 2007;92(4):1283–1288.

Brown TT, Hoy J, Borderi M, et al. Recommendations for evaluation and management of bone disease in HIV. *Clin Infect Dis.* 2015;60:1242–1251.

Brown TT, McComsey GA, King MS, et al. Loss of bone mineral density after antiretroviral therapy initiation, independent of antiretroviral regimen. *J AIDS.* 2009;51:554–561.

Brown TT, Qaqish RB. Antiretroviral therapy and the prevalence of osteopenia and osteoporosis: a meta-analytic review. *AIDS.* November 14, 2006;20(17):2165–2174.

Dave JA, Cohen K, Micklesfield LK, et al. Antiretroviral therapy, especially efavirenz, is associated with low bone mineral density in HIV-infected South Africans. *PLoS One.* December 3, 2015;10(12):e0144286.

Duvivier C, Kolta S, Assoumou L, et al. Greater decrease in bone mineral density with protease inhibitor regimens compared with nonnucleoside reverse transcriptase inhibitor regimens in HIV-1 infected naive patients. *AIDS.* April 27, 2009;23(7):817–824.

Endocrine Society (EOS). Clinical guidelines: evaluation, treatment and prevention of vitamin D deficiency: An Endocrine Society clinical practice guideline 2011. Available at http://press.endocrine.org/doi/pdf/10.1210/jc.2011-0385. Accessed December 14, 2015.

Erlandson KM, Lake JE, Sim M, et al. Bone mineral density declines twice as quickly among HIV-infected women compared with men. *J AIDS.* March 1, 2018;77(3):288–294. PMID: 29140875.

Escota GV, Mondy K, Bush T, et al.; the SUN Study Investigators. *AIDS Research and Human Retroviruses*, 2015. doi: 10.1089/aid.2015.0158.

Escota GV, Mondy K, Bush T, et al. High prevalence of low bone mineral density and substantial bone loss over 4 years among HIV-infected persons in the era of modern antiretroviral therapy. *AIDS Res Human Retrov*, 2016;32(1):59–67.

European AIDS Clinical Society (EACS). Guidelines Version 8.0. October 2015. Available at http://www.eacsociety.org/guidelines/guidelines-archive/archive.html. Accessed December 14, 2015.

Goh SSL, Lai PSM, Tan ATB, Ponnampalavanar S. Reduced bone mineral density in human immunodeficiency virus-infected individuals: a meta-analysis of its prevalence and risk factors. *Osteoporos Int.* March 2018;29(3):595–613. PMID: 29159533.

Grant PM, Kitch D, McComsey GA, Collier AC, et al. Long-term bone mineral density changes in antiretroviral-treated HIV-infected individuals. *J Infect Dis.* August 15, 2016;214(4):607–611. PMID:27330053.

Grant PM, Li X, Jacobson LP, et al. Effect of testosterone use on bone mineral density in HIV-infected men. *AIDS Res Hum Retroviruses.* November 1, 2018. doi: 10.1089/AID.2018.0150. [Epub ahead of print] PMID: 30280921.

Guaraldi G, Orlando G, Madeddu G, et al. Alendronate reduces bone resorption in HIV-associated osteopenia/osteoporosis. *HIV Clin Trials.* September-October 2004;5(5):269–277.

Hansen AB, Gerstoft J, Kronborg G, et al. Incidence of low and high-energy fractures in persons with and without HIV infection: a Danish population-based cohort study. *AIDS.* 2012;26(3):285–293. PMID:22095195

Haskelberg H, Cordery DV, Amin J, et al. HLA alleles association with changes in bone mineral density in HIV-1-infected adults changing treatment to tenofovir–emtricitabine or abacavir–lamivudine. *PLoS One.* March 28, 2014;9(3):e93333.

Haskelberg H, Hoy JF, Amin J, et al. Changes in bone turnover and bone loss in HIV-infected patients changing treatment to tenofovir–emtricitabine or abacavir–lamivudine. *PLoS One.* 2012;7(6):e38377.

Havens PL, Stephensen CB, Van Loan MD; Adolescent Medicine Trials Network for HIV/AIDS Interventions (ATN) 109 Study Team. Vitamin D3 supplementation increases spine bone mineral density in adolescents and young adults with human immunodeficiency virus infection being treated with tenofovir disoproxil fumarate: a randomized, placebo-controlled trial. *Clin Infect Dis.* January 6, 2018a;66(2):220–228. PMID: 29020329.

Havens PL, Long D, Schuster GU; Adolescent Medicine Trials Network for HIV/AIDS Interventions (ATN) 117 and 109 study teams. Tenofovir disoproxil fumarate appears to disrupt the relationship of vitamin D and parathyroid hormone. *Antivir Ther.* September 27, 2018b. doi: 10.3851/IMP3269. [Epub ahead of print] PMID: 30260797.

Hileman CO, Labbato DE, Storer NJ, et al. Is bone loss linked to chronic inflammation in antiretroviral-naïve HIV-infected adults? A 48-week matched cohort study. *AIDS.* July 31, 2014;28(12):1759–1767.

Hoy J, Grund B, Roediger M, et al.; INSIGHT START Bone Mineral Density Substudy Group. Effects of immediate versus deferred initiation of antiretroviral therapy on bone mineral density: a substudy of the INSIGHT Strategic Timing of Antiretroviral Therapy (START) Study. Paper presented at the 15th European AIDS Conference and 17th International Workshop on Co-morbidities and Adverse Drug Reactions in HIV, Barcelona, Spain, October 21–24, 2015. Abstract ADRLH-62.

Hoy JF, Richardson R, Ebeling PR; ZEST Study Investigators. Zoledronic acid is superior to tenofovir disoproxil fumarate-switching for low bone mineral density in adults with HIV. *AIDS.* September 10, 2018;32(14):1967–1975. PMID: 29927785.

Huang J, Meixner L, Fernandez S, et al. A double-blinded, randomized controlled trial of zoledronate therapy for HIV-associated osteopenia and osteoporosis. *AIDS.* January 2, 2009;23(1):51–57.

INSIGHT START Study Group. Initiation of antiretroviral therapy in early asymptomatic HIV infection. *N Engl J Med.* 2015;373:795–807.

Institute of Medicine (IOM). *Dietary Reference Intakes for Calcium and Vitamin D.* Washington, DC: National Academies Press. 2011. Available at http://iom.nationalacademies.org/~/media/Files/Report%20Files/2010/Dietary-Reference-Intakes-for-Calcium-and-Vitamin-D/Vitamin%20D%20and%20Calcium%202010%20Report%20Brief.pdf. Accessed December 14, 2015.

Justice A, Falutz J. Aging and HIV: an evolving understanding. *Curr Opin HIV AIDS.* July 2014;9(4):291–293.

Kalayjian RC, Albert JM, Cremers S, Gupta SK; ACTG A5224s, A5303 Teams. Women have enhanced bone loss associated with phosphaturia and CD4⁺ cell restoration during initial antiretroviral therapy. *AIDS.* November 13, 2018;32(17):2517–2524. PMID: 30134291.

Kanis JA, on behalf of the World Health Organization Scientific Group. *Assessment of Osteoporosis at the Primary Health-Care Level. Technical Report.* World Health Organization Collaborating Centre for Metabolic Bone Diseases, University of Sheffield, UK. 2007: Printed by the University of Sheffield. Available at https://www.shef.ac.uk/FRAX/pdfs/WHO_Technical_Report.pdf). Accessed December 14, 2015.

Llop M, Sifuentes WA, Bañón S, et al. Increased prevalence of asymptomatic vertebral fractures in HIV-infected patients over 50 years of age. *Arch Osteoporos.* May 8, 2018;13(1):56. PMID: 29736771.

Looker AC, Wahner HW, Dunn WL, et al. Updated data on proximal femur bone mineral levels of US adults. *Osteoporosis Int.* 1998;8:468–489.

Maalouf NM, Zhang S, Drechsler H, et al. Hepatitis C co-infection and severity of liver disease as risk factor for osteoporotic fractures among HIV-infected patients. *J Bone Miner Res.* December 2013;28(12):2577–2583.

Martin A, Bloch M, Amin J, et al. Simplification of antiretroviral therapy with tenofovir–emtricitabine or abacavir–lamivudine: a randomized, 96-week trial. *Clin Infect Dis.* November 15, 2009;49(10):1591–1601.

McComsey GA, Kendall MA, Tebas P, et al. Alendronate with calcium and vitamin D supplementation is safe and effective for the treatment of decreased bone mineral density in HIV. *AIDS.* November 30, 2007;21(18):2473–2482.

McComsey GA, Kitch D, Daar ES, et al. Bone mineral density and fractures in antiretroviral-naive persons randomized to receive abacavir–lamivudine or tenofovir disoproxil fumarate–emtricitabine along with efavirenz or atazanavir-ritonavir: Aids Clinical Trials Group A5224s, a substudy of ACTG A5202. *J Infect Dis.* June 15, 2011;203(12):1791–1801.

McComsey GA, Tebas P, Shane E, et al. Bone disease in HIV infection: a practical review and recommendations for HIV care providers. *Clin Infect Dis.* October 15, 2010;51(8):937–946.

Mills A, Arribas JR, Andrade-Villanueva J, et al. Switching from tenofovir disoproxil fumarate to tenofovir alafenamide in antiretroviral regimens for virologically suppressed adults with HIV-1 infection: a randomised, active-controlled, multicentre, open-label, phase 3, non-inferiority study. *Lancet Infect Dis.* January 2016;16(1):43–52.

Mondy K, Powderly WG, Claxton SA, et al. Alendronate, vitamin D, and calcium for the treatment of osteopenia/osteoporosis associated with HIV infection. *J AIDS.* April 1, 2005;38(4):426–431.

National Osteoporosis Foundation (NOF). *Clinician's Guide to Prevention and Treatment of Osteoporosis.* Washington, DC: National Osteoporosis Foundation; 2014.

Ofotokun I, Weitzmann MN. HIV and bone metabolism. *Discov Med.* May 2011;11(60):385–393.

Orwoll ES, Klein RF. Osteoporosis in men. *Endocr Rev.* February 1995;16(1):87–116.

Overton ET, Chan ES, Brown TT, Tebas P, McComsey GA, Melbourne KM, Napoli A, Hardin WR, Ribaudo HJ, Yin MT. Vitamin D and Calcium Attenuate Bone Loss With Antiretroviral Therapy Initiation: A Randomized Trial. *Ann Intern Med.* 2015 Jun 16;162(12):815–24. PMID:26075752

Pitukcheewanont P, Safani D, Church J, et al. Bone measures in HIV-1 infected children and adolescents: disparity between quantitative computed tomography and dual-energy X-ray absorptiometry measurements. *Osteoporosis Int.* November 2005;16(11):1393–1396.

Premaor MO, Compston JE. The hidden burden of fractures in people living with HIV. *JBMR Plus.* June 20, 2018;2(5):247–256. PMID: 30283906.

Raynaud-Messina B, Bracq L, Dupont M, et al. Bone degradation machinery of osteoclasts: An HIV-1 target that contributes to bone loss.

Proc Natl Acad Sci U S A. March 13, 2018;115(11):E2556–E2565. PMID: 29463701.

Rozenberg S, Lanoy E, Bentata M, et al. Effect of alendronate on HIV-associated osteoporosis: a randomized, double-blind, placebo-controlled, 96-week trial (ANRS 120). *AIDS Res Hum Retroviruses.* September 2012;28(9):972–980.

Sax PE, Zolopa A, Brar I, et al. Tenofovir alafenamide vs. tenofovir disoproxil fumarate in single tablet regimens for initial HIV-1 therapy: a randomized phase 2 study. *J AIDS.* 2014;67(1):52–58.

Sharma A, Ma Y, Tien PC, et al. HIV infection is associated with abnormal bone microarchitecture: measurement of trabecular bone score in the Women's Interagency HIV Study. *J AIDS.* August 1, 2018;78(4):441–449. PMID: 29940603.

Shiau S, Brown EC, Arpadi SM, et al. Incident fractures in HIV-infected individuals: a systematic review and meta-analysis. *AIDS.* July 31, 2013;27(12):1949–1957.

Tebas P, Powderly WG, Claxton S, et al. Accelerated bone mineral loss in HIV-infected patients receiving potent antiretroviral therapy. *AIDS.* March 10, 2000;14(4):F63–F67.

Titanji K. Beyond antibodies: B cells and the OPG/RANK-RANKL pathway in health, non-HIV disease and HIV-induced bone loss. *Front Immunol.* December 22, 2017;8:1851. PMID:29312334.

Triant VA, Brown TT, Lee H, et al. Fracture prevalence among human immunodeficiency virus (HIV)-infected versus non-HIV-infected patients in a large US healthcare system. *J Clin Endocrinol Metab.* September 2008;93(9):3499–3504.

US Department of Health and Human Services (USDHHS), Panel on Antiretroviral Guidelines for Adults and Adolescents. Guidelines for the use of antiretroviral agents in HIV-1-infected adults and adolescents. Last Updated October 25, 2018. Available at https://www.aidsinfo.nih.gov/ContentFiles/AdultandAdolescentGL.pdf. Accessed April 2, 2019.

US Food and Drug Administration. Bisphosphonates. August 15, 2013. Available at http://www.fda.gov/drugs/drugsafety/postmarketdrugsafetyinformationforpatientsandproviders/ucm124165.htm. Accessed December 14, 2015.

van den Bergh JP, van Geel TA, Lems WF, et al. Assessment of individual fracture risk: FRAX and beyond. *Curr Osteoporosis Rep.* September 2010;8(3):131–137.

van Vonderen MG, Lips P, van Agtmael MA, et al. First line zidovudine/lamivudine/lopinavir/ritonavir leads to greater bone loss compared to nevirapine/lopinavir/ritonavir. *AIDS.* July 17, 2009;23(11):1367–1376.

Womack JA, Goulet JL, Gibert C, et al. Increased risk of fragility fractures among HIV infected compared to uninfected male veterans. *PloS One.* 2011;6(2):e17217.

Woolf AD, Pfleger B. Burden of major musculoskeletal conditions. *Bull World Health Organization.* 2003;81(9):646–656.

World Health Organization (WHO). WHO manual of diagnostic imaging. 2002. Available at http://apps.who.int/iris/bitstream/10665/42457/1/9241545550_eng.pdf. Accessed December 14, 2015.

World Health Organization (WHO). WHO Technical Report Series 843: assessment of fracture risk and its application to screening for postmenopausal osteoporosis. Report of a WHO Study Group. *World Health Organ Tech Rep Ser.* 1994;843:1–129. PMID: 7941614.

World Health Organization (WHO). Metabolic Bone Disease Group. FRAX tool. 2008. Available at http://www.shef.ac.uk/FRAX. Accessed December 15, 2015.

Yin M. Bone loss in HIV: virus, host or ART. Paper presented at the Conference on Retroviruses and Opportunistic Infections (CROI), March 5–8, 2012a, Seattle, WA.

Yin MT, Overton ET. Increasing clarity on bone loss associated with antiretroviral initiation. *J Infect Dis.* June 15, 2011;203(12):1705–1707.

Yin MT, Shi Q, Hoover DR, et al. Fracture incidence in HIV-infected women: results from the Women's Interagency HIV Study. *AIDS.* November 13, 2010;24(17):2679–2686.

Yin MT, Zhang CA, McMahon DJ, et al. Higher rates of bone loss in postmenopausal HIV-infected women: a longitudinal study. *J Clin Endocrinol Metab.* February 2012b;97(2):554–562.

Young B, Dao CN, Buchacz K, et al. Increased rates of bone fracture among HIV-infected persons in the HIV Outpatient Study (HOPS) compared with the US general population, 2000–2006. *Clin Infect Dis.* April 15, 2011;52(8):1061–1068.

47.

HIV-ASSOCIATED LIPODYSTROPHY AND LIPOATROPHY

Rajagopal V. Sekhar

CHAPTER GOAL

Upon completion of this chapter, the reader should be able to
- Understand about HIV associate lipodystrophy and lipoatrophy.

INTRODUCTION

The advent of combination antiretroviral therapy (ART) in the mid to late 1990s resulted in significant health benefits for patients infected with HIV by reducing AIDS-related mortality and increasing life expectancy. Additional collateral benefits were an improvement in nutritional status and a reduction in HIV-associated opportunistic infections. In parallel with these benefits, HIV patients began to develop unusual changes in body habitus with variable combinations of loss of peripheral fat in the limbs, buttocks, and face (termed *lipoatrophy*) and central fat accumulation in the abdomen (termed *lipohypertrophy*). These changes were described as a lipodystrophic syndrome afflicting HIV patients (Carr, 1998), and the condition was referred to as *HIV-associated lipodystrophy* (HAL).

Although the origins of HAL are unclear, its onset has been associated with several factors. Since improvements in ART regimens have increased the life span of HIV patients, it is possible that the HAL phenotype is simply a representation of HIV as a chronic disease. The specific effects of antiretroviral medications have also been implicated. The initial usage of combination ART in the 1990s was accompanied by multiple reports of abnormalities in body fat distribution linked to the protease inhibitor (PI) and nucleoside reverse transcriptase inhibitor (NRTI) classes of drugs, with terminologies ranging from "protease paunch," "Crixivan belly," and "buffalo hump" to reporting breast enlargement (Munk, 1997; Mishriki, 1998; Vazquez, 1999, Carr, 1998; Herry, 1997; Lo, 1998; Massip, 1997; Miller, 1998). Factors other than ART agents implicated in the pathogenesis of HAL include immune phenomenon and effects mediated directly by HIV itself. However, despite two decades of intensive research to understand the mechanistic underpinnings of HIV lipodystrophy and lipoatrophy, the answers continue to remain elusive (Bacchetti, 2005a, 2005b; Safrin, 1999; Sattler, 2003; Tien, 2004).

LEARNING OBJECTIVE

Discuss the established and evolving science regarding the diagnosis and treatment of HIV-associated lipodystrophy and lipoatrophy.

WHAT'S NEW?

- The incidence of new-onset lipoatrophy is declining.
- There is a greater risk and prevalence of abdominal obesity.

KEY POINTS

- HIV is associated with abnormal fat distribution, which is termed *lipodystrophy*.
- HIV lipodystrophy can manifest as fat loss (lipoatrophy), fat gain (lipohypertrophy), or a mixed pattern.
- Therapeutic options are limited, and treatment is challenging.
- HIV lipodystrophy is associated with increased risk of developing cardiovascular disease (CVD) and also fat accumulation in the liver.

LIPODYSTROPHY, LIPOHYPERTROPHY, AND LIPOATROPHY

"Lipodystrophy" is a broad term that collectively describes a variable combination of accumulation of fat in several regions, such as the abdomen (Engelson, 1999; Miller, 1998; Vigano, 2005; Yin, 2005); interscapular dorsocervical region, termed the "buffalo hump" (Lo, 1998; Roth, 1998; Torres, 1999); and the submental region, where it was termed the "bull neck," Meinrenken, 1998), together with a simultaneous loss of fat from the limbs, face, and buttocks (Bacchetti, 2005a, 2005b; Carr, 1998; Lichtenstein, 2003; Martin, 2005; Parruti, 2005). This "mixed" pattern of lipodystrophy includes a variable and simultaneous expression of both lipoatrophy (fat loss) and lipohypertrophy (fat gain) occurring concomitantly in the same patient. These abnormalities in body habitus are often accompanied by distinct biochemical abnormalities, including dyslipidemia (mainly hypertriglyceridemia) and insulin resistance (Tsiodras, 2000; van der Valk, 2001). The US Cholesterol Education Program Adult Treatment Panel III (ATP III) defines metabolic syndrome to include three of the following five criteria: increased waist circumference (>102 cm men, >88 cm women), increased triglycerides (>150 ng/dL), reduced high-density lipoprotein cholesterol (HDL-C; <40 mg/dL men, <50 mg/dL women), high blood pressure (>130/>85 mm Hg), and elevated fasting glucose (>110 mg/dL) (National Cholesterol Education Program, 2001). A study that evaluated HIV patients reported a 14% prevalence of metabolic syndrome by the International Diabetes Federation criteria and 18% by ATP III criteria (Samaras, 2007). In effect, the changes associated with HIV-associated lipodystrophy, especially with the mixed pattern, resemble an accelerated form of metabolic syndrome.

DEFINITION AND PREVALENCE OF HAL

The initial description of HIV-associated lipodystrophy by Carr et al. in 1998 was followed by a flood of reports of HAL prevalence in the scientific community, but the prevalence varied widely due to the absence of a consensus case definition, leading to wide fluctuations in the clinical diagnosis of HAL (Carter, 2001). Since it became necessary to have a standard and uniformly accepted case definition for HAL, the HIV Lipodystrophy Case Definition Study Group developed a statistical model for the diagnosis of lipodystrophy (including age, sex, duration of HIV infection, HIV disease stage, waist-to-hip ratio [WHR], anion gap, serum HDL-C concentration, trunk-to-peripheral fat ratio, percentage leg fat, and intra- and extra-abdominal fat ratio as variables), with a quantitative scale for identification (Carr, 2003a, 2003b). This model identified HIV lipodystrophy with a fair degree of accuracy, but it required multiple parameters whose measurement was not feasible or practical in a clinical outpatient setting. Thus, the field is still challenged by the lack of a simple, effective, standardized, practical, clinically applicable, and relevant case definition for HIV-associated lipodystrophy. The current practical approach to the patient with mixed lipodystrophy is for the treating physician to document objective evidence of central obesity and peripheral lipoatrophy, with evidence of dyslipidemia, insulin resistance, or both.

Despite these uncertainties, HIV infection was associated with an increased prevalence of lipodystrophy at the turn of the century, with multiple studies reporting peripheral fat wasting, increased central fat accumulation, or both in HIV-infected patients (Worm, 2002; Bergersen, 2004; Bernasconi, 2002; Miller, 2003; Saint-Marc, 2000), with a higher association of lipoatrophy with the use of nucleoside analogue therapy, especially stavudine (Saint-Marc, 1999; Chêne, 2002; Bernasconi, 2002). When fat accumulation and fat loss were analyzed, it was found that the prevalence of fat accumulation was 56%, that of fat loss was 24%, and the mixed form occurred in 83% of patients infected with HIV (Safrin, 1999). More stringent analyses of the relative prevalence of the individual components of lipodystrophy have reported on average 45% central obesity, up to 62% for any lipodystrophy, and 38%

for peripheral lipoatrophy (Lichtenstein, 2004; Paparizos, 2000; Rozenbaum, 1999; Saves, 2002; Tien, 2004). HAL has also been described to affect children. A study from India found that lipodystrophy was observed in 33.7% of children, with lipoatrophy being the most common subtype, followed by lipohypertrophy (Bhutia, 2014). These data confirm a significant presence of the lipodystrophic phenotype in the HIV-infected population. However, since the use of stavudine appeared to be closely linked to lipoatrophy, phasing out the use of stavudine has lowered the incidence of new-onset lipoatrophy (Ribera, 2008; Innes, 2018). Alongside these changes, the risk of abdominal obesity in PLWH appears to be rising for any given body mass index (BMI), and the excess odds of abdominal obesity was stronger with older age, hypertension, and hypertriglyceridemia (Gelpi, 2018). This is also the clinical experience of this author, where the incidence of de novo HAL with a mixed pattern of lipodystrophy has declined significantly over the past decade, especially with almost no patients presenting with lipoatrophy, although the proportion of patients with abdominal obesity has skyrocketed. These observed changes could be due to the advent of improved and newer classes of ART agents, suggesting that older ART drugs may have played a great contributory role in the pathogenesis of HAL than originally suspected. An alternate possibility is that when lipodystrophy was described in the 1990s, it could simply have been a coincidental juxtaposition of nucleoside analogue–induced lipoatrophy, abdominal obesity due to other causes, and a coincidental occurrence of both phenotypes in some patients—this suggestion provides the most parsimonious explanation to link the HAL phenotype from the 1990s to the current phenotype of abdominal obesity with its associated metabolic and cardiovascular risk profile. The lipoatrophic phenotype is rapidly disappearing, whereas the central obesity phenotype persists and is increasing in its prevalence. Clearly, additional studies are needed to understand the dynamic evolution of the HIV body phenotype. Despite these observations, since HAL is linked to an increased risk of metabolic complications, including CVD, diabetes, and liver fat accumulation, it is still important to understand the underlying contributory mechanisms.

DIAGNOSING HAL

The clinical diagnosis of HAL is based on multiple approaches, including self-reporting, use of questionnaires, clinical scales with scores, anthropometric formulas, and radiographic techniques. Standard anthropometric tests have the advantage of being readily available to clinicians (Schwenk, 2001, 2002). Computed tomography, magnetic resonance imaging, and dual-energy X-ray absorptiometry (DXA) scans provide quantifiable data on the location and mass of visceral fat and subcutaneous adipose tissue (Schambelan, 2002) and subcutaneous limb fat (Cavalcanti, 2005). However, the usefulness of these imaging modalities in the outpatient clinical setting is limited due to considerable expense, limited availability, radiation exposure, and dependence on single-slice data instead of whole-body studies. Therefore, they are impractical for use in routine clinical practice. A study of 100 patients on ART used DXA scan for anthropometric measures and proposed a fat mass ratio of 1.26, waist:thigh ratio of 1.74, and arm:trunk ratio of 2.08 to diagnose lipodystrophy (Beraldo, 2015). Routine measurement of waist circumference and/or WHR may be helpful and is recommended for all patients, especially since the phenotype of central fat accumulation is much more prevalent now in HIV patients.

MECHANISMS UNDERLYING THE DEVELOPMENT OF HAL

The notion of fat loss in some regions of the body concomitant with fat accumulation in other regions has led to questions of whether fat is reciprocally "redistributed" from one site to another. However, evidence to support this hypothesis is lacking. A large cross-sectional study of HIV-infected and uninfected patients did not find any correlation between changes in central and peripheral fat in HIV-infected men (Bacchetti, 2005a, 2005b). These data suggest that, in HIV, central fat accumulation and peripheral fat loss are independent of each other, which means that two distinctly separate phenomena were operating in these patients—one to cause lipoatrophy and the other to cause abdominal obesity.

Several mechanistic studies using stable isotope tracer methodologies shed light on some of the fundamental biochemical defects underlying HIV (Reeds, 2003; Sekhar, 2002). It has been shown that HAL is associated with accelerated rates of adipocyte lipolysis. Although there is a significant increase in adipocyte re-esterification, most of the fatty acids released by adipocyte lipolysis are released into the plasma. Since oxidation of plasma fatty acids is blunted, they are available for increased re-esterification and accumulation in the liver and the central compartment, including the abdomen. These fundamental defects may account for the phenotypic appearance of lipodystrophy, where lipoatrophy may be accounted for by the increased lipolysis, and lipohypertrophy in selected sites may be the result of increased adipocyte re-esterification. In addition, the increased delivery of fatty acids to the liver raises the possibility of an increased risk of fatty liver disease, which is increasingly being described in patients with HIV. The factors contributing to these metabolic defects are unclear, but antiretroviral drugs, immune phenomena, adipokines, and HIV itself are involved.

Antiretroviral drugs have been implicated in the mechanistic origins of HAL. Stavudine, in particular, has been linked to the development of lipoatrophy (Saint-Marc, 1999; Chêne, 2002; Bernasconi, 2002), and incidence of lipoatrophy appears to recede significantly after discontinuing stavudine as part of standard ART regimens in recent years (Ribera, 2008; Innes, 2018). PI agents have been linked to the development of lipohypertrophy. A study used a human preadipocyte cell line and found that ritonavir caused massive apoptosis, whereas atazanavir triggered both autophagy and mitophagy (Gibellini, 2012). The progression of HAL has been a dynamic process with a high incidence and prevalence in the late 1990s and early 2000s, but that of decreasing lipoatrophy and increasing central obesity since that time. As patients with HAL are living longer lives and there are continual improvements and changes in the use of ART, it is important to follow and monitor the natural progression of HAL in these patients.

CLINICAL IMPLICATIONS OF HAL

Patients with HAL may experience several clinical complications as a result of lipodystrophy. Abdominal obesity and peripheral lipoatrophy lead to the psychological discomfort of a potentially disfiguring condition (Persson, 2005; Turner, 2006; Peterson, 2008). Abdominal obesity may also produce physical discomfort from abdominal distension, along with the potential for umbilical herniation and gastroesophageal reflux disease (Miller, 2003). Visceral fat accumulation has also been linked to an elevated risk of developing insulin resistance, CVD, and liver fat accumulation and fatty liver. In addition, visceral fat accumulation is a known predictor of all-cause mortality in non–HIV-infected people (Kuk, 2006).

DYSLIPIDEMIA

The increased association of HAL with dyslipidemia and its management are discussed in Chapter 43.

INSULIN RESISTANCE

Patients with HAL have an increased predisposition to insulin resistance and possibly diabetes mellitus. The contributing factors include antiretroviral drugs, lipotoxicity, immunocytokine factors, and hepatic steatosis. An estimated 30–90% of patients receiving PI agents are insulin resistant, although the incidence of diabetes mellitus is less than 10% (van der Valk, 2001). Lipodystrophy (peripheral lipoatrophy and/or lipohypertrophy) and the presence of the dorsocervical fat pad or "buffalo hump" are linked to hyperinsulinemia and insulin resistance (Balasubramanyam, 2004; Calza, 2004; Hadigan, 2006; Miller, 1998).

Antiretroviral drugs also play a role in the development of insulin resistance in HIV. Drugs from the PI class of agents predispose to insulin resistance by inhibiting the insulin-sensitive glucose transporter Glut4 (Mallon, 2005), and 35% of patients in a study were reported to have developed insulin resistance on PI therapy (Murata, 2002). PIs also predispose to impaired glucose tolerance and fasting hyperinsulinemia (Hadigan, 2001). NRTI drugs, especially the thymidine analogs, also promote insulin resistance in HIV, induce lipotoxicity by disrupting mitochondrial oxidative phosphorylation, and cause defective mitochondrial fatty acid oxidation.

Defective lipid kinetics together with impaired fat oxidation (Reeds, 2003; Sekhar, 2002, 2005) promote accumulation of ectopic fat in critical metabolic sites of insulin action (e.g., liver and skeletal muscle), resulting in insulin resistance (Gan, 2002; Sutinen, 2002). Studies in rodents and humans have reported that correcting the deficiency of the endogenous antioxidant glutathione (GSH) significantly improves insulin sensitivity. A study used the gold standard "hyperinsulinemic–euglycemic clamp" to measure insulin sensitivity and found that improving levels of GSH using oral supplementation with N-acetylcysteine and glycine in HIV-infected patients increased insulin sensitivity by 32% within 2 weeks (Nguyen, 2014). HAL is associated with defects in adipocyte function that result in altered secretion of critical adipokines such as adiponectin. Deficiency of adiponectin is strongly linked to insulin resistance, and it also occurs in patients with HAL (Addy, 2003; Kim, 2007; Samaras, 2007).

CARDIOVASCULAR RISKS

HIV-positive patients have an elevated risk of CVD (d'Arminio, 2004; Friis-Moller, 2003) and acute myocardial infarction (Hadigan, 2003; Mary-Krause, 2003; Varriale, 2004; Triant, 2007; Friis-Moller, 2007; Glesby, 2018; Beires, 2018) (see Chapter 42). The mechanistic underpinnings of this increased risk are complex and likely include a combination of factors, including adipocyte dysfunction, excessive lipolysis, hypertriglyceridemia, elevated low-density lipoprotein cholesterol (LDL-C) and decreased HDL-C, proatherogenic lipoprotein particle sizes with small dense LDL-C, postprandial lipemia, diabetes, adipokine, and immunokine factors, and increased carotid intimal thickness.

RENAL COMPLICATIONS

HIV lipodystrophy may adversely affect renal function. Data from the LIPOKID study, a prospective cohort study of HIV patients in Switzerland published in 2018 suggests that HAL is independently associated with chronic kidney disease (CKD) (Bouatou, 2018). It is not clear whether this is unique to HAL since renal complications have also been described in patients with generalized lipodystrophy (Akinci, 2018) (see Chapter 43). Nonetheless, it is important to regularly monitor renal function in the clinical care of HIV patients with features of lipodystrophy.

SYSTEMIC STEATOSIS

There are reports of hepatic and intramyocellular fat accumulation in HAL. In HIV, fatty liver may be induced by a combination of factors, including coinfection with viral hepatitis B or C, chronic inflammation, and metabolic defects in lipid cycling as described previously (Ristig, 2005). Interestingly, in patients with HAL, insulin resistance appears to be related to hepatic fat accumulation more than intra-abdominal fat accumulation (Sutinen, 2002). Excess circulating free fatty acids due to excessive lipolysis can be stored in other ectopic sites and contribute to systemic steatosis. An important site for fat deposition is skeletal muscle, and elevated levels of intramyocellular triglycerides have been reported in the soleus and tibialis anterior muscles (Luzi, 2003). An important consequence of increased myocellular fat is the development of insulin resistance in these patients.

ECTOPIC FAT ACCUMULATION

In patients with HAL, ectopic fat accumulation occurs in the interscapular dorsocervical "buffalo hump" area and the submental "bull neck" area (Lo, 1998). Such patterns of ectopic fat accumulation predispose to other comorbidities, such as obstructive sleep apnea, limited neck motion, and neck and back discomfort (Gold, 2005; Reynolds, 2006).

METABOLIC SYNDROME

Not surprisingly, the combination of the previously discussed defects has led to an increase in metabolic syndrome in many of these HIV patients. A study of HIV-positive Hispanic patients found that the presence of lipodystrophy was associated with a higher prevalence of metabolic syndrome (69%) compared to nonlipodystrophic patients (39%) (Ramirez-Marrero, 2014).

TREATMENT OF HAL PHENOTYPE

Currently, there is no single therapy for all the components of HAL. Medical management has included trials of underlying pathophysiological defects, including the use of thiazolidinedione drugs to increase fat deposition in lipodystrophic sites. Although data from clinical studies are conflicting (Carr, 2004; Hadigan, 2004; Sutinen, 2003), a small stable isotope-based study examining the interplay of kinetic factors suggested that rosiglitazone usage increased fat deposition, but this benefit was offset by elevated rates of lipolysis and the inability of adipocytes to retain triglycerides (Sekhar, 2011).

Growth hormone (GH) has been used in an attempt to lower abdominal fat, but doses used were supraphysiological. Using GH at a physiological dose resulted in a decrease in lipolysis (D'Amico, 2006), and newer approaches using combinations of thiazolidinedione and GH could be useful and should be studied. The GH analog tesamorelin (Egrifta) was approved by the US Food and Drug Administration (FDA) in 2010 and has been shown to have benefits in lowering central fat and improving dyslipidemia (Falutz, 2007). Use of this product has been limited by cost and the need for daily subcutaneous injections. A recent rodent study has shown that farnesyltransferase inhibitors (FTIs) tipifarnib and lonafarnib were successful in preventing lipodystrophy and metabolic syndrome induced by lopinavir/ritonavir in mice (Tanaka, 2018). Further studies are needed to understand the role of FTIs in human patients with HAL.

Surgical treatment of excess fat accumulation has been attempted with liposuction, but long-term success is limited by the tendency of fat to reaccumulate. Facial lipoatrophy has been treated with lipofilling with autologous fat transfer (Uzzan, 2012); polyalkylimide gel (De Santis, 2012) and other artificial fillers including silicone have been tried with psychological improvement in body image perception (Mori, 2006). The treatment of dyslipidemia, insulin resistance, and other complications is discussed elsewhere in this text.

CONCLUSION

HIV infection and ART have been associated with lipodystrophy and lipoatrophy. Although these complications affected many patients in the mid to late 1990s and early 2000s, the relative incidences of lipoatrophy and lipohypertrophy are changing over time, with a decrease in the former and an increase in the latter, especially as seen in the aging HIV population. Nevertheless, these changes in body morphology are complicated by physical symptoms due to the nature of fat accumulation, psychological discomfort due to abnormal body image perception, and metabolic complications such as dyslipidemia and insulin resistance with an increased risk of CVD and fatty liver. Urgent therapies are needed for these complications because current therapeutic options are limited. There is an important need for further research to find effective therapeutic interventions for the metabolic and cardiovascular complications afflicting patients with HAL.

REFERENCES

Addy CL, Gavrila A, Tsiodras S, et al. Hypoadiponectinemia is associated with insulin resistance, hypertriglyceridemia, and fat redistribution in human immunodeficiency virus-infected patients treated with highly active antiretroviral therapy. *J Clin Endocrinol Metab.* 2003;88:627–636.

Akinci B, Unlu SM, Simsir IY, et al. Renal complications of lipodystrophy: a closer look at the natural history of kidney disease. *Clin Endocrinol.* July 2018;89(1):65–75. doi: 10.1111/cen.13732. Epub 2018 May 17.

Bacchetti P, Gripshover B, Grunfeld C, et al.; Study of Fat Redistribution and Metabolic Change in HIV Infection (FRAM). Fat distribution in men with HIV infection. *J AIDS.* 2005a;40(2):121–131.

Bacchetti P, Gripshover B, Grunfeld C, et al. Fat distribution in men with HIV infection. *J AIDS.* 2005b;40:121–131.

Balasubramanyam A, Sekhar RV, Jahoor F, et al. Pathophysiology of dyslipidemia and increased cardiovascular risk in HIV lipodystrophy: a model of "systemic steatosis." *Curr Opin Lipidol.* 2004;15:59–67.

Beires MT, Silva-Pinto A, Santos AC, et al. Visceral adipose tissue and carotid intima-media thickness in HIV-infected patients undergoing cART: a prospective cohort study. *BMC Infect Dis.* January 11, 2018;18(1):32

Beraldo RA, Vassimon HS, Aragon DC, et al. Proposed ratios and cutoffs for the assessment of lipodystrophy in HIV-seropositive individuals. *Eur J Clin Nutr.* February 2015;69(2):274–278.

Bouatou Y, Gayet Ageron A, Bernasconi E et al. Lipodystrophy increases the risk of CKD development in HIV positive patients in Switzerland: the LIPOKID study. *Kidney Int Rep.* May 8, 2018;3(5):1089–1099.

Bergersen BM, Sandvik L, Bruun JN. Body composition changes in 308 Norwegian HIV-positive patients. *Scand J Infect Dis.* 2004;36:186–191.

Bernasconi E, Boubaker K, Junghans C, et al. Abnormalities of body fat distribution in HIV-infected persons treated with antiretroviral drugs: the Swiss HIV Cohort Study. *J AIDS.* 2002;31:50–55.

Bhutia E, Hemal A, Yadav TP, et al. Lipodystrophy syndrome among HIV infected children on highly active antiretroviral therapy in northern India. *Afr Health Sci.* June 2014;14(2):408–413.

Calza L, Manfredi R, Chiodo F. Insulin resistance and diabetes mellitus in HIV infected patients receiving antiretroviral therapy. *Metab Syndr Relat Disord.* 2004;2:241–250.

Carr A, Emery S, Law M, et al. An objective case definition of lipodystrophy in HIV-infected adults: a case–control study. *Lancet.* 2003a;361:726–735.

Carr A, Law M. An objective lipodystrophy severity grading scale derived from the lipodystrophy case definition score. *J AIDS.* 2003b;33:571–576.

Carr A, Samaras K, Burton S, et al. A syndrome of peripheral lipodystrophy, hyperlipidemia and insulin resistance in patients receiving HIV protease inhibitors. *AIDS.* 1998;12:F51–F58.

Carr A, Workman C, Carey D, et al. No effect of rosiglitazone for treatment of HIV-1: randomized, double-blind, placebo-controlled trial. *Lancet.* 2004;363(9407):429–438.

Carter VM, Hoy JF, Bailey M et al. The prevalence of lipodystrophy in an ambulant HIV-infected population: it all depends on the definition. *HIV Med.* July 2001;2(3):174–180.

Cavalcanti RB, Cheung AM, Raboud J, et al. Reproducibility of DXA estimations of body fat in HIV lipodystrophy: implications for clinical research. *J Clin Densitom.* 2005;8:293–297.

Chêne G, Angelini E, Cotte L, et al. Role of long-term nucleoside-analogue therapy in lipodystrophy and metabolic disorders in human immunodeficiency virus-infected patients. *Clin Infect Dis.* March 1, 2002;34(5):649–657.

D'Amico S, Shi J, Sekhar RV, et al. Physiologic growth hormone replacement improves fasting lipid kinetics in patients with HIV lipodystrophy syndrome. *Am J Clin Nutr.* 2006;84(1):204–211.

d'Arminio A, Sabin CA, Phillips AN, et al. Cardio- and cerebrovascular events in HIV-infected persons. *AIDS.* 2004;18(13):1811–1817.

De Santis G, Pignatti M, Baccarani A, et al. Long-term efficacy and safety of polyacrylamide hydrogel injection in the treatment of human immunodeficiency virus-related facial lipoatrophy: a 5-year follow-up. *Plastic Reconstruct Surg.* 2012;129(1):101–109.

Engelson ES, Kotler DP, Tan Y, et al. Fat distribution in HIV-infected patients reporting truncal enlargement quantified by whole-body magnetic resonance imaging. *Am J Clin Nutr.* 1999;69:1162–1169.

Falutz J, Allas S, Blot K, et al. Metabolic effects of a growth hormone-releasing factor in patients with HIV. *N Engl J Med.* 2007;357(23):2359–2370.

Friis-Moller N, Reiss P, Sabin CA, et al. Class of antiretroviral drugs and the risk of myocardial infarction. *N Engl J Med.* 2007;356:1723–1735.

Friis-Moller N, Weber R, Reiss P, et al. Cardiovascular disease risk factors in HIV patients—association with antiretroviral therapy. Results from the D:A:D study. *AIDS.* 2003;17(8):1179–1193.

Gan SK, Samaras K, Thompson CH, et al. Altered myocellular and abdominal fat partitioning predict disturbance in insulin action in HIV protease inhibitor-related lipodystrophy. *Diabetes.* 2002;51:3163–3169.

Gelpi M, Afzal S, Lundgren J, et al. Higher risk of abdominal obesity, elevated LDL cholesterol, hypertriglyceridemia, but not of hypertension in PLWH: results from the Copenhagen Comorbidity in HIV Infection (COCOMO) Study. *Clin Infect Dis.* February 17, 2018. doi: 10.1093/cid/ciy146.

Gibellini L, De Biasi S, Pinto M et al. The protease inhibitor atazanavir triggers autophagy and mitochoagy in human preadipocytes. *AIDS* October 23, 2012;26(16):2017–2026.

Glesby MJ, Hanna DB, Hoover DR, et al. Abdominal fat depots and subclinical carotid artery atherosclerosis in women with and without HIV Infection. *J AIDS.* March 1, 2018;77(3):308–316

Gold DR, Annino DJ, Jr. HIV-associated cervicodorsal lipodystrophy: etiology and management. *Laryngoscope.* 2005;115:791–795.

Hadigan C, Kamin D, Liebau J, et al. Depot-specific regulation of glucose uptake and insulin sensitivity in HIV-lipodystrophy. *Am J Physiol Endocrinol Metab.* 2006;290:E289–E298.

Hadigan C, Meigs JB, Corcoran C, et al. Metabolic abnormalities and cardiovascular disease risk factors in adults with human immunodeficiency virus infection and lipodystrophy. *Clin Infect Dis.* 2001;32:130–139.

Hadigan C, Meigs JB, Wilson PW, et al. Prediction of coronary heart disease risk in HIV-infected patients with fat redistribution. *Clin Infect Dis.* 2003;36:909–916.

Hadigan C, Yawetz S, Thomas A, et al. Metabolic effects of rosiglitazone in HIV lipodystrophy: a randomized, controlled trial. *Ann Intern Med.* 2004;140(10):786–794.

Herry I, Bernard L, de Truchis P, et al. Hypertrophy of the breasts in a patient treated with indinavir. *Clin Infect Dis.* 1997;25:937–938.

Innes S, Harvery J, Collins IJ et al. Lipoatrophy/lipohypertrophy outcomes after antiretroviral therapy switch in children in the UK/Ireland. *PLoS One.* 2018;13(4):e0194132.

Kim RJ, Carlow DC, Rutstein JH, et al. Hypoadiponectinemia, dyslipidemia, and impaired growth in children with HIV-associated facial lipoatrophy. *J Pediatr Endocrinol Metab.* 2007;20:65–74.

Kuk JL, Katzmarzyk PT, Nichaman MZ, et al. Visceral fat is an independent predictor of all-cause mortality in men. *Obesity (Silver Spring).* 2006;14:336–341.

Lichtenstein K, Wanke C, Henry K, et al. Estimated prevalence of HIV-associated adipose redistribution syndrome (HARS): abnormal abdominal fat accumulation in HIV-infected patients. *Antiviral Ther.* 2004;9: L33.

Lichtenstein KA, Delaney KM, Armon C, et al. Incidence of and risk factors for lipoatrophy (abnormal fat loss) in ambulatory HIV-1-infected patients. *J AIDS.* 2003;32:48–56.

Lo JC, Mulligan K, Tai VW, et al. "Buffalo hump" in men with HIV-1 infection. *Lancet.* 1998;351:867–870.

Luzi L, Perseghin G, Tambussi G, et al. Intramyocellular lipid accumulation and reduced whole body lipid oxidation in HIV lipodystrophy. *Am J Physiol Endocrinol Metab.* 2003;284: E274–E280.

Mallon PW, Wand H, Law M, et al.; HIV Lipodystrophy Case Definition Study; Australian Lipodystrophy Prevalence Survey Investigators. Buffalo hump seen in HIV-associated lipodystrophy is associated with hyperinsulinemia but not dyslipidemia. *J AIDS.* 2005;38:156–162.

Martin A, Mallon PW. Therapeutic approaches to combating lipoatrophy: do they work? *J Antimicrob Chemother.* 2005;55:612–615.

Mary-Krause M, Cotte L, Simon A, et al. Increased risk of myocardial infarction with duration of protease inhibitor therapy in HIV-infected men. *AIDS.* 2003;17(17):2479–2486.

Massip P, Marchou B, Bonnet E, et al. Lipodystrophy with protease inhibitors in HIV patients. *Thérapie.* 1997;52:615.

Meinrenken S. "Bull-neck" in HIV-positive patients: result of therapy? *Disch Med Wochenschr.* May 22, 1998;22:123(21):A9.

Miller J, Carr A, Emery S, et al. HIV lipodystrophy: prevalence, severity and correlates of risk in Australia. *HIV Med.* 2003;4:293–301.

Miller KD, Jones E, Yanovski JA, et al. Visceral abdominal-fat accumulation associated with use of indinavir. *Lancet.* 1998;351:871–875.

Mishriki YY. A baffling case of bulging belly. Protease paunch. *Postgrad Med.* September 1998;104(3):45–46.

Mori A, Lo Russo G, Agostini T, et al. Treatment of human immunodeficiency virus-associated facial lipoatrophy with lipofilling and submalar silicone implants. *J Plastic Reconstruct Aesthetic Surg.* 2006;59(11):1209–1216.

Munk B. Protease paunch? *Posit Aware.* November-December 1997;8(6):20–21.

Murata H, Hruz PW, Mueckler M. Indinavir inhibits the glucose transporter isoform Glut4 at physiologic concentrations. *AIDS.* 2002;16:859–863.

National Cholesterol Education Program. Executive summary of the third report of the National Cholesterol Education Program (NCEP) Expert Panel on Detection, Evaluation, and Treatment of High Blood Cholesterol in Adults (Adult Treatment Panel III). *JAMA.* 2001;285:2486–2497.

Nguyen D, Hsu JW, Jahoor F, et al. Effect of increasing glutathione with cysteine and glycine supplementation on mitochondrial fuel oxidation, insulin sensitivity, and body composition in older HIV-infected patients. *J Clin Endocrinol Metab.* January 2014;99(1):169–177.

Paparizos VA, Kyriakis KP, Polydorou-Pfandl D, et al. Epidemiologic characteristics of Koebner's phenomenon in AIDS-related Kaposi's sarcoma. *J AIDS.* 2000;25:283–284.

Parruti G, Toro GM. Persistence of lipoatrophy after a four-year long interruption of antiretroviral therapy for HIV1 infection: case report. *BMC Infect Dis.* 2005;5:80.

Persson A. Facing HIV: body shape change and the (in) visibility of illness. *Med Anthropol.* 2005;24:237–264.

Peterson S, Martins CR, Cofranscesci J Jr. Lipodystrophy in the patient with HIV: social, psychological and treatment considerations. *Anesthet Surg J.* July-August 2008;28(4):443–451.

Ramírez-Marrero FA, Santana-Bagur JL, Joyner MJ, et al. Metabolic syndrome in relation to cardiorespiratory fitness, active and sedentary behavior in HIV+ Hispanics with and without lipodystrophy. *P R Health Sci J.* December 2014;33(4):163–169

Reeds DN, Mittendorfer B, Patterson BW, et al. Alterations in lipid kinetics in men with HIV-dyslipidemia. *Am J Physiol Endocrinol Metab.* 2003;285: E490–E497.

Reynolds NR, Neidig JL, Wu AW, et al. Balancing disfigurement and fear of disease progression: patient perceptions of HIV body fat redistribution. *AIDS Care.* 2006;18:663–673.

Ribera E, Paradineiro JC, Curran A, et al. Improvements in subcutaneous fat, lipid profile, and parameters of mitochondrial toxicity in patients with peripheral lipoatrophy when stavudine is switcher to tenofovir (LIPOTEST study). *HIV Clin Trials.* November-December 2008;9(6):407–417.

Ristig M, Drechsler H, Powderly WG. Hepatic steatosis and HIV infection. *AIDS Patient Care STDs.* 2005;19:356–365.

Roth VR, Kravcik S, Angel JB. Development of cervical fat pads following therapy with human immunodeficiency virus type 1 protease inhibitors. *Clin Infect Dis.* 1998;27:65–67.

Rozenbaum W, Gharakhanian S, Salhi Y, et al. Clinical and laboratory characteristics of lipodystrophy in a French cohort of HIV-infected patients treated with protease inhibitors. *Antiviral Ther.* 1999;4(2): L34.

Safrin S, Grunfeld C. Fat distribution and metabolic changes in patients with HIV infection. *AIDS.* 1999;13:2493–2505.

Saint-Marc T, Partisani M, Poizot-Martin I, et al. Fat distribution evaluated by computed tomography and metabolic abnormalities in patients undergoing antiretroviral therapy: preliminary results of the LIPOCO study. *AIDS.* 2000;14:37–49.

Saint-Marc T, Partisani M, Poizot-Martin I, et al. A syndrome of peripheral fat wasting (lipoatrophy) in patients receiving long-term nucleoside analogue therapy. *AIDS.* September 10, 1999;13(13):1659–1667.

Samaras K, Wand H, Law M, et al. Prevalence of metabolic syndrome in HIV-infected patients receiving highly active antiretroviral therapy using International Diabetes Foundation and Adult Treatment Panel III Criteria: associations with insulin resistance, disturbed body fat compartmentalization, elevated C-reactive peptide, and hypoadiponectinemia. *Diabetes Care.* 2007;30:113–119.

Sattler F. Body habitus changes related to lipodystrophy. *Clin Infect Dis.* 2003;36: S84–S90.

Saves M, Raffi F, Capeau J, et al. Factors related to lipodystrophy and metabolic alterations in patients with human immunodeficiency virus infection receiving highly active antiretroviral therapy. *Clin Infect Dis.* 2002;34:1396–1405.

Schambelan M, Benson CA, Carr A, et al. Management of metabolic complications associated with antiretroviral therapy for HIV-1 infection: recommendations of an International AIDS Society–USA panel. *J AIDS.* 2002;31:257–275.

Schwenk A. Methods of assessing body shape and composition in HIV-associated lipodystrophy. *Curr Opin Infect Dis.* 2002;15:9–16.

Schwenk A, Breuer P, Kremer G, et al. Clinical assessment of HIV-associated lipodystrophy syndrome: bioelectrical impedance analysis, anthropometry and clinical scores. *Clin Nutr.* 2001;20:243–249.

Sekhar RV, Jahoor F, Pownall HJ, et al. Severely dysregulated disposal of postprandial triacylglycerols exacerbates hypertriacylglycerolemia in HIV lipodystrophy syndrome. *Am J Clin Nutr.* 2005;81:1405–1410.

Sekhar RV, Jahoor F, White AC, et al. Metabolic basis of HIV lipodystrophy syndrome. *Am J Physiol Endocrinol Metab.* 2002;283: E332–E337.

Sekhar RV, Patel SG, D'Amico S, et al. Effects of rosiglitazone on abnormal lipid kinetics in HIV-associated dyslipidemic lipodystrophy: a stable isotope study. *Metabolism*. 2011;60(6):754–760.

Sutinen, J, Hakkinen, A.M, Westerbacka, J, et al. Increased fat accumulation in the liver in HIV-infected patients with antiretroviral therapy-associated lipodystrophy. *AIDS*. 2002;16:2183–2193.

Sutinen J, Hakkinen AM, Westerbacka J, et al. Rosiglitazone in the treatment of HAART-associated lipodystrophy: a randomized double-blind placebo-controlled study. *Antiviral Ther*. 2003;8(3):199–207.

Tanaka T, Nakazawa H, Kuriyama N et al. Farnesyltransferase inhibitors prevent HIV protease inhibitor (lopinavir/ritonavir) induced lipodystrophy and metabolic syndrome in mice. *Exp Ther Med*. February 2018;15(2):1314–1320.

Tien PC, Grunfeld C. What is HIV-associated lipodystrophy? Defining fat distribution changes in HIV infection. *Curr Opin Infect Dis*. 2004;17:27–32.

Torres RA, Unger KW, Cadman JA, et al. Recombinant human growth hormone improves truncal adiposity and "buffalo humps" in HIV-positive patients on HAART. *AIDS*. 1999;13:2479–2481.

Triant VA, Lee H, Hadigan C, et al. Increased acute myocardial infarction rates and cardiovascular risk factors among patients with HIV disease. *J Clin Endocrinol Metab*. 2007;92:2506–2512.

Tsiodras S, Mantzoros C, Hammer S, et al. Effects of protease inhibitors on hyperglycemia, hyperlipidemia, and lipodystrophy: a 5-year cohort study. *Arch Intern Med*. 2000;160:2050–2056.

Turner R, Testa MA, Su M, et al. The impact of HIV-associated adipose redistribution syndrome (HARS) on health-related quality of life. *Antiviral Ther*. 2006;11:L25.

Uzzan C, Boccara D, Lacheré A, et al. Treatment of facial lipoatrophy by lipofilling in HIV infected patients: retrospective study on 317 patients on 9 years. *Ann Chir Plast Esthet*. 2012;57(3):210–216.

van der Valk M, Bisschop PH, Romijn JA. Lipodystrophy in HIV-1-positive patients is associated with insulin resistance in multiple metabolic pathways. *AIDS*. 2001;15:2093–2100.

Varriale P, Saravi G, Hernandez E, et al. Acute myocardial infarction in patients infected with human immunodeficiency virus. *Am Heart J*. 2004;147(1):55–59.

Vazquez E. Understanding and treating protease paunch. *Posit Aware*. July-August 1999;10(4):59–63.

Vigano A, Mora S, Manzoni P, et al. Effects of recombinant growth hormone on visceral fat accumulation: pilot study in human immunodeficiency virus-infected adolescents. *J Clin Endocrinol Metab*. 2005;90:4075–4080.

Worm D, Kirk O, Anderson O et al. Clinical lipoatrophy in HIV-1 patients on HAART is not associated with increased abdominal girth, hyperlipidemia or glucose intolerance. *HIV Med*. October 2002;3(4):239–246.

Yin MT, Glesby MJ. Recombinant human growth hormone therapy in HIV-associated wasting and visceral adiposity. *Expert Rev Anti-Infect Ther*. 2005;3:727–738.

48.

IMMUNE RECONSTITUTION INFLAMMATORY SYNDROME (IRIS)

Dagan Coppock and William R. Short

CHAPTER GOAL

Upon completion of this chapter, the reader should be able to

- Understand the epidemiology of IRIS and its associated opportunistic infections.

- Recognize the timing considerations regarding opportunistic infection treatment and antiretroviral therapy intiation as related to the risk for IRIS.

- Understand the management approaches to IRIS, based upon its presentation and the underlying opportunistic infection.

INTRODUCTION

The hallmark of HIV pathogenesis is the gradual destruction of the cell-mediated immune system over a period of many years, as evidenced by a progressive and profound decline in $CD4^+$ T-helper lymphocytes, leading to increased susceptibility to opportunistic infections (OIs), malignancies, and the development of acquired immunodeficiency syndrome (AIDS). ART can suppress HIV replication, preventing further deterioration, and it allows for the regeneration of the immune system. Even patients with advanced AIDS have a marked improvement in both quantity and quality of their immune system after starting ART. In a subset of those initiating ART, the harmonious, gradual reconstitution of the immune system does not occur; rather, there is a rapid immunologic recovery with an abrupt transition to a pathologic inflammatory state often causing clinical deterioration. Opportunistic and other infections, previously unrecognized or tolerated by the failing immune system, suddenly become the targets of this overzealous immunologic recovery. In this inflammatory state, patients can clinically worsen despite an otherwise excellent response to ART, as evidenced by a decreased viral load and increased $CD4^+$ T cell counts. This paradoxical inflammatory response has been termed *immune reconstitution inflammatory syndrome* or IRIS (French, 2004), which is used an umbrella term encompassing two clinical entities: (1) Paradoxical IRIS: An exacerbation of a known OI, and (2) Unmasking IRIS: A flare of an undiagnosed (subclinical) OI.

LEARNING OBJECTIVE

Review the current status of research and clinical recommendations regarding immune reconstitution inflammatory syndrome (IRIS).

WHAT'S NEW?

- In contrast to prior observational data, recent clinical trial data suggest that the use of integrase strand transfer inhibitor (INSTI)-based antiretroviral therapy (ART) regimens do not increase the risk for IRIS.

- For patients with HIV/hepatitis C virus (HCV) coinfection and active hepatitis B virus (HBV) infection, the approach to timing ART initiation is important when considering IRIS. Current guidelines recommend the initiation of ART that is active against HBV prior to the initiation of HCV treatment.

KEY POINTS

- IRIS is associated with either worsening of a recognized infection (paradoxical IRIS) or an unrecognized infection (unmasking IRIS), which occurs in the setting of improved immunologic function.

- Most patients presenting with IRIS should be maintained on ART along with treatment for the associated infection.

INCIDENCE AND ASSOCIATED OPPORTUNISTIC INFECTIONS

The incidence of IRIS is dependent on the patient population being studied. It occurs more frequently in persons with specific OIs, a higher viral load, and more significant immunosuppression (Müller, 2010). The HIV Outpatient Study—an eight-city, US-wide, prospective, observational cohort study—evaluated 2,610 patients with 370 cases of IRIS (occurring in 276 patients) who initiated or resumed ART and, during the next 6 months, demonstrated a decline in plasma HIV RNA viral load of at least $0.5 \log_{10}$ copies/mL or had an increase of at least 50% in $CD4^+$ T cell count per microliter; it reported that the incidence of IRIS was 10.6%. The most common IRIS-defining diagnoses were candidiasis (23%), cytomegalovirus (CMV) infection (3.5%), disseminated *Mycobacterium avium* intracellulare (3.2%), *Pneumocystis* pneumonia (2.7%), *Varicella zoster* (2.4%), Kaposi's sarcoma (KS) (2.4%), non-Hodgkin's lymphoma (2.2%), and *Mycobacterium tuberculosis* (0.3%). IRIS was independently associated with CD4+ T cell counts of less than 50 cells/mL versus at least 200 cells/mL (odds ratio [OR], 5.0) and a viral load of at least 5.0 $\log_{10}$ copies/mL versus less than 4.0 $\log_{10}$ copies/mL (OR, 2.3) (Novak, 2012). In contrast, a study from the University of Washington HIV Cohort demonstrated a higher rate of IRIS in patients with Kaposi's sarcoma (29%), with no evident cases in patients with CMV disease or *Candida* esophagitis. In this study, the highest IRIS-associated morbidity was in cases of visceral KS. The differences in clinical characteristics between these two studies alone may reflect population and geographic variability.

IRIS AND ANTIRETROVIRAL THERAPY

In addition to the potential demographic factors that might affect the presentation of IRIS, the choice of ART regimen may also play a role. The AIDS Clinical Trial Group (ACTG) reported the incidence and associations with IRIS in ACTG 5202, which was a phase 3b, randomized clinical trial conducted in the United States that compared the safety, tolerability, and efficacy of four commonly used, once-daily, initial ART regimens. Two dual nucleoside/nucleotide reverse transcriptase inhibitor (NRTI) fixed-dose combinations (tenofovir DF/emtricitabine or abacavir/lamivudine) were compared when used in combination with either the non-nucleoside reverse transcriptase inhibitor (NNRTI) efavirenz or a ritonavir-boosted protease inhibitor, atazanavir/ritonavir. Among 1,848 eligible participants who initiated in this study, IRIS events occurred in 52 participants by week 48, with 4 participants having two events. Incidence rates were 6.05 (95% confidence interval [CI], 4.57–8.00) and 3.30 (95% CI, 2.51–4.33) cases/100 person-years (py) through 24 and 48 weeks, respectively. IRIS occurred 1–298 days after the initiation of ART, with 75% of cases occurring within 67 days and 3 cases after 24 weeks. IRIS events included the following associated OIs or other clinical diagnoses: *Mycobacterium avium* complex (MAC) ($n = 11$); *Varicella zoster* virus ($n = 11$); herpes simplex virus ($n = 8$); KS ($n = 5$); HCV, tuberculosis (TB), and *Pneumocystis jirovecii* pneumonia (PCP) ($n = 4$ each); toxoplasmosis and cryptococcosis ($n = 2$ each); and CMV-associated colitis, progressive multifocal leukoencephalopathy (PML), *Mycobacterium kansasii*, eosinophilic folliculitis, and swollen lymph node ($n = 1$ each). The most commonly reported symptoms were fever and pain. There were no deaths from IRIS in this cohort. Among participants with IRIS, median baseline HIV RNA was 4.9 $\log_{10}$ copies/mL, median CD4+ T cell count was 49 cells/mm^3, and 50% had prior AIDS illness. In univariate Cox proportional hazards models, an increased risk of IRIS was associated with baseline prior AIDS illness, higher HIV RNA level, lower CD4+ T cell count and percentage, lower CD8+ T cell count and higher percentage, and lower CD4+:CD8+ T cell ratio (all $p \leq 0.01$). No significant association was observed with sex, age, or race/

ethnicity ($p > 0.19$). Of note, IRIS events were more common with abacavir/lamivudine relative to tenofovir/emtricitabine for participants with low CD4+ T cell counts. This finding may reflect the observed more rapid CD4+ T cell increases with abacavir/lamivudine regimens (Fischl, 2010).

Recently, observational data have raised concerns regarding INSTI-based regimens and their associations with IRIS, although subsequent clinical trial data do not bear out these findings. In a retrospective cohort trial, 2,287 patients with CD4+ T-cell counts below 200/mm^3 were evaluated by ART regimen. Cohorts consisted of participants receiving either INSTI-based or non-INSTI-based ART regimens. The odds ratio for developing IRIS was 1.99 (1.09–3.47) ($P = 0.04$) for the INSTI-based group (Dutertre, 2017). Similarly, a Dutch observational study evaluated the association of INSTI initiation with the development of IRIS, as defined either by previously established criteria (French, 2004) or the French criteria plus clinical diagnosis. The study found that the use of INSTI-based treatment was independently associated with IRIS based on the French criteria (HR 2.6, 1.3-5.1, $p = 0.004$) as well as IRIS based on the French criteria plus clinical diagnosis (HR 2.6, 95%CI 1.6-4.4, $p = 0.0001$) (Wijting, 2017). However, a subsequent clinical trial demonstrated no significant risk of IRIS despite the use of INSTI-based therapy. In this trial, 1,805 participants were randomized to receive either standard therapy (2NRTI + NRTI) or standard therapy plus raltegravir. Looking at an outcome of fatal/nonfatal IRIS-compatible events, there was no significant difference between the standard arm compared with the standard plus raltegravir arm (9.5% vs, 9.9%, $p = 0.79$) (Gibb, 2018).

ETIOLOGY AND PATHOGENESIS

Recovery of pathogen-specific T cell responses and an increased production of pro-inflammatory chemokines and cytokines produced by the innate immune response after commencing ART may contribute to the immunopathogenesis of IRIS. Higher T cell responses to nonstructural antigens of HCV in enzyme-linked immunosorbent spot assays and higher serum levels of antibodies to a mixture of virus proteins were demonstrated in patients with HIV and HCV coinfection who experienced an increase in serum liver enzyme levels after commencing ART (Cameron, 2011). Patients who develop TB-IRIS have lower plasma levels of the chemokine CCL2 before commencing ART (Oliver, 2010).

The identification of biomarkers could be used to diagnose IRIS in the future and predict which patients might be at risk. A cohort of 45 HIV-1–infected, treatment-naïve patients with baseline CD4+ T cell counts of 100 cells/µL or less who were started on ART, suppressed HIV RNA to less than 50 copies/mL, and seen every 1–3 months for 1 year were retrospectively evaluated for suspected or confirmed IRIS. Pre-ART levels of both D-dimer and the inflammatory biomarker C-reactive protein (CRP) were higher in IRIS cases versus controls (Porter, 2010). In another study, individuals with elevated baseline levels of CRP and the fibrosis biomarker hyaluronic acid were more likely to progress to AIDS, develop IRIS, or die within the first month after starting ART (Boulware,

2011). Large prospective studies to elucidate the predictive and diagnostic values of IRIS biomarkers are needed.

GUIDELINES FOR ART INITIATION

Current guidelines recommend the early initiation of ART with the exception of select clinical scenarios. US Department of Health and Human Services (USDHHS) guidelines recommend early initiation of ART despite the presence of OIs, with the exception of cryptococcal and tuberculous meningitis, for which a "short delay" may be warranted (USDHHS, 2018). Recommendations of the International Antiviral Society (IAS)-USA Panel agree that, in the setting of most OIs, ART should be initiated within 2 weeks (Saag, 2018). However, the guidelines go on to elaborate that for pulmonary TB, ART can be initiated within 2 weeks of starting TB treatment for patients with a CD4$^+$ T cell count less than 50 cells/mm^3 and between 2 to 8 weeks for patients with a CD4$^+$ T cell count greater than 50 cells/mm^3. Ther IAS-USA guidelines go on to state that, in cases of cryptococcal meningitis in resource-rich areas, ART can be initiated within 2 weeks albeit with careful monitoring and aggressive management of intracranial pressure.

ART INITIATION AND THE RISK OF NON–TUBERCULOSIS- ASSOCIATED IRIS

The timing of ART initiation and its association with OI-specific IRIS remains a concern for clinicians In the ACTG 5164 study, 282 participants with an acute OI and a baseline median CD4$^+$ T cell count of 29 cells/mm^3 were prospectively randomized to immediate (<14 days) versus delayed (>28 days) initiation of ART. In this study, which included participants diagnosed with PCP (63%), cryptococcal meningitis (12%), and bacterial infections (12%), earlier initiation of ART resulted in less progression to AIDS and/or death and no increase in adverse events or loss of virologic response compared to deferred ART. Participants with or on treatment for TB were excluded. Rates of IRIS in this study were low (7%) and did not differ by timing of ART (Zolopa, 2009). IRIS was reported in 23 cases and confirmed in 20:8 participants in the immediate arm and 12 in the deferred arm. There was no evidence of an association of IRIS with the entry OI/bacterial infection: 13 (65%) IRIS cases were in participants with PCP who comprised 63% of the study population. IRIS developed a median of 33 days (interquartile range, 26–72 days) after initiation of ART. There was no significant difference in the frequency of IRIS between participants who received corticosteroids during the treatment of their OI and those who did not receive corticosteroids: 9/150 (6%) versus 11/112 (9.8%), respectively ($p = 0.35$).

The optimal timing of ART initiation in cryptococcal meningitis is controversial. Approximately 25% of patients with HIV and treated cryptococcal meningitis will experience IRIS after commencing ART (Haddow, 2010). It is associated with mortality in more than 25% of patients from resource-poor countries, and it is an important cause of early mortality after starting ART in patients with HIV from these countries. Early initiation of ART (within 72 hours) in patients with treated cryptococcal meningitis was associated with a higher rate of mortality compared to those who waited for at least 10 weeks in one study (Makadzange, 2010). However, a more recent study suggested that, in high-resource areas, there is no significant difference in mortality for patients who initiate ART within 2 weeks of beginning antifungal treatment (Ingle, 2015). Based on the studies completed and expert opinion, it is prudent to delay initiation of ART until after the completion of induction therapy (the first 2 weeks) and possibly until the total induction/consolidation (10 weeks) phase has been completed. There are certain scenarios where a delay in ART may be important, such as when there is evidence of increased intracranial pressure or in those with low cerebrospinal fluid (CSF) white cell counts.

IRIS related to JC polyoma virus infection remains a clinical challenge as ART initiation and immune reconstitution is the only available treatment. Prior to ART, JC virus infection can lead to PML in patients with advanced HIV infection. However, approximately 15% of patients experience an exacerbation of PML after ART is commenced (Martin-Blondel, 2011). A review of 54 cases of PML IRIS evaluated the mortality of patients as stratified by steroid use. Five of the 12 patients receiving steroids and 14 of the 42 patients not receiving steroids died, suggesting a high mortality of PML IRIS, regardless of steroid use (Tan, 2009).

In patients coinfected with HIV and viral hepatitides, IRIS is a frequent concern. Up to 25% of patients with HIV and HBV or HCV coinfection experience a flare of hepatitis and/or elevation of serum liver enzyme levels after commencing ART (Cameron, 2011; Crane, 2009). Hepatitis flares in patients with HIV and HBV coinfection are associated with a higher plasma HBV DNA level before ART (Crane, 2009), suggesting that pathogen load is an important determinant of disease. Even when ART with activity against HBV is selected for treatment, HBV IRIS can still occur, complicating the differential of a hepatitis flare (Crane, 2008). In recent years, the use of direct-acting antivirals (DAAs) for treating HCV has further complicated the differential. The use of DAAs has been associated with HBV reactivation (Bersoff-Matcha, 2017). This has led to changes in guidelines regarding the timing of ART initiation in patients with viral hepatitis. For patients who are both coinfected with HIV/HCV and who have active HBV infection, USDHHS guidelines now recommend first initiating ART with activity against HBV prior to the initiation of DAAs.

TUBERCULOSIS IRIS AND ART INITIATION

For individuals with HIV and TB coinfection, unmasking and paradoxical IRIS can lead to two distinct clinical scenarios. In the context of TB, unmasking IRIS is the development of overt TB in patients who initially screened negative for this infection, typically seen within the first 60 days following ART initiation (Dheda, 2004; Shelburne, 2006). It is thought to be due to an increase in circulating memory T cells that were sequestered in lymphatic tissue prior to therapy. Alternatively, paradoxical IRIS involves worsening of signs and symptoms of TB in individuals with a known history of TB after they have been started on ART.

The HIV-CAUSAL Collaboration demonstrated that the incidence of TB decreased after ART initiation but not among persons older than age 50 years or those with a CD4+ T cell count of less than 50 cells/mm³. Despite an overall decrease in TB incidence, the increased rate during 3 months of ART suggests unmasking IRIS. This is a multinational cohort study among HIV-positive patients from high-income countries. Among 65,121 individuals, 712 developed TB during 28 months of median follow-up (incidence, 3.0 cases per 1,000 py). The hazard ratio (HR) for TB for ART versus no ART was 0.56 (95% CI, 0.44–0.72) overall, 1.04 (95% CI, 0.64–1.68) for individuals aged older than 50 years, and 1.46 (95% CI, 0.70–3.04) for people with a CD4+ T cell count of less than 50 cells/mm³. Compared with people who had not started ART, HRs differed by time since ART initiation: 1.36 (95% CI, 0.98–1.89) for initiation less than 3 months previously and 0.44 (95% CI, 0.34–0.58) for initiation 3 months or more previously. Compared with people who had not initiated ART, HRs less than 3 months after ART initiation were 0.67 (95% CI, 0.38–1.18), 1.51 (95% CI, 0.98–2.31), and 3.20 (95% CI, 1.34–7.60) for people younger than age 35, 35–50, and older than age 50 years, respectively, and 2.30 (95% CI, 1.03–5.14) for people with a CD4+ T cell counts of less than 50 cells/mm³ (HIV-CAUSAL Collaboration, 2012).

In a South African cohort of 498 persons with advanced HIV, symptomatic patients were screened for TB by chest X-ray and/or sputum examination. Patients who screened positive were initiated on anti-TB therapy prior to starting ART. Individuals who screened negative and went on to develop unmasking IRIS were found to have significantly elevated levels of interferon-γ (IFN-γ) and CRP at baseline prior to ART compared to non-IRIS, non-TB controls. These results suggest the presence of subclinical TB infection despite negative screening that was done prior to the initiation of ART (Haddow, 2009). Persons who exhibit paradoxical IRIS have been reported to have elevated tuberculin-specific effector memory CD4+ T cells prior to initiation of ART. Following the commencement of ART, increased levels of Th1-associated cytokines, IFN-γ, and tumor necrosis factor-α most likely contribute to the overwhelming inflammatory reaction to the TB antigen present (Bourgarit, 2009). Persons with HIV and latent TB (defined as >5 mm skin test induration or positive IFN-γ release assay) are at increased risk for progression to active TB compared to the HIV-negative population, which underscores the need to identify and treat patients with latent disease. Active TB in HIV-infected patients requires immediate treatment. However, optimal timing of ART has yet to be established. Potential for multiple adverse drug reactions, drug–drug interactions, and IRIS reactions has led to increased difficulty in defining the proper timing of ART.

TIMING OF ART WITH TB IRIS

In recent years, there has been debate on the timing of ART initiation relative to the initiation of TB treatment in known coinfected patients. However, based on a number of trials, as discussed here, current USDHHS guidelines recommend an early, integrative approach to ART and TB treatment initiation.

In the SAPiT trial, there were no differences in rates of AIDS or death between patients who started ART within 4 weeks after initiating TB treatment and those who started ART at 8–12 weeks (i.e., within 4 weeks after completing the intensive phase of TB treatment) (Abdool Karim, 2010). However, in patients with baseline CD4+ T cell counts of less than 50 cells/mm³, the rate of AIDS or death was lower in the earlier therapy group than in the later therapy group (8.5 vs. 26.3 cases per 100 py, a strong trend favoring the earlier treatment arm [$p = 0.06$]). For all patients, regardless of CD4+ T cell count, earlier therapy was associated with a higher incidence of IRIS and of adverse events that required a switch in antiretroviral drugs compared to those who started therapy later. In this study, two deaths were attributed to IRIS.

In the CAMELIA study, patients who had CD4+ T cell counts of less than 200 cells/mm³ were randomized to initiate ART at 2 or 8 weeks after initiation of TB treatment (Blanc, 2011). Study participants had a median CD4+ T cell count of 25 cells/mm³ and high rates of disseminated TB disease. ART initiated at 2 weeks resulted in a 38% reduction in mortality ($p = 0.006$) compared with that of therapy initiated at 8 weeks. A significant reduction in mortality was seen in patients with CD4+ T cell counts of 50 cells/mm³ or less and in patients with CD4+ T cell counts of 51–200 cells/mm³. Overall, six deaths were associated with TB IRIS.

The ACTG 5221 (STRIDE) trial, a multinational study, randomized ART-naïve patients with confirmed or probable TB and CD4+ T cell counts of less than 250 cells/mm³ to earlier (<2 weeks) or later (8–12 weeks) ART (Havlir, 2011). At study entry, the participants' median CD4+ T cell count was 77 cells/mm³. The rates of mortality and AIDS diagnoses were not different between the earlier and later arms, although higher rates of IRIS were seen in the earlier arm. However, a significant reduction in AIDS or death was seen in the subset of patients with CD4+ T cell counts of less than 50 cells/mm³ who were randomized to the earlier ART arm ($p = 0.02$).

Given the previously discussed data, USDHHS guidelines recommend the initiation of HAART within 2 weeks when an individual's CD4+ T cell count is less than 50 cells/mm³ and by 8–12 weeks for all others. This reflects the observation that earlier ART initiation in TB-infected patients improves mortality.

TREATMENT OF IRIS

Although the nonsteroidal anti-inflammatory agents or steroids are commonly used in clinical practice, the dosage and timing have not been well-established in the medical literature. A double-blind, placebo-controlled, randomized clinical trial, including patients receiving both ART and anti-TB therapy and experiencing paradoxical IRIS, evaluated a tapering course of prednisone over 4 weeks. Individuals on steroid therapy had a significantly decreased length of hospitalization and marked improvement of symptoms related to IRIS, suggesting a potential role for steroids in the management of paradoxical IRIS (Meintjes, 2010). In the previously described ACTG 5164 study, 63% of participants reported having *Pneumocystis* pneumonia as an OI. There was no significant difference in the frequency of IRIS between participants who received corticosteroids during the treatment and those who did not receive corticosteroids: 9/150 (6%) versus 11/112 (9.8%), respectively ($p = 0.35$).

In other forms of IRIS, such as MAC, surgical drainage of necrotic lymphadenitis may be of benefit. In patients with cryptococcal meningitis IRIS, CSF drainage may provide relief of increased intracranial pressure. While the data to support the use of corticosteroids in cryptococcal meningitis IRIS are sparse, Infectious Disease Society of America guidelines recommend considering their use in the setting of CNS inflammation and increased intracranial pressure (Perfect, 2010). Corticosteroid or other anti-inflammatory therapies may also be effective for treating some forms of IRIS, such as PML-associated IRIS (Martin-Blondel, 2011).

As a general approach, in unmasking IRIS, management should focus on diagnosis of the OI and instituting appropriate treatment. Screening for latent TB infection should be undertaken in all HIV-infected patients. In paradoxical IRIS, it is crucial to exclude alternate diagnoses and ensure the patient is receiving appropriate treatment for the condition. In the majority of cases, ART is continued, but on rare occasions, cessation of ART is warranted in severe IRIS, particularly when it is life-threatening.

REFERENCES

Abdool Karim SS. Timing of initiation of antiretroviral drugs during tuberculosis therapy. *N Engl J Med*. February 5, 2010;362(8):697–706.

Bersoff-Matcha SJ, Cao K, et al. Hepatitis B virus reactivation associated with direct-acting antiviral therapy for chronic hepatitis C virus: a review of cases reported to the US Food and Drug Administration adverse event reporting system. *Ann Intern Med*. 2017;166(11):792–798.

Blanc FX, Sok T, Laureillard D, et al. Earlier versus later start of antiretroviral therapy in HIV-infected adults with tuberculosis. *N Engl J Med*. October 20, 2011;365(16):1471–1481.

Boulware DR, Hullsiek KH, Puronen CE, et al.; INSIGHT Study Group. Higher levels of CRP, D-dimer, IL-6, and hyaluronic acid before initiation of antiretroviral therapy (ART) are associated with increased risk of AIDS or death. *J Infect Dis*. June 1, 2011;203(11):1637–1646.

Bourgarit A, Carcelain G, Samri A, et al. TB-associated immune restoration syndrome in HIV-1-infected patients involves tuberculin-specific CD4 Th1 cells and can be predicted by KIR-negative gammadelta T cells. Paper presented at the 16th Conference on Retroviruses and Opportunistic Infections, February 8–11, 2009, Montréal, Canada. Abstract 772.

Cameron BA, Emerson CR, Workman C, et al. Alterations in immune function are associated with liver enzyme elevation in HIV and HCV co-infection after commencement of combination antiretroviral therapy. *J Clin Immunol*. 2011;31:1079–1083.

Crane M, Oliver B, Matthews G, et al. Immunopathogenesis of hepatic flare in HIV/hepatitis B virus (HBV)-coinfected individuals after the initiation of HBV-active antiretroviral therapy. *J Infect Dis*. 2009;199:974–981.

Crane M, Matthews G, Lewin SR. Hepatitis virus immune restoration disease of the liver. *Curr Opin HIV AIDS*. 2008;3(4):446–452.

Dheda K, Lampe FC, Johnson MA, et al. Outcome of HIV-associated tuberculosis in the era of highly active antiretroviral therapy. *J Infect Dis*. 2004;190(9):1670.

Dutertre M, Cuzin L, Demonchy E, et al. Initiation of antiretroviral therapy containing integrase inhibitors increases the risk of IRIS requiring hospitalization. *JAIDS*. 2017;76(1):e23–e26.

Fischl M, Mollan K, Pahwa S, et al. IRIS among US subjects starting ART in AIDS Clinical Trials Group Study A5202. Paper presented at the 15th Conference on Retroviruses and Opportunistic infections, February 16–19, 2010, San Francisco, CA. Abstract 791.

French MA, Price P, Stone SF. Immune restoration disease after antiretroviral therapy. *AIDS*. 2004;18:1615–1627.

Gibb D, Szubert AJ, Chidziva E, et al. Impact of raltegravir intensification of first-line ART on IRIS in the REALITY trial. Paper presented at the 25th Conference on Retroviruses and Opportunistic Infections, March 4–7, 2018. Abstract 23.

Haddow L, Borrow P, Dibben O, et al. Cytokine profiles predict unmasking TB immune reconstitution inflammatory syndrome and are associated with unmasking and paradoxical presentations of TB immune reconstitution inflammatory syndrome. Paper presented at the 16th Conference on Retroviruses and Opportunistic Infections, February 8–11, 2009, Montréal, Canada. Abstract 773.

Haddow LJ, Colebunders R, Meintjes G, et al. Cryptococcal immune reconstitution inflammatory syndrome in HIV-1-infected individuals: proposed clinical case definitions. *Lancet Infect Dis*. 2010;10:791–802.

Havlir DV, Kendall MA, Ive P, et al. Timing of antiretroviral therapy for HIV-1 infection and tuberculosis. *N Engl J Med*. October 20, 2011;365(16):1482–1491.

HIV-CAUSAL Collaboration. Impact of antiretroviral therapy on tuberculosis incidence among HIV-positive patients in high-income countries. *Clin Infect Dis*. May 2012;54(9):1364–1372.

Ingle SM, Miro JM, Furrer H, et al. Impact of ART on mortality in cryptococcal meningitis patients: high-income settings. Paper presented at 22nd Conference on Retroviruses and Opportunistic Infections. February 23–26, 2015, Seattle, WA. Abstract 837.

Makadzange AT, Ndhlovu CE, Takarinda K, et al. Early versus delayed initiation of antiretroviral therapy for concurrent HIV infection and cryptococcal meningitis in sub-Saharan Africa. *Clin Infect Dis*. 2010;50:1532–1538.

Martin-Blondel G, Delobel P, Blancher A, et al. Pathogenesis of the immune reconstitution inflammatory syndrome affecting the central nervous system in patients infected with HIV. *Brain*. 2011;134:928–946.

Meintjes G, Wilkinson RJ, Morroni C, et al. Randomized placebo-controlled trial of prednisone for paradoxical tuberculosis-associated immune reconstitution inflammatory syndrome. *AIDS*. September 24, 2010;24(15):2381–2390.

Müller M, Wandel S, Colebunders R, et al. Immune reconstitution inflammatory syndrome in patients starting antiretroviral therapy for HIV infection: a systematic review and meta-analysis. *Lancet Infect Dis*. 2010;10:251–261.

Novak RM, Richardson JT, Buchacz K, et al.; HIV Outpatient Study (HOPS) Investigators. Immune reconstitution inflammatory syndrome: Incidence and implications for mortality. *AIDS*. March 27, 2012;26(6):721–730.

Oliver BG, Elliott JH, Price P, et al. Mediators of innate and adaptive immune responses differentially affect immune restoration disease associated with *Mycobacterium tuberculosis* in HIV patients beginning antiretroviral therapy. *J Infect Dis.* 2010;202:1728–1737.

Porter BO, Ouedraogo GL, Hodge JN, et al. d-Dimer and CRP levels are elevated prior to antiretroviral treatment in patients who develop IRIS. *Clin Immunol.* July 2010;136(1):42–50.

Perfect JR, Clinical practice guidelines for the management of cryptococcal disease: 2010 update by the Infectious Diseases Society of America. *Clin Infect Dis.* 2010;50(3):291–322.

Saag M, Benson CA, Gandhi RT, et al. Antiretroviral drugs for treatment and prevention of HIV infection in adults: 2018 recommendations of the International Antiviral Society–USA Panel. *JAMA.* 2018;320(4):379–396.

Shelburne SA, Montes M, Hamill RJ. Immune reconstitution inflammatory syndrome: more answers, more questions. *J Antimicrob Chemother.* 2006;57(2):167.

Tan K, Roda R, Ostrow L, McArthur J, Nath A. PML-IRIS in patients with HIV infection: clinical manifestations and treatment with steroids. *Neurology.* 2009;72(17):1458–1464.

US Department of Health and Human Services (USDHHS). Guidelines for the use of antiretroviral agents in adults and adolescents living with HIV. Available at https://aidsinfo.nih.gov/guidelines. 2018.

Wijting I, Rokx C, Wit F, et al. Integrase inhibitors are an independent risk factor for IRIS: an ATHENA-Cohort study. Paper presented at the 24th Conference on Retroviruses and Opportunistic Infections, February 13–16, 2017. Abstract 731.

Zolopa AR, Anderson J, Komarow L, et al. Early antiretroviral therapy reduces AIDS progression/death in individuals with acute opportunistic infections: a multicenter randomized strategy trial. *PLoS One.* 2009;4(5):e5575.

49.

US HEALTHCARE SYSTEMS, HIV PROGRAMS, AND COVERAGE POLICY ISSUES

Anna Forbes and Bruce J. Packett, II

CHAPTER GOAL

Upon completion of this chapter, the reader should be able to
- Broadly understand the landscape of the US healthcare systems and payers as they relate to the provision of HIV care, treatment, prevention and medical coding.

INTRODUCTION

HIV-related healthcare services have historically been covered or provided by a patchwork of federal, state, and local programs, such as Medicare, Medicaid, the Ryan White Program, and state and local health programs. HIV/AIDS service organizations (H/ASOs) and private and charitable health organizations also provided services for HIV patients without coverage. These programs represent the long-standing pathways to insurance coverage, access to care, and access to treatment for people living with HIV (PLWH). Some of these programs also supply coverage for, or access to, medications that treat co-occurring conditions for PLWH.

LEARNING OBJECTIVE

Discuss the issues related to the coverage and reimbursement for HIV services with regard to private insurance, Medicaid, Medicare, and the Ryan White Program.

WHAT'S NEW?

Implementation of the Affordable Care Act (ACA), primarily in 2014, greatly expanded the availability of health coverage for people living with HIV in the United States. However, challenges such as affordability and access to treatment still remain, especially in those states that have chosen not to expand Medicaid coverage. The landscape of coverage options, including Medicaid, now varies widely among states.

KEY POINTS

- Under the ACA since 2014, all US citizens were required by law to have some form of health coverage, although the nature of that coverage varied widely. However, the Tax Cuts and Jobs has repealed the individual mandate beginning in 2019.

- Coverage and reimbursement for HIV services vary widely based on payer, coverage source, and state of residence.

- Access to treatment varies greatly among payers, as does affordability.

- The majority of states in the United States now offer Medicaid coverage to all citizens at or under 138% federal poverty level (FPL). However, several still do not, and some states are considering, but have not yet implemented, Medicaid expansion. Health coverage systems are evolving rapidly based largely on politics.

- The Ryan White Program is a federal "wrap-around" or "payer of last resort" program designed to provide services to HIV patients with insufficient coverage and benefits.

In 2010, the Patient Protection and Affordable Care Act (the "Affordable Care Act" or "ACA") was passed by Congress and signed into law by President Obama (Levy, 2015). The law, aimed at reforming healthcare coverage in the United States, represents the broadest reform to the US healthcare systems since the 1960s. The law has many aspects. Among the reforms with greatest impact for PLWH are:

1. Prohibition of discrimination by insurers against individuals with preexisting conditions

2. A requirement for all US citizens to obtain health insurance coverage (although this has been effectively repealed)

3. The expansion of the Medicaid program to cover all individuals under 138% of FPL (although this was made optional for states by a 2012 Supreme court ruling; see later discussion)

4. The creation of individual and small-group insurance markets (exchanges) in each state along with federal tax credits to enable low-income individuals to purchase insurance affordably

More recent public policy maneuvers, however, have brought about significant changes in availability and affordability of private insurance coverage to PLWH.

The constitutionality of the law was challenged in several cases that reached the US Supreme Court (Duignan, "Affordable Care Act Cases"). In 2012, a key provision of the law was struck down by the Court in part, effectively making Medicaid expansion optional to states. In states that have not instituted Medicaid expansion, access to the ACA is virtually nonexistent. Adults who do not qualify for Medicaid (i.e., are not disabled, elderly, caring for children, or pregnant) do not meet the requirements for Medicaid access—leaving those states with a pool of very poor adults with little to no access to affordable health coverage options whatsoever.

The lack of universal Medicaid expansion, coupled with significant flexibility provided to state lawmakers and insurers in the state insurance markets, has created high variability among coverage options available to HIV patients in each state. Because the Ryan White Program is a safety net program designed to wrap around other forms of health coverage, these changes result in challenges for that program as well.

Since the 2016 Presidential election, opponents of the ACA have expended considerable political and financial clout in efforts to overturn it, thus repudiating a hallmark of the Obama administration. The ACA's repeal by Congress in 2018 was narrowly avoided, and future attempts to repeal it legislatively could be expected. Meanwhile, the executive branch continues taking steps to limit and/or undermine it.

By the 2018 ACA enrollment cycle, for example, the Centers for Medicare and Medicaid Services (CMS, a part of DHHS) had reduced funding to hire ACA Market Navigators by up to 96% in some states. These Navigators work to educate ACA applicants about their various insurance options and then help them select the plan that matches their needs and enroll in it successfully (Politz, 2018). Their utility was so evident in the first year of ACA that the Obama administration increased the number hired for the second year. However, funding has been cut and virtually eliminated in 2017 and 2018.

The CMS also issued a final rule in 2018 to increase the maximum use of ACA-noncompliant "short-term" insurance policies from 3 months to 364 days, thus facilitating uptake of these policies by people who want or need to buy their insurance as cheaply as possible. Often referred to as "junk insurance," these policies usually do not cover prescription drugs, maternity care, or care for people with preexisting medical conditions. Purchasers are often not fully aware of their very limited utility.

PRIVATE INSURANCE

Private health insurance in the United States is typically offered by private for-profit or nonprofit companies to various markets. In 2008, employment-based health insurance was the primary source of coverage for American workers (Rho and Schmitt, 2010), offered as benefits or in the form of other compensation to employees by their employer. Individual insurance plans were less common before the healthcare law in 2014.

Some common forms of private insurance are indemnity plans, preferred provider plans, and health maintenance organizations. With indemnity plans, individuals can generally choose any healthcare provider and have a portion of the fees paid by the insurance. With preferred provider plans, individuals must choose from a defined network of clinicians, but the clinicians are generally employed by different groups. With health maintenance plans, individuals receive care from one or a small number of clinician groups.

Reimbursement to clinicians varies widely with private insurance policies, with lower rates generally paid by managed care organizations. The provider networks within insurance plans can affect reimbursement levels, as can plan benefits, co-pays, and cost-sharing mechanisms. Coverage of particular medications and treatments for patients varies widely under private insurance plans.

The ACA prohibits health insurance discrimination based on health status or gender, as well as lifetime limits on coverage, preexisting condition exclusions, and charging higher premiums based on gender or health status (Obamacare Facts, "Obamacare Pre-Existing Conditions"; Obamacare Facts, "Obamacare No Discrimination"). The ACA created a so-called individual mandate requiring all US citizens to obtain health coverage beginning in 2014 or face federal tax penalties (Obamacare Facts, "Obamacare Individual Mandate"; HealthCare.gov, "If You Don't Have Health Insurance: How Much You'll Pay"), though—as noted earlier—the individual mandate (in the form of tax penalties) effectively disappeared beginning in 2019. Individuals who do not have access to employer-based insurance or other insurance coverage and do not qualify for public health coverage programs such as Medicaid, could purchase individual insurance through the state insurance exchanges (marketplaces), assuming they can afford to do so.

STATE INSURANCE EXCHANGES (MARKETPLACES)

One of the most significant accomplishments of the ACA was the creation of marketplaces for individual and small-group insurance plans in each state (Center for Consumer Information & Oversight, "State Health Insurance Marketplaces"). Each state insurance exchange (marketplace) is simply a market forum where private insurance companies offer various qualified health plans (QHPs) to residents of that state. Individuals can access the marketplace online, by phone, or in person through assisters, and they can also use the marketplace to determine eligibility for Medicaid or CHIP benefits (HealthCare.gov, "Medicaid and CHIP Coverage Health Insurance Marketplace").

The ACA also makes tax credit subsidies available to some low- and medium-income individuals in order to purchase insurance through the state exchanges. Tax credits of gradated amounts are available to those with income levels between 138% and 400% FPL, and they are taken as upfront subsidies to the plan premium (HealthCare.gov, "Premium Tax Credit").

The plans offered within the markets vary in cost as well as coverage and benefit design. The Essential Health Benefits (EHBs) include services within the following 10 categories: ambulatory patient services, emergency services, hospitalization, maternity and newborn care, mental health and substance use disorder services (including behavioral health treatment), prescription drugs, rehabilitative and habilitative services and devices, laboratory services, preventive and wellness services and chronic disease management, and pediatric services (including oral and vision care) (HealthCare.gov, "Essential Health Benefits"; HealthCare.gov, "10 Health Care Benefits Covered in the Health Insurance Marketplace").

In addition, all plans in the state exchanges are required to include a minimum percentage of all the Essential Community Providers (ECPs) in a geographic area in their provider networks. ECPs are providers that serve predominately low-income medically underserved individuals. This includes Ryan White HIV/AIDS providers.

MEDICAID

The Medicaid program has long been the nation's public health insurance program for those with low-income status, limited resources, and disability. Originally, the program covered only certain populations, such as the medically disabled and pregnant women, infants, and children living in poverty.

The ACA sought to expand the program's coverage to include all citizens below 138% FPL regardless of other categorizations. However (as discussed earlier), this was not accepted by all states. Some states have partially expanded their Medicaid program in a variety of ways, and others have declined expansion altogether, for political reasons. Individuals in those states are exempt from the tax penalties under the individual mandate (Obamacare Facts, "Obamacare Mandate: Exemption and Tax Penalty") but many are also left with little or no access to healthcare whatever except through free clinics or community health departments where they are available.

Medicaid is the single largest source of coverage for people with HIV in the United States. Medicaid and/or Medicare provide healthcare to over half of PLWH (Henry J. Kaiser Family Foundation, "Medicaid's Role for Individuals with HIV") in the US. Medicaid covers inpatient, ambulatory care, and skilled nursing care. Medicaid also covers prescription medications except for persons who also have Medicare (dual eligibles). Coverage levels, eligibility criteria, and program benefits vary widely from state to state (Medicaid.gov, "Benefits").

Medicaid is financed jointly by the federal government and states. It is administered by state governments in accordance with certain basic federal eligibility and benefit standards (Medicaid.gov, "Financing & Reimbursement"). At the federal level, the Medicaid program is run by the Centers for Medicare and Medicaid Services (CMS) under the USDHHS. Medicaid is the third largest domestic program in the federal budget, after Social Security and Medicare (Rudowitz, 2015a, 2015b). It is also the second largest program in most state budgets. The federal government matches state spending in Medicaid, paying for 56% of the program's spending overall (Rudowitz, 2015a, 2015b). The ACA law initially paid for 100% of the cost of a state's expansion of Medicaid, with that amount decreasing over time.

In recent years, some states have tried to mitigate Medicaid budgetary costs through reductions of benefits, limitations to drug formularies, and other efforts. Many states also offer managed care–type programs to particular populations in efforts to reduce costs.

Medicaid managed care has grown significantly in recent decades, with more than half of Medicaid beneficiaries now receiving care and services through Medicaid managed care organizations (MCOs). MCOs contract directly with the state to provide services and benefits in a variety of capacities (Henry J. Kaiser Family Foundation, "Medicaid Managed Care Market Tracker"). Some MCOs are operated by a parent firm that also participates in the private insurance market.

Traditional Medicaid programs offer provider reimbursement through fee-for-service rates that are determined by the state. MCOs make agreements for provider reimbursement based on monthly capitation rates.

MEDICARE

Medicare is the federal health insurance program for seniors older than age 65 years and also for people younger than age 65 years with permanent disabilities, including PLWH. The Medicare program is administered by the CMS. About one-quarter of PLWH receive their medical care through Medicare (Henry J. Kaiser Family Foundation, "Medicare and HIV").

Eligibility is tied to work history and contributions to Medicare through employment-based withholding. Some individuals are eligible for both Medicare and Medicaid (dual eligibles), given their income and disability status. The number of PLWH who use Medicare has increased due to increased survival rates from antiretroviral therapies and the aging of the population living with HIV/AIDS. Medicare covers inpatient and outpatient care, some skilled nursing and home care, and medications. Medicare also covers HIV testing for beneficiaries.

In 2006, Medicare began providing prescription drug coverage under the Medicare Part D drug benefit. Most Medicare-eligible individuals can decide whether to participate through enrollment in one of several prescription drug plans that are marketed as stand-alone coverage or to rely on managed care plans (called Medicare Advantage). Medicare requires that each plan cover six categories of drugs, one of which is anti-retroviral drugs. Medicare Part D includes an "exceptions and appeals" process that can be used to request coverage of drugs not covered by the plan.

Individual Medicare Part D plans differ widely in terms of premiums and other cost-sharing requirements. Medicare Part D includes a sequence of cost-sharing requirements, including an initial deductible and subsequent "out-of-pocket" costs. Most Medicare Part D plans also have a coverage gap (or "donut hole") in which, after a certain amount of costs have been paid through the coverage plan, any additional costs become the responsibility of the individual (Medicare.gov, "Costs in the Coverage Gap") until the costs reach the catastrophic coverage threshold (Medicare.gov, "Catastrophic Coverage"). At that point, nearly all costs are then covered by Medicare. The ACA is closing the "donut hole" gap in coverage gradually by 2020, and it provides some rebates for those who encounter the coverage gap in the interim (Medicare.gov, "Costs in the Coverage Gap").

Medicare reimbursement rates are similar to those of private insurance. Clinicians who accept Medicare reimbursement are subject to federal audits of their charts to check billed amounts against services documented.

THE RYAN WHITE PROGRAM

The Ryan White HIV/AIDS Program is a federal program designed specifically to ensure provision of care, treatment, and supportive services for people with HIV/AIDS in the United States. The Ryan White Program was first enacted in 1990, and it is administered by the Health Resources and Services Administration under the US Department of Health and Human Services (USDHHS) (HRSA HIV AIDS Programs, "About the Ryan White HIV/AIDS Program").

The Ryan White Program is a "safety net" for people with HIV/AIDS who have no other source of coverage or face coverage limits (HRSA HIV AIDS Programs HRSA, "About the Ryan White Program"). The program is designed to wrap around other forms of coverage and is "payer of last resort," as required by law. This designation means that if an individual is eligible for any other program, he or she must access its coverage and benefits before accessing the Ryan White Program (HRSA.gov, "Eligible Individuals & Allowable Uses of Funds for Discretely Defined Categories of Services,").

As the third largest source of federal funding for HIV care in the United States after Medicare and Medicaid, the Ryan White Program is estimated to reach more than half a million PLWH each year (Health Resources and Services Administration, Published 2018, Accessed March 19, 2019). Funding for the Ryan White Program is subject to Congressional appropriations each year. In addition to federal funding, some states and localities also provide funding to their Ryan White services through state matching funds requirements.

Part A of the Ryan White Program provides funding to Eligible Metropolitan Areas and Transitional Grant Areas hardest hit by the HIV/AIDS epidemic for a wide range of services and efforts. Part B of the program provides funding to states and territories ("HRSA HIV AIDS Programs About the Ryan White HIV/AIDS Program").

A vitally important part of the program for HIV patients is the AIDS Drug Assistance Program (ADAP), which is funded through allocations to the states under Part B of the program along with state funding contributions. The ADAP in each state provides HIV-related prescription drugs to low-income individuals with limited or no prescription drug coverage (Henry J. Kaiser Family Foundation, "AIDS Drug Assistance Programs"). Many states also use ADAP funding to purchase health insurance and/or pay insurance premiums, copayments, or deductibles for people with HIV/AIDS. All ADAPs participate in the 340B program, enabling them to purchase drugs at or below the statutorily defined 340B ceiling price.

Part C of the Ryan White Program funds providers and medical clinics that deliver comprehensive medical care and treatment to PLWH who have no other source for care ("About the Ryan White HIV/AIDS Program"). Part C also funds early intervention services, ambulatory care, and primary healthcare services for people with HIV in underserved or rural communities and communities of color. Finally, Part C also provides planning grants and capacity grants to support organizations in the delivery of high-quality, effective HIV care ("The Ryan White Program").

Part D of the program grants support services for women, infants, children, and youth ("About the Ryan White HIV/AIDS Program").

Part F of the program provides funding for a variety of programs, including the Special Projects of National Significance, AIDS Education & Training Centers, dental programs, and the Minority AIDS Initiative ("About the Ryan White HIV/AIDS Program").

The Ryan White Program is a "payer of last resort," meaning that patients who have access to other forms of coverage must access those benefits first. For this reason, the implementation of ACA, even given its more recent rollbacks, has had an effect on uptake of Ryan White services, particularly in states that are maximizing their residents' uptake of ACA-available insurance. But the Kaiser Family Foundation nevertheless asserts in a 2017 fact sheet that "the Ryan White Program remains a critical component of the nation's response to HIV in the ACA era" (The Ryan White HIV/AIDS Program: The Basics").

NETWORKS OF CARE

For HIV providers, inclusion in networks of care for health programs is of great importance. Most patients' health coverage limits them to either to seeing only certain providers who are "in network" or to being charged substantially higher fees or being declined payment for services by providers not included in the network.

The ACA requires that all plans in the state exchanges include a minimum percentage of all the Essential Community Providers (ECPs) in a geographic area in their provider network. ECPs are providers that serve predominately low-income, medically underserved individuals (Henry J. Kaiser Family Foundation, "Definition of Essential Community Providers in Marketplaces"). This includes Ryan White HIV/AIDS providers.

Reimbursement rates and schedules for providers who are part of the network are set by or negotiated with health coverage issuers and entities.

PROVIDER REIMBURSEMENT

Reimbursement for medical procedures highly depends on thorough and accurate documentation of the medical encounter, diagnosis, treatment, and services as recorded and submitted through coding claims. The level of complexity and severity of the medical encounter—and thus the level of reimbursement owed—is defined by the complexity of the problem(s), the number of problems at issue, the amount of time spent with the patient, and other factors.

Careful documentation of these factors is required to ensure adequate and appropriate reimbursement. Other factors that are essential to document are the specific elements of the medical history, the physical examination, and the medical decision-making. Documenting time spent on prevention efforts (e.g., counseling the patient about consistent condom use and disclosure to partners) and promoting other behavioral changes (e.g., quitting smoking or avoiding substance abuse) is also essential for accurate reimbursement of these services.

CODING

Standardized coding systems are used in the United States to process billing claims to private and public insurers. The two principal systems used for coding medical information in the United States are the International Classification of Diseases (ICD) and the Current Procedural Terminology (CPT) codes that make up the Healthcare Common Procedure Coding System (HCPCS). In general, CPT/HCPCS codes identify the services rendered, whereas ICD codes focus more on the diagnosis.

The CPT codes are created, maintained, and trademarked by the American Medical Association (AMA) (AMA, "Coding with CPT for Proper Reimbursement").

The HCPCS was created by the federal CMS. The HCPCS is based on the CPT codes but provides for two levels of coding. Level I consists of AMA's CPT codes and provides for medical services and procedures furnished by clinicians. Level I codes are numeric. Level II codes are alphanumeric and apply primarily to medical devices and non-clinician services, such as ambulatory care, immunizations, diagnostic procedures, family counseling, and services provided by other health professionals (e.g., clinical nurses, psychologists, and pharmacists) (Center for Medicare and Medicaid Services, "HCPCS—General Information"). Medicaid and Medicare services are reimbursed by CMS on the basis of the HCPCS codes for clinician activities.

The ICD is the international standard diagnostic classification for all epidemiological, health, and clinical usage. It is a coding and classification system of diseases, symptoms, injuries, and abnormal findings. It also documents the social circumstances and external causes of injury or diseases, as classified by the World Health Organization (WHO). The most recent iteration of these codes, ICD-11, is set for endorsement by the World Health Assembly in 2019. With its 11th update, many technological and infrastructural improvements with the 11th update are expected to enhance transition and usability.

Though it was first used by World Health Assembly member states as early as 1994, the United States did not fully transition to the ICD-10 system until October 2015 (Centers for Disease Control and Prevention, "International Classification of Diseases, Tenth Revision, Clinical Modification [ICD-10-CM]").

In the context of reimbursement, ICD codes are used in conjunction with CPT codes to classify vital records and health condition codes associated with outpatient, inpatient, medical office utilization, and hospital charges.

REFERENCES

American Medical Association. Coding with CPT for proper reimbursement. Available at http://www.ama-assn.org/ama/pub/physician-resources/solutions-managing-your-practice/coding-billing-insurance/cpt.page. Accessed January 14, 2016.

Center for Consumer Information & Oversight. State health insurance marketplaces. Available at https://www.cms.gov/cciio/resources/fact-sheets-and-faqs/state-marketplaces.html. Accessed January 14, 2016.

Centers for Disease Control and Prevention (CDC). International Classification of Diseases, Tenth Revision, Clinical Modification (ICD-10-CM). National Center for Health Statistics. Available at https://www.cdc.gov/nchs/icd/icd10cm.htm. Accessed November 16, 2018.

Centers for Medicare and Medicaid Services. HCPCS—general information. Available at https://www.cms.gov/medicare/coding/medhcpcsgeninfo/index.html. Accessed January 14, 2016.

Centers for Medicare and Medicaid Services. ICD 10. Available at https://www.cms.gov/medicare/Coding/ICD10/index.html. Accessed January 14, 2016.

Duignan B. Affordable Care Act Cases. Encyclopedia Britannica. Available at http://www.britannica.com/event/Affordable-Care-Act-cases. Accessed January 14, 2016.

HealthCare.gov. 10 Health care benefits covered in the health insurance marketplace blog. August 22, 2013. Available at https://www.healthcare.gov/blog/10-health-care-benefits-covered-in-the-health-insurance-marketplace. Accessed March 19, 2019.

HealthCare.gov. Health Insurance Marketplace. HealthCare.gov. Available at https://www.healthcare.gov/glossary/health-insurance-marketplace-glossary. Accessed January 14, 2016.

HealthCare.gov. If you don't have health insurance: how much you'll pay. Available at https://www.healthcare.gov/fees. Accessed January 14, 2016.

Healthcare.gov. Essential health benefits glossary. Available at https://www.healthcare.gov/glossary/essential-health-benefits. Accessed January 14, 2016.

HealthCare.gov. Medicaid and CHIP Coverage Health Insurance Marketplace. Accessed March 19, 2019.

Healthcare.gov. Premium tax credit glossary. Available at https://www.healthcare.gov/glossary/premium-tax-credit. Accessed January 14, 2016.

Henry J. Kaiser Family Foundation. AIDS drug assistance programs. April 8, 2014. Available at http://kff.org/hivaids/fact-sheet/aids-drug-assistance-programs/

Henry J. Kaiser Family Foundation. Definition of essential community providers (ECPs) in Marketplaces. Available at http://kff.org/other/state-indicator/definition-of-essential-community-providers-ecps-in-marketplaces. Accessed January 14, 2016.

Henry J. Kaiser Family Foundation. Medicaid Managed Care Market Tracker. Available at http://kff.org/data-collection/medicaid-managed-care-market-tracker. Accessed January 14, 2016.

Henry J. Kaiser Family Foundation. Medicaid's role for individuals with HIV. April 18, 2017. Available at https://www.kff.org/infographic/medicaids-role-for-individuals-with-hiv/. Accessed November 16, 2018.

Henry J. Kaiser Family Foundation. Medicare and HIV. October 14, 2016. Available at https://www.kff.org/hivaids/fact-sheet/medicare-and-hiv/. Accessed November 16, 2018.

HRSA HIV AIDS Programs. About the Ryan White HIV/AIDS Program. Available at http://hab.hrsa.gov/abouthab/aboutprogram.html. Accessed January 14, 2016.

HRSA.gov. Eligible individuals & allowable uses of funds for discretely defined categories of services. Available at http://hab.hrsa.gov/manageyourgrant/pinspals/eligible1002.html. Accessed January 14, 2016.

HRSA.gov. Annual Client-Level Data Report: Ryan White HIV/AIDS Program Services Report 2017. http://hab.hrsa.gov/data/data-reports. Accessed March 19, 2019.

Kates J. Medicaid and HIV: A national analysis. Henry J. Kaiser Family Foundation. October 2011. Available at http://kff.org/hivaids/report/medicaid-and-hiv-a-national-analysis.

Levy M. Patient Protection and Affordable Care Act (PPACA). Encyclopedia Britannica, June 26, 2015. Available at https://www.britannica.com/topic/Patient-Protection-and-Affordable-Care-Act. Accessed January 14, 2016.

Macsata B. Taking a deeper dive into the Ryan White HIV/AIDS Program. February 8, 2018. Available at http://adapadvocacyassociation.blogspot.com/2018/02/taking-deeper-dive-into-ryan-white.html. Accessed November 16, 2018.

Medicaid.gov. Benefits. Available at https://www.medicaid.gov/medicaid-chip-program-information/by-topics/benefits/medicaid-benefits.html. Accessed January 14, 2016.

Medicaid.gov. Dual eligibles. Available at https://www.medicaid.gov/affordablecareact/provisions/dual-eligibles.html. Accessed January 14, 2016.

Medicaid.gov. Financing & reimbursement. Available at https://www.medicaid.gov/medicaid-chip-program-information/by-topics/financing-and-reimbursement/financing-and-reimbursement.html. Accessed January 14, 2016.

Medicare.gov. Catastrophic coverage. Available at https://www.medicare.gov/part-d/costs/catastrophic-coverage/drug-plan-catastrophic-coverage.html. Accessed January 14, 2016.

Medicare.gov. Costs in the coverage gap. Available at https://www.medicare.gov/part-d/costs/coverage-gap/part-d-coverage-gap.html. Accessed January 14, 2016.

Obamacare Facts. Health care reform timeline. Available at http://obamacarefacts.com/health-care-reform-timeline. Accessed January 14, 2016.

Obamacare Facts. No discrimination. Available at http://obamacarefacts.com/no-discrimination. Accessed January 14, 2016.

Obamacare Facts. Obamacare individual mandate. Available at http://obamacarefacts.com/obamacare-individual-mandate. Accessed January 14, 2016.

Obamacare Facts. Obamacare mandate: exemption and tax penalty. Available at http://obamacarefacts.com/obamacare-mandate-exemption-penalty. Accessed January 14, 2016.

Obamacare Facts. Pre-existing conditions. Available at http://obamacarefacts.com/pre-existing-conditions. Accessed January 14, 2016.

Pollitz JT, Diaz M. Data note: further reductions in navigator funding for Federal Marketplace States. Available at https://www.kff.org/health-reform/issue-brief/data-note-further-reductions-in-navigator-funding-for-federal-marketplace-states/. Published September 14, 2018. Accessed November 18, 2018.

Rho, HJ, Schmitt J. Health-Insurance Coverage Rates for US Workers, 1979-2008. Available at http://cepr.net/documents/publications/hc-coverage-2010-03.pdf. Published March 2010. Accessed March 19, 2019.

Rudowitz R, Snyder L. The ACA and medicaid expansion waivers. The Henry J. Kaiser Family Foundation, May 20, 2015a. Available at http://kff.org/medicaid/issue-brief/medicaid-financing-how-does-it-work-and-what-are-the-implications/.

Rudowitz R, Musumeci M. The ACA and medicaid expansion waivers. The Henry J. Kaiser Family Foundation. November 20, 2015b. Available at http://kff.org/medicaid/issue-brief/the-aca-and-medicaid-expansion-waivers.

Ryan White HIV/AIDS Program. The Basics. Kaiser Family Foundation. February 2017. Available at http://files.kff.org/attachment/fact-sheet-pdf-the-ryan-white-program. Accessed November 16, 2018.

Ryan White Program. The Henry J. Kaiser Family Foundation, March 5, 2013. Available at http://kff.org/hivaids/fact-sheet/the-ryan-white-program.

World Health Organization. International Classification of Diseases (ICD). Available at http://www.who.int/classifications/icd/en. Accessed January 14, 2016.

50.

LEGAL ISSUES

Jeffrey T. Schouten

CHAPTER GOALS

Upon completion of this chapter, the reader should be able to

- Demonstrate knowledge about legal issues surrounding HIV health care and to interact more effectively, professionally, and sensitively with patients and their families.

ROUTINE HIV TESTING (WITH CONSENT)

LEARNING OBJECTIVE

Discuss the Centers for Disease Control and Prevention's (CDC) recommendations for routine HIV testing in various health care settings.

WHAT'S NEW?

- The CDC published in September 2006 revised recommendations concerning routine HIV testing in healthcare settings. However, in 2015, an estimated 15% of persons living with HIV were unaware of their infection, and they accounted for approximately 40% of annual HIV transmissions in the United States. Approximately half of unaware men who have sex with men (MSM) and PWID who reported not having been tested in the past year reported not being offered HIV testing by any clinician despite having seen one.

- An MMWR report from the Centers for Disease Control and Prevention (CDC) in June 2018 evaluated a sample of 333 healthcare-seeking, heterosexual adults at increased risk for acquiring HIV infection: 194 (58%) reported not receiving an HIV test offer at a recent medical visit(s), and men (vs. women) had a significantly lower prevalence of provider-initiated HIV test offers (32% vs. 48%). Recent HIV testing was higher among recipients of provider-initiated offers compared with nonrecipients (71% vs. 16%). Provider-initiated HIV test offers are an important strategy for increasing HIV testing among heterosexual populations. More provider-initiated HIV

screening among heterosexual adults at increased risk for acquiring HIV infection, especially men, is needed.

KEY POINTS

- It is estimated that the 15% of people who do not know they are HIV-infected account for 40% of new cases of HIV infection.

- The CDC recommends that all people aged 13–65 years receive an HIV test at least once as part of routine healthcare. Persons identified as high risk for HIV infection should be retested at least annually.

- Routine testing delinks pre- and posttest counseling from testing.

- Both in routine and emergency care settings, many opportunities for routine HIV testing are missed.

The CDC estimates that more than 1.2 million people in the United States are living with HIV infection. About one in seven (15%) of those people are unaware of their infection (CDC, 2015). A meta-analysis of 11 independent studies showed that the prevalence of high-risk sexual behavior is reduced substantially after people become aware that they are HIV-infected (Marks, 2006). Estimated transmission is 3.5 times higher among persons who are unaware of their infection than among persons who are aware of their infection, which contributes disproportionately to the number of new HIV infections each year in the United States (Marks, 2006). Updated modeling data showed that an estimated 49% of transmissions were from the 20% of persons living with HIV unaware of their infection (Hall, 2012).

A study in South Carolina found that among the persons identified as late testers (persons who received an AIDS diagnosis within 1 year of HIV diagnosis), approximately three-fourths had visited a South Carolina healthcare facility prior to their HIV diagnosis. In addition, most of the late testers had made multiple visits, and most of their visits occurred 1 year or more before diagnosis of HIV infection. According to the report, the majority of diagnoses for these previous visits probably would not have prompted HIV testing under a risk-based testing strategy (CDC, 2006). The CDC published revised recommendations concerning routine HIV testing in healthcare settings in September 2006. The major revisions in the recommendations are as follows:

- For patients in all healthcare settings
  - HIV screening is recommended for patients in all healthcare settings after patients are notified that testing will be performed, unless patients decline (opt-out screening).
  - Persons at high risk for HIV infection should be screened for HIV at least annually.
  - Separate written consent for HIV testing should not be required; general consent for medical care should be considered sufficient to encompass consent for HIV testing.
  - Prevention counseling should *not* be required as part of HIV diagnostic testing or HIV screening programs in healthcare settings.

- For pregnant women
  - HIV screening should be included in the routine panel of prenatal screening tests for all pregnant women.
  - HIV screening is recommended after the patient is notified that testing will be performed unless the patient declines (opt-out screening).
  - Separate written consent for HIV testing should not be required; general consent for medical care should be considered sufficient to encompass consent for HIV testing.
  - Repeat screening in the third trimester is recommended in certain jurisdictions with elevated rates of HIV infection among pregnant women.

Although the CDC recommends that prevention counseling should not be required with HIV diagnostic testing in healthcare settings, the elements of informed consent include some of the information communicated during pretest counseling. Also, risk assessment is needed to identify patients at high risk for HIV infection who should be screened at least annually. The CDC recommendations define informed consent as follows (CDC, 2006):

A process of communication between patient and provider, through which, an informed patient can choose whether to undergo HIV testing or decline to do so. Elements of informed consent typically include providing oral or written information regarding HIV, the risks and benefits of testing, the implications of HIV test results, how test results will be communicated, and the opportunity to ask questions.

Routine testing means that HIV testing is offered to all patients. Testing requires informed consent, but that consent can be included in the general consent to care agreements. Patients can choose to "opt out" of routine testing if they do not want to be tested.

The CDC revisited its recommendations for HIV Screening of Gay, Bisexual, and Other Men Who Have Sex

with Men in August 2017 and concluded that the "CDC's 2006 recommendation for HIV screening of MSM is unchanged; providers in clinical settings should offer HIV screening at least annually to all sexually active MSM. Clinicians can also consider the potential benefits of more frequent HIV screening (e.g., every 3 or 6 months) for some asymptomatic sexually active MSM based on their individual risk factors, local HIV epidemiology, and local policies" (DiNenno, 2017). The CDC also noted that "additional research is needed to establish the individual- or community-level factors that might increase the risk for HIV acquisition for MSM and merit more frequent HIV screening. For MSM who are prescribed preexposure prophylaxis, HIV testing every 3 months and immediate testing whenever signs and symptoms of acute HIV infection are reported is indicated" (DiNenno, 2017).

Laws governing consent for HIV testing are state specific. Although all states require consent for an HIV test, most states that had required explicit written consent prior to the 2006 CDC revised HIV testing recommendations have changed their laws (*JAMA*, 2011). This remains a dynamic area of law and regulation. A good resource is the Compendium of State HIV Testing Laws maintained by the Nations HIV/AIDS Clinicians' Consultation Center, although it is no longer updated.

Challenges in implementing routine HIV testing include cost of testing, follow-up notification of positive results in emergency departments and in-patient settings, and adoption of rapid testing. The US Preventive Services Task Force (USPSTF) recommends that clinicians screen for HIV infection in adolescents and adults aged 15–65 years. Younger adolescents and older adults who are at increased risk should also be screened.

RECOMMENDED READING

American Medical Association (AMA). AMA Code of Ethics: Opinion 2.23—HIV Testing. Available at http://www.ama-assn.org/ama/pub/physician-resources/medical-ethics/code-medical-ethics/opinion223.page. Accessed August 12, 2018.

Centers for Disease Control and Prevention (CDC). Revised recommendations for HIV testing of adults, adolescents, and pregnant women in health-care settings. *MMWR Morbid Mortal Wkly Rep.* 2006;55(RR14):1–17. Available at www.cdc.gov/mmwr/preview/mmwrhtml/rr5514a1.htm. Accessed August 12, 2018

Cossarini F, Hanna DB, Ginsberg MS, et al. Missed opportunities for HIV prevention: individuals who HIV seroconverted despite accessing healthcare. *AIDS Behav.* November 2018;22(11):3519–3524.

Dailey AF, Hoots BE, Hall HI, et al. Vital signs: human immunodeficiency virus testing and diagnosis delays—United States. *MMWR Morb Mortal Rep.* 2017;66(47):1300–1306.

Diepstra KL, Cunningham T, Rhodes AG, et al. Prevalence and predictors of provider-initiated HIV Test offers among heterosexual persons at increased risk for acquiring HIV infection—Virginia, 2016. *MMWR Morb Mortal Wkly Rep.* June 29, 2018;67(25):714–717.

DiNenno EA, Prejean J, Irwin K, et al. Recommendations for HIV screening of gay, bisexual, and other men who have sex with men—United States, 2017. *MMWR Morb Mortal Wkly Rep.* August 11, 2017;66(31):830–832.

Hughes C. ICD-10 simplifies preventive care coding, sort of. *Fam Pract Manag.* July-August 2014;21(4): OA1–OA4. Available at http://www.aafp.org/fpm/2014/0700/oa1.html. Accessed August 12, 2018.

Wejnert C, et al. Prevalence of missed opportunities for HIV testing among persons unaware of their infection. *JAMA.* 2018;319(24):2555–2557.

HIV TESTING WITHOUT CONSENT

LEARNING OBJECTIVE

Discuss the circumstances under which it is allowable to test a patient for HIV without consent, including reference to applicable legal regulations.

WHAT'S NEW?

The information on HIV testing without consent has remained consistent during the past few years.

KEY POINTS

- Many states allow nonconsented HIV testing in limited situations, such as emergency situations or when a healthcare worker or public safety officer has had a potential exposure to HIV.

- Some states require HIV testing of convicted sex offenders, and some states allow testing of persons charged with a crime capable of transmitting HIV, such as rape.

Although all states require consent for HIV testing (Halpern, 2005), there are situations in which it is possible to obtain an HIV test without the consent of the person to be tested. In some cases, nonconsented HIV testing may be standard practice. For example, in New York, newborn infants are tested without parental consent if their mother did not consent to HIV testing during pregnancy. Some states require HIV testing of convicted sexual offenders (e.g., Revised Code of Washington RCW 70.24.340).

A minority of states provide explicit exceptions for consent for HIV testing in emergency medical situations (Halpern, 2005). Some states allow for testing of source patients when there has been a potential exposure to HIV in a healthcare setting or when a public safety officer has had potential exposure. California allows for nonconsented testing of blood samples but will not permit the ordering of a blood draw specifically for HIV testing after an occupational exposure without the consent of the local public health officer or a court (California Health and Safety Code 120260-120263). In most healthcare settings, when there has been an occupational exposure capable of transmitting blood-borne pathogens, the source patient will consent to testing and allow access to his or her medical record (Maryland Department of Health and Mental Hygiene, 2003).

California and several other states allow for HIV testing of persons accused of a criminal act capable of transmitting HIV. California requires a court hearing showing there is probable cause to believe that the accused committed the offense and that blood, semen, or another bodily fluid capable of transmitting HIV (as identified in State Department of Health Services regulations) has been transferred from the accused to the victim (California Penal Code 1524.1(b)(3)(A)). A major challenge with nonconsented testing is getting the required order from the appropriate authority so that testing and initiation of postexposure prophylaxis can take place in a timely manner (see Chapter 3). A survey showed that intensivists' decisions to pursue nonconsented testing, a not uncommon situation, are associated with their personal ethics and often erroneous perceptions of state laws but not with the laws themselves (Halpern, 2007). Because laws and regulations vary by state, the clinician is responsible for knowing the appropriate rules in the state in which he or she practices. Consultation with the local public health officer is advised whenever nonconsented HIV testing is believed to be necessary.

RECOMMENDED READING

Halpern SD. HIV testing without consent in critically ill patients. *JAMA.* 2005;294(6):734–737.

Halpern SD, Metkus TS, Fuchs BD, et al. Nonconsented human immunodeficiency virus testing among critically ill patients: intensivists' practices and the influence of state laws. *Arch Intern Med.* November 26, 2007;167(21):2323–2328.

DISEASE REPORTING SYSTEM

LEARNING OBJECTIVE

Discuss the system of disease reporting in the United States and identify reportable conditions related to HIV care.

WHAT'S NEW?

- All states use name-based HIV case surveillance reporting. Lab-based reporting of CD4 counts and HIV RNA for surveillance have become helpful tools to assess engagement, linkage, and retention in care.

- The CDC updated its HIV Surveillance Case Definition for HIV Infection in 2014.

KEY POINTS

- All state and local departments of health use HIV diagnosis and AIDS reporting to track HIV infection.

- HIV case reporting laws vary by state and generally require that a diagnosis of HIV infection or a related illness and the patient's name be reported.

AIDS SURVEILLANCE

Since HIV/AIDS was first recognized as a disease, most state and city departments of health have used the reporting of AIDS cases to track the incidence and prevalence of HIV infections and HIV-related complications. Data on AIDS cases are reported in a standardized format to the CDC by all 50 states, the District of Columbia, and US dependencies and possessions.

HIV/AIDS SURVEILLANCE

In 1991, some states began implementing standardized HIV case reporting in addition to AIDS case reporting. The reauthorization of the Ryan White CARE Act in 2000 gave states 6 years to adopt name-based HIV reporting or risk losing federal funds. Most states complied with this mandate. Integrated AIDS and HIV case reporting among adults, adolescents, and children had been implemented in 33 states, the Virgin Islands, and Guam by July 2005. Seven states (California, Hawaii, Illinois, Maryland, Massachusetts, Rhode Island, and Vermont) and the District of Columbia implemented a code-based system to conduct case surveillance for HIV infection (not AIDS); five other states (Delaware, Maine, Montana, Oregon, and Washington) implemented a name-to-code system. In 2005, the CDC recommended that name-based HIV reporting be implemented using the same approach that is used for nationwide AIDS surveillance. All states successfully implemented confidential name-based HIV infection reporting by April 2008.

The 2014 Revisions to Surveillance Case Definition revised the laboratory criteria for a confirmed case, which addressed new diagnostic testing algorithms that do not use the western blot or immunofluorescence HIV antibody assays. Another significant change was the addition of "stage 0" based on a sequence of negative and positive test results indicative of early HIV infection (MMWR, 2014).

BENEFITS OF HIV SURVEILLANCE

The rationale frequently cited for using HIV rather than AIDS case surveillance is that it allows for a more thorough and accurate characterization of the populations in which HIV infection has been newly diagnosed and helps in the prioritization of prevention services (CDC, 2005b; Holtgrave, 2004). Significant changes in HIV transmission and behavior can be achieved by appropriate programs. For example, aggressive efforts to prevent maternal–fetal transmission have been credited with the steep decline in mother-to-child HIV transmission, the increase in the proportion of HIV-infected pregnant women who have been tested prior to delivery, and the high proportion of HIV-infected pregnant women who accept antiretroviral prophylaxis (Wortley, 2001). Lab-based reporting of CD4 counts and HIV RNA for surveillance has become a helpful tool to assess engagement, linkage, and retention in care (Lubelchek, 2015; Wiewel, 2015).

ANONYMOUS AND CONFIDENTIAL HIV TESTING

Although most studies have not shown a decrease in HIV testing in states that have adopted name-based reporting, data indicate that some people prefer anonymous HIV testing to name-based confidential testing (CDC, 1998; Charlebois, 2005). Many people are understandably reluctant to have their name entered in a database of persons with HIV infection. Although the states have established elaborate precautions to prevent breaches of security, the risk of revelation of HIV status can be intimidating. Therefore, in many areas, individuals can choose to be tested for HIV either anonymously (without giving any identifying information) or confidentially (with the HIV test result linked to identifying information, such as patient name).

In states that require HIV case reporting, only confidential testing results must be reported to public health authorities. Test results from anonymous testing are not reportable. However, they do provide the clinician with an important opportunity for educating and counseling patients about reducing high-risk behaviors and seeking HIV treatments.

REPORTABLE HIV-RELATED DISEASES

Most states require reporting of conditions that commonly occur or are associated with HIV infection, including syphilis and other sexually transmitted diseases (STDs), tuberculosis, acute hepatitis (A, B, or C), histoplasmosis, and HIV-related opportunistic infections. Certain microbiologic diagnoses that are made by culture or serology are reported directly by the laboratory to the appropriate state or local health authority.

THE CLINICIAN'S ROLE

Healthcare providers should know which illnesses and complications must be reported to their state health departments and the time frame within which reporting is required. They should understand that reporting of notifiable conditions is dependent on the jurisdiction, that a legal obligation is imposed upon practitioners by those states, and that sanctions (e.g., fines) can be imposed upon practitioners for failure to report (CDC, 2014).

RECOMMENDED READING

Centers for Disease, C. and Prevention (2014). "Revised surveillance case definition for HIV infection—United States, 2014." MMWR Recomm Rep 63(RR-03): 1

Lubelchek RJ, Finnegan KJ, Hotton AL, et al. Assessing the use of HIV surveillance data to help gauge patient retention-in-care. *J AIDS.* 2015;69:S25–S30.

US Department of Health and Human Services (USDHHS), Office for Civil Rights. HIPAA. Medical Privacy—National standards to protect the privacy of personal health information. Washington, DC: US Department of Health and Human Services. Available at http://www.hhs.gov/ocr/privacy/index.html.

Wiewel E, Braunstein SL, Xiaet Q, et al. Monitoring outcomes for newly diagnosed and prevalent HIV cases using a care continuum created with New York City surveillance data. *J AIDS.* 2015;68:217–226.

Wortley PM, Lindegren ML, Fleming PL. Successful implementation of perinatal HIV prevention guidelines: a multistate surveillance evaluation. *MMWR Morbid Mortal Wkly Rep.* 2001;50(RR-6):17–28.

PARTNER NOTIFICATION AND PREVENTION FOR HIV-POSITIVE PATIENTS

LEARNING OBJECTIVE

Describe the requirements for partner notification practices in HIV disease.

WHAT'S NEW?

Major efforts are ongoing at the national, state, and local levels in many communities to encourage HIV-infected individuals to take a proactive approach to preventing the spread of HIV. These include immediate antiretroviral therapy (ART) for persons newly diagnosed with HIV and the use of preexposure prophylaxis (PrEP) by at-risk, HIV negative people.

KEY POINTS

- Many states require healthcare providers to discuss partner notification options with their HIV-infected patients. The federal 1996 Ryan White CARE Act requires all states to adopt laws requiring notification of spouses of HIV-infected patients.

- Many HIV-infected individuals do not disclose their HIV status to their partners out of fear of rejection, loss of financial support, and/or abuse. Their partners then remain unaware of their potential HIV exposure.

- Partner notification programs typically allow HIV-infected persons to anonymously inform their sexual and needle-sharing partners that they may have been exposed to HIV.

PARTNER NOTIFICATION LEGAL REQUIREMENTS

In many states, healthcare providers are required to discuss partner notification options with HIV-infected patients. This is not only a legal requirement, carrying the possibility of civil and/or legal sanctions for violation of partner notification laws, but also an ethical issue. Amendments to the federal Ryan White CARE Act in 1996 require states to take "administrative or legislative action to require that a good faith effort" is made to notify the spouse of a known HIV-infected patient of the spouse's potential exposure to HIV. This action must be taken by states in order to be eligible for CARE Act funds (Webber, 2004).

States can be categorized into three groups based on their rules and regulations for partner notification programs: (1) states that require healthcare providers to give the contact's name to the local health officer, and the public health official then notifies the contact; (2) states that give the healthcare provider the choice of notifying either the local health officer or the contacts named by the source patient directly; and (3) states that make such disclosures to a state agency discretionary or optional (Lin, 2005). Healthcare providers should seek advice from local public health departments and their own attorneys to specifically understand their legal responsibilities.

THE CLINICIAN'S ROLE

Preventing harm not only to the patient but also to others should be the goal of every clinician. The CDC has recommended an increased emphasis on prevention efforts in the primary care of HIV-infected people (Box 50.1).

In general, an HIV-infected person should be given the option of directly informing his or her sexual or needle-sharing contacts. A study of MSM found that knowledge of HIV status resulted in a significant decrease in behaviors capable of transmitting HIV; however, the behavioral changes were not permanent (Colfax, 2002).

Many HIV-infected individuals do not disclose their HIV status to their partners, fearing that they would be threatened, harmed, or abandoned. Nondisclosers, however, are not more likely than disclosers to use condoms or other disease prevention measures (Stein, 1998; Wolitski, 1998). When individuals are reluctant to disclose their HIV status to their partners themselves, partner notification programs can assist (CDC, 2008).

PARTNER NOTIFICATION PROGRAMS

Partner notification programs are designed to allow HIV-infected individuals to inform their sexual and needle-sharing partners that they may have been exposed to HIV. For HIV-infected persons who opt not to inform their partners themselves, these programs typically provide counselors who will inform the at-risk persons of possible HIV exposure without revealing the identity of the HIV-infected person who may have exposed them.

Partner notification programs maximize the opportunity for persons to become aware of their HIV exposure and to access HIV testing and counseling. Partner notification may prevent an at-risk individual from acquiring HIV or, if he or she already has HIV, allow him or her to receive appropriate

---

Box 50.1 **METHODS FOR HEALTHCARE PROVIDERS TO HELP REDUCE HIV INFECTION**

- HIV testing and linkage to care

- HIV medications

- Access to condoms

- Prevention programs for people with HIV and their partners

- Prevention programs for people at high risk for HIV infection

- Substance abuse treatment and access to sterile needles and syringes

- STI screening and treatment

SOURCE: CDC (2016).

treatment and learn how to prevent the transmission of HIV infection to others.

RECOMMENDED READING

Centers for Disease Control and Prevention (CDC). Recommendations for partner services programs for HIV infection, syphilis, gonorrhea, and chlamydial infection. 2008 MMWR Recomm Rep 57(Rr-9):1–83; quiz CE81–84. Available at https://www.cdc.gov/mmwr/preview/mmwrhtml/rr5709a1.htm

Centers for Disease Control and Prevention (CDC). Incorporating HIV prevention into the medical care of persons living with HIV. Recommendations of CDC, the Health Resources and Services Administration, the National Institutes of Health, and HIV Medicine Association of the IDSA. *MMWR Morbid Mortal Wkly Rep.* 2003;52:1–24. Available at http://www.cdc.gov/mmwr/preview/mmwrhtml/rr5212a1.htm.

Colfax GN, Buchbinder SP, Cornelisse PGA, et al. Sexual risk behaviors and implications for secondary HIV transmission during and after HIV seroconversion. *AIDS.* 2002;16:1529–1535.

Laar AK, DeBruin DA, Craddock S. Partner notification in the context of HIV: an interest-analysis. *AIDS Res Ther.* 2015;12:15. Available at http://www.biomedcentral.com/content/pdf/s12981-015-0057-8.pdf. Accessed November 30, 2015.

Lin L, Liang BA. HIV and health law: striking the balance between legal mandates and medical ethics. *Virtual Mentor AMA J Ethics.* 2005;7(10). Available at http://journalofethics.ama-assn.org/2005/10/hlaw1-0510.html.

Stein MD, Freedberg KA, Sullivan LM, et al. Sexual ethics: disclosure of HIV-positive status to partners. *Arch Intern Med.* 1998;158:253–257.

Webber DW. Self-incrimination, partner notification, and the criminal law: negatives for the CDC's "prevention for positives" initiative. *AIDS Public Policy J.* 2004;19:54–66.

Wejnert C, et al. Prevalence of missed opportunities for HIV testing among persons unaware of their infection. *JAMA.* 2018;319(24):2555–2557

Available at http://www.hivlawandpolicy.org/resources/self-incrimination-partner-notification-and-criminal-law-negatives-cdc%E2%80%99s-%E2%80%9Cprevention. Accessed November 30, 2015.

ISSUES IN DISCLOSURE

LEARNING OBJECTIVE

Discuss the healthcare provider's legal responsibilities to HIV-infected patients who do not disclose their HIV status to sexual and needle-sharing partners.

WHAT'S NEW?

Information regarding disclosure issues has remained consistent during the past several years.

KEY POINTS

- The obligation of healthcare providers to maintain patient confidentiality may be overridden to protect the public health or individuals who are endangered by HIV-infected persons.

- Healthcare providers should consult an attorney or their state laws and regulations before making any such disclosures.

- Healthcare providers may have a "duty to warn" if there is an ongoing exposure to potential HIV infection. Conversely, there may be criminal actions brought against patients based on information provided to local health departments about ongoing behaviors endangering the public health.

Information disclosed by a patient to a healthcare provider during the course of the provider–patient relationship is considered confidential. This confidentiality is essential for a full and free disclosure of information so that effective counseling and therapy can be provided. In general, unless required by the law to do so, a healthcare provider is ethically barred from revealing confidential communications or information without the patient's consent.

The obligation to maintain patient confidence is not without limits, however, and it may be overridden by exceptions that are ethically and legally justified. Such justification may occur when a patient threatens to inflict bodily harm to another person or to him- or herself and there is a reasonable probability that the patient may carry out the threat, and also when reports are required by law, such as with communicable diseases and gunshot and knife wounds. California established a physician's duty to warn third parties if there is an imminent threat of serious harm to a known third party (Tarasoff, 1976). Subsequent to the *Tarasoff* case, many other states have adopted this duty-to-warn requirement and even expanded it to the unknown third parties. However, it is still not clear whether the duty to warn as identified in the *Tarasoff* case would apply to a sexual or needle-sharing partner of an HIV-infected patient who had not disclosed his or her HIV status.

It is important to differentiate "permissive" disclosures allowed under state laws, usually to local public health officers, from "mandatory" disclosures as required by law. A mandatory disclosure is one that a healthcare provider must make, such as disclosure of reportable diseases or suspected child abuse. In a permissive disclosure, local regulations allow a healthcare provider to discuss a specific patient with local public health officials (e.g., to seek their assistance in modifying a patient's behavior).

It is within this legal and ethical framework that providers should consider their obligations when they are aware that an HIV-infected patient is endangering others by engaging in acts that may lead to transmission of HIV. American Medical Association (AMA) guidelines issued in 1992 and updated in 1994, while recognizing a physician's obligation to protect the patient's confidentiality whenever possible, acknowledge that there are exceptions to this confidentiality:

When necessary to protect the public health or when necessary to protect individuals, including healthcare workers, who are endangered by persons infected with HIV. If a physician knows that a seropositive individual is endangering a third party, the physician should, within the constraints of the law: (1) attempt to persuade the infected patient to cease endangering the third party; (2) if persuasion fails, notify authorities; and (3) if the authorities take no action, notify the endangered third party.

Given the legal implications of divulging a person's HIV status, healthcare providers should consult an attorney or become familiar with state laws and regulations before making any such disclosures.

RECOMMENDED READING

AIDS.gov. HIV disclosure policies and procedures. Available at AIDS.gov/hiv-aids-basics. Accessed August 12, 2018.

Downs L. The duty to protect a patient's right to confidentiality: Tarasoff, HIV, and confusion. *J Forensic Psychol Pract.* 2015;15(2):160–170. Available at http://dx.doi.org/10.1080/15228932.2015.1007776.

Lin L, Liang BA. HIV and health law: striking the balance between legal mandates and medical ethics. *Virtual Mentor Am Med Assoc J Ethics.* 2005;7(10). Available at http://journalofethics.ama-assn.org/2005/10/hlaw1-0510.html.

Obermeyer CM, Baijal P, Pegurri E. Facilitating HIV disclosure across diverse settings: a review. *Am J Pub Health.* 2011;101(6):1011–1023.

Richardson R, Golden S, Hanssens C. *Ending & defending against HIV criminalization—A manual for advocates: Vol. 1. State and federal laws and prosecutions,* 2nd ed., Winter 2015. Available at http://www.hivlawandpolicy.org/sites/www.hivlawandpolicy.org/files/HIV%20Crim%20Manual%20%28updated%205.4.15%29.pdf.

Webber DW. Self-incrimination, partner notification, and the criminal law: negatives for the CDC's "prevention for positives" initiative. *AIDS Public Policy J.* 2004;19:54–66.

HIV CRIMINALIZATION

LEARNING OBJECTIVE

Describe the scientific rationale of the International AIDS Society's expert consensus statement on the science of HIV in the context of criminal law and the recommendations from the National HIV/AIDS Strategy (NHAS) concerning criminal laws regarding HIV transmission and prevention.

WHAT'S NEW?

This section has been separated from the Issues in Disclosure section due to the increased concerns about criminalization of HIV nondisclosure and/or exposure.

KEY POINTS

- Stigma and discrimination continue to be major challenges to the comprehensive response necessary to address the HIV public health crisis.

- The NHAS recommends that evidence-based public health approaches to HIV prevention and care be implemented and that state legislatures should review HIV-specific criminal statutes to ensure that they are consistent with current scientific knowledge of HIV transmission and support public health approaches to preventing and treating HIV.

- The International AIDS Society recommends that those working in legal and judicial systems pay close attention to the significant advances in HIV science that have occurred over the past three decades to ensure that current scientific knowledge informs application of the law in cases related to HIV.

In an attempt to limit the spread of HIV, many states have enacted laws that criminalize willful or knowing exposure of another person to HIV infection (Gostin, 1989). Some statutes do not require proof of intent to harm—only proof that the person knew that he or she was HIV-infected and, despite that knowledge, failed to inform at-risk contacts or use appropriate precautions (e.g., safer sex or clean needles) to prevent contacts from becoming infected. These laws have also been applied to HIV-positive people who solicited sex for money, a prisoner who bit a prison guard, and individuals who spat on another person. Although these statutes have been challenged on the alleged grounds of unconstitutional vagueness or violations of free speech or free association, most have been upheld. In addition to these laws, prosecutors have brought other criminal charges against HIV-infected individuals who unreasonably risk transmission of HIV through such acts as attempted murder, assault or assault with a dangerous or deadly weapon, and reckless endangerment (Gostin, 1989; Webber, 2004). The tension between the public health approach versus a criminal justice approach and the effect on disclosure continues as applied to HIV transmission (Csete, 2011; Obermeyer, 2011).

Criminalization of potential HIV exposure is largely a matter of state law. An analysis by CDC and US Department of Justice researchers found that, through 2011, a total of 67 laws explicitly focused on persons living with HIV had been enacted in 33 states. These laws vary as to what behaviors are criminalized or result in additional penalties. In 24 states, laws require persons who are aware that they have HIV to disclose their status to sexual partners, and 14 states require disclosure to needle-sharing partners. Twenty-five states have laws that criminalize one or more behaviors that, as noted by Lehman et al., pose low or negligible risk for HIV transmission (Lehman, 2014). The majority of laws were passed before studies showed that ART reduces HIV transmission risk, and most laws do not account for HIV prevention measures that reduce transmission risk, such as condom use, ART, or PrEP. Punishing people for behavior that is either consensual or poses no risk of HIV transmission only serves to further stigmatize already marginalized communities while missing opportunities for prevention education.

The American Academy of HIV Medicine (AAHIVM) and its members are opposed to laws that distinguish HIV disease from other comparable diseases or that create disproportionate penalties for disclosure, exposure, or transmission of HIV disease beyond normal public health ordinances.

The AAHIVM supports nonpunitive prevention approaches to HIV centered on current scientific understanding and evidence-based research. The HIV Medicine Association (HIVMA) urged repeal of HIV-specific criminal statutes and noted that stigma and discrimination continue to be major impediments to the comprehensive response necessary to address the HIV public health crisis. HIVMA noted that policies and laws that create HIV-specific crimes or that impose penalties for persons who are HIV-infected are unjust and harmful to public health throughout the world.

The NHAS, released by the White House in July 2010 and updated in 2015 with goals through 2020, recommends that federal and state governments should ensure that federal and state criminal laws reflect current scientific information regarding HIV transmission and prevention. The NHAS document also recommends evidence-based public health approaches to HIV prevention and care. The document notes that state legislatures should review HIV-specific criminal statutes to ensure that they are consistent with current scientific knowledge of HIV transmission and support public health approaches to preventing and treating HIV.

An expert consensus statement on the science of HIV in the context of criminal law was published in July 2018. The statement concluded that

> we strongly recommend that more caution be exercised when considering criminal prosecution, including careful appraisal of current scientific evidence on HIV-related risks and harms. This is instrumental to reduce stigma and discrimination and to avoid miscarriages of justice. In this context, we hope this Consensus Statement will encourage governments and those working in the legal and judicial system to pay close attention to the significant advances in HIV science that have occurred over the last three decades, and make all efforts to ensure that a correct and complete understanding of current scientific knowledge informs any application of the criminal law in cases related to HIV. (Barre-Sinoussi, 2018)

The Sero Project is a network of persons living with HIV and their allies fighting for freedom from stigma and injustice. Sero is particularly focused on ending inappropriate criminal prosecutions of people with HIV, including for nondisclosure of their HIV status and potential or perceived HIV exposure or HIV transmission. Iowa and California have both revised their HIV criminalization laws to better reflect the current scientific information about HIV transmission.

RECOMMENDED READING

Adam BD, Corriveau P, Elliott R, et al. HIV disclosure as practice and public policy. *Crit Public Health*. 2015;25(4):386–397. Available at http://dx.doi.org/10.1080/09581596.2014.980395.

American Civil Liberties Union. State criminal statutes on HIV transmission—2008. Available at https://www.aclu.org/state-criminal-statutes-hiv-transmission?redirect=lgbt-rights_hiv-aids/state-criminal-statutes-hiv-transmission. Accessed December 2, 2015.

Barre-Sinoussi F, Abdool Karim SS, Albert J, et al. Expert consensus statement on the science of HIV in the context of criminal law. *J Int AIDS Soc*. July 2018;21(7):e25161.

Center for HIV Law & Policy: HIV Criminalization in the United States: an overview of the variety and prevalence of laws used to prosecute and punish people living with HIV (PLHIV) in the US. June 2018. Available at https://www.hivlawandpolicy.org/sites/default/files/CHLP%20HIV%20Crim%20Map%20061418.pdf.

Francis LP, Francis JG. Criminalizing health-related behaviors dangerous to others? Disease transmission, transmission-facilitation, and the importance of trust. *Criminal Law Philosophy*. 2012;6:47–63.

Haire B, Kaldor J. HIV transmission law in the age of treatment-as-prevention. *J Med Ethics*. 2015;41:982–986.

HIV Criminalization Resources. Available at http://www.seroproject.com/resources. Accessed August 12, 2018.

HIV Law and Policy. State HIV laws HIV-specific criminal laws, state guidelines for health care workers with HIV, youth access to STI and HIV testing and treatment, HIV testing. Available at http://www.hivlawandpolicy.org/state-hiv-laws.

HIV.gov. National HIV/AIDS Strategy for the United States. Updated to 2020. Available at https://files.hiv.gov/s3fs-public/nhas-update.pdf.

HIVMA urges repeal of HIV-specific criminal statutes. Available at http://www.hivma.org/uploadedFiles/HIVMA/FINAL%20HIVMA%20Policy%20Statement%20on%20HIV%20Criminalization.pdf.

Lehman JS, Carr MH, Nichol AJ, et al. Prevalence and public health implications of state laws that criminalize potential HIV exposure in the United States. *AIDS Behav* 2014;18(6):997–1006. Available at http://rd.springer.com/article/10.1007/s10461-014-0724-0/fulltext.html.

Mykhalovskiy E. The public health implications of HIV criminalization: past, current, and future research directions. *Crit Public Health*. 2015;25(4):373–385. Available at http://dx.doi.org/10.1080/09581596.2015.1052731.

TREATING MINORS

LEARNING OBJECTIVE

Describe legal issues related to treatment of minors with HIV infection.

WHAT'S NEW?

On May 15, 2018, the US Food and Drug Administration (FDA) approved an indication for Truvada for PrEP in adults and adolescents who weigh at least 35 kg (77 lb). The approval of PrEP for adolescents has refocused attention on consent for minors for HIV prevention interventions.

KEY POINTS

- Medical treatment of minors (persons younger than age 18 years) must generally be authorized by a parent or legal guardian, with specific exceptions that vary across states.

- This area of law is often complex and variable. Healthcare providers unsure of their state laws and regulations should seek legal advice before treating minors for HIV.

The medical care of a minor—defined in most states as a person younger than age 18 years—must generally be authorized by his or her parent or legal guardian. This usually means that a parent or guardian of a minor is required to give informed consent on behalf of the minor for most medical decisions. However, there are exceptions to this rule, and certain minors can consent to certain types of medical care without the authority of a parent or legal guardian.

CONSENT FOR STD SERVICES AND MEDICAL TREATMENT

STD Services

All 50 states and the District of Columbia explicitly allow minors to consent to STD services, although 11 states require that a minor be of a certain age (generally ages 12–14 years) before being allowed to consent. Thirty-two states explicitly include HIV testing and treatment in the package of STD services to which minors may consent.

Medical Treatment

Most states have laws that authorize minors to consent to certain types of medical treatment, such as care for pregnancy; contraception and abortion care; treatment for contagious diseases, STDs, rape, sexual assault, mental health, and drug or alcohol abuse; and HIV testing. In many states, absent exceptional circumstances, a minor is not able to consent to HIV treatment, and consent must be obtained from the parent or legal guardian (e.g., see New York State Public Health Law 2504).

Exceptions

Almost all states have laws that authorize minors who have attained a certain status to make the majority of their own healthcare decisions. These may include minors who are married (or divorced), on active duty with the US Armed Forces, emancipated by a court order, or self-sufficient such that they have attained a designated age and live away from home and manage their own financial affairs.

LAWS RELATED TO INFORMING PARENTS

Eighteen states allow healthcare providers to inform a minor's parents that he or she is seeking or receiving STD services. With the exception of one state (Iowa requires parental notification in the case of a positive HIV test), no state requires that providers notify parents (Guttmacher Institute, 2007; Ho, 2005). In some states, healthcare providers are prohibited from telling the minor's parent(s) or legal guardian about any test-related medical care unless the minor authorizes it (e.g., see New York State Public Health Law 2780.5).

SEEKING LEGAL ADVICE

Healthcare providers should be aware that this area of the law is very complex, highly variable by state, and rife with legal risks and exposure if an incorrect decision regarding treatment is made. Therefore, it is highly advisable that healthcare providers who are unsure of the law in their state consult a lawyer before providing HIV testing or treatment to a minor. Healthcare providers must be acutely aware of the importance of consulting and obtaining the informed consent of a parent or legal guardian of the minor when required by law.

RECOMMENDED READING

Guttmacher Institute. Minors' access to STD services. Available at http://www.guttmacher.org/statecenter/spibs/spib_MASS.pdf. Accessed August 12, 2018
Ho WW, Brandfield J, Retkin R, et al. Complexities in HIV consent in adolescents. *Clin Pediatr (Phil)*. 2005;44:473–478.
HIV.gov. National HIV/AIDS Strategy for the United States: Updated to 2020. Available at https://files.hiv.gov/s3fs-public/nhas-update.pdf.
HIV Law and Policy. State HIV laws HIV-specific criminal laws, state guidelines for health care workers with HIV, youth access to STI and HIV testing and treatment, HIV testing. Available at http://www.hivlawandpolicy.org/state-hiv-laws
HIV Law and Policy. Services. Available at https://www.cdc.gov/hiv/policies/law/states/minors.html

CONFIDENTIALITY

LEARNING OBJECTIVE

Discuss legal issues related to confidentiality and HIV, including health information protected under the Health Insurance Portability and Accountability Act of 1996 (HIPAA). along with HIPAA's Privacy Rule and its impact on communicating a patient's personal health information.

KEY POINTS

- There are many reasons for maintaining strict confidentiality in the medical setting, including the need to maintain effective clinician–patient relationships.

- Various state and federal regulations govern confidentiality of medical information. Noncompliance carries the risk of civil and/or criminal penalties.

- Federal provisions governing confidentiality were established in HIPAA. The act defines which health entities are covered, the types of medical information covered, how information can be used, and requirements for notifying patients. The deadline for compliance with the HIPAA Privacy Rule was April 14, 2003.

- The HIPAA Security Standards dictate that "administrative, physical, and technical" safeguards must be in place to protect confidential information and its transmission and storage. Healthcare providers had to comply with the HIPAA Security Standards by April 21, 2005, with a 1-year extension permitted for small health plans.

- Available resources may assist clinicians in complying with HIPPA and other confidentiality provisions.

The rationale for confidentiality in the medical setting is that an effective clinician–patient relationship is based on trust and strict confidentiality regarding the patient's medical information. Maintaining patient confidentiality has particular importance when the patient is infected with HIV. The patient may choose to keep his or her status private in order to avoid significant emotional, social, and financial stigmatization, isolation, and loss that many HIV-infected persons encounter when their status becomes known. Therefore, every clinician should seek to respect the privacy of his or her patients, including persons living with HIV, and their wishes not to have personal information about themselves made available to others.

The Hippocratic Oath and other ethical guidelines instruct providers that information gained through the provider–patient relationship is confidential. Confidentiality requirements are also underscored by various state laws and federal provisions. HIPAA has implications for nearly all healthcare providers and facilities, including federally funded facilities that provide substance abuse treatment services.

In general, both state and federal confidentiality requirements address the areas discussed in the following sections.

HANDLING OF MEDICAL INFORMATION

State laws require patient consent for releasing information to all or only certain requestors. The HIPAA provide criteria to oversee transmission of information within the current interrelated healthcare system for purposes of treatment, payment, or other healthcare functions. HIPAA regulates the sharing of information among multiple providers and payers.

PROCEDURES FOR HANDLING EXCEPTIONAL SITUATIONS

State laws typically provide for disclosure of information for public health purposes, such as the "duty to warn" an individual facing imminent harm from a patient. Assaults and communicable diseases are reportable, and their reporting may be legally mandated (AMA, 2005). Physician–patient confidentiality is not absolute under the law of most states. The courts and legislators in many states have attempted to strike a balance between competing rights: those of patients to confidentiality and those of others to information about the significant dangers they may face. It seems reasonable that the patient's right to privacy should be breached only when it is necessary to avoid imminent and serious harm. If the chance of contracting HIV from contact with the patient is remote (i.e., a household contact), then the right to confidentiality should be considered paramount. However, if the chance of contracting HIV is high (i.e., through sexual contact), then the duty to warn may take precedence (see Objective 60.5, Issues in Disclosure).

PENALTIES

Providers treating HIV-infected patients must seek to balance these legal and ethical obligations. There is no guarantee that the balance struck by the clinician will be the same struck by a court should the matter end up in litigation. Almost half of the states have provisions for revoking a healthcare provider's medical license or exercising other disciplinary action when confidential patient information is inappropriately or unlawfully disclosed. HIPAA also contains penalty provisions. When in doubt, the clinician should consult an attorney before taking any action or making any disclosure without consent.

HIPAA

In 2003, Boyle and colleagues described the HIPAA regulations on privacy and disclosure of medical information (i.e., the "Privacy Rule"). HIPAA places the burden on healthcare providers and others who have access to confidential medical information to keep that information private and protected. HIPAA outlines who must comply, what information is protected, and what providers must do to comply. Similar state laws take precedence if they are more stringent than HIPAA.

The Privacy Rule definition of who must comply ("covered entities") covers most clinicians and health plans because it essentially applies to anyone who bills for services electronically. "Protected health information" (PHI) also is broadly defined (i.e., medical records and other identifying information). Covered entities were required to comply with the Privacy Rule by April 14, 2003.

The Privacy Rule stipulates in great detail how information may be used and disclosed. A key example of allowed uses is the release of information to the patient in question. Patients must have access to their medical records along with information about who has been granted access to them. Information also can be used in treatment and payment processes. HIPAA contains provisions for special circumstances in which medical information can be released, such as the "duty to warn" provisions cited previously.

Patient consent must be obtained for most disclosures of medical information. Covered entities are also required to provide patients with a written "Notice of Privacy Practices" that clearly explains the provider's privacy policy—and they must document that their patients received it (Boyle, 2003). In general, healthcare providers must institute reasonable measures to prevent incidental disclosure of patient information. Such measures include ensuring that unauthorized persons cannot wander into record rooms, access computer databases, or overhear names during in-person or telephone communications. However, HIPAA is not intended to impede customary communications, nor does it require protection against any conceivable incidental disclosure, such as when a visitor glimpses patient names on a sign-in sheet.

In addition to the Privacy Rule, HIPAA also requires clinicians and health plans to protect the security of patients' medical information that is stored or transmitted electronically (the "Security Standards"). The Security Standards call for all covered entities to enact administrative, physical, and technical safeguards for electronic data. Examples of such safeguards in an office setting are policies that limit access to

Table 50.1 WEB-BASED HIPAA AND PRIVACY COMPLIANCE RESOURCES FOR HEALTHCARE PROVIDERS

ORGANIZATION	URL	CONTENTS
American Medical Association	http://www.ama-assn.org/ama/pub/physician-resources/solutions-managing-your-practice/coding-billing-insurance/hipaahealth-insurance-portability-accountability-act.page?	HIPAA information FAQ page Sample documents Links to other resources Complaint form for out-of-compliance health plans and other payers
US Department of Health and Human Services Office of Civil Rights	www.hhs.gov/ocr/hipaa	HIPAA information for clinicians and patients Fact sheets Sample documents Educational materials
Centers for Medicare and Medicaid Services	https://www.cms.gov/Regulations-and-Guidance/Administrative-Simplification/HIPAA-ACA/index.html	Standards Educational materials

database software to those who require it (physical safeguard), sanctions for employees who violate the standards (administrative safeguard), and the maintenance of electronic "audit logs" on computer systems that are equipped to access PHI (technical safeguard).

The compliance date for the Security Standards was April 21, 2005. Small health plans had an additional year to comply with the rules.

IDEAS FOR COMPLIANCE

Clinicians should establish compliance provisions not only to fulfill HIPAA requirements but also to be prepared to handle confidentiality in a responsible manner. Among the methods used is the securing of written informed consent from patients (required by HIPAA for certain situations) and formulation of clear procedures for handling patient information (e.g., secure storage, definitions of what information is to be protected and with whom it can be shared, and strategies for handling special circumstances). Other options include designating a privacy officer who is knowledgeable about the details of HIPAA and providing staff training on confidentiality.

For handling situations in which a "duty to warn" another individual arises, such as a sex partner or injection drug-using partner, clinicians can seek assistance. Most local or state health departments have partner notification programs that do this work. A number of Internet resources can assist clinicians in complying with HIPAA and other confidentiality provisions (Table 50.1).

The Patient Safety and Quality Improvement Act of 2005 (PSQIA) establishes a voluntary reporting system to enhance the data available to assess and resolve patient safety and healthcare quality issues. To encourage the reporting and analysis of medical errors, PSQIA provides federal privilege and confidentiality protections for patient safety information called *patient safety work product*. The patient safety work product includes information collected and created during the reporting and analysis of patient safety events. The regulation

implementing the PSQIA became effective on January 19, 2009 (42 C.F.R. Part 3).

PSQIA authorizes the US Department of Health and Human Services (USDHHS) to impose civil money penalties for violations of patient safety confidentiality. PSQIA also authorizes the Agency for Healthcare Research and Quality (AHRQ) to list patient safety organizations (PSOs). PSOs are the external experts that collect and review patient safety information.

The Administrative Simplification provisions of HIPPA (Title II) require the USDHHS to adopt national standards for electronic healthcare transactions and national identifiers from providers, health plans, and employers. To date, the implementation of HIPPA standards has increased the use of electronic data interchange. Provisions under the Affordable Care Act of 2010 include requirements to adopt the following:

- Operating rules for each of the HIPPA-covered transactions

- A unique, standard Health Plan Identifier (HPID)

- Standard and operating rules for electronic funds transfer and electronic remittance advice and claims attachments

In addition, health plans will be required to certify their compliance. The Act provides for substantial penalties for failures to comply with the new standards and operation rules.

RECOMMENDED READING

American Medical Association (AMA). The AMA Code of Medical Ethics' opinions on confidentiality of patient information. Available at http://journalofethics.ama-assn.org/2012/09/coet1-1209.html.

American Medical Association (AMA). The AMA Code of Medical Ethics' opinions on confidentiality of patient information. Opinion 9.124—Professionalism in the use of social media. Available at http://journalofethics.ama-assn.org/2011/07/coet1-1107.html.

ADVANCE PLANNING

LEARNING OBJECTIVE

Discuss the use of advance directives, durable power of attorney, health proxy, and arranging for custody of minors for HIV-infected patients.

WHAT'S NEW?

Information regarding advance planning has remained consistent during the past few years.

People newly diagnosed with HIV infection (or any potentially life-threatening illness) face a myriad of legal concerns that affect almost every facet of their lives. At times, this may seem overwhelming to patient and provider alike. However, legal planning can greatly benefit HIV-infected patients and their families. Providers can play an important role in informing patients of the benefits of planning ahead.

All providers should advise their patients to investigate and prepare three essential tools of effective legal planning:

1. A durable power of attorney for medical decision-making

2. An advance directive ("living will")

3. A will

DURABLE POWER OF ATTORNEY

A durable power of attorney makes legal provision for someone to make decisions in a patient's stead if he or she is no longer able to do so. Patients should consider two such documents to best protect their legal interests: one for healthcare decisions and one for legal and financial decisions. A patient may choose a single person to fill both roles, but the responsibilities are different. A durable power of attorney for financial issues may cover any and all financial concerns or may stipulate only specific tasks, such as paying standard household expenses or filing tax returns (Nolo, 2002a). A durable power of attorney for healthcare may cover any and all medical decisions or may stipulate only specific decisions can be made, such as consenting to or refusing any medical treatment. These documents are particularly important for couples who are not legally married, including gay and lesbian couples, because without a durable power of attorney, hospitals and courts usually defer to the closest biological relative to make medical decisions.

A power of attorney may take effect immediately when a patient signs it, or it may become effective only at a time or circumstance that the patient designates—for example, upon the patient's incapacity or other disability that hinders medical or financial decision-making (Nolo, 2002a). Patients must state in the document that a power of attorney is durable, or it will automatically end if the patient becomes incapacitated. In all cases, a power of attorney ends when the patient dies. Patients may choose to revoke the power of attorney at any time. If married patients grant power of attorney to a spouse,

in some states (e.g., California, Illinois, and Texas) the power terminates if the couple divorces (Nolo, 2002a). Patients should consult an attorney in drafting a durable power of attorney to ensure that it is drawn up correctly.

ADVANCE DIRECTIVES

An advance directive is a document in which patients provide specific instructions about the kind of healthcare they do or do not want in the event that they have an incapacity that makes them unable to make or communicate medical decisions. These instructions are commonly referred to as a "living will." However, there is an important distinction: living wills generally are limited to cases of terminal illness, whereas advance directives may apply to any situation in which a patient is incapacitated, even temporarily. This distinction is especially compelling regarding HIV-infected patients, who may experience AIDS-related dementia or other complications that may impair rational decision-making, but they may subsequently have improved executive function as a result of ART. Patients should know that an advance directive "may be the most convincing evidence of your wishes you can create" (American Association of Retired Persons, 1995). However, in a large national study of HIV-infected patients, fewer than half reported having advance directives. The most important factor associated with having an advance directive was whether their practitioner had discussed end-of-life issues (Wenger, 2001). As the HIV population ages, these discussions should routinely be part of each medical visit.

Advance directives are valid in every US state and the District of Columbia, but the specifics of the law vary from state to state. Therefore, patients who spend significant time in more than one state or who move to another state should have directives adjusted to follow each state's guidelines (Caring Connections, 2006). In creating an advance directive, the patient should consult an expert and should attempt to answer three important questions:

- What are my goals for treatment? Among other things, patients should consider their values relative to independence and their environment and their religious beliefs.

- How specific should I be? No directive can cover all eventualities, but it is suggested that patients address anything that is especially important to them.

- How can I make sure that healthcare providers will follow my advance directive?

Most states give healthcare providers the right to refuse to honor directives on grounds of conscience. In such cases, healthcare providers generally are obligated to refer patients to other healthcare providers who will honor the directive. It is important to ask patients about their wishes. Generally, patients need both a durable power of attorney and an advance directive. In essence, the advance directive expresses a patient's specific wishes, and the durable power of attorney grants someone the authority to execute those wishes or to make healthcare decisions that could not be anticipated by the advance directive.

Although patients are urged to draft durable powers of attorney and advance directives in every state, legal arrangements are especially critical in New York, Michigan, and Massachusetts. In New York, families are not authorized to make medical decisions for patients who cannot make decisions for themselves (New York State Department of Health, 1991). Therefore, an incapacitated patient may have healthcare decisions made for him or her by healthcare providers or lawyers. To avoid that situation, patients in New York must have a healthcare proxy. The healthcare proxy combines elements of an advance directive and a durable power of attorney; the proxy is a form that patients must sign. Two witnesses (other than the person named in the proxy to make decisions on the patient's behalf) are required (New York State Department of Health, 2003).

Massachusetts and Michigan do not have statutes allowing for living wills, but they do allow for healthcare proxies, which can serve a similar function (FindLaw, 2006). Massachusetts requires a specific healthcare proxy form which clinicians should make available to patients.

A 2001 study by Stein and Bonuck found that gay men and lesbians were more likely than the general population to have executed advance directives (Stein, 2001). However, given the importance of these documents to HIV-infected patients, and because fewer than half of those studied had executed formal directives, healthcare providers are urged to assume a larger role in educating patients about advance care planning. Another study in 2000 affirmed previous results that intervention in an outpatient setting significantly increased the likelihood that HIV-infected patients would execute advance care planning (Ho, 2000).

Although the focus of advance care planning is usually on the healthcare and legal value of the process, another study showed that advance care planning also increased patients' sense of control and strengthened their relationships with their loved ones (Martin, 1999). However, more than 75% of all respondents in the Stein and Bonuck study said that their healthcare provider had never asked who should make medical decisions if patients were unable to do so themselves (Stein, 2001). Healthcare providers are encouraged to discuss these issues with patients.

PHYSICIAN ORDER FOR LIFE-SUSTAINING TREATMENT

A physician order for life-sustaining treatment (POLST) form is becoming more commonly implemented as a part of advance care planning in many states. This form should be done with the healthcare provider, and it specifies medical treatments that a patient may or may not want in the event of a medical emergency or life-threatening event. In many cases it can complement the advanced directive and may be more appropriate for persons with a serious illness or advanced frailty near the end of life.

WILLS

A will determines what happens to a person's property after his or her death. Despite considerable attention to wills in the popular press, do not assume that your patients have one—half of all Americans die without one (Met Life Consumer Education Center, 2006). Without a will, the courts will distribute a person's assets according to state laws. Wills are particularly important for people with minor children because, without a will, the state will decide the children's guardianship (Nolo, 2002b). Wills are also important in situations in which the person is not legally married to his or her partner (e.g., common law marriage and unmarried gay and lesbian couples) because, without a will, a survivor may inherit nothing and, worse, may lose personal property because he or she cannot prove ownership (Human Rights Campaign, 2004).

Many people mistakenly believe that they do not need wills because they do not have large estates. In truth, everyone needs a will to ensure that their wishes are followed when their assets are distributed. Handwritten, unwitnessed wills (called *holographic wills*) are valid in approximately 25 states, but more formal wills are preferable. A valid, legal will must include the following elements:

- It must be typewritten or computer generated (except holographic wills, described previously).

- The document must expressly state that it is a "Will."

- The person making the will must date and sign it.

- The will must be signed by at least two or, in some states, three witnesses who will not inherit anything under the terms of the will.

Healthcare providers should be aware that legal planning is vital for all patients but especially for HIV-infected patients. By focusing on the documents discussed previously (durable power of attorney, advance directives, POLST form, and wills) and by obtaining appropriate legal advice, the planning should not be difficult or confusing.

ARRANGING FOR CUSTODY OF MINORS

A major concern for HIV-infected parents is the welfare of their children (or grandchildren) in the event of the death of the parents. Several legal mechanisms help to address this concern, but the underlying principle is that the court will look to the best interest of the child, considering the parent's desires. A statement in a will about child custody will help inform the court of the parent's wishes. In addition, guardianships with a *springing clause for incapacity* (standby guardianship) can be used to appoint a guardian if a single parent becomes incapacitated. Adoption is a less attractive choice because it requires the parent(s) to surrender all parental rights. Because it is common for parents not to make formal legal arrangements for custody of their children in the event of the parents' death, providers can be helpful in urging patients to consider custody arrangements in advance.

ACKNOWLEDGMENTS

The author wrote or revised text from previous editions and takes responsibility for it; however, the work represents a group product including previous authors.

RECOMMENDED READING

American Association of Retired Persons, American Bar Association Commission on Legal Problems of the Elderly, and American Medical Association. Shape your health care future with health care advance directives. 1995. Available at http://www.americanbar.org/content/dam/aba/migrated/publiced/practical/books/wills/appendix_b.authcheckdam.pdf.

Human Rights Campaign. Last will and testament. Available at http://www.hrc.org/resources/entry/last-will-and-testament.

Human Rights Campaign. Health care proxy. Available at http://www.hrc.org/resources/entry/health-care-proxy.

Nolo. Website. http://www.nolo.com/about.html.

Simoni JM, Davis ML, Drossman JA, et al. Mothers with HIV/AIDS and their children: disclosure and guardianship issues. *Women Health*. 2000;31:39–54.

REFERENCES

American Academy for HIV Medicine. HIV criminalization. Available at http://www.aahivm.org/hivcriminalization. Accessed December 2, 2015.

American Association of Retired Persons, American Bar Association Commission on Legal Problems of the Elderly, and American Medical Association. Shape your health care future with health care advance directives. 1995. Available at http://www.americanbar.org/content/dam/aba/migrated/publiced/practical/books/wills/appendix_b.authcheckdam.pdf.

Boyle BA, Bradley T, Bradley H, et al. Health Insurance Portability and Accountability Act of 1996: new national medical privacy standards. *AIDS Read*. 2003;13:261–262, 265–266.

Caring Connections. Advance Care Planning. Caring Connections web site. www.caringinfo.org/i4a/pages/index.cfm?pageid=3278. Accessed March 14, 2006.

Center for HIV Law and Policy. Criminal law. Available at http://www.hivlawandpolicy.org/issues/criminal-law. Accessed November 30, 2015.

Centers for Disease Control and Prevention (CDC). HIV testing among populations at risk for HIV infection—nine states. November 1995–December 1996. *MMWR*. 1998;47(50):1086–1091.

Centers for Disease Control and Prevention (CDC). HIV surveillance report. Available at http://www.cdc.gov/hiv/library/reports/surveillance/index.htmlpanel0. Accessed November 30, 2015.

Centers for Disease Control and Prevention (CDC). HIV/AIDS statistics overview. Available at http://www.cdc.gov/hiv/statistics/overview/index.html. Accessed November 28, 2015.

Centers for Disease Control and Prevention (CDC). HIV-specific criminal law. Available at http://www.cdc.gov/hiv/policies/law/states/exposure.html. Accessed November 30, 2015.

Centers for Disease Control and Prevention (CDC). Revised recommendations for HIV testing of adults, adolescents, and pregnant women in health-care settings. *MMWR*. 2006;55(RR14):1–17. Available at www.cdc.gov/mmwr/preview/mmwrhtml/rr5514a1.htm. Accessed November 30, 2015.

Centers for Disease Control and Prevention (CDC). State HIV laws. Available at http://www.cdc.gov/hiv/policies/law/states/index.html. Accessed November 28, 2015.

Centers for Disease Control and Prevention (CDC). Trends in HIV/AIDS diagnosis-33 States, 2001–2004. *MMWR*. 2005b;54(45):1149–1153.

Centers for Disease Control and Prevention (CDC). Revised surveillance case definition for HIV infection–United States, 2014." *MMWR Recomm Rep*. 2014;63(RR-03):1–10.

Charlebois ED, Maiorana A, McLaughlin M, et al. Potential deterrent effect of name-based HIV infection surveillance. *J AIDS*. 2005;39:219–227.

Colfax GN, Buchbinder SP, Cornelisse PGA, et al. Sexual risk behaviors and implications for secondary HIV transmission during and after HIV seroconversion. *AIDS*. 2002;16:1529–1535.

Csete J, Elliott R. Criminalization of HIV transmission and exposure: in search of rights-based public health alternatives to criminal law. *Future Virol*. 62011:941.

DiNenno EA, et al. Recommendations for HIV screening of gay, bisexual, and other men who have sex with men—United States, 2017. *MMWR*. 2017;66(31):830–832.

FindLaw. State laws: living wills. FindLaw Web site. Available at http://estate.findlaw.com/estate-planning/living-wills/estate-planning-law-state-living-wills.html. Accessed December 1, 2015.

Gostin L. The politics of AIDS: compulsory state powers, public health and civil liberties. *Ohio State Law J*. 1989;49:1017–1058.

Guttmacher Institute. Minors' access to STD services. State Polices in Brief. April 1, 2007. Available at http://www.guttmacher.org/statecenter/spibs/spib_MASS.pdf.

Hall HI, Holtgrave D, Maulsby C. HIV transmission rates from persons living with HIV who are aware and unaware of their infection. *AIDS*. 2012;26:893–896.

Halpern SD. HIV testing without consent in critically ill patients. *JAMA*. 2005;294(6):734–737.

Halpern SD, Metkus TS, Fuchs BD, et al. Nonconsented human immunodeficiency virus testing among critically ill patients: intensivists' practices and the influence of state laws. *Arch Intern Med*. November 26, 2007;167(21):2323–2328.

HIV Medicine Association. HIVMA urges repeal of HIV-specific criminal statutes. Available at http://www.hivma.org/uploadedFiles/IDSA/Careers_and_Training/Opportunities_for_Students_Residents/ID_Career_Paths/HIVMA%20Policy%20Statement%20on%20HIV%20Criminalization.pdf. Accessed December 2, 2015.

Ho VW, Thiel EC, Rubin HR, et al. The effect of advance care planning on completion of advance directives and patient satisfaction in people with HIV/AIDS. *AIDS Care*. 2000;12:97–108.

Ho WW, Brandfield J, Retkin R, et al. Complexities in HIV consent in adolescents. *Clin Pediatr (Phil)*. 2005;44:473–478.

Holtgrave DR, Anderson T. Utilizing HIV transmission rates to assist in prioritizing HIV prevention services. *Int J STD AIDS*. 2004;15:7890792.

Human Rights Campaign (HRC), Last will and testament. Human Rights Campaign Web site. 2004. Available at www.hrc.org/Template.cfm?Section=Home&Template=/ContentManagement/ContentDisplay.cfm&ContentID=18673. Accessed December 1, 2015.

Kaiser Foundation. Minors' authority to consent to STI services. Available at http://kff.org/hivaids/state-indicator/minors-right-to-consent. Accessed November 28, 2015.

Lehman JS, Carr MH, Nichol AJ, et al. Prevalence and public health implications of state laws that criminalize potential HIV exposure in the United States. *AIDS Behav* 2014;18(6):997–1006. Available at http://rd.springer.com/article/10.1007/s10461-014-0724-0/fulltext.html.

Lin L, Liang BA. HIV and health law: striking the balance between legal mandates and medical ethics. *Virtual Mentor AMA J Ethics.* 2005;7(10). Available at http://journalofethics.ama-assn.org/2005/10/hlaw1-0510.html.

Lubelchek RJ, Finnegan KJ, Hotton AL, et al. Assessing the use of HIV surveillance data to help gauge patient retention-in-care. *J AIDS.* 2015;69: S25–S30.

Marks G, Crepaz N, Janssen RS. Estimating sexual transmission of HIV from persons aware and unaware that they are infected with the virus in the USA. *AIDS.* 2006;20:1447–1450.

Martin DK, Thiel EC, Singer PA. A new model of advance care planning: observations from people with HIV. *Arch Intern Med.* 1999;159:86–92.

Massachusetts Medical Society. Health care proxies and end of life care. Available at http://www.massmed.org/Patient-Care/Health-Topics/Health-Care-Proxies-and-End-of-Life-Care/Health-Care-Proxies-and-End-of-Life-Care/.Vl9Xmzfru70. Accessed December 2, 2015.

Met Life Consumer Education Center (MCEC). Making a will. Available at www.thebody.com/metlife/will.html. Accessed December 1, 2015.

Neff S, Goldschmidt R. Centers for Disease Control and Prevention 2006 human immunodeficiency virus testing recommendations and state testing laws. *JAMA.* 2011;305(17):1767–1768.

New York State Department of Health (NYSDOH). Frequently asked questions: why should I choose a health care agent? January 2003. Available at www.health.state.ny.us/nysdoh/hospital/healthcareproxy/faq/htm. Accessed December 1, 2015.

New York State Department of Health (NYSDOH). New York State Task Force on Life and the Law. The Health Care Proxy Law: A Guidebook for Health Professionals. New York: New York State Department of Health. 1991. Revised October 2001. Available at www.health.state.ny.us.nysdoh/consumer/patient/hcproxy.htm. Accessed December 1, 2015.

Nolo. How a financial power of attorney works. 2002a. Available at www.nolo.com/lawcenter/ency/article.cfm/objectID/8DB3E0EC-D6CA-4479-B3FA7E9174E0827A/catID/EDC82D5A-7723-4A77-9E10DDB947D1F801. Published 2002a. Accessed December 1, 2015.

Nolo. Wills FAQ. 2002b. Available at www.nolo.com/lawcenter/ency/article.cfm/objectid/10689FA1-E24C-4849-BEA73FE77F295A5F/

catID/F251EA55-13A9-4EE0-85D21CEB27636030C6722A8D-33C5-4A8E-A49D330568AACE2F. Accessed December 1, 2015.

Obermeyer CM, Baijal P, Pegurri E. Facilitating HIV disclosure across diverse settings: A review. *Am J Pub Health.* 2011;101(6):1011–1023.

Stein GL, Bonuck KA. Attitudes on end-of-life care and advance care planning in the lesbian and gay community. *J Palliat Med.* 2001;4:173–190.

Stein MD, Freedberg KA, Sullivan LM, et al. Sexual ethics: disclosure of HIV-positive status to partners. *Arch Intern Med.* 1998;158:253–257.

Tarasoff v. Regents of U. of California, 131 Cal. Rptr. 14, 551 P.2d 334 (1976).

University of California San Francisco Clinical Consultation Center. State testing laws. Available at http://www.cdc.gov/hiv/policies/law/states/index.html. Accessed November 30, 2015.

US Department of Health and Human Services (USDHHS), Office for Civil Rights Privacy Rule. Available at http://www.hhs.gov/ocr/privacy/psa/understanding/index.html. Accessed December 2, 2015.

US Preventative Services Task Force (USPSTF). Recommendations for screening. Available at http://www.uspreventiveservicestaskforce.org/BrowseRec/Search?s=hiv+screening. Accessed November 30, 2015.

Webber DW. Self-incrimination, partner notification, and the criminal law: negatives for the CDC's "prevention for positives" initiative. *AIDS Public Policy J.* 2004;19:54–66. Available at http://www.hivlawandpolicy.org/resources/self-incrimination-partner-notification-and-criminal-law-negatives-cdc%E2%80%99s-%E2%80%9Cprevention. Accessed November 30, 2015.

Wenger NS, Kanouse DE, Collins RL, et al. End-of-life discussions and preferences among persons with HIV. *JAMA.* 2001;285:2880–2887.

Wiewel E, Braunstein SL, Xiaet Q, et al. Monitoring outcomes for newly diagnosed and prevalent HIV cases using a care continuum created with New York City surveillance data. *J AIDS.* 2015;68:217–226.

Wolitski RJ, Rietmeijer CA, Goldbaum GM, et al. HIV serostatus disclosure among gay and bisexual men in four American cities: general patterns and relation to sexual practices. *AIDS Care.* 1998;10:599–610.

Wortley PM, Lindegren ML, Fleming PL. Successful implementation of perinatal HIV prevention guidelines: a multistate surveillance evaluation. *MMWR.* 2001;50(RR-6):17–28.

51

RESEARCH DESIGN AND ANALYSIS

Christian B. Ramers

CHAPTER GOAL

Upon completion of this chapter, the reader should be able to

- Demonstrate basic knowledge regarding the interpretation of results of medical research related to HIV in order to better incorporate emerging scientific concepts into the provision of optimal patient care.

EVALUATING THE STATISTICAL ANALYSIS OF CLINICAL TRIALS

LEARNING OBJECTIVES

- Differentiate between on-treatment (OT) and intent-to-treat (ITT) analyses and between time-to-loss of virologic response (TLOVR) analysis and a US Food and Drug Administration (FDA) SNAPSHOT analysis.

- Give an example of when noninferiority analysis might be used.

KEY POINTS

- Because of inherent differences in approach, the OT analysis will frequently report better outcomes than will the ITT analysis due to exclusion of study drop-out and loss to follow-up (LTFU).

- Therapeutic responses to antiretroviral therapy (ART) regimens may be evaluated using various approaches, such as TLOVR and SNAPSHOT analyses; each method may be more appropriate in certain study populations than in others.

- New ART regimens are usually compared to existing standard-of-care regimens using a type of statistical comparison called a *noninferiority analysis*.

- A common error in reporting clinical trial results is not correctly distinguishing between clinical and statistical significance.

- To properly interpret the results of scientific studies, the reader must understand the difference between a statistical association and causality.

ON-TREATMENT (OT) VERSUS INTENT-TO-TREAT (ITT)

In randomized trials, an OT analysis (also known as "as-treated analysis" or "observed analysis") examines outcomes in only those patients who remain on their assigned study regimen for the duration of the trial or, in the case of an interim analysis, up to a particular time point. An ITT analysis evaluates each patient according to the treatment group to which he or she was originally randomized, regardless of whether that patient received the treatment or completed the study. Both ITT and OT analyses are valuable in understanding the findings of a clinical trial.

By removing from the analysis those patients who are lost to follow-up, do not complete the study (for any reason), drop out due to side effects, or do not stay on their prescribed regimen, the OT analysis selects for those patients who have been able to tolerate study medication(s). This analysis method is intrinsically biased toward a best-case scenario, and it may systematically bias results such that bad outcomes associated with a treatment that is not well tolerated may be hidden. The value of the ITT analysis is that it limits bias by evaluating the entire population of patients randomized to a given drug regimen. ITT analyses more completely encompass efficacy, tolerability, adverse events, and the myriad other reasons why patients do not remain on or deviate from the prescribed drug regimen; therefore, it accounts for the influence of these factors on outcomes (Lang, 1997). The more rigorous ITT approach conveys a truer sense of a regimen's overall effectiveness and is considered to be less subject to bias.

Because of the inherent differences in these approaches, the OT analysis will frequently report better outcomes than will the ITT analysis (e.g., a higher proportion of patients achieving undetectable HIV-1 RNA). OT analyses exclude patients who are noncompliant with study medications, procedures, and/or study visits and also those who drop out due to intolerance of the assigned regimen. If more patients are excluded from one treatment arm than another, the OT analysis may report a clinical difference that is quite different from the actual treatment difference obtained when all subjects are analyzed. Conversely, an OT analysis may find no difference between two treatments, whereas an ITT analysis, which better accounts for tolerability, may find a superior outcome for a treatment due to less study drop-out or discontinuation.

TIME TO LOSS OF VIROLOGIC RESPONSE VERSUS SNAPSHOT ANALYSIS

Achieving undetectable HIV RNA levels (viral load) is the most widely accepted endpoint for antiretroviral clinical trials as it is felt to serve as a clinically relevant surrogate marker for end points that may be rare or take years to occur (e.g., progression to AIDS and death). As such, antiretroviral drug regimens are frequently evaluated by assessing the percentage of subjects achieving low (suppressed) plasma levels of HIV-1 RNA. Because assays that detect HIV RNA have different limits of detection, it is important to know which prespecified level of HIV RNA was considered "suppressed" or "undetectable." Often, trials will allow some "forgiveness" in statistical analysis to account for small elevations or "blips" in viral load that likely do not affect ultimate clinical outcome. In addition to measuring the failure to achieve or maintain HIV-1 RNA suppression, the TLOVR analysis also considers the introduction of a new antiretroviral drug, death, or loss to follow-up as failures (US Food and Drug Administration [FDA], 2002). More recently, FDA introduced the SNAPSHOT method of analyzing results with the goal of simplifying the evaluation of study results. SNAPSHOT differs from TLOVR in that it primarily focuses on a visit of interest (e.g., only if a subject is a responder with an HIV RNA <50 copies/mL at week 48, +/− a 1- to 2-week window) (Qaqish, 2010). Both methods of analysis have value, and clinical trials often report results in both forms, although more recent analyses have favored the SNAPSHOT analysis.

NONINFERIORITY ANALYSIS

In contrast to statistical analyses used to demonstrate superiority, new drug regimens may be evaluated with the aim of demonstrating equivalence or noninferior efficacy relative to a standard drug regimen. The noninferiority trial is used mainly when the added value of a new drug/regimen is due to issues such as improved convenience, better tolerability, simpler dosing schedule, lower toxicity, or lower cost (Wittkop, 2010). Guidance given by the FDA to industry regarding procedures for accelerated and traditional new drug approval has helped to standardize the statistical methods used in clinical trials. The proportion of treatment responders at 48 weeks is often used to assess noninferiority using a specific margin of difference that is acceptable between study arms (FDA, 2002). In practical terms, a noninferiority analysis is a statistically rigorous way in which a clinical trial can show that a new regimen is at least as good as a currently available option. Often, efficacy results may appear numerically different, with one regimen achieving a slightly higher proportion of patients with undetectable viral loads at week 48, for example. In a noninferiority trial, numerical difference is less important than whether efficacy of both regimens falls within the prespecified "noninferiority margin," to determine clinical equivalence. Trials are often powered differently, with larger numbers of participants if they aim to show superiority of one regimen over another rather than noninferiority. Recently, the FDA has tightened this noninferiority margin to ensure that new drugs are truly equivalent to existing therapies before coming to market.

CLINICAL VERSUS STATISTICAL SIGNIFICANCE

When evaluating research findings, it is important to be aware of the difference between a statistically significant difference and a clinically significant difference. One of the most common errors in interpreting and reporting clinical trial results is not correctly distinguishing between clinical and statistical significance (Braitman, 1991). A clinically significant finding is one that has important implications for patient care. A statistically significant finding, in pure statistical terms, is a conclusion that there is evidence against the null hypothesis; that is, a low probability exists of getting a result as extreme or more extreme than the one observed in the data by chance alone. Statistical significance, when applied to the terms noninferiority or superiority, means that the result of a clinical trial would be unlikely to occur by chance. It does not necessarily mean that the result will be important for treating patients (Braitman, 1991; Lang, 1997). Clinically significant findings typically must involve outcomes with particular relevance to clinical medicine and must have an effect size that is large enough to influence clinical decision-making.

RECOMMENDED READING

Friedman LM, Furberg CD, DeMets DL. *Fundamentals of clinical trials*, 5th ed. New York: Springer; 2015.
Pocock SJ. *Clinical trials: a practical approach*. New York: Wiley; 1991.

DETERMINING CAUSE-AND-EFFECT ASSOCIATIONS

LEARNING OBJECTIVE

Discuss the difficulties of drawing cause-and-effect conclusions about associations identified in research studies, including the limitations of observational studies and cross-study comparisons.

KEY POINTS

- Randomized clinical trials and observational cohorts provide different but equally valuable information.

- Cohort studies frequently follow large numbers of HIV-infected people for prolonged periods and have greater representation of "real-world" populations (e.g., women and minorities) than do typical randomized studies.

- Cohort studies lack randomization and controls but are useful in generating hypotheses and demonstrating long-term associations that can be further evaluated in randomized, prospective trials.

Randomized controlled trials (RCTs) are the gold standard of modern clinical research because they randomly assign equivalent groups of patients to different treatments, thus eliminating many types of bias that might influence outcome. If randomization works, the different arms of an RCT should be equivalent in all aspects except for the treatment administered, allowing conclusions to be drawn regarding the causality of the intervention and a given outcome. However, RCTs are expensive, time-consuming, and typically must include a large number of patients in order to show results that are generalizable across patient populations. Although considered to provide a less rigorous level of evidence, observational cohort studies, cross-sectional analyses, and case–control studies have also played a major role in HIV research and can add value to our general scientific understanding of a particular problem.

From the earliest findings of the Multicenter AIDS Cohort Study (MACS) to other ongoing national and international cohorts, these databases have provided crucial insights into the natural history of HIV and the efficacy and toxicity of HIV treatment. Lipodystrophy, cardiovascular disease, renal and bone complications, treatment interruptions, and the timing of initiation of ART are areas with recent contributions from observational studies. Compared to randomized clinical trials, cohort analyses are no more or less valuable; rather, they are simply different methodologies designed to answer different types of questions.

Cohort studies are able to follow large numbers of patients for prolonged periods of time and often better reflect the "real world" of HIV-infected patients, in contrast to patients who are able and willing to participate in randomized trials. While randomized trials will typically measure 48-, 96-, or rarely 192-week data, cohort studies run for much longer and frequently have greater representation of women, minorities, and those with comorbid conditions than do typical randomized studies.

Cohort studies, however, do have biases. First, the quality of the results is only as good as the quality, consistency, and completeness of the data from participants in the cohort. Second, a lack of randomization or control of treatments administered to patients can significantly impact interpretation of the results through introduction of selection bias. For example, patients starting a particular treatment in a cohort study may be selected by clinicians to avoid a perceived toxicity or selected to gain a perceived benefit, and this in turn could lead to results favoring one agent over another that may or may not be correct. Similarly, large changes in policy, availability of treatment advances, or other confounding disease states—so-called historical bias—can influence outcomes and may be more important than the specific variables being assessed. Cohort studies are useful for observing events and outcomes that only occur many years after exposure that might be missed by a 1- to 3-year randomized clinical trial. They also may find associations which can generate hypotheses, where an observation may lead to the undertaking of a randomized clinical trial to confirm or refute the observations made in the cohort analysis.

Cohort studies may detect associations between certain treatments or factors with an outcome that prompts a more rigorous evaluation to help determine causality. They can provide preliminary information about long-term clinical end points, survival, complications, and the role of comorbid conditions that may be tested later in an RCT. Thus, the observational cohort study and the RCT are complementary rather than competitive.

Focused observational studies can be valuable for evaluating factors associated with rare diseases or outcomes. In a case–control study, a set of individuals (cases) with the condition of interest is assembled (Schulz, 2002). A corresponding set of individuals (controls) without the condition is then selected. Controls are frequently matched to be similar to the cases, and they should be selected from the same population.

Information on risk factors is then collected and analyzed to identify factors that are more (or less) common in the cases compared to the controls. For example, thresholds used to define the appropriate use of prophylaxis for opportunistic infections are largely derived from case–control studies that showed increased risk for these infections in groups of patients with lower CD4+ counts than those patients with higher counts. Careful design and implementation are needed to minimize bias in case–control studies, particularly to select appropriate controls and to collect unbiased information on risk factors.

Cross-study comparisons of randomized trials—that is, trying to relate efficacy of one particular treatment to that of another when they have not been directly compared—must be undertaken with caution because patient characteristics, study protocols, and extrinsic factors may differ considerably between studies that share the same primary end point. A meta-analysis of related studies is more reliable than a simplistic comparison because researchers can carefully analyze data to avoid misleading conclusions, and they can thoroughly explain what they did and why.

In summary, when attempting to determine causality between an intervention or risk factor and an outcome, RCTs provide the highest level of evidence. Observational studies such as cohort, case–control, and cross-sectional studies are useful to generate hypothesis, to show preliminary associations, and to guide the design of future clinical trials. Most of what is known about HIV natural history, treatment response, and associated clinical risk factors for progression or virologic control is derived from these types of studies.

RECOMMENDED READING

Collins R, MacMahon S. Reliable assessment of the effects of treatment on mortality and major morbidity: I. Clinical trials. *Lancet*. 2001;357:373–380.

Ioannidis JPA, Haidich A, Pappa M, et al. Comparison of evidence of treatment effects in randomized and nonrandomized studies. *JAMA*. 2001;286:821–830.

MacMahon S, Collins R. Reliable assessment of the effects of treatment on mortality and major morbidity: II. Observational studies. *Lancet*. 2001;357:455–462.

REFERENCES

Braitman LE. Confidence intervals assess both clinical significance and statistical significance. *Ann Intern Med.* 1991;114:515–517.

Lang TA, Secic M. *How to report statistics in medicine: annotated guidelines for authors, editors, and reviewers.* Philadelphia, PA: American College of Physicians; 1997.

Qaqish R, van Wyk J, King M. *JIAS.* 2010;13:P58. doi:10.1186/1758-2652-13-S4-P58.

Schulz KF, Grimes DA. Case–control studies: research in reverse. *Lancet.* 2002;359:431–434.

US Food and Drug Administration (FDA). *Guidance for industry submitting select clinical trial data sets for drugs intended to treat human immunodeficiency virus-1 infection.* Washington, DC: US Department of Health and Human Services. 2018. Available at https://www.fda.gov/downloads/forindustry/datastandards/studydatastandards/ucm603323.pdf Accessed August 12, 2018.

Wittkop L, Smith C, Fox Z, et al. Methodological issues in the use of composite endpoints in clinical trials: examples from the HIV field. *Clin Trials.* February 2010;7(1):19–35.

52.

ETHICAL CONDUCT OF CLINICAL TRIALS, INSTITUTIONAL REVIEW BOARDS, INFORMED CONSENT, AND FINANCIAL CONFLICTS OF INTEREST

Christian B. Ramers

LEARNING OBJECTIVE

Describe the essential components of the ethical conduct of research, the role of the institutional review board, the process of informed consent, the potential areas of conflict of interest for clinicians participating in research, and other ethical issues related to research in HIV medicine.

INTRODUCTION

Treatment advances in the management of HIV-infected patients have been a direct result of decades of research initiatives involving tens of thousands of patients. The ethical considerations when performing research include basic ethical principles (e.g., autonomy, confidentiality, nonmaleficence, informed consent, beneficence, justice, and utility), as well as nuances such as appropriate study designs, investigator conflict of interests, and bias in all its forms. To help guide clinicians, a number of professional and governmental organizations have posted guidelines and recommendations on various aspects of clinical research (e.g., the American Medical Association, the National Institutes of Health, and the US Food and Drug Administration [FDA]).

The *Declaration of Helsinki* and the *Belmont Report* are important historical benchmarks that have laid the foundation of currently accepted ethical standards in the treatment of patients participating in clinical trials. The Declaration of Helsinki, first adopted in 1964 and updated in 2013, stresses that it is the duty of the physician to promote and safeguard the health of patients and that the well-being of the individual research participants must take precedence over all other interests (World Medical Association, 2013). Although the document does not highlight individual diseases or research initiatives, the following points have particular importance to HIV-infected patients: (1) participation in clinical trials must be completely voluntary and without undue coercion or influence, (2) it is the duty of the physician to maintain privacy and confidentiality of personal information, and (3) populations that are underrepresented in medical research should be provided appropriate access to participation in research. Similarly, the Belmont Report (US Department of Health and Welfare, 1979) highlights three fundamental ethical principles relating specifically to the conduct of research: (1) the principle of *respect for persons* acknowledges the dignity and autonomy of individuals, (2) the principle of *beneficence* protects individuals by maximizing anticipated benefits and minimizing possible harms, and (3) the principle of *justice* requires that all subjects are treated fairly.

There are seven requirements for determining whether a research trial is ethical; these are discussed next.

SEVEN REQUIREMENTS FOR DETERMINING WHETHER A RESEARCH TRIAL IS ETHICAL

Emanuel and colleagues described the following requirements for determining whether a clinical trial is ethical (Emanuel, 2000):

1. *Value*: Enhancements of health or knowledge must be derived from the research.

2. *Scientific validity*: The research must be methodologically rigorous.

3. *Fair subject selection*: Scientific objective, not vulnerability or privilege, and the potential for and distribution of risks and benefits should determine the communities selected for study sites and the inclusion criteria for individual subjects.

4. *Favorable risk–benefit ratio*: Within the context of standard clinical practices and the research protocol, risk must be minimized and potential benefits enhanced, and the potential benefits to individuals and the knowledge gained for society must outweigh the risks.

5. *Independent review*: Unaffiliated individuals must review the research and approve, amend, or terminate it.

6. *Informed consent*: Individuals should be informed about the research and provide their voluntary consent.

7. *Respect for enrolled subjects*: Participants should have their privacy protected, the opportunity to withdraw from the research without penalty, and their well-being monitored.

Facing ethical dilemmas during the conduct of a clinical trial is not uncommon. A survey of physicians engaged in clinical research found that almost all of them had recently faced such issues (DuVal, 2005). They can arise at any stage of the research process, from trial design through execution to the final publication of the research report. Notably, this survey found that most ethical dilemmas occurred after institutional review board (IRB) approval, suggesting that ethical consideration should be continuous rather than a one-time process. Approximately half of the physicians requested an ethical consultation before resolving the issue, and many institutions are beginning to offer such services outside of the IRB process.

INSTITUTIONAL REVIEW BOARDS

IRBs are charged with (1) the review of protocols and consent documents and any modifications to them prior to their implementation and (2) monitoring those trials on a periodic basis to ensure ethical conduct. IRBs do not have primary responsibility for the safety issues of a trial; that responsibility resides with the principal investigator(s), the safety officer designated by the study sponsor, and the regulatory affairs office responsible for adverse event reporting to the FDA and other regulatory agencies. However, IRBs must be informed of safety concerns as they arise because safety issues may impact the ethical conduct of the trial. Multicenter trials may utilize an independent, central IRB chosen by the trial sponsor as well as local IRBs established by participating research centers. IRB composition and responsibilities are guided by the *US Code of Federal Regulations* (21 CFR 56.107-111), which provides minimum standards for subject safety and information. Although some forms of research (e.g., retrospective chart reviews) may be considered "low risk" and thus eligible for an IRB exemption or waiver, when in doubt regarding the ethical merits of a particular research effort, an investigator or clinician should always err on the side of caution and engage a local IRB or ethics committee.

INFORMED CONSENT

The FDA provides a comprehensive review on the informed consent process and guidance for development of the informed consent document (FDA, 2016). The informed consent procedure is more than just a signature on a form; it is a process of information exchange that may include, in addition to reading and signing the informed consent document,

participant recruitment materials, verbal instructions, a question–answer session, and measures of participant understanding. Researchers must provide potential participants with full disclosure of anticipated benefits, risks, and alternatives to the study intervention. That obligation extends throughout the course of the study to include updating volunteer participants in a timely manner on emerging knowledge that might change their perception of the risks and benefits of continued participation in the trial. The informed consent document should be in a language and at a level understandable to the subject (or subject's representative) and provide the subject with sufficient opportunity to consider whether or not to participate without the possibility of coercion or undue influence. In addition, the document must state that participation is completely voluntary and that subjects can withdrawal from the study at any point in time without loss of benefits or penalty.

CONFLICTS OF INTERESTS IN THE CONDUCT OF CLINICAL TRIALS

As research has expanded to include centers outside academic health institutions, partnerships between pharmaceutical companies and private practice research sites have grown. As such, physicians may play dual roles of both investigator and clinician. This could lead to a conflict of interest to enroll participants in trials when financial incentives are in place. The American Medical Association (AMA) has posted recommendations to safeguard against conflict of interests during clinical trials. Only physicians with medical expertise in the areas of the research being performed should be investigators. When financial compensation is offered from trial sponsors, it should be at fair market value, with the rate commensurate with the efforts of the physician performing the research; should not vary according to the volume of participants enrolled by the physician; and must be disclosed to a potential participant as part of the informed consent process. In addition, the AMA states that it is unethical for physicians to accept payment solely for referring patients to research studies. Finally, both the AMA and the Declaration of Helsinki (2008) make specific statements about the publication of study results. The AMA states that physicians should ensure that the publications of study results not be unduly delayed or otherwise obstructed by the sponsoring company, and the most recent update of the Declaration of Helsinki highlights that negative and inconclusive as well as positive results should be published or otherwise be made publicly available.

PERCEPTIONS AND MISPERCEPTIONS

Altruism often is a core but seldom a sole reason for volunteering to participate in a study (Kass, 1996). Many people participate in clinical trials for very pragmatic reasons, such as having inadequate or no health insurance, or they may have exhausted or found no relief from currently approved therapies (Council of Public Representatives, 2001; Kass, 1996). A trial may represent their only perceived access to care or hope for relief. These mixed motives can exacerbate the "therapeutic misconception," wherein volunteers believe that they are receiving care rather than engaging in research.

With an increasing number of clinical trials being performed and the expansion of their conduct from research medical centers to private practice settings, the distinction between research and care can become blurred (Morin, 2002). It may be difficult for individual physicians to separate their roles of healthcare provider and researcher (Miller, 1998), both within their own minds and in communicating with patients who are potential participants in a study. This also may lead investigators to circumvent strict enrollment criteria or bypass the randomization process (Morin, 2002). This can heighten the potential for a volunteer's "therapeutic misconception." The two roles that the physician plays often result in a tension that is ethically complex and ambiguous, and, if it cannot be avoided, it must be managed (Miller, 1998).

The AMA has taken the position that the physician who has treated a patient on an ongoing basis should not be responsible for obtaining informed consent. Rather, once a patient has been identified as meeting trial eligibility, a nontreating person should conduct the formal consent procedure (Morin, 2002). This is particularly important when studies are performed in institutional settings, including correctional facilities, in which broad supervision may impact on the free will and autonomy of the potential volunteer.

Clinicians must be mindful of the trust that patients place in them in helping to make healthcare decisions, including participation in a clinical research trial, and clinicians must be clear in distinguishing between providing care and offering participation in a clinical trial (Kass, 1996). Many clinician-researchers find it helpful to separate clinical care visits temporally and geographically from research study visits in order to clearly separate the goals of each interaction.

ETHICAL CONSIDERATIONS IN INTERNATIONAL RESEARCH

Advances in the treatment of HIV have produced antiretroviral regimens that are highly potent, well-tolerated, and easy to take. As a result, the interest in patient participation in clinical trials of novel agents and regimens in industrialized countries has declined. This in turn has caused many biotechnology and pharmaceutical companies to shift a large portion of their research initiatives to regions of the world that are lacking in infrastructure and/or resources to provide standard of care treatments. In an editorial in *The New England Journal of Medicine* in 2001, Shapiro and Meslin highlighted the following key issues regarding research in developing countries (Shapiro, 2001):

1. Clinical trials conducted abroad should meet all ethical standards for trials based in the United States.

2. Studies should be sensitive to the local customs, conditions, and culture of the region.

3. Careful consideration must be undertaken in areas that have high rates of illiteracy or where signing a form may be considered dangerous in countries with oppressive political regimes.

4. It is unethical to ask persons to participate in a trial in which the intervention being tested is not likely affordable in the host country or where the healthcare infrastructure cannot support its proper distribution and use.

5. The experimental intervention should be normally compared with an established, effective treatment.

6. Research participants should not be made worse off by their inability to have continued access to a successful intervention after the trial has ended.

7. A review by ethics committees in both host and sponsoring countries should be performed.

CONCLUSION

HIV-related biomedical research has resulted in a large body of therapeutic advancements and vast improvements in our scientific knowledge and understanding of the biology, pathogenesis, natural history, and epidemiology of HIV infection. Foundational ethical principles such as autonomy, confidentiality, nonmaleficence, informed consent, beneficence, justice, and utility must be continually applied to the conduct of research in order to maintain ethically sound research programs. IRBs and ethics consultation services can serve as resources for researchers and clinicians in need of consultation.

REFERENCES

Council of Public Representatives. *Human research protections in clinical trials: a public perspective.* Report to the Director of the National Institutes of Health. Bethesda, MD: National Institutes of Health; October 2001.

DuVal G, Gensler G, Danis M. Ethical dilemmas encountered by clinical researchers. *J Clin Ethics.* 2005;16(3):267–276.

Emanuel EJ, Wendler D, Grady C. What makes clinical research ethical? *JAMA.* 2000;283(20):2701–2711.

Kass NE, Sugarman J, Faden R, et al. Trust, the fragile foundation of contemporary biomedical research. *Hastings Cent Rep.* 1996;26(5):25–29.

Miller FG, Rosenstein DL, DeRenzo EG. Professional integrity in clinical research. *JAMA.* 1998;280(16):1449–1454.

Morin K, Rakatansky H, Riddick FA, et al. Managing conflicts of interest in the conduct of clinical trials. *JAMA.* 2002;287:78–84.

Shapiro HT, Mesline EM. Ethical issues in the design and conduct of clinical trials in developing countries. *N Engl J Med.* 2001;345(2):139–142.

US Department of Health and Welfare, National Commission for the Protection of Human Subjects of Biomedical and Behavioral Research. The Belmont report: ethical principles and guidelines for the protection of human subjects of research. April 18, 1979. Available at http://www.hhs.gov/ohrp/humansubjects/guidance/belmont.html.

US Food and Drug Administration. A guide to informed consent—Information sheet: Guidance for institutional review boards and clinical investigators. 2016. Available at www.fda.gov/RegulatoryInformation/Guidances/ucm126431.htm.

World Medical Association. World Medical Association Declaration of Helsinki: ethical principles for medical research involving human subjects. *JAMA.* 2013;310(20):2191–2194.

INDEX

Tables, figures, and boxes are indicated by an italic *t, f,* and *b,* respectively, following the page number.